THE EPILEPSIES

Seizures, Syndromes and Management

Based on the ILAE classifications and practice parameter guidelines

CD ROM with patient videos and EEGs

C P Panayiotopoulos MD PhD FRCP

BLADON
MEDICAL
PUBLISHING

12 New Street, Chipping Norton, Oxfordshire
OX7 5LJ, UK

First published 2005

Always refer to the manufacturer's Prescribing Information before prescribing drugs cited in this book.

British Library Cataloguing in Publication Data. A catalogue record for this title is available from the British Library

ISBN 1-904218-34-2

C P Panayiotopoulos. THE EPILEPSIES: Seizures, Syndromes and Management

Design and production:
Design Online Limited, 21 Cave Street, Oxford OX4 1BA, UK

Printed by
Talleres Gráficos Hostench s.a., Venezuela 87–93, Barcelona, Spain

Distributed by
NBN International Ltd., Estover Road, Plymouth PL6 7PY, UK

To my wife Thalia

because

she is a beautiful woman

my muse

the flower, the smile and the angel in my life

ACKNOWLEDGEMENTS

I am gratefu l to the following eminent experts who gave him valuable advise over the last 4 years during the preparation of this book:
Adachi,N.
Akanuma,N.
Benbadis, S.
Berkovic,S.F.
Covanis, A.
Eeg-Olofsson,O.
Dravet,C.
Duncan,J.S.
Engel,J,Jr.
Fejerman, N.
Ferrie,C.D.
Genton,P.
Grünewald,R.A.
Kasteleijn-Nolst Trenite,D.G.A.
Koutroumanidis,M.
Kuzniecky, R.
Oguni,H.
Ohtahara,S.
Patsalos, P.
Plouin,P.
Sander,J.W.A.S.
Scott,R.C.
Shorvon,S.D.
Stephenson,J.B.R.
Watanabe,K.
Whitehouse, W.
Wilkins, A.
Zifkin,B.G.

I am also grateful to Thalai Valeta for writing the section on 'Parental attitude, reaction and education in benign childhood focal seizures'

The over 12 years assistance of S. Rowlinson and S. Sanders, expert EEG technologists, is greatly appreciated.

John Harrison, perfectionist publisher, Design Online – Steve Millar, exceptional book designer and John Nicholson, creator of the CD ROM – worked very hard to publish this book within 2 months of receiving the manuscript.

CONTENTS

PREFACE

The epilepsies manifest with various types of epileptic seizures and comprise a broad family of many common syndromes of diverse age at onset, symptomatology, aetiology, severity, prognosis and specific management requirements.

Outstanding achievements in addressing the scientific and social aspects of epilepsies in the last 50 years should be largely attributed to the leaders and committee members of the International League Against Epilepsy (ILAE). The ILAE standardised classification and terminology for epileptic seizures and syndromes provides a fundamental framework for organising and differentiating the epilepsies. This categorisation is essential in clinical practice, randomised controlled trials of antiepileptic drugs (AEDs), epidemiology and research into these disorders. The currently valid *Classification of Epileptic Seizures* was published in 1981 and the last revision of the *Classification of Epilepsies and Epileptic Syndromes* in 1989. In June 2001, the ILAE Task Force on Classification and Terminology under the tireless and wise leadership of Pete Engel and Natalio Fejerman proposed a "diagnostic scheme for people with epileptic seizures and with epilepsy" to incorporate the significant progress that has been made in the last decade. This is planned to be a flexible and dynamic classification that will be revised periodically based on emerging new information and resolution of problems that will inevitably be identified through use. The basic concepts of the new diagnostic scheme were accepted by the ILAE General Assembly, but "none of these proposals are yet complete, nor are any intended to constitute a classification". The different methodologies, approaches, targets and philosophies of these classifications have been authoritatively detailed in a multi-authored editorial entitled 'Cabbages and Kings in the Classification of Seizures and the Epilepsies' in *Epilepsia* (January 2003), the official journal of the ILAE, which is achieving miraculous high standards and objectivity with Bob Fisher as its Editor. The lead editorial was by Peter Wolf, the newly elected ILAE President, who is an immensely valued and respected clinician, scientist and philosopher, and he will undoubtedly make his mark in the classifications.

My previous concise book, *A Clinical Guide to Epileptic Syndromes and their Treatment*, was based on the new ILAE diagnostic scheme. Its success, as reflected in scientific reviews of eminent colleagues and the sale of over 10,000 copies, is a tribute to the ILAE Task Force and emphasises the need for their colossal assignment to be completed.

This new book, *The Epilepsies*, details the most recent advances in epileptic seizures, epileptic syndromes and their management. It is based on the ILAE classification, and practice parameter and guidelines issued by the ILAE and other recognised medical authorities. Seizures and syndromes are explored in their scientific context and also include newly described seizures, syndromes and methodologies that, in my opinion, should be appreciated by practising physicians and should be considered in future ILAE revisions and practice parameters. This is in accord with the ILAE Task Force invitation to physicians to contribute to the shaping of future revisions.

Updated to December 2004, this book encompasses: new and developing aspects and concepts about epilepsy; information about old and new developments; diagnostic approaches and methods, and factors leading to diagnostic error and misconceptions; management; and critical analysis of the relevant literature. The most appropriate modern therapies are presented objectively for everyday clinical practice. The literature, including research and pathophysiology, is critically evaluated, but priority is given only to the facts that are useful to the practitioner. The content serves as a bridge from practice to research. The text is further reinforced by the use of illustrative case reports.

The CD-ROM that accompanies this book contains clips of video EEG and reviews of patients, which provide an extremely powerful tool for documentation and teaching. In particular, clips that refer to areas of existing diagnostic uncertainty over which expert opinion differs, such as autonomic status epilepticus, Panayiotopoulos syndrome, eyelid myoclonia with absences and self-induced epilepsy, are included.

The EEG illustrations have been sourced mainly from video-EEG recordings from my personal files. High quality figures of modern brain imaging have been provided thanks to the courtesy of cited eminent colleagues.

The first chapter details the diagnostic steps necessary to establish a precise seizure and syndrome classification of patients. It is my conviction that this book serves no purpose without emphasising that "inappropriate generalisations regarding terminology, diagnosis and treatment is the single most important cause of mismanagement in epilepsies". Effective classification of epileptic seizures and syndromes is indispensable for appropriate management and prognosis. Patients with epileptic seizures and their families are entitled to a diagnosis, prognosis and management that are specific and precise. The inclusive, monolectic diagnostic label 'epilepsy' is unsatisfactory for both patient and physician alike, and may result in avoidable morbidity and mortality.

The second chapter is devoted to the optimal use of EEG in the diagnosis of epilepsy. Although not a substitute for a clinical examination, EEG is the most important investigation in the diagnosis and management of epilepsy provided that it is properly performed by experienced technicians, and carefully studied and interpreted in the context of a well-described clinical setting by experienced physicians.

The third chapter is a brief account of various brain imaging methodologies and their optimal use in the diagnosis and management of epilepsies. Current optimal magnetic resonance imaging (MRI) allows in vivo visualisation of structural causes of epilepsy in over 80% of patients with focal symptomatic seizures. MRI is much superior to X-ray computed tomography in terms of its sensitivity and specificity for identifying lesional epilepsies. Functional brain imaging including magnetoencephalography is currently supplementary to MRI in clinical practice and principally in the evaluation of possible neurosurgical treatment.

The fourth chapter details the principles of therapy in the epilepsies with AEDs, surgical and other non-pharmacological treatments. The aim of therapy is total freedom from seizures without clinically significant adverse effects. This is achievable in more than two-thirds of patients with epileptic seizures. New AEDs are thoroughly reviewed and pragmatic recommendations made as to their correct indications and contraindications. The evaluation of the AEDs has been the most demanding and difficult task. Ideally, AED prescribing should be entirely evidence-based, but this is often sparse, selective and primarily designed for justifying regulatory licence requirements rather than addressing the needs of clinical practice. My recommendations are pragmatic in that they are based on a thorough review of the efficacy, tolerability, safety and interactions of AEDs after examining evidence-based reports, post-marketing reports and expert physicians' experience of the AED in clinical use. Controlled trial data would never have been obtained for certain recommendations, such as the fact that vigabatrin and tiagabine are deleterious in absence seizures. Pragmatic and rational AED treatment is detailed in the management section of every syndrome.

In Chapters 5–13, each syndrome is analysed with respect to its clinical manifestations, epidemiology, aetiology, investigative procedures and EEG, prognosis and management.

Chapter 5 is a thorough review of epileptic seizures and epileptic syndromes, and their management, in the neonatal period. The neonatal period is the most vulnerable period of life for developing seizures. Neonatal seizures demand special clinical and investigative skills in their recognition and differentiation from normal or abnormal behaviours. They may be short-lived events lasting for only a few days or signify serious malfunction or damage of the immature brain, and constitute a neurological emergency demanding urgent diagnosis and management. Recognised epileptic syndromes range from the mild and age-limited, such as benign familial neonatal seizures and benign neonatal seizures (non-familial), to the devastating early myoclonic encephalopathy and Ohtahara syndrome.

Chapter 6 describes idiopathic seizures and syndromes in infancy. These include: epileptic seizures, such as febrile seizures that do not require a diagnosis of epilepsy; idiopathic epileptic syndromes, such as benign myoclonic epilepsy in infancy, which is the earliest form of IGE; and 'autosomal dominant epilepsy with febrile seizures plus', which is one of the most fascinating and most common genetic epileptic disorders that is linked to many other benign and severe epileptic conditions.

Chapter 7 provides a comprehensive modern review of all aspects of the devastating epileptic encephalopathies in infancy and early childhood. These comprise West syndrome, Dravet syndrome, Lennox–Gastaut syndrome, Landau–Kleffner syndrome, epilepsy with continuous spike-and-waves during slow-wave sleep and myoclonic status in non-progressive encephalopathies. The tremendous progress that has been made in our understanding of the genetics of the epilepsies is well illustrated by Dravet syndrome. Surgical achievements are exemplified by the treatment of hypothalamic (gelastic) epilepsy, which is also included in this chapter.

Chapter 8 deals with the severe neocortical epileptic syndromes with onset in infancy and childhood, which are Kozhevnikov-Rasmussen syndrome (chronic epileptic encephalitis), hemiconvulsion-hemiplegia syndrome and migrating partial epilepsy of early childhood. As in other parts of this book, I have also explored certain myths and misconceptions, which in this case refer to the historical aspects and nomenclature of chronic encephalitis with epilepsy.

Chapter 9 is concerned with benign childhood focal seizures and related epileptic syndromes, to which I have devoted two previous monographs: *Benign childhood partial seizures and related epileptic syndromes* and *Panayiotopoulos syndrome*. Benign childhood focal seizures are the most common and probably the most fascinating and rewarding topic in paediatric epileptology. They form a significant part of the everyday practice of paediatricians, neurologists and clinical neurophysiologists who care for children with seizures. Yet, only Rolandic seizures are widely known. Panayiotopoulos syndrome, which affects around 13% of children aged 3–6 years with non-febrile seizures, remains grossly underdiagnosed, though with its acceptance into the ILAE classification, independent reports of eminent physicians from around the world and recent editorials in *Neurology*, the *Lancet* and *British Medical Journal*, it may become more readily recognised by clinicians. Again, I must particularly emphasise autonomic seizures and autonomic status epilepticus, which appear to be specific to childhood and may be disguised as non-epileptic symptoms of other diseases, such as encephalitis, migraine, gastroenteritis or syncope. The result is avoidable morbidity and costly medical treatments. Despite the fact that I described them 20 years ago, autonomic seizures and autonomic status epilepticus in children are still missing in a significant proportion of the literature on paediatric clinical and EEG epileptology. Searching for autonomic status epilepticus in *Pediatrics*, and other major paediatric journals and reputable Web sites of epilepsy foundations and associations brings *"zero results"*.

It appears that Rolandic seizures, Panayiotopoulos syndrome, Gastaut-type idiopathic childhood occipital epilepsy and other benign childhood clinical-EEG phenotypes are linked together in a broad age-related and age-limited benign childhood seizure susceptibility syndrome (BCSSS), which may also constitute a biological continuum with febrile seizures and benign infantile and neonatal seizures. It is my thesis that the clinical, EEG, pathophysiological and management aspects of BCSSS should be properly re-examined and redefined. Once more, I take this opportunity to repeat my plea to the relevant medical committees that practice parameters for these common epileptic disorders are urgently needed.

The IGEs, which constitute one-third of all epilepsies, are comprehensively and extensively dealt with in Chapter 10. IGEs manifest with typical absences, myoclonic jerks and GTCS, alone or in varying combinations and severity. Absence status epilepticus is common. Most syndromes of IGE start in childhood or adolescence, but some have an adult onset. They are usually life long, though a few are age related. The EEG is the most sensitive test in the diagnosis and confirmation of IGE. Childhood absence epilepsy, juvenile absence epilepsy, juvenile myoclonic epilepsy and epilepsy with GTCS are well-established and well-recognised syndromes of IGE. Other syndromes, such as IGE with phantom absences may exist, and are also described. Irrespective, of whether all the syndromes of IGE constitute a biological continuum or not, the most important practical aspect is that IGEs require meticulous diagnostic precision to differentiate between absence seizures and focal seizures, primarily and secondarily GTCS, and absence status epilepticus and non-epileptic confusion or epileptic prodrome. Failure to make this differentiation results in therapeutic disasters, which is why these matters are discussed at length. Another equally crucial matter refers to continuing errors in the treatment of IGE. The fact that nearly 50% of patients with IGE are currently taking *"ill-advised AED"* medication is a grave problem. I have tried to identify the main reasons for this mismanagement, so that they may be properly addressed and a remedy found. Reasons include: (a). diagnostic misclassification; (b). sparse or methodologically ambiguous randomised controlled trials of AEDs; (c). official guidelines and publications paying scant attention to important aspects of the management of IGE; (d). a *'one size fits all'* policy with regard to *'how to treat epilepsy'*; and (e). formal national formularies that are conspicuously devoid of warnings about the established pro-epileptic action of certain AEDs in certain types of seizures and syndromes of IGE.

Chapter 11 incorporates the significant progress in molecular and statistical genetics that has led to breakthroughs in the mapping and identification of gene variants of genetic diseases, such as familial (autosomal dominant) focal epilepsy syndromes. Autosomal dominant nocturnal frontal lobe epilepsy, mesial and lateral familial temporal lobe epilepsy and familial focal epilepsy with variable foci are extensively described. Others, such as benign familial neonatal, and neonatal-infantile and infantile seizures, are covered in Chapters 5 and 6. These disorders are caused by mutations in genes encoding subunits of ion channels or neurotransmitter receptors. Although these findings concern only a few families, they are of immense potential importance, because these genes are implicated in a wide range of more common epileptic disorders.

Chapter 12 describes focal seizures and focal syndromes with respect to their anatomical origins in the frontal, temporal, parietal and occipital lobes. Current optimal MRI allows in-vivo visualisation of structural causes in 80% of patients with symptomatic focal epilepsies, such as hippocampal sclerosis and malformations of cortical development. Tuberculomas and cysticercosis are the main causes in developing countries. Functional brain imaging offers valuable insights and is useful in the presurgical evaluation of these patients. With so many new choices, AED treatment either as monotherapy or rational polytherapy is demanding and requires a thorough knowledge and consideration of the available medications. Medical treatment with AEDs is effective in 80% of patients; in the remaining 20% and probably many more with intractable seizures, neurosurgical resection of the offending epileptogenic region is usually successful. There is now concrete evidence to accept, diagnose and treat certain focal epilepsies on the basis of aetiology rather than simply localisation. Mesial temporal lobe epilepsy with hippocampal sclerosis, which is one of the more common and most distinct epileptic syndromes, is a striking example of this. There is now Class I evidence that 64% of those who received surgery were free of disabling seizures compared with 8% in the group randomised to continued medical therapy. This chapter also details the differential diagnosis of visual occipital lobe seizures from migraine, which is a source of considerable and continuing misunderstanding and misdiagnosis between these two distinct classes of disorder that is perpetuated in classical textbooks on epilepsies.

Reflex seizures and syndromes of reflex epilepsy are the topic of Chapter 13. Photic, pattern, fixation-off, somatosensory, reading and other modes of precipitation are described in depth. Of the recognised syndromes, idiopathic occipital lobe epilepsy, and startle and reading epilepsy are thoroughly reviewed together with others such as Jeavons syndrome (eyelid myoclonia with absences) which, based on concrete evidence, also constitute reflex epileptic syndromes awaiting formal recognition.

Chapter 14 comprises a pharmacopoeia of AEDs used in prophylactic treatment, with particular emphasis on the new AEDs.

Realistically, I have to accept that despite all my efforts, omissions and errors may be unavoidable. I regret if I have unintentionally undermined, omitted or misunderstood the work of some colleagues, and I would be grateful if this is brought to my attention. Certain statements that I have made may not meet with universal approval, but I would urge readers to give these assertions ample consideration before rejecting them.

My intention is that this book serves as: (a). a primary source of information and reference for neurologists, clinical neurophysiologists and epileptologists; and (b). as a practical guide for any clinician who treats children or adults with epileptic seizures, and any electroencephalographer who compiles their EEG reports. Other health professionals with an interest in epilepsies, and even patients and their relatives, may also find this book interesting and useful.

C P Panayiotopoulos MD PhD FRCP
London 2nd December 2004

ABBREVIATIONS

ACTH	adrenocorticotropin hormone
ADCME	autosomal dominant cortical myoclonus and epilepsy
ADNFLE	autosomal dominant nocturnal frontal lobe epilepsy
AED	anti-epileptic drug
ASE	absence status epilepticus
BCSSS	benign childhood seizure susceptibility syndrome
CAE	childhood absence epilepsy
CD	coeliac disease
CFSAAP	Committee on Quality Improvement, Subcommittee on Febrile Seizures, of the American Academy of Pediatrics
CHES	Child Health and Education Study
CNS	central nervous system
COE	childhood occipital epilepsy
CRH	corticotropin-releasing hormone
CSE	convulsive status epilepticus
CSF	cerebrospinal fluid
CSWS	continuous spikes and waves during slow-wave sleep
CT	computed tomography
CTS	centrotemporal spikes
DDI	drug–drug interaction
DNET	dysembryoplastic neuroepithelial tumours
ECG	electrocardiography/electrocardiogram
ECSWS	epilepsy with continuous spikes and waves during slow-wave sleep
EEG	electroencephalography/electroencephalogram
EGTCSA	epilepsy with generalised tonic-clonic seizures on awakening
EMA	eyelid myoclonia with absences (Jeavons syndrome)
EM-AS	epilepsy with myoclonic astatic seizures (Doose syndrome)
EMG	electromyography
ESES	extreme somatosensory-evoked spikes
ESESS	electrical status epilepticus during slow-wave sleep
FAME	familial adult myoclonic epilepsy
FDG	^{18}F fluoro-deoxyglucose
fMRI	functional magnetic resonance imaging
FOS	fixation-off sensitivity
FS	febrile seizures
FS+	febrile seizures plus
GABA	gamma-aminobutyric acid
GEFS+	generalised epilepsy with febrile seizures plus
GFD	gluten-free diet
G-ICOE	Gastaut-type idiopathic childhood occipital epilepsy
GnRH	gonadotrophin-releasing hormone
GSWD	generalised spike and wave discharge
GTCS	generalised tonic clonic seizures
JAE	juvenile absence epilepsy
JME	juvenile myoclonic epilepsy (Janz syndrome)
HS	hippocampal sclerosis
ICEGTC	intractable childhood epilepsy with generalised tonic-clonic seizures
ICOE	idiopathic childhood occipital epilepsy
IGE	idiopathic generalised epilepsy
ILAE	International League Against Epilepsy
IPOE	idiopathic photosensitive occipital lobe epilepsy
IPS	intermittent photic stimulation
LFTLE	lateral familial temporal lobe epilepsy
LGI1	leucine-rich, glioma inactivated 1

MAE	epilepsy with myoclonic absences
MEG	magnetoencephalography
MELAS	mitochondrial encephalomyopathy, lactic acidosis, and stroke-like episodes
MFTLE	Mesial familial temporal lobe epilepsy
MHD	10-hydroxy-10,11-dihydro-5H-dibenzazepine-5-carboxamide
MSI	magnetic source imaging
MRI	magnetic resonance imaging
MRS	magnetic resonance spectroscopy
MRSI	magnetic resonance spectroscopic imaging
MTLE	mesial temporal lobe epilepsy
MTLE-HS	mesial temporal lobe epilepsy with hippocampal sclerosis
NAA	*N*-acetyl aspartate
NADH	reduced nicotinamide adenine dinucleotide
NICE	National Institute for Clinical Excellence
NMDA	*N*-methyl-D-aspartate
NREM	non-rapid eye movement
OPL	oro-pharyngo-laryngeal
OPS	occipital seizures precipitated by photic stimuli
PET	positron emission tomography
PMA	perioral myoclonia with absences
PNES	psychogenic nonepileptic seizure
PPR	photoparoxysmal responses
PS	Panayiotopoulos syndrome
QS&TTA	Quality Standards and the Therapeutic and Technology Assessment Subcommittee of the American Academy of Neurology and the American Epilepsy Society
RCT	randomised clinical trial
REM	rapid eye movement
RS	Rolandic seizures
SANAD	Standard and New Antiepileptic Drugs Project
S1po	perioral region of the primary somatosensory cortex
SMA	supplementary sensorimotor area
SPECT	single photon emission computed tomography
SV2A	synaptic vesicle protein 2A
SWI	spike–wave index
TDS	therapeutic drug monitoring
TLE	temporal lobe epilepsy
UGT	uridine diphosphate glucuronosyltransferase
VER	visual evoked response
VGS	video game-induced seizures
VNS	vagal nerve stimulation

1 CLINICAL ASPECTS OF THE DIAGNOSIS OF EPILEPTIC SEIZURES AND EPILEPTIC SYNDROMES

Patients with epileptic seizures and their families are entitled to a diagnosis, prognosis and management that are specific and precise. The inclusive, monolectic diagnostic label 'epilepsy' is unsatisfactory to patient and physician alike and may result in avoidable morbidity and mortality. 'Epilepsy' is not a single disease entity. Epilepsies are many syndromes and diseases that have a multitude of different manifestations and causes. Effective classification of epileptic seizures and syndromes is indispensable for appropriate management and prognosis. The short- and long-term management of epilepsies is often syndrome related and differs markedly between various disorders manifesting with seizures, thereby emphasising the need for accurate diagnosis.

There are three important diagnostic steps towards this aim.

- **First step: are the paroxysmal events epileptic seizures?** This is detailed in the differential diagnosis of epileptic from nonepileptic seizures (pages 2-7)
- **Second step: what type of epileptic seizures?** This is detailed in epileptic seizures and their classification (pages 8-14)
- **Third step: what is their cause and what is the epileptic syndrome or epileptic disease?** This is detailed in epileptic syndromes and their classification (pages 15-26)

ILAE definitions of epilepsy and seizures

There is no uniform definition of 'epilepsy'. The following are definitions of the ILAE [1-4] for epileptic seizures and epileptic syndromes/diseases, some of which are not satisfactory. It is expected that any new ILAE proposal will solve the problem of better defining our topic of study.

Epilepsy: a liability to clinically manifested seizures of any type (would be my proposal).

Epileptic disorder: a chronic neurological condition characterised by recurrent epileptic seizures.[4]

Epilepsies: those conditions involving chronic recurrent epileptic seizures that can be considered epileptic disorders.[4]

Epilepsy: a condition characterised by recurrent (two or more) epileptic seizures, unprovoked by any immediate identified cause (operational definition for epidemiological purposes). [1;2] Multiple seizures occurring in a 24-h period are considered a single event. An episode of status epilepticus is considered a single event. Persons who have had only febrile seizures or only neonatal seizures as herein defined are excluded from this category.[1;2]

Author's note: in this definition the type of 'epileptic seizures' is not defined, but this probably refers to generalised tonic clonic seizures (GTCS).[1;2]

"Active" epilepsy: a prevalent case of active epilepsy is defined as a person with epilepsy who has had at least one epileptic seizure in the previous 5 years, regardless of antiepileptic drug (AED) treatment. A case under treatment is someone with the correct diagnosis of epilepsy receiving (or having received) AEDs on prevalence day.[1;2]

Epilepsy in remission with treatment: a prevalent case of epilepsy with no seizures for ≥ 5 years and receiving AED treatment at the time of ascertainment.[1;2]

Epilepsy in remission without treatment: a prevalent case of epilepsy with no seizures for ≥ 5 years and no receiving AED treatment at the time of ascertainment.[1;2]

Epileptic seizure: manifestation(s) of epileptic (excessive and/or hypersynchronous) usually self-limited activity of neurones in the brain.[4]

Epileptic seizure: a clinical manifestation presumed to result from an abnormal and excessive discharge of a set of neurones in the brain. The clinical manifestation consists of a sudden and transitory abnormal phenomena which may include alterations of consciousness, motor, sensory, autonomic, or psychic events perceived by the patient or an observer.[1;2]

Epileptic seizure type: an ictal event believed to represent a unique pathophysiological mechanism and anatomic substrate. This is a diagnostic entity with aetiologic, therapeutic and prognostic implications (new concept).[3]

Single or isolated seizure: one or more epileptic seizures occurring in a 24-h period. [1;2]

DIFFERENTIAL DIAGNOSIS OF PAROXYSMAL EVENTS: EPILEPTIC AND NONEPILEPTIC SEIZURES

The first step towards the *correct* diagnosis of epilepsies is to establish whether a paroxysmal clinical event was actually an epileptic seizure or something else. The differential diagnosis includes all causes of episodic impairment of awareness, aberrations of mental function, falls, sensory/motor phenomena and generalised convulsive movements, which are common presenting symptoms of epileptic seizures. This is often easy for physicians adequately trained in the recognition of the various forms of epileptic seizures, who are able to obtain a clear history of the events from the patient and witnesses. However, even the most experienced epileptologists time and again have great difficulties in reaching an unequivocal diagnosis for reasons such as atypical seizure presentations, inadequate historical data or overlapping symptom manifestations.

Misdiagnosis in epilepsies, when considering its dimensions and consequences, is a colossal medical problem. Common disorders and even normal phenomena may imitate epileptic seizures and, conversely, certain types of epileptic seizures may imitate symptoms of other diseases. Misdiagnosis has serious repercussions. Patients with nonepileptic disorders incorrectly diagnosed as having epileptic seizures are likely to be mistreated with antiepileptic drugs and also denied specific and possibly life-saving treatment (Figure 1.1). Similarly, patients with epileptic seizures erroneously diagnosed as migraine, encephalitis or other nonepileptic paroxysmal events are likely to be mismanaged with inappropriate treatments and also deprived of specific therapies.

FITS, FAINTS AND FUNNY TURNS

The differentiation between seizures and other causes of transient neurological disturbance and collapse is epitomised by the familiar theme 'fits, faints and funny turns'.[5,6] Distinguishing epileptic *(fits)* from paroxysmal symptoms of nonepileptic disorders, particularly syncopal *(faints)*[5,7,8] or psychogenic attacks *(funny turns)*[9-13] should be a core skill of all trained physicians as detailed in any textbook of medicine. However, this is often simplistic and frequently perpetuates certain myths such as that incontinence of urine or postsyncopal confusion are rare in syncopes (Figure 1.1) or tongue biting and injuries are exceptional features in psychogenic nonepileptic seizures.

The presence or absence of a single symptom is not sufficiently diagnostic of one or another disease and may be misleading. The clinical diagnosis is often easy and secured only if individual elements of clinical events are meaningfully assessed regarding quantity, quality, location, onset, chronological sequence, development, speed of progress and duration.

PAROXYSMAL NONEPILEPTIC EVENTS MISDIAGNOSED AS EPILEPTIC SEIZURES

Paroxysmal nonepileptic events misdiagnosed as epileptic seizures affect as many as 20–30% of patients diagnosed and often treated for many years as epilepsy or admitted in tertiary care epilepsy units.[11,12] The problem is complicated by the fact that approximately 30% of patients with genuine epileptic seizures also suffer from nonepileptic mainly psychogenic seizures. In one study, the mean time-lapse between the first attack and the correct diagnosis of nonepileptic seizures was over 9 years.[14] In financial terms the annual cost of such a misdiagnosis can be estimated at between \$650 000 000 and \$4 000 000 000.[15]

Nonepileptic seizure is the currently preferred descriptive name for common and numerous paroxysmal clinical events of diverse aetiologies that mimic or look like but are not epileptic seizures.[11,13,16,17] These are divided into two groups.

- **Physiological or organic nonepileptic seizures.**
- **Psychogenic nonepileptic seizures.**

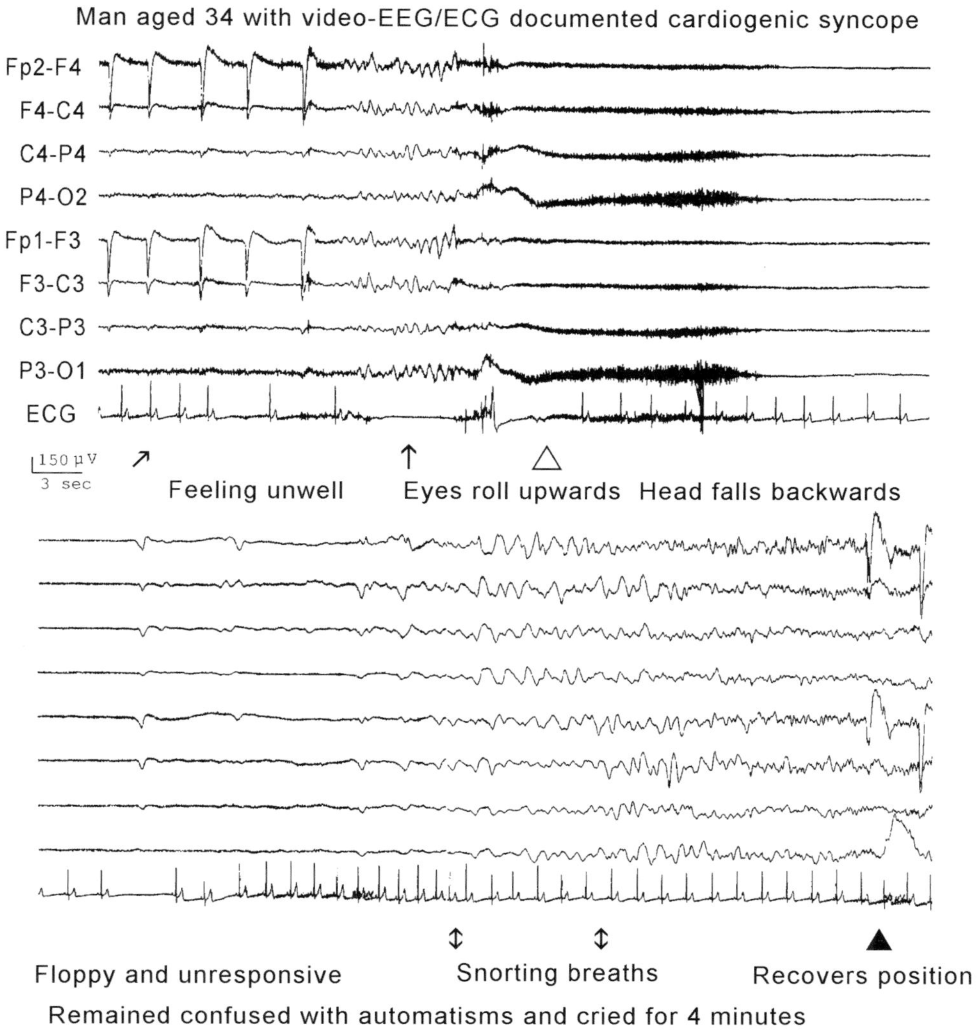

Figure 1.1 Potentially life-threatening cardiogenic syncopes imitating epileptic generalised convulsive seizures.

A 34-year-old man was referred for routine EEG because of 'two episodes of GTCS in the last 2 months. The first occurred on his way home after college. He does not recall events until waking in the ambulance with the paramedics telling him that he had a seizure. He has no memory of the preceding 30 minutes. He did bite his tongue but there was no incontinence… This is likely to be generalised epilepsy… Treatment with valproate was initiated.'

In accordance with our policy this was a video EEG recording (page. 39). A few minutes after the start of the recording he developed sinus bradycardia and then ventricular standstill for 9 s with one escape ectopic beat as documented with ECG (bottom trace). Clinically, at the oblique arrow the technologist asked him if he felt okay and he said no. At the vertical arrow his eyes rolled slowly upwards to the extreme. At the open arrow, he became flaccid and unresponsive and his head dropped backwards. Some recovery started at the double-headed arrows when he took two snorting breaths. At the black arrowhead, he resumed his position as before the syncope. Afterwards he was confused, he could not answer questions and, when asked again what happened to him, he was distressed and cried. He did not come back to normal until after more than 4 min from the start of the syncope.

A cardiac pacemaker has been implanted and the patient remained well in the next 6 months of follow-up.

PHYSIOLOGICAL OR ORGANIC NONEPILEPTIC SEIZURES

The physiological or organic nonepileptic seizures are a broad spectrum of episodic manifestations ranging from normal phenomena such as hypnagogic jerks, hallucinations or illusions to a galaxy of abnormal paroxysmal symptoms of a variety of brain and systemic disorders. These include syncope, vertigo and dizziness, migraine attacks, transient ischaemic attacks, transient global amnesia and other manifestations of cerebrovascular disease, paroxysmal movement disorders,[18] paroxysmal symptoms of endocrine or metabolic diseases and paroxysmal toxic phenomena. In sleep the parasomnias, including bruxism (teeth gnashing), pavor nocturnus (night terrors), somnambulism (sleep walking) and rapid eye movement (REM) behaviour disorders, are frequently mistaken for epileptic seizures.[19-24] The differential diagnosis is much more demanding in neonates, babies, toddlers and young children in whom there are many different causes and seizure imitators such as normal and abnormal behaviours of neonates, hyperekplexia, reflex anoxic epileptic seizures,[25] cyanotic breath-holding attacks, gastro-oesophageal reflux, nonepileptic myoclonus, parasomnias, benign paroxysmal vertigo,[26] cyclic vomiting syndrome,[27,28] episodic ataxias, tics, staring, Munchausen syndrome by proxy (a term used to describe the situation in which one person, usually a mother on behalf of her child, persistently fabricates illness on behalf of another)[29-32] and self-gratification.[5,16,25,33-38]

Syncopal attacks

Syncopal attacks are frequently associated with myoclonic jerking, rolling of the eyes and brief automatisms[5,39-41] and, conversely, epileptic seizures may manifest with syncopal-like attacks.

Occasionally, but more often than has been reported, true epileptic seizures are triggered by nonepileptic syncopes in children and adults.[5,25,42-44] This combination of syncope and epileptic seizure has been called an anoxic epileptic seizure. This phenomenon is not considered in any international classification despite significant diagnostic and management implications. Recently, anoxic epileptic seizures have been reported and documented with home video recordings.[43] Examples include the following:

- Neurally mediated syncope, probably mediated by prolonged expiratory apnoea (breath-holding attacks), inducing a long, clonic epileptic seizure with some features of myoclonic absence.
- A compulsive Valsalva in an older autistic child provoking a vibratory tonic epileptic seizure.
- Spontaneous epileptic seizures with features of myoclonic absence in a child who had both epilepsy and identical episodes induced by syncopes.[43]

Important points in the differential diagnosis of syncope from epileptic seizures

Convulsions occur in 70–90% of neurocardiogenic syncopes and symptoms include myoclonus, tonic flexion or extension, more complex movements and automatisms such as lip licking, chewing or fumbling.

Eyes are always open during syncope and the most consistent ocular motor sign is an upward turning of the eyes early in the course of syncope (Figure 1.1), which may be followed by lateral eye deviation.[45]

Visual hallucinations (a perception of grey haze, coloured patches, glaring lights or more complex scenes involving landscapes, familiar situations or people) and, less often, auditory hallucinations (rushing and roaring sounds, traffic and machine noises and talking and screaming human voices, but never intelligible speech) are frequent (60%) in both convulsive and nonconvulsive syncope.[46]

PSYCHOGENIC NONEPILEPTIC SEIZURES

Psychogenic nonepileptic seizures are amongst the commoner recurrent paroxysmal seizure-imitating events that result from a variety of psychological disturbances.[9-13] Psychogenic nonepileptic seizures is the currently preferred name rather than their synonym *pseudoseizures*, which is considered prejudicial. These are not *'pseudo'* in that they are extremely real episodes and pseudo implies a disparaging element to the events. Like epileptic seizures, psychogenic nonepileptic seizures can be very troublesome to a person's life and have their own stigma.

Patients with psychogenic nonepileptic seizures are often experiencing severe depression, anxiety, emotional stress, rage, fear, panic and other mental disturbances. Conversion disorder is the most common cause of psychogenic nonepileptic seizures.[47] Others, with natural histories and treatments different from those of conversion disorder, include anxiety, dissociative, depersonalisation, somatisation, panic or psychotic disorders.[9-13] Factitious psychogenic nonepileptic seizures, including Munchausen syndrome, are sometimes difficult to diagnose and prove.

Pseudostatus epilepticus is common in patients with psychogenic nonepileptic seizures and it is often misdiagnosed as genuine and life-threatening convulsive status epilepticus.[48] These patients commonly have multiple episodes of *'status'* and receive intensive care unit management. They usually have a history of other unexplained illness and of deliberate self-poisoning. Episodes of anticonvulsant-induced respiratory arrest may occur.[48]

Diagnostic clues for convulsive psychogenic nonepileptic seizures (the commoner of all psychogenic nonepileptic seizures)

Often precipitated by stressful circumstances and in response to suggestion.

Occur in wakefulness and in the presence of witnesses.

Lack stereotypicity.

'Convulsions' consist of asynchronous, asymmetrical, waxing and waning, accelerating and decelerating, convulsive-like movements often with pelvic thrusts, flailing and tremors. These may be interrupted or resistant to restraint. Attempts to open the eyes passively often result in tightening of the eyelids.

Consciousness may be retained throughout or shows marked fluctuations.

There is no actual postictal confusion. The patient may become emotional and cry after the end of the nonepileptic seizure.

Intractable to antiepileptic medication.

Diagnostic traps

At least one of the usual signs associated with a GTCS (tongue biting, falling or incontinence) is reported by more than half (66%) of patients with nonepileptic seizures.[14]
An ictal EEG is not always abnormal during epileptic seizures.

Psychogenic nonepileptic seizures including staring[49,50] are often extremely difficult to differentiate from epileptic seizures[9-13,16] and, conversely, certain types of epileptic seizures such as of mesial frontal lobe origin masquerade as psychogenic-like attacks.

Psychogenic nonepileptic seizures need urgent and skilful treatment, which is often successful particularly if recognised and managed at an early stage.[11-13] The role of the physician is not just simply to announce to the patient *'you do not suffer from epileptic seizures'*. At this stage, the patient requires a thorough and tactful explanation of what this new diagnosis of psychogenic nonepileptic seizures means and the appropriate management procedures. These patients were allowed to believe for many years that they suffered from 'epilepsy' that was intractable to medication. Their reaction and that of their family to a new diagnosis of 'psychogenic seizures' (also taking into consideration the negative social implications and attitudes to this term) should be thoroughly considered. Patients' understanding and reactions to a diagnosis of these nonepileptic attacks are important factors that should contribute to the development of more tailored treatment approaches.[51]

> Many neurologists and epileptologists, those steeped in the organic tradition, are dreadfully uncomfortable with psychologically mediated disorders … Obviously, sensitivity to the patient, utilization of a multidisciplinary team, and recognition that psychogenic nonepileptic seizures are as devastating as medically refractory epilepsy are critical to a successful treatment outcome.[12]

Diagnostic clues for staring
Staring is a frequent epileptic or nonepileptic manifestation.[49] During a spell of unresponsiveness, documenting an increase in heart rate > 30% over baseline has a positive predictive value of 97% in favour of epileptic rather than psychogenic nonepileptic seizures.[50]

EPILEPTIC SEIZURES IMITATING NONEPILEPTIC ATTACKS

Epileptic seizures may imitate syncope, psychogenic attacks, migraine, sleep disorders or sinister acute brain insults

Their diagnosis is also demanding as documented by the fact that, until recently, (1) frontal seizures from the supplementary sensorimotor area were considered as sleep disorders, (2) ictus emeticus and autonomic status epilepticus, common in children, were dismissed as nonepileptic events or misdiagnosed as migraine or encephalitis and (3) visual seizures were confused with basilar migraine or migraine with visual aura.

Simple focal seizures of epigastric aura and 'panic attacks' are unlikely to raise suspicion of epilepsy either by the patient or the general physician (Figure 2.2). These patients are often investigated for gastroenterological and psychological disorders[52] or hypoglycaemia until more salient seizure features appear with the development of complex focal seizures and secondarily GTCS.

DIAGNOSING EPILEPTIC AND NONEPILEPTIC SEIZURES

The diagnosis of epileptic and nonepileptic seizures is almost always based solely on the clinical history, which should be masterly obtained, often requiring lengthy interrogation(s) of the patient and witnesses. Sometimes the diagnosis is easy based on clinical history alone, while at other times it is necessary to ask for video recordings of the events. More difficult cases need video EEG documentation.

In taking the medical history, every piece of information should be patiently gathered in order to assess the whole pattern of these transient events from the time that these started to their end and up to normality. The medical history should include the circumstances under which the paroxysmal events occurred, timing, awake or sleep, standing or sitting, at rest or during exercise, possible triggering, precipitating or facilitating factors and personal and family medical history. A second interview frequently provides more observations and recollections after learning what is desired during the initial consultation. Lengthy medical interviews may seem luxury medicine, but this by far outweighs the benefits to patients, their families and their physicians. Constraints on the physicians' time should not be an excuse for allowing misdiagnosis and mismanagement to occur. With experience the time required to take an appropriate medical history is significantly shortened. Personally, I devote more time to eliciting the events preceding a GTCS than detailing what happened during the convulsive phase (if I am satisfied that this was a genuine GTCS) and directing the witnesses to portray what they saw rather than allocate time for endless descriptions of how they felt and what they did (though I fully respect it).

Circadian distribution (on awakening, nocturnal and diurnal) and precipitating factors (flickering lights, sleep deprivation, alcohol indulgence, stress and reading) often provide invaluable clues for the correct diagnosis and may also prompt the appropriate EEG procedure to be performed.

'That's it!' phenomenon

It is often necessary for the physician to imitate and demonstrate physically or, when in doubt, to show videotaped examples of different epileptic or nonepileptic seizures in order to discover which resemble the events under investigation: the 'that's it!' phenomenon (as Stephenson[4] called it).

Home video recording should be routinely requested if the diagnosis is uncertain. Videotaping the clinical events is the only practical means of demonstrating and objectively documenting the symptoms of paroxysmal disorders. Camcorders are widely available, cheap and easy to use. Genuine epileptic or nonepileptic seizures are often frequent, sometimes predictable and can be recorded reliably by relatives or friends and sometimes by the patients themselves.

INVESTIGATIVE PROCEDURES

Laboratory procedures (blood and urine tests, ECG, EEG, brain imaging and others) should be tailored to the particular clinical problem and aim to provide supplementary evidence of the clinical suspicion and may be diagnostic of specific disorders. In epilepsies EEG is mandatory for all patients (but often misleading in nonepileptic seizures without video-recorded symptoms). Brain imaging is for documenting or excluding suspected structural abnormalities.

Ideally, epileptic or nonepileptic seizures should be recorded during out-patient video EEG or in-patient video EEG monitoring, if the diagnosis is questionable.[35,36,38,53] An ambulatory EEG is of significance only if recorded habitual seizures (epileptic or nonepileptic) are void of significant muscle and movement artefacts that may obscure genuine brain activity.

Postictal prolactin levels can be used for differentiating between epileptic and nonepileptic seizures, but their value is often limited.[12,53] Prolactin levels are elevated at approximately 20 min postictally of a convulsive or complex focal seizure. Prolactin fails to rise after nonepileptic seizures. However, the prolactin levels do not elevate after all complex focal seizures and may decrease after repetitive epileptic fits. Further, prolactin may be elevated in convulsive syncope, nipple manipulation in females and patients on psychotropic drugs.

The significance of the EEG and its optimal use in the diagnosis of the epilepsies is detailed in Chapter 2. Brain imaging in the diagnosis and management of epilepsies is outlined in Chapter 3. Molecular genetics are already making decisive discoveries in the identification of epilepsies and these are mainly described in Chapter 11.

EPILEPTIC SEIZURES AND THEIR CLASSIFICATION

Having established that a paroxysmal event is genuinely epileptic , the next step, not the final step, is to define the type of seizure or seizures, which is a prerequisite for the correct diagnosis and management.

There are numerous types of epileptic seizures, which in their presentation may be minor or dramatic, brief or long, frequent or sparse or singular. Clinical manifestations of seizures range from the dramatic events of a GTCS to the mild myoclonic flickering of the eyelids or a focal numbness of the thumb and mouth. Minor seizures are often overlooked although they are more important than a GTCS in the diagnosis of epilepsies.[54] The same patient may suffer from different types of minor and major seizures, independently or evolving from one to the other.

Minor seizures are more important than major seizures for diagnostic procedures, correct diagnosis and appropriate management strategies

Minor seizures include myoclonic jerks, absences and simple or complex focal seizures. Minor seizures should be thoroughly sought during the clinical evaluation (Figure 1.2). Patients are unlikely to report minor seizures because they do not appreciate that these are epileptic events and their significance. It is the physician's responsibility to detect and evaluate them.

A single GTCS does not require medication, but if the patient also has other even minor seizures treatment is usually mandatory (Figure 1.2). Similarly, it is a medical error to advise the withdrawal of medication for a patient with minor seizures even if free of convulsive seizures for many years.

Clarification on the ILAE seizure and syndrome classifications

The standardised classification and terminology for epileptic seizures[56] and syndromes [57] by the ILAE provides a fundamental framework for organising and differentiating them. This categorisation is essential in clinical practice and research on epilepsies. The currently valid classification of Epileptic Seizures is used from 1981[56] and the last revision of the Classification of Epilepsies and Epileptic Syndromes was in 1989.[57] The ILAE Task Force recently proposed a new diagnostic scheme[3] the basic concepts of which were accepted by the ILAE General Assembly in 2001 but "none of these proposals are yet complete, nor are any intended to constitute a classification… ".[58] The relevant editorials in *Epilepsia* on 'Cabbages and Kings in the Classification of Seizures and the Epilepsies' are authoritative and well-presented views on the different methodologies, approaches, targets and philosophies of these classifications.[58-63]

Definitions

Focal (synonym = partial) seizure: a seizure that has an initial semiology which indicates or is consistent with initial activation of only part of one cerebral hemisphere.[4] See also another ILAE definition in page 10.

Generalised (synonym = bilateral) seizure: a seizure that has an initial semiology which indicates or is consistent with more than minimal involvement of both cerebral hemispheres.[4] .

Aura: a subjective ictal phenomenon that, in a given patient, may precede an observable seizure; if alone it constitutes a sensory seizure.[4]

Prodrome: a preictal phenomenon, i.e. a subjective or objective clinical alteration (e.g. ill-localised sensation or agitation) that heralds the onset of an epileptic seizure but does not form part of it.[4]

Aura is not synonymous to prodrome: aura is a seizure itself while prodrome is not a seizure.

Ictus: a sudden neurological occurrence such as a stroke or an epileptic seizure.[4]

Ictal: the seizure period or events due to a seizure.

Interictal: the interval between seizures.

Postictal: a transient clinical abnormality of central nervous system function that appears or becomes accentuated when clinical signs of the ictus have ended.[4]

Impaired consciousness is defined as the inability to respond normally to exogenous stimuli by virtue of altered awareness and/or responsiveness. Aberrations of behaviour (automatisms) may occur in patients with impaired consciousness. There is considerable evidence that simple partial seizures usually have unilateral hemispheric involvement and only rarely have bilateral hemispheric involvement; however, complex partial seizures frequently have bilateral hemispheric involvement.[56]

Minor seizures, such as brief myoclonic jerks, mild absences and simple or even complex focal seizures, may go unnoticed for many years or be ignored as normal

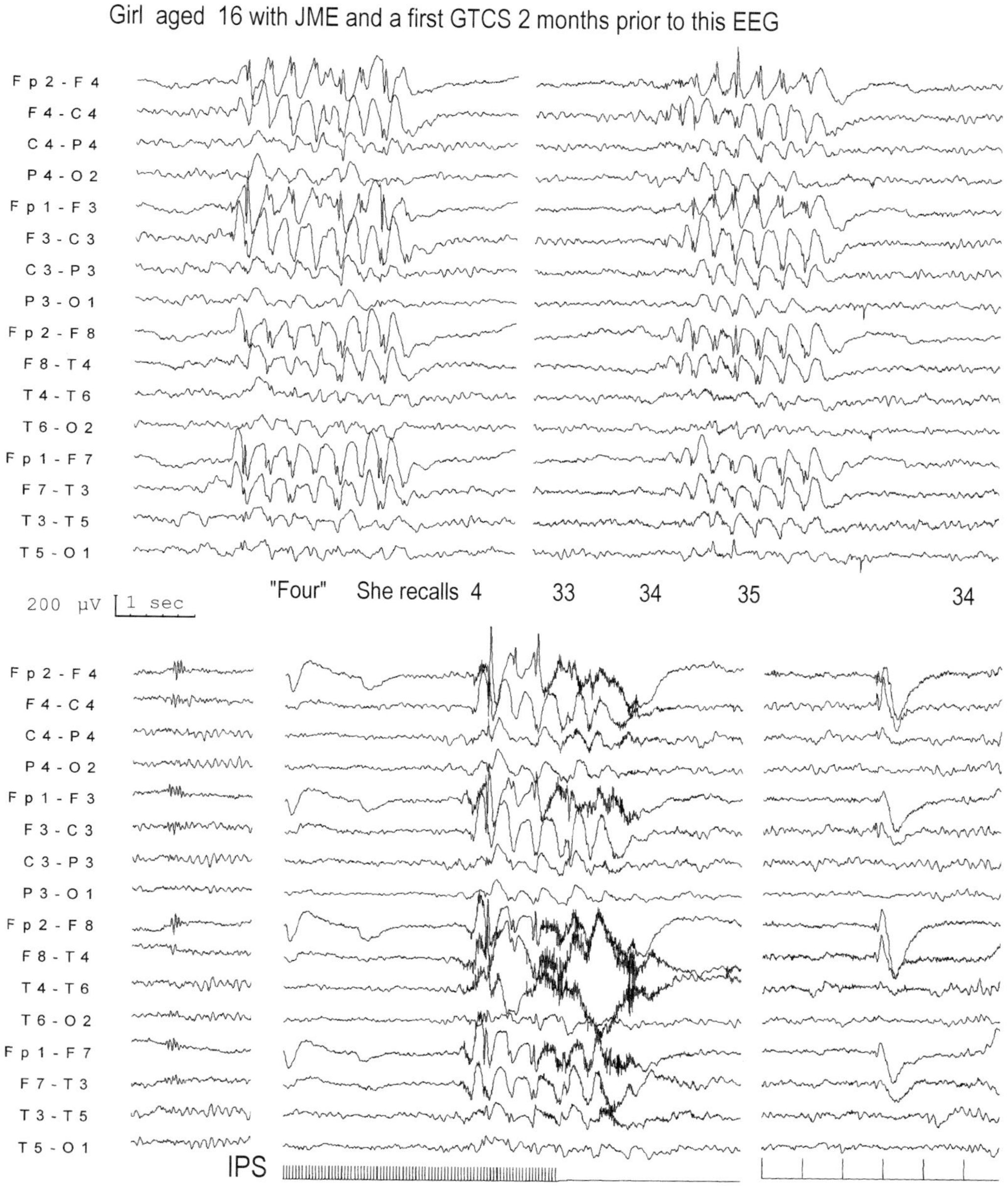

Figure 1.2 Video EEG of a 16-year-old girl referred for an EEG because of 'a first generalised tonic clonic seizure' at age 16 years.

This happened in the morning on her way to school for examinations. She suddenly became vague and nearly simultaneously she fell on the ground with generalised convulsions. On questioning by the EEG technologist, it was revealed that 1 year before the GTCS she had mild jerks of the fingers in the morning interpreted as clumsiness. The EEG had generalised discharges of 3–4 Hz spike/multiple spike and slow wave. The girl recalled the number shouted to her during the discharge. However, breath counting during hyperventilation was disturbed during a similar discharge (annotated numbers). In addition there were photoparoxysmal discharges. Brief frontal bursts of polyspikes or spike and slow wave could be erroneously interpreted as 'frontal lobe epilepsy with secondary bilateral synchrony' (page 166). On clinical and EEG grounds the diagnosis of juvenile myoclonic epilepsy was established and appropriate treatment was initiated because she had many more seizures (myoclonic jerks) prior and in addition to the single GTCS.

variations in a person's life. Typical examples in this respect are patients with juvenile myoclonic epilepsy who may have frequent myoclonic jerks many years prior to a GTCS (Figure 1.2) or patients with temporal lobe epilepsy who may have frequent classical simple focal seizures (auras) many years prior to a GTCS. Even if frequent, these seizure events are unlikely to raise concerns and promote a medical consultation. Conversely, a major seizure such as a GTCS invariably draws medical attention.

Patients may often suffer many minor seizures long before the reported 'first seizure' or long after what is considered as their 'last seizure'.[54]

Three-quarters (74%) of patients with 'newly identified unprovoked seizures' (mainly GTCS) had experienced multiple seizure episodes prior to their first medical contact.[55] Yet, studies on the prognosis and treatment of the 'first seizure' mainly refer to a GTCS although this may not be the first seizure in the patient's life.

EPILEPTIC SEIZURES IN ACCORDANCE WITH THE ILAE CLASSIFICATION OF 1981[56]

The currently valid ILAE seizure classification of 1981[56] is an old updated version of the classification proposed by Gastaut in 1970.[64] It is based on clinical and EEG (ictal and interictal) manifestations (Tables 1.1 and 1.2). Seizures are primarily divided into the following types.

- **Partial (focal or local) seizures** (with great variation in clinical expression and severity).
- **Generalised seizures (tonic, clonic or tonic-clonic, myoclonic and typical or atypical absences).**

Such a dichotomy is necessary because an abnormal paroxysmal discharge of cerebral neurons may be localised (partial seizures) or simultaneously affect the whole cerebral cortex from onset to termination (generalised seizures).[56]

This classification also recognises the following types of seizure.

- **Unclassified epileptic seizures**, which cannot be classified because of inadequate or incomplete data and some that defy classification in hitherto described categories. This includes some neonatal seizures, e.g. rhythmic eye movements, chewing and swimming movements.[56]
- **Prolonged or repetitive seizures (status epilepticus).**

PARTIAL (OR FOCAL) SEIZURES (Table 1.1)

Partial seizures are those in which, in general, the first clinical and EEG changes indicate initial activation of a system of neurons limited to a part of one cerebral hemisphere.[56]

Terminological changes in the new diagnostic scheme[3]

The old term 'focal' is reintroduced to replace 'partial' and 'localisation-related' epileptic seizures, which is understandable.

However, this new scheme abandons the division of focal seizures into 'simple' (without impairment of consciousness) and 'complex' (with impairment of consciousness).[3] The reason given is that this 'inappropriately created the impression that impairment of consciousness had certain mechanistic implications related to limbic system involvement' and that 'complex partial seizures' has been erroneously used as a synonym of 'temporal lobe epilepsy'.[3] Though these are correct, there are significant practical reasons (medico-legal cases, driving and job-related performance) for distinguishing seizures with or without impairment of consciousness.

Therefore, I keep using the terms 'simple' and 'complex' focal seizures in this book, while emphasising that (1) ictal impairment of consciousness is a symptom of either neocortical or limbic seizures and (2) complex focal seizures may originate from any cerebral lobe and therefore they are not synonymous with temporal lobe epilepsy.

The scheme also introduces the terms 'continuous seizure types' for status epilepticus and 'self-limited seizure types' for briefer seizures. These terms are unlikely to find any support and I do not use them in this book.

Table 1.1 ILAE Classification of partial (focal, local) seizures[56]

Clinical seizure type	EEG seizure type	EEG interictal expression
A. Simple partial seizures (consciousness not impaired) 1. With motor signs a) Focal motor without march b) Focal motor with march (Jacksonian) c) Versive d) Postural e) Phonatory (vocalization or arrest of speech) 2. With somatosensory or special-sensory symptoms (simple hallucinations, e.g., tingling, light flashes, buzzing) a) Somatosensory b) Visual c) Auditory d) Olfactory c) Gustatory f)) Vertiginous 3. With autonomic symptoms or signs (including epigastric sensation, pallor, sweating, flushing, piloerection, and pupillary dilatation). 4. With psychic symptoms (disturbance of higher cerebral function). These symptoms rarely occur without impairment of consciousness and are much more commonly experienced as complex partial seizures. a) Dysphasic b) Dysmnesic (e.g., déjà-vu) c) Cognitive (e.g., dreamy states, distortions of time sense). d) Affective (fear, anger, etc.) e) Illusions (e.g., macropsia) f) Structured hallucinations (e.g., music, scenes)	Local contralateral discharge starting over the corresponding area of cortical representation (not always recorded on the scale)	Local contralateral discharge
B. Complex partial seizures (with impairment of consciousness; may sometimes begin with simple symptomatology) 1. Simple partial onset followed by impairment of consciousness a) With simple partial features (Al to A4) followed by impaired consciousness b) With automatisms 2. With impairment of consciousness at onset a) With impairment of consciousness only b) With automatisms	Unilateral or, frequently, bilateral discharge, diffuse or focal in temporal or fronto-temporal regions	Unilateral or bilateral generally asynchronous focus; usually in the temporal or frontal regions
C. Partial seizures evolving to secondarily generalized seizures (this may be generalized tonic-clonic tonic. or clonic) (above discharges becomes secondarily and rapidly generalised) 1. Simple partial seizures (A) evolving to generalised seizure 2. Complex partial (B) evolving to generalised seizure 3. Simple partial seizures evolving to complex partial seizures evolving to generalised seizure		

From: The Commission on Classification and Terminology of the International League Against Epilepsy. Proposal for revised clinical and electroencephalographic classification of epileptic seizures. With the permission of the Editor of Epilepsia.[55]

Partial seizures are classified primarily on the basis of whether or not consciousness is impaired during the attack and whether or not progression to generalised convulsions occurs.

A. Simple partial seizures (when consciousness is not impaired).

B. Complex partial seizures (when consciousness is impaired). Impairment of consciousness may be the first clinical sign or simple partial seizures may evolve into complex partial seizures.

A partial seizure may not terminate, but instead progress to a generalised motor seizure.

C. Partial seizures evolving to secondarily generalised (tonic-clonic or tonic or clonic) seizures.

GENERALISED SEIZURES (Table 1.2)

'Generalised seizures are those in which the first clinical changes indicate initial involvement of both hemispheres. Consciousness may be impaired and this impairment may be the initial manifestation. Motor manifestations are bilateral. The ictal EEG patterns initially are bilateral and presumably reflect neuronal discharge, which is widespread in both hemispheres'. [56]

Generalised seizures may be convulsive or nonconvulsive and vary considerably: mild or severe myoclonic jerks, inconspicuous or severe typical and atypical absences and generalised clonic, tonic or tonic clonic convulsions. [56]

Generalised seizures may be primarily or secondarily generalised.

- *Primarily* generalised seizures are generalised from the onset.
- *Secondarily* generalised seizures are partial (focal) at onset but do not remain localised. They spread and trigger a generalised fit.

Important note on the terminology of *primarily* and *secondarily* generalised seizures

I purposely highlighted the words *primarily* and *secondarily* generalised seizures because these are often confused with primary (= idiopathic) and secondary (= symptomatic or cryptogenic) which are often used as adjuncts to 'epilepsy' (see also page. 281).

The ILAE classification of generalised seizures is presented in Table 1.2 with the following broad categories.[56]

A1. Absence seizures.

A2. Atypical absence seizures.

B. Myoclonic seizures.

C. Clonic seizures.

D. Tonic seizures.

E. Tonic-clonic seizures.

F. Atonic seizures.

PRECIPITATED (REFLEX) SEIZURES

Reflex epileptic seizures are detailed in Chapter 13.

They are consistently precipitated by environmental or internal stimuli and are differentiated from spontaneous epileptic attacks in which precipitating factors cannot be identified. In individual patients, the precipitating stimuli are usually limited to a single specific stimulus or a limited number of closely related stimuli.

Reflex seizures may, like spontaneous seizures, be:

- generalised, primarily or secondarily
- focal, simple or complex.

SEIZURE CLASSIFICATION IN THE NEW DIAGNOSTIC ILAE SCHEME

The new diagnostic scheme of the ILAE Task Force is divided into five parts or axes, organised to facilitate a logical clinical approach to the development of hypotheses necessary to determine the diagnostic studies and therapeutic strategies to be undertaken in individual patients (Table 1.3).[3,65]

Table 1.4 is the list of seizures as provided by the ILAE Task Force.[3]

For didactic purposes, I describe the various types of seizures when appropriate in the relevant epileptic syndromes.

Table 1.2 ILAE Classification of generalised seizures (convulsive and nonconvulsive)[56]

Clinical seizure type	EEG seizure type	EEG interictal expression
A1. Absence seizures a) Impairment of consciousness only b) With mild clonic components c) With atonic components d) With tonic components e) With automatisms f) With autonomic components *(b through f may be used alone or in combination)*	Usually regular and symmetrical 3 Hz but may be 2–4 Hz spike-and-slow wave complexes and may have multiple spike-and-slow wave complexes. Abnormalities are bilateral	Background activity usually normal although paroxysmal activity (such as spikes or spike-and-slow wave complexes) may occur. This activity is usually regular and symmetrical
A2. Atypical absence May have: a) Changes in tone which are more pronounced than in A1 b) Onset and/or cessation which is not abrupt	EEG more heterogeneous, may include irregular spike-and-wave complexes. fast activity or other paroxysmal actions. Abnormalities are bilateral but often irregular and asymmetrical	Background usually abnormal paroxysmal activity (such as spikes or spike-and-slow wave complexes) frequently irregular and asymmetrical
B. Myoclonic seizures Myoclonic jerks (single or multiple)	Polyspike and wave or sometimes spike and wave or sharp and slow waves	Same as ictal
C. Clonic seizures	Fast activity (10 cycles/s or more) and slow waves or occasional spike and wave patterns	Spike and wave or polyspike and wave discharges
D. Tonic seizures	Low voltage fast activity or a fast rhythm 9–10 cycles/s or more decreasing in frequency and increasing in amplitude	More or less rhythmic discharges of sharp and slow waves, sometimes asymmetrical, background is often abnormal for age
E. Tonic-clonic seizures	Rhythm at 10 or more cycles/s decreasing in frequency and increasing in amplitude during tonic phase. Interrupted by slow waves during clonic phase	Polyspike and waves or spike and wave or, sometimes, sharp- and slow-wave discharges
F. Atonic seizures (astatic) *Combinations of the above may occur, e.g. B and F, B and D*	Polyspikes and wave or flattening or low-voltage fast activity	Polyspikes and slow wave

From: The Commission on Classification and Terminology of the International League Against Epilepsy. Proposal for revised clinical and electroencephalographic classification of epileptic seizures. With the permission of the Editor of Epilepsia.[55]

Table 1.3 Proposed diagnostic scheme for people with epileptic seizures and with epilepsy [3]

Epileptic seizures and epilepsy syndromes are to be described and categorized according to a system that uses standardized terminology, and that is sufficiently flexible to take into account the following practical and dynamic aspects of epilepsy diagnosis:

1. Some patients cannot be given a recognized syndromic diagnosis.
2. Seizure types and syndromes change as new information is obtained.
3. Complete and detailed descriptions of ictal phenomenology are not always necessary.
4. Multiple classification schemes can, and should, be designed for specific purposes (e.g., communication and teaching; therapeutic trials; epidemiologic investigations; selection of surgical candidates; basic research; genetic characterizations).

This diagnostic scheme is divided into five parts, or axes, organized to facilitate a logical clinical approach to the development of hypotheses necessary to determine the diagnostic studies and therapeutic strategies to be undertaken in individual patients:

Axis 1: Ictal phenomenology, from the Glossary of Descriptive Ictal Terminology, can be used to describe ictal events with any degree of detail needed.

Axis 2: Seizure type, from the List of Epileptic Seizures. Localization within the brain and precipitating stimuli for reflex seizures should be specified when appropriate.

Axis 3: Syndrome, from the List of Epilepsy Syndromes, with the understanding that a syndromic diagnosis may not always be possible.

Axis 4: Etiology, from a Classification of Diseases Frequently Associated with Epileptic Seizures or Epilepsy Syndromes when possible, genetic defects, or specific pathologic substrates for symptomatic focal epilepsies.

Axis 5: Impairment, this optional, but often useful, additional diagnostic parameter can be derived from an impairment classification adapted from the WHO ICIDH-2.

From Engel (2001)[3] with permission of the author and the editor of *Epilepsia.*

Table 1.4 Epileptic seizure types and precipitating stimuli for reflex seizures [3]

Self-limited seizure types
- Generalized seizures
  - Tonic-clonic seizures (includes variations beginning with a clonic or myoclonic phase)
  - Clonic seizures
    - Without tonic features
    - With tonic features
  - Typical absence seizures
  - Atypical absence seizures
  - Myoclonic absence seizures
  - Tonic seizures
  - Spasms
  - Myoclonic seizures
  - Eyelid myoclonia
    - Without absences
    - With absences
  - Myoclonic atonic seizures
  - Negative myoclonus
  - Atonic seizures
  - Reflex seizures in generalized epilepsy syndromes
- Focal seizures
  - Focal sensory seizures
    - With elementary sensory symptoms (e.g., occipital and parietal lobe seizures)
    - With experiential sensory symptoms (e.g., temporo-parieto-occipital junction seizures)

Focal seizures cont.
  - Focal motor seizures
    - With elementary clonic motor signs
    - With asymmetric tonic motor seizures (e.g., supplementary motor seizures)
    - With typical (temporal lobe) automatisms (e.g., mesial temporal lobe seizures)
    - With hyperkinetic automatisms
    - With focal negative myoclonus
    - With inhibitory motor seizures
  - Gelastic seizures
  - Hemiclonic seizures
  - Secondarily generalized seizures
  - Reflex seizures in focal epilepsy syndromes

Continuous seizure types
- Generalized status epilepticus
  - Generalized tonic-clonic status epilepticus
  - Clonic status epilepticus
  - Absence status epilepticus
  - Tonic status epilepticus
  - Myoclonic status epilepticus
- Focal status epilepticus
  - Epilepsia partialis continua of Kozhevnikov
  - Aura continua
  - Limbic status epilepticus (psychomotor status)
  - Hemiconvulsive status with hemiparesis

Precipitating stimuli for reflex seizures
- Visual stimuli
  - Flickering light: colour to be specified when possible
  - Patterns
  - Other visual stimuli
- Thinking
- Music
- Eating
- Praxis
- Somatosensory
- Proprioceptive
- Reading
- Hot water
- Startle

From Engel (2001)[3] with permission of the author and the editor of *Epilepsia.*

EPILEPTIC SYNDROMES AND THEIR CLASSIFICATION

Having established that a paroxysmal event is epileptic, the diagnosis by the non-specialist is often limited to excluding structural abnormalities of the brain or predisposing medical disease. However, simply diagnosing 'epilepsy' or 'seizures, is insufficient. Symptom/seizure diagnosis cannot provide guidance on important items such as severity of the disease, prognosis, short- and long-term therapeutic decisions and genetics (research and counselling), which are all factors that crucially affect family and social life and the education and career choices of patients. Defining the type of epilepsy should now be considered mandatory as it offers the best guide to both management and prognosis.[66-69]

Syndromic diagnosis of epilepsies provides a firm foundation for short- and long-term therapeutic decisions and enables natural history, inheritance, treatment efficacy and prognosis of epilepsies to be studied scientifically. The benefits of syndromic diagnosis over seizure/symptom diagnosis or an inclusive diagnosis such as 'epilepsy' far outweigh any morbidity from miscategorisation that may arise in difficult cases.

Imprecise syndromic diagnosis commonly results in avoidable morbidity and sometimes mortality.[57]

The most important milestone in modern epileptology has been the recognition of epileptic syndromes and diseases, most of which are well defined and easy to diagnose. The concept of epilepsies as specific syndromes is old (see for example *pyknolepsy = childhood absence epilepsy*)[70] and the first attempt to formalise them in an international classification was published in 1970.[71] The current classification[57] originated from a meeting in the Centre Saint-Paul, Marseilles, France, in July 1983 and has been the basis of the book *Epileptic Syndromes in Infancy, Childhood and Adolescence*, also known as *Guide Bleu*, which is now published as an updated third edition.[72]

The classification and definitions from this meeting were adopted in 1985 by the Commission on Classification and Terminology of the ILAE[74] and remained essentially the same in the revised proposal of 1989.[57]

ILAE definitions

An epileptic syndrome: is an epileptic disorder characterized by a cluster of signs and symptoms customarily occurring together; these include such items as type of seizure, etiology, anatomy, precipitating factors, age of onset, severity, chronicity, diurnal and circadian cycling, and sometimes prognosis. However, in contradistinction to a disease, a syndrome does not necessarily have a common aetiology and prognosis. [57]

Epilepsy syndrome: a complex of signs and symptoms that define a unique epilepsy condition. This must involve more than just the seizure type; thus frontal lobe seizures *per se*, for instance, do not constitute a syndrome (changed concept).[3]

Epilepsy disease: a pathological condition with a single specific, well-defined aetiology. Thus, progressive myoclonus epilepsy is a syndrome, but Unverricht–Lundborg is a disease (new concept).[3]

Idiopathic epilepsy syndrome: a syndrome that is only epilepsy, with no underlying structural brain lesion or other neurological signs or symptoms. These are presumed to be genetic and are usually age dependent (unchanged term).[3]

Idiopathic comes from the Greek words *idios* (meaning self, own and personal) and *pathic* (suffer, see also pathology and pathological).[73] Idiopathic is not synonymous with being. There are idiopathic epilepsies with bad prognosis or lifelong duration and, conversely, there are symptomatic epilepsies with a few seizures that may not even need treatment.

Symptomatic epilepsy syndrome: a syndrome in which the epileptic seizures are the result of one or more identifiable structural lesions of the brain (unchanged term).[3]

Probably symptomatic epilepsy syndrome: synonymous with but preferred to the term cryptogenic used for defining syndromes that are believed to be symptomatic, but no aetiology has been identified (new term).[3]

The number of cryptogenic epilepsies is decreasing in favour of the symptomatic ones with the use of high-resolution magnetic resonance imaging (MRI), which demonstrates structural cortical lesions previously undetected by a computed tomography brain scan or first generation MRI scanners.

Benign epilepsy syndrome: a syndrome characterised by epileptic seizures that are easily treated or require no treatment and remit without sequelae (clarified concept).[3]

Medical diagnosis is defined as 'The identification of a disease by investigation of its symptoms and history, which provides a solid basis for the treatment and prognosis of the individual patient'.[70]

Similarly, in the epilepsies the recognition of non-fortuitous clustering of symptoms and signs requires the study of detailed clinical and laboratory data.

Important clinical features of a syndrome include the type of seizures, their localisation, frequency, sequence of events, circadian distribution, precipitating factors, response to treatment, age at onset, mode of inheritance and physical or mental symptoms and signs.

Although some symptoms predominate and may indicate the underlying disease, no single symptom or sign can be considered entirely pathognomonic. The process of differential diagnosis requires close scrutiny of the clinical data before a list of possible diagnoses can be drawn up and the final diagnosis reached. It should be realised that some epilepsies are easy to diagnose and some more difficult, but this is not unusual in medicine. Molecular genetics are already making decisive discoveries in the identification of epilepsies (Chapter 11).

Some parts of the current ILEA classification[3,57] remain contentious and some syndromes are ill or broadly defined and require further clarification.[59,67-69,75] There are patients whose clinical and EEG features do not appear to fit neatly into any recognised category or erroneously appear to evolve from one syndrome to another. Some may represent new or 'overlap' syndromes, others may be unusual or atypical forms of known syndromes or cases where clinical history is misleading. However, many syndromes are common, well characterised and easily diagnosed.

EPILEPTIC SYNDROMES IN ACCORDANCE WITH CURRENTLY VALID ILAE CLASSIFICATION OF 1989[57]

The currently valid 1989 syndromic classification of the ILAE[57] is presented in Table 1.5.

Two divisions are widely used to shape the major classes.

- The first separates epilepsies with generalised seizures (*generalised epilepsy*) from epilepsies with partial seizures (*localisation related, partial* or *focal epilepsies*).
- The other separates epilepsies of known aetiology (*symptomatic* or *'secondary' epilepsies*) from those that are *idiopathic* (or *'primary'*) and those that are *cryptogenic*.

The following are the four major classes in this 1989 classification as defined by the ILAE;[57]

1. **Localisation-related (focal, local and partial) epilepsies and syndromes**
2. **Generalised epilepsies and syndromes**
3. **Epilepsies and syndromes undetermined as to whether they are focal or generalised**
4. **Special syndromes**

The description and definitions of epileptic seizures and syndromes in this chapter are based entirely on the currently valid ILEA proposals.[56, 57]

Clarification on primary/primarily and secondary/secondarily seizures or syndromes

There is significant confusion regarding the words primary and secondary as adjuncts to seizures or syndromes.
In syndromes, primary is synonymous to idiopathic and secondary is synonymous to symptomatic or probably symptomatic (cryptogenic).
In seizures, primary denotes seizures that are generalised from onset (primarily generalised) while secondary denotes generalised seizures that are generated from a cortical focus (secondarily generalised seizures).
In this book these terms primary/primarily and secondary/secondarily are used only in relation to seizures. In syndromes, only the terms idiopathic, symptomatic and cryptogenic (or probably symptomatic) are used.

LOCALISATION-RELATED EPILEPSIES AND SYNDROMES

Localisation-related epilepsies and syndromes are epileptic disorders in which seizure semiology or findings at investigation disclose a localised origin of the seizures. This includes not only patients with small, circumscribed, constant epileptogenic lesions (anatomic or functional), i.e. true focal epilepsies, but also patients with less well-defined lesions, whose seizures may originate from variable loci. In most symptomatic localisation-related epilepsies, the epileptogenic lesions can be traced to one part of one cerebral hemisphere, but in idiopathic age-related epilepsies with focal seizures corresponding regions of both hemispheres may be functionally involved.[57]

Table 1.5 Syndromic Classification of the ILAE [57]

1. Localization-related (focal, local, partial) epilepsies and syndromes

1.1 Idiopathic (with age-related onset)
At present, the following syndromes are established, but more may be identified in the future:
- Benign childhood epilepsy with centrotemporal spike
- Childhood epilepsy with occipital paroxysms
- Primary reading epilepsy

1.2 Symptomatic
- Chronic progressive epilepsia partialis continua of childhood (Kozhevnikov syndrome)
- Syndromes characterized by seizures with specific modes of precipitation
- Temporal lobe epilepsies
- Frontal lobe epilepsies
- Parietal lobe epilepsies
- Occipital lobe epilepsies

1.3 Cryptogenic
Cryptogenic epilepsies are presumed to be symptomatic and the aetiology is unknown. This category thus differs from the previous one by the lack of etiologic evidence (See definitions).

2. Generalized epilepsies and syndromes

2.1 Idiopathic (with age-related onset – listed in order of age)
- Benign neonatal familial convulsions
- Benign neonatal convulsions
- Benign myoclonic epilepsy in infancy
- Childhood absence epilepsy (pyknolepsy)
- Juvenile absence epilepsy
- Juvenile myoclonic epilepsy (impulsive petit mal)
- Epilepsy with grand mal (GTCS) seizures on awakening
- Other generalized idiopathic epilepsies not defined above
- Epilepsies with seizures precipitated by specific modes of activation

2.2 Cryptogenic or symptomatic (in order of age)
- West syndrome (infantile spasms, Blitz-Nick-Salaam Krampfe)
- Lennox-Gastaut syndrome
- Epilepsy with myoclonic-astatic seizures
- Epilepsy with myoclonic absences

2.3 Symptomatic

2.3.1 Non-specific aetiology
- Early myoclonic encephalopathy
- Early infantile epileptic encephalopathy with suppression burst
- Other symptomatic generalized epilepsies not defined above

2.3.2 Specific syndromes
- Epileptic seizures may complicate many disease states. Under this heading are included diseases in which seizures are a presenting or predominant feature

3. Epilepsies and syndromes undetermined whether focal or generalized

3.1 With both generalized and focal seizures
- Neonatal seizures
- Severe myoclonic epilepsy in infancy
- Epilepsy with continuous spike-waves during slow wave sleep
- Acquired epileptic aphasia (Landau-Kleffner syndrome)
- Other undetermined epilepsies not defined above

3.2 Without unequivocal generalized or focal features. All cases with generalized tonic-clonic seizures in which clinical and EEG findings do not permit classification as clearly generalized or localization related, e.g., many cases of sleep-grand mal (GTCS) are considered not to have unequivocal generalized or focal features

4. Special syndromes

4.1 Situation-related seizures (Gelegenheitsanfälle)
- Febrile convulsions
- Isolated seizures or isolated status epilepticus
- Seizures occurring only when there is an acute metabolic or toxic event due to factors such as alcohol, drugs, eclampsia, nonketotic hyperglycaemia

From: The Commission on Classification and Terminology of the International League Against Epilepsy. Proposal for revised clinical and electroencephalographic classification of epileptic seizures. With the permission of the Editor of Epilepsia.[55]

Localisation-related (focal, local and partial) epilepsies and syndromes are

1.1 Idiopathic

1.2 Symptomatic

1.3 Cryptogenic

The symptomatic sydromes are anatomically classified as:

– Temporal lobe epilepsies – Frontal lobe epilepsies
– Parietal lobe epilepsies – Occipital lobe epilepsies

Idiopathic localisation-related epilepsies are childhood epilepsies with partial seizures and focal EEG abnormalities. They are age related, without demonstrable anatomic lesions and are subject to spontaneous remission. Clinically, patients have neither neurological nor intellectual deficit nor a history of antecedent illness, but frequently have a family history of benign epilepsy. The seizures are usually brief and rare, but may be frequent early in the course of the disorder. The seizure patterns may vary from case to case, but usually remain constant in the same child. The EEG is characterised by normal background activity and localised high voltage repetitive spikes, which are sometimes independently multifocal. Brief bursts of generalised spike and wave can occur. Focal abnormalities are increased by sleep and are without change in morphology.[57]

Symptomatic localisation-related epilepsies: apart from the rare conditions of Kozhevnikov–Rasmussen syndrome and focal reflex epilepsies, the symptomatic

Table 1.6 Epilepsy syndromes and related conditions[3]

- Benign familial neonatal seizures
- Early myoclonic encephalopathy
- Ohtahara syndrome
- [a]Migrating partial seizures of infancy
- West syndrome
- Benign myoclonic epilepsy in infancy
- Benign familial infantile seizures
- Benign infantile seizures (nonfamilial)
- Dravet syndrome
- Hemiconvulsion-hemiplegia syndrome
- [a]Myoclonic status in nonprogressive encephalopathies
- Benign childhood epilepsy with centrotemporal spikes
- Early-onset benign childhood occipital epilepsy (Panayiotopoulos type)
- Late-onset childhood occipital epilepsy (Gastaut type)
- Epilepsy with myoclonic absences
- Epilepsy with myoclonic-astatic seizures

- Lennox-Gastaut syndrome
- Landau-Kleffner syndrome (LKS)
- Epilepsy with continuous spike-and-waves during slow-wave sleep (other than LKS)
- Childhood absence epilepsy
- Progressive myoclonus epilepsies
- Idiopathic generalized epilepsies with variable phenotypes
    - Juvenile absence epilepsy
    - Juvenile myoclonic epilepsy
    - Epilepsy with generalized tonic-clonic seizures only
- Reflex epilepsies
    - Idiopathic photosensitive occipital lobe epilepsy
    - Other visual sensitive epilepsies
    - Primary reading epilepsy
    - Startle epilepsy
- Autosomal dominant nocturnal frontal lobe epilepsy
- Familial temporal lobe epilepsies
- [a]Generalized epilepsies with febrile seizures plus
- [a]Familial focal epilepsy with variable foci

- Symptomatic (or probably symptomatic) focal epilepsies
    - Limbic epilepsies
        - Mesial temporal lobe epilepsy with hippocampal sclerosis
        - Mesial temporal lobe epilepsy defined by specific etiologies
        - Other types defined by location and etiology
    - Neocortical epilepsies
        - Rasmussen syndrome
        - Other types defined by location and etiology
- Conditions with epileptic seizures that do not require a diagnosis of epilepsy
    - Benign neonatal seizures
    - Febrile seizures
    - Reflex seizures
    - Alcohol-withdrawal seizures
    - Drug or other chemically induced seizures
    - Immediate and early posttraumatic seizures
    - Single seizures or isolated clusters of seizures
    - Rarely repeated seizures (oligoepilepsy)

[a] *Syndromes in development*

From Engel (2001)[3] with permission of the author and the editor of *Epilepsia*

category comprises syndromes of great individual variability which are based mainly on seizure types and other clinical features as well as anatomic localisation and aetiology – as far as these are known. The seizure types refer to the ILAE classification. Inferences regarding anatomic localisation must be drawn carefully. The scalp EEG (both interictal and ictal) may be misleading and even local morphological findings detected by neuroimaging techniques are not necessarily identical with an epileptogenic lesion. Seizure symptomatology and, sometimes, additional clinical features often provide important clues. The first sign or symptom of a seizure is often the most important indicator of the site of origin of seizure discharge, whereas the following sequence of ictal events can reflect its further propagation through the brain. However, this sequence can still be of high localising importance. One must bear in mind that a seizure may start in a clinically silent region, so that the first clinical event occurs only after spread to a site more or less distant from the locus of initial discharge. The tentative descriptions of syndromes related to anatomic localisations are based on data that include findings in studies with depth electrodes.[57]

GENERALISED EPILEPSIES AND SYNDROMES

Generalised epilepsies and syndromes are epileptic disorders with generalised seizures, i.e. seizures in which the first clinical changes indicate initial involvement of both hemispheres. The ictal encephalographic patterns initially are bilateral.[57] Generalised epilepsies and syndromes are

2.1 Idiopathic

2.2 Cryptogenic

2.3 Symptomatic

2.3.1 Non-specific aetiology

2.3.2 Specific syndrome

Idiopathic generalised epilepsies are forms of generalised epilepsies in which all seizures are initially generalised, with an EEG expression that is a generalised, bilateral, synchronous, symmetrical discharge (such as is described in the seizure classification of the corresponding type). The patient usually has a normal interictal state, without neurological or neuroradiological signs. In general, interictal EEGs show normal background activity and generalised discharges, such as spikes, polyspike, spike and wave and polyspike waves of about 3 Hz. The discharges are increased by non-REM sleep. The various syndromes of idiopathic generalised epilepsies differ mainly in age of onset.[57]

Symptomatic generalised epilepsies, most often occurring in infancy and childhood, are characterised by generalised seizures with clinical and EEG features different from those of idiopathic generalised epilepsies. There may be only one type, but more often there are several types, including myoclonic jerks, tonic seizures, atonic seizures and atypical absences. EEG expression is bilateral but less rhythmical than in idiopathic generalised epilepsies and is more or less asymmetrical. Interictal EEG abnormalities differ from idiopathic generalised epilepsies, appearing as suppression bursts, hypsarrhythmia, slow spike and wave or generalised fast rhythms. Focal abnormalities may be associated with any of the above. There are clinical, neuropsychological and neuroradiological signs of a usually diffuse, specific or nonspecific encephalopathy.[57]

Symptomatic generalised epilepsies of specific aetiologies are "only diseases in which epileptic seizures are the presenting or a prominent feature". [57] These diseases often have epileptic features that resemble symptomatic generalised epilepsies without specific aetiology, appearing at similar ages and include diseases such as Aicardi syndrome, Lissencephaly-pachygyria, Sturge-Webber syndrome, hypothalamic hamartomas, disorders of inborn error of metabolism, Lafora disease and others.

EPILEPSIES AND SYNDROMES UNDETERMINED AS TO WHETHER THEY ARE FOCAL OR GENERALISED

There may be two reasons why a determination of whether seizures are focal or generalised cannot be made. [57]

- The patient has both focal and generalised seizures together or in succession (e.g. partial seizures plus absences) and has both focal and generalised EEG seizure discharges (e.g. temporal spike focus plus independent bilateral spike and wave discharges). [57]
- There are no positive signs of either focal or generalised seizure onset. The most common reasons for this are that the seizures occur during sleep, the patient recalls no aura and ancillary investigations ir revealing.[57]

Therefore, epilepsies and syndromes undetermined as to or generalised may be:

3.1 With both generalised and focal seizures

3.2 Without unequivocal generalised or focal features

SPECIAL SYNDROMES

These manifest with situation-related seizures (*Gelegenhei*

- febrile seizures
- isolated seizures or isolated status epilepticus
- seizures occurring only when there is an acute metaboli factors such as alcohol, drugs, eclampsia and nonketotic

EPILEPSIES WITH SEIZURES PRECIPITATED BY S OF ACTIVATION

Reflex epileptic syndromes are detailed in Chapter 13. The reflex seizures which are consistently related to specific m such as primary reading epilepsy. Seizures also occur sponta epilepsies. [57]

DISEASES AND SYNDROMES OF SPECIFIC AETIOL

The ILAE classification also recognises certain diseases a epileptic seizures are the presenting or a prominent feature such as progressive myoclonic epilepsies and inherited metabolic disorders.

SYNDROMIC CLASSIFICATION OF THE NEW DIAGNOSTIC ILAE SCHEME[3]

Recent advances in the clinical EEG manifestations of previously recognised and newly described syndromes, video EEG information, functional and structural imaging, investigative procedures and genetics mandated a new thorough and realistic revision of this classification and the definitions of epileptic syndromes.[3] The proposed diagnostic scheme for people with epileptic seizures and with epilepsy is such an attempt by the ILAE Task Force.[3] Table 1.6 shows the epileptic syndromes and related conditions as listed in the new diagnostic scheme[3] and Table 1.7 is an example of their group classification. Table 1.8 lists diseases which are frequently associated with epileptic seizures.

Table 1.7 An example of a classification of epilepsy syndromes [3]

Groups of syndromes	Specific syndromes
Idiopathic focal epilepsies of infancy and childhood	Benign infantile seizures (nonfamilial) Benign childhood epilepsy with centrotemporal spikes Early-onset benign childhood occipital epilepsy (Panayiotopoulos type) Late-onset childhood occipital epilepsy (Gastaut type)
Familial (autosomal dominant) focal epilepsies	Benign familial neonatal seizures Benign familial infantile seizures Autosomal dominant nocturnal frontal lobe epilepsy Familial temporal lobe epilepsy Familial focal epilepsy with variable foci[a]
Symptomatic and probably symptomatic focal epilepsies	Limbic epilepsies Mesial temporal lobe epilepsy with hippocampal sclerosis Mesial temporal lobe epilepsy defined by specific etiologies Other types defined by location and etiology Neocortical epilepsies Rasmussen syndrome Hemiconvulsion-hemiplegia syndrome Other types defined by location and etiology Migrating partial seizures of early infancy[a]
Idiopathic generalized epilepsies	Benign myoclonic epilepsy in infancy Epilepsy with myoclonic astatic seizures Childhood absence epilepsy Epilepsy with myoclonic absences Idiopathic generalized epilepsies with variable phenotypes Juvenile absence epilepsy Juvenile myoclonic epilepsy Epilepsy with generalized tonic-clonic seizures only Generalized epilepsies with febrile seizures plus[a]
Reflex epilepsies	Idiopathic photosensitive occipital lobe epilepsy Other visual sensitive epilepsies Primary reading epilepsy Startle epilepsy
Epileptic encephalopathies (in which the epileptiform abnormalities may contribute to progressive dysfunction)	Early myoclonic encephalopathy Ohtahara syndrome West syndrome Dravet syndrome (previously known as severe myoclonic epilepsy in infancy) Myoclonic status in nonprogressive encephalopathies[a] Lennox-Gastaut syndrome Landau-Kleffner syndrome Epilepsy with continuous spike-waves during slow-wave sleep
Progressive myoclonus epilepsies	See specific diseases
Seizures not necessarily requiring a diagnosis of epilepsy	Benign neonatal seizures Febrile seizures Reflex seizures Alcohol-withdrawal seizures Drug or other chemically induced seizures Immediate and early post traumatic seizures Single seizures or isolated clusters of seizures Rarely repeated seizures (oligoepilepsy)

[a] *Syndromes in development*

From Engel (2001)[3] with permission of the author and the editor of *Epilepsia*

Table 1.8 An example of a classification of diseases frequently associated with epileptic seizures or syndromes[3]

Groups of diseases
Specific diseases

Progressive myoclonic epilepsies
- Ceroid lipofuscinosis
- Sialidosis
- Lafora disease
- Unverricht-Lundborg disease
- Neuroaxonal dystrophy
- MERRF
- Dentatorubropallidoluysian atrophy
- Other

Neurocutaneous disorders
- Tuberous sclerosis complex
- Neurofibromatosis
- Hypomelanosis of Ito
- Epidermal nevus syndrome
- Sturge-Weber syndrome

Malformations due to abnormal cortical developments
- Isolated lissencephaly sequence
- Miller-Dieker syndrome
- X-linked lissencephaly
- Subcortical band heterotopia
- Periventricular nodular heterotopia
- Focal heterotopia
- Hemimegalencephaly
- Bilateral perisylvian syndrome
- Unilateral polymicrogyria
- Schizencephalies
- Focal or multifocal cortical dysplasia
- Microdysgenesis

Other cerebral malformations
- Aicardi syndrome
- PEHO syndrome
- Acrocallosal syndrome
- Other

Tumors
- DNET
- Gangliocytoma
- Ganglioglioma
- Cavernous angiomas
- Astrocytomas
- Hypothalamic hamartoma (with gelastic seizures)
- Other

Chromosomal abnormalities
- Partial monosomy 4P or Wolf-Hirschhorn syndrome
- Trisomy 12p
- Inversion duplication 15 syndrome
- Ring 20 chromosome
- Other

Monogenic mendelian diseases with complex pathogenetic mechanisms
- Fragile X syndrome
- Angelman syndrome
- Rett syndrome
- Other

Groups of diseases
Specific diseases

Inherited metabolic disorders
- Nonketotic hyperglycinemia
- D-glyceric acidemia
- Propionic acidemia
- Sulphite-oxidase deficiency
- Fructose 1-6 diphosphatase deficiency
- Other organic acidurias
- Pyridoxine dependency
- Aminoacidopathies (maple syrup urine disease, phenylketonuria, other)
- Urea cycle disorders
- Disorders of carbohydrate metabolism
- Disorders of biotin metabolism
- Disorders of folic acid and B12 metabolism
- Glucose transport protein deficiency
- Menkes' disease
- Glycogen-storage disorders
- Krabbe disease
- Fumarase deficiency
- Peroxisomal disorders
- Sanfilippo syndrome
- Mitochondrial diseases (pyruvate dehydrogenase deficiency, respiratory chain defects, MELAS)

Prenatal or perinatal ischemic or anoxic lesions or cerebral infections causing nonprogressive encephalopathies
- Porencephaly
- Periventricular leukomalacia
- Microcephaly
- Cerebral calcifications and other lesions due to toxoplasmosis, CVI, HIV, etc.

Postnatal infections
- Cysticercosis
- Herpes encephalitis
- Bacterial meningitis
- Other

Other postnatal factors
- Head injury
- Alcohol and drug abuse
- Stroke
- Other

Miscellaneous
- Celiac disease (epilepsy with occipital calcifications and celiac disease)
- Northern epilepsy syndrome
- Coffin-Lowry syndrome
- Alzheimer's disease
- Huntington disease
- Alpers' disease

MERRF, myoclonus epilepsy with ragged red fibers;
PEHO, progressive encephalopathy with oedema, hypsarrhythmia and optic atrophy
DNET, dysembryoplastic neuroepithelial tumor;
MELAS, mitochondrial encephalomyopathy, lactic acidosis, and stroke-like symptoms;
CVI, cerebrovascular incident;

From Engel (2001)[3] with permission of the author and the editor of *Epilepsia*

GARDENERS AND BOTANISTS, SPLITTERS AND LUMPERS

In epileptological literature there is frequent comparison of physicians and classifications to gardeners and botanists or splitters and lumbers. This should not be misunderstood. Neither of these paradigms advocates or justifies a unification of all epilepsies under a single diagnostic category.

GARDENERS AND BOTANISTS

An outstanding scientific account of the principles and terminology of classification systems is the recent lead Editorial by Peter Wolf in *Epilepsia.*[60] He also refers to Johns Hughlings Jackson who is the first to compare the classification systems needed for epilepsies to the classification of plants for botanists and gardeners.[76] The botanists, like all scientists, need a taxonomy, while the gardeners, like all practising physicians need something to use in daily work.

> "There are two ways of investigating diseases, and two kinds of classification corresponding thereto, the empirical and the scientific. The former is to be illustrated by the way in which a gardener classifies plants, the latter by the way in which a botanist classifies them. The former is, strictly speaking, only an arrangement. The gardener arranges his plants as they are fit for food, for ornament, etc. One of his classifications of ornamental plants is into trees, shrubs, and flowers. His object is the direct application of knowledge to utilitarian purposes. It is, so to speak, practical. The other kind of classification (the classification properly so-called) is rather for the better organization of existing knowledge, and for discovering the relations of new facts; its principles are methodical guides to further investigation. It is of great utilitarian value, but not directly."
>
> Johns Hughlings Jackson (1874)[76]

SPLITTERS AND LUMPERS

There are two main schools of thought in the classifications. The 'splitters' try to identify specific epileptic syndromes while recognising the existence of borderline cases. The 'lumpers' do not recognise specific syndromes within the spectrum of epilepsies.

Berg and Blackstone[62] have provided an excellent and objective debate on classification systems and I quote them regarding lumping and splitting in epilepsies:

> "Related to differentiation is the debate about lumping together what may or may not be similar forms of epilepsy or splitting apart groups that may represent minor variations of the same form of epilepsy. Ideally any method for classifying the epilepsies should require identification and measurement of all potentially relevant characteristics (be they phenotypic characteristics, gene mutations, etc.) and appropriate analyses to determine which characteristics truly define and differentiate between 'syndromes'. Implicitly, one must be prepared to split before one can lump. Thus we must always be on guard against unwittingly lumping because we are unaware of certain characteristics on which we should have split." [62]

THE SIGNIFICANCE OF SPECIFYING THE TYPE OF 'EPILEPSY'

The significance of the syndromic diagnosis of epilepsies has been emphasised on many occasions.[67-69] The results to be expected of syndromic diagnosis of epilepsies can be compared with the advances, which have accrued from the

Terminological changes in the new diagnostic scheme[3]

The new diagnostic scheme maintains focal and generalised epilepsies, does not specify on syndromes of uncertain origin and replaces 'seizures with a specific situation' to 'seizures that do not require the diagnosis of epilepsy'.[3] In addition, the scheme rightly maintains and lists the 'diseases frequently associated with epileptic seizures or syndromes' (Table 1.8).

widespread acceptance of syndromic diagnosis of other medical disorders such as neuromuscular diseases. If diagnosed on a few symptoms alone, distinction would be impossible even between the broad categories of muscular dystrophies, inflammatory myopathies and motor neurone diseases which all manifest with muscle weakness and muscle atrophy. Similarly, if diagnosed on a few symptoms alone, distinction would be often impossible even between the broad categories of focal or generalised, idiopathic or symptomatic epilepsies which all manifest with seizures. Despite the occasional occurrence of 'overlap syndromes', syndromic classification allows the scientific analysis of the underlying disease processes and their specific clinicopathological features and genetics and provides a framework for clinical trials aimed at optimising treatment.[77,78]

Traditional medical teaching and attitudes to the diagnosis and management of epilepsies often differ from those applied in other medical conditions.[54,66]

Accurate diagnosis is the golden rule in medicine and epilepsies should not be an exception to this.

Physicians who rightly seek bedside confirmation of muscle fatigability in a patient with a clear-cut history of myasthenia gravis, should also request to view the seizures which if frequent can be easily captured with modern digital recorders. Physicians who rightly emphasise the differential diagnosis between spinal muscular atrophy and polymyositis should give the same emphasis to the differentiation between absences of idiopathic generalised epilepsies and complex focal seizures. Major paediatric journals which often emphasise rare disease should at least give the same space to highlight that childhood autonomic status epilepticus is a common and costly cause of misdiagnosis and mismanagement adversely affecting thousands of children around the world (page 240).[79]

The danger of a unified diagnosis of 'epilepsy' or a symptomatic diagnosis of 'seizures' is exemplified by three common epileptic syndromes: benign childhood focal seizures, juvenile myoclonic epilepsy (JME) and hippocampal epilepsy, which comprise more than one-third of all epilepsies. They are entirely different in presentation, causes, investigative procedures, short- and long-term treatment strategies and prognosis.

Benign childhood focal seizures (Chapter 9), like febrile seizures, are age-related, show genetic predisposition, may manifest as a single seizure, remit within a few years of onset and may or may not require a short course of antiepileptic drug (AED) treatment. The risk of recurrent seizures in adult life (1–2%) is less than in febrile seizures (4%). Recognition of the characteristic clinical and EEG features of benign childhood focal epilepsies will enable the parents to be reassured of the invariably benign prognosis with spontaneous resolution of the disorder by the middle teens.

Juvenile myoclonic epilepsy, an easy to diagnose syndrome of idiopathic generalised epilepsies, has a prevalence of 8–10% among adult patients with seizures. It manifests with myoclonic jerks on awakening, GTCS and, more rarely, absences. The management of JME differs from standard medical practice for the treatment of seizures in several important respects. Recommendations not to treat after the first seizure are usually inappropriate, not only because affected patients have usually experienced other epileptic events (e.g. myoclonic jerks and absences) for many months or years before their first GTCS, but also because JME is a lifelong disease with a high risk of major and minor seizures, particularly after sleep deprivation, fatigue and alcohol indulgence. Emphasising avoidance of precipitating factors in JME is part of the management strategy. Many AED such as carbamazepine or gabapentin worsen JME. Withdrawal of appropriate AED after 2–3 years seizure free is inappropriate because relapses are inevitable.

Hippocampal epilepsy is the commoner focal epileptic disorder affecting around 20% of patients with epilepsies. It is of defined pathology that can be documented in vivo with high resolution MRI in nearly all patients. If carbamazepine alone or in combination with another one or two of the main AEDs fails, the chances of achieving medical control are negligible. These patients, even in childhood, need urgent evaluation for neurosurgical treatment for which they are the best candidates and the most likely to have excellent and sustained benefit.[80,81]

EPILEPSY OR EPILEPSIES?

Even the most sceptical physicians among those who doubt the clinical or practical significance of the syndromic diagnosis of epilepsies have to accept that benign childhood focal epilepsies, JME and hippocampal epilepsy have nothing in common other than the fact that they may all be complicated by GTCS, which are primarily GTCS in JME and secondarily GTCS in benign childhood focal epilepsies and hippocampal epilepsy. Furthermore, the short- and long-term treatment strategies are entirely different for each disorder: benign childhood focal epilepsies may or may not require medication for a few years, appropriate AED treatment is lifelong in JME while neurosurgery may be life saving for patients with hippocampal epilepsy. What may be a saviour drug for one may be deleterious for another type of epilepsy.

It should not be difficult to distinguish an intelligent child with benign focal seizures or childhood absence epilepsy from a child with Kozhevnikov–Rasmussen, Lennox–Gastaut, Down or Sturge–Weber syndrome or a child with severe post-traumatic cerebral damage, brain anoxia or catastrophic progressive myoclonic epilepsy. Diagnosing all these children as simply having epilepsy just because they have seizures offers no more benefit than a diagnosis of a febrile illness irrespective of cause, which may be a mild viral illness, bacterial meningitis or malignancy. Describing all these children as simply having epilepsy just because they have seizures offers no more benefit than a diagnosis of muscle atrophy, irrespective of whether it is localised or generalised, post-traumatic or genetically determined, static, reversible or progressive, or whether the underlying cause is in the muscle, nerve or spinal cord, and is treatable or untreatable.

The treatment of epilepsies will change, but their correct diagnosis will always be the golden rule. We should discourage randomised control trials that lump all

The Web and new avenues for information and communication

There has been an explosive growth of the Internet and Web as tools for seeking and communicating health and medical information. An increasing number of physicians and patients use Web search engines to seek very detailed advice and solicit or share specific medical and health information. More specialised medical or health websites, such as WebMD, are becoming available.

There is a rapid growth in the literature addressing the role of the Internet in medicine and in particular patient education, patient support networks, education and communication among health providers, and communication between providers and patients.

In this shared-decision-making medical environment, immediate access to such information has been of great benefit to health-care professionals and patients. However, there is growing concern that a substantial proportion of clinical information on the Web might be inaccurate, erroneous, misleading, or fraudulent, and thereby pose a threat to public health. Medical website quality is being tested through many sources and guidelines for quality criteria are being developed. With e-mail use patients also have easy, direct and fast access to experts around the world. Parents and patients often use the wide information provided on the Internet for formulating their own opinion regarding diagnosis and management. They are entitled to do so and this is often useful. The following is an example from many e-mails that I receive from non-medically qualified parents and patients:

... For years her condition has gone undiagnosed and to this day it still is. I have searched extensively on the Web and PubMed for vomiting and seizures because I understand that the aura and the way a seizure starts can be very informative.....I finally found out about Panayiotopoulos syndrome which perfectly matched her symptoms. Upon forwarding the articles to our neurologist, I was told that her EEG did not fit the pattern. Author's note: the EEG was a typical example of multifocal EEG in this syndrome.

patients with any type of seizures as a 'universe of epilepsy' or recommendations such as 'start with valproate and if this does not work change it to carbamazepine', 'an EEG is not needed after the first seizure because treatment is after the second seizure' (not even specifying the type of seizure and the need to specifically inquire for minor fits).

Significant progress is expected if emphasis is directed on 'how to diagnose the epilepsies' rather than the current theme of 'how to treat epilepsy'.

Inappropriate generalisations regarding terminology, diagnosis and treatment is the single most important cause of mismanagement in epilepsies.

REFERENCES

1. Commission on Epidemiology and Prognosis, International League Against Epilepsy. Guidelines for epidemiologic studies on epilepsy. *Epilepsia* 1993;**34**:592-6.
2. ILAE Commission Report. The epidemiology of the epilepsies: future directions. International League Against Epilepsy. *Epilepsia* 1997;**38**:614-8.
3. Engel J, Jr. A proposed diagnostic scheme for people with epileptic seizures and with epilepsy: Report of the ILAE Task Force on Classification and Terminology. *Epilepsia* 2001;**42**:796-803.
4. Blume WT, Luders HO, Mizrahi E, Tassinari C, van Emde BW, Engel J, Jr. Glossary of descriptive terminology for ictal semiology: report of the ILAE task force on classification and terminology. *Epilepsia* 2001;**42**:1212-8.
5. Stephenson JB. Fits and faints. London: MacKeith Press, 1990.
6. Murtagh J. Fits, faints and funny turns. A general diagnostic approach. *Aust Fam Physician* 2003;**32**:203-6.
7. Benditt D, Blanc JJ, Brignole M, Sutton R. Evaluation and Treatment of Syncope. London: Blackwell Publishing, 2003.
8. Brignole M, Alboni P, Benditt D, Bergfeldt L, Blanc JJ, Bloch Thomsen PE *et al.* Guidelines on management (diagnosis and treatment) of syncope. *Eur Heart J.* 2001;**22**:1256-306.
9. Lesser RP. Psychogenic seizures. *Neurology* 1996;**46**:1499-507.
10. Gumnit RJ. Psychogenic seizures. In Wyllie E, ed. *The treatment of epilepsy: Principles and practices*, pp 699-703. Philadelphia: Lippincott Williams & Wilkins, 2001.
11. Gates JR, Rowan AJ. Nonepileptic seizures. Boston: Butterworth-Heinemann, 2000.
12. Gates JR. Nonepileptic seizures:Classification, coexistence with epilepsy, diagnosis, therapeutic approaches, and consensus. *Epilepsy Behav.* 2002;**3**:28-33.
13. Reuber M, Elger CE. Psychogenic nonepileptic seizures: review and update. *Epilepsy Behav.* 2003;**4**:205-16.
14. de Timary P, Fouchet P, Sylin M, Indriets JP, De Barsy T, Lefebvre A *et al.* Non-epileptic seizures: delayed diagnosis in patients presenting with electroencephalographic (EEG) or clinical signs of epileptic seizures. *Seizure* 2002;**11**:193-7.
15. Nowack WJ. Epilepsy: a costly misdiagnosis. *Clin Electroencephalogr.* 1997;**28**:225-8.
16. Fisher RS. Imitators of epilepsy. New York: Demos Publications, Inc., 1994.
17. Francis P, Baker GA. Non-epileptic attack disorder (NEAD): a comprehensive review. *Seizure.* 1999;**8**:53-61.
18. Guerrini R, Aicardi J, Andermann F, Hallett M. Epilepsy and movement disorder. Cambridge: Cambridge University Press, 2001.
19. Foldvary N. Sleep and Epilepsy. *Curr Treat Options Neurol.* 2002;**4**:129-35.
20. Beran RG, Plunkett MJ, Holland GJ. Interface of epilepsy and sleep disorders. *Seizure* 1999;**8**:97-102.
21. Scher MS. Applying classifications of sleep disorders to children with neurologic conditions. *J Child Neurol* 1998;**13**:525-36.
22. Shouse MN, da Silva AM, Sammaritano M. Sleep. In Engel JJ, Pedley TA, eds. *Epilepsy: A comprehensive Textbook*, pp 1929-42. Philadelphia: Lippincott-Raven Publishers, 1997.
23. Bourgeois B. The relationship between sleep and epilepsy in children. *Semin Pediatr Neurol* 1996;**3**:29-35.
24. Barthlen GM, Stacy C. Dyssomnias, parasomnias, and sleep disorders associated with medical and psychiatric diseases. *Mt Sinai J Med* 1994;**61**:139-59.
25. Stephenson JB. Anoxic seizures: self-terminating syncopes. *Epileptic Disord.* 2001;**3**:3-6.
26. Drigo P, Carli G, Laverda AM. Benign paroxysmal vertigo of childhood. *Brain Dev.* 2001;**23**:38-41.
27. Li BU. Cyclic vomiting syndrome: age-old syndrome and new insights. *Semin.Pediatr Neurol* 2001;**8**:13-21.
28. Li BU, Balint JP. Cyclic vomiting syndrome: evolution in our understanding of a brain-gut disorder. *Adv Pediatr* 2000;**47**:117-60.
29. Meadow R. Different interpretations of Munchausen Syndrome by Proxy. *Child Abuse Negl.* 2002;**26**:501-8.
30. Meadow R. What is, and what is not, 'Munchausen syndrome by proxy'? *Arch Dis Child* 1995;**72**:534-8.
31. Schreier H. Munchausen by proxy defined. *Pediatrics* 2002;**110**:985-8.
32. Thomas K. Munchausen syndrome by proxy: identification and diagnosis. *J Pediatr Nurs.* 2003;**18**:174-80.
33. Golden GS. Nonepileptic paroxysmal events in childhood. *Pediatr Clin North Am.* 1992;**39**:715-25.
34. Andriola MR,.Ettinger AB. Pseudoseizures and other nonepileptic paroxysmal disorders in children and adolescents. *Neurology* 1999;**53**:S89-S95.
35. Bye AM, Kok DJ, Ferenschild FT, Vles JS. Paroxysmal non-epileptic events in children: a retrospective study over a period of 10 years. *J Paediatr Child Health* 2000;**36**:244-8.
36. Villanueva-Gomez F. A video-EEG description of non-epileptic paroxysmal seizures. *Rev Neurol.* 2000;**30 Suppl 1**:S9-15.
37. Pellock JM. Other nonepileptic paroxysmal disorders. In Wyllie E, ed. *The treatment of epilepsy: Principles and practices*, pp 705-16. Philadelphia: Lippincott Williams & Wilkins, 2001.
38. Kotagal P, Costa M, Wyllie E, Wolgamuth B. Paroxysmal nonepileptic events in children and adolescents. *Pediatrics* 2002;**110**:e46.
39. Lempert T. Recognizing syncope: pitfalls and surprises. *J R Soc Med* 1996;**89**:372-5.
40. Kapoor WN. Syncope. *N Engl J Med* 2000;**343**:1856-62.
41. McLeod KA. Syncope in childhood. *Arch Dis Child* 2003;**88**:350-3.
42. Stephenson JB. Differentiating convulsive syncope and epilepsy. *Ann Intern Med* 1992;**116**:777-8.
43. Stephenson J, Breningstall G, Steer C, Kirkpatrick M, Horrocks I, Nechay A *et al.* Anoxic-epileptic seizures: home video recordings of epileptic seizures induced by syncopes. *Epileptic Disord.* 2004;**6**:15-9.
44. Ferrie CD. Reflex anoxic seizures. In Gilman S, ed. *Medlink Neurology*, San Diego SA: 2005.
45. Lempert T, von Brevern M. The eye movements of syncope. *Neurology* 1996;**46**:1086-8.
46. Lempert T, Bauer M, Schmidt D. Syncope: a videometric analysis of 56 episodes of transient cerebral hypoxia. *Ann Neurol* 1994;**36**:233-7.
47. Alper K, Devinsky O, Perrine K, Vazquez B, Luciano D. Psychiatric classification of nonconversion nonepileptic seizures. *Arch Neurol.* 1995;**52**:199-201.
48. Howell SJ, Owen L, Chadwick DW. Pseudostatus epilepticus. *Q J Med.* 1989;**71**:507-19.
49. Carmant L, Kramer U, Holmes GL, Mikati MA, Riviello JJ, Helmers SL. Differential diagnosis of staring spells in children: a video- EEG study. *Pediat Neurol* 1996;**14**:199-202.
50. Opherk C, Hirsch LJ. Ictal heart rate differentiates epileptic from non-epileptic seizures. *Neurology* 2002;**58**:636-8.
51. Carton S, Thompson PJ, Duncan JS. Non-epileptic seizures: patients' understanding and reaction to the diagnosis and impact on outcome. *Seizure* 2003;**12**:287-94.
52. Meyer MA, Zimmerman AW, Miller CA. Temporal lobe epilepsy presenting as panic attacks: detection of interictal hypometabolism with positron emission tomography. *J Neuroimaging* 2000;**10**:120-2.
53. Cragar DE, Berry DT, Fakhoury TA, Cibula JE, Schmitt FA. A review of diagnostic techniques in the differential diagnosis of epileptic and nonepileptic seizures. *Neuropsychol Rev.* 2002;**12**:31-64.
54. Panayiotopoulos CP. Benign childhood partial seizures and related epileptic syndromes. London: John Libbey & Company Ltd, 1999.
55. Hauser WA, Rich SS, Annegers JF, Anderson VE. Seizure recurrence after a 1st unprovoked seizure: an extended follow-up. *Neurology* 1990;**40**:1163-70.
56. Commission of Classification and Terminology of the International League Against Epilepsy. Proposal for revised clinical and electroencephalographic classification of epileptic seizures. *Epilepsia* 1981;**22**:489-501.
57. Commission on Classification and Terminology of the International League Against Epilepsy. Proposal for revised classification of epilepsies and epileptic syndromes. *Epilepsia* 1989;**30**:389-99.
58. Engel JJr. Reply to " Cabbages and Kings in the classification of seizures and the epilepsies ". *Epilepsia* 2003;**44**:4-6.

59. Fisher RS, Wolf P, Engel JJr, Luders H, Najm I, Wyllie E *et al.* Cabbages and Kings in the classification of seizures and the epilepsies. *Epilepsia* 2003;**44**:1-13.
60. Wolf P. Of cabbages and kings: some considerations on classifications, diagnostic schemes, semiology, and concepts. *Epilepsia* 2003;**44**:1-4.
61. Luders HO, Najm I, Wyllie E. Reply to " Cabbages and Kings in the classification of seizures and the epilepsies ". *Epilepsia* 2003;**44**:6-8.
62. Berg A,Blackstone NW. Reply to "Cabbages and Kings in the classification of seizures and the epilepsies ". *Epilepsia* 2003;**44**:8-12.
63. Avanzini G. Reply to " Cabbages and Kings in the classification of seizures and the epilepsies ". *Epilepsia* 2003;**44**:12-3.
64. Gastaut H. Clinical and electroencephalographical classification of epileptic seizures. *Epilepsia* 1970;**11**:102-13.
65. Nicholl JS. Of Cabbages and Kings: Some considerations on classifications, diagnostic schemes, semiology, and concepts. *Epilepsia* 2003;**44**:988.
66. Panayiotopoulos CP. Importance of specifying the type of epilepsy. *Lancet* 1999;**354**:2002-3.
67. Grunewald RA, Panayiotopoulos CP. The diagnosis of epilepsies. *JRCPhys London* 1996;**30**:122-7.
68. Benbadis SR, Luders HO. Epileptic syndromes: an underutilized concept [editorial]. *Epilepsia* 1996;**37**:1029-34.
69. Nordli DR, Jr. Diagnostic difficulty in infants and children. *J Child Neurol.* 2002;**17 Suppl 1**:S28-S35.
70. Adie WJ. Pyknolepsy:a form of epilepsy occurring in children with a good prognosis. *Brain* 1924;**47**:96-102.
71. Merlis JK. Proposal for an international classification of the epilepsies. *Epilepsia* 1970;**11**:114-9.
72. Roger J, Bureau M, Dravet C, Genton P, Tassinari CA, Wolf P *et al,* eds. Epileptic syndromes in infancy, childhood and adolescence (3rd edn). London: John Libbey & Co Ltd, 2002.
73. Wolf P. Historical aspects: the concept of idiopathy. In Malafose A, Genton P, Hirsch E, Marescaux C, Broglin D, Bernasconi R, eds. *Idiopathic generalised epilepsies:clinical, experimental and genetic aspects*, pp 3-6. London: John Libbey & Company, 1994.
74. Commission on Classification and Terminology of the International League Against Epilepsy. Proposal for classification of epilepsy and epileptic syndromes. Epilepsia 26, 268-278. 1985.
75. Camfield P, Camfield C. Childhood epilepsy: what is the evidence for what we think and what we do? *J Child Neurol.* 2003;**18**:272-87.
76. Jackson HJ. On Classification and on Methods of Investigation (1874). In Taylor J, ed. *Selected writing of John Hughlings Jackson*, London: Hodder and Stoughton, 1952.
77. Commission on Antiepileptic Drugs of the International League Against Epilepsy. Guidelines for clinical evaluation of antiepileptic drugs. *Epilepsia* 1989;**30**:400-8.
78. Commission on Antiepileptic Drugs of the International League Against Epilepsy. Guidelines for antiepileptic drug trials in children. *Epilepsia* 1994;**35**:94-100.
79. Panayiotopoulos CP. Autonomic seizures and autonomic status epilepticus peculiar to childhood: diagnosis and management. *Epilepsy Behav.* 2004;**5**:286-95.
80. Engel J, Jr., Wiebe S, French J, Sperling M, Williamson P, Spencer D *et al.* Practice parameter: temporal lobe and localized neocortical resections for epilepsy. *Epilepsia* 2003;**44**:741-51.
81. Wieser HG. ILAE Commission Report. Mesial temporal lobe epilepsy with hippocampal sclerosis. *Epilepsia* 2004;**45**:695-714.

2 OPTIMAL USE OF THE EEG IN THE DIAGNOSIS AND MANAGEMENT OF EPILEPSIES

The EEG,[1–5] which is entirely harmless and relatively inexpensive, is the most important investigation in the diagnosis and management of epilepsies providing that it is properly performed by experienced technicians and carefully studied and interpreted in the context of a well-described clinical setting by experienced physicians.

Although not a substitute for a clinical examination, EEG is an integral part of the diagnostic process in epilepsies and this should not be underrated.

More than one-half of children and adults currently referred for a routine EEG are suspected of suffering from or do suffer from epilepsies. The EEG is indispensable in the correct syndromic diagnosis of these patients.

Epilepsies are usually easy to diagnose. However, as with any other medical condition, they are sometimes difficult and challenging. I use the EEG as an integral part of the diagnostic process. In this sense, there is more than enough justification for performing an EEG after the first seizure or in patients suspected of having epilepsy. The EEG may be the only means of an incontrovertible syndromic diagnosis. That the patient may not need treatment[6] is not a convincing argument against such a practice. The prime aim in medicine is the diagnosis, which determines the prognosis and management strategies.

The role of the EEG is to help the physician to establish an accurate diagnosis. In most conditions (infantile spasms, myoclonic epilepsies, idiopathic generalised epilepsy (IGE), symptomatic generalised epilepsy, temporal lobe epilepsy (TLE), Landau–Kleffner syndrome, benign childhood focal seizures and photosensitive and other reflex epilepsies) the EEG may specifically confirm or may specifically direct towards such a diagnosis if this is clinically uncertain. In other situations it may not be helpful with normal rhythms or some non-specific diffuse or paroxysmal slow activity. These cases may need an EEG during sleep, on awakening or both and again it may not reveal specific changes in approximately 10% of patients. However, even a normal EEG in an untreated patient may be useful as it may exclude some of the above conditions where EEG abnormalities are expected to be high, such as in IGE with absence seizures.

An EEG in chronic epilepsies or treated patients may be uninformative and misleading. Obtaining previous medical and EEG reports is essential.

A request for an EEG should describe the clinical problem well but, because this is rarely the reality, the EEG technologist should also obtain the relevant clinical information.

THE VALUE OF ROUTINE INTER-ICTAL OR ICTAL EXTRACRANIAL EEG IN EPILEPSIES SHOULD NEITHER BE OVERRATED NOR UNDERVALUED

EEG in epilepsies is overrated by some and undervalued by others. The truth is in between.

REASONS WHY EEG SHOULD NOT BE UNDERVALUED

- An EEG is the only available investigation for recording and evaluating the paroxysmal discharges of cerebral neurons causing seizures. The appropriate evaluation of patients with epileptic disorders is often impossible without an

EEG. In the majority of cases the clinical diagnosis is concordant with the EEG findings. However, it is often with the help of an EEG that the correct diagnosis is established, particularly if the clinical information is inadequate or misleading (Figure 2.1). On other occasions, the clinical data are sounder than the EEG findings, particularly if these are non-specific or in chronic cases of treated epilepsies.

- The seizure and epileptic syndrome classifications are based on combined clinico-EEG manifestations. Epileptic syndromes, the most important advance of recent epileptology, were mainly identified because of their EEG manifestations.
- Focal and generalised epilepsies are often difficult to differentiate without an EEG even by the most experienced epileptologists (Figure 2.1).
- It is the EEG which will often document beyond any doubt that the 'daydreaming' of a child is due to absence seizures (Figure 2.2), that long-lasting episodes of behavioural changes are due to non-convulsive status epilepticus, that the 'eyelid ticks' are due to eyelid myoclonia with photosensitivity, that the clumsiness on awakening is due to myoclonic jerks and that periodic bedwetting is due to nocturnal seizures.
- The EEG in neonatal seizures is the most powerful investigative tool (p. 93).

REASONS WHY EEG SHOULD NOT BE OVERVALUED

- The EEG may be oversensitive in conditions such as the benign childhood seizure susceptibility syndrome and sightless in others such as frontal epilepsies or often TLEs. On rare occasions even ictal events may be undetected in a surface EEG (some frontal seizures are a typical example of this). Patients with mainly focal epilepsies may have a series of normal EEGs and the EEG localisation is not always concordant with ictal intracranial recordings. More than 40% of patients with epileptic disorders may have one normal inter-ictal EEG although this percentage falls dramatically to 8% with series of EEGs and appropriate activating procedures, particularly sleep.[7]
- The frequency of seizures is not proportional to the EEG paroxysmal 'epileptogenic' discharges. Severely 'epileptogenic' EEGs may be recorded from patients with infrequent or controlled clinical seizures and vice versa. The EEG abnormalities do not reflect the severity of the epileptic disorder.[3]
- More than 10% of normal people may have non-specific EEG abnormalities and approximately 1% may have 'epileptiform paroxysmal activity' without seizures.[4] The prevalence of these abnormalities is higher in children, with 2–4% having functional spike discharges.[3]
- Paroxysmal epileptiform activity is high in patients with non-epileptic, neurological or medical disorders or with neurological deficits. For example, children with congenital visual deficits frequently have occipital spikes and patients with migraine have a high incidence of sharp paroxysmal activity and other abnormalities.[3,8]

SOURCES OF ERROR IN EEG

Even the most reliable investigative tools in medicine cannot escape severe errors because of poor technical quality (equipment, personnel or both), interpretation by poorly qualified physicians or both. A competent report should not only describe the EEG abnormality accurately, but also provide its significance and meaning in accordance with a well-described clinical setting.[3]

Failing to achieve this leads to severe errors and erroneous criticism such as 'a routine inter-ictal EEG is one of the most abused investigations in clinical medicine and is unquestionably responsible for great human suffering'.[9] Anything in medicine, clinical or laboratory, may be harmful if misinterpreted. Raising standards, not abandoning the service, is the proper response (Figure 2.1).[10]

That a patient with a brain tumour may not have clinical signs does not invalidate the clinical examination and the same is true for the EEG.

The main cause of concern and suffering is that physicians, including a few epilepsy authorities, have misunderstood the EEG, its value and its limitations.

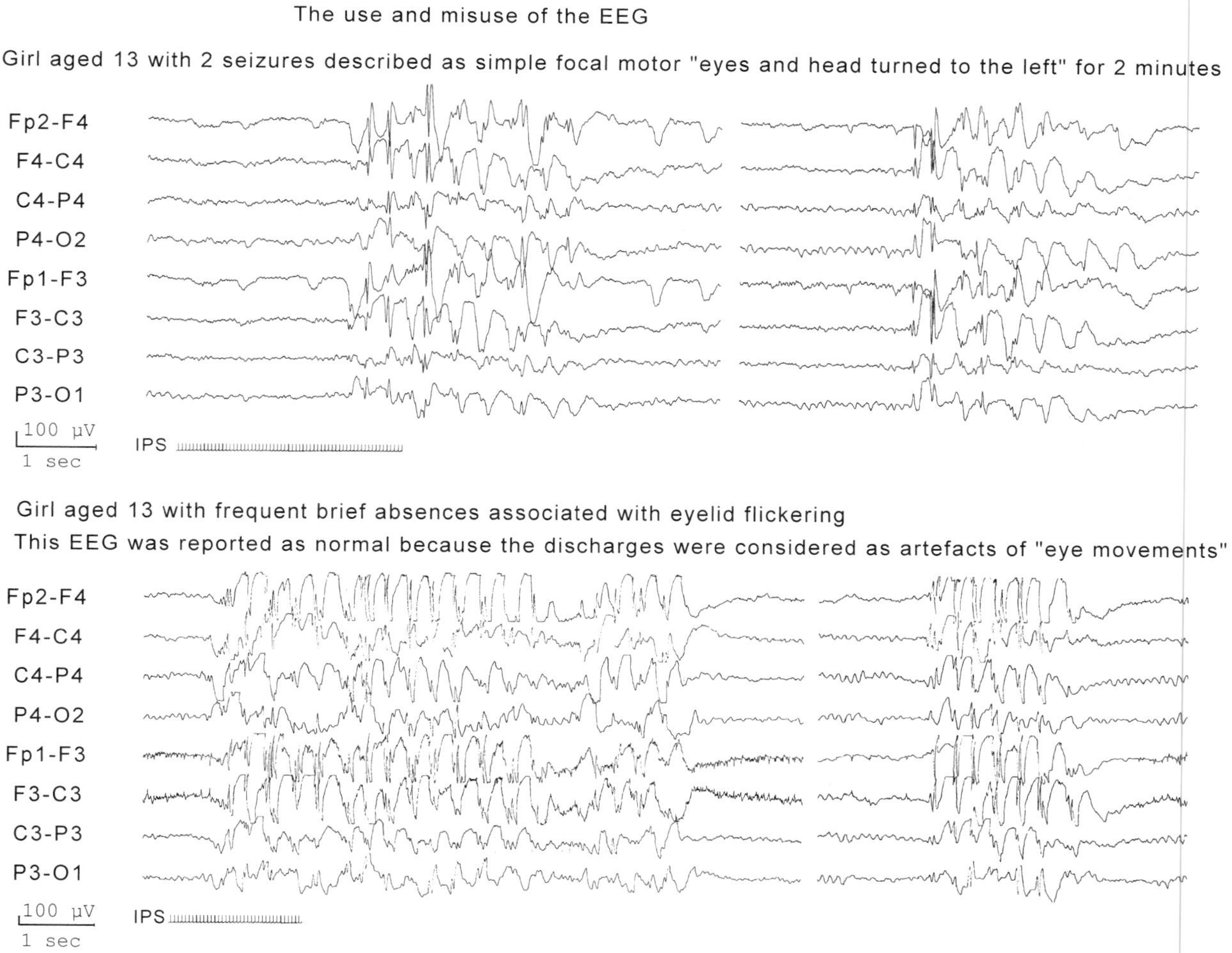

Figure 2.1 Use and misuse of EEGs. Two girls with similar EEG abnormalities of generalised spike/multiple spike and slow wave discharges either spontaneous or elicited by intermittent photic stimulation.

Top: proper use of EEGs. This girl gave a clear-cut history of two seizures that, on clinical grounds, had all the elements of focal motor seizures. Her eyes first and then her head turned to the left and 'I could not bring them back to normal' for 2 min. The EEG clearly documented that she had generalised not focal epilepsy.

Bottom: misuse of the EEG. A 26-year-old woman with JME had the onset of seizures at age 13 years. These consisted of brief absences with eyelid jerking. Her first EEG documented the epileptic nature of the attacks, but the reporting physician and the EEG technologist considered the discharges as artefacts produced by the concurrent eyelid jerking. The EEG was erroneously reported as normal.

Providing that the EEG is technically correct, the following are in my opinion the most important sources of error listed in order of significance.

1. *The single most significant source of error is that the EEG is often interpreted out of the clinical context.* There are two reasons for this. Firstly, the referring physician provides inadequate information regarding the events ('patient with loss of consciousness or grand mal seizures', 'black-outs: epilepsy?' and 'unexplained aggressiveness: TLE?') and often fails to mention other medical conditions or drugs that may significantly affect the EEG and its interpretation. Secondly, the reporting clinical neurophysiologist prefers a convenient but rather unhelpful and uncommitted abbreviation of the factual report ('normal EEG', 'an abnormal EEG with generalised discharges of frontal origin' and so forth). In St Thomas' Hospital, I am in the advantageous position to be the referring and reporting physician and this practice may expand to other clinics for epilepsies. Further, our EEG technologists are well trained in obtaining the missing clinical information (see page 38).[11]

2. *Non-specific EEG abnormalities are overemphasised without suggesting means of clarifying their significance, with a sleep-deprived EEG for example or after obtaining more clinical data.* Episodic focal slow waves are non-specific and may occur in a normal person or a patient with migraine, with mild cerebrovascular disease or even cerebral tumours. They may be of lateralising significance even if they are infrequent and of small amplitude in a patient with a well-established clinical history of temporal lobe seizures.[12]

3. *An EEG during hyperventilation, drowsiness and sleep may produce significant changes, which are often difficult to interpret even by experienced neurophysiologists.* EEGs in babies and children are even more complex and demanding. Non-epileptic episodic transients such as benign epileptiform transients of sleep, six and 14 positive spikes per second and rhythmic mid-temporal discharges may often be misinterpreted as evidence of 'epilepsy'.[4]

4. *Previous EEG records and results are lost, destroyed or not sought.* EEGs recorded at the initial stages of the disease and particularly before treatment are significant not only at the first medical presentation of the patients, but also in the re-evaluation of those with long-standing epilepsy. These patients are mainly referred for treatment modifications because they are free of seizures and still on medication, they had a recent convulsion after a long seizure-free period, their seizures are not controlled with long-standing medication, they have adverse reactions to their medication or it is appropriate to change to new anti-epileptic drugs (AEDs), anticipated pregnancy in women and so forth. The answer in all these cases is difficult. It requires a thorough clinical evaluation, review of previous medical and EEG records and the establishment of the appropriate epileptic syndrome. It does not depend on the findings of a new EEG, which may be misleading; for example, it may be normal in a patient with IGE who is on sodium valproate or may show focal slow wave paroxysms in patients with well-documented generalised spike and wave discharges (GSWDs) in an early EEG. However, on other occasions a recent EEG may prompt towards the correct advice documenting mild epileptic seizures such as myoclonic jerks or absences in a patient 'free of seizures' or of 'continuing focal seizures' inadequately treated with carbamazepine.

5. *Alteration of the EEG by drugs* (such as neuroleptics or anti-epileptics) or co-existing medical conditions (cerebrovascular disease, electrolyte disturbances or a previous head injury).

ACTIVATING PROCEDURES

Activating procedures are intended to improve the EEG diagnostic yield by inducing or enhancing epileptogenic paroxysms. Hyperventilation and intermittent photic stimulation are routinely applied in awake stage EEGs. Drowsiness, sleep and awakening are also very important activating procedures.

HYPERVENTILATION

Hyperventilation often induces EEG changes such as diffuse and paroxysmal slow activity in normal people and particularly in young persons who overbreathe well. These changes do not last for more than 30 s after cessation of hyperventilation and they should not be confused with abnormal epileptogenic disturbances, which are also activated by hyperventilation.

Current practice in EEG departments is usually to ask the patient to hyperventilate for 3 min. Patients are instructed to breathe deeply rather than quickly at a rate of 20 deep breaths/min.[13,14] This will cause an air exchange of 20–50 l/min in adults and a drop in pCO_2 of 4–7ml%.[15] Young children are encouraged to hyperventilate by asking them to blow on a brightly coloured pinwheel or a balloon. Infants often hyperventilate while sobbing.

Breath counting for the detection of cognitive impairment during GSWDs of 3–4 Hz

Breath counting is the most effective and practical means of reliably testing transient cognitive impairment during GSWDs induced by hyperventilation.[16,17] Breath counting should be used routinely during overbreathing in patients with GSWDs. Physicians and EEG technologists cannot appreciate its value prior to using and experiencing the benefits of this technique in their clinical practice.

A GSWD of 3–4 Hz, which is the electrical accompaniment of typical absences, is nearly invariably (more than 90% of untreated patients) induced or enhanced by hyperventilation. In current routine practice, if a GSWD occurs the technician is expected to detect possible associated ictal clinical symptoms such as eye opening, staring, cessation of overbreathing, myoclonic jerks, abnormal eye movements, automatisms and so forth. A verbal test stimulus (a phrase, number or rhyme) during the discharge, which the patient is asked to recall, is used for assessing cognitive impairment. Thus, cognitive impairment is examined in an *all or none* fashion or *recall or not recall* fashion. Marked impairment of consciousness is unlikely to be missed even in routine non-video EEG recordings. However, in less severe cases, where impairment of consciousness is mild, the patient often successfully recalls the verbal test stimulus given by the technician during the discharge (Figure 1.2). This results in misinterpretation of the electrical event as a larval or subclinical event. Further, in brief discharges the verbal test stimulus is often given at the end or after the discharge has terminated. It is practically impossible to make an accurate judgement on this without appropriate video–EEG recordings.

It is well documented that, with appropriate psychological testing, brief generalised spike or polyspike and slow wave discharges of 3–4 Hz are often

---

Commentary on the guidelines for the use of EEG methodology in the diagnosis of epilepsy[21]

The recently published *Guidelines for the Use of EEG Methodology in the Diagnosis of Epilepsy* by the International League Against Epilepsy (ILAE) Commission on European Affairs: Subcommission on European Guidelines[21] is of doubtful significance. Firstly, it emphasises aspects relevant to the old paper EEG recordings paying little attention to digital EEG. Secondly, it recommends all-night sleep deprivation for adults and recording during sleep only. Thirdly, no emphasis is placed on the significance and means of detecting clinical events during EEG discharges. Finally, it does not provide a contribution on the significance of video–EEG recording in epilepsies.

associated with momentary impairment of cognitive function, even when absences are not clinically apparent.[18–20] However, these psychological tests are in general not user-friendly and therefore unsuitable for routine clinical practice, which is the reason that they are not used in clinical EEG departments.

Breath counting is a simple modification of the routine EEG technique of hyperventilation, which is easily performed by any patient who can count irrespective of age and intelligence. The technician demonstrates the technique to the patient. The patient counts each deep breath at its expiration phase loudly and consecutively.

Breath counting allows accurate identification of even mild transient cognitive impairment during GSWDs.[17] This is manifested as slurring of the speech, cessation, delay, hesitation, errors in counting with repetitions and counting out of sequence (Figures 1.2 and 2.1–2.3). Some patients may take two consecutive breaths during or immediately after the GSWD, but they count only the last of the two breaths.

Breath counting is powerful in detecting transient cognitive abnormalities because of simultaneously testing attention, concentration, memory, sequential precision and language function. The patient's performance during breath counting acts as its own control.

INTERMITTENT PHOTIC STIMULATION

Intermittent photic stimulation is significant for the detection of photosensitive patients (as detailed in Chapter 13. Photoparoxysmal discharges, which are often generated in the occipital regions, indicate a genetically determined photosensitivity and may occur in more than 1% of healthy subjects.

OTHER FORMS OF APPROPRIATE ACTIVATION OF REFLEX SEIZURES

Other forms of appropriate activation should be used and they are as much fascinating as rewarding in patients with reflex seizures such as reading, pattern, musicogenic, proprioceptive and noogenic epilepsy. Their detection is of significance with regard to diagnosis and management. The avoidance of precipitating factors may be all that is needed in certain patients with reflex seizures.

DROWSINESS, SLEEP AND AWAKENING

Drowsiness, sleep and awakening are important to study with an EEG in patients with epileptic disorders, particularly in those who produce a normal routine awake

Figure 2.2 The significance of EEG in the diagnosis of epilepsies; EEG of four patients with epileptic seizures. *(Facing page).*

Top: Ictal EEG of a 4-year-old boy who had frequent brief episodes of 'panic' without impairment of consciousness or convulsive features. The resting EEG was normal but a 'panic' attack was video-EEG recorded with ictal EEG changes of 2 min on the right, mainly involving the right temporal regions. The child accurately answered all questions and communicated well with the technician during the ictus. This EEG unequivocally established the diagnosis and dictated the appropriate management. MRI showed right hippocampal sclerosis.
Middle: Video-EEG of a child aged 8 years with frequent episodes of "blanks and day dreaming" for 2 years. Frequent typical absence seizures were recorded and appropriate treatment was initiated with complete control of the seizures.
Bottom left. Interictal EEG of a 5-year-old girl 2 days after a prolonged autonomic status epilepticus who was treated for suspected encephalitis (case 47 in ref 23). EEG showed scattered right central and bi-occipital spikes. The diagnosis of Panayiotopoulos syndrome was established and the child was discharged home.
Lower right: Video-EEG of a 32-year-old man with 3-4 GTCS every year from age 16 (case 1 in ref 24). All GTCS were preceded by absence status diagnosed as 'prodrome' or 'temporal lobe aura'. Treatment included inappropriate use of phenytoin and even vigabatrin. Brief generalised discharges of 3-4 Hz spike-multiple spikes and slow waves were recorded during hyperventilation. These were associated with brief rhythmic myoclonic jerks of the eyelids (which would be impossible to detect without video) and minor errors in breath counting. The correct diagnosis of IGE with phantom absences was established and treatment changed to sodium valproate. No further seizures occurred in the next 5 years of follow-up.

stage EEG or in those where their seizures are consistently associated with these physiological stages. However, drowsiness and sleep are associated with dramatic physiological EEG changes, which may imitate epileptogenic paroxysms. Their interpretation should be left only to highly experienced clinical neurophysiologists,

Boy aged 4 with "panic attacks"

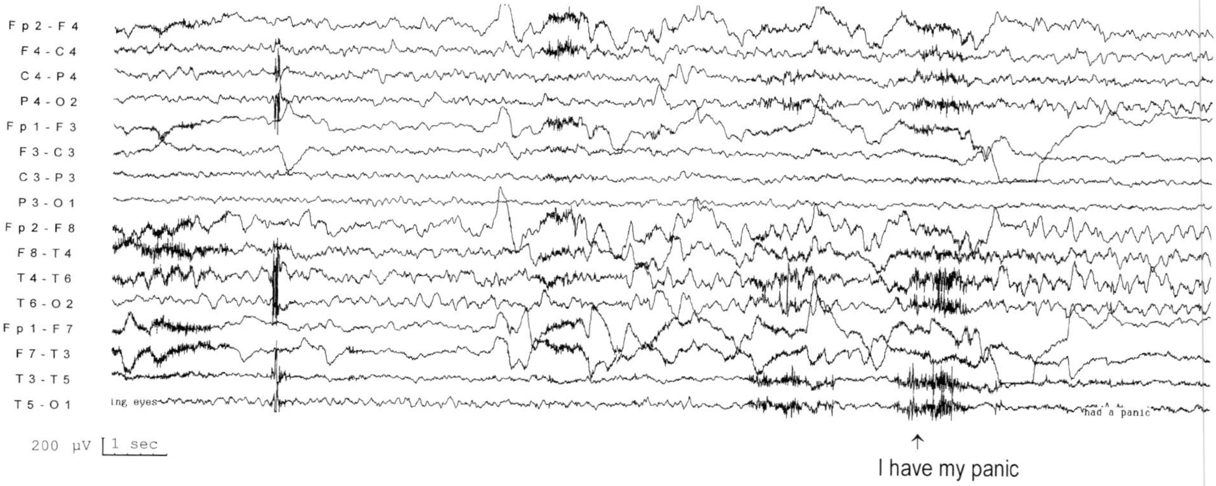

Boy aged 8 with "day dreaming" attacks

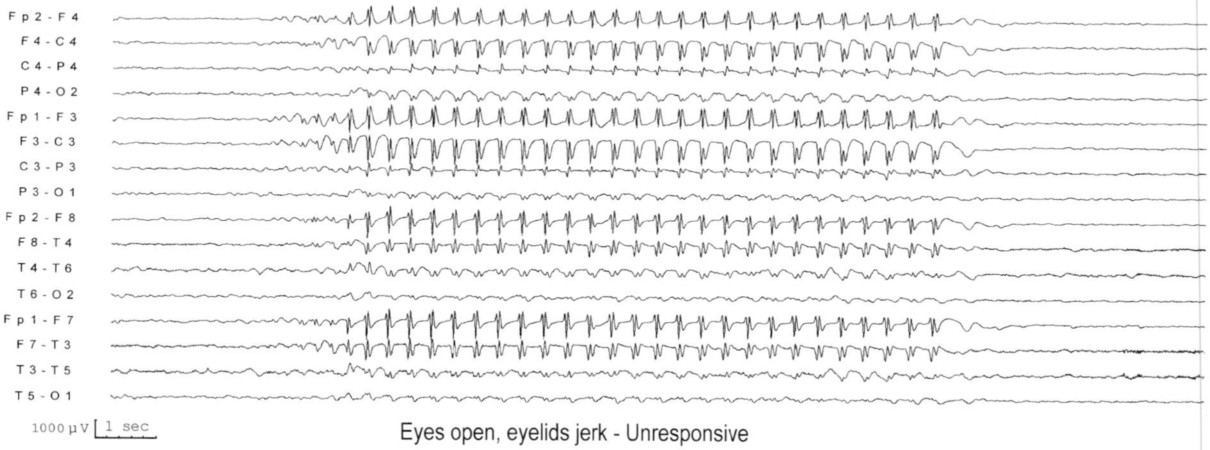

Eyes open, eyelids jerk - Unresponsive

Girl aged 5 suspected for encephalitis

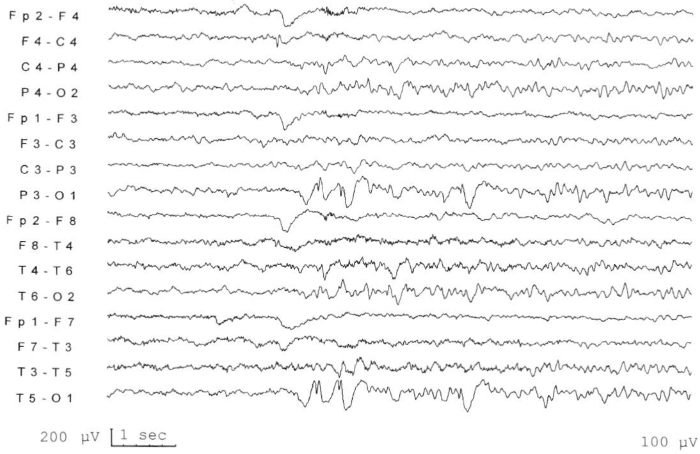

Man aged 32 with GTCS preceded by "temporal lobe aura"

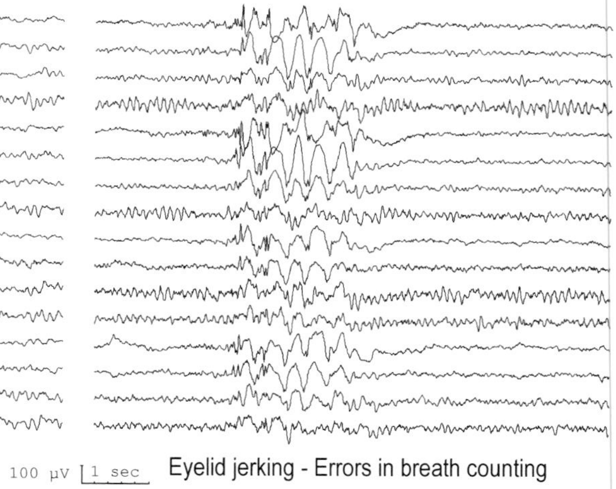

Eyelid jerking - Errors in breath counting

otherwise significant errors are inevitable. In sleep stage EEGs, recording should always continue to include the awakening stage. It is well known that seizures and EEG paroxysms may only occur at this stage in certain epileptic syndromes such as IGE.

Partial instead of all-night sleep deprivation should be preferred.
The recording should continue to include the awakening stage, which is an uncommon practice in most EEG laboratories.

Sleep stage EEG recording is routinely applied for the investigation of patients with a suspected or established diagnosis of epileptic seizures. This is mainly performed because of (1) an alert EEG being normal or equivocal, (2) suspected nocturnal epileptic seizures or (3) possible activation by sleep that may be important in diagnosis, such as in benign childhood focal seizures or suspected electrical status epilepticus during sleep.

The routine practice in most EEG departments is to ask for an all-night sleep deprivation EEG. The EEG is performed the next morning with the aim of obtaining a good sleep stage EEG. As soon as this is achieved the recording is stopped, the patient is awakened and allowed to go home. This practice surprisingly is also recommended in ILAE guidelines.[21] However, all-night sleep deprivation is inconvenient for the patient and often for the whole family and may induce seizures in susceptible individuals, particularly after leaving the EEG department in the awakening period. Patients with juvenile myoclonic epilepsy (JME) are particularly vulnerable because seizures mainly occur on awakening after sleep deprivation.

Drug-induced sleep is also applied in some departments as a substitute for all-night sleep deprivation. Usually, quinalbarbitone, chloral hydrate and, more recently, melatonin is given to the patient prior to or during electrode placement, with the aim of obtaining a sleep stage EEG after which the same procedure as above is followed. There is no requirement for an EEG on awakening. However, drugs that induce sleep may interfere with normal patterns and patients may find it difficult to be sufficiently alert for the rest of the day. They may also have a seizure on awakening as above.

My practice is to perform a sleep EEG that is as close as possible to the natural state and habits of the patient and thereby achieve best results with minimal discomfort and minimal risk to the patient. This is achieved with partial sleep deprivation, which is a practical, more natural, less disturbing and equally rewarding approach.[22] The EEG is recorded during the awake, sleep and awakening stages.

In order to achieve satisfactory results, we ask patients to go to sleep 1–2 h later and wake 1–2 h earlier than their routine practice. However, we do not apply this rigidly, but try to adjust it to each patient's sleep habits. Some patients find it easy

Figure 2.3 The significance of recording the EEG in the awakening stage. *(Facing page)*

From a video–EEG recording of a 23-year-old woman with IGE and absence seizures. She was thought to be free of seizures. A long EEG the previous day, including two sessions of well-performed overbreathing was normal. She slept for 5 h the same night (not an unusual situation for a young person of her age) and the EEG was recorded in the middle of the next day. This showed numerous absence seizures upon awakening that ended with GTCS.
Top: one of the brief typical absences that occurred during hyperventilation with breath counting after awakening. Numbers annotate breath counts. Note the time gap between 3 and 4 when the absence occurred.
Middle: a typical absence seizure progressing to GTCS. Note the smooth transformation from spike and wave discharges of the absence to fast spike discharges of the GTCS.
Bottom: onset of GTCS as in the middle of the figure but at different montage and slower speed.

Modified from Panayiotopoulos (2000)[25] with the permission of the Editor of *Epilepsia*.

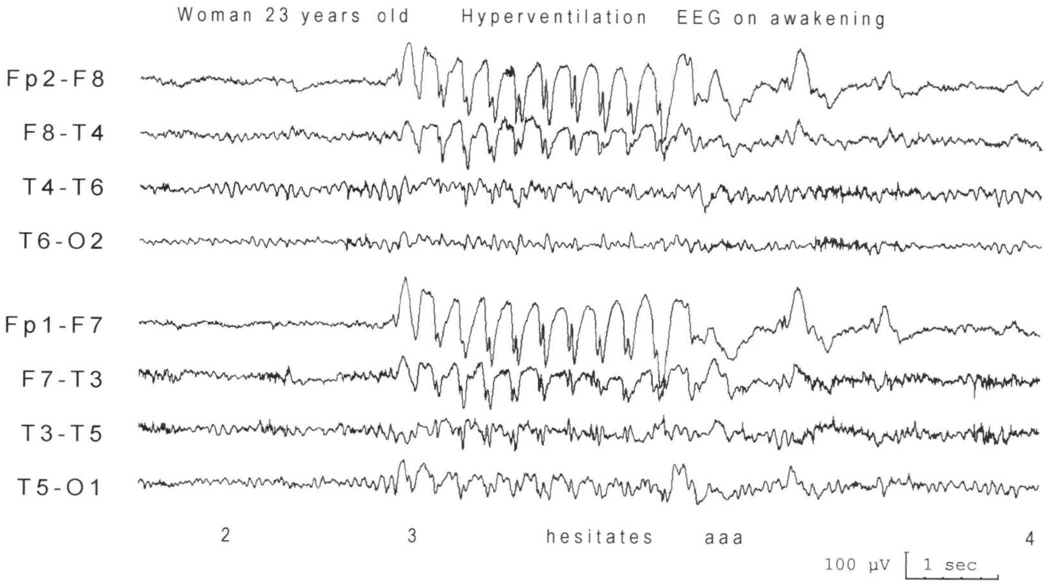
Woman 23 years old
Hyperventilation
EEG on awakening
Fp2-F8
F8-T4
T4-T6
T6-O2
Fp1-F7
F7-T3
T3-T5
T5-O1
2
3
hesitates
aaa
4
100 μV
1 sec

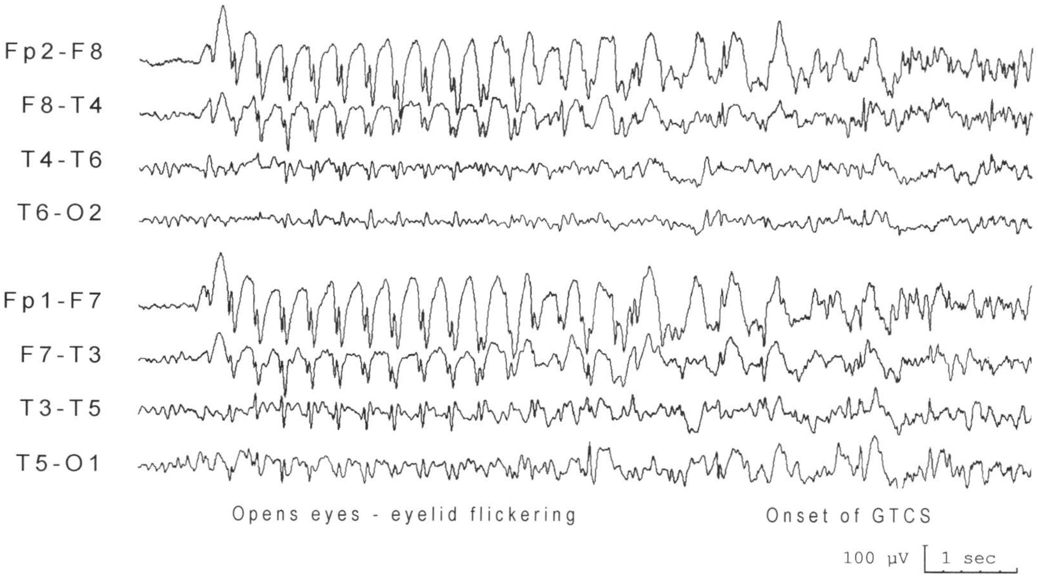
Fp2-F8
F8-T4
T4-T6
T6-O2
Fp1-F7
F7-T3
T3-T5
T5-O1
Opens eyes - eyelid flickering
Onset of GTCS
100 μV
1 sec

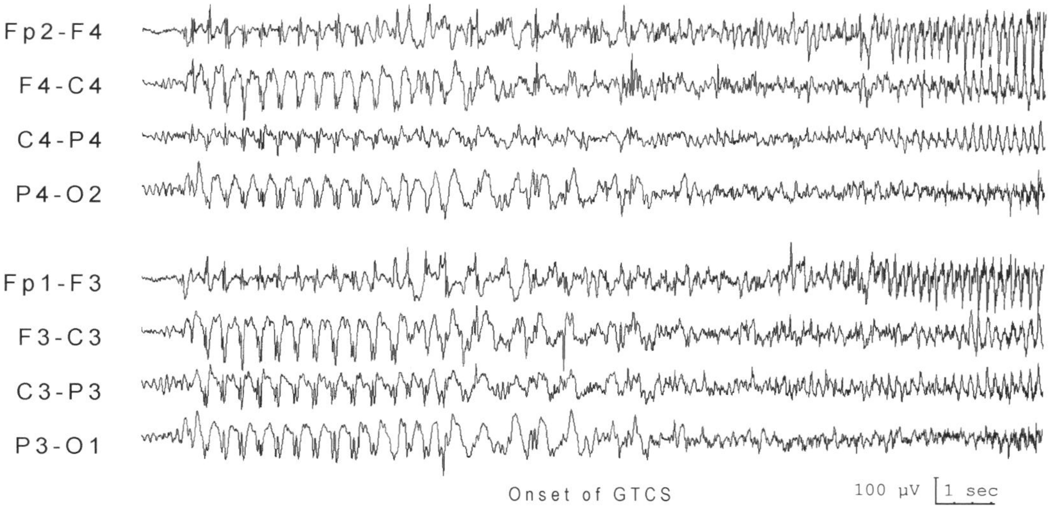
Fp2-F4
F4-C4
C4-P4
P4-O2
Fp1-F3
F3-C3
C3-P3
P3-O1
Onset of GTCS
100 μV
1 sec

to go to sleep whereas others find it difficult. We tell them that our aim is to obtain a natural sleep stage EEG and ask them to go to bed later than usual and wake up very early in the morning and remain awake until their appointment time, which we organise at 13:30 h for adults and at 11:30 h for children. The patient is asked to lie down and relax in a darkened and quiet recording room after application of the EEG electrodes. We allow 30–60 min sleep recording depending on the depth of sleep and EEG abnormalities. Subsequently, the patient is awakened and when alerted sat up and the EEG continues, also including hyperventilation and intermittent photic stimulation. This last phase on awakening lasts for approximately 15 min also depending on EEG interictal and ictal abnormalities. The whole procedure is performed with video–EEG recording, particularly for patients in whom minor or major seizures are expected on clinical or previous EEG grounds.

We have audited this method and found that 93.3% of the patients reached stage II–III and occasionally stage IV of sleep and in all patients EEG recording successfully continued on awakening. The other 6.7% failed to sleep although in some of them stage I was achieved.

In our practice, we have numerous examples of patients with clinical, mainly brief, minor seizures documented only in the awakening state, while their sleep stage video–EEG recording was normal or showed clinically asymptomatic generalised discharges.

THE EEG RECORDING SHOULD BE TAILORED TO THE SPECIFIC CIRCUMSTANCES OF THE INDIVIDUAL PATIENT

- The technician should be alerted to apply the appropriate stimulus when reading or other forms of reflex epilepsy are clinically suspected.
- Patients with IGE may have a normal or non-specifically abnormal routine EEG. In these patients an EEG after partial sleep deprivation with video–EEG recording during sleep and on awakening frequently reveals clinical and EEG ictal events.

The same applies to patients with nocturnal seizures who may have a normal EEG while awake.

- Women with catamenial seizures should have an EEG during their vulnerable periods if EEGs at other times are inconclusive.

THE ROLE OF EEG TECHNOLOGISTS

The principal responsibility of EEG technologists is a competent EEG recording and a factual report. However, their role should be more than this, when considering the following.

- Currently approximately 70% of EEG referrals are for epileptic disorders.
- Referrals commonly come from general paediatricians/general physicians who may not be familiar with the syndromic diagnosis of epilepsies.
- Information in the request form is usually inadequate.
- An EEG technologist spends 15–20 min preparing the patient for the recording, which may be valuably used for obtaining information about such things as minor seizures, precipitating factors and the circadian distribution and other aspects of the particular individual. The interpretation of the EEG depends on a patient's clinical history, which often is poor or missing.
- Currently non-medical health professionals such as nurses are rightly involved in the management of epilepsies.

A well-qualified EEG technician is expected and should be trained to have a thorough knowledge of seizures and epileptic syndromes.[11]

In my department the EEG technologists often provide me with the correct syndromic diagnosis of our patients based on such a dual approach. Even interpretation of a normal EEG may be significantly different according to clinical information (see the illustrative cases on page 40).

DIGITAL EEG

Digital EEG is the paperless recording of an EEG using computer-based instrumentation. The data are stored on electronic media, such as magnetic drives or optical disks and displayed on a monitor. Digital EEG recording has many advantages compared to analogue and paper EEGs, including retrospective reformatting (without the need for recording new data), storage, automatic event detection, quantification and networking capabilities.[26–30] Reading of the EEG record with user-selected montages, filters, vertical scaling (gain/sensitivity) and horizontal scaling (time resolution or compression) allows for more accurate interpretation. Digital EEG replaces the need to warehouse or microfilm paper records, enables optional additional EEG signal processing and allows for electronic exchange of EEGs. Producing EEG figures is also notoriously difficult from paper EEGs particularly if blue ink was used. Most of the figures in this book were easily reproduced from digital EEGs.

VIDEO–EEG RECORDING SHOULD BE MADE ROUTINE PRACTICE

Video–EEG recording should be mandatory in the evaluation of patients suspected of having seizures because it is the only means of reaching an incontrovertible diagnosis if clinical events occur during the recording. These may incidentally occur during the EEG or be predictably recorded based on their circadian distribution and the precipitating factors. Video–EEG machines are relatively inexpensive today with advances in digital compression and storage technology. Cost can be reduced to a minimum by using a commercially available camcorder synchronised with the EEG.

An EEG discharge is of great diagnostic and management significance if it is associated with clinical manifestations. However, these symptoms may be minor and escape recognition in routine EEGs without video recordings (Figures 1.2 and 2.1–2.3). Video–EEG recordings are particularly important in the identification and categorisation of absences, which are easily elicited by hyperventilation, myoclonic jerks or focal seizures which may be inconspicuous and psychogenic or other non-epilepic seizures (Figure 1.1) particularly those of the hyperventilation syndrome.[31]

Seizures or other paroxysmal events may occur at any stage during the EEG. Therefore, it is advisable to start and continue video recording during the whole EEG procedure. Vasovagal attacks often occur during EEG electrode placement. Psychogenic or fraudulent non-epileptic seizures often happen at the end of an EEG while removing the electrodes, particularly when the patient is told that the EEG is normal. Other types of non-epileptic seizures such as paroxysmal kinesiogenic choreoathetosis may also be captured with video–EEG recording and prompt the correct diagnosis.

AN EEG REPORT SHOULD BE HELPFUL AND COMMITTED: IT SHOULD NOT BE AN ABBREVIATED FACTUAL REPORT

One of the most important sources of error in EEGs is that the reporting clinical neurophysiologist prefers a convenient but rather unhelpful and uncommitted approach, which is often an abbreviation of the factual technical report: 'normal EEG', 'an abnormal EEG with generalised discharges of frontal origin', 'there is an active spike in the occipital regions', 'focal episodic left temporal slowing without genuine epileptiform activity' and so forth. This is inadequate, often uninformative and sometimes misleading. The receiving physician is often unfamiliar with these EEG terms and their significance. My approach is to provide as much information as possible supplementing the traditional conclusion with an opinion and often a comment, which improves the EEG contribution.

ILLUSTRATIVE CASES WITH A NORMAL ROUTINE EEG WHERE THE CLINICAL INFORMATION REQUIRES A NEW APPROPRIATELY TAILORED EEG

- The normal routine EEG of a teenager with a single GTCS on awakening after significant sleep deprivation, fatigue and unaccustomed alcohol consumption.

  Conclusion: the EEG is normal but, because the patient's seizure occurred on awakening after significant precipitating factors, we have arranged an EEG after partial sleep deprivation.

  The EEG was normal again, but after awakening there were brief (1–2 s), asymptomatic, GSWDs of 3–4 Hz during hyperventilation. These were consistent with the clinical impression of a low threshold to IGE. The patient was advised regarding precipitating factors and no drug treatment was given.

- The normal routine EEG of an 8-year-old child with GTCS during sleep.

  Conclusion: the routine awake EEG is normal, but because this is a child with a nocturnal convulsive seizure, a sleep EEG is indicated.

  The sleep EEG showed centro-temporal spikes thus documenting the diagnosis of Rolandic epilepsy and securing an excellent prognosis.

- The normal ictal and inter-ictal EEG of a 20-year-old man referred for frequent brief clusters of bizarre movements, which 'sounds like pseudo-seizures'.

  Conclusion: the routine awake EEG is normal. However, in view of the history that the paroxysmal events mainly occurred during sleep, the technician allowed time for the patient to go to sleep, during which several of his habitual attacks were recorded with video–EEG recording. These were typical hypermotor epileptic seizures thus documenting the diagnosis of mesial frontal lobe epilepsy (supplementary sensory motor epilepsy).

- The normal EEG of a 50-year-old man with 'GTCS from age 12 years, but on remission for 10 years. Stop anti-epileptic medication?'

  Conclusion: the EEG is within normal limits. However, stopping medication is not recommended because, according to the information provided to the EEG technologist, the patient continues to have brief seizures. These consist of unilateral multicoloured and spherical visual hallucinations lasting for a few seconds to a minute often progressing to deviation of the eyes and head. They are identical to those occurring prior to his GTCS. The patient suffers from occipital epilepsy with visual seizures and secondarily GTCS, a situation frequently misdiagnosed as migra-lepsy.

  Despite this report medication was discontinued. Two months later the patient had GTCS at work and he lost his job.

ILLUSTRATIVE CASES WITH ABNORMAL EEGS SHOWING THAT THE REPORTING PHYSICIAN MAY MAKE A SIGNIFICANT CONTRIBUTION TO THE CORRECT DIAGNOSIS AND MANAGEMENT

- An EEG with brief generalised discharges of spikes and waves in a 30-year-old man referred because of a first GTCS.

  Conclusion: the EEG is of good organisation with a well-formed alpha rhythm. It is abnormal because of brief generalised discharges of small spikes and waves of 3–4 Hz, which are facilitated by hyperventilation. These are not associated with any ictal clinical manifestations tested with video–EEG recording and breath counting.

Opinion: the EEG abnormality indicates a low threshold to IGE. This is consistent with the clinical information that the recent GTCS occurred in the morning after sleep deprivation and alcohol consumption. The patient is not aware of absences or myoclonic jerks. There is a remote possibility that these abnormalities are due to frontal lesions[32] or subependymal heterotopia (a distinct neuronal migration disorder associated with epilepsy).[33] This may indicate the need for high-resolution MRI though I expect it to be normal.

Comment: this patient may not need any drug treatment, but he should be advised regarding precipitating factors.

MRI was normal and the patient did not have any other seizures in the next 10 years of follow-up.

- A 35-year-old woman was referred because of prolonged confusional premenstrual episodes.

  Conclusion: the EEG is of good organisation with a well-formed alpha rhythm. It is suspiciously but not definitely abnormal because of a brief and inconspicuous generalised burst of larval spikes and theta waves.

  Opinion: the EEG abnormality is mild and not conclusive. We have organised an EEG during her vulnerable premenstrual period because the confusional episodes may be non-convulsive status epilepticus.

  This was performed and showed definite and frequent generalised discharges of spikes/multiple spikes and slow waves of 3–4 Hz associated with impairment of consciousness and eyelid flickering. No further confusional episodes occurred after treatment with valproate.

- A 17-year-old man was referred because of a 'single episode of loss of consciousness and convulsions. Epilepsy?'

  Conclusion: the EEG is of good organisation with a well-formed alpha rhythm. It is abnormal because of brief runs of monomorphic theta waves around the left anterior temporal regions.

  Opinion: the EEG abnormality is mild but definite, although it does not show conventional epileptogenic features. However, because it is strictly unilateral a high-resolution MRI is indicated. This is also mandated because, according to the information gathered by our EEG technologist, the recent convulsive episode was preceded by an ascending epigastric sensation and fear, which had also occurred in isolation several times over the previous 2 years. These raise the possibility of hippocampal epilepsy.

  MRI confirmed left hippocampal sclerosis and a sleep stage EEG showed a clear-cut sharp and slow wave focus in the left anterior temporal electrode.

- An EEG with occipital spikes from a 6-year-old child referred because of 'a prolonged episode of loss of consciousness with convulsions'.

  Conclusion: the EEG is of good organisation with a well-formed alpha rhythm, which is often interrupted by clusters of high-amplitude bi-occipital sharp and slow waves.

  Opinion: the EEG abnormality of occipital spikes is often associated with benign seizures in this age group. From the clinical description, this child may suffer from 'Panayiotopoulos syndrome', whereby seizures are often solitary or infrequent as detailed in the attached paper (I enclose a brief report if the referring physician is not aware of the condition). However, occipital paroxysms may also occur in 1% of normal children and even more frequently in children with congenital visual abnormalities (strabismus and amblyopia) and other conditions with or without seizures.

  Comment: this EEG should be interpreted in accordance with the clinical manifestations in this child.* In particular was the event nocturnal or diurnal? What were the symptoms that preceded the convulsions and what was their duration? Did he have autonomic disturbances, vomiting or eye deviation? Is this a normal child with normal vision and development? Please, let me know, as treatment may not be needed.

---

*Note: The EEG technologist should have obtained this information (p. 38).

- A 19-year-old student was referred because of 'infrequent GTCS from age 13 but now in remission for 2 years. Stop medication?'

  Conclusion: the resting EEG is within normal limits, but hyperventilation elicited high-amplitude generalised spike and slow wave discharges of 3–4 Hz with a duration of 3–5 s. These were associated with significant errors during breath counting as documented with video–EEG recording.

  Opinion: the EEG documents that the patient suffers from IGE with active mild absence seizures.

  Comment: according to the information provided by the patient, she also occasionally has mild myoclonic jerks on awakening particularly during examination periods. These indicate that she suffers from JME and treatment should continue for many years to come.

- A 5-year-old child was referred for an EEG because of 'learning difficulties and absence seizures'.

  Conclusion: this is a long video–EEG recording during an awake period and naturally occurring sleep stages I–IV. The awake stage EEG shows frequent high-amplitude sharp and slow wave complexes mainly around the right central and right posterior parietal electrode. Frequently, this occurs simultaneously with a left-sided similar sharp and slow wave complex, but this is always of higher amplitude on the right. In sleep, these discharges appear continuously as in electrical status epilepticus.

  Opinion: this is a very abnormal EEG, which raises the possibility of Landau–Kleffner syndrome. There is not the slightest evidence of absence seizures.

  On the basis of this EEG the child was appropriately assessed and found to suffer from Landau–Kleffner syndrome.

There are numerous similar examples that this type of communication between electroencephalographers and clinicians is essential for a better diagnosis and management of patients with epilepsies. The problems become even more complicated and demanding in the interpretation of EEGs from patients referred for possible epileptic seizures who also suffer from co-morbid conditions such as migraine, psychiatric diseases, cerebrovascular insufficiency and so forth and who may also be on various medications. In these cases it is often important to admit that 'the EEG, although abnormal, may be misleading in view of the migraine and psychiatric or previous head injuries of the patient. The EEG abnormality cannot be taken as evidence or not of epilepsy'.

THE SIGNIFICANCE OF THE EEG AFTER THE FIRST AFEBRILE SEIZURE

Routine EEG recording is a standard recommendation of the diagnostic evaluation of a child after a first afebrile seizure.[34] This comes from the Quality Standards Subcommittee of the American Academy of Neurology based on analysis of evidence.[34] However, in the UK an EEG is not recommended after the first afebrile seizure, a practice that may have significant adverse implications in the correct diagnosis and management (see Panayiotopoulos[10] and associated commentary[6]).

THE FIRST SEIZURE

Most of the epilepsies manifest with primarily or secondarily GTCS, which may herald the onset or occur long after the beginning of the disease. Studies on the prognosis and treatment of the 'first seizure' mainly refer to GTCS, although this may not be the first seizure in the patient's life.[35] Myoclonic jerks, absences and focal seizures are less dramatic but more important than GTCS for diagnosis. In one study, 74% of patients with newly identified unprovoked seizures had experienced multiple seizure episodes prior to their first medical contact.[36]

The recurrence rate after a first convulsive seizure varies from 27 to 81%, thereby reflecting significant differences in selection, treatment and methodological criteria.[3,10]

An abnormal EEG and particularly GSWDs have been reported as a consistent predictor of recurrence in all[36–40] but one study which was in adults[41] (see Panayiotopoulos[3,10] for reviews). In a meta-analysis of 16 publications on the risk of recurrence after a first fit, seizure aetiology and EEG findings were the stronger predictors of recurrence.[37] This was confirmed in another study of 407 children with a first unprovoked afebrile seizure.[40] In idiopathic and cryptogenic seizures the EEG was the most important predictor of outcome with 52% risk of recurrence at 2 years in those with an abnormal EEG versus 28% in those with a normal EEG.[40] The EEG showed specific abnormalities of focal spikes or GSWDs in 32.5% of 268 children after their first idiopathic seizure.[39]

Numerous studies of homogeneous patients have established markedly different remission rates and prognosis depending on the syndromic classification. For example, consider the excellent prognosis in febrile seizures, benign childhood focal seizures such as Rolandic or Panayiotopoulos syndrome, the lifelong liability to seizures or their worsening in JME, mesial TLE with hippocampal sclerosis, epileptic encephalopathies and so forth.

WHY AN EEG AFTER THE FIRST AFEBRILE SEIZURE?

A convulsive seizure is a dramatic event in a child's life and that of their family.[42] As in all other fields of medicine, they are entitled to a diagnosis, prognosis and management, which is specific and precise.[3,35] Aiming to this goal, an EEG after the first seizure is essential.[34]

That an epileptiform EEG is associated with a two to three times higher risk for recurrence than a normal EEG is well established.[3,10,36–40] However, the most significant reasons for having an EEG after a single afebrile convulsion are fourfold.

Firstly, it is possible to recognise children with the features of specific epileptic syndromes. Between 10% and 40% of children with benign childhood focal seizures may not have had more than a single fit, thus depriving them of a precise diagnosis and prognosis under the current practice, in some counties, of not having an EEG after the first seizure. On other occasions, symptomatic epilepsies may be established requiring early attention.

Secondly, minor seizures such as absences, myoclonic jerks or focal fits may be recorded, which have immense diagnostic and treatment implications.

Thirdly, the EEG is essential in establishing seizure-precipitating factors such as video games or television, thus leading to early and appropriate advice.

Fourthly, an EEG in an untreated stage of an epileptic syndrome is imperative. This is most likely to happen if the EEG is requested after the first seizure. Many paediatricians would be reluctant to withhold treatment after a second or more seizures which are expected to occur in one-quarter of children within 3 months after their first fit. Requesting an EEG at that stage may be too late, considering that EEG waiting lists may sometimes be lengthy. Masking or altering the EEG with AEDs may prevent a correct seizure or syndrome diagnosis. This in turn will be detrimental for management, which may be long term, and expensive in terms of medication, which is often seizure specific.

REFERENCES

1. Haas LF. Hans Berger (1873–1941), Richard Caton (1842–1926), and electroencephalography. *J Neurol Neurosurg Psychiatry* 2003; **74**: 9.
2. Binnie CD,.Stefan H. Modern electroencephalography: its role in epilepsy management. *Clin Neurophysiol* 1999; **110**: 1671–97.
3. Panayiotopoulos CP. *Benign Childhood Partial Seizures and Related Epileptic Syndromes.* London: John Libbey & Company Ltd; 1999.
4. Niedermeyer E, Lopes da Silva, F. *Electroencephalography. Basic Principles, Clinical Applications, and Related Fields*, 4th edn. Baltimore: Williams & Wilkins; 1999.
5. Blume WT. Current trends in electroencephalography. *Curr.Opin Neurol* 2001; **14**: 193–7.
6. Cross J. Significance of the EEG after the first afebrile seizure: commentary. *Arch Dis Child* 1998; **78**: 576–7.
7. Binnie CD. Prior PF. Electroencephalography. *J Neurol Neurosurg Psychiatr* 1994; **57**: 1308–19.
8. Sand T. Electroencephalography in migraine: a review with focus on quantitative electroencephalography and the migraine vs. epilepsy relationship. *Cephalalgia* 2003; **23** (Suppl 1): 5–11.
9. Chadwick D. Diagnosis of epilepsy. *Lancet* 1990; **336**: 291–5.
10. Panayiotopoulos CP. Significance of the EEG after the first afebrile seizure. *Arch Dis Child* 1998; **78**: 575–6.
11. Sanders S, Rowlinson S, Manidakis I, Ferrie CD, Koutroumanidis M. The contribution of the EEG technologists in the diagnosis of Panayiotopoulos syndrome (susceptibility to early onset benign childhood autonomic seizures). *Seizure* 2004; **13**:567-73.
12. Koutroumanidis M, Binnie CD, Elwes RD *et al.* Interictal regional slow activity in temporal lobe epilepsy correlates with lateral temporal hypometabolism as imaged with 18FDG PET: neurophysiological and metabolic implications. *J Neurol Neurosurg Psychiatry* 1998; **65**: 170–6.
13. American Electroencephalographic Society. Guideline one: minimum technical requirements for performing clinical electroencephalography. *J Clin Neurophysiol* 1994; **11**: 2–5.
14. American Electroencephalographic Society. Guideline two: minimum technical standards for pediatric electroencephalography. *J Clin Neurophysiol* 1994; **11**: 6–9.
15. Takahashi T. Activation methods. In Niedermeyer E, Lopes da Silva F (editors). *Electroencephalography. Basic Principles, Clinical Applications, and Related Fields.* Baltimore, MD: Williams & Wilkins; 1999: pp. 261–84.
16. Panayiotopoulos CP, Baker A, Grunewald RA, Rowlinson S. Breath counting during 3 Hz generalized spike and wave discharges. *J Electrophysiol Technol* 1993; **19**: 15–23.
17. Giannakodimos S, Ferrie CD, Panayiotopoulos CP. Qualitative and quantitative abnormalities of breath counting during brief generalized 3 Hz spike and slow wave 'subclinical' discharges. *Clin Electroencephalogr* 1995; **26**: 200–3.
18. Aarts JH, Binnie CD, Smit AM, Wilkins AJ. Selective cognitive impairment during focal and generalized epileptiform EEG activity. *Brain* 1984; **107**: 293–308.
19. Provinciali L, Signorino M, Censori B, Ceravolo G, Del Pesce, M. Recognition impairment correlated with bisynchronous epileptic discharges. *Epilepsia* 1991; **32**: 684–9.
20. Mirsky AF, Duncan CC, Levav LM. Neuropsychological and psychophysiological aspects of absence epilepsy. In Duncan JS, Panayiotopoulos CP (editors). *Typical Absences and Related Epileptic Syndromes.* London: Churchill Communications Europe; 1995: pp. 112–21.
21. Flink R, Pedersen B, Guekht AB *et al.* Guidelines for the use of EEG methodology in the diagnosis of epilepsy. International League Against Epilepsy: commission report. Commission on European Affairs: Subcommission on European Guidelines. *Acta Neurol.Scand.* 2002; **106**: 1–7.
22. Peraita-Adrados R, Gutierrez-Solana L, Ruiz-Falco ML, Garcia-Penas JJ. Nap polygraphic recordings after partial sleep deprivation in patients with suspected epileptic seizures. *Neurophysiol Clin* 2001; **31**: 34–9.
23. Panayiotopoulos CP. *Panayiotopoulos Syndrome: A Common and Benign Childhood Epileptic Syndrome.* London: John Libbey & Company; 2002.
24. Panayiotopoulos CP, Agathonikou A, Sharoqi IA, Parker AP. Vigabatrin aggravates absences and absence status. *Neurology* 1997; **49**: 1467.
25. Panayiotopoulos CP. Efficacy of lamotrigine monotherapy. *Epilepsia* 2000; **41**: 357–9.
26. American Electroencephalographic Society. Guideline fourteen: guidelines for recording clinical EEG on digital media. *J Clin Neurophysiol* 1994; **11**: 114–15.
27. Levy SR, Berg AT, Testa FM, Novotny EJ, Chiappa KH. Comparison of digital and conventional EEG interpretation. *J Clin Neurophysiol* 1998; **15**: 476–80.
28. Blum DE. Computer-based electroencephalography: technical basics, basis for new applications, and potential pitfalls. *Electroencephalogr Clin Neurophysiol* 1998; **106**: 118–26.
29. Nuwer MR, Comi G, Emerson R *et al.* IFCN standards for digital recording of clinical EEG. The International Federation of Clinical Neurophysiology. *Electroencephalogr.Clin Neurophysiol Suppl* 1999; **52**: 11–14.
30. Scherg M, Ille N, Bornfleth H, Berg P. Advanced tools for digital EEG review: virtual source montages, whole-head mapping, correlation, and phase analysis. *J Clin Neurophysiol* 2002; **19**: 91–112.
31. Ferrie CD, Agathonikou A, Panayiotopoulos CP. Electroencephalography and video–electroencephalography in the classification of childhood epilepsy syndromes. *J R Soc Med* 1998; **91**: 251–9.
32. Ferrie CD, Giannakodimos S, Robinson RO, Panayiotopoulos CP. Symptomatic typical absence seizures. In Duncan JS, Panayiotopoulos CP (editors). *Typical Absences and Related Epileptic Syndromes.* London: Churchill Communications Europe; 1995: pp. 241–52.
33. Raymond AA, Fish DR, Stevens JM, Sisodiya SM, Alsanjari N, Shorvon SD. Subependymal heterotopia: a distinct neuronal migration disorder associated with epilepsy. *J Neurol Neurosurg Psychiatry* 1994; **57**: 1195–202.
34. Hirtz D, Ashwal S, Berg A *et al.* Practice parameter: evaluating a first nonfebrile seizure in children: report of the quality standards subcommittee of the American Academy of Neurology, The Child Neurology Society, and The American Epilepsy Society. *Neurology* 2000; **55**: 616–23.
35. King MA, Newton MR, Jackson GD, Berkovic SF. Epileptology of the first-seizure presentation: a clinical, electroencephalographic, and magnetic imaging study of 300 consecutive patients. *Lancet* 1998; **352**: 1007–11.
36. Hauser WA, Rich SS, Annegers JF, Anderson VE. Seizure recurrence after a 1st unprovoked seizure: an extended follow-up. *Neurology* 1990; **40**: 1163–70.
37. Berg AT, Shinnar S. The risk of seizure recurrence following a first unprovoked seizure: a quantitative review. *Neurology* 1991; **41**: 965–72.
38. Hart YM, Sander JW, Johnson AL, Shorvon SD. National General Practice Study of Epilepsy: recurrence after a first seizure [see comments]. *Lancet* 1990; **336**: 1271–4.
39. Shinnar S, Kang H, Berg AT, Goldensohn ES, Hauser WA, Moshe SL. EEG abnormalities in children with a first unprovoked seizure. *Epilepsia* 1994; **35**: 471–6.
40. Shinnar S, Berg AT, Moshe SL *et al.* The risk of seizure recurrence after a first unprovoked afebrile seizure in childhood: an extended follow-up. *Pediatrics* 1996; **98**: 216–25.
41. Hopkins A, Garman A, Clarke C. The first seizure in adult life. Value of clinical features, electroencephalography, and computerised tomographic scanning in prediction of seizure recurrence. *Lancet* 1988; **1**: 721–6.
42. Hoekelman RA. A pediatrician's view. The first seizure – a terrifying event [editorial]. *Pediatr Ann* 1991; **20**: 9–10.

3 BRAIN IMAGING IN THE DIAGNOSIS AND MANAGEMENT OF EPILEPSIES

Current optimal magnetic resonance imaging (MRI) scanning allows *in vivo* visualisation of structural causes of epilepsies such as hippocampal sclerosis and malformations of cortical development. The sensitivity for detecting subtle abnormalities is increasing with improvements in scanner hardware, acquisition sequences and post-acquisition processing. Relevant abnormalities are identified in 80% of patients with refractory focal seizures and in approximately 20% of patients with single unprovoked seizures or epilepsy in remission.

Modern structural and functional brain imaging methodologies have made a colossal impact in the diagnosis and management of epilepsies.[1-24] High levels of anatomical and metabolic data are now provided by different brain imaging techniques.

MRI is much superior to X-ray computed tomography (CT) in terms of its sensitivity and specificity for identifying lesional epilepsies, which commonly include hippocampal sclerosis and malformations of cortical development. Identification of a structural lesion is often but not always a reliable indicator of the site of seizure onset. MRI can offer the prediction of surgical outcome and may hold promise in the future for dimensional localisation of seizure focus.

Functional neuroimaging has been used for localising cerebral dysfunction, predominantly through disturbances in an individual's metabolism or blood flow. The techniques available include single photon emission computed tomography (SPECT), positron emission tomography (PET) and functional MRI (fMRI). In clinical practice and principally in the evaluation of possible neurosurgical treatment, functional brain imaging is currently supplementary to MRI.

Combining appropriate new imaging techniques has led to greater insights into the pathophysiology underlying symptomatic epilepsy and can contribute greatly to elucidating the basic mechanisms of the various forms of epileptic disorders. Investigations of larger, more homogenous genetic disorders and longitudinal rather than cross-sectional neuroimaging studies have advanced our knowledge about the cause and effect of epileptic disorders.[1]

This chapter is based on the recommendations of the International League Against Epilepsy (ILAE) for the neuroimaging of persons with epilepsy in general,[2] the neuroimaging of persons with intractable seizures in their pre-surgical evaluation[3] and, more recently, for functional neuroimaging.[4]

The current status of the neuroimaging of epilepsy has recently been reviewed by Professor John S. Duncan [15,25] who also edited this Chapter.

RECOMMENDATIONS FOR NEUROIMAGING OF PATIENTS WITH EPILEPSY

AIMS AND RATIONALE OF NEUROIMAGING

- To identify underlying pathologies such as tumours, granulomas, vascular malformations, traumatic lesions or strokes that merit specific treatment.
- To aid the formulation of syndromic and aetiological diagnoses and thereby provide an accurate prognosis for patients, their relatives and physicians.

TECHNIQUES

Scans must be interpreted in the context of the entire clinical situation. A specialist in neuroimaging, who has training and expertise in the neuroimaging of epilepsy, must review the images.

Magnetic resonance imaging is the structural imaging tool of choice.[2,3] It is superior to radiographic CT in terms of both sensitivity and specificity for the identification of small lesions and abnormalities of the cerebral cortex. Even when a CT scan reveals an epileptogenic lesion, MRI often adds new and important data in terms of characterising the nature and extent of the underlying pathology and identifying other lesions.

The principle role of MRI is in the definition of the structural abnormalities that underlie seizure disorders. Hippocampal sclerosis may be reliably identified (Figure 3.1), while quantitative studies are useful for research and, in equivocal cases, for clinical purposes. A range of malformations of cortical development may be determined (Figures 3.2–3.4). The proportion of cryptogenic cases of epilepsy has decreased with improvements in MRI hardware, signal acquisition techniques and post-processing methodologies (Figure 3.5).

Both T1-weighted and T2-weighted images should be obtained, with slices as thin as possible. Three-dimensional volume acquisition is preferable, but coronal as well as axial slices should be obtained in all cases. Gadolinium contrast enhancement is not necessary in routine cases, but may be helpful in selected cases if the non-contrast-enhanced MRI scan is not definitive. Myelination is incomplete in the first 2 years of life, thereby resulting in a poor contrast between white and grey matter and, thus, producing difficulties in detecting cortical abnormalities. In contrast, white matter disorders are recognised better, since the normal signal of myelin (which varies according to age) and the topography of the brain are well known. In such young patients, MRI scans may not reveal lesions and scans may have to be repeated again after 1–2 years.[2]

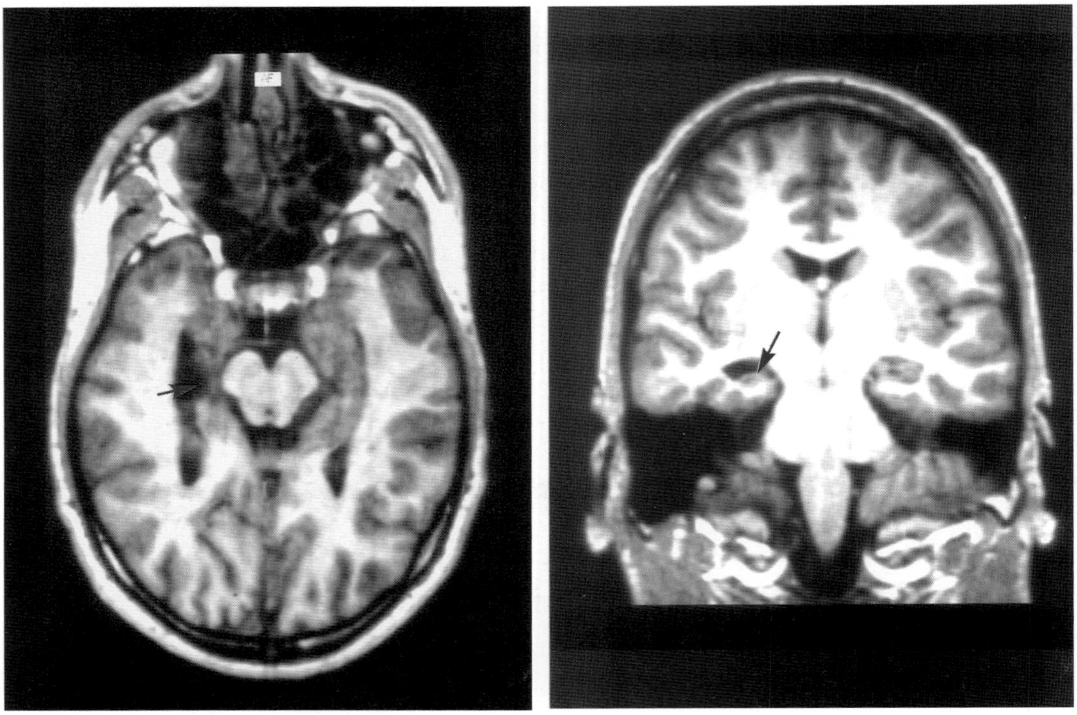

Figure 3.1 Coronal and axial T1-weighted MRI scan showing right hippocampal sclerosis (arrow).

Figure courtesy of Dr Rod C. Scott, Institute of Child Health, London.

However, it should be emphasised that certain lesions such as focal cortical dysplasia are not always identified with conventional MRI and may be more easily identified on a fluid-attenuated inversion recovery (FLAIR) sequence by reconstructing the imaging data set in curvilinear planes and by quantitative assessment of the signal and texture.[15,25]

A fluid-attenuated inversion recovery sequence increases the conspicuity of lesions (Figure 3.6) that may not otherwise be identified and this sequence should be part of a standard MRI protocol for patients with epilepsy. Other sequences, such as T2, may reveal abnormalities such as small cavernous angiomas.

In addition to careful qualitative evaluation of the hippocampus, quantitative assessment can be useful. Hippocampal volumetry requires absolute volumes corrected for the intracranial volume, which must be compared with appropriate controls from the same laboratory, as well as side-to-side ratios. T2 relaxometry also quantitates hippocampal abnormalities and may show evidence of bilateral disease.[2]

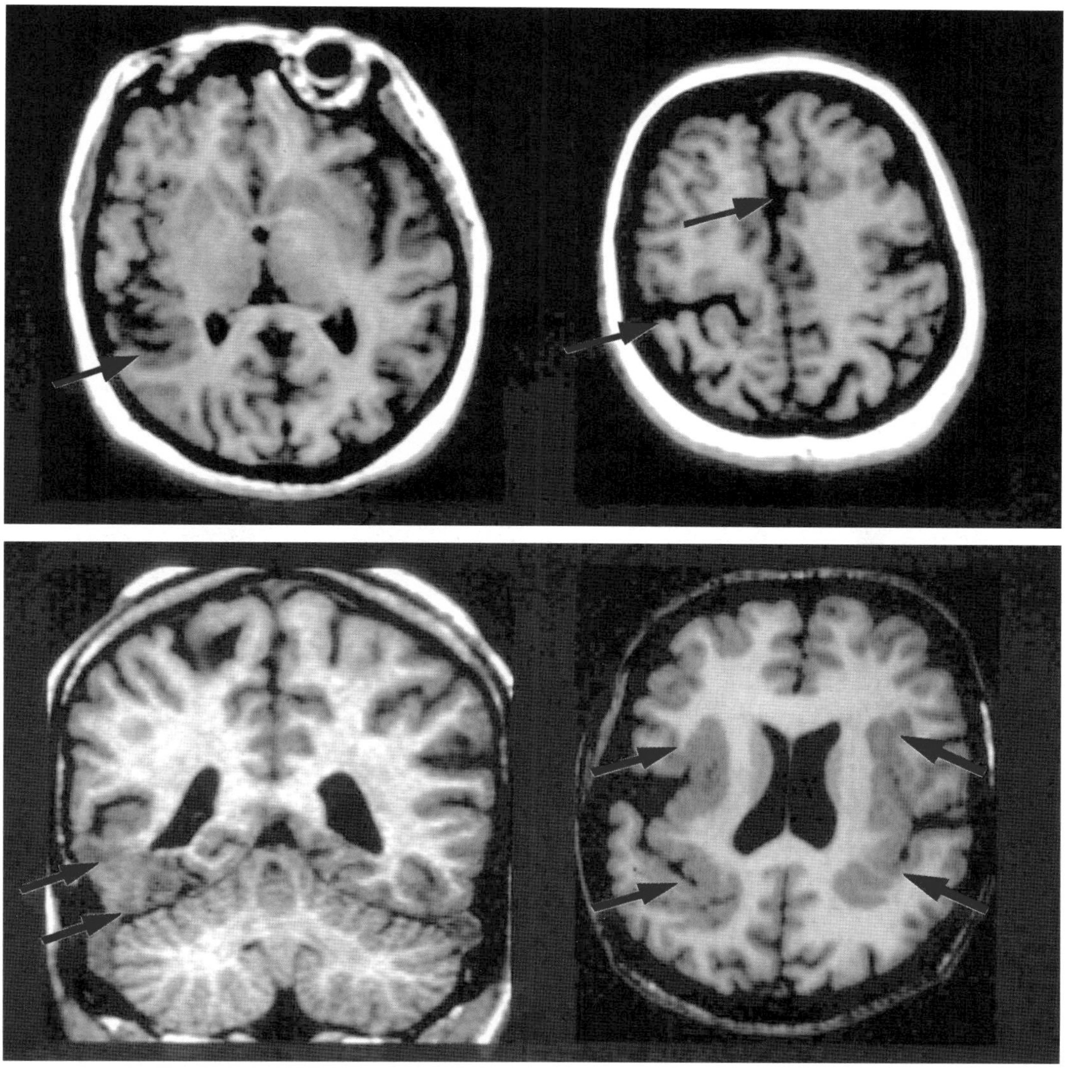

Figure 3.2 Examples of malformations of cortical development documented with MRI

Top: Axial T1-weighted MRI scan showing bilateral schizencephaly (arrows).
Bottom left: Coronal T1-weighted MRI scan showing right focal cortical dysplasia (arrows).
Bottom right: Axial T1-weighted MRI scan showing bilateral perisylvian polymicrogyria (arrows).

Figure courtesy of Professor John S. Duncan and the National Society for Epilepsy MRI Unit.

Suboptimal MRI application in clinical practice

Current knowledge is still not being optimally applied in clinical practice.[26] For example, a recent study in Germany showed that, in patients with focal seizures who had unremarkable MRI scans at general hospitals, a focal lesion was found in 85% of cases when they later underwent MRI at a specialised centre.[27]

X-ray CT scanning can detect gross structural lesions, but will miss many small mass lesions including tumours, vascular malformations, hippocampal sclerosis and most malformations of cortical development.[2] A negative CT scan conveys little information. For this reason CT should not be relied on and usually does not need to be performed when MRI is available. Occasionally CT may be useful as a complementary imaging technique in the detection of cortical calcifications,

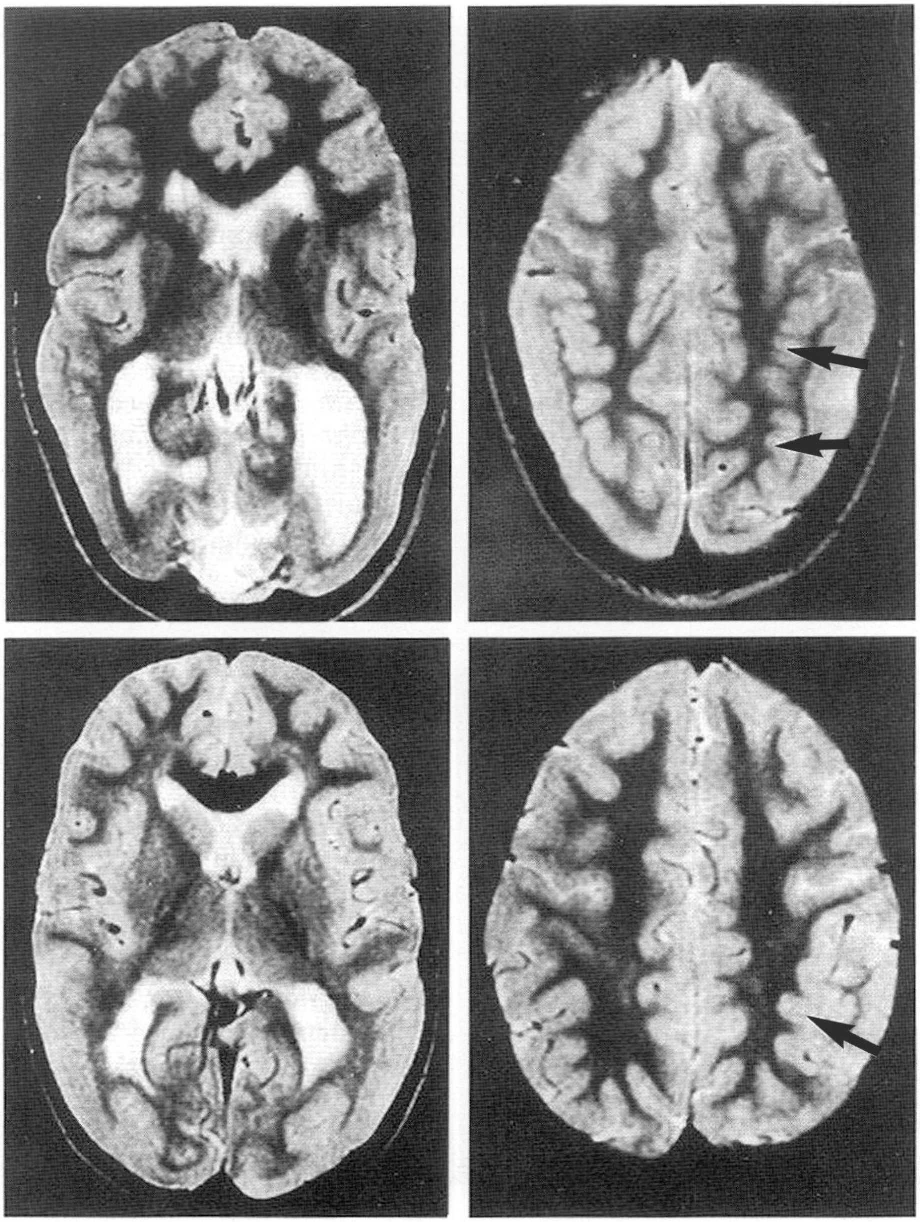

Figure 3.3 Posterior agyria–pachygyria with polymicrogyria documented with MRI scan in two brothers.[28]

Axial T2-weighted MRI scans from the older (top) and younger (bottom) brothers. There is marked posterior agyria–pachygyria with areas of polymicrogyria mainly in the parietal cortex.

From Ferrie et al. (1995)[28] with the permission of the editor of *Neurology*.

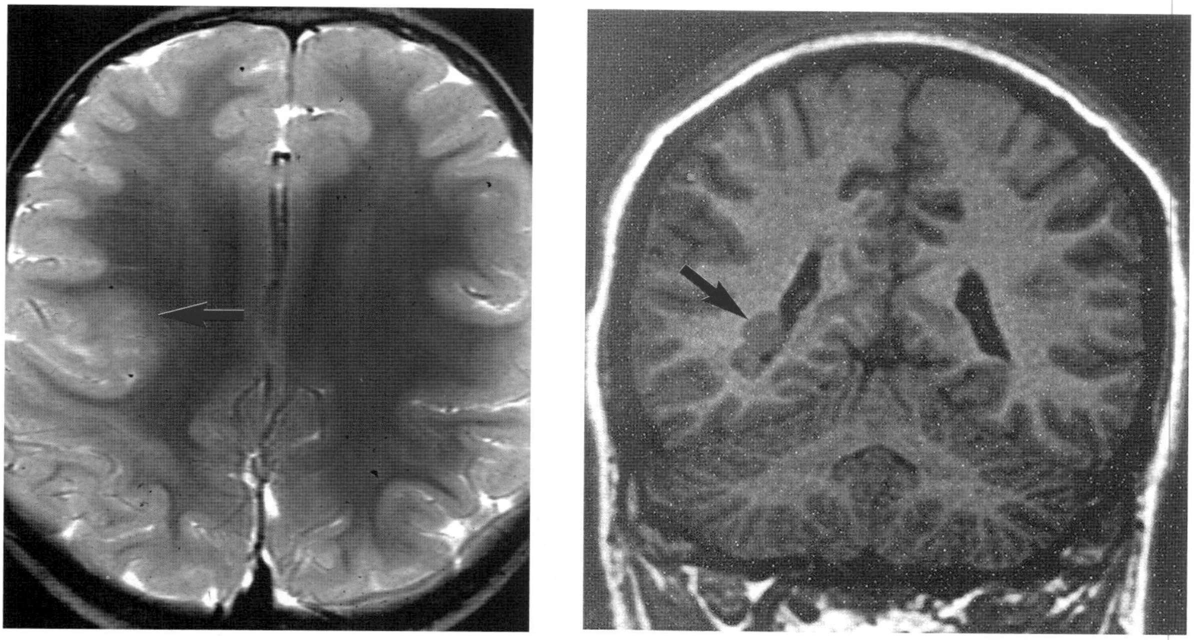

Figure 3.4 Small malformations of cortical development documented with MRI.

Left: coronal T2-weighted MRI scan showing frontal focal cortical dysplasia (arrow).

Figure courtesy of Dr Rod C. Scott, Institute of Child Health, London.

Right: coronal T1-weighted MRI showing nodular subependymal heterotopia in the inferior lateral wall of the right lateral ventricle (arrow).

From Duncan (1997)[5] with the permission of the author and the Editor of the *Brain.*

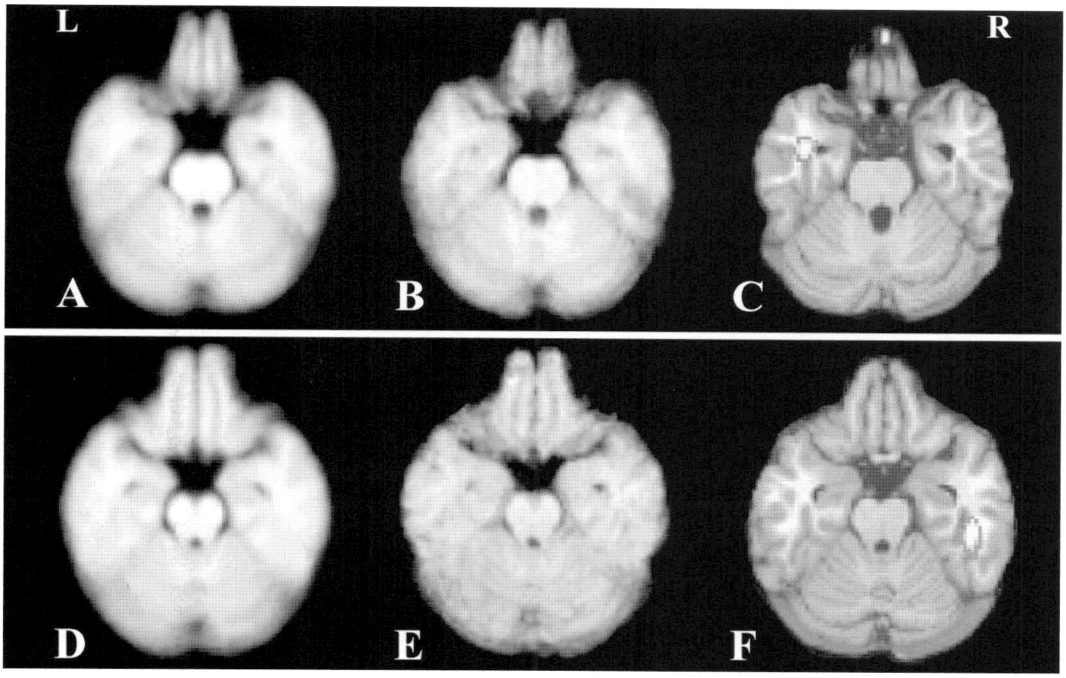

Figure 3.5 Magnetisation transfer ratio maps.

Axial images. Magnetisation transfer ratio maps for 30 control subjects (A and D) and patients with normal conventional MRI and left temporal lobe epilepsy (B) and right temporal lobe epilepsy (E). Statistical analysis showing areas of a significantly reduced magnetisation transfer ratio in patient groups (C) and (F).

Figure courtesy of Professor John S. Duncan and the National Society for Epilepsy MRI Unit.

particularly in patients with congenital or acquired infections (e.g. cysticercosis) or tumours such as oligodendrogliomas.[2]

If MRI is not readily available or cannot be performed for technical reasons (e.g. a patient who has a cardiac pacemaker or a cochlear implant) then an X-ray CT scan is an appropriate initial investigation.

An X-ray CT scan is also useful in the acute situation of seizures developing in the context of a neurological insult such as head injury, intracranial haemorrhage or encephalitis, particularly if there is a need to have ready access to the patient during scanning.[2]

Conventional isotope brain scans do not provide sufficient information about the brain structure for identifying many lesions associated with seizures and their use is not recommended.[2]

Single photon emission computed tomography and positron emission tomography are also inadequate for assessment of the brain structure.[2]

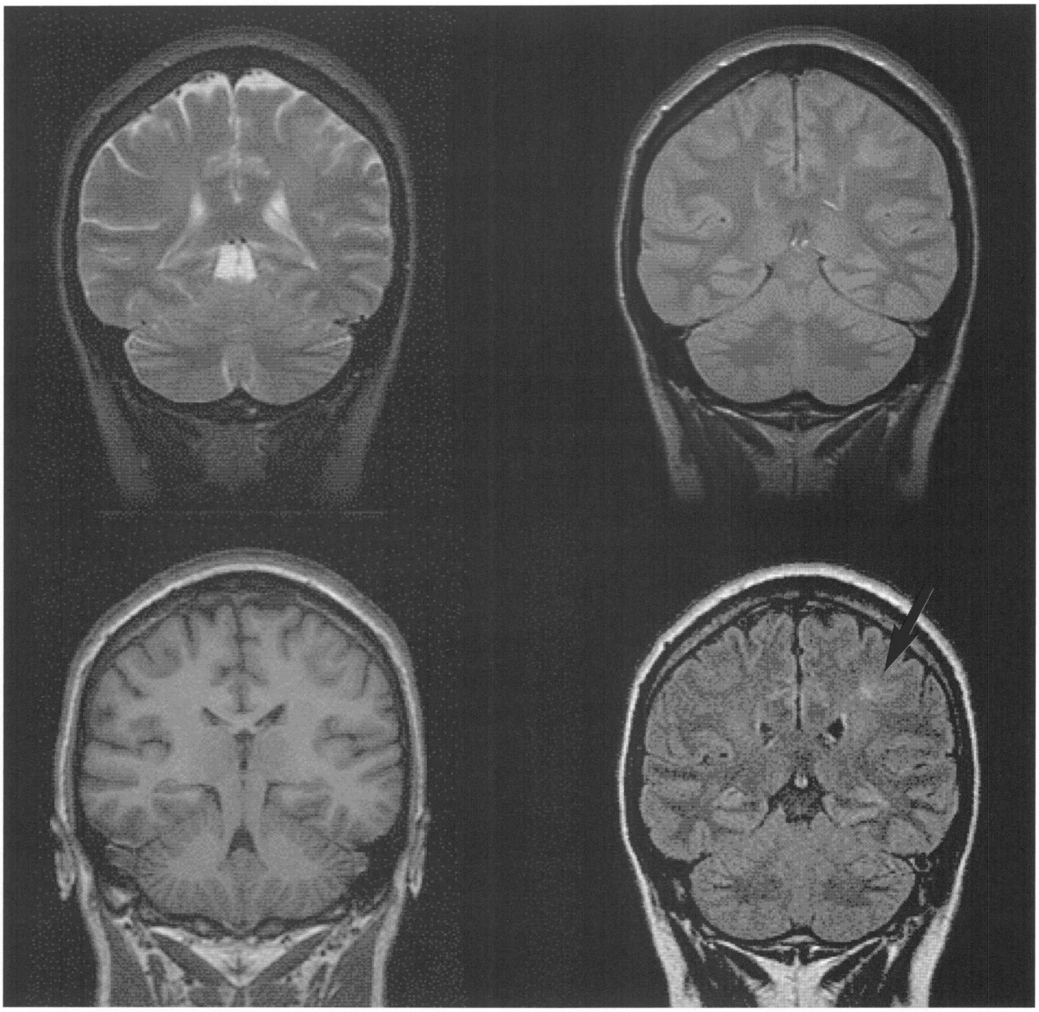

Figure 3.6 Series of coronal MRI scans showing increased lesion conspicuity with FLAIR.

The patient's left is on the right of the images. The patient is a 50-year-old man with a 25-year history of focal motor seizures involving the right hand. The T1-weighted (bottom left), T2-weighted (top left), and proton density (top right) images were read as normal. On the FLAIR scan (bottom right) it is evident that there is an area of increased signal in the brain parenchyma in the left primary sensorimotor cortex (arrow).

Figure courtesy of Professor John S. Duncan and the National Society for Epilepsy MRI Unit.

BRAIN IMAGING IN THE NON-ACUTE SITUATION

IDEAL PRACTICE

In the non-acute situation the ideal practice is to obtain structural neuroimaging with MRI in all patients with epilepsy, except in patients with a definite electroclinical diagnosis of idiopathic generalised epilepsy or benign focal epilepsy of childhood.[2]

MRI is particularly indicated in patients with one or more of the following.

- Onset of seizures at any age with evidence of focal onset in history or EEG.
- Onset of unclassified or apparently generalised seizures in the first year of life or in adulthood.
- Evidence of a focal fixed deficit on neurological or neuropsychological examination.
- Difficulty in obtaining control of seizures with first-line anti-epileptic drug treatment.
- Loss of control of seizures with anti-epileptic drugs or a change in the seizure pattern that may imply a progressive underlying lesion.

MINIMUM STANDARDS

Appropriate minimum standards vary between different countries and societies, according to economic and geographical factors and the system for providing health care.[2]

- Radiographic CT scanning is an alternative procedure if MRI is not available or cannot be performed for technical reasons.
- An MRI scan is essential in the patient with: (a). focal or secondarily generalised seizures and apparently generalised seizures that do not remit with anti-epileptic drug treatment and (b). the development of progressive neurological or neuropsychological deficits.

FUNCTIONAL NEUROIMAGING IN CLINICAL PRACTICE[4]

The Neuroimaging Subcommission of the ILAE has reassessed the roles of the traditional functional imaging techniques of PET and SPECT in clinical practice and research.[4] The place of these methods and of the emerging magnetic resonance-based functional imaging methods of fMRI and magnetic resonance spectroscopy (MRS) also need to be considered in the light of the advances in structural imaging with MRI.

The Neuroimaging Subcommission of the ILAE[4] considered fMRI, MRS, SPECT and PET in turn, according to the following format.

- Indications in clinical practice and research potential.
- Relation to structural imaging.
- Minimum and optimal standards if the investigation is to be carried out, with regard to equipment, clinical protocol and logistics, and reporting and interpretation.
- Misuse and pitfalls.

The conclusions regarding clinical applications of functional neuroimaging are as follows.[4]

Functional magnetic resonance imaging. There is no currently approved or universally accepted clinical indication for fMRI.[4] However, this situation is changing and in many epilepsy surgery centres fMRI is being used for localising the primary motor cortex and lateralising language function (Figure 3.7). Furthermore, continuous recording of an EEG and fMRI is now possible following the introduction of methods for removing the artefact on the EEG trace caused by the fMRI acquisition, resulting in much more detail and analysis of the time course of haemodynamic changes.[29-32] Clinically, these methods will aid EEG interpretation and understanding of the pathophysiological basis of epileptic activity.[15,30]

Magnetic resonance spectroscopy. MRS has been evaluated primarily in temporal lobe epilepsy. Proton MRS provides a useful lateralisation of metabolic

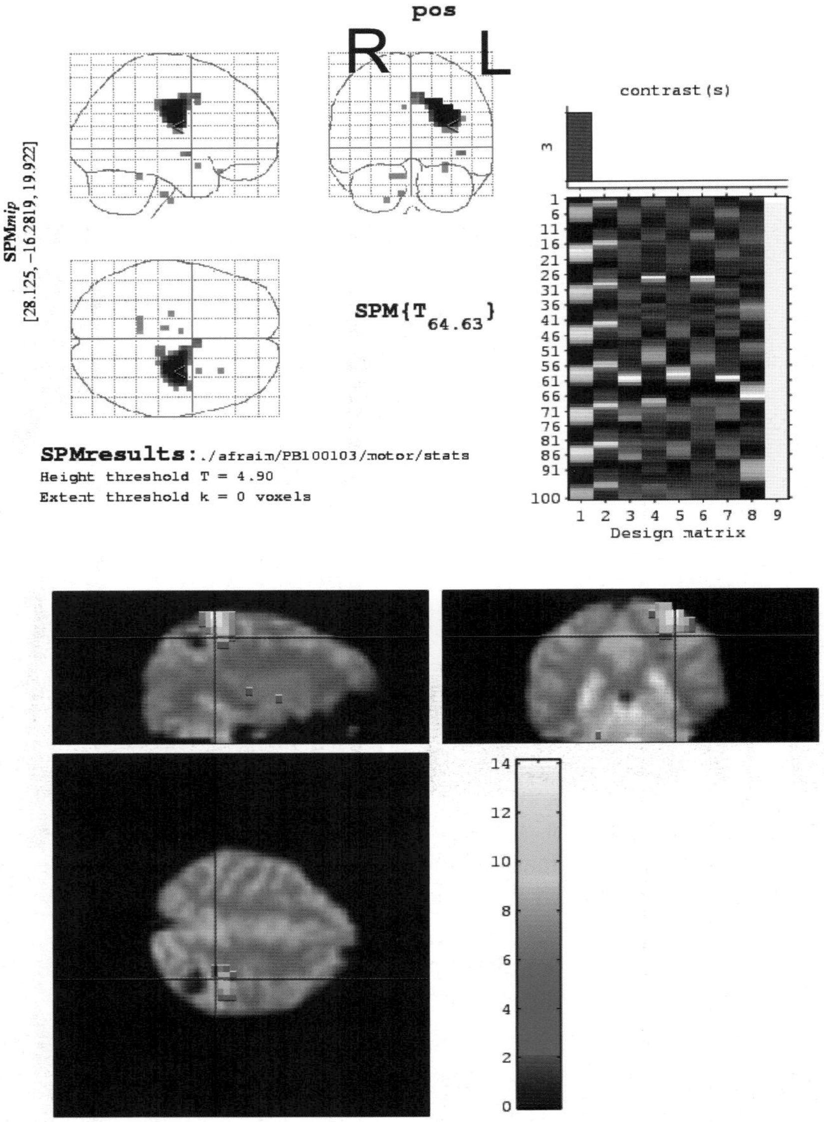

Figure 3.7 fMRI scan showing an area of cerebral activation in relation to right-hand movement that is anterior to structural lesion (dysembryoplastic neuroepithelial tumour).

Figure courtesy of Professor John S. Duncan and the National Society for Epilepsy MRI Unit.

dysfunction. Sensitivity is in the order of 90%, but bilateral temporal abnormalities are common and abnormalities may be reversible. MRS may be useful in patients who have otherwise normal MRI studies. Phosphate (^{35}P) MRS has moderate sensitivity for lateralisation based on abnormal elevations of inorganic phosphate. Abnormalities of pH have been controversial and so cannot be considered to be reliable for lateralisation. MRS has been reported to be useful in extratemporal epilepsies, but the present limitation of spatial coverage limits its clinical utility.[4] It is evident from studies of malformation of cortical development that metabolic derangements are frequently more extensive than the structural lesion seen on MRI.[33]

Single photon emission computed tomography. SPECT with cerebral blood flow agents is useful for supporting the localisation of focal epilepsy when it is performed in a carefully monitored ictal (Figure 3.8) or early post-ictal examination compared with an inter-ictal scan. This may be used as part of pre-surgical evaluation and help to guide the placement of intracranial electrodes if other data including structural imaging are equivocal or non-concordant. In apparently generalised epilepsies, ictal SPECT may be helpful for identifying a focal component.[4] Recent developments allow patients to inject the isotope themselves at the first warning of a seizure, thus increasing the possibility of

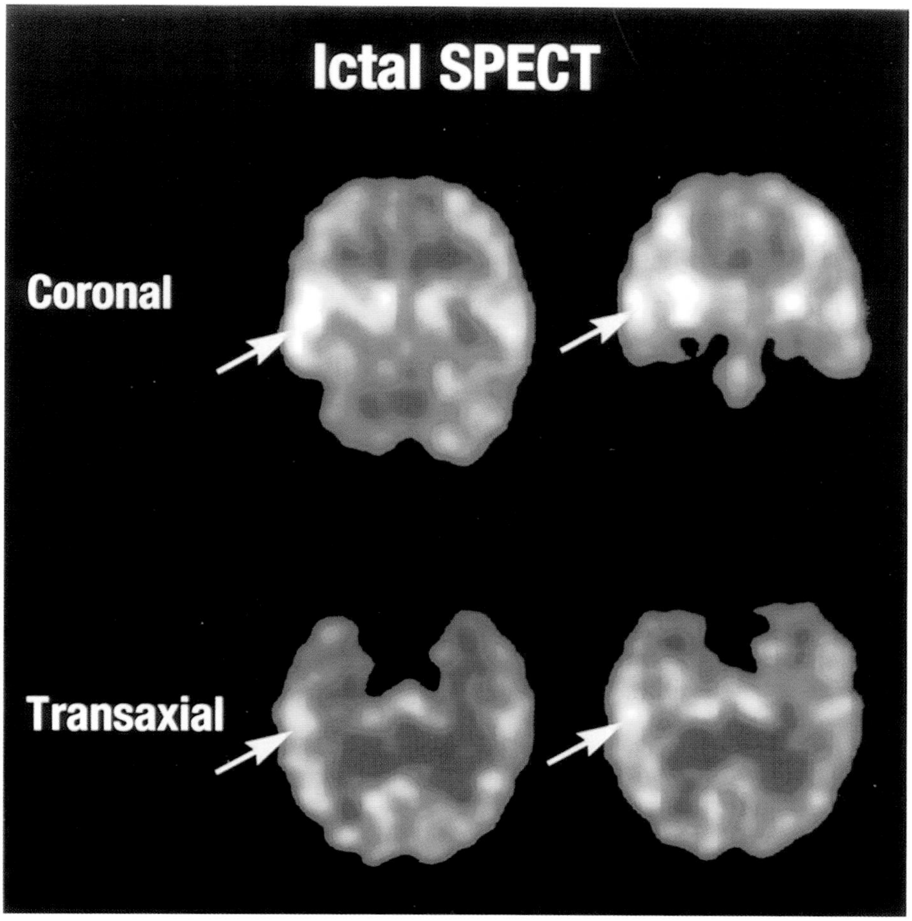

Figure 3.8 Ictal SPECT in a child with right hippocampal epilepsy.

Coronal (top) and axial (bottom) ^{99}Tc HMPAO SPECT images show increased perfusion in the right anterior temporal lobe (arrows).

Figure courtesy of Dr Rod C. Scott, Institute of Child Health, London capturing a seizure as well as reducing the interval between seizure onset and trapping of the tracer in the brain.[34]

Positron emission tomography with ^{18}F fluorodeoxyglucose (FDG) and ^{15}O water ($H_2{}^{15}O$). Inter-ictal FDG-PET may have a role in determining the lateralisation of temporal lobe epilepsy, without intracranial EEG recording of seizures, in patients in whom there is not good concordance between MRI, an EEG and other data (Figure 3.9). This role has decreased with the wider availability of high-quality MRI. In patients with normal or equivocal MRI or discordance between MRI and other data, such that intracranial electrodes are required, FDG-PET may be useful for planning the sites of intracranial electrode placement for recording ictal onsets in temporal and extratemporal epilepsies. However, caution is needed as the ictal onset zone may be at the border of the hypometabolic area and not at the most hypometabolic area. FDG-PET may have a useful role in apparently generalised epilepsies in trying to define a focal abnormality and when resection may be contemplated. For practical purposes, the clinical and research uses of $H_2{}^{15}O$ PET for mapping areas of cerebral activation have been superseded by fMRI.[4]

Positron emission tomography with specific ligands. There are no proven indications for ligand PET in clinical epileptological practice. A role that is being evaluated is in the pre-surgical evaluation of patients with refractory focal seizures. In patients with mesial temporal lobe epilepsy and negative MRI, ^{11}C flumazenil (FMZ) PET may have some advantages over FDG, offering more precise localisation of the epileptogenic region, but it does not appear to be superior for lateralisation. In MRI-negative patients with neocortical seizures, the identification of focal abnormalities using FMZ-PET may be useful for guiding

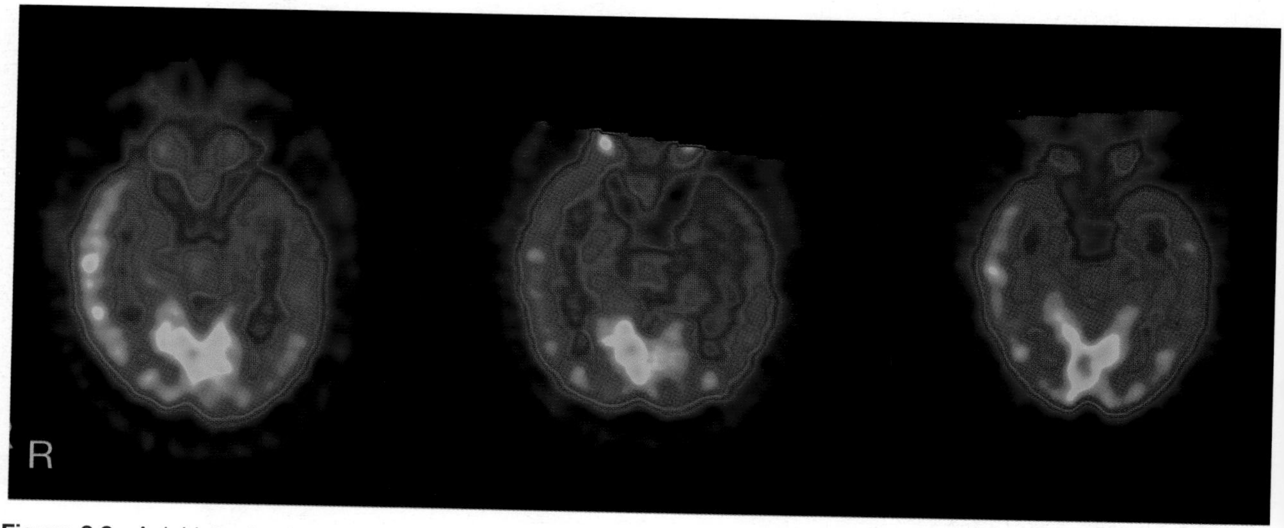

Figure 3.9 Axial inter-ictal FDG-PET images in three patients with left mesial temporal screlosis: all had a left anterior temporal lobectomy and became free of seizures.

Left: Unilateral glucose hypometabolism in a 22-year-old male. FDG uptake is reduced in mesial temporal lobe structures and the tip and anterior portion of the temporal neocortex in the left hemisphere.
Middle: bilateral asymmetrical glucose hypometabolism in a 19-year-old male. Reduction of FDG uptake is observed in both temporal areas, being more remarkable in the left hemisphere.
Right: equivocal symmetrical glucose metabolism in a 34-year-old female. There was no laterality in FDG uptake. Semi-quantitative analysis with regions of interest methods showed that the asymmetry indices of the mesial and lateral temporal areas were within normal range.

Figure courtesy of Dr Nozomi Akanuma, Department of Clinical Neurosciences, Guy's, King's and St Thomas' School of Medicine.

the placement of intracranial EEG electrodes.[4] However, caution is needed as the ictal onset zone may be at the border of the area of abnormal binding and not at the area of maximal abnormality. Co-registration with high-quality MRI is essential (Figure 9.10).

Co-registration of SPECT/PET with MRI. The co-registration of post-ictal SPECT images with a patient's MRI improves the anatomical determination of abnormalities of the cerebral blood flow.[35] The objectivity and accuracy of data interpretation is enhanced with co-registration of inter-ictal with ictal or post-ictal SPECT images, resulting in an 'ictal difference image' that may be co-registered with the individual's MRI. The co-registration of PET images with high-resolution MRI structural images from the same individual has practical value in the anatomical interpretation of functional abnormalities in PET with account been taken for potential partial volume artefacts. Together with an MRI image, PET images with different tracers, for example FDG and FMZ, can be co-registered, which enables a direct comparison of the location, pattern and extent of each abnormality (Figure 3.10).

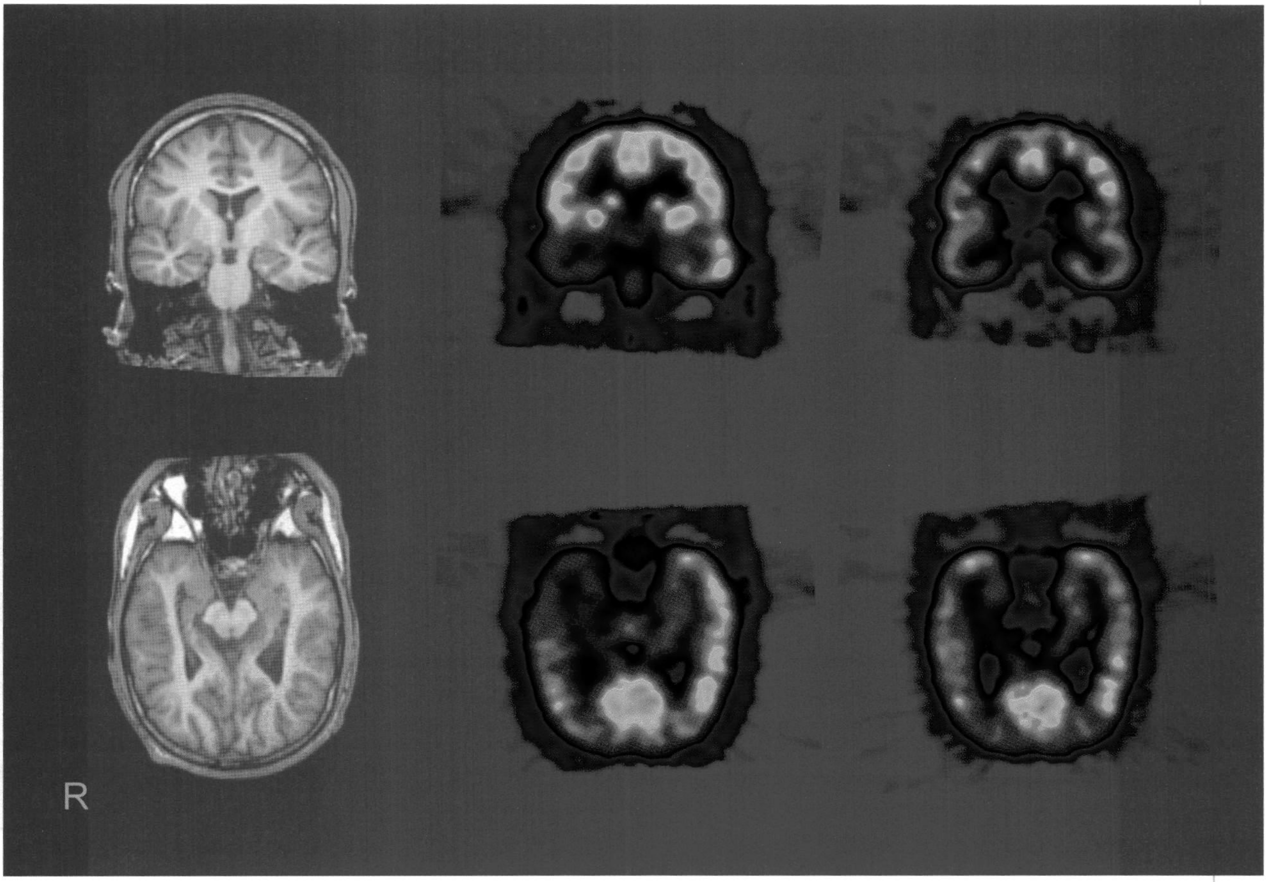

Figure 3.10 Coronal (upper rows) and axial (lower rows) views of structural and functional neuroimages of a 21-year-old male with right mesial temporal sclerosis. A right anterior temporal lobectomy rendered him free of seizures.

FDG-PET (middle) and FMZ-PET (right) images were co-registered with a T1-weighted MRI scan (left). The T1-weighted MRI scan demonstrates hippocampal atrophy on the right. FDG uptake is reduced in the corresponding region extending to the ipsilateral lateral temporal cortex and parietal area. In contrast, the reduction in gamma-aminobutyric acid ($GABA_A$) receptor binding is fairly restricted within the right mesial temporal lobe structures.

Figure courtesy of Dr Nozomi Akanuma, Department of Clinical Neurosciences, Guy's, King's and St Thomas' School of Medicine.

MAGNETOENCEPHALOGRAPHY

Magnetoencephalography (MEG) is a promising but still in development non-invasive and non-hazardous technology of functional brain mapping.[36-45] It is used to identify both normal and abnormal brain function "in action". MEG records externally from the scalp the weak magnetic forces associated with the electrical activity of the brain. It provides good spatial resolution of 2 mm and an excellent high temporal resolution on the order of 1 ms.

The primary advantage of MEG over EEG is that the magnetic fields are not altered by the skull and other surrounding brain structures, thus permitting greater accuracy owing to the minimal distortion of the signal. This allows for more usable and reliable localisation of brain function though MEG is better at detecting more superficially than deep mesial temporal lobe epileptogenic foci.

MEG is usually performed with simultaneous EEG recording. Superimposing MEG with X-ray CT and MRI scans produces functional/anatomic images of the brain, referred to as magnetic source imaging (MSI).

The most thoroughly studied clinical applications of MEG/MSI are to detect and localise (a) epileptogenic foci and (b) eloquent cortex.

The exact localisation of the epileptogenic area is crucial for screening of surgical candidates and surgical planning. MSI has principally been investigated as an alternative to invasive pre-surgical monitoring when clinical, EEG and MRI findings are not concordant. Additionally, in patients who have had past brain surgery, the electrical field measured by EEG may be distorted by the changes in the scalp and brain anatomy. If further surgery is needed, MEG may be able to provide the necessary information without invasive EEG studies.

Localisation of the "eloquent" brain areas such as sensorimotor regions is critical for their preservation during any type of brain surgery. MEG/MSI are used to map the exact location of the normally functioning areas near the lesion that should be avoided in planning surgical resection thus minimising postoperative significant neurological deficits. Such use might also obviate the need for other forms of invasive mapping techniques.

There is no currently approved or universally accepted clinical application for MEG and MSI on epilepsies

In a recent technological report (2003) MEG and MSI have been assessed on whether they provide additional diagnostic information that improves the management and outcomes of patients who are being evaluated for neurosurgical treatment in two main clinical uses:

- MEG/MSI would be used to characterise the location of the epileptic zone for resection in the hopes of either identifying additional surgical candidates or avoiding the need for invasive confirmatory testing.
- MEG/MSI would be used to identify the locations of important functional anatomical regions of the brain that should be avoided in planning surgical resection of the lesion. Such use might obviate the need for other forms of invasive mapping techniques.

No other uses of MEG/MSI were considered in this assessment.

Based on the available evidence, the Blue Cross and Blue Shield Association Medical Advisory Panel made the judgment that currently MEG/MSI for presurgical localisation of seizure foci or presurgical functional mapping does not meet the technological criteria of this Association.

Further, MEG and MSI are of high cost and low availability. Currently, there are no more than 100 centres around the world using these techniques.

REFERENCES

1. Koepp MJ,.Duncan JS. Epilepsy. *Curr Opin Neurol* 2004;**17**:467-74.
2. Recommendations for neuroimaging of patients with epilepsy. Commission on Neuroimaging of the International League Against Epilepsy. *Epilepsia* 1997;**38**:1255-6.
3. Guidelines for neuroimaging evaluation of patients with uncontrolled epilepsy considered for surgery. Commission on Neuroimaging of the International League Against Epilepsy. *Epilepsia* 1998;**39**:1375-6.
4. Commission on Diagnostic Strategies: recommendations for functional neuroimaging of persons with epilepsy. *Epilepsia* 2000;**41**:1350-6.
5. Duncan JS. Imaging and epilepsy. *Brain* 1997;**120 (Pt 2)**:339-77.
6. Jackson GD,.Connelly A. New NMR measurements in epilepsy. T2 relaxometry and magnetic resonance spectroscopy. *Adv Neurol* 1999;**79**:931-7.
7. Chiron C,.Hertz-Pannier L. [Cerebral imaging in childhood epilepsy: what's new?]. *Epil Disord.* 2001;**3 Spec No 2**:SI25-SI36.
8. Kuzniecky RI. Neuroimaging in pediatric epileptology. In Pellock JM, Dodson WE, Bourgeois BFD, eds. *Pediatric epilepsy*, pp 133-43. New York: Demos, 2001.
9. Ruggieri PM,.Najm IM. MR imaging in epilepsy. *Neurol Clin.* 2001;**19**:477-89.
10. Wright NB. Imaging in epilepsy: a paediatric perspective. *Br J Radiol.* 2001;**74**:575-89.
11. Briellmann RS, Kalnins R, Berkovic S, Jackson GD. Hippocampal pathology in refractory temporal lobe epilepsy;T2-weighted signal change reflects dentate gliosis. *Neurology* 2002;**58**:265-71.
12. Chuang NA, Otsubo H, Chuang SH. Magnetic resonance imaging in pediatric epilepsy. *Top Magn Reson Imaging* 2002;**13**:39-60.
13. Meiners LC. Role of MR imaging in epilepsy. *Eur Radiol.* 2002;**12**:499-501.
14. Juhasz C,.Chugani HT. Imaging the epileptic brain with positron emission tomography. *Neuroimaging Clin N Am.* 2003;**13**:705-16, viii.
15. Duncan JS. Neuroimaging of epilepsy. In Sander JW, Walker MC, Smalls JE, eds. *Epilepsy 2003. From synapse to society* pp 203-26. Oxford: Meritus Communications, 2003. *(http://www.e-epilepsy.org.uk),*
16. Bernal B,.Altman NR. Evidence-based medicine: neuroimaging of seizures. *Neuroimaging Clin N Am.* 2003;**13**:211-24.
17. Colombo N, Citterio A, Galli C, Tassi L, Lo RG, Scialfa G *et al.* Neuroimaging of focal cortical dysplasia: neuropathological correlations. *Epil Disord.* 2003;**5 Suppl 2**:S67-S72.
18. Duncan J. The current status of neuroimaging for epilepsy: editorial review. *Curr Opin Neurol* 2003;**16**:163-4.
19. Schauble B,.Cascino GD. Advances in neuroimaging: management of partial epileptic syndromes. *Neurosurg Rev.* 2003;**26**:233-46.
20. Theodore WH. Implications of neuroimaging for the treatment of epilepsy. *Ann Neurol* 2003;**53**:286-8.
21. Wieshmann UC. Clinical application of neuroimaging in epilepsy. *J Neurol Neurosurg Psychiatry* 2003;**74**:466-70.
22. Barkovich AJ,.Raybaud CA. Neuroimaging in disorders of cortical development. *Neuroimaging Clin N Am* 2004;**14**:231-54, viii.
23. Kelley RE, DellaBadia J, Minagar A, Kelley BJ, Brunson R. Neuroimaging of the complications of epilepsy surgery. *J Neuroimaging* 2004;**14**:33-41.
24. Knowlton RC, Lawn ND, Mountz JM, Kuzniecky RI. Ictal SPECT analysis in epilepsy: subtraction and statistical parametric mapping techniques. *Neurology* 2004;**63**:10-5.
25. Duncan JS. Neuroimaging Clinics of North America – Epilepsy. Philadelphia. North America: Elsevier, 2004.
26. Duncan JS. Neuroimaging for epilepsy: quality and not just quantity is important. *J Neurol Neurosurg Psychiatry* 2002;**73**:612-3.
27. Von Oertzen J, Urbach H, Jungbluth S, Kurthen M, Reuber M, Fernandez G *et al.* Standard magnetic resonance imaging is inadequate for patients with refractory focal epilepsy. *J Neurol Neurosurg Psychiatry* 2002;**73**:643-7.
28. Ferrie CD, Jackson GD, Giannakodimos S, Panayiotopoulos CP. Posterior agyria-pachygyria with polymicrogyria: evidence for an inherited neuronal migration disorder. *Neurology* 1995;**45**:150-3.
29. Lemieux L, Salek-Haddadi A, Josephs O, Allen P, Toms N, Scott C *et al.* Event-related fMRI with simultaneous and continuous EEG: description of the method and initial case report. *Neuroimage.* 2001;**14**:780-7.
30. Archer JS, Briellmann RS, Syngeniotis A, Abbott DF, Jackson GD. Spike-triggered fMRI in reading epilepsy: involvement of left frontal cortex working memory area. *Neurology* 2003;**60**:415-21.
31. Nersesyan H, Hyder F, Rothman DL, Blumenfeld H. Dynamic fMRI and EEG recordings during spike-wave seizures and generalized tonic-clonic seizures in WAG/Rij rats. *J Cereb Blood Flow Metab* 2004;**24**:589-99.
32. Bagshaw AP, Aghakhani Y, Benar CG, Kobayashi E, Hawco C, Dubeau F *et al.* EEG-fMRI of focal epileptic spikes: analysis with multiple haemodynamic functions and comparison with gadolinium-enhanced MR angiograms. *Hum.Brain Mapp.* 2004;**22**:179-92.
33. Woermann FG, McLean MA, Bartlett PA, Barker GJ, Duncan JS. Quantitative short echo time proton magnetic resonance spectroscopic imaging study of malformations of cortical development causing epilepsy. *Brain* 2001;**124**:427-36.
34. van Paesschen W, Dupont P, Van Heerden B, Vanbilloen H, Mesotten L, Maes A *et al.* Self-injection ictal SPECT during partial seizures. *Neurology* 2000;**54**:1994-7.
35. Hogan RE, Cook MJ, Binns DW, Desmond PM, Kilpatrick CJ, Murrie VL *et al.* Perfusion patterns in postictal 99mTc-HMPAO SPECT after coregistration with MRI in patients with mesial temporal lobe epilepsy. *J Neurol Neurosurg Psychiatr.* 1997;**63**:235-9.
36. Ko DY, Kufta C, Scaffidi D, Sato S. Source localization determined by magnetoencephalography and electroencephalography in temporal lobe epilepsy: comparison with electrocorticography: technical case report. *Neurosurgery* 1998;**42**:414-21.
37. Paetau R, Granstrom ML, Blomstedt G, Jousmaki V, Korkman M, Liukkonen E. Magnetoencephalography in presurgical evaluation of children with the Landau-Kleffner syndrome. *Epilepsia* 1999;**40**:326-35.
38. Baumgartner C, Pataraia E, Lindinger G, Deecke L. Magnetoencephalography in focal epilepsy. *Epilepsia* 2000;**41 Suppl 3**:S39-S47.
39. Otsubo H,.Snead OC, III. Magnetoencephalography and magnetic source imaging in children. *J.Child Neurol.* 2001;**16**:227-35.
40. Assaf BA, Karkar KM, Laxer KD, Garcia PA, Austin EJ, Barbaro NM *et al.* Ictal magnetoencephalography in temporal and extratemporal lobe epilepsy. *Epilepsia* 2003;**44**:1320-7.
41. Lutkenhoner B. Magnetoencephalography and its Achilles' heel. *J Physiol Paris* 2003;**97**:641-58.
42. Tang L, Mantle M, Ferrari P, Schiffbauer H, Rowley HA, Barbaro NM *et al.* Consistency of interictal and ictal onset localization using magnetoencephalography in patients with partial epilepsy. *J Neurosurg.* 2003;**98**:837-45.
43. Parra J, Kalitzin SN, Da Silva FH. Magnetoencephalography: an investigational tool or a routine clinical technique? *Epilepsy Behav.* 2004;**5**:277-85.
44. Pataraia E, Simos PG, Castillo EM, Billingsley RL, Sarkari S, Wheless JW *et al.* Does magnetoencephalography add to scalp video-EEG as a diagnostic tool in epilepsy surgery? *Neurology* 2004;**62**:943-8.
45. Wheless JW, Castillo E, Maggio V, Kim HL, Breier JI, Simos PG *et al.* Magnetoencephalography (MEG) and magnetic source imaging (MSI). *Neurologist.* 2004;**10**:138-53.
46. Blue Cross and Blue Shield Association Technology Evaluation Center (TEC). MEG and MSI: Presurgical Localization of Epileptic Lesions and Presurgical Function Mapping. www.bcbs.com/tec/vol18/18_06.html . 2003.

PRINCIPLES OF THERAPY IN EPILEPSIES

4

The aim of therapy in epilepsies is total seizure freedom without clinically significant adverse effects. This is achievable in more than two-thirds of patients with epileptic seizures. Correct seizure and often syndrome diagnosis is a precondition for the success of therapeutic decisions. A major group of patients, mainly children, encompassed under 'conditions with epileptic seizures that do not require a diagnosis of epilepsy' do not usually need any prophylactic therapy. For others, such as most of the syndromes of idiopathic generalised epilepsy (IGE) or non-surgically suitable symptomatic focal epilepsies, antiepileptic drug (AED) treatment may be lifelong.

Therapeutic treatments are usually with AEDs in continuous prophylactic schemes. These may be brief if the active seizure state is age dependent or long if remission is not expected to happen, which also refers to patients who have been rendered seizure free with AEDs. Certain epileptic seizures and syndromes respond extremely well to appropriate AEDs, but even these patients with otherwise well-responding conditions may get worse and enter into vicious circles if medicated with badly chosen AEDs.

It is well documented that pharmacological treatments are ineffective for approximately 20% of patients with epileptic disorders, who have an unacceptable quality of life because of continuing seizures and adverse reactions to AEDs.

These patients are candidates for non-pharmacological treatments such as the following:

- neurosurgical interventions
- stimulation techniques, mainly vagus nerve stimulation
- a ketogenic diet (described on page 174-175).

PRINCIPLES OF ANTIEPILEPTIC DRUG TREATMENT IN EPILEPSIES

Antiepileptic drug treatment is the mainstay of management of epilepsies. The decision to treat is based on a careful evaluation of the balance between the likelihood of further seizures and the risk of adverse effects of treatment. The laudable goal of AED treatment in epilepsies is to abolish seizures completely (freedom of seizures) with minimal if any drug-related adverse reactions. This is achieved in around 50-70% of patients with a single appropriately selected AED at target therapeutic doses. This seizure-free rate varies significantly with the type of seizure and epileptic syndrome. Polytherapy should be avoided if possible, but it is inevitable in approximately 30–50% of patients who fail to respond to single-drug therapy. Freedom of seizures should not be pursued at any cost and, in particular, at the expense of drug-induced adverse reactions. For some patients a few minor and often harmless seizures (mild myoclonic jerks, simple focal seizures or absences) may be allowed to occur instead of increasing AED numbers and dosages, which may jeopardise the otherwise social and mental well-being of the patient. Identifying drug-induced adverse effects in out-patient clinic visits is often neglected because of time constraints, confounding factors and the multiplicity of potential symptoms. Patients may also be reluctant to report them or they may confuse them with a consequence of their illness.

The drug treatment of epilepsies requires thorough knowledge of the AEDs with regard to mechanisms, pharmacokinetics, doses, indications, drug interactions and acute and chronic adverse effects. These are widely available through books, journal reviews, the prescribing information sheets of the manufacturers and credible Internet sources.

Important note

The "package insert" (USA) and "summary of product characteristics" (European Medicines Evaluation Agency and UK) that accompanies AED products is the most complete single source of information on the drug. These can be obtained through Web search engines. Simply search for:

x (name of the AED) package insert or

x (name of the AED) summary of product characteristics.

Also, these may often be found on the drug manufacturer's website.

The European Medicines Evaluation Agency (EMEA) Web site is particularly important because the information is in all European languages:

http://www.emea.eu.int/humandocs/Humans/EPAR

The *"package insert"* is reprinted in the *Physician's Desk Reference*, which can be found in many libraries. Labelling for Food and Drug Administration (FDA) drugs approved after 1998 may often be found on the FDA approval page at: http://www.fda.gov/cder/approval or http://www.accessdata.fda.gov/scripts/cder/drugsatfda/

Additional information on a drug's adverse effects can be requested through the FDA's Freedom of Information Office: http://www.fda.gov/foi/foia2.htm

It is also fundamental to remember that special groups of patients with epileptic disorders require particular attention and management.[1] Children,[2-8] the elderly,[9-12] women (particularly of childbearing age)[12-23] and people with mental and physical disabilities[12,24] are vulnerable and their treatment is more demanding.

Cost should not be an issue in medicine, but with the majority of the global population in poverty and often in starvation, options are frequently limited to the old AEDs, which are often life-saving agents.

STARTING ANTIEPILEPTIC DRUG TREATMENT

The decision to commence AED treatment needs thorough consideration and should not be a knee-jerk reaction to a crisis about a dramatic convulsive event (not necessarily an epileptic seizure).[25-27] One-quarter of patients on AEDs do not

Definitions of pharmacokinetics and pharmacodynamics

Clinical pharmacokinetics is the study of the time course of a drug and its metabolites in humans. This is a quantitative description of what happens to the drug once it enters the human body. To simplify, pharmacokinetics is the study of the effect of the human body on a drug. The primary parameters are absorption, distribution, metabolism and excretion.

Oral bioavailability is the proportion of a drug taken orally that reaches the systemic circulation. Most AEDs have nearly total bioavailabilty (80%–90%). Some like gabapentin are absorbed in a saturable fashion so that at higher doses their oral bioavailabilty may drop.

Of clinical significance is that different formulations of the same drug may have different bioavailabilties, which explains the loss of efficacy or emerging signs of toxicity when switching from one preparation to another. This is also the case with some controlled-release formulations such as carbamazepine, which has a lower bioavailabilty than the conventional forms.

Half-life of a drug (T1/2) is the length of time for its plasma concentration to decline by half. This determines time to steady state (approximately 5 half-lives) and provides indications of dosing intervals (usually less than one half-life).

Steady state: equilibrium (after initiation of continuous AED treatment) is achieved when the rate of clearance equals the rate of administration that is the amount of drug ingested equals the amount of drug eliminated at the same time.

A drug reaches the steady state when its clearance equals its dosing rate in other words when the rate of drug input equals the rate of drug output.

Protein binding: drugs are either free (unbound) or bound to serum protein. The active agent is usually the free drug. For extensively bound AEDs, clinically important alterations may occur as a result of physiological (pregnancy), pathological (hepatic, renal disease) or concomitant administration of drugs with higher or lower affinity for protein binding. A protein displaced drug (increase of free levels) may cause toxicity without elevation of its total plasma concentrations. Valproate and phenytoin are the main AEDs subjected to clinically important protein binding changes.

Pharmacodynamics refer to the biochemical and physiological effects of drugs and their mechanisms of action. Within clinical pharmacodynamics attempts are made to describe the relationship of both concentration and time to effect.

Pharmacodynamics is the study of the effect of a drug on humans.

suffer from epilepsy. Of those with genuine epileptic seizures, these are newly identified ictal manifestations, usually convulsions, of an epileptic syndrome which has been previously undiagnosed or dismissed (either by the patient or the physician) or which may just have started. The aim of AED medication should be truly to *treat* and not just to medicate those in need of AEDs. Starting on an AED often implies continuous daily medication for many years, which is sometimes lifelong. Therefore, this should be strictly initiated for those with an unacceptably high rate of seizure recurrence or high risk of seizure injury. Some patients do not need prophylactic treatment as in febrile and benign childhood focal seizures. In others the avoidance of precipitating factors may be sufficiently prophylactic as in some reflex seizures or individuals with a low threshold to seizures. For those in need of prophylactic treatment, the first choice AED should primarily be in accord with the seizure type (Tables 4.1 and 4.2). Certain epileptic seizures are aggravated by some AEDs, which are beneficial in other epileptic seizures. A minimal requirement is to recognise the fundamental differences between focal epilepsy and IGE, since AEDs beneficial for focal epilepsy may be detrimental in IGE (Tables 4.1 and 4.2).[28-31] Indeed, even amongst IGEs, an AED beneficial in one type may be ineffective or aggravate another type of the triad of idiopathic generalised seizures (absences, myoclonic jerks and generalised tonic clonic seizures [GTCS]).[28-31] For example, tiagabine, vigabatrin, carbamazepine, oxcarbazepine and gabapentin may aggravate or be ineffective in absences or myoclonic jerks irrespective of their effect on GTCS (see details in the treatment of IGE page 333–7).

Table 4.1 Efficacy of main AEDs in seizure types

AED	Focal simple or complex seizures	Secondarily GTCS	Primarily GTCS	Myoclonic jerks	Absence seizures
Carbamazepine	*Effective*	*Effective*	*Effective*	*Exaggerates*	*Exaggerates*
Clobazam	Effective	Effective	Effective ?	Effective ?	Effective?
Clonazepam	Effective?	Effective?	Exaggerates?	Effective	Effective
Ethosuximide	Ineffective	Exaggerates?	Exaggerates?	Effective	Effective
Gabapentin	*Effective*	*Effective*	*Ineffective*	*Exaggerates*	*Exaggerates*
Lamotrigine	Effective	Effective	Effective	Exaggerates	Effective
Levetiracetam	Effective	Effective	Effective	Effective	Effective
Oxcarbazepine	*Effective*	*Effective*	*Effective*	*Exaggerates*	*Exaggerates*
Phenobarbitone	Effective	Effective	Effective	Effective	Exaggerates?
Phenytoin	*Effective*	*Effective*	*Effective*	*Ineffective*	*Exaggerates*
Tiagabine	*Effective*	*Effective*	*Ineffective*	*Exaggerates*	*Exaggerates*
Topiramate	Effective	Effective	Effective	Effective	Effective?
Valproate	Effective	Effective	Effective	Effective	Effective
Vigabatrin	*Effective*	*Effective*	*Ineffective*	*Exaggerates*	*Exaggerates*
Zonisamide	Effective	Effective	Effective	Effective	Effective?

Note: AEDs in italics are in general inappropriate or contraindicated for the treatment of IEGs. However, carbamazepine, oxcarbazepine and phenytoin may be used in pure forms of primarily GTCS
Pregabalin is a recently licensed AED for adjunctive treatment of intractable focal seizures, which is not included in the tables but it is detailed in the Pharmacopoeia (page 511).

Table 4.2 Recommendations for AED treatment for children and adults when cost is of concern

Seizures/syndromes	First-line AEDs in order of priority	Second-line AEDs
Focal (simple and complex) seizures with or without secondarily GTCS	Carbamazepine, phenytoin, phenobarbitone	Clobazam, valproate
Primarily GTCS only	Valproate, phenobarbitone, phenytoin	Carbamazepine
Myoclonic seizures only	Clonazepam, phenobarbitone	Phenytoin, ethosuximide
Absence seizures only (typical and atypical)	Valproate, ethosuximide	Clonazepam
Negative myoclonic and atonic seizures	Ethosuximide, valproate	Clonazepam
Tonic seizures	Valproate, phenytoin, phenobarbitone	Clonazepam, clobazam
All syndromes of focal epilepsies	Carbamazepine, phenytoin, phenobarbitone	Clobazam, valproate
Childhood absence epilepsy	Ethosuximide, valproate	Clonazepam
Juvenile absence epilepsy	Valproate, ethosuximide	Clonazepam
Juvenile myoclonic epilepsy	Valproate, phenobarbitone	Clonazepam, ethosuximide
Photosensitive seizures and other reflex seizures	Mainly valproate and clonazepam In accordance with the predominant seizure	
Lennox-Gastaut syndrome and other epileptic encephalopathies	In accordance with the predominant seizure	

Clarifications on AED recommendations in 'newly diagnosed epilepsy'

In the current era of evidence-based medicine, there is an accumulating literature on AED randomised control trials (RCTs) and formal recommendations on the treatment of 'newly diagnosed epilepsy' often used synonymously with the less accurate term 'new onset epilepsy'.[30,35,38]

'Newly diagnosed epilepsy' (or newly identified epilepsy) is a general term for encompassing all types of epilepsies that are newly identified and firmly diagnosed by physicians irrespective of the causes and prognoses. It includes any patient of any age with any form of seizure who seeks medical attention for the first time because of paroxysmal events that are diagnosed as epileptic seizures. It embraces idiopathic or symptomatic, focal or generalised, short-lived or lifelong and mild or severe forms of epilepsies. Thus, 'newly diagnosed epilepsy' is not a diagnostic or therapeutic entity. Its purpose should be to emphasise that these patients require meticulous medical support regarding diagnosis and treatment, which is thoroughly demanding. At this stage of first presentation, medical decisions may affect the rest of the patient's life and often those of their families. Social and psychological support regarding the impact that such a diagnosis may have on them is a significant aspect of proper management.

Furthermore, 'newly diagnosed epilepsy' is not synonymous with 'new onset epilepsy' with which it is incorrectly equated.[34-37] It is evidence based that many patients have onset of seizures several years prior to seeking medical attention (see page 10). Whether 'newly diagnosed epilepsy' or 'new onset epilepsy' both terms are imprecise without defining the type of epilepsy,[39] which is possible for the majority of patients.[40] Unifying them as a single therapeutic category discourages diagnostic precision and encourages inappropriate AED trial strategies[30] such as *"inclusion criteria do not specify seizure type or epilepsy syndrome so AED study results are generalised to the universe of patients with newly diagnosed epilepsy"*.[41] In turn, this promotes detrimental indiscriminate use of carbamazepine and valproate because *"neither of them is regarded as the single drug of choice for all patients with newly diagnosed epilepsy"* [41] despite established documentation that these are two different AEDs with different indications and contraindications in partial and generalised epilepsies.[30]

Rating classification system for evidence-based medicine and clarification for the ratings of the so-called "therapeutics articles"[34-37]

The American Academy of Neurology has introduced a rating classification system for evidence-based medicine.

Class I: Prospective, randomised, controlled clinical trial with masked outcome assessment, in a representative population. The following are required: a) primary outcome(s) is/are clearly defined, b) exclusion/inclusion criteria are clearly defined, c) adequate accounting for drop-outs and cross-overs with numbers sufficiently low to have minimal potential for bias and d) relevant baseline characteristics are presented and substantially equivalent among treatment groups or there is appropriate statistical adjustment for differences.

Class II: Prospective matched group cohort study in a representative population with masked outcome assessment that meets a-d above OR a RCT in a representative population that lacks one criterion a-d.

Class III: All other controlled trials (including well-defined natural history, controls or patients serving as own controls) in a representative population, where outcome assessment is independent of patient treatment

Class IV: Evidence from uncontrolled studies, case series, case reports, or expert opinion

In the so-called "therapeutics articles" [34-37] these schemes "have the sole purpose of eliminating bias in studies. They do not address whether the study results are clinically valid."[38]

AEDs, like all drugs, may be therapeutic when used appropriately, but they also possess toxic properties (Table 4.3).[32,33] Patients and parents should be well informed concerning the purpose of AED medication, efficacy, side effects and possible length of treatment. Otherwise, there are failures in compliance, disillusionment and erosion of patient/physician trust.

To be meaningful, evidence-based AED management should be precise and respect an evidence-based diagnosis.
AED efficacy and adverse reactions are not determined by how long a diagnosis of seizures has been established prior to the onset of treatment.[30]

Prior to starting prophylactic antiepileptic medication in a patient with newly diagnosed seizures a physician should be confident of the following.

1 The patient unequivocally has epileptic seizures. This requires definite exclusion of imitators of seizures (non-epileptic psychogenic seizures, migraine, normal episodic events and cardiogenic, metabolic, cerebral or other neurological disorders that may produce transient and intermittent symptoms mimicking epileptic seizures).

One-quarter of patients treated for 'epilepsy' do not suffer from genuine epileptic seizures.[49]

2 The epileptic seizures of the patient need treatment. This requires thorough investigation of the type of seizures, their frequency and severity, their likelihood of relapse or remission, precipitating factors and the patient/family concerns and understanding of the risks versus benefits of the antiepileptic medication. Hard and fast rules are not always applicable. For example, the general clinical practice that 'a patient with more than two epileptic seizures needs antiepileptic drug treatment' is often inappropriate. AEDs are not needed for most febrile and benign childhood focal seizures and this is also true for all other types of 'conditions with epileptic seizures that do not require a diagnosis of epilepsy', such as alcohol withdrawal or drug-induced seizures, single seizures or isolated clusters of seizures and immediate and early post-traumatic seizures (see Table 1.6 and page 18). Conversely, AED treatment is mandated for recurring seizures in symptomatic epilepsies and most syndromes of IGE such as juvenile myoclonic epilepsy (JME).

Treatment should be initiated if the risks of further seizures outweigh the risks of adverse reactions induced from AED medication.

3 The most appropriate AED is selected for a particular patient with a particular type of seizure(s). This is an extremely demanding task particularly now there are so many choices amongst old and new AEDs (Tables 4.1 and 4.2). Thorough knowledge of AEDs is a prerequisite of any attempt to start AED treatment. We should have passed the time of the late 1980s when the hazardous advice was 'start with valproate and if this fails change it to carbamazepine'. The appropriate drug is that which is the most likely of all others to be truly prophylactic as monotherapy (single-drug treatment) for the seizures without causing undue side effects interfering with the everyday performance and physical and mental well-being of the treated individual. Balancing between the therapeutic (Table 4.1) and toxic effects (Table 4.3) of an AED is a primary responsibility and the crux of epilepsy management. There is no point in treating epilepsy at the expense of drug-induced disease. This cannot be achieved satisfactorily without thorough evaluation of the patient's seizures, medical history, possible co-medication for other diseases and circumstances of the individual patient.

- Some AEDs may be very effective in some epileptic seizures and syndromes, but contra-indicated in others as emphasised in this book on many occasions.

Table 4.3 Main adverse reactions of AED, which may be serious and sometimes life-threatening

AED	Main adverse reactions	Serious and sometimes life threatening reactions[35,37]
Carbamazepine	Idiosyncratic (rash)*, sedation, headache, ataxia, nystagmus, diplopia, tremor, impotence, hyponatraemia, cardiac arrhythmia	Stevens-Johnson syndrome, AHS, hepatic failure, haematological
Clobazam	Severe sedation, fatigue, drowsiness, behavioural and cognitive impairment, restlessness, aggressiveness, hypersalivation and coordination disturbances. Tolerance and withdrawal syndrome	No
Clonazepam	As of clobazam	No
Ethosuximide	Idiosyncratic (rash)*, gastro-intestinal disturbances, anorexia, weight loss, drowsiness, photophobia and headache	Stevens-Johnson syndrome, AHS, renal and hepatic failure, haematological
Gabapentin	Weight gain,** peripheral oedema, behavioural changes	No
Lamotrigine	Idiosyncratic (rash)*, tics, insomnia, dizziness, diplopia, headache, ataxia, asthenia	Stevens-Johnson syndrome, AHS, hepatic failure
Levetiracetam	Irritability, behavioural changes, insomnia, asthenia, dizziness.	No
Oxcarbazepine	Idiosyncratic (rash)*, headache, dizziness, weakness, nausea, somnolence, ataxia and diplopia, hyponatraemia	AHS, haematological
Phenobarbitone	Idiosyncratic (rash)*, severe drowsiness, sedation, impairment of cognition and concentration, hyperkinesia and agitation in children, shoulder-hand syndrome	Stevens-Johnson syndrome, AHS, haematological
Phenytoin	Idiosyncratic (rash)*, ataxia, drowsiness, lethargy, sedation, encephalopathy, gingival hyperplasia, hirsutism, dysmorphism, rickets, osteomalacia	Stevens-Johnson syndrome, AHS, renal and hepatic failure, haematological
Tiagabine	Stupor or spike-wave stupor, weakness	No
Topiramate	Somnolence, anorexia, fatigue, nervousness, difficulty with concentration/attention, memory impairment, psychomotor slowing, metabolic acidosis, weight loss,** language dysfunction, renal calculi, acute angle-closure glaucoma and other ocular abnormalities, paraesthesia	Hepatic failure, anhidrosis***
Valproate	Nausea, vomiting, dyspepsia, weight gain,** tremor, hair loss, hormonal in women.	Hepatic and pancreatic failure
Vigabatrin	Fatigue, drowsiness, weight gain,** behavioural changes	Irreversible visual field defects
Zonisamide	Idiosyncratic*, drowsiness, anorexia, irritability, photosensitivity, weight loss,** renal calculi	Stevens-Johnson syndrome, AHS, anhidrosis***

AHS= Anticonvulsant hypersensitivity syndrome which is a potentially fatal but rare reaction, manifests as rash, fever, tender lymphadenopathy, hepatitis, and eosinophilia.[42-44] There is usually cross-sensitivity between AEDs, which have the potential to cause AHS; these AEDs should be avoided in patients who have developed idiosyncratic reactions to one or another drug.

* The appearance of skin rash mandates immediate discontinuation of the responsible agent because it may progress to Stevens-Johnson syndrome and anticonvulsant hypersensitive syndrome.

**The risks of obesity are emphasised routinely in the media in the United States and other industrialized countries where obesity has become epidemic. Patients and particularly women should be informed of AEDs that are likely to cause weight gain (gabapentin, pregabalin, valproate and vigabatrin). Conversely, topiramate and zonisamide may cause significant weight loss, which can be relentless. Lamotrigine, levetiracetam and phenytoin are weight neutral AEDs.[45]

*** Hypohidrosis (in most cases anhidrosis=inability to sweat) is a rare but serious adverse effect of topiramate and zonisamide probably due to a reduction in carbonic anhydrase isoenzymes II and IV. Children particularly in warm environments are at higher risk.[46-48]

- Some AEDs are very effective in controlling seizures, but may be unsuitable for particular groups of patients because of side effects (Table 4.3) such as valproate in women, particularly women of childbearing age. Hepatic enzyme-modifiers have lower priority over others in the elderly and patients who are medicated with other drugs for systemic or other comorbid disorders.
- Some AEDs may be effective in one or two but not all multiple types of seizures that a patient may have (Table 4.1). For example, in JME: valproate and levetiracetam control absences, jerks and GTCS, lamotrigine controls GTCS and absences but often exaggerates jerks; clonazepam is the main anti-myoclonic agent but does not control GTCS; and ethosuximide controls absences but not GTCS.
- Providing that the physician is confident of his/her decision regarding the suitability of an AED, this should be thoroughly explained to the patient/carer and ensure that this is well understood.

An antiepileptic drug appropriate for one type of seizure may be deleterious for another type of seizure.
The selected antiepileptic drug should be the most likely to be effective and the most unlikely to cause adverse reactions.

4. The starting dose and titration of the selected drug should be in accordance with the appropriate recommendations (Table 4.4) and the age and primarily the particular needs of the treated patient. Starting with small doses and with a slow titration rate is mandated for certain drugs such as lamotrigine (increased risk of skin rash) and topiramate (increased risk of cognitive impairment) and of less concern in others such as levetiracetam (Table 4.4). The disadvantage of AEDs demanding slow titration is that patients may not be initially protected against potentially hazardous seizures until therapeutic doses have been achieved.

The aim is to achieve seizure control in a possibly shorter time with or without minimal adverse reactions.
The correct dose is the smallest one that achieves seizure control without adverse effects.

The following should also be taken into consideration in deciding how to start and escalate the selected AED.

- Patients, particularly with newly identified epilepsy, are prone to develop adverse reactions (biological, cognitive or behavioural), which in 15% of cases lead to AED discontinuation.
- Some patients develop adverse reactions easily even at an AED dose below the minimal limit of the target (therapeutic) range, while others are resistant to AED adverse reactions even at the maximum limit of the target range.
- Even for patients with the same type of seizures and for the same AED, seizure control may be achieved with a drug concentration below, within or above the target range.

My practice is to allow the patient to self-regulate the rate of escalation both in terms of the dose and dosing intervals of the AED. I explain to the patient and give in writing the recommended dose and the rate of escalation of the AED to use. I clarify that minor adverse reactions such as fatigue or somnolence are usually dose related and should not discourage escalation unless they interfere with the patient's daily activities. I also warn the patient that any type of idiosyncratic reactions such as rash (even if mild) should be reported immediately so as to prevent escalation to more serious and sometimes life-threatening events.

- *Adverse reactions.* I ask that the first dose (*test dose*) be taken at night before sleep and then the planned scheme be continued if there are no adverse reactions. If adverse reactions cause significant discomfort then the test dose should be decreased to half and tried again the next night. Similarly, the patient is at liberty to prolong the escalation time and reduce the escalation dose to suit his/her own reaction to the AED.

Exceptions apply particularly to patients at high risk from ongoing seizures. These patients need appropriate AEDs, which preferably do not require slow titration (Table 4.4). Other AEDs should be introduced faster at the expense of possible adverse reactions. A small dose or very slow escalation in these patients is often insufficient for controlling seizures and their impact on the patient.

- *Control of seizures.* If seizures are controlled at some stage during the escalation, I ask the patient to continue with the same scheme with which seizure control was achieved without further increasing the AED dose.

For many AEDs and for many patients there is a ceiling dose of optimal efficacy, which may be lost by further dose increments. This may be due to a particular efficacy-related property of the AED or the introduction of adverse reactions that may exaggerate seizures.

5. The selected drug should not be abandoned prior to achieving recommended target doses unless unacceptable side effects occur, it is ineffective or

Table 4.4 Recommendations for slow titration and laboratory testing

AED	Needs slow titration (weeks to reach therapeutic dose)*	Needs for laboratory testing**	Therapeutic drug monitoring ***
Carbamazepine	Yes (~4 weeks)	Maximal	Useful
Clobazam	Yes (~4 weeks)	Minimal	Not generally useful
Clonazepam	Yes (~4 weeks)	Minimal	Not generally useful
Ethosuximide	Yes (~4 weeks)	Minimal	Useful
Gabapentin	No or minimal (0-2 weeks)	Minimal	Not recommended
Lamotrigine	Yes (~8 weeks)	Maximal	Very useful in pregnancy and hormonal contraception
Levetiracetam	No or minimal (0-2 weeks)	Minimal	Not recommended
Oxcarbazepine	Yes (~4 weeks)	Maximal	Not generally useful
Phenobarbitone	Yes (~6 weeks)	Minimal	Useful
Phenytoin	Yes (~4 weeks)	Maximal	Very useful
Tiagabine	Yes (~4 weeks)	Minimal	Not needed
Topiramate	Yes (~6 weeks)	Maximal	Useful particularly in co-medication
Valproate	Yes (~6 weeks)	Maximal	Not generally useful
Vigabatrin	Yes (~4 weeks)	Maximal	Not needed
Zonisamide	Yes (~4 weeks)	Maximal	Useful

* Values are approximate and indicative only. Some patients may need slower titration and larger doses while others may need smaller doses and can tolerate faster titration.

** This refers to monitoring of the serum AED levels of the added AED or the co-medications that may be affected as well as blood or other tests needed for detecting possible adverse drug reactions such as hypernatraemia with oxcarbazepine or metabolic acidosis with topiramate.

*** See text for individual AEDs.

exaggeration of seizures occurs. In either of these cases a second drug fulfilling therapeutic expectations for success should be initiated. If the seizures are controlled, the first drug should be gradually withdrawn so as to re-establish monotherapy again.

Start monotherapy with the chosen first-line AED, initially at low doses titrating up to the low maintenance dose.[50] If seizures continue, titrate to the limit of tolerability, which will achieve additional seizure control in approximately 20% of patients. If, as in many patients, dosing to the limit of tolerability is not beneficial, the dose should be reduced.[50] Switching to an average dose of another first-line AED is another option for preventing over-treatment.[50]

MONOTHERAPY VERSUS POLYTHERAPY

Monotherapy with an appropriately selected AED at an appropriate target dose achieves complete control of seizures in 50-70% of patients.[51-55] In a recent study, nearly one-half of newly diagnosed patients of any type (symptomatic or idiopathic) became seizure free on the first-ever AED, with >90% doing so at moderate or even modest dosing.[56] The advantage of monotherapy is to minimise side effects and interactions with other AEDs or non-AEDs as well as achieving better compliance. The risks of polytherapy include more side effects, frequent unwanted interactions with other AEDs or non-AEDs, an increased risk of teratogenicity, an inability to evaluate the efficacy and side effects of individual AED agents and bad compliance.

However, monotherapy should also be rationalised. The paradox is that occasionally polytherapy is more desirable than monotherapy. An example of this is a patient with JME who continues having disturbing myoclonic jerks despite complete control of GTCS and absences on a moderate dose of valproate (1000 mg daily). In this case adding a small dose of 0.5 mg of clonazepam at night may be more efficacious than doubling the dose of valproate. Similarly, in a patient with juvenile absence epilepsy who is moderately controlled with valproate it is better to add small doses of lamotrigine (50 mg in the morning) than increase the dose of valproate.

Patients should be treated with a single AED (monotherapy) wherever possible. If the initial treatment is unsuccessful, then monotherapy using another drug can be tried. Caution is needed during the changeover period. Switching between AEDs must be carried out cautiously, slowly withdrawing the first drug only after the second drug has reached an adequate therapeutic dosage.

Polytherapy (combination, adjunctive or 'add-on' therapy) should only be considered when attempts at monotherapy with AEDs have not resulted in freedom from seizures. If trials of combination therapy do not bring about worthwhile benefits, treatment should revert to the regimen (monotherapy or polytherapy) that has proved most acceptable to the patient in terms of providing the best balance between effectiveness in reducing seizure frequency and the tolerability of side effects.

RATIONAL POLYTHERAPY

Rational polytherapy is often needed for 30–50% of patients with epilepsies who are unsatisfactorily controlled with a single AED.[57-59] This is much higher in patients with symptomatic focal epilepsies than patients with IGE. Nearly all epileptic encephalopathies such as Lennox–Gastaut syndrome require polytherapy.

Initially, a second drug is added to the agent that showed better efficacy and tolerability in monotherapy. The choice of a second or sometimes a third drug depends on many factors such as efficacy, adverse effects, interactions with other drugs, mode of action and the need for laboratory testing. Polytherapy with more than three drugs is discouraged because adverse reactions become more prominent, with little if any seizure improvement.

*The word *"rational"* has been used in conjunction with "polytherapy" in order to emphasise that this can also be *irrational* and *hazardous* if a diagnosis is incorrect and anti-epileptic drug indications/contraindications are violated.

The decision for polytherapy should first scrutinise the possible/probable reasons why the monotherapy failed. The following possibilities should be thoroughly examined, which often requires re-evaluation of the diagnosis (genuine epileptic seizures? and what type of seizures?).

- The patient does not suffer from epileptic seizures.
- The patient has both genuine epileptic and non-epileptic seizures.
- The patient has focal and no generalised seizures or vice versa.
- The AED used as monotherapy was not suitable for the particular type of seizures in this patient either because of contra-indications (tiagabine or carbamazepine in absences or myoclonic jerks, lamotrigine in myoclonic epilepsies), weak efficacy (valproate or gabapentin in focal seizures) or total ineffectiveness (gabapentin in primarily GTCS).
- Non-compliance can vary from unwillingness to take medication to occasionally forgetting or missing the AED dose. The latter is often improved with the use of AED-monitored dosage systems, which are widely available through pharmacies. These usually come in small boxes with a week or longer supply of each individual patient's tablets or capsules to be taken at the time and date shown. These are useful even for patients who comply well, but who often may be uncertain whether or not they have taken their medication.
- Patients may violate instructions to avoid particularly eminent seizure-precipitating factors such as photic stimulation, sleep deprivation and alcohol or drug abuse.

Adding a new AED with another one to three AEDs that have already partially or totally failed or have made the situation worse is a formidable physician's task for a disappointed and frustrated patient. Guidance that gives the physician just a list of options without prioritising them is unsatisfactory. For example, all new AEDs are licensed in polytherapy for focal seizures with or without secondarily GTCS. The priority of an AED over another AED depends on a number of characteristics

Terminogical clarifications on efficacy, efficiency, safety and tolerability

In randomised control trial reports *efficacy* is often not used synonymously with *effectiveness*: 'Efficacy is a relative term defined by the designers of a study, but is usually a specific effect of a treatment. In contrast, effectiveness has many potential components including tolerability, cognition, mood, or quality of life.'[60]

Safety is not synonymous with tolerability. An AED may be well tolerated with regard to cognitive or other adverse effects but with a low safety margin. A typical example of this is vigabatrin, which had excellent tolerability according to all relevant controlled AED trials despite the fact that it was extremely unsafe as documented later in clinical practice with a high incidence of irreversible visual field defects. Similarly, there are significant differences between the safety and tolerability of lamotrigine.

Useful definitions and notes on drug-drug interactions

Drug interactions: refer to phamacokinetic and pharmacodynamic changes that occur with concomitant use of drugs.

Drug interactions may be beneficial (increased effectiveness, reduced risk of unwanted adverse reactions or both) but more often are detrimental (decreased efficiency, increased side effects or both). Pharmacokinetic AED interactions are more frequently the consequence of drug-induced changes in hepatic metabolism through enzyme inhibition or induction. Changes of plasma protein binding are less common.

In enzyme inhibition, the added drug inhibits or blocks drug-metabolising enzymes which in turn decreases the rate of metabolism of the other drug thus resulting in higher plasma concentrations.

In enzyme induction, prolonged administration of another a drug increases (induces) the activity of drug metabolising enzymes. This in turn increases the rate of metabolism of the parent drug thus resulting in lower serum concentrations.

If the affected drug has an active metabolite the impact of an inhibitor or inducer may be reduced but this depends on the subsequent metabolism of the metabolites. Induction for example may increase metabolite concentrations and enhance toxicity without elevation of the parent drug.

Pharmacodynamic interactions may be additive, synergistic or antagonistic.

as detailed in Chapter 12 for focal seizures (Table 12.4, page 431). Briefly, the criteria to determine the order of priority of the AED to be added are:

1. *Efficacy.* The more efficacious a drug is the more likely it is to control seizures and, if successful, withdrawal of other concomitant antiepileptic medications may be possible.
2. *Safety.* Adverse reactions may outweigh any beneficial effect achieved by reduction of the seizures.
3. *Interactions with other AEDs* are particularly unwanted in polytherapy. Raising levels of concomitant AEDs may lead to toxic effects. Conversely, decreasing their levels may increase and worsen seizures causing a vicious circle in clinical management.
4. *Different mechanisms of action in relation to other concurrent AEDs* (Table 4.5). An AED is unlikely to have better success and more likely to have additive adverse reactions if added to another AED with the same mechanisms of action.
5. *Need for less laboratory monitoring.*[34-37] This refers to monitoring of the serum levels of the added AED or the co-medications that may be affected as well as blood or other tests needed for detecting possible adverse drug reactions such as hypernatraemia with oxcarbazepine (Table 4.4)

CONVERTING FROM POLYTHERAPY TO MONOTHERAPY

Evidence from studies with old and new AEDs shows that a significant number of patients can be converted successfully from polytherapy to monotherapy without losing seizure control and, in some cases, with improved seizure control.[63] In these cases the AED that appears, after careful consideration, less effective is gradually withdrawn. 'Gradually' sometimes means in steps of weeks or months. This should be particularly slow for certain AEDs such as phenobarbitone and benzodiazepines in order to avoid withdrawal seizures.

Important notes on antiepileptic drug management

Withdraw of AEDs that are ineffective or contraindicated. Great benefits, without loss of seizure control, are often gained by slowly reducing the overall drug load.[50]

More than three AEDs are pointless and probably harmful, with 70% of patients becoming seizure free on appropriate monotherapy or conservative rational polytherapy. A second AED may be very effective, even in minute doses.

Compliance and avoidance of precipitating factors are essential aspects of success.

ANTIEPILEPTIC DRUG WITHDRAWAL

Consideration of total withdrawal of AEDs is needed in the following patients.

- Patients who do not suffer from epileptic seizures.
- Patients suffering from age-related and age-limited epileptic syndromes who have reached appropriate age of remission. These are detailed in Chapters 5, 6 and 9.
- Patients who are seizure free for more than 3–5 years provided that they do not suffer from epileptic syndromes requiring long-term treatment such as JME.

Discontinuation of AEDs should be extremely slow, in small doses and in long steps of weeks or months. The rate of relapse increases with a faster rate of AED discontinuation.[7] Further, with fast discontinuation of AEDs there is a risk of

Definitions

Intractable or refractory epilepsy: there is no satisfactory definition of refractory epilepsy. Patients are often referred to as refractory or treatment resistant when they have failed to respond to three or more AEDs. Others consider that epilepsy becomes intractable when seizures continue beyond 2–3 years despite optimal drug treatment.[34,36]

Over-treatment is defined as an unnecessary and excessive drug load in the management of epilepsy leading to a suboptimal risk-to-benefit balance.[50]

seizures that are directly related to the withdrawal effects of certain AEDs (phenobarbitone and benzodiazepimes).

Prior to AED withdrawal, there is a need for a thorough re-evaluation of the patient. The presence of even minor and infrequent seizures specifies active disease. Conversely, the occurrence of such seizures in the process of AED discontinuation mandates restoration of AED medication.

Over-medication in the number of AEDs and dosages and length of exposure is undesirable but common. Treatment should be reviewed at regular intervals to ensure that patients are not maintained for long periods on treatment that is ineffective, poorly tolerated or not needed and that concordance with prescribed medication is maintained.[50,64]

THERAPEUTIC DRUG MONITORING

Therapeutic drug monitoring (TDM) or the therapeutic target range of AEDs is a statistical standard of the AED concentration derived from population studies, which represents the balance between drug anti-seizure efficacy and dose-related side effects.[65,66] The quoted target range is a set of odds (measured as trough levels) to give an indication of the drug concentration at which the majority of

Table 4.5 Main mode of action of AEDs and seizure efficacy spectrum

AED	Main mode of action	Broad spectrum
Carbamazepine	Blocks voltage-dependent Na^+ channels (↓Na^+)	No
Clobazam	Increases inhibition by $GABA_A$ (↑$GABA_A$)	No
Clonazepam	Increases inhibition by $GABA_A$ (↑$GABA_A$)	No
Ethosuximide	Blocks T-type $Ca2^+$ channels (↓$Ca2^+$)	No
Gabapentin	Multiple (modifies $Ca2^+$ channels and neurotransmitter release)	No
Lamotrigine	Blocks voltage-dependent Na^+ channels (↓Na^+)	Yes
Levetiracetam*	Novel. Binds to synaptic vesicle protein SV2A	Yes
Oxcarbazepine	Blocks voltage-dependent Na^+ channels (↓Na^+)	No
Phenobarbitone	Multiple (↓Na^+;↓$Ca2^+$; ↑$GABA_A$;↓Glutamate)	Yes
Phenytoin	Blocks voltage-dependent Na^+ channels (↓Na^+)	No
Tiagabine	Increases inhibition by $GABA_A$ (↑$GABA_A$)- potent inhibitor of GAB_A uptake into neurons and glial cells	No
Topiramate	Multiple (↓Na^+;↓$Ca2^+$; ↑$GABA_A$;↓Glutamate)	Yes
Valproate	Multiple (↓Na^+;↓$Ca2^+$; ↑$GABA_A$;↓Glutamate)	Yes
Vigabatrin	Increases inhibition by $GABA_A$ (↑$GABA_A$)- selective and irreversible $GABA_A$-transaminase inhibitor thus increasing whole-brain levels of $GABA_A$	No
Zonisamide	Multiple (↓Na^+;↓$Ca2^+$)	Yes

The main mechanisms of action of the available antiepileptic drugs[61] are thought to be
1. blockading voltage-dependent ion channels (sodium, potassium and calcium channels)
2. increasing the activity of the inhibitory GAB_A (gamma-aminobutyric acid)-ergic system and
3. decreasing the activity of the excitatory glutamatergic system

*Levetiracetam possesses a mechanism of action distinct from that of all other AEDs.[62] It has been recently shown that the synaptic vesicle protein SV2A is the binding site of levetiracetam in the brain and that levetiracetam acts by modulating the function of SV2A (figure 12.21, page 436).[62]

patients achieve optimal seizure control. Above the upper limit of this range dose-related adverse effects are more likely to occur. In other words, TDM is the optimal drug concentration range at which most patients achieve the desired therapeutic effect with no undesirable side effects.[67]

TDM usually measures the total (free and protein bound) AED concentrations in the serum. The free drug may also be assayed. Saliva TDM approximates to the free concentrations of the AED that enters the saliva. Measurements of free AED concentrations are not useful in clinical practice except in cases where protein binding may be affected by other drugs and cases involving pregnancy, liver and renal disease and hypoalbuminaemia. Saliva TDM is rarely used in clinical practice because samples are often contaminated in the mouth, thereby making the results unreliable.

TDM is a useful guideline, but the real goal of effective AED dosing should be based mainly on clinical criteria because the inter-patient variability is considerable. Some patients are well controlled below the target range while others achieve seizure freedom above the therapeutic range. Some patients are free of adverse reactions even at 'toxic' target levels, while others may develop adverse reactions that are unacceptable for them at trough levels, which are just measurable.

Rule of thumb for individual patients

The level is 'therapeutic' when and only when the patient is free of seizures and free of side effects regardless of where the numbers fall along the therapeutic range.[68]

The dose of an AED is adequate if seizures are controlled and if adverse reactions are not present or these are mild.

The dose is high if intolerable adverse reactions are present irrespective of seizure control.

Although monitoring the plasma levels of AEDs may be in decline, TDM is useful in clinical practice for maximising seizure control and minimising adverse reactions providing that it is selectively and appropriately used in response to a patient-specific pharmacokinetic or pharmacodynamic issue or a problem.[67]

Of the old AEDs phenytoin, phenobarbitone and carbamazepine (Table 4.4) are more likely to need TDM.

Considered initially unnecessary for the new AEDs, TDM is of great significance for lamotrigine (in conjunction with pregnancy[69-71] or hormonal contraception[72]), topiramate [73] and zonisamide[74,75] (in polytherapy). However. TDM is less valuable and not widely practised for most new AEDs because a wide range of serum concentrations is associated with clinical efficacy and no useful or considerable overlap is reported between 'concentration–effect' and 'concentration–toxicity'. Current tentative target ranges for each of the new AEDs have been reported. [75]

In general TDM is useful in the following situations:[67]

- establishing 'baseline' effective concentrations in patients successfully stabilised for future comparisons if seizures recur, in pregnancy or in patients in need of concomitant medication for other medical conditions
- evaluating potential causes of lack of efficacy such as suspected non-compliance
- evaluating potential causes of toxicity
- evaluating potential causes of loss of efficacy
- judging 'room to move' or when to change AEDs
- minimising predictable problems.

TDM is complicated in polytherapy because it is unlikely that the therapeutic target range is the same when an AED is taken alone or in combination with other

AEDs. For example, the toxicity from carbamazepine or valproate appears at higher plasma levels when these AEDs are used in monotherapy than when they are combined.

In a class 1 controlled study of children and adults, there was no clear benefit of dose adjustments according to TDM versus clinical response.[76]

TIME OF SAMPLING

For AEDs with a short half-life such as carbamazepine blood samples are obtained prior to the first dose when the concentration is at its trough (which is useful for assessing ineffectiveness) and/or at a time of expected peak concentrations (which is useful for assessing toxicity). For AEDs with a long half-life such as phenobarbitone timing is not important because fluctuations in plasma concentration are negligible in the course of a day.

Useful notes on therapeutic drug monitoring

Regularly repeating TDM in patients who are controlled and with no sign of adverse reactions 'just to make sure that everything is ok' is totally discouraged.

Trough AED plasma levels are important with regard to efficacy while peak AED plasma levels (measured at a time determined by the absorption rate of the AED) are important with regard to toxicity.

In treatment with carbamazepine, inform the patient that diplopia is a sign of exceeding the drug dosage, which should be adjusted below this level.

Lamotrigine needs TDM in conjunction with initiation or withdrawal of hormonal contraception[69] and before, during and after pregnancy.[69-71] The reason for this is that pregnancy[69-71] and hormonal contraception[72] significantly lower (more than half) lamotrigine levels. Patients may suffer breakthrough seizures mainly during the first trimester of pregnancy (if lamotrigine levels are not corrected) or toxic effects postpartum (if lamotrigine levels had been adjusted during pregnancy but not after delivery).

PRAGMATIC RECOMMENDATIONS ON NEW AEDS

The drug treatments with old and new AEDs in individual seizure types and individual epileptic syndromes are detailed in the relevant chapters of this book. Recent reviews,[7,25,75,77-92] the practice parameters of the American Academy of Neurology,[34-37] the guidelines of the British National Institute for Clinical Excellence (http://www.nice.org.uk) [93-96] and ongoing experience and information mandate pragmatic recommendations on the use of new AEDs in epilepsies.

Evidence-based prescribing has become a necessary part of treating epilepsies. However, there are major problems with this. A particular issue with evidence-based RCTs is that these are nearly exclusively used for new AEDs. Diagnostic uncertainties and methodological pressures confound analysis of these studies, which are primarily designed for justifying regulatory licence requirements rather than addressing clinical practice needs.[97-99] These issues may compromise purely evidence-based recommendations[34-37] as happened recently.[30] Partly as a result, such influential recommendations may mislead physicians in the appropriate use of new AEDs and inadvertently perpetuate suboptimal practice in new clinical trials. For multiple reasons, there are significant difficulties in extrapolating data from RCTs into clinical practice[97,98] as also indicated by the discrepancies between guidelines derived from such data.[96]

> "New AED trials can determine the appropriate use of AEDs, but ultimately fail to determine the best use of AEDs and their exact role in treating patients. New AED trials rarely use clinically applicable measures of efficacy and it is difficult to extrapolate the data from populations used in AED trials to the wider population of patients with epilepsy. Furthermore, AED trials ignore the factors that are most likely to determine prognosis: the aetiology, seizure types and epilepsy syndrome. To resolve these issues, we need large multicentre studies in well-defined populations with well-characterised seizures, epilepsy syndromes and aetiologies. Being seizure free should be the primary measure of efficacy rather than meta-analyses and guidelines based upon incomplete data."[97]

> "The studies performed to demonstrate the effectiveness of new AEDs in monotherapy in refractory partial seizure patients are difficult to interpret, because they are driven by FDA requirements to show superiority over placebo or pseudo-placebo rather than by clinical questions. The dosages used in the trials are often higher than those that might be used in practice, because the goal is to retain as many patients as possible and achieve a significant result. Most importantly, the goal of these studies is not to determine whether patients improve after they are converted to monotherapy. Rather, the goal is to determine whether they deteriorate less than the comparison group."[98]

My recommendations in this book are pragmatic in that they are based on a thorough review of the efficacy, tolerability, safety and interactions of new AEDs after examining the following:

1. **Evidence-based reports, reviews and expert assessments of the treatment of children and adults with newly diagnosed or intractable focal and generalised seizures of symptomatic and idiopathic epilepsies.**
2. **Post-marketing open studies and case reports that have appeared as full papers or abstracts.**
3. **Expert physicians' experience of the AED in clinical use that I obtained through critical discussions or correspondence with them.**
4. **Mechanisms of actions in animal models as supportive rather than conclusive evidence of clinical usefulness.**

In these recommendations I also take into account the following.

- Investigators and practising physicians often use these agents beyond their FDA or other formally approved specific indications and specified groups of patients. It is often the case that through this undesired but pragmatically necessary practice of *'trial by success or error'* that an AED finds its true therapeutic potential or its unsuitability in the treatment of epilepsies. This practice of off-label prescribing AEDs is encouraged in all official recommendations.[34-37,93-96] Therefore, it is fundamental that physicians are informed regarding existing evidence (established, probable or possible but not necessarily of class 1 studies that may never be performed to provide such evidence) indicating which of the AEDs and for what type of seizures are effective or potentially useful or ineffective, contra-indicated and harmful. Table 4.1 provides a list of old and new AEDs and their indications/contra-indications for common seizure types.
- The seizure-related efficacy of each new AED is a significant factor in preferring one drug over another when both may be indicated for the same type of seizure. Table 12.4 (p. 431) provides a list of new AEDs according to their efficacy and other properties in intractable focal seizures. Figure 12.20 (p. 435) compares the efficacy versus tolerability of new AEDs in patients with intractable focal seizures.[100]
- Physicians and patients are concerned about the quality of adverse reactions and in particular potentially disabling or even fatal risks. These risks, even if of low frequency, weigh significantly in my recommendations for or against an AED. Table 4.3 provides a list of serious and common non-serious adverse events. Note that some of the serious adverse events are potentially fatal.
- Pharmacokinetics and interactions with commonly used medications or other AEDs are particularly important in monotherapy (which may also fail) and more importantly in AED polytherapy (Tables 4.6 and 4.7).[88,89] After all, one of the requirements for new AEDs was necessitated by the complex pharmacokinetics and frequent drug interactions of old AEDs. On this I quote from a recent clinical parameter:[35,37]

> "The older AEDs as a class have complex pharmacokinetics. Four of the six AEDs available prior to 1990 (phenytoin, carbamazepine, phenobarbital and primidone) are hepatic enzyme inducers. Induction not only complicates combination AED therapy but also changes internal hormonal milieu in possibly important ways. Intrinsic compounds, such as sex steroids and vitamin D, are hypermetabolised. This can lead to reproductive dysfunction and osteopenia. Enzyme-inducing AEDs produce important interactions with many commonly used medications, such as warfarin, oral contraceptives, calcium channel antagonists and chemotherapeutic agents, to name a few. Valproate, in contrast, is a potent hepatic inhibitor. There is controversy about the impact of valproate on the hormonal milieu and inhibition leads to important drug interactions with AEDs as well as other classes. The newer agents are involved in many fewer drug interactions. Many of the newer agents have little if any effect on the CYP450 enzyme system and other metabolic pathways." [35,37]

However, such a generalisation, although correct if old and new AEDs are considered as two different 'classes', is inadequate without specifying that certain new AEDs have similar or even worse drug–drug interactions in relation to certain old AEDs. Tables 4.6 and 4.7 provide lists of comparative pharmacokinetic parameters, drug–drug interactions and metabolic pathways of elimination for new and some common old AEDs. It should be noted that new AEDs are not innocent. All but levetiracetam (characterised as ideal)[101,104] and gabapentin exhibit sometimes complex undesirable drug–drug interactions.

- The speed of titration and the need for less laboratory testing are additional factors that may influence the choice of the AED to be used. Very slow titration may mean more seizures, which may also be traumatic. More laboratory testing means less compliance, more expense and more uncomfortable situations for patients.

Table 4.4 provides a list of AEDs and recommendations regarding titration and the need for laboratory testing.

Table 4.8 provides a guide to clinical practice dosage schemes for AEDs. Details can be found in Chapter 14.

Table 4.6 Pharmacokinetics: Comparisons between new and important old AEDs.

					Drug-drug interactions		
AED	**Oral absorption**	**Dosing**	**Kinetics**	**Metabolisn**	**Affected by others**	**Affects others**	**% of perfect score**
Carbamazepine	3	3	2	1	1	1	61
Gabapentin	3	1-2	2	3	3	3	86
Lamotrigine	3	3	2	1	1	2	67
Levetiracetam	3	3	3	2	3	3	94
Phenytoin	3	3	1	1	1	1	56
Tiagabine	2	2	3	1	2	1	61
Topiramate	2	3	3	3	1	1	72
Valproate	3	3	2	1	2	1	67
Vigabatrin	3	3	3	3	3	2	94

From Patsalos [101] with the permission of the author and the Editor of *Pharmacology & Therapeutics*

Table 4.7 Metabolic pathway, effect of AEDs on hepatic enzymes and drug-drug interactions (DDI)

AED	Metabolic pathway	Hepatic enzyme-inducers and hepatic enzyme-inhibitors[27,102]	DDI
Carbamazepine*	Hepatic	Enzyme-inducer (CYP2C,CYP3A,CYP1A2, microsomal epoxide hydrolases, UGTs) ****	Yes
Clobazam	Hepatic	No	No
Clonazepam	Hepatic	No	No
Ethosuximide	Hepatic	No	Yes
Gabapentin	Renal	No	No
Lamotrigine**	Hepatic	Enzyme-inducer (UGTs)***	Yes
Levetiracetam	Renal	No	No
Oxcarbazepine*	Hepatic	Enzyme-inducer (CYP3A4 , UGTs) and enzyme-inhibitor CYP2C19)	Yes
Phenobarbitone*	Hepatic	Enzyme-inducer (CYP2C,CYP3A, microsomal epoxide hydrolases, UGTs)	Yes
Phenytoin*	Hepatic (90%)	Enzyme-inducer (CYP2C,CYP3A, microsomal epoxide hydrolases, UGTs)	Yes
Tiagabine***	Hepatic	No	Yes
Topiramate*	Hepatic <Renal	Enzyme-inducer (CYP3A4, b-oxidation) and enzyme-inhibitor (CYP2C19)	Yes
Valproate	Hepatic	Enzyme-inhibitor (CYP2C9, microsomal epoxide hydrolases, UGTs)	Yes
Vigabatrin	Renal	No	No
Zonisamide	Hepatic	No	Yes

*These AEDs are CYP3A4 enzyme-inducers, and increase clearance of the oestrogen and also the progestogen component of hormonal contraception, thus decreasing their plasma levels and their effectiveness. Topiramate is a dose-dependent CYP3A4 enzyme-inducer. Also, long use of hepatic enzyme-inducers can lead to significant changes in sex hormones in women and may potentially result in long-term endocrine effects in children.[102]

**Lamotrigine has a reciprocal interaction with hormonal contraception, which decreases plasma concentrations of lamotrigine (see text). Valproate is a potent inhibitor of UGT-dependent metabolism of lamotrigine while enzyme-inducer AEDS are potent inducers of UGT-dependent metabolism of lamotrigine, which is the reason for different schemes of lamotrigine dosage and titration when combined with these AEDS.

***Tiagabine is neither hepatic enzyme inducer nor an inhibitor and therefore does not affect other AEDs or hormonal contraception. However, enzyme inducing drugs significantly lower the plasma concentrations of tiagabine and shorten its half life. Valproate displaces tiagabine from its protein binding sites.

****CYP (cytochrome P450 system) is a superfamily of isoenzymes which are responsible for the oxiative metabolism of many drugs, exogenous compounds and endogenous substrates. They are located in the membranes of the smooth endoplasmic reticulum mainly of the liver. CYP enzymes are classified into families (designated by the first Arabic number), subfamilies (designated by the capital letter following the Arabic number) and isoenzymes according to their similarities in their amino acid sequences.[103]

****UGTs (uridine diphosphate glucuronosyltransferases) are a superfamily of enzymes which are responsible for the formation of hydrophylic drug metabolites that are mainly excreted by renal or biliary routes. They catalyse the glucuronidation of drugs and endogenous substrates. They are located in the endoplasmic reticulum of cells in the liver, kidneys and other organs including the brain. Hepatic glucuronidation is most important.

Autor's note: AEDs with DDIs are undesirable when polytherapy is needed for the control of seizures and also in patients treated with other drugs for other systemic or co-morbid diseases and particularly elderly people (who are often co-medicated with other drugs).[102] In women, use of enzyme inducers can lead to significant changes in sex hormones and can decrease the efficacy of oral contraception.[102]

SURGERY FOR EPILEPSIES

The surgical treatment of drug-resistant epilepsy has become increasingly more valuable and often life saving due to major advances in structural and functional neuroimaging, EEG monitoring and surgical techniques.[105-113]

- The outcome from current surgical methods has improved dramatically both in classical resective surgery and new methodologies being introduced.
- Paediatric surgical outcomes have become similar to those reported for adults.
- A class 1 RCT of surgery for mesial temporal lobe epilepsy[114] found that 64% of those who received surgery were free of disabling seizures compared with 8% free in the group randomised to continued medical therapy. Quality-of-life and social function significantly improved in the operated patients; morbidity was infrequent and there was no mortality.
- Early surgical intervention, when successful, might also prevent or reverse the disabling psychosocial consequences of uncontrolled seizures during critical periods of development.

The spectacular progress in this field is indicated by the fact that one-third (over 300 pages) of a recent book on 'the treatment of epilepsy' is devoted to neurosurgical approaches.[92] Despite all this progress in the safety and outcome of these procedures, surgery in epilepsies is underused[110,115] and appropriate candidates continue to be referred to epilepsy surgery programmes late in the

Table 4.8 Typical comparative single AED dosage schemes in children, adults and elderly patients in clinical practice

	Children 2-12 years Daily dose (mg/kg/day)			Adults Daily dose (mg/day)			Elderly Daily dose (mg/day)		
AED	**Low**	**Average**	**High**	**Low**	**Average**	**High**	**Low**	**Average**	**High**
Carbamazepine	10	20	30	400	800	1800	400	600	1000
*Clobazam**	*0.4*	*0.8*	*1.2*	*10*	*20*	*40*	*10*	*20*	*30*
*Clonazepam**	*0.05*	*0.1*	*0.2*	*0.5*	*4*	*10*	*0.5*	*1*	*2*
*Ethosuximide**	*10*	*20*	*35*	*750*	*1000*	*1500*	*750*	*1000*	*1500*
*Gabapentin**	*30*	*50*	*100*	*900*	*1800*	*3000*	*900*	*1800*	*2700*
Lamotrigine	3	7	10	60	250	500	100	200	300
*Levetiracetam**	*15*	*30*	*45*	*1000*	*2000*	*3000*	*500*	*1000*	*1500*
Oxcarbazepine	20	30	45	800	1000	2200	600	800	1500
Phenobarbitone	3	5	8	100	200	350	50	100	150
Phenytoin	5	10	15	200	400	600	100	300	400
Tiagabine	0.5	1.5	2	20	35	50	15	25	35
Topiramate	3	5	9	200	300	500	100	150	200
Valproate	10	20	30	500	1500	3000	500	1000	2000
*Viagabatrin**	*50*	*100*	*200*	*1000*	*2000*	*3000*	*500*	*1500*	*2000*
Zonisamide	4	7	12	200	400	600	100	300	400

*AEDs in italics (clobazam, clonazepam, ethosuximide, gabapentin, levetiracetam and viagabatrin) are the only ones that do not have clinically meaningful drug–drug interactions. All others, if used in polytherapy, sometimes need very significant dosage adjustments (lamotrigine and tiagabine for example).

course of their disorder or not at all.[115,116] The reasons for this delay include the fears of the patients and physicians about surgery and undue reliability on new AEDs and vagus nerve stimulation in patients who failed to respond to appropriate medical treatment for years.[115]

The applications and outcomes of surgical interventions in certain types of intractable seizures and epileptic syndromes are detailed in the relevant chapters of this book. This section refers to general aspects of surgery in epilepsies.

Surgical treatment for epilepsy need not be a last resort
Often successful surgery, particularly in children, is too late to reverse the crippling psychological and social consequences of repeated epileptic seizures at ages critical for the acquisition of interpersonal and vocational skills and seizure-free patients remain disabled indefinitely.[115]

CRITERIA FOR SURGERY REFERRAL

A candidate for epilepsy surgery must have failed to attain adequate seizure control with appropriate trials of anticonvulsant drugs (drug-resistant epilepsy) and/or suffer from surgically remediable syndromes and have a reasonable chance of benefiting from surgery. An adequate medication trial must be considered within the context of the individual and the individual's epilepsy.

DRUG-RESISTANT EPILEPSY FOR THE PURPOSES OF SURGICAL REFERRAL

The ILAE subcommittee on Surgery proposed (in the year 2000) that drug-resistant epilesy should be defined by inadequate response to a minimum of two first-line AEDs, either as monotherapy or in combination, as appropriate for the epileptic syndrome.[105] They recommended at least 2 years of treatment in adults but this may be too long for children with regard to the consequences of continuing seizures on their development.[105] Engel[91] proposed that, when there is failure of phenytoin, carbamazepine and valproate to control these patients' seizures, their cases should be considered medically refractory because additional medications have little chance of producing significant benefit.

This concept has been revised recently because, with the introduction of new AEDs, it would now literally take a lifetime to prove that epileptic seizures are unresponsive to every AED in every possible combination.[117] Therefore, medical refractoriness can no longer be a prerequisite for surgical referral

The concept of surgically remediable epileptic syndromes

The concept of surgically remediable epileptic syndromes was introduced in order to promote early surgical intervention for certain forms of epilepsy with well-defined pathophysiological substrates that are known to have a poor prognosis after failure of a few AEDs and an excellent surgical prognosis.[117]

The main surgically remediable epileptic syndromes are as follows.

- Mesial temporal lobe epilepsy with hippocampal sclerosis, which is their prototype (Chapter 12).[115] This is the commonest form of human epilepsy, the most refractory to AEDs, the easiest to diagnose non-invasively and has an excellent outcome if treated surgically.[114,115,118,119]

Following temporal lobe surgery, approximately one in four adult patients and approximately one in three children or adolescents can currently be shown to be seizure free for 5 years without AEDs.[119]

- Certain other temporal or extra-temporal neocortical symptomatic focal syndromes with discrete easily resectable structural lesions.[115]
- Epilepsies of infants and small children that can be treated by hemispherectomy.

STRATEGY OF A SURGICAL WORK-UP

A pre-surgical evaluation and surgery should be carried out in designated centres specialised in these procedures, which also may be different in children and adults with epilepsies.

A pre-surgical evaluation of candidates for surgery includes clinical, neuroimaging, neurophysiological and neuropsychological investigations.

- An accurate diagnosis based on a meticulous ictal and inter-ictal clinical history.
- Neuroradiological investigations and particularly high-resolution MRI often supplemented with functional brain imaging.
- Neurophysiological identification of the epileptogenic brain region.
- Neuropsychological evaluation to reveal possible cognitive and linguistic deficits and to predict the effect of cortical resection.
- Quality of life and psychiatric assessment.

Subsequently, a decision is taken on the most appropriate surgical strategy and the potential outcome is estimated.

Resective surgery is most likely to be successful if the findings from different modalities are concordant regarding epileptogenic localisation.

Patients referred to specialised surgery centres should be warned of the following:

- waiting lists may be long
- evaluation procedures are often lengthy lasting for months
- they may not be suitable for surgery.

TYPES OF SURGICAL PROCEDURES

Surgery can be either:

- *curative* (also known as definitive), aiming at a suppression of the epileptogenic focus through a resective or a disconnective surgical procedure
- *palliative*, with the purpose of reducing the intensity and/or the frequency of a certain seizure type (callosotomy and multiple subpial transections).

CURATIVE (DEFINITIVE) SURGERY

In general, curative surgery physically removes seizure-producing brain tissue. Examples are lesionectomy of *small* epileptogenic lesions such as mesial temporal lobe sclerosis, tumours or vascular abnormalities and malformations of cortical development. Curative surgery has a significant chance of producing complete or at least a 90% improvement in seizures.

Focal resective procedure (lesionectomy)

This is the most common, important and rewarding of all surgical treatments for focal epilepsies. The aim is to resect the total irritative zone to a sufficient extent as to lead to the elimination of seizures.

Mesial temporal lobe epilepsy with hippocampal sclerosis benefits most from this procedure (see page 390). A class 1 randomised controlled trial of surgery for mesial temporal lobe epilepsy[114] found that 64% of those who received surgery were free of disabling seizures compared with 8% free in the group randomised to continued medical therapy. There was a significant improvement in quantitative quality-of-life scores and a trend towards better social function at the end of 1 year for patients in the surgical group, no surgical mortality and infrequent morbidity. Complications are rare, probably less than 1–2% overall and vary with the experience of the surgical team rather than the procedure.

Other temporal and extra-temporal resective surgery also produces excellent results (see the surgical treatment of relevant focal epilepsies). In these cases the discreteness of the lesion and its relationship to eloquent cortical areas are major determinants of surgical management and outcome.

The most difficult part of these operations is to define the whole area of this irritative brain tissue exactly, which frequently extends beyond the structural lesion visualised on neuroimaging or the epileptogenic cortical area generating inter-ictal spikes. Where there is no discrete lesion (probably focal symptomatic epilepsies) functional MRI (fMRI) and both acute and chronic electrophysiological recordings may be helpful in determining the extent of the resection.

Often surgical problems may be difficult, needing complex investigative tools such as fMRI or magnetoencephalography, invasive recording and operating with neuronavigation and possibly intra-operative MRI.[113]

Resective surgery in hypothalamic (gelastic) epilepsy has now improved but still has high operative risks.

Cerebral hemispherectomy

Cerebral hemispherectomy for intractable seizures has evolved over the past 50 years and current operations focus less on brain resection and more on disconnection.[120-123]

The main indications are intractable seizures secondary to gross unilateral hemispheric pathology with severe contralateral (to the lesion) neurological deficit including hemianopia. Common conditions where hemispherectomy is recommended are Kozhevnikov–Rasmussen syndrome (p. 207), hemiconvulsion–hemiplegia syndrome (p. 215), hemimegalencephaly and miscellaneous hemispheric residual atrophic or other lesions including Sturge–Weber disease. The structural and functional integrity of the other hemisphere should be appropriately verified.

Seizure outcome is excellent with three-quarters (58–78%) of patients becoming seizure free and it is generally perceived that behaviour and intellectual performance improve in these patients. Outcome is related to the completeness of disconnection and less so to aetiology, although those with malformations of cortical development appear to do worse than others. Operative mortality is low (0–6%).

FUNCTIONAL (PALLIATIVE) SURGERY

Functional surgery is designed to improve seizures by modification of the neuronal pathways responsible for their generation and spread. Its purpose is to reduce the intensity and frequency of certain seizure types. It rarely (3–5%) results in freedom from seizures. Procedures comprise corpus callosotomy and multiple subpial transactions.

Corpus callosotomy

Corpus callosotomy,[124-128] that is surgical division of the corpus callosum, is the only procedure for devastating atonic seizures with traumatic falls (drop attacks) of epileptic encephalopathies (Chapter 7). A favourable outcome, from a >50% reduction to occasional complete cessation of these seizures, is obtained in 60–80% of patients. Improvements (40–80%) have also been reported in symptomatic tonic seizures and less often secondarily GTCS according to the extension of the section. These are cases of symptomatic secondarily generalised epilepsy with EEG bifrontal epileptic foci with secondary bilateral synchrony. Global behavioural and intellectual improvement may occur particularly if surgery is performed early. Other types of seizures are not indicated for callosotomy even though some improvement may be observed.

Despite improvements and modifications of corpus callosotomy with sequential radiofrequency lesions and stereotactic radiosurgery, morbidity is relatively high and there is a tendency for seizures to return after 2 years. More intense focal seizures may occur post-operatively.

Multiple subpial transections

Multiple subpial transactions[129-136] is a novel surgical technique invented by F. Morrell[129,137] for intractable focal epilepsies involving eloquent motor-, sensory- or language-important cortex and Landau–Kleffner syndrome. This technique eliminates the capacity of cortical tissue for generating seizures while preserving the normal cortical physiological function.

The rationale of the technique is based on the observation that horizontal fibres of the cortex facilitate the propagation of epileptic discharge while the vertical fibres subserve function. Thus, surgical division of the tangential fibres at regular intervals in a cortical epileptogenic area would permanently disrupt side-to-side intracortical synchronising neural networks and curtail the epileptic discharges. Function is preserved because these right-angle cuts to the pial surface should not disrupt cortex–subcortical input–output interactions.

The success of the technique depends on selection of cases with a severe epileptogenic abnormality that can be demonstrated to be unilateral in origin despite a bilateral electrographic manifestation.

STIMULATION TECHNIQUES

Neural stimulation is a new technology for the treatment of medically and/or surgically intractable seizures.[138,139] Vagus nerve stimulation (VNS) is the only method currently licensed in several countries as an adjunctive therapy.

Direct deep brain stimulation is being evaluated for clinical purposes in a number of centres. The rationale is that it has been applied with some success to the cerebellum, caudate nucleus, centromedian thalamus, anterior thalamus, subthalamus, hippocampus and directly to the neocortical seizure foci. Some preliminary results are encouraging, but not conclusive and the methods are still at experimental stages.[138,139]

Furthermore, systems are being developed to apply a stimulus when a seizure is impending with the aim to terminate the electrical discharge prior to serious clinical events. The hardware and software of such 'closed loop' systems are complex and impractical for long-term use but have still shown promise.[140]

Transcranial magnetic stimulation is simple and non-invasive, but the therapeutic results in patients with epilepsies are equivocal at best.[141-143]

VAGUS NERVE STIMULATION

VNS is an invasive non-pharmacological treatment licensed since 1997 for drug-resistant focal epilepsy with or without secondarily GTCS in patients over the age of 12 years.[108,144-163]

EFFICACY

In two pivotal well-controlled trials of patients with focal seizures, there was an ~28% reduction in the total seizure frequency during treatment relative to baseline. This refers to high VNS groups, which did significantly better than low stimulation groups. Subsequent unblinded studies concluded that efficacy improved further with continuing VNS treatment over 1 year and that one in five patients had at least a >75% seizure reduction at 12 months.

Systematic reviews of the current evidence for the effects of VNS in intractable focal seizures have concluded that this is an effective and well-tolerated treatment.[149] In general, one-third of patients show a >50% reduction in seizure frequency (but seizure freedom is exceptional), one-third show a 30–50% seizure reduction and one-third of patients show no response.[145] Concomitant AEDs may be reduced, but I am not aware of any reports of patients where all drugs were withdrawn, thereby using VNS as monotherapy. All patients stay on at least one medication in addition to the VNS. On anecdotal evidence, improvement is not immediate but increases over 18–24 months of treatment.[144] Most studies report subjective improvements in various quality-of-life measurements during treatment with VNS and objective trials have confirmed this observation.[144]

In practice VNS has been used for a variety of intractable epilepsies including young children with epileptic encephalopathies, but the results are often conflicting, ranging from good to no effect. In one of the best controlled studies, 16 children with epileptic encephalopathies were treated with VNS and followed up for 3 years.[155,161] There were significant fluctuations in effectiveness, but at the end of the study all children were no better than their pre-VNS baselines regarding seizures and parameters of quality of life.[155]

ADVERSE REACTIONS

- *Surgery-related complications.* Infection (3%), which may demand the removal of the device (1%), vocal cord dysfunction (hoarseness and dysphagia) (1%), facial nerve palsy, Horners' syndrome, bradycardia and exceptionally asystole (0.1%), wound haematoma and lead breakage (0.1%) and aesthetic complications from the incisions (prevalence unknown).
- *Peri-operative adverse reactions.* Pain (29%), coughing (14%), voice alteration (13%), chest pain (12%) and nausea (10%).
- *During treatment.* Hoarseness (37%), throat pain (11%), coughing (7%), dyspnoea (6%), paraesthesia (6%), muscle pain (6%) and discomfort in the face or neck when the stimulator is activated. All are related to the intensity of stimulation, can often be reduced by adjusting the generator's programme and may habituate in most subjects.

There are no apparent effects of VNS on vagally mediated visceral functions or AED serum concentrations. No adverse cognitive or systemic effects are associated with the use of the implanted vagus nerve stimulator.

TECHNICAL ASPECTS

The VNS device (manufactured by Cyberonics, Inc., Houston, Texas, USA) consists of a small (52 mm in diameter and 6.9 mm thick) battery-powered electrical pulse generator implanted under the skin of the left chest. This is linked to the stimulating spring-shaped electrodes (2 mm or 3 mm in diameter) that are wrapped around the main trunk of the left vagus nerve via an under-the-skin insulated cable.

The pulse generator is individually programmed to stimulate the nerve automatically at varying frequencies, typically for 30 s every 5 min, through a computer and a hand-held 'wand'. The frequency is adjusted to the patient's needs.

The treating physician makes readjustments to the programming and stimulus output.

In addition, the patient or carer can activate extra-stimulation at pre-programmed settings through a magnet passed over the generator. This is to shorten or terminate a seizure as soon as possible after its onset. Keeping the magnet over the generator turns off the stimulation.

SURGICAL PROCEDURE

The implantation of the VNS therapeutic device is a surgical procedure requiring general anaesthesia. It is usually performed by an experienced neurosurgeon and it takes approximately 1–2 h. The generator is inserted in the hollow below the clavicle through an incision in the left axilla. The electrodes are inserted through an incision in the left side of the neck. Patients usually go home the same day the VNS device is implanted.

The cost is substantial. In addition to the cost for hospitalisation and the operation, the cost of the VNS device is approximately $15 600. The battery lasts between 3 and 5 years (10 years in the current versions) and is replaced by a small operation under local anaesthesia. A replacement VNS device with new battery is $11 600.

ENVIRONMENTAL PRECAUTIONS FOR THOSE TREATED WITH VAGUS NERVE STIMULATION

Strong magnets such those as of MRI, loudspeakers and hair clippers may interfere with the stimulator or the electrode leads. Body MRI is contra-indicated, while head MRI should only be done with transmit-and-receive head coils.

In general 'avoid areas where pacemaker warning signs are posted'.

The magnet provided for manual stimulation may damage credit cards, mobile phones, computer disks, televisions and other items affected by strong magnetic fields. Care should be taken to store the magnet away from these types of equipment.

WHAT IS THE PLACE OF VAGUS NERVE STIMULATION IN THE TREATMENT OF EPILEPSIES?

This is a question I have tried to answer by studying the following.

- Reports fulfilling the requirements of evidence-based medicine. These document that VNS is effective in intractable focal epilepsies (when multiple polytherapy has failed) and may improve quality of life.[164-166] Similar studies on the effect of VNS in epileptic encephalopathies have been disappointing.[155,161]
- Reports from uncontrolled studies, case reports and their reviews. These are also in favour of VNS in a number of intractable epileptic disorders including epileptic encephalopathies.[144,145,151,154,167,168]
- Patients in my own clinic and the opinion of expert paediatric and adult epileptologists. This is far less enthusiastic.

  'a few patients may improve'.

  'some patients have fewer hospital admissions'.

  'I would try it in patients who had failed AED therapy and are not suitable for operation but I would not give great hope to the patient who may also have to meet a significant cost'.

  'an expensive and useless exercise in epileptic encephalopathies'.

The truth may be somewhere in between these views.

REFERENCES

1. Faught E, Pellock JM,eds. Matching the medicine to the patient. *Epilepsia* 2001;**42 Suppl 8**:1-38.
2. Bourgeois BF. New antiepileptic drugs in children: which ones for which seizures? *Clin Neuropharmacol.* 2000;**23**:119-32.
3. Camfield PR, Camfield CS. Treatment of children with "ordinary" epilepsy. *Epileptic Disord.* 2000;**2**:45-51.
4. Kaminska A. New antiepileptic drugs in childhood epilepsies: indications and limits. *Epileptic Disord.* 2001;**3 Suppl 2**:SI37-SI46.
5. Kopec K. New anticonvulsants for use in pediatric patients (part I). *J Pediat Health Care* 2001;**15**:81-6.
6. Pellock JM, Dodson WE, Bourgeois BFD, eds. Pediatric epilepsy. New York: Demos, 2001.
7. Camfield P, Camfield C. Childhood epilepsy: what is the evidence for what we think and what we do? *J Child Neurol.* 2003;**18**:272-87.
8. Pellock JM. Antiepileptic Drugs in Children with Developmental Delays and Behavioral Problems. *Curr Treat Options Neurol.* 2003;**5**:121-8.
9. Willmore LJ. Choice and use of newer anticonvulsant drugs in older patients. *Drugs Aging* 2000;**17**:441-52.
10. Tallis RC. Management of epilepsy in the elderly person. In Shorvon S, Perucca E, Fish D, Dodson E, eds. *The treatment of epilepsy (2nd edition)*, pp 201-14. Oxford: Blackwell Publishing, 2004.
11. Bergey GK. Initial treatment of epilepsy: special issues in treating the elderly. *Neurology* 2004;**63**:S40-S48.
12. Briggs DE, French JA. Levetiracetam safety profiles and tolerability in epilepsy patients. *Expert Opin Drug Saf* 2004;**3**:415-24.
13. Crawford P, Appleton R, Betts T, Duncan J, Guthrie E, Morrow J. Best practice guidelines for the management of women with epilepsy. The Women with Epilepsy Guidelines Development Group. *Seizure* 1999;**8**:201-17.
14. Morrell MJ. Epilepsy in women: the science of why it is special. *Neurology* 1999;**53**:S42-8.
15. Bauer J, Isojarvi JI, Herzog AG, Reuber M, Polson D, Tauboll E *et al.* Reproductive dysfunction in women with epilepsy: recommendations for evaluation and management. *J Neurol Neurosurg Psychiatry* 2002;**73**:121-5.
16. Bruno MK, Harden CL. Epilepsy in Pregnant Women. *Curr Treat Options Neurol.* 2002;**4**:31-40.
17. Karceski S, Morrell MJ. Women with epilepsy: current treatment strategies. *J Gend Specif Med.* 2002;**5**:22-6.
18. McAuley JW,Anderson GD. Treatment of epilepsy in women of reproductive age: pharmacokinetic considerations. *Clin Pharmacokinet.* 2002;**41**:559-79.
19. Yerby MS. Management issues for women with epilepsy: neural tube defects and folic acid supplementation. *Neurology* 2003;**61**:S23-S26.
20. Yerby MS. Clinical care of pregnant women with epilepsy: neural tube defects and folic acid supplementation. *Epilepsia* 2003;**44 Suppl 3**:33-40.
21. Boon P, Hauman H, Legros B, Sadzot B, van Rijckevorsel K, Van Zandycke M. Belgian consensus on recommendations for standards of care for women with epilepsy before, during and after pregnancy. *Acta Neurol Belg.* 2004;**104**:6-12.
22. Tatum WO, Liporace J, Benbadis SR, Kaplan PW. Updates on the treatment of epilepsy in women. *Arch Intern Med.* 2004;**164**:137-45.
23. Kaplan PW. Reproductive health effects and teratogenicity of antiepileptic drugs. *Neurology* 2004;**63**:S13-S23.
24. Brobtkorb E. Management of epilepsy in people with learning difficulties. In Shorvon S, Perucca E, Fish D, Dodson E, eds. *The treatment of epilepsy (2nd edition)*, pp 215-26. Oxford: Blackwell Publishing, 2004.
25. Gil-Nagel A. Review of new antiepileptic drugs as initial therapy. *Epilepsia* 2003;**44 Suppl 4**:3-10.
26. Hart YM. Management of newly diagnosed epilepsy. In Shorvon S, Perucca E, Fish D, Dodson E, eds. *The treatment of epilepsy (2nd edition)*, pp 161-73. Oxford: Blackwell Publishing, 2004.
27. Perucca E. General principles of medical treatment. In Shorvon S, Perucca E, Fish D, Dodson E, eds. *The treatment of epilepsy (2nd edition)*, pp 139-59. Oxford: Blackwell Publishing, 2004.
28. Genton P, Gelisse P, Thomas P, Dravet C. Do carbamazepine and phenytoin aggravate juvenile myoclonic epilepsy? *Neurology* 2000;**55**:1106-9.
29. Benbadis SR, Tatum WO, Gieron M. Idiopathic generalized epilepsy and choice of antiepileptic drugs. *Neurology* 2003;**61**:1793-5.
30. Panayiotopoulos CP, Benbadis SR, Covanis A, Dulac O, Duncan JS, Eeg-Olofsson O *et al.* Efficacy and tolerability of the new antiepileptic drugs; commentary on the recently published practice parameters. *Epilepsia* 2004;**45**:1646-9.
31. Gelisse P, Genton P, Kuate D, Pesenti A, Baldy-Moulinier M, Crespel A. Worsening of seizures by oxcarbazepine in juvenile idiopathic generalized epilepsies. *Epilepsia* 2004;**45**:1282-8.
32. Greenwood RS. Adverse effects of antiepileptic drugs. *Epilepsia* 2000;**41 Suppl 2**:S42-S52.
33. Gilliam FG, Fessler AJ, Baker G, Vahle V, Carter J, Attarian H. Systematic screening allows reduction of adverse antiepileptic drug effects: a randomized trial. *Neurology* 2004;**62**:23-7.
34. French JA, Kanner AM, Bautista J, Abou-Khalil B, Browne T, Harden CL *et al.* Efficacy and tolerability of the new antiepileptic drugs II: treatment of refractory epilepsy: report of the Therapeutics and Technology Assessment Subcommittee and Quality Standards Subcommittee of the American Academy of Neurology and the American Epilepsy Society. *Neurology* 2004;**62**:1261-73.
35. French JA, Kanner AM, Bautista J, Abou-Khalil B, Browne T, Harden CL *et al.* Efficacy and tolerability of the new antiepileptic drugs I: treatment of new onset epilepsy: report of the Therapeutics and Technology Assessment Subcommittee and Quality Standards Subcommittee of the American Academy of Neurology and the American Epilepsy Society. *Neurology* 2004;**62**:1252-60.
36. French JA, Kanner AM, Bautista J, Abou-Khalil B, Browne T, Harden CL *et al.* Efficacy and Tolerability of the New Antiepileptic Drugs, II: Treatment of Refractory Epilepsy: Report of the TTA and QSS Subcommittees of the American Academy of Neurology and the American Epilepsy Society. *Epilepsia* 2004;**45**:410-23.
37. French JA, Kanner AM, Bautista J, Abou-Khalil B, Browne T, Harden CL *et al.* Efficacy and Tolerability of the New Antiepileptic Drugs, I: Treatment of New-Onset Epilepsy: Report of the TTA and QSS Subcommittees of the American Academy of Neurology and the American Epilepsy Society. *Epilepsia* 2004;**45**:401-9.
38. French JA. Response: efficacy and tolerability of the new antiepileptic drugs. *Epilepsia* 2004;**45**:1649-51.
39. Panayiotopoulos CP. Importance of specifying the type of epilepsy. *Lancet* 1999;**354**:2002-3.
40. King MA, Newton MR, Jackson GD, Berkovic SF. Epileptology of the first-seizure presentation: a clinical, electroencephalographic, and magnetic imaging study of 300 consecutive patients. *Lancet* 1998;**352**:1007-11.
41. Privitera MD, Brodie MJ, Mattson RH, Chadwick DW, Neto W, Wang S. Topiramate, carbamazepine and valproate monotherapy: double-blind comparison in newly diagnosed epilepsy. *Acta Neurol Scand.* 2003;**107**:165-75.
42. Hamer HM, Morris HH. Hypersensitivity syndrome to antiepileptic drugs: a review including new anticonvulsants. *Cleve Clin J.Med.* 1999;**66**:239-45.
43. Beller TC, Boyce JA. Prolonged anticonvulsant hypersensitivity syndrome related to lamotrigine in a patient with human immunodeficiency virus. *Allergy Asthma Proc.* 2002;**23**:415-9.

44. Baba M, Karakas M, Aksungur VL, Homan S, Yucel A, Acar MA *et al.* The anticonvulsant hypersensitivity syndrome. *J Eur Acad Dermatol Venereol.* 2003;**17**:399-401.

45. Sheth RD. Metabolic concerns associated with antiepileptic medications. *Neurology* 2004;**63**:S24-S29.

46. Nieto-Barrera M, Nieto-Jimenez M, Candau R, Ruiz dP. Anhidrosis and hyperthermia associated with treatment with topiramate. *Rev Neurol.* 2002;**34**:114-6.

47. de Carolis P, Magnifico F, Pierangeli G, Rinaldi R, Galeotti M, Cevoli S *et al.* Transient hypohidrosis induced by topiramate. *Epilepsia* 2003;**44**:974-6.

48. French JA. Antiepileptic Drugs: Don't Sweat It! *Epilepsy Curr.* 2004;**4**:33-4.

49. Lesser RP. Psychogenic seizures. *Neurology* 1996;**46**:1499-507.

50. Schmidt D. Strategies to prevent overtreatment with antiepileptic drugs in patients with epilepsy. *Epilepsy Res.* 2002;**52**:61-9.

51. Chadwick D. Monotherapy comparative trials: equivalence and differences in clinical trials. *Epilepsy Res.* 2001;**45**:101-3.

52. Taylor S, Tudur S, Williamson PR, Marson AG. Phenobarbitone versus phenytoin monotherapy for partial onset seizures and generalized onset tonic-clonic seizures. *Cochrane.Database.Syst.Rev.* 2001;CD002217.

53. French JA,.Schachter S. A workshop on antiepileptic drug monotherapy indications. *Epilepsia* 2002;**43 Suppl 10**:3-27.

54. Gilliam FG. Limitations of monotherapy trials in epilepsy. *Neurology* 2003;**60**:S26-S30.

55. Gates JR. Using New Antiepileptic Drugs As Monotherapy. *Curr Treat Options Neurol* 2004;**6**:223-30.

56. Kwan P, Brodie MJ. Effectiveness of first antiepileptic drug. *Epilepsia* 2001;**42**:1255-60.

57. The renaissance of rational polytherapy: the new generation of antiepileptic medications. *Neurology* 1995;**45**:S35-S38.

58. Schmidt D. Modern management of epilepsy: Rational polytherapy. *Baillieres Clin Neurol* 1996;**5**:757-63.

59. Deckers CL, Czuczwar SJ, Hekster YA, Keyser A, Kubova H, Meinardi H *et al.* Selection of antiepileptic drug polytherapy based on mechanisms of action: the evidence reviewed. *Epilepsia* 2000;**41**:1364-74.

60. Gilliam F, Vazquez B, Sackellares JC, Chang GY, Messenheimer J, Nyberg J *et al.* An active-control trial of lamotrigine monotherapy for partial seizures (a reply). *Neurology* 2000;**54**:777-8.

61. Kwan P, Sills GJ, Brodie MJ. The mechanisms of action of commonly used antiepileptic drugs. *Pharmacol Ther.* 2001;**90**:21-34.

62. Lynch BA, Lambeng N, Nocka K, Kensel-Hammes P, Bajjalieh SM, Matagne A *et al.* The synaptic vesicle protein SV2A is the binding site for the antiepileptic drug levetiracetam. *Proc Natl Acad.Sci.U.S.A* 2004;**101**:9861-6.

63. Baulac M. Rational conversion from antiepileptic polytherapy to monotherapy. *Epileptic Disord.* 2003;**5**:125-32.

64. Schmidt D, Elger C, Holmes GL. Pharmacological overtreatment in epilepsy: mechanisms and management. *Epilepsy Res.* 2002;**52**:3-14.

65. Commission on Antiepileptic Drugs, International League Against Epilepsy. Guidelines for therapeutic monitoring on antiepileptic drugs. *Epilepsia* 1993;**34**:585-7.

66. Glauser TA. Expanding first-line therapy options for children with partial seizures. *Neurology* 2000;**55**:S30-S37.

67. Glauser TA, Pippenger CE. Controversies in blood-level monitoring: reexamining its role in the treatment of epilepsy. *Epilepsia* 2000;**41 Suppl 8**:S6-15.

68. Troupin AS. Antiepileptic drug therapy: A clinical overview. In Wyllie E, ed. *The treatment of epilepsy:Principles and practice*, pp 785-90. Philadelphia: Lea & Febiger, 1993.

69. Tran TA, Leppik IE, Blesi K, Sathanandan ST, Remmel R. Lamotrigine clearance during pregnancy. *Neurology* 2002;**59**:251-5.

70. de Haan GJ, Edelbroek P, Segers J, Engelsman M, Lindhout D, Devile-Notschaele M *et al.* Gestation-induced changes in lamotrigine pharmacokinetics: a monotherapy study. *Neurology* 2004;**63**:571-3.

71. Pennell PB, Newport DJ, Stowe ZN, Helmers SL, Montgomery JQ, Henry TR. The impact of pregnancy and childbirth on the metabolism of lamotrigine. *Neurology* 2004;**62**:292-5.

72. Sabers A, Ohman I, Christensen J, Tomson T. Oral contraceptives reduce lamotrigine plasma levels. *Neurology* 2003;**61**:570-1.

73. Contin M, Riva R, Albani F, Avoni P, Baruzzi A. Topiramate therapeutic monitoring in patients with epilepsy: effect of concomitant antiepileptic drugs. *Ther Drug Monit.* 2002;**24**:332-7.

74. Chong E, Dupuis LL. Therapeutic drug monitoring of lamotrigine. *Ann Pharmacother.* 2002;**36**:917-20.

75. Johannessen SI, Battino D, Berry DJ, Bialer M, Kramer G, Tomson T *et al.* Therapeutic drug monitoring of the newer antiepileptic drugs. *Ther Drug Monit.* 2003;**25**:347-63.

76. Jannuzzi G, Cian P, Fattore C, Gatti G, Bartoli A, Monaco F *et al.* A multicenter randomized controlled trial on the clinical impact of therapeutic drug monitoring in patients with newly diagnosed epilepsy. The Italian TDM Study Group in Epilepsy. *Epilepsia* 2000;**41**:222-30.

77. Bauer J, Reuber M. Medical treatment of epilepsy. *Expert Opin Emerg Drugs* 2003;**8**:457-67.

78. Bourgeois BF. Chronic management of seizures in the syndromes of idiopathic generalized epilepsy. *Epilepsia* 2003;**44 Suppl 2**:27-32.

79. Coppola G. Treatment of partial seizures in childhood : an overview. *CNS Drugs* 2004;**18**:133-56.

80. Brodie MJ,.French JA. Role of levetiracetam in the treatment of epilepsy. *Epileptic Disord.* 2003;**5 Suppl 1**:S65-S72.

81. Faught E. Clinical trials for treatment of primary generalized epilepsies. *Epilepsia* 2003;**44 Suppl 7**:44-50.

82. Nguyen DK, Spencer SS. Recent advances in the treatment of epilepsy. *Arch Neurol.* 2003;**60**:929-35.

83. Ryvlin P, Kahane P, Semah F, Hirsch E, Arzimanoglou A, Thomas P. Should new generation antiepileptic drugs be prescribed as first-line treatment of newly diagnosed epilepsy in adolescents and adults?. *Rev Neurol.(Paris)* 2003;**159**:936-41.

84. Sander JW. The natural history of epilepsy in the era of new antiepileptic drugs and surgical treatment. *Epilepsia* 2003;**44 Suppl 1**:17-20.

85. Sirven JI. The current treatment of epilepsy: a challenge of choices. *Curr Neurol Neurosci Rep.* 2003;**3**:349-56.

86. Wheless JW. Acute management of seizures in the syndromes of idiopathic generalized epilepsies. *Epilepsia* 2003;**44 Suppl 2**:22-6.

87. Wheless JW, Sankar R. Treatment Strategies for Myoclonic Seizures and Epilepsy Syndromes with Myoclonic Seizures. *Epilepsia* 2003;**44 Suppl 11**:27-37.

88. Patsalos PN, Perucca E. Clinically important drug interactions in epilepsy: general features and interactions between antiepileptic drugs. *Lancet Neurol* 2003;**2**:347-56.

89. Patsalos PN, Perucca E. Clinically important drug interactions in epilepsy: interactions between antiepileptic drugs and other drugs. *Lancet Neurol.* 2003;**2**:473-81.

90. Tidwell A, Swims M. Review of the newer antiepileptic drugs. *Am J Manag Care* 2003;**9**:253-76.

91. LaRoche SM,.Helmers SL. The new antiepileptic drugs: scientific review. *JAMA* 2004;**291**:605-14.

92. Shorvon S, Perucca E, Fish D, Dodson E, eds. The treatment of epilepsy (2nd edition). *The treatment of epilepsy (2nd edition)*, pp 1-913. Oxford: Blackwell Publishing, 2004.

93. Perucca E. NICE guidance on newer drugs for epilepsy in adults. *BMJ* 2004;**328**:1273-4.

94. Mayor S. NICE gives guidance on use of new antiepileptic drugs in children. *BMJ* 2004;**328**:1093.

95. Langley PC. The NICE reference case requirement: implications for drug manufacturers and health systems. *Pharmacoeconomics.* 2004;**22**:267-71.

96. Beghi E. Efficacy and tolerability of the new antiepileptic drugs: comparison of two recent guidelines. *Lancet Neurol.* 2004;**3**:618-21.

97. Walker MC, Sander JW. Difficulties in extrapolating from clinical trial data to clinical practice: the case of antiepileptic drugs. *Neurology* 1997;**49**:333-7.

98. Shorvon SD. The choice of drugs and approach to drug treatments in partial epilepsy. In Shorvon S, Perucca E, Fish D, Dodson E, eds. *The treatment of epilepsy (2nd edition)*, pp 317-33. Oxford: Blackwell Publishing, 2004.

99. Mohanraj R, Brodie MJ. Measuring the efficacy of antiepileptic drugs. *Seizure.* 2003;**12**:413-43.

100. Hovinga CA. Levetiracetam: a novel antiepileptic drug. *Pharmacotherapy* 2001;**21**:1375-88.

101. Patsalos PN. Pharmacokinetic profile of levetiracetam: toward ideal characteristics. *Pharmacol.Ther.* 2000;**85**:77-85.

102. Anderson GD. Pharmacogenetics and enzyme induction/inhibition properties of antiepileptic drugs. *Neurology* 2004;**63**:S3-S8.

103. Danielson PB. The cytochrome P450 superfamily: biochemistry, evolution and drug metabolism in humans. *Curr Drug Metab* 2002;**3**:561-97.

104. Patsalos PN. The pharmacokinetic characteristics of levetiracetam. *Methods Find Exp Clin Pharmacol.* 2003;**25**:123-9.

105. Binnie CD, Polkey CE, eds. Commission on Neurosurgery of the International League Against Epilepsy (ILAE) 1993-1997: recommended standards. *Epilepsia* 2000;**41**:1346-9.

106. Jones MW, Andermann F. Temporal lobe epilepsy surgery: definition of candidacy. *Can J Neurol Sci.* 2000;**27 Suppl 1**:S11-S13.

107. Wieser HG, Blume WT, Fish D, Goldensohn E, Hufnagel A, King D *et al.* ILAE Commission Report. Proposal for a new classification of outcome with respect to epileptic seizures following epilepsy surgery. *Epilepsia* 2001;**42**:282-6.

108. Buchhalter JR, Jarrar RG. Therapeutics in pediatric epilepsy, Part 2: Epilepsy surgery and vagus nerve stimulation. *Mayo Clin Proc.* 2003;**78**:371-8.

109. Hardy SG, Miller JW, Holmes MD, Born DE, Ojemann GA, Dodrill CB *et al.* Factors predicting outcome of surgery for intractable epilepsy with pathologically verified mesial temporal sclerosis. *Epilepsia* 2003;**44**:565-8.

110. Shaefi S, Harkness W. Current status of surgery in the management of epilepsy. *Epilepsia* 2003;**44 Suppl 1**:43-7.

111. Zimmerman RS, Sirven JI. An overview of surgery for chronic seizures. *Mayo Clin Proc.* 2003;**78**:109-17.

112. Schmidt D, Baumgartner C, Loscher W. Seizure recurrence after planned discontinuation of antiepileptic drugs in seizure-free patients after epilepsy surgery: a review of current clinical experience. *Epilepsia* 2004;**45**:179-86.

113. Polkey CE. Clinical outcome of epilepsy surgery. *Curr Opin Neurol.* 2004;**17**:173-8.

114. Wiebe S, Blume WT, Girvin JP, Eliasziw M. A randomized, controlled trial of surgery for temporal-lobe epilepsy. *N Engl J Med.* 2001;**345**:311-8.

115. Engel J, Jr., Wiebe S, French J, Sperling M, Williamson P, Spencer D *et al.* Practice parameter: temporal lobe and localized neocortical resections for epilepsy. *Epilepsia* 2003;**44**:741-51.

116. Berg AT. Understanding the delay before epilepsy surgery: who develops intractable focal epilepsy and when? *CNS Spectr.* 2004;**9**:136-44.

117. Engel J, Jr. Surgery for seizures. *N Engl J Med* 1996;**334**:647-52.

118. Wieser HG. ILAE Commission Report. Mesial temporal lobe epilepsy with hippocampal sclerosis. *Epilepsia* 2004;**45**:695-714.

119. Schmidt D, Baumgartner C, Loscher W. The chance of cure following surgery for drug-resistant temporal lobe epilepsy What do we know and do we need to revise our expectations? *Epilepsy Res.* 2004;**60**:187-201.

120. Villemure JG, Rasmussen T. Functional hemispherectomy in children. *Neuropediatrics* 1993;**24**:53-5.

121. Devlin AM, Cross JH, Harkness W, Chong WK, Harding B, Vargha-Khadem F *et al.* Clinical outcomes of hemispherectomy for epilepsy in childhood and adolescence. *Brain* 2003;**126**:556-66.

122. Cook SW, Nguyen ST, Hu B, Yudovin S, Shields WD, Vinters HV *et al.* Cerebral hemispherectomy in pediatric patients with epilepsy: comparison of three techniques by pathological substrate in 115 patients. *J Neurosurg.* 2004;**100**:125-41.

123. Pulsifer MB, Brandt J, Salorio CF, Vining EP, Carson BS, Freeman JM. The cognitive outcome of hemispherectomy in 71 children. *Epilepsia* 2004;**45**:243-54.

124. Rougier A, Claverie B, Pedespan JM, Marchal C, Loiseau P. Callosotomy for intractable epilepsy: overall outcome. *J Neurosurg Sci.* 1997;**41**:51-7.

125. Pendl G, Eder HG, Schroettner O, Leber KA. Corpus callosotomy with radiosurgery. *Neurosurgery* 1999;**45**:303-7.

126. Pinard JM, Delalande O, Chiron C, Soufflet C, Plouin P, Kim Y *et al.* Callosotomy for epilepsy after West syndrome. *Epilepsia* 1999;**40**:1727-34.

127. Pressler RM, Binnie CD, Elwes RD, Polkey CE. Return of generalized seizures and discharges after callosotomy. *Adv Neurol* 1999;**81**:171-82.

128. Kwan SY, Wong TT, Chang KP, Yang TF, Lee YC, Guo WY *et al.* Postoperative seizure outcome after corpus callosotomy in reflex epilepsy. *Chung Hua I Hsueh Tsa Chih (Taipei)* 2000;**63**:240-6.

129. Morrell F, Whisler WW, Bleck TP. Multiple subpial transection: a new approach to the surgical treatment of focal epilepsy. *J Neurosurg.* 1989;**70**:231-9.

130. Smith MC, Byrne R. Multiple subpial transection in neocortical epilepsy: Part I. *Adv Neurol.* 2000;**84**:621-34.

131. Wyler AR. Multiple subpial transections in neocortical epilepsy: Part II. *Adv Neurol.* 2000;**84**:635-42.

132. Mulligan LP, Spencer DD, Spencer SS. Multiple subpial transections: the Yale experience. *Epilepsia* 2001;**42**:226-9.

133. Polkey CE. Multiple subpial transection: a clinical assessment. *Int Rev Neurobiol.* 2001;**45**:547-69.

134. Shimizu T, Maehara T, Hino T, Komori T, Shimizu H, Yagishita A *et al.* Effect of multiple subpial transection on motor cortical excitability in cortical dysgenesis. *Brain* 2001;**124**:1336-49.

135. Faught E. Collective Data Supports Efficacy of Multiple Subpial Transection. *Epilepsy Curr.* 2002;**2**:108.

136. Spencer SS, Schramm J, Wyler A, O'Connor M, Orbach D, Krauss G *et al.* Multiple subpial transection for intractable partial epilepsy: an international meta-analysis. *Epilepsia* 2002;**43**:141-5.

137. Morrell F, Whisler WW, Smith MC, Hoeppner TJ, de Toledo-Morrell L, Pierre-Louis SJ *et al.* Landau-Kleffner syndrome. Treatment with subpial intracortical transection. *Brain* 1995;**118**:1529-46.

138. Theodore WH,.Fisher RS. Brain stimulation for epilepsy. *Lancet Neurol.* 2004;**3**:111-8.

139. Chkhenkeli SA, Sramka M, Lortkipanidze GS, Rakviashvili TN, Bregvadze ES, Magalashvili GE *et al.* Electrophysiological effects and clinical results of direct brain stimulation for intractable epilepsy. *Clin Neurol Neurosurg.* 2004;**106**:318-29.

140. Goodman JH. Brain stimulation as a therapy for epilepsy. *Adv Exp Med Biol.* 2004;**548**:239-47.

141. Tassinari CA, Cincotta M, Zaccara G, Michelucci R. Transcranial magnetic stimulation and epilepsy. *Clin Neurophysiol.* 2003;**114**:777-98.

142. Theodore WH. Transcranial Magnetic Stimulation in Epilepsy. *Epilepsy Curr.* 2003;**3**:191-7.

143. Brasil-Neto JP, de Araujo DP, Teixeira WA, Araujo VP, Boechat-Barros R. Experimental therapy of epilepsy with transcranial magnetic stimulation: lack of additional benefit with prolonged treatment. *Arq Neuropsiquiatr.* 2004;**62**:21-5.

144. Ben Menachem E. Vagus-nerve stimulation for the treatment of epilepsy. *Lancet Neurol.* 2002;**1**:477-82.

145. Boon P, Vonck K, De Reuck J, Caemaert J. Vagus nerve stimulation for refractory epilepsy. *Seizure* 2002;**11 Suppl A**:448-55.

146. George MS, Nahas Z, Bohning DE, Kozel FA, Anderson B, Chae JH *et al.* Vagus nerve stimulation therapy: a research update. *Neurology* 2002;**59**:S56-S61.

147. Heck C, Helmers SL, DeGiorgio CM. Vagus nerve stimulation therapy, epilepsy, and device parameters: scientific basis and recommendations for use. *Neurology* 2002;**59**:S31-S37.

148. Henry TR. Therapeutic mechanisms of vagus nerve stimulation. *Neurology* 2002;**59**:S3-14.

149. Privitera MD, Welty TE, Ficker DM, Welge J. Vagus nerve stimulation for partial seizures. *Cochrane.Database.Syst.Rev.* 2002;CD002896.

150. Schachter SC. Vagus nerve stimulation: where are we? *Curr Opin Neurol.* 2002;**15**:201-6.

151. Schachter SC. Vagus nerve stimulation therapy summary: five years after FDA approval. *Neurology* 2002;**59**:S15-S20.

152. Wilber DJ, Morton JB. Vagal stimulation and atrial fibrillation: experimental models and clinical uncertainties. *J Cardiovasc Electrophysiol.* 2002;**13**:1280-2.

153. Frost M, Gates J, Helmers SL, Wheless JW, Levisohn P, Tardo C *et al.* Vagus nerve stimulation in children with refractory seizures associated with Lennox-Gastaut syndrome. *Epilepsia* 2001;**42**:1148-52.

154. Helmers SL, Wheless JW, Frost M, Gates J, Levisohn P, Tardo C *et al.* Vagus nerve stimulation therapy in pediatric patients with refractory epilepsy: retrospective study. *J Child Neurol.* 2001;**16**:843-8.

155. Parker AP, Polkey CE, Robinson RO. Vagal nerve stimulation in the epileptic encephalopathies: 3-year follow-up. *Pediatrics* 2001;**108**:221.

156. Winston KR, Levisohn P, Miller BR, Freeman J. Vagal nerve stimulation for status epilepticus. *Pediatr Neurosurg.* 2001;**34**:190-2.

157. Binnie CD. Vagus nerve stimulation for epilepsy: a review. *Seizure* 2000;**9**:161-9.

158. Murphy JV, Wheless JW, Schmoll CM. Left vagal nerve stimulation in six patients with hypothalamic hamartomas. *Pediatr Neurol* 2000;**23**:167-8.

159. Aicardi J. Vagal nerve stimulation in epileptic encephalopathies. *Pediatrics* 1999;**103**:821-2.

160. Camfield PR, Camfield CS. Vagal nerve stimulation for treatment of children with epilepsy [editorial]. *J Pediatr.* 1999;**134**:532-3.

161. Parker AP, Polkey CE, Binnie CD, Madigan C, Ferrie CD, Robinson RO. Vagal nerve stimulation in epileptic encephalopathies. *Pediatrics* 1999;**103**:778-82.

162. Fisher RS, Krauss GL, Ramsay E, Laxer K, Gates J. Assessment of vagus nerve stimulation for epilepsy: report of the Therapeutics and Technology Assessment Subcommittee of the American Academy of Neurology. *Neurology* 1997;**49**:293-7.

163. McLachlan RS. Vagus nerve stimulation for intractable epilepsy: a review. *J Clin Neurophysiol.* 1997;**14**:358-68.

164. Buoni S, Mariottini A, Pieri S, Zalaffi A, Farnetani MA, Strambi M *et al.* Vagus nerve stimulation for drug-resistant epilepsy in children and young adults. *Brain Dev.* 2004;**26**:158-63.

165. Holmes MD, Silbergeld DL, Drouhard D, Wilensky AJ, Ojemann LM. Effect of vagus nerve stimulation on adults with pharmacoresistant generalized epilepsy syndromes. *Seizure* 2004;**13**:340-5.

166. Uthman BM, Reichl AM, Dean JC, Eisenschenk S, Gilmore R, Reid S *et al.* Effectiveness of vagus nerve stimulation in epilepsy patients: a 12-year observation. *Neurology* 2004;**63**:1124-6.

167. Park YD. The effects of vagus nerve stimulation therapy on patients with intractable seizures and either Landau-Kleffner syndrome or autism. *Epilepsy Behav.* 2003;**4**:286-90.

168. Sheth RD, Stafstrom CE. Intractable pediatric epilepsy: vagal nerve stimulation and the ketogenic diet. *Neurol.Clin.* 2002;**20**:1183-94.

NEONATAL SEIZURES AND NEONATAL SYNDROMES

5

NEONATAL SEIZURES

Neonatal seizures or neonatal convulsions are epileptic fits occurring from birth to the end of the neonatal period. [1-18] The neonatal period is the most vulnerable of all periods of life for developing seizures, particularly in the first 1–2 days to the first week from birth. They may be short-lived events lasting for a few days only. However, they often signify serious malfunction of or damage to the immature brain and constitute a neurological emergency demanding urgent diagnosis and management.

DEMOGRAPHIC DATA

The prevalence is approximately 1.5% and overall incidence approximately 3 per 1000 live births. The incidence in pre-term infants is very high (57–132 per 1000 live births). Most (80%) neonatal seizures occur in the first 1–2 days to the first week of life.

CLINICAL MANIFESTATIONS

Neonatal seizures, as with any other type of seizure, are paroxysmal, repetitive and stereotypical events. They are usually clinically subtle, inconspicuous and difficult to recognise from the normal behaviours of the inter-ictal periods or physiological phenomena. There is no recognisable post-ictal state. Generalised tonic clonic seizures (GTCS) are exceptional. The most widely used scheme is by Volpe[20] of five main types of neonatal seizure.

- **Subtle seizures (50%)**
- **Tonic seizures (5%)**
- **Clonic seizures (25%)**
- **Myoclonic seizures (20%)**
- **Non-paroxysmal repetitive behaviours**

Useful definitions

The neonatal period is defined as the first 28 days of life of a full-term infant.

Neonatal seizures are those that occur from birth to the end of the neonatal period.

Gestational age is defined as the duration of pregnancy.

Chronological age is the actual legal age of the infant from the time of birth.

Conceptional age is the combined gestational and chronological ages.

Full-term infants are those of 40 weeks gestational age.

ILAE classification and definitions

The ILAE Commission (1989)[19] broadly classifies neonatal seizures amongst 'epilepsies and syndromes undetermined as to whether they are focal or generalised' under the subheading 'with both generalised and focal seizures'.

Neonatal seizures differ from those of older children and adults. The most frequent neonatal seizures are described as subtle because the clinical manifestations are frequently overlooked. These include tonic, horizontal deviation of the eyes with or without jerking, eyelid blinking or fluttering, sucking, smacking or other oral–buccal–lingual movements, swimming or pedalling movements and, occasionally, apnoeic spells. Other neonatal seizures occur as tonic extension of the limbs, mimicking decerebrate or decorticate posturing. These occur particularly in premature infants. Multifocal clonic seizures characterised by clonic movements of a limb, which may migrate to other body parts or other limbs or focal clonic seizures, which are much more localised, may occur. In the latter, the infant is usually not unconscious. Rarely, myoclonic seizures may occur and the EEG pattern is frequently that of suppression–burst activity. The tonic seizures have a poor prognosis because they frequently accompany intraventricular haemorrhage. The myoclonic seizures also have a poor prognosis because they are frequently a part of the early myoclonic encephalopathy syndrome.[19]

In another scheme by Mizrahi[12] neonatal seizures are classified as follows: focal clonic, focal tonic, generalised tonic, myoclonic, spasms and motor automatisms (which include occular signs, oral–buccal–lingual movements, progression movements and complex purposeless movements).

Nearly one-quarter of infants experience several seizure types and the same seizure may manifest with subtle, clonic, myoclonic, autonomic or other symptoms (Figure 5.1).

SUBTLE SEIZURES

Subtle seizures are far more common than other types of neonatal seizures. They are described as *subtle* because the clinical manifestations are frequently overlooked. They imitate normal behaviours and reactions. These include the following.

a *Ocular movements,* which range from random and roving eye movements to sustained conjugate tonic deviation with or without jerking. Eyelid blinking or fluttering, eyes rolling up, eye opening, fixation of a gaze or nystagmus may occur alone or with other ictal manifestations.

b *Oral–buccal–lingual movements* (sucking, smacking, chewing and tongue protrusions).

c *Progression movements* (rowing, swimming, pedalling, bicycling, thrashing or struggling movements).

d *Complex purposeless movements* (sudden arousal with episodic limb hyperactivity and crying).[15]

MOTOR SEIZURES

Clonic seizures are rhythmic jerks that may localise in a small part of the face or limbs, axial muscles and the diaphragm or be multifocal or hemiconvulsive. Todd's paresis follows prolonged hemiconvulsions.

Tonic seizures manifest with sustained contraction of facial, limb, axial and other muscles. They may be focal, multifocal or generalised, symmetrical or asymmetrical. Truncal or limb tonic extension imitates decerebrate or decorticate posturing.

Myoclonic seizures are rapid, single or arrhythmic repetitive jerks. They may affect a finger, a limb or the whole body. They may mimic the Moro reflex and startling responses. They are more frequent in pre-term than full-term infants indicating, if massive, major brain injury and poor prognosis. Myoclonic seizures are associated with the most severe brain damage.[21] However, healthy pre-term and rarely full-term neonates may have abundant myoclonic movements during sleep. Neonates have cortical, reticular and segmental types of myoclonus, similar to adult forms.[22]

Spasms producing flexion or extension similar to those of West syndrome are rare. They are slower than myoclonic seizures and faster than tonic seizures.

AUTONOMIC ICTAL MANIFESTATIONS

Autonomic ictal manifestations commonly occur with motor manifestations in 37% of subtle seizures.[23,24] These are paroxysmal changes of heart rate, respiration and systemic blood pressure.[25,26] Apnoea as an isolated seizure phenomenon unaccompanied by other clinical epileptic features is probably exceptional.[26] Salivation and pupillary changes are common.

DURATION OF NEONATAL SEIZURES

The duration of neonatal seizures is usually brief (10 s to 1–2 min) and repetitive with a median of 8 min in between each seizure. Longer seizures and status epilepticus develop more readily at this age, but convulsive neonatal status epilepticus is not as severe as that of older infants and children.

NON-EPILEPTIC NEONATAL SEIZURES

By definition all neonatal seizures are epileptic in origin, generated by abnormal, paroxysmal and hypersynchronous neuronal discharges characteristic of epileptogenesis.

The characterisation of neonatal seizures as epileptic and non-epileptic by Kellaway and Mizrahi[4,10,27] is a topic of considerable debate.

Epileptic neonatal seizures. Focal clonic, focal tonic and some types of myoclonic jerks are genuine epileptic seizures documented with ictal EEG changes and they have a high correlation with focal brain lesions and a favourable short-term outcome.[4,10,27]

Non-epileptic neonatal seizures. Many of the subtle seizures, generalised tonic posturing and some myoclonic symptoms may be non-epileptic seizures. These show clinical similarities to reflex behaviours of the neonates, they are not associated with ictal EEG discharges and are commonly correlated with diffuse abnormal brain processes such as hypoxic–ischaemic encephalopathy and a poor short-term outcome.[4,10,27] They are considered as exaggerated reflex behaviours due to abnormal release of brain stem tonic mechanisms from cortical control. Hence, the term *brain stem release phenomena*:[4,27] *"They most typically occur in neonates with clinical and EEG evidence of forebrain depression that may release brain stem facilitatory centres for generating reflex behaviours without cortical inhibition"*.[4,10,27]

The argument to support the non-epileptic nature of these episodic clinical events is that they have the following characteristics.[4,10,27]

- They are suppressed by restraint or repositioning of the infant.
- They are elicited by tactile stimulation and their intensity is proportional to the rate, intensity and number of sites of stimulation. Stimulation at one site can provoke paroxysmal movements at another site.
- They are not associated with ictal EEG discharges.

Reservations about these features are based on the following reasons.

- The electrical seizure activity may occur deep within brain structures that are inaccessible to an EEG. This is well documented in neurosurgical patients with simultaneous surface and deep EEG recordings.
- The responses to stimulation and restraint are also well-known phenomena of genuine epileptic seizures (see photic and tactile stimulation and inhibition).

AETIOLOGY

Aetiology of neonatal seizures is extensive and diverse (Table 5.1). Severe causes predominate. The prevalence and significance of aetiological factors are continuously changing and differ between developed and developing countries depending on available improved neonatal and obstetric care.

By far the commonest cause is hypoxic–ischaemic encephalopathy. It may be responsible for 80% of all seizures in the first 2 days of life.[28] Brain damage due to prenatal distress and malformations of cortical development is being increasingly recognised . Intracranial haemorrhage and infarction, stroke[29] and prenatal and neonatal infections are common. Most previously common acute metabolic disturbances such as electrolyte and glucose abnormalities have been minimised

Table 5.1 Main causes of neonatal seizures

Cause	*Frequency*
Hypoxia-ischaemia – prenatal (toxaemia, fetal distress, abruptio placentae, cord compression) – perinatal (iatrogenic, maternal haemorrhage, fetal distress) – postnatal (cardio-respiratory causes such as hyaline membrane disease, congenital heart disease, pulmonary hypertension)	+++++++
Haemorrhage and intracerebral infarction – intraventricular and periventricular (mainly preterm neonates) – intracerebral (spontaneous, traumatic) – subarachnoid – subdural haematoma – cerebral artery and vein infarction	++++
Trauma – intracranial haemorrhage – cortical vein thrombosis	++++
Infections – encephalitis, meningitis, brain abscess – intrauterine (rubella, toxoplasmosis, syphilis, viral – such as cytomegalovirus, herpes simplex virus, human immunodeficiency virus, coxsackie virus B) – postnatal (beta-haemolytic streptococci, *Escherichia coli* infection, herpes simplex virus, *Mycoplasma*)	++++
Metabolic – hypoglycaemia (glucose levels <20 mg/d in preterm and, <30 mg/d in full-term babies indicating hypoglycaemia; mainly associated with prenatal or perinatal insults) – neonates of diabetic and toxaemic mothers – pancreatic disease – glucogen storage disease (idiopathic) – hypocalcaemia (early, in first 2–3 days, mainly in preterm neonates with prenatal or perinatal insults; late, at 5–14 days, is mainly nutritional; maternal hyperparathyroidism; DiGeorge's syndrome) – hypomagnesaemia (may accompany or occur independently of hypocalcaemia) – hyponatraemia (mainly associated with prenatal or perinatal insults; inappropriate secretion of antidiuretic hormone) – hypernatraemia (mainly nutritional or iatrogenic) – inborn errors of metabolism (amino acid and organic acid disorders, hyperammonaemias; they usually manifest with peculiar odours, protein intolerance, acidosis, alkalosis, lethargy, or stupor) – pyridoxine dependency	++
Malformations of cerebral development – all disorders of neuronal induction, segmentation, migration, myelination and synaptogenesis such as polymicrogyria, neuronal heterotopias, lissencephaly, holoprosencephaly, and hydranencephaly	++
Neurocutaneous syndromes – tuberous sclerosis, incontinentia pigmenti	++++
Drug withdrawal and toxic – withdrawal from narcotic-analgesics, sedative-hypnotics, and alcohol; heroin- and methadone-addicted mothers; barbiturates	+++
Inadvertent injections of local anaesthetics during delivery	++
Idiopathic benign neonatal seizures (familial and non-familial)	++

because of improved neonatal intensive care and awareness of nutritional hazards. Late hypocalcaemia is virtually eliminated, while electrolytic derangement and hypoglycaemia are now rare.

Inborn errors of metabolism such as urea cycle disorders are rare.[10,20,30,31]

Pyridoxine dependency, with seizures in the first days of life (which are reversible with treatment), is exceptional.

Exogenous causes of neonatal convulsions may be iatrogenic or due to drug withdrawal in babies born to mothers on drugs.[24]

In most cases, the neonate may present with a combination of different neurological disturbances, each of which can cause seizures.

PATHOPHYSIOLOGY

The early postnatal development time is a period of increased susceptibility to seizures in relation to other ages. This may be due to a combination of factors specific to the developing brain that enhance excitation and diminish inhibition. There is an unequal distribution of anticonvulsant and proconvulsant neurotransmitters and networks.[13,32,33]

Animal studies are contradictory regarding the effect of prolonged epileptic seizures on the developing immature brain.[34-36]

See also the pathophysiology of individual neonatal syndromes detailed in this section.

DIAGNOSTIC PROCEDURES

Neonatal seizures represent one of the very few emergencies in the newborn. Abnormal, repetitive and stereotypic behaviours of neonates should be suspected and evaluated as possible seizures. Polygraphic video–EEG recording of suspected events is probably mandatory for an incontrovertible seizure diagnosis. Confirmation of neonatal seizures should initiate urgent and appropriate clinical and laboratory evaluation for the aetiological cause (Table 5.1) and treatment. Family and prenatal history is important. A thorough physical examination of the neonate should be coupled with urgent and comprehensive biochemical tests for correctable metabolic disturbances. Although rare, more severe inborn errors of metabolism should be considered for diagnosis and treatment.

BRAIN IMAGING

Cranial ultrasonography, brain imaging with X-ray computed tomography (CT) scan and preferably magnetic resonance imaging (MRI)[37]should be used for the detection of structural abnormalities such as malformations of cortical development, intracranial haemorrhage, hydrocephalus and cerebral infarction.

Cranial ultrasonograghy is the main imaging modality of premature neonates and well suited for the study of neonates in general. It is performed at the bedside and provides effective assessment of ventricular size and other fluid-containing lesions as well as effective viewing of haemorrhagic and ischaemic lesions and their evolution. Cranial ultrasonography is limited in resolution and the type of lesions that it can identify.

A CT brain scan is often of secondary or adjunctive importance to ultrasound. Last-generation CT brain scan images are of high resolution, can be generated within seconds and can accurately detect haemorrhage, infarction, gross malformations and ventricular and other pathological conditions. A CT scan has low sensitivity in many other brain conditions such as abnormalities of cortical development where *MRI is much superior*. However, MRI interpretation should take into consideration the normal developmental and maturational states of

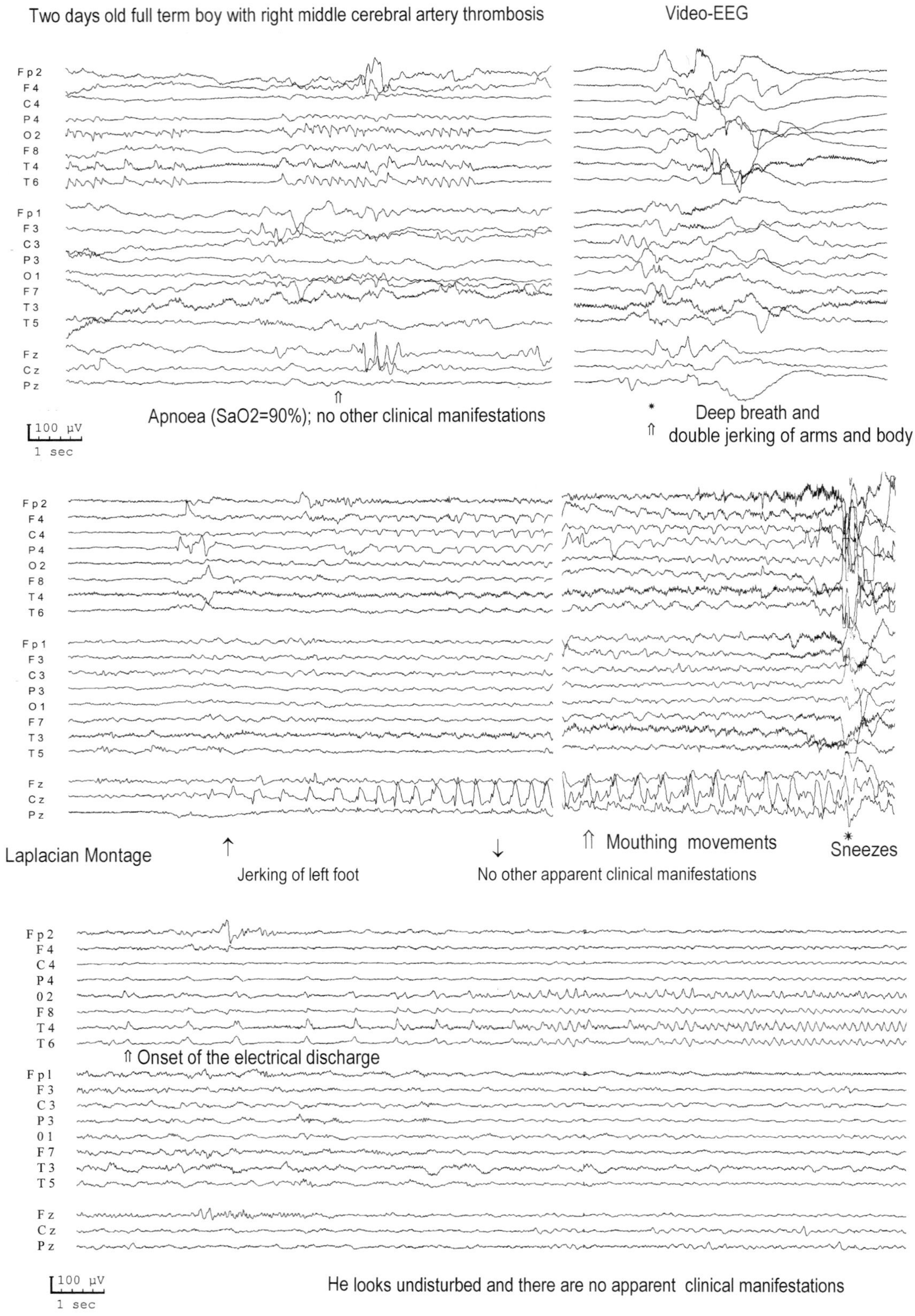

Figure 5.1 Ictal EEG patterns in a 2-day-old boy with right middle cerebral artery thrombosis

Top and middle: Apnoeic, myoclonic, clonic and subtle seizure of motor automatisms associated with various ictal EEG patterns and locations.

Bottom: "Electroclinical dissociation": the electrical discharge is not associated with apparent clinical manifestations.

neonates and infants. In infants younger than 6 months, cortical abnormalities are detected with T2-weighted images, whereas T1-weighted images are needed for the evaluation of brain maturation.[37]

ELECTROENCEPHALOGRAPHY

The neonatal EEG is probably one of the best and most useful of EEG applications.[10,38-45] However, neonatal EEG recordings and interpretations require the special skills of well-trained technologists and physicians. Polygraphic studies with simultaneous video–EEG recording are essential.[46]

Only 10% of neonates with suspected seizures have EEG confirmation. Suspected clonic movements have the highest yield of 44% but this is only 17% for 'subtle' movements.[47]

Inter-ictal EEG

Inter-ictal EEG epileptogenic spikes or sharp slow wave foci are not reliable markers at this age.

Certain inter-ictal EEG patterns may have diagnostic significance (Figure 5.2 and 5.3.)[4,10]

- Electrocerebral inactivity of a flat or near-flat EEG of severe brain damage.
- The suppression–burst pattern of neonatal epileptic encephalopathies (Figure 5.4).
- Theta pointu alternant of benign neonatal convulsions (Figure 5.3).
- Persistently focal sharp or slow waves in localised lesions.
- Quasi-periodic focal or multifocal pattern in neonatal herpes simplex encephalitis.[48]
- Periodic complexes in glycine encephalopathy.[31,49]
- Inter-hemispheric or intra-hemispheric abnormalities.

Background EEG activity, mainly in serial EEGs, often provides objective evidence of the degree and severity of the underlying cause.[4,10,31,49]

Important note on the suppression–burst pattern

The suppression–burst pattern is relatively frequent in the neonatal period. It is associated with heterogeneous seizures and can be induced by drugs.[50,51] It is common in neonatal ischaemic encephalopathy where it is usually transient and short lived.[50] Conversely, the suppression–burst pattern is relatively stable lasting for more than 2 weeks in Ohtahara syndrome and early myoclonic encephalopathy.[52]

Ictal EEG

Documentation of seizures with an ictal EEG is often mandatory in view of the subtle clinical seizure manifestations (Figures 5.1 and 5.2). EEG ictal activity may be focal or multifocal appearing in a normal or abnormal background. The electrical ictal seizure EEG patterns of neonatal seizures vary significantly even in the same neonate and in the same EEG recording (Figure 5.1). The same EEG may show focal or multifocal ictal discharges that may occur simultaneously or independently in different brain locations.

Ictal EEG paroxysms consist of repetitive waves with a predominant beta, alpha, theta and delta range or a mixture of all that may accelerate in speed, decelerate in speed or both (Figures 5.1 and 5.2). These are spikes, sharp or saw tooth or sinusoidal waves (monomorphic or polymorphic) ranging in amplitude from very low to very high. The patterns may be synchronous or asynchronous, focal or multifocal and, less frequently, generalised. They may appear and disappear suddenly or build up from accelerating localised repetitive waves. Ictal discharges may gradually or abruptly change in frequency, amplitude and

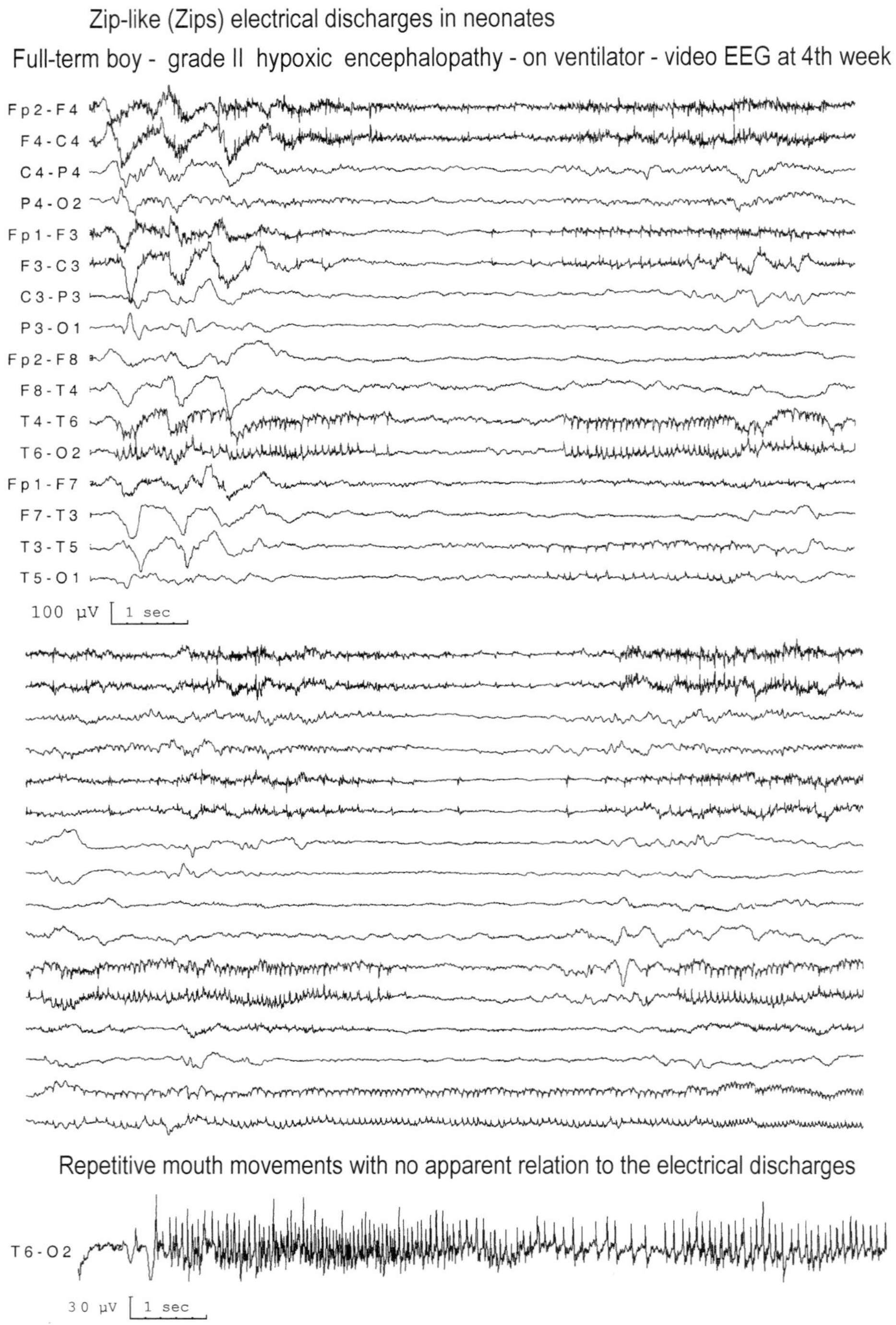

Figure 5.2 Zip-like electrical discharges

Top and middle: Continuous recording in a neonate with severe brain hypoxia. Zip-like electrical discharges consist of high frequency rapid spikes of accelerating and decelerating speed. They start from various locations, terminating in one while continuing in another.

Bottom: Amplification of zips with high sensitivity in T6-O2 derivation.

Definition of zips

Zips. This is a descriptive term I coined for a common ictal EEG pattern in neonates which consists of localised episodic rapid spikes of accelerating and decelerating speed that look like zips (Figure 5.2). Zips may be associated with subtle and focal clonic/tonic seizures or remain clinically silent. Zips of subtle seizures are often multifocal and of shifting localisation.

morphology in the course of the same or subsequent seizures. Conversely, they may remain virtually unchanged from onset to termination. The background EEG may be normal or abnormal.

Focal EEG ictal discharges are usually associated with subtle, clonic or tonic seizures. The most common locations are the centrotemporal followed by the occipital regions. Midline (Cz) and temporal regions may be involved but frontal localisations are exceptional. The same infant may have unifocal or multifocal ictal discharges that may be simultaneous, develop one from the other or occur independently in different brain sites. Neonates do not show the clinical or EEG Jacksonian march of older children. There may be abrupt changes of location in the progress of the seizure.

Seizures with consistently focal EEG paroxysms are highly correlated with focal brain lesions. Seizures that lack or have an inconstant relationship with EEG discharges correlate with diffuse pathological conditions.

Generalised manifestations are more likely to occur with myoclonic jerks and neonatal spasms.

Two specific electrical seizure patterns of neonates usually carry a poor prognosis because they are 'typically associated with severe encephalopathies'.[10,27,53,54]

1 *Alpha seizure discharges* are characterised by sustained and rhythmic activity of 12 Hz and 20–70 μV in the centrotemporal regions.
2 *Electrical seizure activity of the depressed brain* is of low voltage and long duration. It is highly localised on one side and shows little tendency to spread.

Post-ictal EEG

Post-ictally, the EEG usually returns to the pre-ictal state immediately (Figure 5.1). Transient slowing or depression of EEG activity may occur following frequent or prolonged seizures.

Stimulus-evoked electrographic patterns

Stimulus-evoked electrographic patterns with or without concomitant clinical ictal manifestations usually occur in pre-term neonates or neonates with significant diffuse or multifocal brain damage.[55] The electrographic seizures are elicited by tactile or painful stimulation. The majority of neonates die or have significant neurological handicaps.

ELECTROCLINICAL DISSOCIATION OR DECOUPLING RESPONSE

Only one-fifth (21%) of electrical ictal EEG patterns (*electrical or electrographic seizures*) associate with distinctive clinical manifestations (*electroclinical seizures*). All others are occult, that is they are clinically silent or subclinical.[56]

Electrographic or electrical seizures, namely EEG electrical seizure activity without apparent clinical manifestations, are more common after initiation of anti-epileptic drugs (AEDs). This is because AEDs may suppress the clinical manifestations of seizures but not the EEG ictal discharge. This phenomenon is named the *'decoupling response'*[10,27,53] or *'electroclinical dissociation'*.[57,58] Electroclinical dissociation may arise from foci not consistently reflected in surface electrodes.[57]

Neonates with electrographic seizures do not differ from those with exclusively electroclinical seizures regarding peri-natal factors, aetiology or outcome, though the background EEG is more abnormal in the electrographic group.[57] Movements of the limbs occur at a statistically significant higher rate during electroclinical seizures. Electrographic seizures, like electroclinical seizures, are also associated with disturbed cerebral metabolism.[59]

PROGNOSIS

This is cause dependent because the main factor that determines outcome is the underlying cause and not the seizures themselves. Despite high mortality (approximately 15%) and morbidity (approximately 30%), one-half of neonates with seizures achieve a normal or near normal state. One-third of the survivors develop epilepsy.[60] Table 5.2 provides indicators of good, bad or intermediate prognosis.

DIFFERENTIAL DIAGNOSIS

Neonatal seizures often impose significant difficulties in their recognition and differentiation from normal or abnormal behaviours of the pre-term and full-term neonate.[4,10]

As a rule any suspicious repetitive and stereotypical events should be considered as possible seizures requiring video–EEG recording confirmation.

Normal behaviours. Amongst normal behaviours neonates may stretch, exhibit spontaneous sucking movements and have random and non-specific movements of the limbs. Intense physiological myoclonus may occur during rapid eye movement sleep. Jitteriness or tremulousness of the extremities or facial muscles is frequent in normal or abnormal neonates.

Tremor has a symmetrical 'to and fro' motion, is faster than clonic seizures, mainly affects all four limbs and will stop when the limb is restrained or repositioned. Conversely, clonic seizures are mainly focal, usually have a rate of 3–4 Hz or slower, decelerate in the progress of the attack and they are not interrupted by passive movements.

Abnormal behaviours. Amongst abnormal behaviours of neonates with CNS disorders are episodic and repetitive oral–buccal–lingual movements. These are often reproducible with tactile or other stimuli and are interrupted by restraint. Conversely, neonatal seizures persist despite restraint and they are rarely stimulus sensitive.

Non-epileptic movement disorders. Neonatal seizures should be differentiated from benign neonatal sleep myoclonus, hyperekplexia and other non-epileptic movement disorders.

Table 5.2 Indicators of prognosis

Indicators of bad prognosis

- Severe hypoxia–ischaemia
- Severe congenital malformations of cortical development and meningoencephalitis
- Subtle and generalised tonic seizures
- Nearly flat EEG or of very low voltage and discontinuous EEG with bursts of high-voltage spikes and slow activity

Indicators of good prognosis

- Hypocalcaemia (alimentary type) and other transient metabolic changes
- Extracranial infections with seizures (otitis, pneumonia, gastroenteritis, etc.)
- Benign familial and non-familial convulsions
- Clonic seizures that are short and infrequent
- Normal inter-ictal EEG

Indicators of intermediate or guarded prognosis

- Moderately severe central nervous system (CNS) infections or malformations
- Most of the intracranial haemorrhages or infarctions
- More serious metabolic CNS disturbances
- EEG persistence of immature patterns
- Frequent or prolonged clonic seizures and clonic status epilepticus

Significant impairment of vital signs, which may be periodic, is mainly due to non-neurological causes. Changes in respiration, heart rate and blood pressure are exceptional sole manifestations of neonatal seizures.

Inborn errors of metabolism manifest with neonatal subtle seizures or abnormal movements that may not be genuine epileptic seizures. Their identity is often revealed by other associated significant symptoms, such as peculiar odours, protein intolerance, acidosis, alkalosis, lethargy or stupor. In most cases, pregnancy, labour and delivery are normal. Food intolerance may be the earliest indication of a systemic abnormality. If untreated, metabolic disorders commonly lead to lethargy, coma and death. In surviving infants weight loss, poor growth and failure to thrive are common.

MANAGEMENT [14,17,61]

This demands accurate aetiological diagnosis and treatment of the cause of the seizures. The principles of general medical management and cardiovascular and respiratory stabilisation should be early and appropriately applied. Cardiorespiratory symptoms may result from the underlying disease, the seizures and the anti-epileptic medication.

Neonatal seizures of metabolic disturbances need correction of the underlying cause and not anti-epileptic medication. A trial of pyridoxine may be justifiable.

The drug treatment of neonatal seizures is *empirical* with significant practice variations amongst physicians. Phenobarbitone first and then phenytoin are the most commonly used AEDs, although short-acting benzodiazepines are gaining ground. Large loading doses are followed by a maintenance scheme for a variable period.

Facts and requirements for the treatment of neonatal seizures

Neonatal seizures have a high prevalence and their response to anti-epileptic drugs (AEDs) is likely to be different to that of other specified groups of patients. Yet, current treatment of neonatal seizures is entirely empirical. Neonatologists rely on their medical judgment and "trials by success and error" with off-label use of new and old AEDs.

The authorities, including formal regulatory agents, should urgently address these issues.

Phenobarbitone and phenytoin. Phenobarbitone and phenytoin are equally but incompletely effective as anticonvulsants in neonates. Phenobarbitone in a loading dose of 15–20 mg/kg and a maintenance dose of 3–4 mg/kg daily controls one-third of neonatal seizures.[62] Efficacy may improve to 85% with stepwise increments to 40 mg/kg.[63] The serum levels required are between 16 and 40 μg/ml. Phenytoin may be equally as effective as phenobarbitone at a loading dose of 15–20 mg/kg.[64] With either drug given alone, the seizures are controlled in fewer than half of the neonates.[64] The severity of the seizures appears to be a stronger predictor of the success of treatment than the assigned AED. Mild seizures or seizures decreasing in severity before treatment are more likely to respond regardless of the treatment assignment.

Fosphenytoin. Fosphenytoin is an attractive alternative to phenytoin because of less potential for adverse reactions at the infusion site and the facility for intramuscular administration.[15] This needs further evaluation.

Other drugs. Intravenous benzodiazepines such as diazepam, lorazepam,[65] clonazepam and midazolam[66] are used particularly in Europe for acute neonatal seizures. They may be used as the first anti-seizure AED. However, in a recent randomised trial of second-line anticonvulsant treatments for neonates,[67] 11 out of 22 subjects responded to phenobarbitone at a dose of 40 mg/kg as first-line treatment. Three of five neonates treated with lignocaine responded. However, of 6 neonates treated with benzodiazepines as second-line treatment, none responded and their neurodevelopmental outcome was poor.[67]

Primidone, valproate, lignocaine,[68] *carbamazepine*[69] and *paraldehyde* (now not available in the USA) are also used mainly as adjunctive AEDs if others fail. Of the new AEDs *vigabatrin*[70] *and lamotrigine*[71] may be effective.

Maintenance treatment

Maintenance treatment may not be needed or be brief as the active seizure period in neonates is usually short. Less than 15% of infants with neonatal seizures will have recurrent seizures after the newborn period.[72] A normal EEG[73] and other predictors of good outcome[74] may encourage early discontinuation of treatment. The current trend is to withdraw the AED 2 weeks after the last seizure.

Do electrographic (electrical) seizures need treatment?

There is significant difference of opinion as to whether EEG electrical seizure activity that may persist despite drug control of clinical seizures needs more vigorous treatment. Electrical seizures may be highly resistant to drug treatment and attempts to eliminate them may require high doses of usually multiple drugs with significant adverse reactions such as CNS or respiratory depression and systemic hypotension. The risks should be weighed against the benefits while also remembering that these will eventual subside in time.

NEONATAL SYNDROMES

Despite the high prevalence of neonatal seizures, epileptic syndromes in neonates are rare. Four syndromes have been recognised by the ILAE.[19,75]

- **Benign familial neonatal seizures**
- **Benign neonatal seizures (non-familial)**
- **Early myoclonic encephalopathy**
- **Ohtahara syndrome**

BENIGN FAMILIAL NEONATAL SEIZURES

Benign familial neonatal seizures [76-80] constitute a rare autosomal dominant epileptic syndrome characterised by frequent brief seizures within the first days of life.

DEMOGRAPHIC DATA

Onset is commonly in the first week of life, mainly on the second or third day.[81] All 116 affected individuals in one study had seizures by 2–8 days of life.[81] The strict age dependence of the syndrome is indicated by the fact that affected premature babies develop seizures later.[6] Contrary to this, in one-third of patients seizures may start as late as 3 months of age.[82] Boys and girls are equally affected.

Changes in the new ILAE diagnostic scheme regarding the nomenclature and classification of neonatal syndromes

The 1989 ILAE classification considers 'benign familial neonatal convulsions' and 'benign neonatal convulsions (non-familial)' as 'idiopathic generalised epilepsies (age related)'.[19] The ILAE new diagnostic scheme abandons the name convulsions using instead seizures, thus also emphasising that these are 'conditions with epileptic seizures that do not require a diagnosis of epilepsy'.[75]

'Early myoclonic encephalopathy' and 'Ohtahara syndrome' are considered as 'generalised symptomatic epilepsies of non-specific aetiology (age related)'[19] by the 1989 ILAE classification. The new ILAE diagnostic scheme classified them as 'epileptic encephalopathies (in which the epileptiform abnormalities may contribute to progressive dysfunction)' (Chapter 7).

ILAE definition for benign neonatal familial convulsions

Benign neonatal familial convulsions are a rare, dominantly inherited disorder manifesting mostly on the second and third days of life, with clonic or apnoeic seizures and no specific EEG criteria. History and investigations reveal no aetiological factors. Approximately 14% of these patients later develop epilepsy.[19]

The syndrome appears to be rare but this may be under-recognised or not reported by the families who know its benign character from their own experience. So far 44 families with 355 affected members have been reported.[76] The incidence is 14.4 per 100 000 live births.[6]

CLINICAL MANIFESTATIONS

Seizures mainly occur in full-term normal neonates after a normal pregnancy and delivery and without precipitating factors. Seizures are brief, of 1–2 min and may be as frequent as 20–30 per day.

Most seizures start with tonic motor activity and posturing with apnoea followed by vocalisations, ocular symptoms, other autonomic features, motor automatisms, chewing and focal or generalised clonic movements.[76,77,83,84] The clonic components of the later phase are usually asymmetrical and unilateral. The post-ictal state is brief and inter-ictally the neonates are normal.

Pure clonic or focal seizures are considered rare.

AETIOLOGY

This is a genetically determined channelopathy of an autosomal dominant pattern of inheritance and a high degree (approximately 85%) of penetrance. Thus, 15% of those with a mutant gene are not clinically affected. The disease is caused by mutations in the voltage-gated potassium channel subunit gene *KCNQ2* on chromosome 20q 13.3[84,85] and *KCNQ3* on chromosome 8q.13.3.[86-91] More than 11 mutations have been identified in *KCNQ2*, but only two have been identified in *KCNQ3*.[92,93] Mutations in either *KCNQ2* or *KCNQ3* can produce the same phenotype.

Mutations in the sodium channel subunit gene *SCN2A* appear specific to 'benign familial neonatal-infantile seizures'*.[94]

PATHOPHYSIOLOGY

It appears that benign familial neonatal seizures are caused by a small loss of function of heteromeric voltage-gated potassium channels that decrease the potassium current. This impairs repolarisation of the neuronal cell membrane resulting in hyperexcitability of the brain that can produce seizures. It has also been postulated that a slight reduction in KCNQ channels alone cannot produce seizure activity, but can facilitate it under conditions of unbalanced neurotransmission, either by an increase in excitation or decrease in inhibition.[96] Thus, this unbalance in excitation and inhibition could be one possible explanation as to why the neonatal period is a vulnerable time for the seizures to occur. Another possibility is the differential expression of potassium channels during different stages of maturation.[80]

DIAGNOSTIC PROCEDURES

All relevant biochemical, haematological and metabolic screenings and brain imaging are normal.

ELECTROENCEPHALOGRAPHY

The inter-ictal EEG may be normal, discontinuous, have focal or multifocal abnormalities or have a theta pointu alternant pattern (Figure 5.3). The inter-ictal EEG is of limited value though it may exclude other causes of serious neonatal seizures.

Note on a recent development

'Benign familial neonatal–infantile seizures' is a newly described clinically intermediate variant between benign familial neonatal seizures and benign familial infantile seizures. The disorder can now be strongly suspected clinically and the families can be given an excellent prognosis.[94,95]

The ictal EEG commonly starts with a synchronous and bilateral flattening of 5–19 s coinciding with apnoea and tonic motor activity. This is followed by bilateral and often asymmetrical discharges of spikes and sharp waves with a duration of 1–2 min, which coincide with vocalisations, chewing and focal or generalised clonic activity.[76,77]

Conversely, seizure manifestations and the ictal EEG indicated focal seizures in a neonate,[97] had both focal and generalised features in another neonate[98] and had right frontal onset with or without generalisation in a third neonate.[99]

DIFFERENTIAL DIAGNOSIS

A family history of similar convulsions, a prerequisite for the diagnosis of benign familial neonatal seizures, eliminates the possibility of other diseases. However, other causes of neonatal seizures should be excluded.

Despite artificially similar names[3,75] benign familial neonatal seizures are entirely different from benign neonatal seizures (non-familial) (Table 5.3).

PROGNOSIS

Seizures remit between 1 and 6 months from onset; in 68% during the first 6 weeks. However, 10–14% may later develop other types of febrile (5%) or afebrile seizures. Afebrile seizures are not well defined in the relevant reports but they are probably heterogeneous. Idiopathic generalised seizures are more common. There have also been accounts of Rolandic seizures.

In some families none of the patients had seizures after the first 10 months of life, with long-term follow-up ranging from 10 months to 56 years.[100] In other reports a few patients[101] or 20%[102] continued having seizures in adult life. The subsequent risk of a recurrent seizure disorder depends on whether other affected relatives developed a seizure disorder later in life.[102]

The prevalence of mental retardation and learning disability is reported to be approximately 2.5%, which is not significantly different from the expected rate for the general population.[81]

Deaths during neonatal seizures are exceptional but they have been reported.[101]

MANAGEMENT

There is no consensus regarding treatment. Convulsions usually remit spontaneously without medication. The use of anti-epileptic medication does not influence the eventual outcome. Prolonged seizures may be shortened or terminated with benzodiazepines, phenobarbitone or phenytoin.

Table 5.3 Benign (non-familial) neonatal seizures versus benign familial neonatal seizures

	Benign (non-familial) neonatal seizures	Benign familial neonatal seizures
Main seizures	Mostly clonic	Tonic-clonic
Onset	Fifth day of life	Second or third day of life
Duration of seizures	Status epilepticus (median 20 hours)	Repetitive isolated seizures
Main causes	Unknown, probably environmental	Autosomal dominant
Subsequent seizures	Practically nil (0.5%)	Relatively high (11%)
Psychomotor deficits	Minor	Practically non-existent
Ictal EEG	Usually localised spikes	Usually generalised flattening
Interictal EEG	Usually theta pointu alternant	Normal or focal abnormalities

The family's reaction to and their fears about this inherited disease as well as means of appropriate consultations in order to reduce their magnitude should be appropriately considered.[103]

A normal boy started having frequent seizures at age 3 days. He had 4-8 stereotyped fits per 24 hours, awake or asleep. All seizures started with tonic motor activity and posturing with apnoea for 5-10 s followed by vocalisations, ocular symptoms, other autonomic features, motor automatisms, chewing and focal or generalised, asymmetrical, occasionally unilateral clonic movements.

All relevant tests including an inter-ictal EEG were normal.

Recommended treatment with valproate was vigorously rejected by the grandmother, a dominant member of the family, who herself, her father and two of her 4 children had similar neonatal seizures without any residuals or consequences in their successful lives. The boy continued having his habitual seizures up to the age of 6 weeks. He was normal in between the fits. On last follow-up at age 2 years he is an entirely normal child for his age. "The granny was right again" the family admitted.

BENIGN NEONATAL SEIZURES (NON-FAMILIAL)

Benign neonatal seizures (non-familial)[76,79,104-106] constitute a short-lived and self-limited benign epileptic syndrome. It manifests with a single episode of repetitive lengthy seizures, which constitutes clonic status epilepticus.

DEMOGRAPHIC DATA

The age at onset is characteristically between the first and seventh days of life. It is by far more common (90%) between the fourth and sixth days, for which the synonym *'fifth day fits'* was coined.[104] Boys (62%) are slightly more affected than girls. The prevalence is 7% of neonatal seizures, but this has declined significantly in recent years.[76,105]

CLINICAL MANIFESTATIONS

There is a one-off event of a repetitive lengthy seizure which constitutes clonic status epilepticus, which occurs in otherwise normal full-term neonates. This consists of successive unilateral clonic convulsions affecting the face and the limbs. Convulsions may change side and may also less often be bilateral. Apnoea is a common concomitant in one-third of these clonic fits. Each seizure lasts for 1–3 min repeating at frequent intervals and cumulating to discontinuous or continuous clonic status epilepticus. The whole seizure–status event lasts for 2 h to 3 days with a median of approximately 20 h. It does not recur again. Tonic seizures are incompatible with this syndrome.

AETIOLOGY

This is unknown but is probably environmental. There is no genetic background and there are various other propositions:

- Environmental causes because of significant periodic variations in the prevalence of the syndrome.

ILAE definition and corrections[19]

Benign neonatal seizures (non-familial) are defined as follows in the 1989 ILAE classification.[19]

Benign neonatal convulsions are very frequently repeated clonic or apnoeic seizures occurring at about the fifth day of life, without known aetiology or concomitant metabolic disturbance. The inter-ictal EEG often shows alternating sharp theta waves. There is no recurrence of seizures and the psychomotor development is not affected.[19]

Comment. In the 1989 ILAE classification, benign neonatal seizures (non-familial) were classified as idiopathic generalised epilepsy (IGE) (age related).[19] However, many authors have emphasised that this is a predominantly focal (and not generalised) seizure syndrome[8,107] and this should be considered in future revisions. This syndrome most likely belongs to the category of "conditions with epileptic seizures that do not require a diagnosis of epilepsy".[75]

- Acute zinc deficiency detected in the cerebrospinal fluid of affected neonates.
- Viral illness, mainly rotavirus.
- Type of feeding.

PATHOPHYSIOLOGY

The pathophysiology is unknown. However, this syndrome provides firm evidence that even prolonged seizures in early life may not produce hippocampal damage in the absence of other complicating factors.[108]

DIAGNOSTIC PROCEDURES

By definition all tests other than EEG are normal.

ELECTROENCEPHALOGRAPHY

The inter-ictal EEG shows a 'theta pointu alternant pattern' in one-half of cases (Figure 5.3).[76,79] In the others the EEG may show focal or multifocal, non-specific abnormalities or a discontinuous pattern or it may be normal in approximately 10%.

The theta pointu alternant pattern consists of runs of a dominant theta wave activity of 4–7 Hz intermixed with sharp waves often of alternating side.[76] It is not reactive to various stimuli. It may occur on awakening and during sleep. It may persist for 12 days after the cessation of convulsions. However, the theta pointu alternant pattern is not specific as it may be recorded in other conditions such as hypocalcaemia, meningitis, subarachnoid haemorrhage, in neonatal encephalopathies including hypoxic–ischaemic encephalopathy and benign familial neonatal seizures.

In follow-up studies, centrotemporal spikes are found at a later age in otherwise asymptomatic cases.

The ictal EEG consists of rhythmic spikes or slow waves mainly in the Rolandic regions though they can also localise anywhere else.[76,105,107] The EEG ictal paroxysms may be unilateral, generalised or first localised and then generalised. The duration of the ictal discharges is 1–3 min and this may be followed by subclinical discharges for many hours.

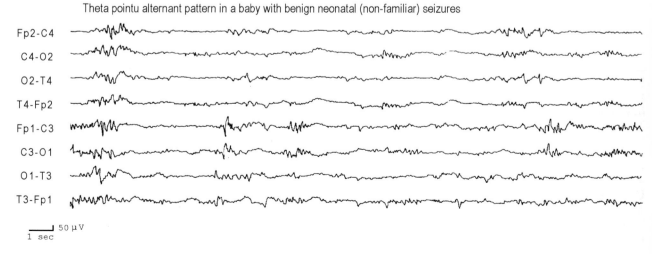

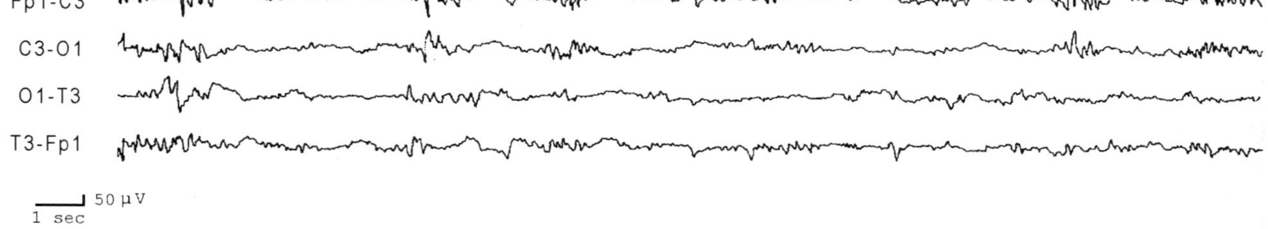

Figure 5.3 Inter-ictal EEG in a neonate with benign neonatal (non-familial) seizures.

The theta pointu alternant pattern is usually associated with a good prognosis.

From Plouin (1992)[102] with the permission of the author and the publisher John Libbey.

DIFFERENTIAL DIAGNOSIS

The diagnosis can be made only after other causes of neonatal seizures have been excluded. The aetiologies of neonatal seizures with favourable outcomes include late hypocalcaemia, subarachnoid haemorrhage and certain meningitides (Table 5.2).[76,105,107] There are significant differences between benign neonatal seizures (non-familial) and benign familial neonatal seizures despite the artificially similar names[3,75] and the fact that they have a similar age at onset (Table 5.3).

Diagnostic tips for benign neonatal seizures (non-familial)

A single episode of repetitive clonic seizures that are mainly unilateral, often of alternating side and lasting for around 20 h in a full-term neonate that was normal up to that stage. All relevant investigations other than EEG are normal.

PROGNOSIS

The prognosis is commonly excellent with normal development and no recurrence of seizures. Minor psychomotor deficits and occasional febrile or afebrile seizures (0.5%) have been reported.[76,79,107] However, North et al.[109] had less optimistic results. Afebrile seizures or developmental delay occurred in one-half of their patients and there was a single case of sudden infant death.[109]

MANAGEMENT

Convulsions usually remit spontaneously without medication. Prolonged seizures may be shortened or terminated by intravenous administration of benzodiazepines, phenobarbitone or phenytoin. If medications are used they are discontinued soon after the seizures subside.

EARLY MYOCLONIC ENCEPHALOPATHY

Early myoclonic encephalopathy is a dreadful but fortunately rare epileptic encephalopathy of the first days and weeks of life. [50,52,110-113]

DEMOGRAPHIC DATA

Early myoclonic encephalopathy usually starts in the first days of life, sometimes immediately after birth. More than 60% start before 10 days of age and rarely after the second month. Boys and girls are equally affected. The prevalence and incidence is unknown. There are approximately 80 reported cases, but this may be an underestimation because neonates with such a severe disease and early death may escape clinico-EEG diagnosis.

ILAE definitions

Early myoclonic encephalopathy is defined as follows by the ILAE Commission (1989).[19]

The principal features of early myoclonic encephalopathy are onset occurring before age 3 months, initially fragmentary myoclonus and then erratic focal seizures, massive myoclonias or tonic spasms. The EEG is characterised by suppression–burst activity, which may evolve into hypsarrhythmia. The course is severe, psychomotor development is arrested and death may occur in the first year. Familial cases are frequent and suggest the influence of one or several congenital metabolic errors, but there is no specific genetic pattern.[19]

Clarifications on myoclonus

There is no generally accepted, precise definition of "myoclonus" and there is a long-standing source of confusion and debate regarding the term and concept of epileptic and non-epileptic "myoclonus"[114-116] "Myoclonus" is a descriptive term for heterogeneous phenomena such as "sudden brief jerk caused by involuntary muscle activity", "quick muscle regular or irregular jerks"," a sudden brief , shock-like muscle contraction arising from the central nervous system", "abrupt, jerky, involuntary movements unassociated with loss of consciousness". Clinically myoclonus is divided into physiological, essential, epileptic, and symptomatic. [116] Symptomatic causes are more common and include post-hypoxia, toxic-metabolic disorders, reactions to drugs, storage disease, and neurodegenerative disorders.

For definitions of myoclonus, myoclonic and other seizures see Chapter 7 (page 138).

CLINICAL MANIFESTATIONS

The syndrome manifests with a triad of intractable seizures. Erratic myoclonus appears first followed by simple focal seizures and later by tonic epileptic (infantile) spasms.

Erratic or fragmentary myoclonus is the defining seizure type that sometimes may appear immediately after birth. The term *erratic* is because the myoclonias shift typically from one part of the body to another in a random and asynchronous fashion. Erratic myoclonus affects the face or limbs. It is often restricted in a finger, a toe, the eyebrows, eyelids or lips occurring in the same muscle group and often migrating elsewhere usually in an asynchronous and asymmetrical fashion. Myoclonias are brief, single or repetitive, very frequent and nearly continuous. It is exceptional for a baby with early myoclonic encephalopathy to have mild and infrequent jerks.

Massive usually bisynchronous axial myoclonic jerks may start from the onset of the disease or occur later, often interspersed with erratic myoclonias.

Simple focal seizures, often clinically inconspicuous, manifest with eye deviation or autonomic symptoms such as flushing of the face or apnoea. Focal clonic seizures affect any part of the body. Asymmetric tonic posturing also occurs.

Tonic seizures occur frequently and usually appear in the first month of life. They manifest with truncal tonic contraction which usually also involves the limbs. They occur during wakefulness and sleep.

Genuine tonic epileptic spasms are rare and generally appear later. They usually develop within 2–4 months from the onset of myoclonias, they are solitary or in clusters and are more frequent during alert stages than sleep stages.

Psychomotor development may be abnormal from the onset of seizures or arrests and deteriorates rapidly afterwards. There may be marked truncal hypotonia, limb hypertonia, disconjugate eye movements, dyspnoea, opisthotonic or decerebrate posturing. All patients have bilateral pyramidal signs. Practically, there is no trace of intelligent activity. Patients are unable to follow moving objects with their eyes. One patient developed peripheral neuropathy.[110]

AETIOLOGY

Early myoclonic encephalopathy is a multi-factorial disease with a high incidence of familial cases.[52,113] Some may be due to an autosomal recessive inheritance. Inborn errors of metabolism are the most common causes. These are non-ketotic hyperglycinaemia, propionic aciduria, methylmalonic acidaemia, D-glyceric acidaemia, sulphite and xanthine oxidase deficiency, Menkes disease and Zellweger syndrome and molybdenum co-factor deficiency.[113] Metabolic causes explain the high incidence of siblings with this disorder.

A case with a clinical picture of early myoclonic encephalopathy and an atypical suppression–burst pattern had full recovery after administration of pyridoxine.[119] Lesional brain abnormalities are rare.

Neuropathological findings when available are not consistent. These include depletion of cortical neurones and astrocytic proliferation, severe multifocal spongy changes in the white matter, peri-vascular concentric bodies, demyelination in cerebral hemispheres, imperfect lamination of the deeper cortical layers and unilateral enlargement of the cerebral hemisphere with astrocytic proliferation.[120] No pathological abnormalities have been reported in two cases.[110]

PATHOPHYSIOLOGY

It is apparent from the various and diverse causes of early myoclonic encephalopathy that no one single factor appears to be responsible. Most likely early myoclonic encephalopathy and Ohtahara syndrome are the earliest forms of epileptic encephalopathies as detailed in Chapter 7.

Spreafico et al. [121] proposed a common neuropathological basis irrespective of aetiology. They assumed that numerous large spiny neurones scattered in the white matter along the axons of the cortical gyri represent interstitial cells of neocortical histogenesis that failed to follow their natural programming to die at the end of gestation or soon after birth.[121]

DIAGNOSTIC PROCEDURES

These are the same as those for neonatal seizures, attempting to find an aetiological cause. Brain imaging is usually normal at the onset of the disease but progressive cortical and peri-ventricular atrophy often develops. Asymmetrical enlargement of one hemisphere, dilatation of the corresponding lateral ventricle, cortical and peri-ventricular atrophy and exceptionally malformations of cortical development have been reported.

When considering the relatively high rate of inborn errors of metabolism and mainly non-ketotic hyperglycinaemia a thorough metabolic screening is mandatory. This should include serum levels of amino acids and particularly glycine and glycerol metabolites, organic acids and amino acids in the cerebrospinal fluid.

ELECTROENCEPHALOGRAPHY

The inter-ictal EEG of early myoclonic encephalopathy is a repetitive suppression–burst pattern without physiological rhythms (Figure 5.4). The bursts of high-amplitude spikes and sharp and slow waves last for 1–5 s and alternate with periods of a flat or almost flat EEG lasting 3–10 s. In most cases the suppression–burst pattern becomes more apparent during deep sleep and may not occur in the EEG of wakefulness.[113] The suppression–burst pattern may appear late at 1–5 months of age in some cases and characteristically persists for a prolonged period.[122]

Erratic myoclonias usually do not have an ictal EEG expression and may follow the bursts.

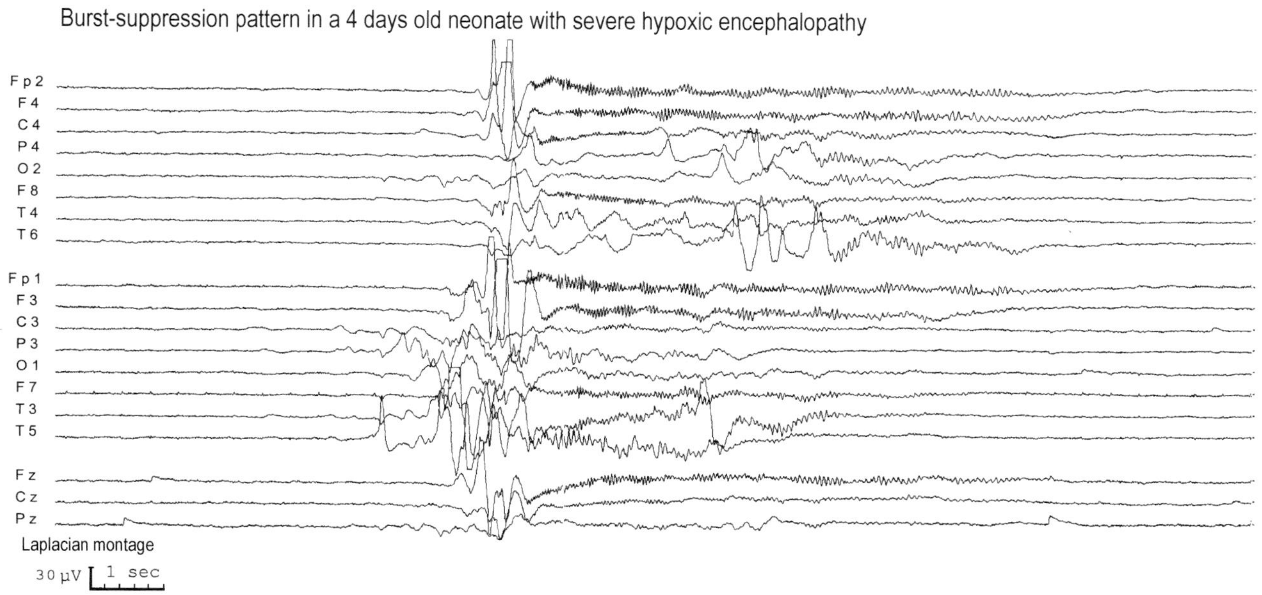

Figure 5.4 The burst–suppression pattern in a neonate with severe hypoxic encephalopathy.

The suppression–burst pattern evolves to atypical hypsarrhythmia or multifocal spikes and sharp waves 3–4 months from onset of the disease. However, this EEG state of atypical hypsarrhythmia is transient and returns to the suppression–burst pattern, which persists for a long time.

PROGNOSIS

Early myoclonic encephalopathy is one of the most dreadful diseases. More than half of patients die within weeks or months from onset and the others develop permanent severe mental and neurological deficits.

MANAGEMENT

There is no effective treatment. Adrenocorticotropic hormone therapy and antiepileptic medication (clonazepam, nitrazepam, valproate, phenobarbitone and others) are of no benefit. Patients with non-ketotic hyperglycinaemia may benefit from a reduction in dietary protein and administration of 120 mg/kg of sodium benzoate daily though the outcome is commonly very poor.[123]

A trial with pyridoxine is justifiable.

Diagnostic tips for early myoclonic encephalopathy
Segmental and erratic myoclonias affecting the face and limbs, usually restricted to a finger, the eyebrows and peri-oral muscles, that is nearly continuous and often shifting from place to place. A persistent EEG suppression–burst pattern.

OHTAHARA SYNDROME

Ohtahara syndrome[52,112,113,124,125] is a rare and devastating form of severe epileptic encephalopathy of very early life.

DEMOGRAPHIC DATA

Onset is mainly around the first 10 days of life, sometimes intra-uterinely or up to 3 months of age. There may be a slight male predominance. The prevalence and incidence are unknown. There are approximately 100 reported cases but this may be an underestimation as many newborn babies with such a severe disease and early death may escape clinico-EEG diagnosis. According to one report 'attacks of cerebral spasms occur in 1.5–5 per 1000 newborn post-partum'.[126]

CLINICAL MANIFESTATIONS

Ohtahara syndrome manifests with clinico-EEG features of mainly tonic spasms and suppression–burst EEG patterns that consistently occur in the sleeping and waking states.

Tonic spasms usually consist of a forwards tonic flexion lasting 1–10 s that is singular or in long clusters 10–300 times every 24 h. They may be generalised and symmetrical or lateralised. They occur in both the wake and sleep stages. Less often, one-third of the neonates may have erratic focal motor clonic seizures or hemiconvulsions. Alternating hemiconvulsions or GTCS are exceptional. Myoclonic seizures are rare. Erratic myoclonias are not featured.

ILAE definition of Ohtahara syndrome [19]

Ohtahara syndrome or 'early infantile epileptic encephalopathy with suppression–burst' is defined by the ILAE Commission as follows.[19]

This syndrome, as described by Ohtahara et al.,[127] is defined by very early onset, within the first few months of life, frequent tonic spasms and a suppression–burst EEG pattern in both the waking and sleeping states. Partial seizures may occur. Myoclonic seizures are rare. The aetiology and underlying pathology are obscure. The prognosis is serious with severe psychomotor retardation and seizure intractability. Often there is evolution to West syndrome at age 4–6 months.[19]

AETIOLOGY

The most common cause is malformations of cerebral development such as hemimegalencephaly, porencephaly, Aicardi syndrome, olivary-dentate dysplasia, agenesis of mamillary bodies, linear sebaceous naevus syndrome, cerebral dysgenesis and focal cortical dysplasia.[113] Rarely, other lesional brain or metabolic disorders may also be responsible.[52,113] There are no familial cases.

In neuropathological studies, patients with Ohtahara syndrome had the most severe lesions in comparison with early myoclonic encephalopathy and West syndrome.[128]

PATHOPHYSIOLOGY

Ohtahara syndrome is likely to be the earliest age-related specific epileptic reaction of the developing brain to heterogeneous insults similar to those of other epileptic encephalopathies that occur at a later brain maturity age (Chapter 7). This is supported by the fact that, between 2 and 6 months of age, the clinico-EEG features often change to those of West syndrome and later to Lennox–Gastaut syndrome.

There may be a dysfunction of the catecholaminergic and serotonergic systems that may be responsible for this type of neonatal epileptic encephalopathy.[128]

DIAGNOSTIC PROCEDURES

These are the same as for neonatal seizures, involving attempts at detecting an aetiological cause and possible treatment. Brain imaging usually shows severe abnormalities and malformations of cortical development. Metabolic screening is mandatory if brain imaging is normal.

ELECTROENCEPHALOGRAPHY

The EEG suppression–burst pattern has a pseudo-rhythmic periodicity. The bursts consist of high-amplitude slow waves intermixed with spikes lasting for 2–6 s. The suppression period of a flat or near flat EEG lasts for 3–5 s. The interval between the onsets of two successive bursts is in the range of 5–10 s. This pattern occurs during both the waking and sleeping stages.

According to Ohtahara et al.[129] the pseudo-rhythmic appearance of the suppression–burst pattern during wakefulness and sleep distinguishes Ohtahara syndrome from the periodic type of hypsarrhythmia in which periodicity becomes clear during sleep and from the burst–suppression EEGs of severely abnormal neonates.

The burst–suppression pattern in Ohtahara syndrome versus early myoclonic encephalopathy

There are certain differentiating features of burst–suppression pattern between Ohtahara syndrome and early myoclonic encephalopathy. According to Ohtahara[122] the suppression–burst pattern of early myoclonic encephalopathy is accentuated during sleep and often may not occur in the awake state while this is continuous in Ohtahara syndrome.[122] Furthermore, the suppression–burst pattern appears at the onset of the disease and disappears within the first 6 months of life in Ohtahara syndrome, whereas in early myoclonic encephalopathy the suppression–burst pattern appears at 1–5 months of age in some cases and characteristically persists for a prolonged period.[122]

On video–EEG and polymyographic recordings, the suppression–burst pattern is associated with tonic spasms of variable duration concomitant with the burst phase.[124] Tonic spasms may also occur with the following EEG features.

- Diffuse desynchronisation with disappearance of suppression–burst activity when tonic spasms cluster in intervals of 5–10 s.
- A pattern in which the suppression–burst pattern becomes more frequent, more diffuse and of higher amplitude compared to the inter-ictal pattern.

Progression of clinical and electroencephalogram features to West syndrome and Lennox–Gastaut syndrome

There is an age-related evolution of clinical and EEG patterns from Ohtahara syndrome, first to West syndrome and then to Lennox–Gastaut syndrome.

In EEG, a characteristic development is the gradual disappearance of the suppression–burst pattern and the emergence of hypsarrhythmia within 3–6 months from onset. This may again progress later to the slow spike-wave EEG patterns of Lennox–Gastaut syndrome.

The suppression–burst transformation to hypsarrhythmia starts with the gradual emergence of higher amplitude rhythms in the suppression phase, followed by disappearance of the suppression–burst pattern in the awake stage EEG and finally in the sleep stage EEG.[129] Changing from hypsarrhythmia to diffuse slow spike-wave, the hypsarrhythmic patterns gradually become fragmented and disappear. They are replaced initially in the awake and subsequently in the sleep EEG by the slow spike-wave patterns of Lennox-Gastaut syndrome.[129]

Some survivors may show highly localised or entirely unilateral spikes and these patients may frequently have severe focal seizures. Multifocal spikes are frequent while an EEG void of spikes is rather exceptional. Asymmetrical suppression–burst patterns are more likely to develop spike foci and less likely to progress to hypsarrhythmia.

DIFFERENTIAL DIAGNOSIS

The main differential diagnosis of Ohtahara syndrome is from early myoclonic encephalopathy (Table 5.4).[52,130]

PROGNOSIS

This is a devastating syndrome associated with high mortality and morbidity. Half of patients die within weeks or months from onset and the others soon develop permanent severe mental and neurological deficits. Psychomotor development relentlessly deteriorates. The babies become inactive with spastic diplegia,

Table 5.4 Early myoclonic encephalopathy versus Ohtahara syndrome

	Ohtahara syndrome	**Early myoclonic encephalopathy**
Main seizures	Tonic spasms	Erratic myoclonias, focal seizures, clusters of spasms
Main causes	Malformations of cerebral development	Genetic and metabolic
Suppression-burst	Sleep and awake – shorter lifespan	Probably accentuated by sleep – longer lifespan
Paroxysmal bursts	Longer	Shorter
Suppression	Shorter	Longer
Transformation to West syndrome	As a rule	Common but transient

hemiplegia, tetraplegia, ataxia or dystonia. In survivors, the clinical and EEG patterns change to that of West syndrome within a few months from onset and this may also change to Lennox–Gastaut syndrome features if patients reach 2–3 years of age.

According to Ohtahara et al.[129] patients with suppression–burst patterns evolving to hypsarrhythmia and then to slow spike-wave EEG have the worse prognosis and a high mortality rate. Conversely, those who develop spike foci, have fewer seizures and less mortality despite severe psychomotor handicaps.

MANAGEMENT

There is no effective treatment. Adrenocorticotropic hormone therapy and anti-epileptic medication of any type are of no benefit. An excellent response to zonisamide was reported in a single case.[131] A short-lived beneficial effect of vigabatrin has been reported. Newer drugs have not been tested. Neurosurgery in focal cerebral dysplasia is sometimes beneficial.[132]

Diagnostic tips for Ohtahara syndrome

Tonic seizures during the awake and sleep stages in the early days or weeks of life are nearly pathognomonic of Ohtahara syndrome. The EEG has a burst–suppression pattern with a pseudo-rhythmic appearance occurring during the awake and sleep stages.

NON-EPILEPTIC MOVEMENT DISORDERS IN NEONATES AND INFANTS IMITATING SEIZURES

Non-epileptic movement disorders in neonates and infants may be misdiagnosed as epileptic seizures. The commoner of these are:

- **Benign neonatal sleep myoclonus**
- **Benign non-epileptic myoclonus of early infancy (benign non-epileptic infantile spasms)**
- **Hyperekplexia (familial startle disease)**

BENIGN NEONATAL SLEEP MYOCLONUS

Benign neonatal sleep myoclonus[133-136] is a common non-epileptic condition misdiagnosed as epileptic seizures and even as infantile spasms.

DEMOGRAPHIC DATA

Onset is from the first day to 3 weeks of life with a peak at the seventh day. Boys and girls are equally affected. Though common the exact prevalence is unknown.

CLINICAL MANIFESTATIONS

The myoclonus occurs during non-REM sleep in otherwise normal neonates. It mainly affects the distal parts of the upper extremities. The lower limbs and axial muscles are less often involved. The myoclonic jerks, synchronous or asynchronous, unilateral or bilateral, mild or violent, usually last for 10–20 s. Occasionally they may occur in repetitive clusters of 2–3 s for 30 min or longer imitating myoclonic status epilepticus or a series of epileptic fits. The myoclonic jerks may get worse with gentle restraint. They abruptly stop when the child is awakened. Sleep is not disturbed.

There are no other clinical manifestations like those accompanying neonatal seizures such as apnoea, autonomic disturbances, automatisms, eye deviation, oral–buccal–lingual movements or crying.

Neurological mental state and development are normal.

AETIOLOGY

This is unknown and the condition does not appear to be familial. The myoclonus is likely to be generated in the brain stem.

DIAGNOSTIC PROCEDURES

The diagnosis is based on clinical features. All relevant laboratory studies including sleep EEG during the myoclonus are normal.

DIFFERENTIAL DIAGNOSIS

Benign neonatal sleep myoclonus should be easy to differentiate from relevant epileptic disorders in this age group by its occurrence in normal neonates and only during sleep. When in doubt, a normal sleep EEG during the myoclonus is confirmatory of this non-epileptic condition.

PROGNOSIS

The prognosis is excellent with the myoclonus commonly remitting by the age of 2–7 months.

TREATMENT

There is no need for any treatment though minute doses of clonazepam before bed are often beneficial. Other anti-epileptic drugs are contraindicated.

BENIGN NON-EPILEPTIC MYOCLONUS OF EARLY INFANCY

BENIGN NON-EPILEPTIC INFANTILE SPASMS

Benign non-epileptic myoclonus of early infancy,[137-140] as described by Fejerman and Lombroso,[137] is a paroxysmal, non-epileptic movement disorder of otherwise healthy infants who have normal EEG and development. Its synonym of *'benign non-epileptic infantile spasms'* is descriptively more accurate than myoclonus.[141] It is probably the same disease as *'shuddering attacks'*.[142]

DEMOGRAPHIC DATA

Onset is from around 4–12 months of age. Both sexes are probably equally affected.

CLINICAL MANIFESTATIONS

The attacks are sudden and brief symmetrical axial flexor spasms mainly of the trunk and often the head. Less frequently, there may be flexion, abduction or adduction of the elbows and knees and extension or elevation of the arms. The spasms do not involve localised muscle groups and there are no focal or lateralising features. Clinically, each spasm lasts for 1–2 s.

The attacks are more likely to occur in clusters, sometimes recurring at frequent and brief intervals several times a day. The intensity of the spasms varies. They are usually mild and inconspicuous but may at times become severe and imitate infantile spasms. They occur in the awake state and are also elicited by excitement, fear, anger, frustration or the need to move the bowels or to void.

AETIOLOGY

This is unknown. Benign non-epileptic infantile spasms may result from an exaggeration of physiological myoclonus.[139]

DIAGNOSTIC PROCEDURES

The diagnosis is based on clinical features. All relevant laboratory studies including sleep and awake stage EEGs during the spasms are normal.

DIFFERENTIAL DIAGNOSIS

The main differential diagnosis is from epileptic spasms that may share similar clinical features. A normal ictal and inter-ictal EEG in benign non-epileptic infantile spasms is of decisive significance.

PROGNOSIS

Benign non-epileptic myoclonus of early infancy has a good prognosis with spontaneous remission in the first 5 years of life, usually by age 2–3 years.

TREATMENT

There is no convincing evidence of any beneficial treatment. Anti-epileptic drugs are unnecessary and potentially harmful.[139]

HYPEREKPLEXIA

FAMILIAL STARTLE DISEASE

Hyperekplexia or familial startle diseases[143-149] is the first human disease shown to result from mutations within a neurotransmitter gene.

DEMOGRAPHIC DATA

Onset is from intra-uterine life or birth or later at any time from the neonatal period to adulthood. Both sexes are equally affected. It is a rare disorder. Only approximately 150 cases have been reported.

CLINICAL MANIFESTATIONS

Clinically hyperekplexia is characterised by:

- pathological and excessive startle responses to unexpected auditory or tactile stimuli (sudden noise, movement or touch)
- severe generalised stiffness (hypertonia in flexion which disappears in sleep).

The startle response is characterised by sudden generalised muscular rigidity and resistance to habituation. In babies the muscle stiffening often causes respiratory impairment and apnoea that may be fatal. In older patients the startle response causes frequent falls, like a log, without loss of consciousness.

If an unborn baby is affected the mother may first notice abnormal intra-uterine movements. In newborn neonates apnoea and sluggish feeding efforts occur as a consequence of episodic extreme stiffening during the first 24 h of life. After the first 24 h surviving infants exhibit the hyperekplexic startle response to nose tapping, which is a useful diagnostic test (page 112).

Clinical phenotypic expression varies from mild to very severe forms.[150,151]

The minor forms manifest with excessive startle responses only, which are often mild and inconsistent. In infancy these are facilitated by febrile illness whereas in adults these are facilitated by emotional stress.

In the major forms affected neonates occasionally have fatal hypertonia and startle responses result in falls that may be traumatic. There is no impairment of consciousness, but the patient remains temporarily stiff after the attack.

Sleep episodic shaking of the limbs (nocturnal or sleep myoclonus) resembling generalised clonus or repetitive myoclonus is often prominent, lasting for minutes with no impairment of consciousness. The jerks are spontaneous arousal reactions.[152]

Neurologically, there is generalised muscle hypertonia–stiffness hence the term *stiff baby syndrome* (which is probably the same disease is hyperekplexia).[153] Gait may be unstable, insecure and puppet like. Brain stem and tendon reflexes are exaggerated.

Umbilical and inguinal hernias, presumably due to increased intra-abdominal pressure, are common.

AETIOLOGY

Hyperekplexia is usually inherited as an autosomal dominant and less often recessive trait. It is due to mutations within the *GLRA1* gene in chromosome 5q33-35, encoding the alpha 1 subunit of the glycine receptor.[147,148,154-157] The minor form of hyperekplexia is seldom due to a genetic defect in the *GLRA1* gene.[151]

DIAGNOSTIC PROCEDURES

The nose tap test is the most useful test. Tapping the tip of the nose of an unaffected baby will elicit a blink response or no response, but in hyperekplexia there is an obvious startle response, which is repeated each time the nose is tapped.

The EEG of startle responses in hyperekplexia is normal.[158] Slowing of background activity with eventual flattening may occur, but this corresponds to the phase of apnoea, bradycardia and cyanosis.[158]

DIFFERENTIAL DIAGNOSIS

Hyperekplexia in the neonatal period may be misdiagnosed as congenital stiff-man syndrome, startle epilepsy, myoclonic seizures, neonatal tetany, cerebral palsy and drug (phenothiazine) toxicity. Accurate recognition of hyperekplexia in a newborn is important so as to initiate early and appropriate treatment, which may be life saving.

PROGNOSIS

This is generally good in treated patients. Untreated infants experience recurring apnoea until 1 year of age. The exaggerated startle response persists to adulthood. Hypertonia diminished during the course of the first and second year of life and tone is usually almost normal by the age of 3 years. Hypertonia may recur in adult life.

TREATMENT

There is a dramatic response to clonazepam (0.1–0.2 mg/kg/day).[144] A simple manoeuvre to terminate the startle response is forcibly flexing the baby by pressing the head towards the knees. This may be life saving when prolonged stiffness impedes respiration. Affected families are advised to seek genetic counselling.

REFERENCES

1. Volpe JJ. Neonatal seizures. Philadelphia: W B Saunders, 1995.
2. Lombroso CT. Neonatal seizures: historic note and present controversies. *Epilepsia* 1996;**37 Suppl 3**:5-13.
3. Mizrahi EM. Treatment of neonatal seizures. In Engel J, Pedley TA, eds. *Epilepsy. A comprehensive textbook*, pp 1295-303. Lippincott-Raven, 1997.
4. Mizrahi EM, Plouin P, Kellaway P. Neonatal seizures. In Engel J, Pedley TA, eds. *Epilepsy. A comprehensive textbook*, pp 647-63. Lippincott-Raven, 1997.
5. Rennie JM. Neonatal seizures. *Eur J Pediatr.* 1997;**156**:83-7.
6. Ronen GM, Penney S, Andrews W. The epidemiology of clinical neonatal seizures in Newfoundland: a population-based study. *J Pediatr.* 1999;**134**:71-5.
7. Schmid R, Tandon P, Stafstrom CE, Holmes GL. Effects of neonatal seizures on subsequent seizure-induced brain injury. *Neurology* 1999;**53**:1754-61.
8. Watanabe K, Miura K, Natsume J, Hayakawa F, Furune S, Okumura A. Epilepsies of neonatal onset: seizure type and evolution. *Dev Med Child Neurol* 1999;**41**:318-22.
9. Levene M. The clinical conundrum of neonatal seizures. *Arch Dis Child Fetal Neonatal Ed* 2002;**86**:F75-F77.
10. Mizrahi EM, Kellaway P. Diagnosis and management of neonatal seizures. Hagerstown: Lippincott Williams & Wilkins, 1999.
11. Hill A. Neonatal seizures. *Pediatr Rev.* 2000;**21**:117-21.
12. Mizrahi EM, Kellaway P. Neonatal seizures. In Pellock JM, Dodson WE, Bourgeois BFD, eds. *Pediatric epilepsy*, pp 145-61. New York: Demos, 2001.
13. Holmes GL, Khazipov R, Ben Ari Y. New concepts in neonatal seizures. *Neuroreport* 2002;**13**:A3-A8.
14. Scher MS. Controversies regarding neonatal seizure recognition. *Epileptic Disord.* 2002;**4**:139-58.
15. Mizrahi E, Watanabe K. Symptomatic neonatal seizures. In Roger J, Bureau M, Dravet C, Genton P, Tassinari CA, Wolf P, eds. *Epileptic syndromes in infancy, childhood and adolescence (3rd edn)*, pp 15-31. London: John Libbey & Co Ltd, 2002.
16. Tharp BR. Neonatal seizures and syndromes. *Epilepsia* 2002;**43 Suppl 3**:2-10.
17. Mizrahi EM. Seizures in the neonate. In Wallace SJ, Farrell K, eds. *Epilepsy in childen*, pp 111-22. London: Arnold, 2004.
18. Arzimanoglou A, Guerrini R, Aicardi J. Neonatal seizures. In Arzimanoglou A, Guerrini R, Aicardi J, eds. *Aicardi's epilepsy in children*, pp 188-209. Philadelphia: Lippincott Williams & Wilkins, 2004.
19. Commission on Classification and Terminology of the International League Against Epilepsy. Proposal for revised classification of epilepsies and epileptic syndromes. *Epilepsia* 1989;**30**:389-99.
20. Volpe JJ. Neonatal seizures: current concepts and revised classification. *Pediatrics* 1989;**84**:422-8.
21. Watanabe K, Hara K, Miyazaki S, Hakamada S, Kuroyanagi M. Apneic seizures in the newborn. *Am J Dis Child* 1982;**136**:980-4.
22. Scher MS. Pathologic myoclonus of the newborn: electrographic and clinical correlations. *Pediatr Neurol* 1985;**1**:342-8.
23. Fenichel GM, Olson BJ, Fitzpatrick JE. Heart rate changes in convulsive and nonconvulsive neonatal apnea. *Ann Neurol* 1980;**7**:577-82.
24. Scher MS. Seizures in the newborn infant. Diagnosis, treatment, and outcome. *Clin Perinatol.* 1997;**24**:735-72.
25. Perlman JM,.Volpe JJ. Seizures in the preterm infant: effects on cerebral blood flow velocity, intracranial pressure, and arterial blood pressure. *J Pediatr.* 1983;**102**:288-93.
26. Watanabe K, Hara K, Hakamada S, Negoro T, Sugiura M, Matsumoto A *et al.* Seizures with apnea in children. *Pediatrics* 1982;**70**:87-90.
27. Mizrahi EM, Kellaway P. Characterization and classification of neonatal seizures. *Neurology* 1987;**37**:1837-44.
28. Minchom P, Niswander K, Chalmers I, Dauncey M, Newcombe R, Elbourne D *et al.* Antecedents and outcome of very early neonatal seizures in infants born at or after term. *Br J Obstet Gynaecol.* 1987;**94**:431-9.
29. Nelson KB, Lynch JK. Stroke in newborn infants. *Lancet Neurol.* 2004;**3**:150-8.
30. Aicardi J. Neonatal seizures. In Dam M, Gram L, eds. *Comprehensive epileptology*, pp 99-112. New York: Raven Press, 1991.
31. Aicardi J. Epilepsy in Children. New York: Raven Press, 1994.
32. Moshe SL. Seizures in the developing brain. *Neurology* 1993;**43**:S3-S7.
33. Velisek L, Moshe SL. Pathophysiology of seizures and epilepsy in the immature brain:Cells, synapses and circuits. In Pellock JM, Dodson WE, Bourgeois BFD, eds. *Pediatric epilepsy*, pp 1-23. New York: Demos, 2001.
34. Holmes GL, Ben Ari Y. Seizures in the developing brain: perhaps not so benign after all. *Neuron* 1998;**21**:1231-4.
35. Jensen FE. Acute and chronic effects of seizures in the developing brain: experimental models. *Epilepsia* 1999;**40 Suppl 1**:S51-S58.
36. Mizrahi EM. Acute and chronic effects of seizures in the developing brain: lessons from clinical experience. *Epilepsia* 1999;**40 Suppl 1**:S42-S50.
37. Kuzniecky RI. Neuroimaging in pediatric epileptology. In Pellock JM, Dodson WE, Bourgeois BFD, eds. *Pediatric epilepsy*, pp 133-43. New York: Demos, 2001.
38. Aso K, Abdab-Barmada M, Scher MS. EEG and the neuropathology in premature neonates with intraventricular hemorrhage. *J Clin Neurophysiol.* 1993;**10**:304-13.
39. Holmes GL,.Lombroso CT. Prognostic value of background patterns in the neonatal EEG. *J Clin Neurophysiol.* 1993;**10**:323-52.
40. Scher MS. Neonatal encephalopathies as classified by EEG-sleep criteria: severity and timing based on clinical/pathologic correlations. *Pediatr Neurol* 1994;**11**:189-200.
41. Clancy RR. The contribution of EEG to the understanding of neonatal seizures. *Epilepsia* 1996;**37 Suppl 1**:S52-S59.
42. Ortibus EL, Sum JM, Hahn JS. Predictive value of EEG for outcome and epilepsy following neonatal seizures. *Electroencephalogr Clin Neurophysiol.* 1996;**98**:175-85.
43. Marret S, Parain D, Menard JF, Blanc T, Devaux AM, Ensel P *et al.* Prognostic value of neonatal electroencephalography in premature newborns less than 33 weeks of gestational age. *Electroencephalogr Clin Neurophysiol* 1997;**102**:178-85.
44. de Weerd AW, Despland PA, Plouin P. Neonatal EEG. The International Federation of Clinical Neurophysiology. *Electroencephalogr Clin Neurophysiol Suppl* 1999;**52**:149-57.
45. Patrizi S, Holmes GL, Orzalesi M, Allemand F. Neonatal seizures: characteristics of EEG ictal activity in preterm and fullterm infants. *Brain Dev.* 2003;**25**:427-37.
46. Bednarek N. Video-EEG monitoring in neonates: indications. *Epileptic Disord.* 2001;**3 Spec No 2**:SI21-SI24.
47. Scher MS, Aso K, Beggarly ME, Hamid MY, Steppe DA, Painter MJ. Electrographic seizures in preterm and full-term neonates: clinical correlates, associated brain lesions, and risk for neurologic sequelae. *Pediatrics* 1993;**91**:128-34.
48. Mizrahi EM,.Tharp BR. A characteristic EEG pattern in neonatal herpes simplex encephalitis. *Neurology* 1982;**32**:1215-20.
49. Arzimanoglou A, Guerrini R, Aicardi J. Aicardi's epilepsy in children. Philadelphia: Lippincott Williams & Wilkins, 2004.
50. Lombroso CT. Early myoclonic encephalopathy, early infantile epileptic encephalopathy, and benign and severe infantile myoclonic epilepsies: a critical review and personal contributions. *J Clin Neurophysiol.* 1990;**7**:380-408.
51. Tendero GA, Lopez M, V, Arcas MJ, Roche Herrero MC, Martinez BA. Neonatal EEG trace of burst suppression. Etiological and evolutionary factors. *Rev Neurol.* 2001;**33**:514-8.
52. Aicardi J, Ohtahara S. Severe neonatal epilepsies with suppression-burst pattern. In Roger J, Bureau M, Dravet C, Genton P, Tassinari CA, Wolf P, eds. *Epileptic syndromes in infancy, childhood and adolescence (3rd edn)*, pp 33-44. London: John Libbey & Co Ltd, 2002.
53. Kellaway P, Mizrahi EM. Neonatal seizures. In Luders H, Lesser RP, eds. *Epilepsy. Electroclinical syndromes*, pp 13-47. Berlin: Springer-Verlag, 1987.
54. Mizrahi EM. Clinical and neurophysiologic correlates of

neonatal seizures. *Cleve Clin J Med.* 1989;**56 Suppl Pt 1**:S100-S104.

55. Scher MS. Stimulus-evoked electrographic patterns in neonates: an abnormal form of reactivity. *Electroencephalogr Clin Neurophysiol.* 1997;**103**:679-91.

56. Clancy RR, Legido A, Lewis D. Occult neonatal seizures. *Epilepsia* 1988;**29**:256-61.

57. Weiner SP, Painter MJ, Geva D, Guthrie RD, Scher MS. Neonatal seizures: electroclinical dissociation. *Pediatr Neurol.* 1991;**7**:363-8.

58. Biagioni E, Ferrari F, Boldrini A, Roversi MF, Cioni G. Electroclinical correlation in neonatal seizures. *Europ J Paediatr Neurol.* 1998;**2**:117-25.

59. Boylan GB, Panerai RB, Rennie JM, Evans DH, Rabe-Hesketh S, Binnie CD. Cerebral blood flow velocity during neonatal seizures. *Arch Dis Child Fetal Neonatal Ed* 1999;**80**:F105-F110.

60. Garcias Da Silva LF, Nunes ML, da Costa JC. Risk factors for developing epilepsy after neonatal seizures. *Pediatr Neurol.* 2004;**30**:271-7.

61. Rennie JM,Boylan GB. Neonatal seizures and their treatment. *Curr Opin Neurol.* 2003;**16**:177-81.

62. Fischer JH, Lockman LA, Zaske D, Kriel R. Phenobarbital maintenance dose requirements in treating neonatal seizures. *Neurology* 1981;**31**:1042-4.

63. Donn SM, Grasela TH, Goldstein GW. Safety of a higher loading dose of phenobarbital in the term newborn. *Pediatrics* 1985;**75**:1061-4.

64. Painter MJ, Scher MS, Stein AD, Armatti S, Wang Z, Gardiner JC *et al.* Phenobarbital compared with phenytoin for the treatment of neonatal seizures. *N Engl J Med.* 1999;**341**:485-9.

65. Maytal J, Novak GP, King KC. Lorazepam in the treatment of refractory neonatal seizures. *J Child Neurol.* 1991;**6**:319-23.

66. Sheth RD, Buckley DJ, Gutierrez AR, Gingold M, Bodensteiner JB, Penney S. Midazolam in the treatment of refractory neonatal seizures. *Clin Neuropharmacol.* 1996;**19**:165-70.

67. Boylan GB, Rennie JM, Chorley G, Pressler RM, Fox GF, Farrer K *et al.* Second-line anticonvulsant treatment of neonatal seizures: a video-EEG monitoring study. *Neurology* 2004;**62**:486-8.

68. Wallin A, Nergardh A, Hynning PA. Lidocaine treatment of neonatal convulsions, a therapeutic dilemma. *Eur J Clin Pharmacol.* 1989;**36**:583-6.

69. Singh B, Singh P H I, Khan M, Majeed-Saidan M. Treatment of neonatal seizures with carbamazepine. *J Child Neurol.* 1996;**11**:378-82.

70. Baxter PS, Gardner-Medwin D, Barwick DD, Ince P, Livingston J, Murdoch-Eaton D. Vigabatrin monotherapy in resistant neonatal seizures. *Seizure.* 1995;**4**:57-9.

71. Barr PA, Buettiker VE, Antony JH. Efficacy of lamotrigine in refractory neonatal seizures. *Pediatr Neurol.* 1999;**20**:161-3.

72. Massingale TW,.Buttross S. Survey of treatment practices for neonatal seizures. *J Perinatol.* 1993;**13**:107-10.

73. Brod SA, Ment LR, Ehrenkranz RA, Bridgers S. Predictors of success for drug discontinuation following neonatal seizures. *Pediatr Neurol.* 1988;**4**:13-7.

74. Ellison PH, Horn JL, Franklin S, Jones MG. The results of checking a scoring system for neonatal seizures. *Neuropediatrics* 1986;**17**:152-7.

75. Engel J, Jr. A proposed diagnostic scheme for people with epileptic seizures and with epilepsy: Report of the ILAE Task Force on Classification and Terminology. *Epilepsia* 2001;**42**:796-803.

76. Plouin P. Benign familial neonatal convulsions and benign idiopathic neonatal convulsions. In Engel J.jr., Pedley T.A, eds. *Epilepsy. A comprehensive textbook*, pp 2247-55. Lippincott-Raven, 1997.

77. Hirsch E, Velez A, Sellal F, Maton B, Grinspan A, Malafosse A *et al.* Electroclinical signs of benign neonatal familial convulsions. *Ann Neurol* 1993;**34**:835-41.

78. Hirsch E, Saint-Martin A, Marescaux C. Benign familial neonatal convulsions: a model of idiopathic epilepsy. *Rev Neurol (Paris)* 1999;**155**:463-7.

79. Plouin P, Anderson VE. Benign familial and non-familial neonatal seizures. In Roger J, Bureau M, Dravet C, Genton P, Tassinari CA, Wolf P, eds. *Epileptic syndromes in infancy, childhood and adolescence (3rd edn)*, pp 3-13. London: John Libbey & Co Ltd, 2002.

80. Vidaurre JA, Ballaban-Gil KR, Plouin P, Moshe SL. Benign neonatal familial seizures. In Gilman S, ed. *Medlink Neurology*, San Diego SA: Arbor Publishing Corp, 2004.

81. Zonana J, Silvey K, Strimling B. Familial neonatal and infantile seizures: an autosomal-dominant disorder. *Am J Med Genet.* 1984;**18**:455-9.

82. Miles DK,Holmes GL. Benign neonatal seizures. *J Clin Neurophysiol.* 1990;**7**:369-79.

83. Ronen GM, Rosales TO, Connolly M, Anderson VE, Leppert M. Seizure characteristics in chromosome 20 benign familial neonatal convulsions. *Neurology* 1993;**43**:1355-60.

84. Ryan SG, Wiznitzer M, Hollman C, Torres MC, Szekeresova M, Schneider *et al.* Benign familial neonatal convulsions: evidence for clinical and genetic heterogeneity. *Ann Neurol* 1991;**29**:469-73.

85. Leppert M, Anderson VE, Quattlebaum T, Stauffer D, O'Connell P, Nakamura Y *et al.* Benign familial neonatal convulsions linked to genetic markers on chromosome 20. *Nature* 1989;**337**:647-8.

86. Lewis TB, Leach RJ, Ward K, O'Connell P, Ryan SG. Genetic heterogeneity in benign familial neonatal convulsions: identification of a new locus on chromosome 8q. *Am J Hum Genet.* 1993;**53**:670-5.

87. Singh NA, Charlier C, Stauffer D, DuPont BR, Leach RJ, Melis R *et al.* A novel potassium channel gene, KCNQ2, is mutated in an inherited epilepsy of newborns. *Nature Genetics* 1998;**18**:25-9.

88. Biervert C, Steinlein OK. Structural and mutational analysis of KCNQ2, the major gene locus for benign familial neonatal convulsions. *Hum Genet.* 1999;**104**:234-40.

89. Lee WL, Biervert C, Hallmann K, Tay A, Dean JC, Steinlein OK. A KCNQ2 splice site mutation causing benign neonatal convulsions in a Scottish family.. *Neuropediatrics* 2000;**31**:9-12.

90. Hirose S, Zenri F, Akiyoshi H, Fukuma G, Iwata H, Inoue T *et al.* A novel mutation of KCNQ3 (c.925T—>C) in a Japanese family with benign familial neonatal convulsions. *Ann Neurol.* 2000;**47**:822-6.

91. Castaldo P, del Giudice EM, Coppola G, Pascotto A, Annunziato L, Taglialatela M. Benign familial neonatal convulsions caused by altered gating of KCNQ2/KCNQ3 potassium channels. *J Neurosci.* 2002;**22**:RC199.

92. Leppert M, Singh N. Benign familial neonatal epilepsy with mutations in two potassium channel genes. *Curr Opin Neurol.* 1999;**12**:143-7.

93. Singh NA, Westenskow P, Charlier C, Pappas C, Leslie J, Dillon J *et al.* KCNQ2 and KCNQ3 potassium channel genes in benign familial neonatal convulsions: expansion of the functional and mutation spectrum. *Brain* 2003;**126**:2726-37.

94. Berkovic SF, Heron SE, Giordano L, Marini C, Guerrini R, Kaplan RE *et al.* Benign familial neonatal-infantile seizures: Characterization of a new sodium channelopathy. *Ann Neurol.* 2004;**55**:550-7.

95. Heron SE, Crossland KM, Andermann E, Phillips HA, Hall AJ, Bleasel A *et al.* Sodium-channel defects in benign familial neonatal-infantile seizures. *Lancet* 2002;**360**:851-2.

96. Okada M, Wada K, Kamata A, Murakami T, Zhu G, Kaneko S. Impaired M-current and neuronal excitability. *Epilepsia* 2002;**43 Suppl 9**:36-8.

97. Aso K,Watanabe K. Benign familial neonatal convulsions: generalized epilepsy? *Pediat Neurol.* 1992;**8**:226-8.

98. Baxter P, Kandler R. Benign familial neonatal convulsions: abnormal intrauterine movements, provocation by feeding and ICTAL EEG. *Seizure* 1997;**6**:485-6.

99. Bye AM. Neonate with benign familial neonatal convulsions: recorded generalized and focal seizures. *Pediatr Neurol.* 1994;**10**:164-5.

100. Shevell MI, Sinclair DB, Metrakos K. Benign familial neonatal seizures: clinical and electroencephalographic characteristics. *Pediatr Neurol.* 1986;**2**:272-5.

101. Pettit RE,.Fenichel GM. Benign familial neonatal seizures. *Arch Neurol.* 1980;**37**:47-8.

102. Kaplan RE, Lacey DJ. Benign familial neonatal-infantile seizures. *Am J Med Genet* 1983;**16**:595-9.

103. Psenka TM, Holden KR. Benign familial neonatal convulsions; psychosocial adjustment to the threat of recurrent seizures. *Seizure* 1996;**5**:243-5.

104. Dehan M, Quilleron D, Navelet Y, et al. Les convulsions du cinquieme jour de vie: un nouveau syndrome? *Arch Fr Pediatr* 1977;**37**:730-42.

105. Plouin P. Benign neonatal convulsions (familial and non-familial). In Roger J, Bureau M, Dravet C, Dreifuss FE, Perret A, Wolf P, eds. *Epileptic syndromes in infancy, childhood and adolescence*, pp 2-11. London: John Libbey & Company, 1992.

106. Ballaban KR, Plouin P, Moshe SL. Benign neonatal familial seizures. In Gilman S, ed. *Medlink Neurology*, San Diego SA: Arbor Publishing Corp, 2004.

107. Vidaurre JA, Ballaban-Gil KR, Plouin P, Moshe SL. Benign neonatal seizures (nonfamilial). In Gilman S, ed. *Medlink Neurology*, San Diego SA: Arbor Publishing Corp, 2004.

108. Sperber EF, Haas KZ, Stanton PK, Moshe SL. Resistance of the immature hippocampus to seizure-induced synaptic reorganization. *Brain Res Dev.* 1991;**60**:88-93.

109. North KN, Storey GN, Henderson-Smart DJ. Fifth day fits in the newborn. *Aust Paediatr J* 1989;**25**:284-7.

110. Dalla Bernardina B, Dulac O, Fejerman N, Dravet C, Capovilla G, Bondavalli S *et al.* Early myoclonic epileptic encephalopathy (E.M.E.E.). *Eur J Pediatr.* 1983;**140**:248-52.

111. Bruel H, Boulloche J, Chabrolle JP, Layet V, Poinsot J. Early myoclonic epileptic encephalopathy and non-ketotic hyperglycemia in the same family. *Arch Pediatr* 1998;**5**:397-9.

112. Ohtahara S, Yamatogi Y. Epileptic encephalopathies in early infancy with suppression-burst. *J.Clin.Neurophysiol.* 2003;**20**:398-407.

113. Ohtahara S, Yamatogi Y, Ohtsuka Y. Early epileptic encephalopathies. In Wallace SJ, Farrell K, eds. *Epilepsy in childen*, pp 133-41. London: Arnold, 2004.

114. Agarwal P, Frucht SJ. Myoclonus. *Curr Opin Neurol.* 2003;**16**:515-21.

115. Faught E. Clinical presentations and phenomenology of myoclonus. *Epilepsia* 2003;**44 Suppl 11**:7-12.

116. Caviness JN, Brown P. Myoclonus: current concepts and recent advances. *Lancet Neurol.* 2004;**3**:598-607.

117. Blume WT, Luders HO, Mizrahi E, Tassinari C, van Emde BW, Engel J, Jr. Glossary of descriptive terminology for ictal semiology: report of the ILAE task force on classification and terminology. *Epilepsia* 2001;**42**:1212-8.

118. Janz D, Inoue Y, Seino M. Myoclonic seizures. In Engel JJ, Pedley TA, eds. *Epilepsy: A comprehensive Textbook*, pp 591-603. Philadelphia: Lippincott-Raven Publishers, 1997.

119. Wang PJ, Lee WT, Hwu WL, Young C, Yau KI, Shen YZ. The controversy regarding diagnostic criteria for early myoclonic encephalopathy. *Brain Dev.* 1998;**20**:530-5.

120. Aicardi J. Early myoclonic encephalopathy (neonatal myoclonic encephalopathy). In Roger J, Bureau M, Dravet C, Dreifuss FE, Perret A, Wolf P, eds. *Epileptic syndromes in infancy, childhood and adolescence*, pp 13-23. London: John Libbey & Company, 1992.

121. Spreafico R, Angelini L, Binelli S, Granata T, Rumi V, Rosti D *et al.* Burst suppression and impairment of neocortical ontogenesis: electroclinical and neuropathologic findings in two infants with early myoclonic encephalopathy. *Epilepsia* 1993;**34**:800-8.

122. Ohtahara S, Ohtsuka Y, Oka E. Epileptic encephalopathies in early infancy. *Indian J Pediatr.* 1997;**64**:603-12.

123. Chien YH, Hsu CC, Huang A, Chou SP, Lu FL, Lee WT *et al.* Poor outcome for neonatal-type nonketotic hyperglycinemia treated with high-dose sodium benzoate and dextromethorphan. *J Child Neurol.* 2004;**19**:39-42.

124. Fusco L, Pachatz C, Di Capua M, Vigevano F. Video/EEG aspects of early-infantile epileptic encephalopathy with suppression-bursts (Ohtahara syndrome). *Brain Dev.* 2001;**23**:708-14.

125. Yamatogi Y, Ohtahara S. Early-infantile epileptic encephalopathy with suppression-bursts, Ohtahara syndrome; its overview referring to our 16 cases. *Brain Dev.* 2002;**24**:13-23.

126. Romann D, Golz N, Garbe W. [Ohtahara syndrome]. *Geburtshilfe Frauenheilkd.* 1996;**56**:393-5.

127. Ohtahara S, Ishida T, Oka E, Yamatogy Y, Inoue H. On the specific age-dependent epileptic syndromes: the early-infantile epileptic encephalopathy with suppression-burst. *No To Hattatsu* 1976;**8**:270-80.

128. Itoh M, Hanaoka S, Sasaki M, Ohama E, Takashima S. Neuropathology of early-infantile epileptic encephalopathy with suppression-bursts; comparison with those of early myoclonic encephalopathy and West syndrome. *Brain Dev.* 2001;**23**:721-6.

129. Ohtahara S, Ohtsuka Y, Yamatogi Y, Oka E, Inoue H. Early-infantile epileptic encephalopathy with suppression-bursts. In Roger J, Bureau M, Dravet C, Dreifuss FE, Perret A, Wolf P, eds. *Epileptic syndromes in infancy, childhood and adolescence*, pp 25-34. London: John Libbey & Company, 1992.

130. Murakami N, Ohtsuka Y, Ohtahara S. Early infantile epileptic syndromes with suppression-bursts: early myoclonic encephalopathy vs. Ohtahara syndrome. *Jpn J Psychiatry Neurol.* 1993;**47**:197-200.

131. Ohno M, Shimotsuji Y, Abe J, Shimada M, Tamiya H. Zonisamide treatment of early infantile epileptic encephalopathy. *Pediatr Neurol.* 2000;**23**:341-4.

132. Komaki H, Sugai K, Maehara T, Shimizu H. Surgical treatment of early-infantile epileptic encephalopathy with suppression-bursts associated with focal cortical dysplasia. *Brain Dev.* 2001;**23**:727-31.

133. Di Capua M, Fusco L, Ricci S, Vigevano F. Benign neonatal sleep myoclonus: clinical features and video- polygraphic recordings. *Mov Disord.* 1993;**8**:191-4.

134. Daoust-Roy J,.Seshia SS. Benign neonatal sleep myoclonus. A differential diagnosis of neonatal seizures. *Am J Dis Child.* 1992;**146**:1236-41.

135. Caraballo R, Yepez I, Cersosimo R, Fejerman N. Benign neonatal sleep myoclonus. *Rev Neurol.* 1998;**26**:540-4.

136. Sheldon SH. Benign neonatal sleep myoclonus. In Gilman S, ed. *Medlink Neurology*, San Diego SA: Arbor Publishing Corp, 2004.

137. Lombroso CT, Fejerman N. Benign myoclonus of early infancy. *Ann Neurol.* 1977;**1**:138-43.

138. Pachatz C, Fusco L, Vigevano F. Benign myoclonus of early infancy. *Epilep Disord.* 1999;**1**:57-61.

139. Maydell BV, Berenson F, Rothner AD, Wyllie E, Kotagal P. Benign myoclonus of early infancy: an imitator of West's syndrome. *J Child Neurol.* 2001;**16**:109-12.

140. Wilner AN, Ballaban KR, Moshe SL. Benign nonepileptic infantile spasms. In Gilman S, ed. *Medlink Neurology*, San Diego SA: Arbor Publishing Corp, 2004.

141. Dravet C, Giraud N, Bureau M, Roger J, Gobbi G, Dalla Bernardina B. Benign myoclonus of early infancy or benign non-epileptic infantile spasms. *Neuropediatrics* 1986;**17**:33-8.

142. Kanazawa O. Shuddering attacks-report of four children. *Pediatr Neurol.* 2000;**23**:421-4.

143. Andermann F, Keene DL, Andermann E, Quesney LF. Startle disease or hyperekplexia: further delineation of the syndrome. *Brain* 1980;**103**:985-97.

144. Ryan SG, Sherman SL, Terry JC, Sparkes RS, Torres MC, Mackey RW. Startle disease, or hyperekplexia: response to clonazepam and assignment of the gene (STHE) to chromosome 5q by linkage analysis. *Ann Neurol.* 1992;**31**:663-8.

145. Tijssen MA, Schoemaker HC, Edelbroek PJ, Roos RA, Cohen AF, van Dijk JG. The effects of clonazepam and vigabatrin in hyperekplexia. *J Neurol Sci.* 1997;**149**:63-7.

146. Vergouwe MN, Tijssen MA, Peters AC, Wielaard R, Frants RR. Hyperekplexia phenotype due to compound heterozygosity for GLRA1 gene mutations. *Ann Neurol* 1999;**46**:634-8.

147. Saul B, Kuner T, Sobetzko D, Brune W, Hanefeld F, Meinck HM *et al.* Novel GLRA1 missense mutation (P250T) in dominant hyperekplexia defines an intracellular determinant of glycine receptor channel gating. *J Neurosci.* 1999;**19**:869-77.

148. Shiang R, Ryan SG, Zhu YZ, Fielder TJ, Allen RJ, Fryer A *et al.* Mutational analysis of familial and sporadic hyperekplexia. *Ann Neurol* 1995;**38**:85-91.

149. Praveen V, Patole SK, Whitehall JS. Hyperekplexia in neonates. *Postgrad Med J.* 2001;**77**:570-2.

150. Bernasconi A, Regli F, Schorderet DF, Pescia G. Familial hyperekplexia: startle disease. Clinical, electrophysiological and genetic study of a family. *Rev Neurol (Paris)* 1996;**152**:447-50.

151. Tijssen MA, Vergouwe MN, van Dijk JG, Rees M, Frants RR, Brown P. Major and minor form of hereditary hyperekplexia. *Mov Disord.* 2002;**17**:826-30.

152. de Groen JH,.Kamphuisen HA. Periodic nocturnal myoclonus in a patient with hyperexplexia (startle disease). *J Neurol Sci.* 1978;**38**:207-13.

153. Cioni G, Biagioni E, Bottai P, Castellacci AM, Paolicelli PB. Hyperekplexia and stiff-baby syndrome: an identical neurological disorder? *Ital J Neurol Sci.* 1993;**14**:145-52.

154. Findlay GS, Phelan R, Roberts MT, Homanics GE, Bergeson SE, Lopreato GF *et al.* Glycine receptor knock-in mice and hyperekplexia-like phenotypes: comparisons with the null mutant. *J Neurosci.* 2003;**23**:8051-9.

155. Miraglia DG, Coppola G, Bellini G, Ledaal P, Hertz JM, Pascotto A. A novel mutation (R218Q) at the boundary between the N-terminal and the first transmembrane domain of the glycine receptor in a case of sporadic hyperekplexia. *J Med Genet.* 2003;**40**:e71.

156. Gomeza J, Ohno K, Hulsmann S, Armsen W, Eulenburg V, Richter DW *et al.* Deletion of the mouse glycine transporter 2 results in a hyperekplexia phenotype and postnatal lethality. *Neuron* 2003;**40**:797-806.

157. Castaldo P, Stefanoni P, Miceli F, Coppola G, del Giudice EM, Bellini G *et al.* A novel hyperekplexia-causing mutation in the pre-transmembrane segment 1 of the human glycine receptor alpha1 subunit reduces membrane expression and impairs gating by agonists. *J Biol Chem.* 2004;**279**:25598-604.

158. Brown P. Neurophysiology of the startle syndrome and hyperekplexia. *Adv Neurol.* 2002;**89**:153-9.

IDIOPATHIC EPILEPTIC SEIZURES AND SYNDROMES IN INFANCY

6

The idiopathic epileptic seizures (that do not require a diagnosis of epilepsy) and idiopathic epileptic syndromes, which start mainly in the infantile (or very early childhood) period are listed below:[1,2]

CONDITIONS WITH EPILEPTIC SEIZURES THAT DO NOT REQUIRE A DIAGNOSIS OF EPILEPSY

- **Febrile seizures**
- **Benign familial infantile seizures***
- **Benign infantile seizures (non-familial)***

IDIOPATHIC EPILEPTIC SYNDROMES

- **Generalised epilepsy with febrile seizures plus (GEFS+) (autosomal dominant epilepsy with febrile seizures plus)****
- **Benign myoclonic epilepsy in infancy**

FEBRILE SEIZURES

> Convulsions occur to children if acute fever be present… These complaints occur most readily to children, who are very young up to their seventh year; older children and adults are not equally liable to be seized with convulsions…
>
> Hippocrates in part 24 of *Prognostics* 400 BC.

Febrile seizures[5-20] (a term preferred to its synonym febrile convulsions) are due to an age-related and predominantly genetic benign susceptibility to epileptic fits precipitated by fever of at least 38°C without evidence of intracranial infection or other cause. Children who have suffered a previous non-febrile seizure are excluded.

DEMOGRAPHIC DATA

Febrile seizures are the most common seizure disorder in childhood. The age at onset is from 6 months to 5 years with a peak at 18–22 months.[8,12,13] Onset outside this age range (6 months to 5 years) is not acceptable for the pure forms of febrile seizures (see febrile seizures plus on page 128)

Boys (60%) are slightly more affected than girls.

The prevalence is approximately 3%, but this is higher in certain ethnic groups such as Japan (7%) and Guam (14%). The annual incidence is 460 per 100 000 children in the age group 0–4 years.[21]

---

*These are newly recognised syndromes and, although not specified by the International League Against Epilepsy (ILAE) Task Force, benign infantile seizures (familial and non-familial) are classified by name (seizures) in the group of conditions with 'epileptic seizures that do not require a diagnosis of epilepsy' (Table 1.6).

**'GEFS+' or 'autosomal dominant epilepsy with febrile seizures plus'[3,4] has been recognised by the ILAE Task Force as a new syndrome in development.[2]

CLINICAL MANIFESTATIONS

> One minute he was a little boy with a cold and slight fever, lying on the sofa feeling miserable and the next his body was madly convulsing ... It was very scary.
>
> From an Internet description by a father

The body temperature that is accepted for the term 'febrile' is at least 38°C (others prefer 38.5°C) rectal temperature. Though a rapid rise in temperature is assumed to be a trigger, the temperature level may be more important.[28] One-fifth (21%) of febrile seizures occur within 1 h of the onset of fever, while 57% occur between 1 and 24 h, and 22% after more than 24 h from the onset of fever.[17]

TYPES OF FEBRILE SEIZURES

Generalised tonic clonic seizures (GTCS) are by far the commonest seizure type (80%). Tonic (13%), atonic (3%), and unilateral or focal onset tonic clonic seizures (4%) may occur in the remaining 20%. On rare occasions, seizures consist of staring accompanied by stiffness or floppiness, rhythmic jerking movements without prior stiffening, focal stiffness or jerking only. Myoclonic jerks or absences are not part of febrile seizures. Repetitive seizures in the same febrile illness occur in 16%.

Because of different prognostic implications, febrile seizures are categorised into simple and complex febrile seizures.

Simple febrile seizures

Simple febrile seizures (70% of all) are generalised tonic clonic convulsions with a duration of less than 15 min and without recurrence within the next 24 h (or within the same febrile illness).

According to the 1999 practice parameter of the American Pediatric Academy[12,13] simple febrile convulsions are strictly defined as occurring in

ILAE and other formal definitions for febrile seizures

The 1989 ILAE Classification categorised febrile seizures amongst the 'situation-related seizures' (which is synonymous to 'conditions with epileptic seizures that do not require a diagnosis of epilepsy' of the ILAE Task Force)[2] and defined them as follows.

Febrile convulsions are an age-related disorder almost always characterised by generalised seizures occurring during an acute febrile illness. Most febrile convulsions are brief and uncomplicated, but some may be more prolonged and followed by a transient or permanent neurological sequel, such as the hemiconvulsion–hemiplegia–epilepsy syndrome. Febrile convulsions tend to recur in approximately one-third of affected patients. Controversy about the risks of developing epilepsy later has largely been resolved by some recent large studies. The overall risk is probably no more than 4%. The indications for prolonged drug prophylaxis against recurrence of febrile convulsions are now more clearly defined and most individuals do not require prophylaxis. Essentially, this condition is a relatively benign disorder of early childhood.[1]

In the 1980 Consensus Development Conference on Febrile Seizures, National Institutes of Health, febrile seizures were defined as follows.[22,23]

A febrile seizure (an abnormal, sudden, excessive electrical discharge of neurones (grey matter) which propagates down the neuronal processes (white matter) to effect an end organ in a clinically measurable fashion) is an event in infancy or childhood, usually occurring between 3 months and 5 years of age, associated with fever, but without evidence of intracranial infection or defined cause. Seizures with fever in children who have suffered a previous non-febrile seizure are excluded. Febrile seizures are to be distinguished from epilepsy, which is characterised by recurrent non-febrile seizures.[22]

The working group of the Research Unit of the British Paediatric Association[8] considered that it was proper to use the term 'epileptic' instead of 'event' (used by the Americans)[22,23] and to distinguish 'convulsions with fever' from 'febrile convulsions'. Accordingly, for the purposes of clinical management the term febrile convulsions should be limited to an epileptic seizure occurring in a child aged from 6 months to 5 years, precipitated by fever arising from infection outside the nervous system in a child who is otherwise neurologically normal. The working group considered that it was proper to use the term 'epileptic' insofar as the neurophysiological substrate of a febrile convulsion is a paroxysmal neuronal discharge, as in an epileptic seizure. Among children who have convulsions with fever are those with pyogenic or viral meningitis, herpes simplex encephalitis, other acute encephalitides, cerebral palsy with intercurrent infection and metabolic or neurodegenerative disease with a seizure precipitated by fever. Children who have a prolonged seizure or who have not completely recovered within 1 h should be suspected of having one of these conditions and investigated accordingly.[8]

Febrile status epilepticus of longer than 30 min is either one long-lasting seizure or a series of shorter seizures, without regaining consciousness inter-ictally.[6,24–27]

neurologically healthy children between 6 months and 5 years of age whose seizure is brief (less than 15 min), generalised and occurs only once during a period of 24 h during a fever. Children whose seizures are attributable to a central nervous system (CNS) infection and those who have had a previous non-febrile seizure or CNS abnormality are excluded.

Complex febrile seizures

Complex febrile seizures (also known as *'complicated'* or *'atypical'*) are defined by seizures that may be prolonged or repetitive, or seizures that have focal features. One-third of all febrile seizures may have one, two or all three of these complicating factors. [5,6,29,30]

1 Prolonged febrile seizures are those which last for more than 15 min (8%).[31]

2 Repetitive febrile seizures occur in clusters of two or more within 24 h (11[29]–16%[5]).

3 Focal febrile seizures are those with a focal onset or those occurring in children with perinatal psychomotor deficits (3.5–7%). These also include those with the exceptional Todd's postictal paresis (0.4%).

Complex focal seizures of repetitive or prolonged character are probably easy to diagnose.[32] However, focal elements and particularly lateral eye deviation, staring episodes and motor asymmetries in the context of a bilateral convulsion may not be easy to recognise and categorise.[32]

Duration of febrile seizures

In 92% of cases seizures are brief, lasting 3–6 min or less than 15 min. In the other 8% the convulsions are longer than 15 min and two-thirds of these long seizures progress to febrile status epilepticus. Prolonged febrile seizures may constitute the initial stage of the hemiconvulsion–hemiplegia syndrome[1] (Chapter 8), but this is extremely rare (0.06%)[5,6] and found only among children with a recognisable specific illness (usually infectious) of the CNS.[15]

Post-ictal stage

Post-ictal symptoms other than drowsiness are rare and should raise the suspicion of another diagnosis. Todd's paralysis is exceptional (0.4%).[5,6]

RISK FACTORS FOR FEBRILE SEIZURES

The risk factors for a first febrile seizure have been studied in comparison with age-matched febrile and non-febrile control children.[33,34]

The risk of a first febrile seizure is approximately 30% if a child has two or more of the following independent risk factors:

- a first- or second-degree relative with febrile seizures
- delayed neonatal discharge of greater than 28 days of age
- parental reports of slow development
- day care attendance.

The risk for younger siblings of affected children is approximately 10–20% and this risk is greater if a parent is also affected. Males are more susceptible than females.

One-half of children will have recurrences: 32% have one, 15% have two and 7% have three or more recurrent seizures after a first febrile seizure. Half of those with a second febrile seizure will suffer at least one additional recurrence.

The following predisposing factors make recurrences more likely.[35]

- The first febrile seizure occurs in the first year of life.
- The first febrile seizure occurs during a short and low-grade febrile illness.
- There is a family history of febrile seizures in first-degree relatives.
- There are persistent neurological abnormalities.
- The first febrile seizure is complex.

AETIOLOGY

Genetic predisposition is important, as febrile seizures are often familial.[36,37] Children with siblings or parents with febrile seizures have a four- to fivefold higher risk than the general population. The reported concordance rates range up to as high as 70% in monozygotic twins and 20% in dizygotic twins. The mode of inheritance is unknown though this is likely polygenic. Autosomal recessive inheritance is unlikely, as there is an excess of parents affected and the risk to siblings is less than 25%.[6] Large autosomal dominant kindreds of febrile seizures made it possible to identify at least four different genetic loci mapped on chromosomes 8q13-21,[38,39] 19p13.3 and 19q13.1,[40,41] 5q14-q15[42] and 6q22–q24,[43] thereby assuring genetic heterogeneity.[37] No definitive gene or locus for febrile seizure has yet been established. However, genetic defects have been identified in a new genetically important syndrome of GEFS+ characterised by heterogeneous phenotypes of focal and generalised epileptic seizures[3,37,44] as detailed on page 128. Evidence suggests the involvement of various sodium channels, $GABA_A$ receptors and additional auxiliary proteins in the pathogenesis of febrile seizures plus and even in simple febrile seizures.[36]

PATHOPHYSIOLOGY

The pathophysiology of febrile seizures is unknown. They constitute a specific response to fever irrespective of cause. Circulating toxins and immune reaction products and viral or bacterial invasion of the CNS have been implicated, together with a relative lack of myelination in the immature brain and increased oxygen consumption during the febrile episode. Immaturity of thermoregulatory mechanisms and a limited capacity to increase cellular energy metabolism at elevated temperatures have been suggested as contributory factors.

The central histaminergic neuronal system may be involved in inhibition of the seizures associated with febrile illnesses in childhood. Children in whom the cerebrospinal fluid histamine does not rise during febrile illnesses may be susceptible to febrile seizures.[45]

Viral diseases are commoner, but this may reflect their higher prevalence in children. A specific association between acute human herpesvirus 6 infection (roseola infantum) and febrile seizures has been postulated.[46] The causes of fever vary and include upper respiratory tract infection or pharyngitis (38%), otitis media (23%), pneumonia (15%), gastroenteritis (7%), roseola infantum (5%) and non-infectious illness (12%).

Seizures occurring soon after immunisation with diphtheria/pertussis/tetanus and measles vaccines are due to fever and not to an adverse effect of the vaccine.

DIAGNOSTIC PROCEDURES

Febrile seizures do not need any investigation if the diagnosis is secure. EEG and brain imaging are unhelpful.

However, it is important to distinguish 'febrile convulsions' from 'convulsions with fever' such as in meningitis, encephalitis, cerebral palsy with inter-current infection and metabolic or neurodegenerative disease. Lumbar puncture may be mandatory in children who have a convulsion with fever in their first year of life (though this is still debated).

ELECTROENCEPHALOGRAPHY

EEG in straightforward cases is not needed.[10] EEG is more likely to be normal or show non-specific abnormalities that may be overemphasised by inexperienced neurophysiologists.

The reported incidence of EEG abnormalities in children with febrile seizures varies from 2 to 86%.[47] Such a wide difference is due in part to the definition of the EEG abnormalities, the time elapsed since the febrile seizure and the age of the patient at the time of the EEG.

Some authors have suggested that 'hypnagogic paroxysmal spike wave activity' is a special EEG feature seen in many children with febrile seizures.[48-50] This involves brief (1–2 s) generalised bursts of slow waves intermixed with small larval spikes as the child drifts to sleep. However, this is not specific and of no predictive significance.

Other authors have found that 20–50% of children who have serial EEGs starting at least 2 years after the initial febrile seizure demonstrate spikes or spike and wave abnormalities and photosensitivity.[20,51] In addition, there appears to be a high incidence of Rolandic spikes in children with febrile seizures.[52,53]

The American Academy of Paediatrics emphasises that, "*No published study demonstrates that an EEG performed either at the time of presentation after a simple febrile seizure or within the following month will predict the occurrence of future non-febrile seizures. Although the incidence of abnormal EEGs increases over time after a simple febrile seizure, no evidence exists that abnormal EEGs after the first febrile seizure are predictive for either the risk of recurrence of febrile seizures or the development of epilepsy. Even studies that have included children with complex febrile seizures and/or those with pre-existing neurological disease (a group at higher risk of having epilepsy develop) have not shown EEGs to be predictive of the development of epilepsy.*"[10]

PROGNOSIS

Overall, children with febrile seizures have a sixfold excess (3%) of subsequent non-febrile seizures and epilepsy compared with controls (Table 6.1).[5,29,54] Simple febrile seizures without any of these risk factors (60%) have only a twofold excess (1%) of unprovoked seizures compared wth controls. The risk after complex febrile seizures increases from 6–8% when a single complex feature is present to 49% if all three elements (prolonged, repetitive and focal febrile seizures) are present. These non-febrile seizures occur a few months to two to three decades after the initial febrile attack, but 85% start within 4 years. The risk is 2% by age 5 years, 4.5% by age 10 years, 5.5% by age 15 years and 7% by age 25 years.[54]

Non-febrile seizures of the subsequent epilepsy are of any type.[54] Generalised seizures are much more common than focal seizures and tend to occur when there is a positive family history of non-febrile seizures and a large number of brief generalised febrile seizures. Focal epilepsies follow prolonged lateralised febrile seizures in approximately 20%. In addition, earlier onset and persisting neurological abnormalities favour the development of focal epilepsy.[54]

The risk factors for later epilepsy are:
(1) abnormal neurological or developmental status prior to the first febrile seizure,
(2) a family history of non-febrile seizures,
(3) complex febrile seizures.
The overall risk is 3%.[5,29,54]

The estimated risk of developing temporal lobe epilepsy (TLE) subsequent to prolonged febrile seizures is negligible, probably 1 in 75 000 children per year.[55,56] Conversely, one-third of patients with hippocampal epilepsy have a previous history of prolonged febrile seizures (see mesial TLE with hippocampal sclerosis on page 378).[57-61]

PREDISPOSITION TO BOTH FEBRILE SEIZURES AND OTHER TYPES OF EPILEPSIES

It is well known that febrile seizures precede the onset of various forms of epilepsies in 10–15% of children.[56,63] There is a predisposition to both febrile seizures and other types of idiopathic generalised epilepsies (IGEs),[54,56,63,64] benign childhood focal seizures[65] and other epilepsies such as Dravet syndrome. There is unanimous agreement that children with benign childhood focal seizures, mainly Rolandic epilepsy and Panayiotopoulos syndrome, have a high prevalence of preceding febrile seizures (10–30%).[65] One-fifth of children with benign myoclonic epilepsy of infancy suffer preceding attacks of febrile seizures.

Contrary to the above are the results of another study of children with epilepsies, 13.9% of whom also had febrile seizures.[56] Children with febrile seizures were less likely to have childhood absence epilepsy and absence seizures compared with children without febrile seizures. This was particularly true for simple febrile seizures. Complex but not simple febrile seizures were associated with a younger age at onset of epilepsy. There was no evidence that focal or prolonged febrile seizures were associated with focal epilepsies or TLE *per se*. Of three children whose initial MRI scans demonstrated hippocampal atrophy, none had a history of febrile seizures.[56]

INTELLECTUAL AND BEHAVIOURAL OUTCOME

Children with febrile seizures perform as well as other children in terms of their academic progress, intellect and behaviour at 10 years of age.[66]

The subsequent psychomotor development of children who were normal prior to the onset of febrile seizures is normal.[66,67] If psychomotor deficits, learning difficulties and behavioural problems are found in children with febrile seizures, they are not related to the febrile seizures, but probably reflect the overall developmental status of the child.[20]

Table 6.1 Rates of epilepsy in children

Epilepsy	Rate (%)
Without febrile seizures	0.4[29]–0.5[5]
With simple febrile seizures	1,[29] 1.5,[5] and 2.6[54]
With complex febrile seizures	4[5]
With multiple febrile seizures	4[29]
With prolonged febrile seizures	6[29]
With focal febrile seizures	29[29]
With a single complex febrile seizure factor	7[54]
With two complex febrile seizure factors	17–22[54]
With all three complex febrile seizure factors	4[54]
The rates are similar irrespective of the type of treatment for febrile seizures.[15,62]	

MANAGEMENT[12,13,15]

This is mainly based on the recent recommendations of the American Academy of Pediatrics. [12,13]

ACUTE MANAGEMENT OF A CHILD WITH A FEBRILE SEIZURE

- Control of the seizures is paramount. Long-lasting febrile seizures (longer than 10 min) or status epilepticus (longer than 30 min) is a genuine paediatric emergency that demands appropriate and vigorous treatment, similar to non-febrile status epilepticus.[15,25] Early, usually parental treatment is more effective than late emergency treatment.[15] The parents of children with recurrent seizures should be advised to place the child on his/her side or stomach on a protected surface and administer a preparation of rectal benzodiazepine. In an emergency facility, the child's airway should be kept clear, oxygenation maintained and intravenous or rectal diazepines given to halt the seizure. *Diazepam* intravenously at a dose of 0.2–0.3 mg/kg or in rectal preparations at a dose of 0.5 mg/kg is probably the first choice. Rectal absorption of liquid diazepam is very rapid, reaches the brain within minutes and has a near-intravenous efficacy. A disadvantage of diazepam is its short duration of action. Rectal tubes containing liquid diazepam are the most widely used formulation. Diazepam rectal gel is now available in the USA. *Lorazepam* administered intravenously (0.1 mg/kg), which is less likely to cause respiratory depression and probably has a longer action than diazepam, is often preferred in medical facilities. *Midazolam* administered by buccal or nasal application may be another alternative for terminating prolonged seizures in the home.[68-70]
- Treatment of the fever and, mainly, the underlying illness is also important. Sponging with tepid water, anti-pyretics or both are usually recommended for reducing high fever. Anti-pyretics have a more sustained action while tepid sponging has a quicker but shorter effect. Anti-pyretic treatment during febrile illnesses does not reduce the recurrence rate and cannot be recommended other than to make the child more comfortable and avoid dehydration. Paracetamol is more widely used than ibuprofen, while aspirin is avoided because it has been associated with the development of Reye's syndrome.

Physical methods such as fanning, cold bathing and sponging are likely to cause discomfort and are not recommended.[8]

PROPHYLACTIC MANAGEMENT

Simple febrile seizures do not need prophylactic treatment. The risks are small and the potential side effects of drugs appear to outweigh the benefits.

Prophylactic treatment may be desired if a child has one or, mainly, a combination of the following features: (1) complex febrile seizures, (2) neurological abnormalities, (3) age less than 1 year and (4) frequent recurrences. Prophylactic treatment may be continuous or intermittent at the time of a febrile illness. Neither of these may be needed for the majority of children with febrile seizures, who nearly invariably do well.

Continuous treatment consists of daily administration of, mainly, phenobarbitone (which at a blood level of 15 μg/ml can effectively reduce the risk of recurrences) and, less often, valproate (fatal hepatitis in this age group or pancreatitis make valproate totally unacceptable). Carbamazepine and phenytoin are ineffective in the prevention of febrile seizures.

Intermittent treatment at the time of a febrile illness, mainly with rectal or oral diazepam, is an alternative to continuous medication (again a debated issue). There is a small reduction in the recurrence risk with a dose of 0.3 mg/kg of diazepam, although one-third of children will have significant side effects of somnolence or ataxia.

Supportive family management

The parents of young children should have general information provided by the family doctor about fever and febrile seizures. Parents who have watched their child during a fit need specific information in order to avoid long-term reactions.

In a study of parental reactions to a child's first febrile convulsion[71] most of the parents knew little about febrile seizures before the fit and most of them thought the child was dying (77%), suffocating or had meningitis (15%). Afterwards, the parental behaviour altered with restless sleep (60%), dyspepsia (29%) and overnight watching of the child (6%) or when feverish (8%). Parents with previous knowledge of febrile seizures took more appropriate measures but only 21% positioned the child correctly during the seizure.

Supportive family management includes education about febrile seizures, specific instructions about anti-pyretic and anti-epileptic prophylaxis and emergency procedures for possible subsequent seizures.

BENIGN INFANTILE SEIZURES (FAMILIAL AND NON-FAMILIAL)

WATANABE–VIGEVANO SYNDROME

Benign infantile (familial and non-familial) seizures[87-98] constitute a benign age-related idiopathic syndrome of infancy. The seizures are focal and the infants are otherwise normal.

DEMOGRAPHIC DATA

Age at onset is 3–20 months with a peak at 5–6 months. The familial form mostly starts between 4 and 7 months. Boys and girls are equally affected in the non-familial form, but more girls are reported in the familial cases. Only small numbers, approximately 100 of all types, have been reported so far but this may increase with improved awareness of the condition.

CLINICAL MANIFESTATIONS

Seizures characteristically occur in clusters of five to ten per day for 1–3 days and may recur after 1–3 months. One-third of patients have single isolated seizures 10–15 days before the clusters occur. The seizures are brief (0.5–3 min) but may be longer (3–6 min) at the beginning of the clusters and in the familial cases. They are predominantly diurnal. Inter-ictally the children remain normal.

The seizures are focal, manifesting with motor arrest, decreased responsiveness, impairment of consciousness, staring, eye and head deviation and mild unilateral clonic convulsions. Simple automatisms are frequent. Alternating from one side to the other is common. The seizures may or may not progress to hemi- or generalised convulsions.

AETIOLOGY

The familial form is most likely autosomal dominant with genetic heterogeneity. Linkage has been found to chromosomes 19q12-13.1,[100] 2q24[101] and 16p12-q12.[102]

Considerations on classification

The new ILAE diagnostic scheme recognises two types of benign infantile seizures (familial and non-familial).[2]

Three types of benign infantile seizures have been described.

1. Benign infantile familial convulsions.[89]
2. Benign infantile epilepsy with complex focal seizures.[87,88]
3. Benign focal epilepsy with secondarily generalised seizures in infancy.[99]

These have more in common than dividing features, as the main protagonists of their description, Watanabe and Vigevano, stated in a joint review.[90] Thus, all these are idiopathic seizures affecting otherwise normal infants, they:

a. are focal with or without secondarily generalised convulsions
b. appear in clusters in around the fifth to sixth months of life
c. have an entirely benign course.

In the dividing line is the familial or sporadic occurrence. Age at onset may be after the first year of life in the sporadic forms, while it is strictly limited to this age group (3 months-12 months) in the familial forms.

Benign familial infantile seizures do not appear to have genetic links with benign neonatal seizures though they may also prove to be channelopathies. In this respect the discovery of familial forms with seizure onset in the intermediate age (1–3 months) between benign neonatal and infantile seizures, for which the term *'benign familial neonatal–infantile seizures'* has been coined (page 126), may be relevant.[103,104] They are caused by mutations in the sodium channel subunit gene *SCN2A*.[103,104] No such mutations were found in ten families with benign familial infantile seizures.[104]

In addition, of significant genetic interest is the description of *'familial infantile convulsions and choreoathetosis'* linked to chromosome 16.[105,106] In this syndrome benign infantile seizures are inherited as an autosomal dominant trait together with variably expressed paroxysmal choreoathetosis.[105,106]

In another familial syndrome there is partial co-segregation of benign familial infantile seizures and familial hemiplegic migraine (which is linked to chromosome 19p13 in 50% of the families tested).[107]

The sporadic cases of benign infantile seizures may be identical to the familial cases, but with reduced expressivity[108] or they may be due to exogenous factors such as rotavirus infections.[109]

DIAGNOSTIC PROCEDURES

All relevant tests performed for infantile seizures are normal. However, they are needed, particularly in sporadic cases, in order to exclude symptomatic infantile seizures.

ELECTROENCEPHALOGRAPHY

The inter-ictal EEG is normal. The ictal EEG demonstrates focal discharges of fast activity intermixed with spikes that usually spread to neighbouring areas or the whole brain (Figure 6.1). Onset may be frontal, temporal, parietal or occipital and may vary in location and side between seizures in the same patient.[98,109]

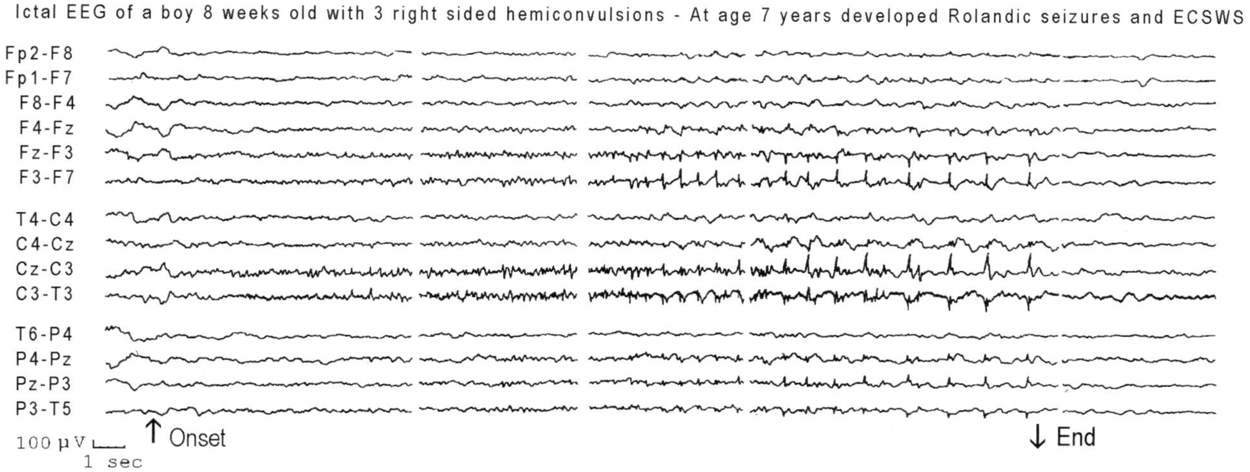

Figure 6.1 Benign infantile seizures (non-familial).

An ictal EEG of a seizure in an 8-week-old baby who, at this age, had three focal seizures of right-sided convulsions involving the face and upper limbs (This is case 17.2 in reference [65]). Brain MRI was normal
The inter-ictal EEG was normal. Subsequent EEGs were normal and treatment stopped at age 10 months. He was well until age 7 years when he started having Rolandic seizures and later developed epilepsy with continuous spike and wave during slow wave sleep (see Figure 7.12). The arrows mark the onset and termination of the seizure. Note the ictal EEG onset with focal left-sided fast spikes of low amplitude.

DIFFERENTIAL DIAGNOSIS

This may be difficult in the sporadic form, which requires a long follow-up before such a diagnosis can be established.[94]

PROGNOSIS

By definition seizures remit within 1–2 years from onset. Development is normal. In untreated cases there can be isolated or brief clusters within this infantile period of life.

MANAGEMENT

In the active seizure period, drug treatment is usually effective. Complete seizure control is achieved in nearly all cases. Recurrences after 1–2 months may occur in one-third of patients, but these are also easily controlled by drug dose adjustments. Anti-epileptic treatment is usually withdrawn after 1–3 years with no relapses.

Watanabe mainly used carbamazepine while Vigevano used valproate or phenobarbitone.

OTHER HEREDITARY SYNDROMES WITH BENIGN INFANTILE SEIZURES

Not yet recognised by the International League Against Epilepsy

BENIGN FAMILIAL NEONATAL–INFANTILE SEIZURES

This syndrome has been described in a small number of families by Berkovic's team.[103,104] The term 'benign familial neonatal–infantile seizures' is used to denote the fact that the onset of seizures is in the intermediate age period of when benign neonatal and benign infantile seizures occur.

Benign familial neonatal–infantile seizures is an autosomal dominant disorder presenting between day 2 and 7 months (mean 11.2 ± 9.2 weeks) with non-febrile secondarily generalised focal seizures: neonatal seizures were not seen in all families. The frequency of seizures varied, with some individuals having only a few attacks without treatment and others having clusters of many per day. Febrile seizures were rare. All cases remitted by 12 months. Ictal recordings in four subjects showed onset from the posterior quadrants.

The disorder is a sodium channelopathy caused by mutations in the sodium channel subunit gene *SCN2A*.[103,104] No such mutations were found in ten families with benign familial infantile seizures.[104]

FAMILIAL INFANTILE CONVULSIONS AND CHOREOATHETOSIS

Familial infantile convulsions and choreoathetosis has been described in four families from France in which benign infantile convulsions were inherited as an autosomal dominant trait together with variably expressed paroxysmal choreoathetosis.[105] The clinical manifestations of infantile seizures are the same as those already described for benign infantile seizures. Choreoathetotic movements start during infancy or childhood, are of dystonic type, occur at rest or can be induced by exertion or anxiety. Strong evidence of linkage for the disease gene was obtained in the peri-centromeric region of chromosome 16.[105]

In another report from Japan, Hamada *et al.*[106] reported 11 patients from five unrelated families. Paroxysmal choreoathetosis started between the ages of 5 and 17 years and was controlled with anti-epileptic drugs (AEDs) or subsided spontaneously. Eight cases also had infantile convulsions with onset between 3 and 8 months and an excellent prognosis. Four had complex focal seizures, which were characterised by staring, eye deviation, apnoea or loss of consciousness. Paroxysmal choreoathetosis was no different between those with or without infantile convulsions.[106]

FAMILIAL HEMIPLEGIC MIGRAINE AND BENIGN FAMILIAL INFANTILE SEIZURES

Terwindt *et al.*[107] reported a large Dutch–Canadian family with familial hemiplegic migraine and benign familial infantile seizures concurring and partially co-segregating. Familial hemiplegic migraine is a dominantly inherited subtype of migraine with attacks of hemiparesis linked to chromosome 19p13 in half of the families tested. Mutations in a brain-specific P/Q-type calcium channel alpha 1 subunit gene (CACNL1A4) were identified in families with chromosome 19-linked familial hemiplegic migraine. Molecular analysis of this family excluded linkage of the infantile convulsions to markers on chromosome 20q13.2, 8q or 19p13.

IDIOPATHIC EPILEPTIC SYNDROMES

GENERALISED EPILEPSY WITH FEBRILE SEIZURES PLUS

AUTOSOMAL DOMINANT EPILEPSY WITH FEBRILE SEIZURES PLUS

GEFS+[3,4,44,72-78] is the most important familial epileptic syndrome because it links febrile seizures with various other epileptic seizures/syndromes and documents genetic relations between (1) benign and severe and (2) focal and generalised epileptic disorders.
GEFS+ has been described by Berkovic and his associates[44,73] and has been recognised as a syndrome in development by the ILAE Task Force.[2]

DEMOGRAPHIC DATA

The age at onset, from the first months of life to childhood, varies considerably between individuals, even individuals of the same family. Both sexes are equally affected. The prevalence is unknown, but may be high considering the increasing numbers of publications and the very broad spectrum of GEFS+.

CLINICAL MANIFESTATIONS

GEFS+ is characterised by heterogeneous clinical phenotypes ranging from classical febrile seizures, 'febrile seizures plus' (FS+), non-febrile generalised convulsions, absences, myoclonic or atonic seizures and, more frequently myoclonic-atonic seizures. Focal frontal and temporal lobe seizures may occur[80] in 13% of affected individuals[4] and these focal seizures may dominate in some members of affected families.[3] Within the GEFS+ spectrum, more severe syndromic phenotypes can occur including Dravet syndrome, epilepsy with myoclonic-astatic seizures (EM-AS) of Doose and TLE.[81,82]

GEFS+ shows marked genetic and phenotypic heterogeneity. There are extreme intra-familial and inter-familial clinical variations regarding seizure type, seizure frequency, severity and prognosis. By definition, in all families some patients suffer from FS+, which are often preceded by classical febrile seizures.

Febrile seizures may occur alone (approximately 75% of patients) or combine with other type of seizures such as the following:

- Brief non-febrile generalised convulsions
- Other generalised seizures, such as absences, myoclonic jerks and tonic seizures
- Focal seizures of mainly frontal or temporal lobe origin
- More severe forms of seizures such as those occurring in Dravet syndrome and epilepsy with myoclonic-astatic seizures.

Definitions and clarifications for febrile seizures plus

Febrile seizures plus' (FS+) is a term used to denote childhood onset febrile seizures, which (unlike the typical febrile seizures) start earlier (less than 6 months with mean 1 year) than the classical febrile seizures. They are often multiple and continue beyond the age of 5 years usually remitting by mid-childhood (median 11 years). Individuals with FS+ may also have additional non-febrile seizures.
According to Berkovic, the critical feature in diagnosing the 'febrile seizures plus' phenotype is the continuity of generalised seizures from early to mid-childhood, not the presence or absence of fever. Indeed, families often do not recognise the absence of a fever, interpreting all attacks as 'febrile seizures'. In some children with FS+, seizures with fever did occur beyond age 6 years, whereas in others, all seizures beyond age 6 years were non-febrile.[79]
Some authors have proposed that the name 'autosomal dominant epilepsy with febrile seizures plus' may be more appropriate than GEFS+ because recent discoveries document that the spectrum of the syndrome includes diverse types of focal and generalised seizures.[3]

Typical febrile seizures and FS+ are the most common clinical phenotypes occurring in approximately 75% of affected patients.

Of nine families identified by probands suffering from myoclonic-atonic seizures genealogical information was available for 799 individuals: 91 had a history of seizures and 63 had seizures consistent with the diagnosis of GEFS+ syndrome.[73] Of these 63 patients 49% had classical febrile seizures only, 29% had FS+, 13% had FS+ with other seizure types such as absences (5%), myoclonic seizures (3%) and temporal lobe seizures (3%) and 14% had myoclonic- atonic seizures.[73] Of other members (not considered to suffer from GEFS+) one had typical childhood absence epilepsy and another three had nocturnal GTCS after a head concussion.

In another family with GEFS+, all 15 patients had typical febrile seizures.[77] Of these 40% had FS+, 13% non-febrile tonic clonic convulsions, 13% atonic seizures, 6% nocturnal tonic seizures and 6% a single focal seizure with orofacial onset.[77]

The high prevalence of GEFS+ amongst patients with Dravet syndrome has only recently been realised (see Chapter 7, page 155).[81,83,84]

In seven recently described families (unrelated to *SCN1A*, *SCN1B* and *GABRG2* gene mutations) of 167 individuals, 41 had epilepsy: 29 had a phenotype consistent with GEFS+, seven had IGE, in three the epilepsy type could not be classified and two were considered phenocopies.[4] The clinical phenotypes included FS+ (29.2%), febrile seizures (29.2%), IGE (18.2%), FS+ with focal seizures (13%) or absence seizures (2.6%) and febrile seizures with absence seizures (2.6%).

AETIOLOGY

GEFS+ is a purely genetic disorder with profound heterogeneity. Inheritance is generally autosomal dominant with incomplete penetrance,[73] but this may not be the only situation.[37]

As Berkovic indicated, "*GEFS+ may follow a more complex inheritance and serve as an entrée to the genetics of common forms of epilepsy. It is likely that the severe phenotypes within GEFS+ are the result of cumulative effects of multiple genes. Thus, finding one gene within a family may form a basis from which other genes may be found, entering the domain of true complex inheritance.*"[37]

GEFS+ is genetically heterogeneous with two loci described on chromosome 19q (GEFS+) and chromosome 2q (GEFS2). Mutations were found in the *SCN1A*, *SCN1B* and *SCN2A* genes (encoding the alpha 1, alpha 2 and beta 1 voltage-gated sodium channel subunits) and the *GABRG2* gene ($GABA_A$–receptor gamma 2 subunit).[85] At least nine mutations that cause GEFS+ have been identified in the *SCN1A* gene encoding the alpha subunit of the Na(v)1.1 voltage-gated sodium channel.[86] More recent studies have indicated that mutations of the *SCN1A*, *SCN2A*, *SCN1B* and *GABRG2* genes in patients with GEFS+ are rare.[4,77]

There may be many mechanisms by which sodium channel alterations cause the various clinical phenotypes of GEFS+. To produce the different seizure types observed in families with GEFS+, seizure predisposition determined by the GEFS+ genes could be modified by other genes and/or by environmental factors.[82]

One of the most significant recent developments is the frequent association of GEFS+ with EM-AS of Doose (Chapter 10, page 291) and Dravet syndrome. (see Chapter 7, page 152).[81,83,84] Dravet syndrome probably represents the very severe end of the spectrum within the GEFS+ phenotype.[82]

DIAGNOSTIC PROCEDURES

Brain MRI when performed is within the normal limits.

EEG findings depend on the clinical phenotype. The EEG is usually normal, particularly in patients with febrile seizures only. The commonest EEG abnormality is sparse and brief generalised discharges of spike and slow wave that might require sleep EEGs for their detection. In clinical phenotypes of EM-AS or Dravet syndrome the EEG abnormalities are severe as described in the relevant chapters. In patients with focal seizures, the EEG shows focal sharp waves, which are mainly localised in the frontal and temporal regions.[3,4]

PROGNOSIS

In most studies, the overall picture is that GEFS+ is usually benign and self-limited.[73,77] Non-febrile seizures occur in only approximately one-quarter of the patients and these are usually infrequent and often remit by mid-childhood (median 11 years). However, this overall good prognosis is now being reconsidered with the inclusion of Dravet syndrome, a devastating epileptic encephalopathy, within the broad spectrum of GEFS+.

DIFFERENTIAL DIAGNOSIS

In a child presenting with recurrent convulsions precipitated by fever, the diagnostic issue is whether they are typical febrile seizures or FS+. This is because, at onset, the FS+ phenotype resembles typical febrile seizures occurring between 6 months and 5 years. [12] The distinguishing features are the persistence of febrile seizures beyond the age of 6 years and/or the occurrence of non-febrile seizures.

Absences when they feature are usually brief and mild. They are easily distinguishable from the severe forms of childhood or juvenile absence epilepsy.

The evolution to other more severe clinical phenotypes such as EM-AS or Dravet syndrome becomes apparent only with the emergence of new types of seizures compatible with these disorders.

MANAGEMENT

Repetitive febrile seizures or FS+ may need prophylactic treatment. Valproate or newer drugs such as lamotrigine, levetiractetam or topiramate should be used for non-febrile generalised seizures, if these are frequent. Treatment of more severe phenotypes has been described in the chapter on Dravet syndrome (page 152) and EM-AS (page 291).

BENIGN MYOCLONIC EPILEPSY IN INFANCY

Benign myoclonic epilepsy in infancy[90,110-116] is probably the earliest form of an age-dependent IGE syndrome manifested mainly or exclusively by myoclonic jerks only. The jerks may be spontaneous, reflex or both.

DEMOGRAPHIC DATA

Onset is between 6 months and 3 years, but in a few infants may start earlier (4 months) or later (2–5 years). Boys are twice as likely to be affected than girls. The prevalence may be around 1–2% of epilepsies starting before the age of 3 years.[115,116] This syndrome is based on retrospective studies and single case reports of approximately 100 patients, sometimes heterogeneous and including those with stimulus-elicited myoclonic jerks.[115,116]

CLINICAL MANIFESTATIONS

Myoclonic seizures are the predominant and often the only type of fits in benign myoclonic epilepsy in infancy.[116]

MYOCLONIC JERKS

Myoclonic jerks mainly affect the head, eyeballs, upper extremities and the diaphragm (Figure 6.2). The jerks are brief and singular or clusters that vary in frequency and violence. They clinically manifest with head nodding and more rarely flexion or extension of the body. The upper limbs usually fling upwards and outwards, while the eyeballs may roll upwards. A brief yell, probably resulting from the contraction of the diaphragm, sometimes accompanies the jerks. Falls may occur in the rare cases in which the lower limbs are affected.

Consciousness is commonly intact but clusters of jerks may be associated with mild clouding.

Myoclonic seizures are usually spontaneous, occurring randomly in alert stages and exaggerated by drowsiness and slow sleep. In some patients they tend to cluster on awakening or during the first hours of sleep. Reflex myoclonic jerks are sometimes prominent. Patients may have spontaneous or reflex-only jerks or both.

The duration of the jerks is usually brief (1–2 s). Vigevano et al.[90] reported that some children have more significant generalised clonic seizures, exclusively during sleep or on awakening, that are prolonged up to 15–20 min and can cause cyanosis without loss of consciousness.[90]

OTHER TYPES OF SEIZURES

One-fifth of patients have simple, brief and infrequent febrile seizures usually preceding the onset of myoclonias.

One-fifth of patients may develop infrequent GTCS usually in their early teens.

Non-febrile convulsions of uncertain categorisation prior to the onset of myoclonic seizures or during the clinical course of the disease have been reported.[112]

In one report six out of 11 children also had non-epileptic myoclonus.[117]

PRECIPITATING FACTORS

One-fifth of patients have clinical and EEG photosensitivity. In 10% the myoclonic jerks are predominantly or exclusively elicited by unexpected acoustic or tactile stimuli and these may have a better prognosis.[111,114,118,119] Single jerks or clusters of two to eight symmetric limb jerks, mainly of the arms, are elicited by sudden noise or tactile stimuli either when awake or asleep. Startle is important. If expected the stimulus is ineffective.[111]

AETIOLOGY

Benign myoclonic epilepsy in infancy is probably the earliest form of IGE. There is no evidence that it is linked with juvenile myoclonic epilepsy or indeed any other type of IGE. A family history of epilepsy or febrile seizures is present in 30% of cases.

Familial benign myoclonic epilepsy in infancy with autosomal recessive inheritance and linkage to chromosome 16p13 has been reported, but in this family myoclonic seizures persisted into adulthood and all patients developed GTCS in their early teens.[120]

DIAGNOSTIC PROCEDURES

All tests other than the EEGs are normal.

ELECTROENCEPHALOGRAPHY

The inter-ictal EEG is normal. Spontaneous inter-ictal generalised polyspike wave discharges without associated jerks are exceptional.

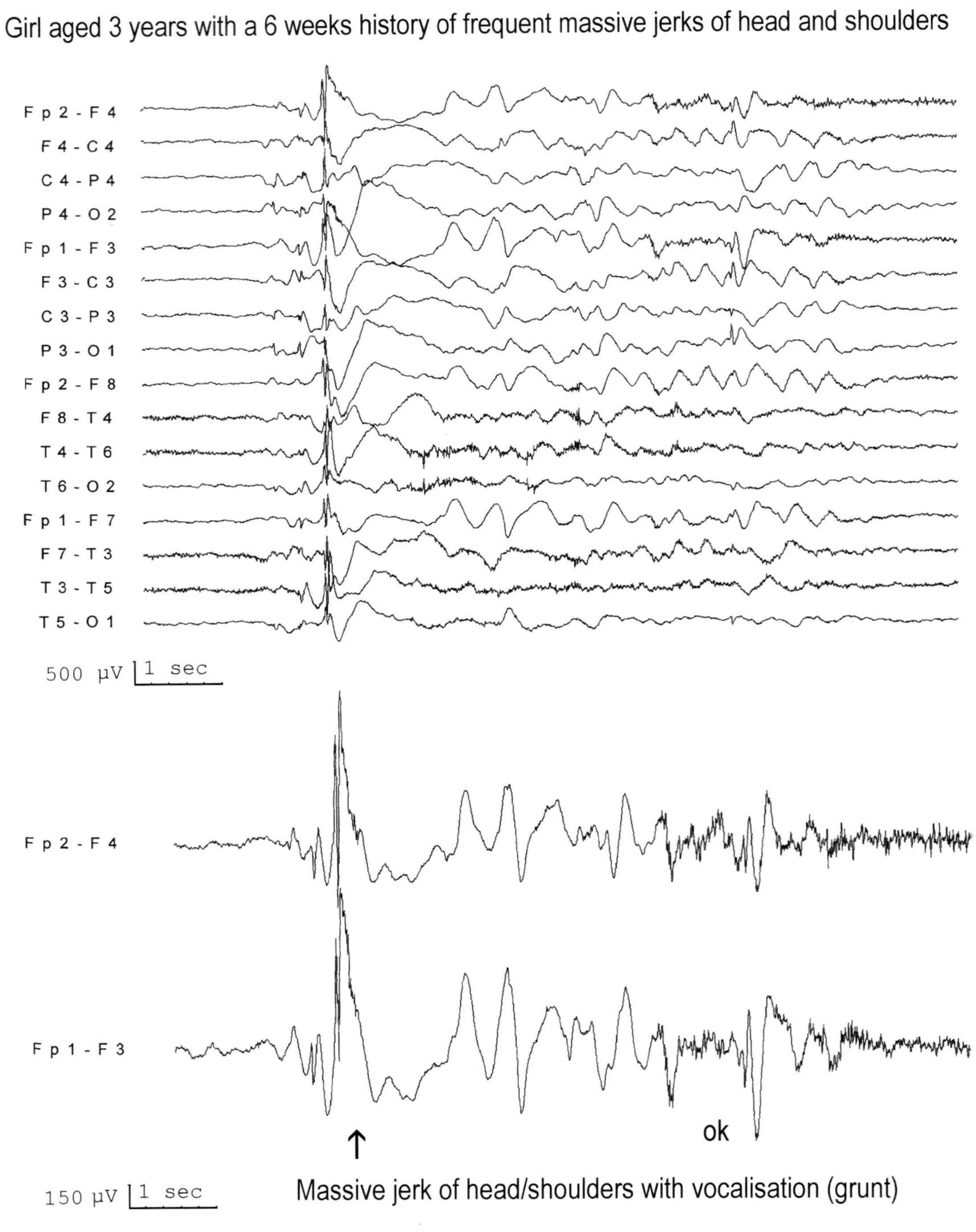

Figure 6.2 Benign myoclonic epilepsy in infancy.

This is a typical case of benign myoclonic epilepsy in infancy with myoclonic jerks only and an excellent prognosis. At age 3 years, she developed frequent and violent myoclonic jerks mainly in the head and shoulders with grunting noises. She was referred for a routine EEG 6 weeks from the onset of the jerks. On the basis of the history, the EEG technologist performed video–EEG recording and purposely extended the recording for clinical events. Two electroclinical seizures were captured, one of which is shown in this figure. Clinically, the first symptom was a sudden jerk of the head and shoulders backwards. This coincided with a giant (approximately 1 mV) spike or multiple spike and slow wave followed by rhythmic slow activity at around 3–5 Hz together with some random spikes and slow waves. The whole discharge lasted for approximately 5–7 s. The seizures only stopped when clonazepam was added to valproate (which probably was not needed). Subsequent serial EEGs were normal. At age 6 years she is not on medication, has developed well, is free of seizures and has a normal EEG.

The ictal EEG during jerks shows generalised polyspike or spike and slow wave discharges with a duration of 1–3 s (Figure 6.2).

Drowsiness and the early stages of sleep exaggerate the EEG discharges that may occur with or without jerks. EEG generalised discharges of mainly multiple spikes with jerks are often stimulus evoked by photic stimulation or unexpected acoustic or tactile stimuli. These occur in awake or sleep stages.

DIFFERENTIAL DIAGNOSIS

Benign myoclonic epilepsy in infancy should first be differentiated from non-epileptic conditions such as hypnagogic jerks and benign non-epileptic myoclonus (page 110). Hypnagogic jerks do not occur in waking states and the EEG is normal. Benign non-epileptic myoclonus resembles epileptic spasms rather than myoclonic jerks of benign myoclonic epilepsy in infancy.

It should not be difficult to differentiate benign myoclonic epilepsy in infancy from epileptic encephalopathies such as West, Dravet or Lennox–Gastaut syndromes with multiform seizures, severe EEG abnormalities and often neurodevelopmental deficits.

PROGNOSIS

Remission usually occurs between 6 months and 5 years from onset. Patients with jerks provoked by auditory or tactile stimuli have a better prognosis and the jerks are easily controlled with anti-epileptic medication or stimulus preventive measures. Conversely, EEG photosensitivity may persist many years after clinical remission.

In general, 10–20% of all patients with benign myoclonic epilepsy in infancy develop infrequent GTCS in their early teens when medication has been withdrawn.

Psychomotor development is often normal, but 10–20% of children may later develop usually mild cognitive, behavioural or motor deficits if untreated.

MANAGEMENT

The response to AED treatment is usually excellent. Patients with photosensitivity are more difficult to control and EEG photosensitivity may persist several years after the remission of seizures. Patients with acoustic- and somatosensory-evoked myoclonus may not need treatment or withdrawal may be initiated after 1 year.

Valproate is considered the drug of choice by all authors. With adequate doses 80% of patients may become seizure free. However, no other suitable AEDs have been tried in this condition. Clonazepam is more effective than valproate in controlling myoclonic jerks. Levetiracetam is the most potent new anti-myoclonic drug, which also significantly suppresses photosensitivity (Table 10,.8 page 317).[121] Therefore, these AEDs may be more effective as monotherapy and probably in smaller doses than valproate.

Gradual and slow withdrawal of drug treatment over 6 months to a year can be initiated 3–5 years from onset.

REFERENCES

1. Commission on Classification and Terminology of the International League Against Epilepsy. Proposal for revised classification of epilepsies and epileptic syndromes. *Epilepsia* 1989;**30**:389-99.
2. Engel J, Jr. A proposed diagnostic scheme for people with epileptic seizures and with epilepsy: Report of the ILAE Task Force on Classification and Terminology. *Epilepsia* 2001;**42**:796-803.
3. Ito M, Nagafuji H, Okazawa H, Yamakawa K, Sugawara T, Mazaki-Miyazaki E *et al.* Autosomal dominant epilepsy with febrile seizures plus with missense mutations of the (Na+)-channel alpha 1 subunit gene, SCN1A. *Epilepsy Res.* 2002;**48**:15-23.
4. Bonanni P, Malcarne M, Moro F, Veggiotti P, Buti D, Ferrari AR *et al.* Generalized epilepsy with febrile seizures plus (GEFS+): clinical spectrum in seven Italian families unrelated to SCN1A, SCN1B, and GABRG2 gene mutations. *Epilepsia* 2004;**45**:149-58.
5. Nelson KB,.Ellenberg JH. Predictors of epilepsy in children who have experienced febrile seizures. *N Engl J Med* 1976;**295**:1029-33.
6. Nelson KB,.Ellenberg JH. Prognosis in children with febrile seizures. *Pediatrics* 1978;**61**:720-7.
7. Wallace SJ. The Child with Febrile Seizures. London: Butterworth, 1988.
8. Joint Working Group of the Research Unit of the Royal College of Physicians and the British Paediatric Association. Guidelines for the management of convulsions with fever. Joint Working Group of the Research Unit of the Royal College of Physicians and the British Paediatric Association. *BMJ* 1991;**303**:634-6.
9. Fukuyama Y, Seki T, Ohtsuka C, Miura H, Hara M. Practical guidelines for physicians in the management of febrile seizures. *Brain Develop* 1996;**18**:479-84.
10. American Academy of Pediatrics. Practice parameter: the neurodiagnostic evaluation of the child with a first simple febrile seizure. American Academy of Pediatrics. Provisional Committee on Quality Improvement, Subcommittee on Febrile Seizures. *Pediatrics* 1996;**97**:769-72.
11. Berg AT, Shinnar S, Darefsky AS, Holford TR, Shapiro ED, Salomon ME *et al.* Predictors of recurrent febrile seizures. A prospective cohort study. *Arch Pediatr Adolesc.Med* 1997;**151**:371-8.
12. American Academy of Pediatrics. Practice parameter: long-term treatment of the child with simple febrile seizures. American Academy of Pediatrics. Committee on Quality Improvement, Subcommittee on Febrile Seizures. *Pediatrics* 1999;**103**:1307-9.
13. Baumann RJ. Technical report: treatment of the child with simple febrile seizures. *Pediatrics* 1999;**103**:e86.
14. Baumann RJ,.Duffner PK. Treatment of children with simple febrile seizures: the AAP practice parameter. American Academy of Pediatrics. *Pediatr Neurol* 2000;**23**:11-7.
15. Knudsen FU. Febrile seizures: treatment and prognosis. *Epilepsia* 2000;**41**:2-9.
16. Baram TZ, Shinnar S (eds). Febrile Seizures. San Diego, California: Academic Press, 2002.
17. Shinnar S,.Glauser TA. Febrile seizures. *J Child Neurol.* 2002;**17 Suppl 1**:S44-S52.
18. Camfield P, Camfield C, Kurlemann G. Febrile seizures. In Roger J, Bureau M, Dravet C, Genton P, Tassinari CA, Wolf P, eds. *Epileptic syndromes in infancy, childhood and adolescence (3rd edn)*, pp 145-52. London: John Libbey & Co Ltd, 2002.
19. Verity CM. Febrile convulsions. In Duncan JS, Walker MC, Smalls JE, eds. *Epilepsy 2003. From synapse to patient*, pp 87-100 (http://www.epilepsynse.org.uk). Oxford: Meritus Communications, 2003.
20. Wallace SJ. Febrile seizures. In Wallace SJ, Farrell K, eds. *Epilepsy in childen*, pp 123-30. London: Arnold, 2004.
21. Forsgren L, Sidenvall R, Blomquist HK, Heijbel J. A prospective incidence study of febrile convulsions. *Acta Paediatr Scand* 1990;**79**:550-7.
22. American Academy of Pediatrics. Consensus statement. Febrile seizures: long-term management of children with fever-associated seizures. *Pediatrics* 1980;**66**:1009-12.
23. Freeman JM. Febrile seizures: a consensus of their significance, evaluation, and treatment. *Pediatrics* 1980;**66**:1009.
24. Maytal J,.Shinnar S. Febrile status epilepticus. *Pediatrics* 1990;**86**:611-6.
25. Mitchell WG. Status epilepticus and acute repetitive seizures in children, adolescents, and young adults: etiology, outcome, and treatment. *Epilepsia* 1996;**37 Suppl 1**:S74-S80.
26. Shinnar S. Prolonged febrile seizures and mesial temporal sclerosis [editorial; comment]. *Ann Neurol* 1998;**43**:411-2.
27. Verity CM, Ross EM, Golding J. Outcome of childhood status epilepticus and lengthy febrile convulsions: findings of national cohort study. *BMJ* 1993;**307**:225-8.
28. Berg AT. Are febrile seizures provoked by a rapid rise in temperature?. *Am J Dis Child* 1993;**147**:1101-3.
29. Verity CM,.Golding J. Risk of epilepsy after febrile convulsions: a national cohort study. *BMJ* 1991;**303**:1373-6.
30. Berg AT,.Shinnar S. Complex febrile seizures. *Epilepsia* 1996;**37**:126-33.
31. Shinnar S, Pellock JM, Berg AT, O'Dell C, Driscoll SM, Maytal J *et al.* Short-term outcomes of children with febrile status epilepticus. *Epilepsia* 2001;**42**:47-53.
32. Berg AT, Steinschneider M, Kang H, Shinnar S. Classification of complex features of febrile seizures: interrater agreement. *Epilepsia* 1992;**33**:661-6.
33. Berg AT, Shinnar S, Hauser WA, Leventhal JM. Predictors of recurrent febrile seizures: a metaanalytic review. *J Pediatr* 1990;**116**:329-37.
34. Berg AT, Shinnar S, Shapiro ED, Salomon ME, Crain EF, Hauser WA. Risk factors for a first febrile seizure: a matched case-control study. *Epilepsia* 1995;**36**:334-41.
35. Offringa M, Bossuyt PM, Lubsen J, Ellenberg JH, Nelson KB, Knudsen *et al.* Risk factors for seizure recurrence in children with febrile seizures: a pooled analysis of individual patient data from five studies. *J Pediatr* 1994;**124**:574-84.
36. Hirose S, Mohney RP, Okada M, Kaneko S, Mitsudome A. The genetics of febrile seizures and related epilepsy syndromes. *Brain Dev.* 2003;**25**:304-12.
37. Berkovic SF,.Scheffer IE. Genetics of the epilepsies. *Epilepsia* 2001;**42 Suppl 5**:16-23.
38. Berkovic SF,.Scheffer IE. Febrile seizures: genetics and relationship to other epilepsy syndromes. *Curr Opin Neurol.* 1998;**11**:129-34.
39. Wallace RH, Berkovic SF, Howell RA, Sutherland GR, Mulley JC. Suggestion of a major gene for familial febrile convulsions mapping to 8q13-21. *J Med Genet.* 1996;**33**:308-12.
40. Johnson EW, Dubovsky J, Rich SS, O'Donovan CA, Orr HT, Anderson VE *et al.* Evidence for a novel gene for familial febrile convulsions, FEB2, linked to chromosome 19p in an extended family from the Midwest. *Hum Mol Genet.* 1998;**7**:63-7.
41. Kugler SL, Stenroos ES, Mandelbaum DE, Lehner T, McKoy VV, Prossick T *et al.* Hereditary febrile seizures: phenotype and evidence for a chromosome 19p locus. *Am J Med Genet.* 1998;**79**:354-61.
42. Nakayama J, Hamano K, Iwasaki N, Nakahara S, Horigome Y, Saitoh H *et al.* Significant evidence for linkage of febrile seizures to chromosome 5q14- q15. *Hum Mol Genet.* 2000;**9**:87-91.
43. Nabbout R, Prud'homme JF, Herman A, Feingold J, Brice A, Dulac O *et al.* A locus for simple pure febrile seizures maps to chromosome 6q22-q24. *Brain* 2002;**125**:2668-80.
44. Scheffer IE,.Berkovic SF. Generalized epilepsy with febrile seizures plus. A genetic disorder with heterogeneous clinical phenotypes. *Brain* 1997;**120**:479-90.
45. Kiviranta T, Tuomisto L, Airaksinen EM. Histamine in cerebrospinal fluid of children with febrile convulsions. *Epilepsia* 1995;**36**:276-80.
46. Barone SR, Kaplan MH, Krilov LR. Human herpesvirus-6 infection in children with first febrile seizures. *J Pediatr* 1995;**127**:95-7.
47. Maytal J, Steele R, Eviatar L, Novak G. The value of early postictal EEG in children with complex febrile seizures. *Epilepsia* 2000;**41**:219-21.
48. Tsuboi T,.Endo S. Febrile convulsions followed by nonfebrile convulsions. A clinical, electroencephalographic and follow-up study. *Neuropadiatrie* 1977;**8**:209-23.
49. Alvarez N, Lombroso CT, Medina C, Cantlon B. Paroxysmal spike and wave activity in drowsiness in young children: its

relationship to febrile convulsions. *Electroencephalogr Clin Neurophysiol* 1983;**56**:406-13.

50. Sofijanov N, Emoto S, Kuturec M, Dukovski M, Duma F, Ellenberg JH *et al.* Febrile seizures: clinical characteristics and initial EEG. *Epilepsia* 1992;**33**:52-7.

51. Doose H, Ritter K, Volzke E. EEG longitudinal studies in febrile convulsions. Genetic aspects. *Neuropediatrics* 1983;**14**:81-7.

52. Kajitani T, Ueoka K, Nakamura M, Kumanomidou Y. Febrile convulsions and rolandic discharges. *Brain Dev.* 1981;**3**:351-9.

53. Kajitani T, Kimura T, Sumita M, Kaneko M. Relationship between benign epilepsy of children with centro-temporal EEG foci and febrile convulsions. *Brain Dev.* 1992;**14**:230-4.

54. Annegers JF, Hauser WA, Shirts SB, Kurland LT. Factors prognostic of unprovoked seizures after febrile convulsions. *N Engl J Med* 1987;**316**:493-8.

55. VanLandingham KE, Heinz ER, Cavazos JE, Lewis DV. Magnetic resonance imaging evidence of hippocampal injury after prolonged focal febrile convulsions. *Ann Neurol* 1998;**43**:413-26.

56. Berg AT, Shinnar S, Levy SR, Testa FM. Childhood-onset epilepsy with and without preceding febrile seizures. *Neurology* 1999;**53**:1742-8.

57. Falconer MA. Genetic and related aetiological factors in temporal lobe epilepsy. A review. *Epilepsia* 1971;**12**:13-31.

58. Maher J,.McLachlan RS. Febrile convulsions. Is seizure duration the most important predictor of temporal lobe epilepsy? *Brain* 1995;**118 (Pt 6)**:1521-8.

59. O'Connor WM, Masukawa L, Freese A, Sperling MR, French JA, O'Connor MJ. Hippocampal cell distributions in temporal lobe epilepsy: a comparison between patients with and without an early risk factor. *Epilepsia* 1996;**37**:440-9.

60. Ohtsu M, Oguni H, Awaya Y, Osawa M. Clinical and EEG analysis of initial status epilepticus during infancy in patients with mesial temporal lobe epilepsy. *Brain Dev.* 2002;**24**:231-8.

61. Cendes F. Febrile seizures and mesial temporal sclerosis. *Curr Opin Neurol.* 2004;**17**:161-4.

62. Knudsen FU, Paerregaard A, Andersen R, Andresen J. Long-term prognosis in febrile convulsions with and without prophylaxis. *Ugeskrift for Laeger* 1997;**159**:3598-602.

63. Camfield P, Camfield C, Gordon K, Dooley J. What types of epilepsy are preceded by febrile seizures? A population-based study of children. *Developmental Medicine & Child Neurology* 1994;**36**:887-92.

64. Rocca WA, Sharbrough FW, Hauser WA, Annegers JF, Schoenberg BS. Risk factors for absence seizures: a population-based case- control study in Rochester, Minnesota. *Neurology* 1987;**37**:1309-14.

65. Panayiotopoulos CP. Benign childhood partial seizures and related epileptic syndromes. London: John Libbey & Company Ltd, 1999.

66. Verity CM, Greenwood R, Golding J. Long-term intellectual and behavioral outcomes of children with febrile convulsions. *N Engl J Med* 1998;**338**:1723-8.

67. Ellenberg JH,.Nelson KB. Febrile seizures and later intellectual performance. *Arch Neurol* 1978;**35**:17-21.

68. Koren G. Intranasal midazolam for febrile seizures. A step forward in treating a common and distressing condition. *BMJ* 2000;**321**:64-5.

69. Lahat E, Goldman M, Barr J, Bistritzer T, Berkovitch M. Comparison of intranasal midazolam with intravenous diazepam for treating febrile seizures in children: prospective randomised study. *BMJ* 2000;**321**:83-6.

70. Scott RC, Besag FM, Neville BG. Intranasal midazolam for treating febrile seizures in children. Buccal midazolam should be preferred to nasal midazolam. *BMJ* 2001;**322**:107.

71. Balslev T. Parental reactions to a child's first febrile convulsion. A follow-up investigation. *Acta Paediatr Scand* 1991;**80**:466-9.

72. Baulac S, Gourfinkel-An I, Picard F, Rosenberg-Bourgin M, Prudhomme JF, Baulac M *et al.* A second locus for familial generalized epilepsy with febrile seizures plus maps to chromosome 2q21-q33. *Am J Hum Genet.* 1999;**65**:1078-85.

73. Singh R, Scheffer IE, Crossland K, Berkovic SF. Generalized epilepsy with febrile seizures plus: a common childhood- onset genetic epilepsy syndrome. *Ann Neurol* 1999;**45**:75-81.

74. Lopes-Cendes I, Scheffer IE, Berkovic SF, Rousseau M, Andermann E, Rouleau GA. A new locus for generalized epilepsy with febrile seizures plus maps to chromosome 2. *Am J Hum Genet.* 2000;**66**:698-701.

75. Escayg A, Heils A, MacDonald BT, Haug K, Sander T, Meisler MH. A novel SCN1A mutation associated with generalized epilepsy with febrile seizures plus—and prevalence of variants in patients with epilepsy. *Am J Hum Genet.* 2001;**68**:866-73.

76. Wallace RH, Scheffer IE, Barnett S, Richards M, Dibbens L, Desai RR *et al.* Neuronal sodium-channel alpha1-subunit mutations in generalized epilepsy with febrile seizures plus. *Am J Hum Genet.* 2001;**68**:859-65.

77. Gerard F, Pereira S, Robaglia-Schlupp A, Genton P, Szepetowski P. Clinical and genetic analysis of a new multigenerational pedigree with GEFS+ (Generalized Epilepsy with Febrile Seizures Plus). *Epilepsia* 2002;**43**:581-6.

78. Annesi G, Gambardella A, Carrideo S, Incorpora G, Labate A, Pasqua AA *et al.* Two novel SCN1A missense mutations in generalized epilepsy with febrile seizures plus. *Epilepsia* 2003;**44**:1257-8.

79. Scheffer IE, Wallace RH, Mulley JC, Berkovic SF. Locus for febrile seizures. *Ann Neurol* 2000;**47**:840-1.

80. Sugawara T, Tsurubuchi Y, Agarwala KL, Ito M, Fukuma G, Mazaki-Miyazaki E *et al.* A missense mutation of the Na+ channel alpha II subunit gene Na(v)1.2 in a patient with febrile and afebrile seizures causes channel dysfunction. *Proc Natl Acad Sci U S A* 2001;**98**:6384-9.

81. Scheffer IE, Wallace R, Mulley JC, Berkovic SF. Clinical and molecular genetics of myoclonic-astatic epilepsy and severe myoclonic epilepsy in infancy (Dravet syndrome). *Brain Dev.* 2001;**23**:732-5.

82. Scheffer IE. Severe infantile epilepsies: molecular genetics challenge clinical classification. *Brain* 2003;**126**:513-4.

83. Dravet C, Bureau M, Oguni H, Fukuyama H, Cokar O. Severe myoclonic epilepsy in infancy (Dravet syndrome). In Roger J, Bureau M, Dravet C, Genton P, Tassinari CA, Wolf P, eds. *Epileptic syndromes in infancy, childhood and adolescence (3rd edn)*, pp 81-103. London: John Libbey & Co Ltd, 2002.

84. Herranz JL. Severe myoclonic epilepsy in infancy (Dravet's syndrome). Some genetic aspects. *Rev Neurol.* 2003;**37**:60-3.

85. Mulley JC, Scheffer IE, Petrou S, Berkovic SF. Channelopathies as a genetic cause of epilepsy. *Curr Opin Neurol.* 2003;**16**:171-6.

86. Spampanato J, Escayg A, Meisler MH, Goldin AL. Generalized epilepsy with febrile seizures plus type 2 mutation W1204R alters voltage-dependent gating of Na(v)1.1 sodium channels. *Neuroscience* 2003;**116**:37-48.

87. Watanabe K, Yamamoto N, Negoro T, Takaesu E, Aso K, Furune S *et al.* Benign complex partial epilepsies in infancy. *Pediatr Neurol* 1987;**3**:208-11.

88. Watanabe K, Yamamoto N, Negoro T, Takahashi I, Aso K, Maehara M. Benign infantile epilepsy with complex partial seizures.. *J Clin Neurophysiol* 1990;**7**:409-16.

89. Vigevano F, Fusco L, Di Capua M, Ricci S, Sebastianelli R, Lucchini *et al.* Benign infantile familial convulsions. *Eur J Pediatr* 1992;**151**:608-12.

90. Vigevano F, Cusmai R, Ricci S, Watanabe K. Benign epilepsies of infancy. In Engel J.jr., Pedley T.A, eds. *Epilepsy. A comprehensive textbook*, pp 2267-76. Lippincott-Raven, 1997.

91. Watanabe K. Benign partial epilepsies in infancy and early childhood:clinical description and genetic background. In Berkovic SF, Genton P, Hirsch E, Plouin P, eds. *Genetics of focal epilepsies*, pp 73-8. London: John Libbey & Company Ltd, 1999.

92. Gennaro E, Malacarne M, Carbone I, Riggio MC, Bianchi A, Bonanni P *et al.* No evidence of a major locus for benign familial infantile convulsions on chromosome 19q12-q13.1. *Epilepsia* 1999;**40**:1799-803.

93. Gautier A, Pouplard F, Bednarek N, Motte J, Berquin P, Billard C *et al.* Benign infantile convulsions. French collaborative study. *Arch Pediatr.* 1999;**6**:32-9.

94. Okumura A, Hayakawa F, Kato T, Kuno K, Negoro T, Watanabe K. Early recognition of benign partial epilepsy in infancy. *Epilepsia* 2000;**41**:714-7.

95. Watanabe K,.Okumura A. Benign partial epilepsies in infancy. *Brain Dev.* 2000;**22**:296-300.

96. Vigevano F, Bureau M. Idiopathic and/or benignlocalization-related epilepsies in infants and young children. In Roger J, Bureau M, Dravet C, Genton P, Tassinari CA, Wolf P, eds.

Epileptic syndromes in infancy, childhood and adolescence (3rd edn), pp 153-60. London: John Libbey & Co Ltd, 2002.

97. Nelson GB, Olson DM, Hahn JS. Short duration of benign partial epilepsy in infancy. *J Child Neurol.* 2002;**17**:440-5.
98. Vigevano F. Benign epilepsy of infancy with partial seizures. In Gilman S, ed. *Medlink Neurology*, San Diego SA: Arbor Publishing Corp, 2004.
99. Watanabe K, Negoro T, Aso K. Benign partial epilepsy with secondarily generalized seizures in infancy. *Epilepsia* 1993;**34**:635-8.
100. Guipponi M, Rivier F, Vigevano F, Beck C, Crespel A, Echenne B *et al.* Linkage mapping of benign familial infantile convulsions (BFIC) to chromosome 19q. *Hum Mol Genet.* 1997;**6**:473-7.
101. Malacarne M, Gennaro E, Madia F, Pozzi S, Vacca D, Barone B *et al.* Benign familial infantile convulsions: mapping of a novel locus on chromosome 2q24 and evidence for genetic heterogeneity. *Am J Hum Genet.* 2001;**68**:1521-6.
102. Caraballo R, Pavek S, Lemainque A, Gastaldi M, Echenne B, Motte J *et al.* Linkage of benign familial infantile convulsions to chromosome 16p12-q12 suggests allelism to the infantile convulsions and choreoathetosis syndrome. *Am J Hum Genet.* 2001;**68**:788-94.
103. Heron SE, Crossland KM, Andermann E, Phillips HA, Hall AJ, Bleasel A *et al.* Sodium-channel defects in benign familial neonatal-infantile seizures. *Lancet* 2002;**360**:851-2.
104. Berkovic SF, Heron SE, Giordano L, Marini C, Guerrini R, Kaplan RE *et al.* Benign familial neonatal-infantile seizures: Characterization of a new sodium channelopathy. *Ann Neurol.* 2004;**55**:550-7.
105. Szepetowski P, Rochette J, Berquin P, Piussan C, Lathrop GM, Monaco *et al.* Familial infantile convulsions and paroxysmal choreoathetosis: a new neurological syndrome linked to the pericentromeric region of human chromosome 16. *Am J Hum Genet* 1997;**61**:889-98.
106. Hamada Y, Hattori H, Okuno T. Eleven cases of paroxysmal kinesigenic choreoathetosis; correlation with benign infantile convulsions. *No To Hattatsu* 1998;**30**:483-8.
107. Terwindt GM, Ophoff RA, Lindhout D, Haan J, Halley DJ, Sandkuijl LA *et al.* Partial cosegregation of familial hemiplegic migraine and a benign familial infantile epileptic syndrome. *Epilepsia* 1997;**38**:915-21.
108. Vigevano F. Benign epilepsy of infancy with partial seizures. In Gilman S, ed. *Medlink Neurology*, San Diego SA: Arbor Publishing Corp, 2004.
109. Imai K, Otani K, Yanagihara K, Li Z, Futagi Y, Ono J *et al.* Ictal video-EEG recording of three partial seizures in a patient with the benign infantile convulsions associated with mild gastroenteritis. *Epilepsia* 1999;**40**:1455-8.
110. Dravet C, Bureau M, Genton P. Benign myoclonic epilepsy of infancy: electroclinical symptomatology and differential diagnosis from the other types of generalized epilepsy of infancy. *Epilepsy Research - Supplement* 1992;**6**:131-5.
111. Ricci S, Cusmai R, Fusco L, Vigevano F. Reflex myoclonic epilepsy in infancy: a new age-dependent idiopathic epileptic syndrome related to startle reaction. *Epilepsia* 1995;**36**:342-8.
112. Lin Y, Itomi K, Takada H, Kuboda T, Okumura A, Aso K *et al.* Benign myoclonic epilepsy in infants: video-EEG features and long-term follow-up. *Neuropediatrics* 1998;**29**:268-71.
113. Prats-Vinas JM, Garaizar C, Ruiz-Espinoza C. Benign myoclonic epilepsy in infant. *Rev Neurol.* 2002;**34**:201-4.
114. Caraballo R, Casar L, Monges S, Yepez I, Galicchio S, Cersosimo R *et al.* Reflex myoclonic epilepsy in infancy: a new reflex epilepsy syndrome or a variant of benign myoclonic epilepsy in infancy. *Rev Neurol.* 2003;**36**:429-32.
115. Fejerman N. Benign myoclonic epilepsy in infancy. In Wallace SJ, Farrell K, eds. *Epilepsy in childen*, pp 153-6. London: Arnold, 2004.
116. Dravet C, Bureau M. Benign myoclonic epilepsy in infancy. In Gilman S, ed. *Medlink Neurology*, San Diego SA: Arbor Publishing Corp, 2004.
117. Rossi PG, Parmeggiani A, Posar A, Santi A, Santucci M. Benign myoclonic epilepsy: long-term follow-up of 11 new cases. *Brain Dev.* 1997;**19**:473-9.
118. Kurian MA,.King MD. An unusual case of benign reflex myoclonic epilepsy of infancy. *Neuropediatrics* 2003;**34**:152-5.
119. Zafeiriou D, Vargiami E, Kontopoulos E. Reflex myoclonic epilepsy in infancy: a benign age-dependent idiopathic startle epilepsy. *Epil Disord.* 2003;**5**:121-2.
120. de Falco FA, Majello L, Santangelo R, Stabile M, Bricarelli FD, Zara F. Familial infantile myoclonic epilepsy: clinical features in a large kindred with autosomal recessive inheritance. *Epilepsia* 2001;**42**:1541-8.
121. Covanis A, Stodieck SR, Wilkins AJ. Treatment of photosensitivity. *Epilepsia* 2004;**45 Suppl 1**:40-5.

7

EPILEPTIC ENCEPHALOPATHIES IN INFANCY AND EARLY CHILDHOOD

IN WHICH THE EPILEPTIFORM ABNORMALITIES MAY CONTRIBUTE TO PROGRESSIVE DYSFUNCTION

Epileptic encephalopathies are severe brain disorders in which the epileptic electrical discharges may contribute to progressive psychomotor dysfunction.[1-14] They are a group of nosologies that are related to early age and manifest with EEG paroxysmal activity that is often aggressive, seizures that are commonly multi-form and intractable, cognitive, behavioural and neurological deficits that may be relentless and sometimes early death. Cognitive deficits and behavioural disturbances are presumed to be the main and sometimes the first and only unique manifestation of electrographic epileptic discharges in epileptic encephalopathies.

The concept of 'epileptic encephalopathies' is based on the assumption that aggressive ictal (seizure) and electrical (electrographic) epileptogenic activity during brain maturation is the main cause of progressive cognitive and neuropsychological deterioration or regression. In other words there is a detrimental effect of continuing seizures and electrographic discharges on the normal function of the developing brain.[15,16] Cognitive and behavioural decline is paralleled by changes in brain connectivity, diminishing excitatory glutamatergic receptor distribution, and decreased neurogenesis.

Conversely, this deleterious epileptic activity is a specific age-related brain reaction of excessive neocortical excitability to different pathological conditions, which are focal or diffuse, and of symptomatic or idiopathic cause. This age-related epileptogenic reaction is peculiar to the immature brain and varies significantly in accordance with the stage of brain maturity at the time that this occurs. Thus, EEG demonstrates primarily burst–suppression patterns in the neonatal period, hypsarrhythmia in infancy and slow generalised spike-wave discharges (GSWD) in early childhood. With advancing age, the seizure and electrographic epileptogenic features may evolve from one to another age-related stage that is from burst–suppression to hypsarrhythmia and then to slow GSWD. All epileptic encephalopthies have a tendency to abate, discontinue or even stop in adolescence but often with serious neurocognitive residual effect.

These features explain certain clinico-EEG phenomena such as the following:

- the age-related similar features of the various epileptic encephalopathies irrespective of cause
- the overlapping clinico-EEG features between the various epileptic encephalopathies
- the evolutional changes from Ohtahara syndrome to West syndrome and from West syndrome to Lennox–Gastaut syndrome with age
- the age-related cessation of the deteriorating progression and some recovery of the neuropsychological consequences that occurred during the active epileptic encephalopathic periods
- the age-related remission of seizures and electrographic manifestations in Landau–Kleffner syndrome and epilepsy with continuous spikes and waves during slow wave sleep (ECSWS).

The aetiopathology of these syndromes has not been fully elucidated. It may be multiple and not necessarily the same for all. The major determinant is the brain functional and structural immaturity, with a 'cause–effect' interaction between abnormal electrical discharges generated by and modifying/acting upon neuronal circuits in development.

Epileptic encephalopathies have recently been authoritatively reviewed by leading experts.[6-9,13,17-20]

The following are syndromes of epileptic encephalopathies with onset in the neonatal period, infancy and early childhood:[1,21]

- **Early myoclonic encephalopathy** (see chapter 5, page 103)
- **Ohtahara syndrome** (see chapter 5, page 106)
- **West syndrome**
- **Dravet syndrome** (severe myoclonic epilepsy in infancy)*
- **Lennox–Gastaut syndrome**
- **Landau–Kleffner syndrome****
- **Epilepsy with continuous spike-and-waves during slow-wave sleep** (other than Landau-Kleffner syndrome)
- **Myoclonic status in non-progressive encephalopathies*****

---

* The descriptive name 'severe myoclonic epilepsy in infancy'[21] has been discarded in favour of the eponymic nomenclature 'Dravet syndrome' in the new ILAE diagnostic scheme.[1]

**The descriptive name 'acquired epileptic aphasia'[21] has been discarded in favour of the eponymic nomenclature 'Landau–Kleffner syndrome' in the new ILAE diagnostic scheme.[1]

***A syndrome in development according to the new ILAE diagnostic scheme.[1]

Nomenclature clarifications on epileptic encephalopathies and catastrophic epilepsies

Epileptic encephalopathies are often cited as catastrophic epilepsies, which as the name "catastrophic" implies (catastrophy in Greek means disaster), they are invariably associated with significant neurological morbidity and often early death. However, catastrophic epilepsies is a broader term to encompass all severe forms of progressive epilepsies including some but not all epileptic encephalopathies and the progressive myoclonic epilepsies.[24-27] Progressive myoclonic epilepsies (Unverricht-Lundborg disease, mitochondrial encephalopathy with ragged-red fibers, Lafora body disease, neuronal ceroid lipofuscinosis, and sialidosis cherry-red spot myoclonus syndrome) are all genetic disorders (most are autosomal recessive) classified by the ILAE as 'diseases frequently associated with epileptic seizures or syndromes' (Table 1.8).[1]

Nomenclature clarifications on slow-wave sleep

I would discourage the use of the term *"slow-wave sleep"* in favour of the formal terminology of sleep stages. "Slow-wave sleep" usually refers to stages III and IV of non-rapid eye movement (NREM) sleep (particularly in humans) but it is also used to denote all stages (I-IV) of NREM sleep (particularly in animals). In the case of 'epilepsy with continuous spike-and-waves during slow-wave sleep' or the EEG finding of 'continuous spike-and-waves during slow-wave sleep, "slow -wave sleep" appears to refer to all stages of NREM sleep. This is documented with all night sleep recordings where 'continuous spike-wave' or 'electrical status epilepticus' appears as soon as the patient falls to sleep and continues through all NREM I-IV sleep stages. It is intrerrupted during random eye movement (REM) stage and repeats the same cycle again in NREM and REM stages.[28,29]

Definitions of seizures commonly occurring in epileptic encephalopathies.[30]

Atonic seizure. A sudden loss or diminution of muscle tone without an apparent preceding myoclonic or tonic event lasting approximately 1–2 s, involving the head, trunk, jaw or limb musculature.[30]

Astatic seizure (synonym: drop attack). A loss of erect posture that results from an atonic, myoclonic or tonic mechanism.[30,31]

Clonic seizure (synonym: rhythmic myoclonus). A myoclonus that is regularly repetitive, involves the same muscle groups, is at a frequency of approximately 2–3 Hz and is prolonged.[30]

Epileptic spasm (formerly infantile spasm). A sudden flexion, extension or mixed extension–flexion of predominantly the proximal and truncal muscles that is usually more sustained than a myoclonic movement, but not so sustained as a tonic seizure (i.e. approximately 1 s). Limited forms may occur, for example grimacing and head nodding. Epileptic spasms frequently occur in clusters.[30,32,33] See also other definitions in page 291.

Myoclonic-atonic seizures. These are characterised by a myoclonic-atonic sequence. Symmetrical myoclonic jerks of the arms or irregular twitching of the face precede the more or less pronounced loss of tone.[30,31,34]

Myoclonic seizure or myoclonus. Sudden, brief (less than 100 ms), involuntary, single or multiple contraction(s) of muscles(s) or muscle groups of variable topography (axial, proximal limb and distal).[30,35]

Negative myoclonic seizure or negative myoclonus. Interruption of tonic muscular activity for less than 500 ms without evidence of preceding myoclonia.[30,36-38]

Tonic seizure. A sustained increase in muscle contraction lasting a few seconds to minutes.[30,39]

I have also included hypothalamic (gelastic) epilepsy (page 193) in this Chapter because many authorities consider it as a form of epileptic encephalopathy with progressive severe seizures and cognitive and behavioural decline.[22] The acquired cognitive and behavioural symptoms probably result from a direct effect of the seizures.[23] Children with hypothalamic hamartomas and precocious puberty, but without seizures do not develop cognitive and behavioural problems.

WEST SYNDROME

West syndrome is an age-related specific epileptic encephalopathy due to multiple and diverse causes. It is characterised by a unique type of seizure called epileptic (infantile) spasms (Figure 7.1) and gross EEG abnormalities of hypsarrhythmia (Figure 7.2).[3,13,32,40-63] An expert consensus on West syndrome has recently been published (November 2004).[63]

DEMOGRAPHIC DATA

This is a remarkably age-dependent syndrome, with the onset of the attacks at between 3 and 12 months of age and a peak at 5 months in 90% of cases. Younger and older children are more likely to have other conditions, and a greater risk of misclassification exists.[63] In 70% of cases onset is in the first 6 months, while an onset under 3 months is uncommon and an onset between 1 and 3 years is rare, probably around 5%. Localisation of focal cortical lesions may influence the age of onset of epileptic spasms.[65]

Boys (60%) are affected more than girls though reports differ, sometimes giving a 2:1 preponderance of males over females.

ILAE classification and nomenclature of West syndrome

The 1989 ILAE Commission[21] categorised West syndrome amongst 'generalised cryptogenic or symptomatic epilepsies (age related)' and defined it as follows.

West syndrome (infantile spasms, Blitz-Nick-Salaam Krampfe): Usually, West syndrome consists of a characteristic triad: infantile spasms, arrest of psychomotor development, and hypsarrhythmia, although one element may be missing. Spasms may be flexor, extensor, lightning, or nods, but most commonly they are mixed. Onset peaks between the ages of 4 and 7 months and always occurs before the age of 1 year. Boys are more commonly affected. The prognosis is generally poor. West syndrome may be separated into two groups. The symptomatic group is characterized by previous existence of brain damage signs (psychomotor retardation, neurologic signs, radiologic signs, or other types of seizures) or by a known etiology. The smaller, cryptogenic group is characterized by a lack of previous signs of brain damage and of known etiology. The prognosis appears to be partly based on early therapy with adrenocorticotropic hormone or oral steroids.[21]

The ILAE new diagnostic scheme[1] classifies West syndrome amongst 'epileptic encephalopathies' and prefers 'epileptic spasms' rather than 'infantile spasms'.

Gibbs and Gibbs[64] described the EEG pattern of infantile spasms and called it *hypsarrhythmia* from the Greek words *hypsos* (=high) and *arrhythmia* (which does not need translation).

Clarifications on terminology

West syndrome is commonly used synonymously with *infantile spasms*. However, officially "infantile spasms" refer to a type of seizures (preferably called "epileptic spasms"), which are common but not exclusive for the West syndrome.[1,30]

In a recent consensus of experts, terminology has become more complex.[63]

Infantile spasms is an inclusive term to describe an epilepsy syndrome of all children with clinical spasms and EEG abnormalities typically, although not necessarily, of hypsarrhythmia or modified hypsarrhythmia provided that the EEG findings do not suggest another specific diagnosis. This syndrome rarely has onset in children older than 2 years and usually has onset in children younger than 1 year. Its main clinical manifestation is clinical spasms that usually occur in clusters. Many potential aetiologies or associated conditions exist. The most characteristic EEG finding is hypsarrhythmia. However, hypsarrhythmia is not found in all cases, nor is it found throughout the clinical course of the condition. Hypsarrhythmia is usually interrupted during a clinical attack of epileptic spasms. The spasms are often associated with developmental arrest or regression.[63]

West syndrome is considered a specific subgroup of the syndrome of infantile spasms to describe the combination of spasms that occur in clusters and hypsarrhythmia on an EEG. Evidence of delayed development before the onset of spasms is not required.[63]

Epileptic spasms describes the seizure type.[63]

Cinical spasms describes the ictal phenomenology irrespective of ictal EEG.[63]

The incidence of West syndrome appears to be approximately 3–5 per 10,000 live births. It was found in 3 per 10,000 in Iceland,[66] 5 per 10,000 in Sweden,[67] 2.9 per 10,000 in the USA[68] and 4.1 per 10,000 in Finland.[69]

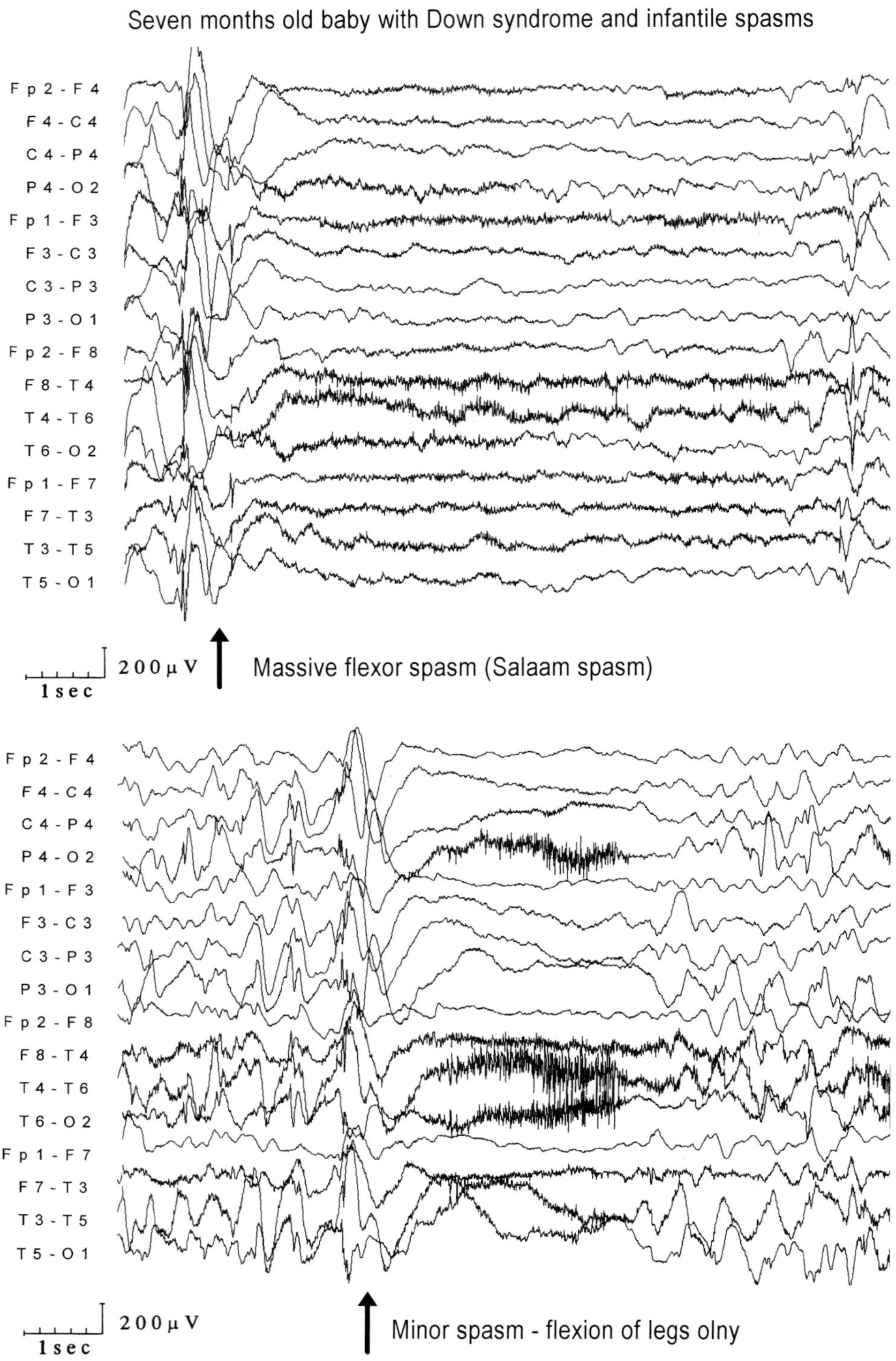

Figure 7.1 Epileptic spasms in Down syndrome.

From video-EEG of a 7-month-old baby with infantile spasms and Down syndrome. There were numerous major (top) or minor (bottom) infantile spasms.

CLINICAL MANIFESTATIONS

Epileptic (infantile) spasms are the defining clinical manifestation of West syndrome.

> ...these bobbings ... they come on whether sitting or lying; just before they come on he is all alive and in motion ... and then all of a sudden down goes his head and upwards his knees; he then appears frightened and screams out. W. J. West (1841)[70]

EPILEPTIC (INFANTILE) SPASMS

The epileptic spasms are clusters of sudden, brief (0.2–2 s), bilateral tonic contractions of the axial and limb muscles. The epileptic spasms are slower than myoclonic jerks and faster than tonic seizures. They may involve widespread muscle groups or be fragmented involving flexion of the neck only (bobbing of the

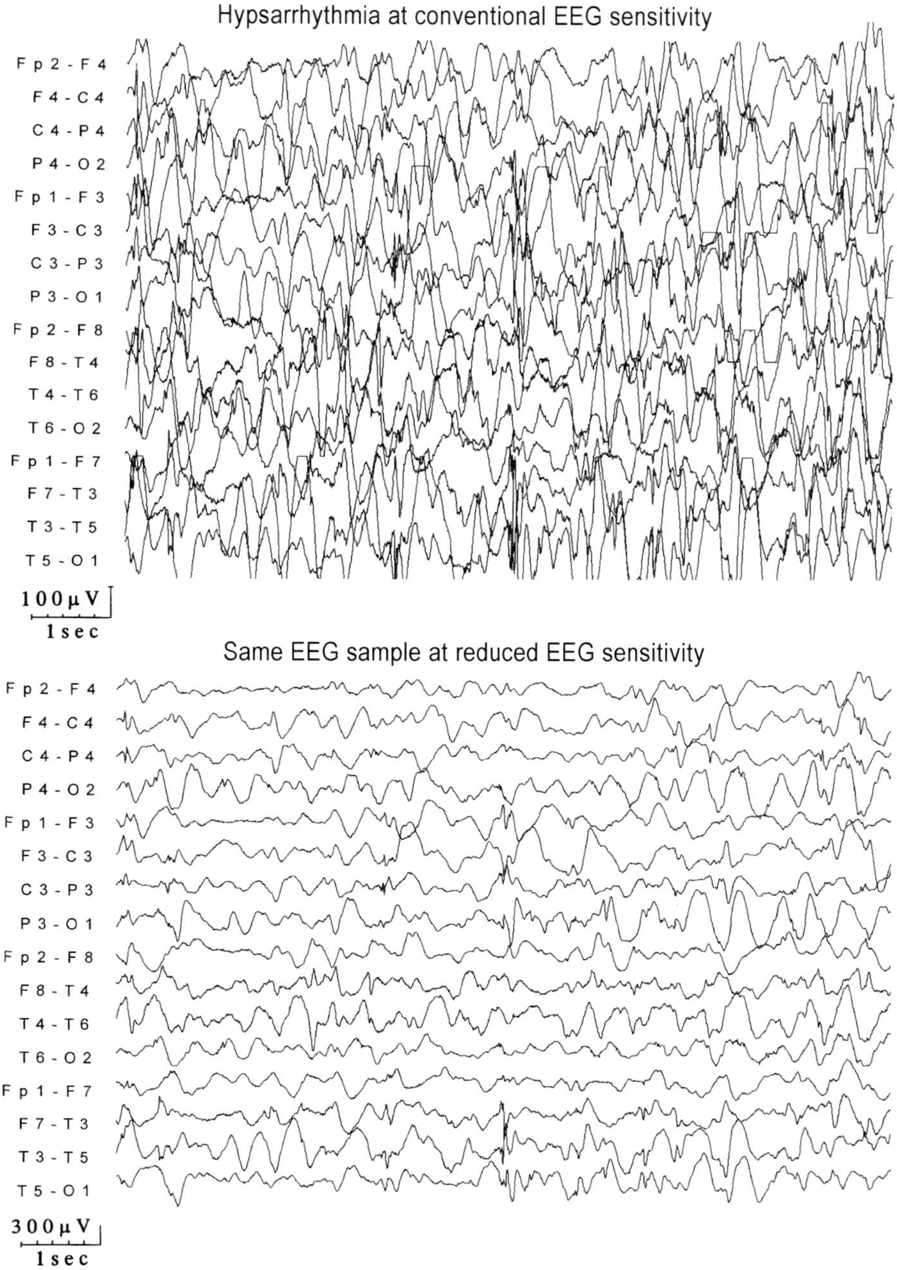

Figure 7.2 Typical hypsarrhythmic pattern seen at routine (top) and reduced (bottom) sensitivity.

head), abdomen (mild bending) or just the shoulders (a shrug-like movement). The force is usually violent but may also be mild or intermediate. The spasm is often followed by motionless and diminished responsiveness lasting up to 90 s. On rare occasions this 'arrest' effect constitutes the entire seizure. Alteration and pauses of respiration during the spasms are common (60%) while changes in heart rate are rare. A cry or laughter often follows the end of the attacks.

Each infant has more than one type of spasm, which may also be influenced by body positions.

Spasms may be flexor, more often flexor extensor and less frequently extensor

Flexor spasms are common (approximately 40% of all epileptic spasms) and are well expressed by the eponyms 'salaam spasms', 'jack-knife spasms', 'spasmes en flexion', 'grusse krampfe' and 'blitz, nick and salaam krampfe' (lightning, nodding and salaam spasms). There is abrupt flexion of the neck and the trunk, the arms raise forwards or sideways sometimes with flexion at the elbows and the legs are elevated with flexion at the hips and knees.

Extensor spasms are less frequent, constituting approximately one-fifth of all epileptic spasms, manifesting with sudden backward movements of the head, hyperextension of the body and extension and abduction of the limbs, similar to that of the Moro reflex.

Flexor–extensor spasms are the most common (half of epileptic spasms), combining sudden contraction of both flexor and extensor muscles with flexion of the neck, trunk and arms, but extension of the legs.

Epileptic spasms may be symmetrical or asymmetrical

Epileptic spasms are usually symmetrical, but 1–30% may have lateralising features with the head or eyes turned to one side or one limb consistently moving more vigorously.[71-73] Eye deviation or nystagmoid movements occur in 60% of epileptic spasms and may be an isolated ictal symptom.

There is no aetiological or prognostic significance to the frequency, violence or flexion–extension of epileptic spasms. However, asymmetrical, lateralised or unilateral spasms are highly correlated with contralateral cerebral lesions of symptomatic West syndrome.

Frequency, distribution and precipitation of epileptic spasms

West syndrome usually starts insidiously with mild spasms occurring two or three times in succession. The full-blown features develop in a few weeks with spasms typically occurring in clusters of one to 30 per day, with each cluster having 20–150 attacks each. Usually the intensity of spasms in a given cluster will peak gradually but, towards the end of a cluster, the interval between spasms lengthens and their severity decreases until they gradually cease, often leaving the child exhausted. Rarely, patients manifest with single rather than clusters of spasms.[63]

The epileptic spasms predominantly occur on arousal and in alert states, less often during NREM sleep (3%) and exceptionally during REM sleep.[18,57] The twilight state, just before sleep or just after waking, often acts as a precipitating factor. Sudden loud noises or tactile stimulation, but not photic stimulation, may precipitate epileptic spasms. Feeding may also provoke the spasms.

Subtle spasms

Epileptic spasms may manifest with subtle movements such as episodes of yawning, gasping, facial grimacing, isolated eye movements, and transient focal motor activity.[63]

OTHER TYPE OF SEIZURES

In symptomatic cases, focal seizures with lateralised motor behaviours occur frequently. These may generate secondarily epileptic spasms in infants with focal cerebral lesions and a poor response to ACTH.

Drop attacks may be the first manifestation of West syndrome with late onset.

PSYCHOMOTOR STATE PRIOR TO THE DEVELOPMENT OF EPILEPTIC SPASMS

Developmental delay, mild or severe, predates the onset of spasms in approximately two-third of cases. In the other one-third the infants are normal before the onset of epileptic spasms. Deterioration of psychomotor development usually occurs with the onset of epileptic spasms and affects head control, reaching for objects and eye tracking. Axial hypotonia, lack of hand grasping or eye contact may have a negative prognostic significance.

AETIOLOGY

The aetiology is multiple and diverse (Table 7.1).

Aetiologically, West syndrome is classified, in order of prevalence, as (1) symptomatic due to discernible organic insults, (2) probably symptomatic

Table 7.1 Main causes of epileptic spasms

Prenatal disorders

- *Neurocutaneous disorders*
  - Tuberous sclerosis
  - Sturge-Weber disease
  - Incontinentia pigmenti (Bloch-Sulzberger syndrome)
  - Neurofibromatosis
- *Chromosomal abnormalities*
  - Down syndrome
  - Miller-Dieker syndrome (17p13 chromosomal deletion)
- *Malformations of cerebral development*
  - Aicardi syndrome
  - Agyria (lissencephaly), pachygyria, polymicrogyria, schizencephaly, laminar heterotopia and other diffuse cortical dysplasias
- *Hypoxic-ischaemic encephalopathies*
- *Congenital infections*
- *Trauma*

Perinatal disorders

- *Hypoxic-ischaemic encephalopathies*
- *Infections* (meningitis, encephalitis)
- *Trauma*
- *Intracranial haemorrhage*

Postnatal disorders

- *Metabolic*
  - Pyridoxine dependency
  - Non-ketotic hyperglycinaemia
  - Phenylketonuria
  - Maple syrup urine disease
  - Mitochondrial encephalopathies
- *Infections (meningitis, encephalitis)*
- *Trauma*
- *Degenerative diseases*
- *Intracranial haemorrhage*
- *Drugs (theophylline and anti-allergic agents of histamine H_1 antagonists such as ketotifen)*

(cryptogenic) and (3) idiopathic. The prevalence of these broad aetiological groups varies significantly in accordance with the methodological investigations.

SYMPTOMATIC WEST SYNDROME

Symptomatic West syndrome is by far the commonest detected cause and probably account for 80% of all cases. Several pre-, peri- and postnatal insults are responsible. These range widely from hypoxia-ischaemia, infections, trauma and intracranial haemorrhage to malformations of cortical development, neurocutaneous diseases, genetic and chromosomal abnormalities and, less often, inborn errors of metabolism.

Pre-, peri- and postnatal brain ischaemia is probably the commonest cause for 20–80% of cases of symptomatic West syndrome.

Brain congenital anomalies are found in one-third of cases.

Half of all patients with tuberous sclerosis have epileptic spasms (constituting 7–25% of cases of West syndrome) and this is significant because of a better response to vigabatrin.

Other common causes of epileptic spasms are malformations of cortical development and include Aicardi syndrome, agyria, pachygyria and laminar heterotopia, hemi-megalencephaly and focal cortical dysplasia, bilateral peri-sylvian microgyria, porencephaly and their variations.

Infants with chromosomal abnormalities are found in all series of West syndrome. Of children with Down's syndrome, 3% may develop epileptic spasms and these appear to have a much better prognosis regarding seizures.

Congenital or acquired infections including viral (cytomegavirus, rubella, herpes simplex virus, enterovirus, adenovirus and pertussis), bacterial (meningococcus and pneumococcus), protozoan (toxoplasmosis) and others, are a significant cause of epileptic spasms. The outcome of epileptic spasms in these children is very poor, signifying the importance of prevention and early treatment of the causative agent.

Inborn errors of metabolism are rare.

PROBABLY SYMPTOMATIC (CRYPTOGENIC) WEST SYNDROME

Probably symptomatic epilepsies may have a prevalence of 10–15%. By definition they are *'presumed to be symptomatic, but the aetiology is unknown, hidden or inconspicuous to available methodology'*.[21] Thus, with improved technology their prevalence is declining as their causes are increasingly documented.

The criteria used for cryptogenic cases vary. The main inclusion criterion is psychomotor deficits prior to the development of the seizures in infants with normal brain imaging and metabolic and other relevant screening.

Cryptogenic versus symptomatic West syndrome

The prevalence of symptomatic versus cryptogenic West syndrome is relevant. For example, in a re-evaluation of 140 infants who had failed to show a structural lesion in major medical centres, 42 (30%) were symptomatic on the basis of a known cause and structural brain imaging and 97 (69%) had a definitely abnormal positron emission tomography (PET) scan, probably indicating dysplastic lesions in 92, thus increasing the prevalence of symptomatic cases from 30 to 95.7%.[74] Only one infant was idiopathic with normal development and a normal PET scan.[74]

Infants with cryptogenic epileptic spasms may differ from those with symptomatic spasms by having different cerebrospinal fluid (CSF) adrenocorticotropin and other hormonal and biochemical contents.[75-77]

IDIOPATHIC WEST SYNDROME

Idiopathic West syndrome, with normal pre-morbid development and possible hereditary predisposition, such as a family history of epilepsy, febrile seizures or EEG genetic patterns, constitutes 5–30% of all cases. Idiopathic West syndrome may have a good prognosis regarding seizures and psychomotor development.

The basic criteria for the diagnosis of the idiopathic forms of West syndrome are as follows:[50,78]

- normal development prior, during and after the active seizure period, with preservation of visual function
- negative functional and structural brain imaging or other symptomatic causes
- symmetrical epileptic spasms and EEG hypsarrhythmia.

The following criteria may also be present:

- a family history of other forms of idiopathic epilepsy or febrile seizures
- EEG genetic traits, such as photoparoxysmal responses or spike-wave discharges or rolandic spikes
- an EEG-identifiable basic activity and sleep spindles despite a hypsarrhythmic pattern
- absence of focal inter-ictal EEG slow wave abnormalities even after intravenous diazepam.

Reappearance of hypsarrhythmia between consecutive spasms of a cluster.

According to Dulac et al.[78] and Vigevano et al.[50] seizures cease and development is normal in all those patients with idiopathic West syndrome who fulfil the above inclusion criteria.

Familial and X-linked West syndrome

Unless the aetiology is a specific genetic disorder, such as tuberous sclerosis or a twin pregnancy, familial occurrence is low at 4–5% of cases.[75]

Family data support a multi-factorial model involving a polygenic determination of susceptibility to epileptic spasms, but requiring environmental factors such as anoxia, birth trauma or febrile illnesses for precipitating seizures.[79] The empiric recurrence risk among siblings was estimated to be 15 ± 3 per 1,000 and that for all first-degree relatives was estimated to be 7 ± 5 per 1,000. These risks should be interpreted with caution since possible heterogeneity of epileptic spasms may result in the occurrence of families in which the cases are presumably totally environmental and other rare families that may be segregating for an autosomal recessive disorder.[79]

A familial idiopathic West syndrome has recently been described.[80]

In rare families, West syndrome occurs in an X-linked recessive mode exclusively in male offspring of asymptomatic mothers. The gene is localised to chromosome Xp21.3-Xp22.[81-83]

IMMUNISATION

Previously there was significant concern that immunisation with various vaccines may cause epileptic spasms, but this appears to be coincidental because the peak age at onset of epileptic spasms corresponds with the immunisation programme of children.

There is evidence against any causative association between epileptic spasms and diphtheria/pertussis/tetanus immunisation or any other immunisation. Goodman et al.[84]examined the time relationship between diphtheria/pertussis/

tetanus immunisation and epileptic spasm onset using three models (association, temporal shift and no effect) and the case–control data from the National Childhood Encephalopathy Study. No data fitted the association model. In addition, cases with abnormalities prior to epileptic spasms showed a no-effect relationship. However, cases who were previously normal suggested a fit to the temporal shift model, i.e. no increase in the number of cases but a shortening of time to onset of seizure.[84]

Reversible causes for epileptic spasms

Drugs such as theophylline[85] or anti-allergic agents of histamine H_1 antagonists and particularly ketotifen[86] may induce epileptic spasms and hypsarrhythmia that are entirely reversible upon drug withdrawal.

Pyridoxine dependency, which is treatable can rarely present with epileptic spasms. This is most likely when other seizure types have occurred before the onset of spasms.[63]

PATHOPHYSIOLOGY

The pathophysiology of West syndrome is unknown but it is probably multiple. The following hypotheses have been proposed:[26,87]

- a very early age-related epileptic encephalopathy in which the epileptiform abnormalities may contribute to progressive dysfunction
- cortical hyperexcitability suggesting over-expression or excessive activation of glutamate and particularly *N*-methyl-D-aspartate (NMDA) receptors
- impaired serotonergic transmission
- alteration of the brain–adrenal axis hormones suggesting that elevated levels of corticotropin-releasing hormone may be responsible for the epileptic spasms and the psychomotor deterioration of the patients
- brain stem dysfunction and abnormal cortical–subcortical interactions
- immunological mechanisms.

DIAGNOSTIC PROCEDURES

A thorough clinical neurodevelopmental assessment and ophthalmological and ultraviolet skin examination may reveal the underlying cause in symptomatic cases, including tuberous sclerosis and Aicardi syndrome. Laboratory screening for electrolyte, metabolic or other disturbances is usually normal. Infectious diseases may be apparent by clinical presentation and suspected infants should have the appropriate investigations including a CSF examination. In infants with frequent vomiting, lethargy, failure to thrive, peculiar odours and unexplained neurological findings, urine and serum amino acid screening, and serum ammonia, organic acid, lactate, pyruvate and liver function tests should be performed. Most paediatricians rightly recommend these neurometabolic tests in all cases unless an alternative cause is clear. Chromosome analysis may lead to a specific diagnosis in infants with unexplained West syndrome.

BRAIN IMAGING

Brain computed tomography (CT) scanning and, more specifically, magnetic resonance imaging (MRI) are indicated. These should be performed prior to steroid treatment, which may lead to apparent atrophy on the CT or MRI scan. Positron emission tomography (PET) of brain glucose use is highly sensitive in detecting focal cortical abnormalities in patients with West syndrome even when the CT scan or MRI are normal. Bilateral hypometabolism of the temporal lobes even in the absence of abnormal CT and MRI scans is a bad prognostic sign.[53]

ELECTROENCEPHALOGRAPHY

Inter-ictal EEG[32,40,55,64,88]

Hypsarrhythmia is the archetypal inter-ictal pattern and occurs in two-thirds of patients. This EEG pattern is anarchy, being a chaotic mixture of giant abnormal, arrhythmic and asynchronous biological brain electrical activity of slow and sharp waves, multi-focal spikes and polyspikes. Because of their high amplitude, individual components and localisation is impossible to detect at routine sensitivity recordings of 100 μV/cm (Figure 7.2). There are no recognisable normal rhythms.

Asymmetrical and other patterns of modified or atypical hypsarrhythmia occur in one-third of cases. Various EEG features have traditionally been labelled modified or atypical hypsarrhythmia. Their presence depends on the stage of West syndrome at which the EEG is performed; it may depend on treatment, and as an aggregate variable, it probably has little practical prognostic significance in randomised studies.[63]

REM sleep shows relative EEG normalisation. In NREM sleep, hypsarrhythmia becomes fragmented and presents with discontinuous repetitive high-amplitude discharges of spikes/polyspikes and slow waves, which are more synchronous than in the awake stage EEG. These are separated by low-amplitude EEG activity that may contain sleep spindles. This sleep EEG pattern may be seen in some infants with a relatively normal awake EEG, mainly at the onset of epileptic spasms.

Certain inter-ictal EEG patterns may contribute to an aetiological diagnosis

Symmetrical hypsarrhythmia is most likely to occur in idiopathic and cryptogenic cases. Asymmetrical and unilateral hypsarrhythmia almost always indicates ipsilateral brain structural lesions. Consistently focal slow waves indicate localised lesions. These become more apparent with intravenous diazepam, which reduces the amount of hypsarrhythmia.

Lissencephaly and Aicardi syndrome may have relative specific EEG patterns with frequent suppression–burst activity. West syndrome of tuberous sclerosis rarely has a typical hypsarrhythmic appearance while spike foci with secondary bilateral synchrony in sleep are frequent.

Ictal EEG

Ictal EEG patterns are variable with at least 11 different types lasting for 0.5 s to 2 min. The commonest and more characteristic pattern in 72% of the attacks is brief (1–5 s) (Figure 7.1) and consists of:

- a high-voltage, generalised slow wave
- episodic, low-amplitude fast activity
- marked diffuse attenuation of EEG electrical activity (*electrodecremental ictal EEG pattern*).

Progress of hypsarrhythmic EEG patterns with age

The chaotic hypsarrhythmic pattern of West syndrome gradually becomes more organised, fragmented and disappears with age. By age 2 and 4 years, this may be replaced by the generalised slow spike-wave pattern of Lennox–Gastaut syndrome. Multi-focal independent spike EEG patterns appear first followed by generalised spike discharges from where the slow GSWD of Lennox–Gastaut syndrome emerges.[89]

DIFFERENTIAL DIAGNOSIS

West syndrome should be easy to diagnose because of the unique characteristic features of each attack and because of their serial and unprovoked clustering. However, parents and physicians often miss this.[47] Erroneous diagnoses include exaggerated startle responses or 'colic and abdominal pain', non-epileptic episodic disorders and gastro-oesophageal reflux.[47]

Benign non-epileptic myoclonus of early infancy (benign non-epileptic infantile spasms)[90-92] is not an epileptic condition, but may cause diagnostic problems because of a similar age at onset and similar spasms (page 110). A normal EEG is of decisive significance in the differential diagnosis.

Benign neonatal sleep myoclonus,[93-95] (page 109) another non-epileptic condition, may also be mistaken as epileptic spasms though myoclonic jerks and not spasms are the main symptom, which occur only during sleep. The EEG is normal.

Sandifer's syndrome of gastro-oesophageal reflux may also be confused with epileptic spasms. Head cocking, torticollis, abnormal dystonic posturing of the body and mainly opisthotonus may imitate epileptic spasms. However, these spells often occur in relation to feeds and the babies often have a history of vomiting, a failure to thrive and respiratory symptoms. Hiatus hernia is common. The EEG is normal. A barium oesophagogram, oesophagoscopy or a pH probe may demonstrate the reflux.

West syndrome is also differentiated from *other benign or severe forms or epilepsies of this age group* because of the unique presentation of epileptic spasms that differ significantly from myoclonic jerks and tonic seizures.

PROGNOSIS

West syndrome is a serious epileptic encephalopathy. The following conclusions probably give a fair account of the overall prognosis irrespective of cause.[41,60,75,96-102]

- Mortality has fallen to approximately 5% in developed countries because of improved medical care. Deaths may be due to the underlying cause and treatment mainly with ACTH and corticosteroids. It is less often due to seizures.
- About 60% of patients develop other types of seizure that are usually resistant to treatment. Lennox–Gastaut type and complex focal seizures are the commonest.
- Half of the patients have permanent motor disabilities and two-thirds have usually severe cognitive and psychological impairment.[41,99,99-102] Autistic behaviour, hyperkinetic syndrome and psychiatric disorders may even be seen in otherwise normal patients with a previous history of epileptic spasms.
- Only approximately 5–12% of patients have normal mental and motor development.

Prognosis is determined nearly exclusively by the causative factors and their severity. The epileptic spasms themselves and their response to treatment may not have prognostic significance.

The consensus is that idiopathic West syndrome and cryptogenic West syndrome have a significant better prognosis than symptomatic cases, with 15–30% of patients achieving relative normality. More optimistic is the view that the seizures cease and development is normal in all patients who fulfil the strict inclusion criteria of idiopathic West syndrome.[50,78]

Spontaneous remissions in untreated patients occur frequently.[103] The cumulative spontaneous remission rates during the first 12 months after the onset of epileptic spasms, as determined by retrospective analysis, are as follows: 2% at 1 month, 2% at 2 months, 5% at 3 months, 7% at 4 months, 9% at 5 months, 11% at 6 months, 11% at 7 months, 14% at 8 months, 16% at 9 months, 18% at 10 months, 25% at 11 months and 25% at 12 months. In 9% of patients, development was normal or only mildly impaired, while the remainder showed various degrees of retardation.[103]

MANAGEMENT

DRUG TREATMENT

ACTH or vigabatrin are the drugs of choice, controlling the epileptic spasms in two-thirds of patients within days of initiating any of these medications.[61,62] However, no treatment has been conclusively shown to improve the long-term intellectual development of these infants.

Lamotrigine, levetiracetam, nitrazepam, pyridoxine, sulthiame, topiramate, valproate and zonisamide are also used as adjunctive medications when ACTH and vigabatrin fail.

Recently, resective neurosurgery has been increasingly recognised as an effective management method in selected medically intractable cases with localised structural lesions.

The drug treatment of West syndrome has been recently (2004) evaluated in a practice parameter report by the American Academy of Neurology and the Child Neurology Society.[61] Recommendations were based on a four-tiered classification scheme and the conclusions are as follows.

- *ACTH* is probably effective for the short-term treatment of epileptic spasms, but there is insufficient evidence to recommend the optimum dosage and duration of treatment.
- There is insufficient evidence to determine whether *oral corticosteroids* are effective.
- *Vigabatrin* is possibly effective for the short-term treatment of epileptic spasms and is possibly also effective for children with West syndrome of tuberous sclerosis. Concerns about retinal toxicity suggest that serial ophthalmological screening is required in patients on vigabatrin. However, the data are insufficient to make recommendations regarding the frequency or type of screening.
- There is insufficient evidence to recommend any other treatment of epileptic spasms.
- There is insufficient evidence to conclude that successful treatment of epileptic spasms improves the long-term prognosis.

The final conclusion is that ACTH is probably an effective agent in the short-term treatment of epileptic spasms. Vigabatrin is possibly effective.[61]

Hormonal therapy

Hormonal therapy with ACTH or corticosteroids has been the most frequent and most effective treatment modality since 1958 (*'Soutraitement Spectaculaire par l'ACTH'*).[104] Hormonal therapy achieves complete control of the epileptic spasms in 50–75% of infants within 2 weeks of initiation.[105] However, there is significant diversity of opinion regarding the dosage, duration of treatment and relative efficacy of ACTH and corticosteroids. The aetiology and treatment lag (within

5 weeks from onset) are not useful predictors of response.[105]

ACTH

There are two main approaches regarding the dosage and duration of treatment.

1. *Small doses (5–40 units/day) and of short duration (1–6 weeks).* The rationale and justification for this is that the response of epileptic spasms to ACTH is *all or none*, the efficacy of small doses is as good as that of large doses and therapy can be discontinued as soon as seizures and EEG hypsarrhythmia cease. One-third who may relapse will benefit from a new course.
2. *High doses (40–150 units/day) and of long duration (3–6 months).* The rationale is that this assures better long-term results, prevents relapses and is superior to corticosteroids.[106]

There may be no difference between the two schemes as the results are conflicting.[105,107]

Corticosteroids

Prednisone and, to a lesser degree, hydrocortisone have been used less often than ACTH. The recommended doses range widely for both prednisone (2–10 mg/kg/day) and hydrocortisone (5–20 mg/kg/day). The duration also varies, from 2–4 weeks to 3–6 months. Corticosteroids may be of equal efficacy to low doses of ACTH,[108] but inferior to high doses of ACTH.[106,109]

Adverse effects of hormonal treatment

There is a high morbidity and 5% mortality rate in infants treated with hormonal medication. The risk of infection is particularly high. The mortality of approximately 5% may be associated with large doses of ACTH.

Vigabatrin

Vigabatrin is a relatively new alternative to hormonal therapy in West syndrome. Its efficacy has been documented in open and control studies.[109-116] The results may be summarised as follows.

- Cessation or amelioration of the seizures and disappearance of the hypsarrhythmic EEG pattern occurs within days of initiating treatment with vigabatrin at a dose of approximately 100 mg/kg/day in 50–70% of the cases.
- Vigabatrin has a quick beneficial effect that usually occurs at the fourth day of treatment with a range of 1–14 days.
- EEG abnormalities and hypsarrhythmia may persist in 10–20% of patients with cessation of clinical seizures. These patients may be more vulnerable to psychomotor deterioration.
- Vigabatrin is more effective by far in epileptic spasms of tuberous sclerosis (approximately 90% of cases).
- The beneficial effect of vigabatrin is sometimes transient, despite continued treatment. Relapses and other types of seizures occur in approximately half of patients who are initially improved.
- In comparison with ACTH, the efficacy of vigabatrin may be slightly less, but its action is faster and there are less acute adverse reactions (10–20%).
- Vigabatrin is effective in some children who are resistant to ACTH or steroids and vice versa. Vigabatrin is definitely superior to hydrocortisone in the treatment of West syndrome of tuberous sclerosis.[109]
- As with steroids and ACTH, there is no evidence that vigabatrin improves the long-term psychomotor development of these children.

- In comparative trials, the incidence of adverse events was statistically lower for vigabatrin than for steroids. Most of the events were relatively mild neuropsychological effects. However, there is still unresolved realistic concern regarding irreversible visual field defects induced by vigabatrin. Some authors support the view that 'the possible benefits of vigabatrin do not justify the risks of the possible irreversible visual changes associated with vigabatrin'.[75,117]

In practice, treatment starts with vigabatrin at doses of 50–100 mg/kg/day in all infants with epileptic spasms. If the seizures are not controlled within 2 weeks, this should be replaced with ACTH. Continuation of the treatment after 3–6 months may be debatable, as with ACTH.

Increasing the vigabatrin dose to more than 100 mg/kg/day may induce more seizures and deterioration in some infants.

Pyridoxine (vitamin B6)

Customarily, children in whom the aetiology of West syndrome cannot be definitely established receive an infusion of 100-200 mg of pyridoxine intravenously during EEG monitoring. Infants with pyridoxine dependency, which is rarely the cause of epileptic spasms, usually improve within minutes.[63] However, intravenous pyridoxine is associated with a risk of apnoea and may not be associated with rapid resolution of hypsarrhythmia.[63] Oral pyridoxine seems to be associated with a median time to response of several days.[63]
Some authors use oral pyridoxine at doses of 150–300 mg/day for 3–14 days prior to initiating any other AED treatments.[75,118] However, there is no firm evidence of a beneficial treatment effect with long term pyridoxine use in West syndrome.[63]

Other drugs and treatments

Valproate benefits 40–70% of patients who fail a trial of ACTH.[119] Nitrazepam is as effective as ACTH in acutely controlling epileptic spasms. However, its long-term effects on the prognosis have not been studied. Lamotrigine, levetiracetam, sulthiame, topiramate, zonisamide, a ketogenic diet, immunoglobulin therapy, felbamate and thyrotropin-releasing hormone have all been used for the treatment of West syndrome with variable results. Improvement is usually temporary. These medications are usually reserved for cases refractory to vigabatrin and/or ACTH.[119]

NEUROSURGERY

Resective neurosurgery may be the desperate solution in selected medically intractable cases with localised structural lesions. However, this is still in the provisional stage provided for hopeless cases that may need multi-lobar resection or hemispherectomy.[120,121] Persistent spasms not amenable to focal surgery and patients who suffer from drop attacks may benefit from total callosotomy, whereas anterior callosotomy is ineffective probably for reasons related to the maturation of the brain.[122]

Diagnostic tips for epileptic spasms

Recognising epileptic (infantile) spasms is easy due to the characteristics of the individual attacks and mainly due to their clustering, often on arousal.

On a practical level it is necessary to ask the parents to demonstrate and imitate the attacks physically rather than merely describe them. If in doubt, demonstrating or showing a video with typical attacks is often conclusive: 'that's it' phenomenon (page 7).

Benign phenomena such as a Moro reflex, attacks of colic or even attempts to sit up may be a cause of confusion that can be avoided by remembering that epileptic spasms occur in clusters. Singular events are rare.

DRAVET SYNDROME
SEVERE MYOCLONIC EPILEPSY IN INFANCY

Dravet syndrome[123-139] is a rare progressive epileptic encephalopathy that is mostly genetically determined. There is significant recent progress in the understanding of the genetics and the diagnostic borders of this syndrome.

DEMOGRAPHIC DATA

Onset is always within the first year of life, with a peak age of 5 months, affecting previously normal children. Twice as many boys are affected. There are approximately 500 reported cases with Dravet syndrome.[132,138] The prevalence is approximately 6% of epilepsies starting before the age of 3 years. The incidence is approximately 1 per 30,000.[140,141]

CLINICAL MANIFESTATIONS

Dravet syndrome is characterised by a tetrad of seizures:[124,128,132,137,138]

1. **Early onset infantile febrile clonic convulsions**
2. **Myoclonic jerks**
3. **Atypical absences**
4. **Complex focal seizures**

Convulsive, myoclonic or absence status epilepticus is common.

The complete tetrad of febrile clonic convulsions, myoclonic jerks, absences and complex focal seizures is seen in more than half of cases. In the others, one or another type of seizure may not occur. Myoclonic jerks, initially considered as the defining seizure type, may not be present in one-fifth of patients or may precede the initial febrile clonic convulsions. Thus, neither myoclonic jerks nor absences are a prerequisite for diagnosis.[128,141-143] Tonic seizures are exceptional if they occur.

The sequence of polymorphic seizures, their resistance to treatment and the progression to mental and neurological deterioration is characteristic of Dravet syndrome.

There are three periods of evolution.

- **The first period is relatively mild (pre-seismic period) with febrile convulsions and febrile convulsive status epilepticus.**
- **The second period is relentlessly aggressive (seismic period) with the appearance of intractable polymorphic seizures.**
- **The third period is static (post-seismic period) with improvement of seizures, but with serious residual mental and neurological abnormalities.**

ILAE classifications and definition

The 1989 ILAE classification used the descriptive nomenclature *'severe myoclonic epilepsy in infancy'*, classified it amongst *'epilepsies and syndromes undetermined as to whether they are focal or generalised'* and defined it as follows.[21]

Severe myoclonic epilepsy in infancy is a recently defined syndrome. The characteristics include a family history of epilepsy or febrile convulsions, normal development before onset, seizures beginning during the first year of life in the form of generalised or unilateral febrile clonic seizures, secondary appearance of myoclonic jerks and often partial seizures. EEGs show generalised spikes and waves and polyspikes and waves, early photosensitivity and focal abnormalities. Psychomotor development is retarded from the second year of life and ataxia, pyramidal signs and inter-ictal myoclonus appear. This type of epilepsy is very resistant to all forms of treatment.

'Dravet syndrome' is the eponymic term assigned by ILAE Task Force to severe myoclonic epilepsy in infancy.[1]

FIRST PERIOD OF MAINLY FEBRILE CONVULSIONS

The first period is relatively mild (pre-seismic period) with seizures usually occurring during febrile illnesses and consisting of clonic convulsions that are unilateral or generalised, brief or prolonged.

Convulsive seizures start before the age of 12 months (with a peak at 5 months) in all patients and these are typically febrile at onset. They consist of unilateral and less often bilateral clonic convulsions intermixed with some tonic components. They are usually long lasting (more than 10 min) and often (in approximately one-quarter of cases) progress to convulsive status epilepticus.

According to Dravet:[124,132,138] "These convulsive seizures, carefully analysed with video-EEG recordings performed along the course, are polymorphic. They can be clearly generalised, clonic and tonic clonic, or unilateral, hemiclonic. More often, they have peculiar clinical and EEG features that do not permit classification under generalised clonic or tonic-clonic seizures. They are characterized by clonic or tonic components, initially predominating in the head and the face, evolving to variable, bilateral localisation, and loss of consciousness. When they are short in duration there are no autonomic symptoms. They were named falsely generalised or unstable." [124,132,138]

In three-quarters of patients seizures are usually provoked by hyperthermia of around 38°C, minor infections, immunisations or hot baths.[124,128,132,138] The remaining one-third of patients have non-febrile convulsive seizures. Isolated episodes of focal myoclonic jerking and, more rarely, focal seizures may predate or appear just before the febrile convulsions.

These seizures recur frequently within 6–8 weeks and later may also be non-febrile.

This period lasts for 2 weeks to 6 months before progressing to the second stage.

SECOND RELENTLESSLY AGGRESSIVE PERIOD

The second period is relentlessly aggressive (seismic period) with the emergence of other multiple-seizure types and severe neurocognitive deterioration. Various forms of febrile and non-febrile convulsive seizures, myoclonic fits, atypical absences and complex focal seizures occur on a daily basis and frequently evolve to status epilepticus.

Convulsive seizures (febrile and non-febrile)

These are similar but more frequent and more prolonged than in the first period.

Myoclonic seizures

Myoclonic seizures usually appear between the ages of 1 and 4 years, after an average of 1–2 years from onset. In some cases myoclonic jerks may also occur at a much earlier age, sometimes clustering prior to the onset of febrile clonic convulsions. Myoclonic seizures may be segmental or generalised. Segmental jerks affect facial muscles and the limbs, mainly distally. Generalised jerks predominantly affect the axial body muscles causing flexion or extension and often falls. Myoclonic jerks are as a rule very frequent several times per day and may cluster in myoclonic status epilepticus without impairment of consciousness. However, other patients may have jerks only hours or days prior to a convulsive seizure. Myoclonic jerks are usually violent, forceful and massive, but they may also be mild and inconspicuous as revealed by appropriate clinical testing or video–EEG monitoring. One-fifth of patients have segmental myoclonic jerks that are not violent.[124,132,138]

Myoclonic seizures may be single or clusters and occur at any time of the day or only on awakening or prior to a generalised convulsion. They persist during drowsiness, but usually disappear during stages III and IV of sleep.[124,132,138]

Atypical absence seizures

Atypical absence seizures occur in 40[124,132,138]–93% of patients.[142,144] They are short (5–6 s) with moderate impairment of consciousness and often with myoclonic jerks of the upper limbs and dropping of the head. The EEG GSWD is slow, usually below 2.5 Hz.

Complex focal seizures

Focal seizures occur in nearly half of patients. They manifest with a number of symptoms such as atonic or adversive components, autonomic phenomena (pallor and peri-oral cyanosis) and automatisms. They occasionally progress to GTCS. One seizure recorded by Dravet[124] may be an illustrative example. This was a 2-year-old girl who, upon awakening, had deviation of the eyes to the right, arrhythmic bilateral myoclonic jerks of the deltoids and loss of consciousness. The seizure ended within 80 s with a hiccup, pallor, cyanosis of the lips and rare myoclonias.

Status epilepticus

Myoclonic, atypical absence, complex focal and convulsive status epilepticus, alone or in combination, are common and frequent.[124,128,132,137,138,145] These various types of status epilepticus may last for hours or days. They may be facilitated or precipitated by photic stimulation, eye-closure or fixation on patterns.

Absence status epilepticus of decreased responsiveness often combines with unsteadiness, dribbling, frank ataxia and with erratic small myoclonias, sometimes associated with hypertonia. More typical complex focal and rarely simple focal status epilepticus occur. Episodes of GSWD EEG interspersed with erratic small myoclonic jerks may also persist for hours or days.

Cognitive and neurological deterioration

All patients show variable but usually severe impairment of cognitive functions, which develops between the second and the sixth years (with a peak at 1 year) and remains stable later.[124,132,138]

This is followed by progressive neurological deficits such as ataxia and pyramidal symptoms. Paroxysmal movement disorders occur.[146]

THIRD STATIC PERIOD OF REGRESSION

The third period is static (post-seismic period). The seizures may improve, but serious mental and neurological abnormalities remain forever.

The relentless worsening and progression of the symptoms usually comes to a halt at around the age of 11–12 years.[124,128,132,137,138] This marks the post-seismic period where seizures improve but do not stop.

- Convulsive seizures are the most persistent type of seizure.[124,128,132,137,138] They are less dramatic and less frequent, mainly occurring at the end of the night. They are still precipitated by fever. These may be generalised tonic clonic or clonic tonic clonic convulsions[124,128,132,137,138] often with focal components at the onset, end or during the course of the seizure. Some diurnal seizures may manifest with clonic convulsions localised to a segment of a limb or the face, followed by hypotonia and sleep. Febrile status epilepticus may continue in adolescence.

- Complex focal seizures with autonomic components and hypotonia tend to disappear but may also persist.
- Myoclonic attacks and segmental myoclonias as well as atypical absence status epilepticus tend to decrease or disappear. They are exacerbated by fever.

Cognitive and neurological deficits and signs persist without worsening.

SEIZURE-PRECIPITATING FACTORS

Febrile illnesses, a raised body temperature and a warm environment (hot baths) are frequent precipitating factors, particularly at the onset of seizures, but this may continue in adolescence ("febrile seizures plus").[124,128,132,137,138] The elevation of body temperature itself rather than its aetiology is the precipitating factor.[128] Photic and pattern stimulation, movements and eye-closure precipitate GSWD, myoclonic jerks and absence seizures.[124,128,132,137,138] One-quarter of patients have self-induced seizures by hand waving or pattern stimulation.

AETIOLOGY

Dravet syndrome is mostly genetically determined, but the mode of inheritance is unknown. Approximately half of the patients have a family history of various epileptic syndromes (including idiopathic generalised epilepsy) and mainly febrile seizures. Rarely, siblings or twins may suffer from this syndrome.

A significant recent development is the genetic discovery that Dravet syndrome is related and may be the most severe phenotype in the *'generalised epilepsy with febrile seizures plus'* (GEFS+) spectrum. GEFS+ is associated with mutations in the *SCN1A*, *SCN1B*, *SCN2A* (genes encoding the alpha 1, alpha 2 and beta 1 sodium channel subunits) and *GABRG2* genes (gamma 2 subunit of the $GABA_A$ receptor) (Chapter 6, page 129).

Mutations of the *SCN1A* gene were found in a high percentage (range 35–100%) of patients with Dravet syndrome.[129-131,134-136,139,147-153] Most cases of Dravet syndrome arise from *de novo* mutations (missense, frame shift and nonsense) of the *SCN1A* gene.[150,152-154] Inherited *SCN1A* gene mutations appear to associate with mild phenotypes in most family members.[153,154] Phenotypes with complete (myoclonic seizures and/or atypical absences) or incomplete (only segmental myoclonias) seizure semiology show no difference in the type or rate of *SCN1A* gene mutations. The differences may be attributed to other genetic mechanisms.[152] The mutant channels show remarkably attenuated or barely detectable inward sodium currents.[135]

More recently, the phenotypic spectrum of *SCN1A* gene defects has been broadened to include *'intractable childhood epilepsy with generalised tonic clonic seizures'*[153] and other borderline cases of Dravet syndrome.[139] *Intractable childhood epilepsy with generalised tonic clonic seizures (GTCS)* is an entity recognised primarily in the Japanese literature[153] and may be the same disorder as the *'severe IGE of infancy with GTCS'* described by Doose.[155] Patients develop febrile seizures by 1 year of age, often recurring in clusters or status epilepticus, with GTCS remaining the predominant seizure type. Cognitive decline is usual and neurological deficits may develop.[153] *Borderline cases* have clinical features similar to those of core Dravet syndrome, but are not necessarily consistent with all the accepted criteria for such a diagnosis.[128,132,139]

Other than sodium channel genes or modifying genes may be involved in the pathogenesis of Dravet syndrome,[139] as suggested by the findings of (1) a family with an individual with Dravet syndrome in whom a third $GABA_A$ receptor gamma 2 subunit mutation was found,[156] (2) a family in which the proband and the healthy father shared the same mutation of the *SCN1A* gene[139] and (3) families with definite Dravet syndrome who are not mutant for the *SCN1A* gene.[151]

The state of affairs in Dravet syndrome is summarised as follows by Scheffer: [154] "Mutational analysis of *SCN1A* gene defects initially seemed straightforward, implicating missense mutations with the milder familial GEFS+ phenotypes and more severe truncation mutations in Dravet syndrome.[154] As more mutations are discovered, the molecular picture is becoming less clear-cut with *de novo* missense, frame shift and nonsense mutations associated with Dravet syndrome. In the case of familial mutations, the *SCN1A* or *GABRG2* gene defects are associated with mild phenotypes in most family members. Thus, the severe myoclonic epilepsy of infancy phenotype is likely to result from the cumulative effects or interaction of a few or several genes, of which the reported GEFS+ gene is merely one player".[154]

DIAGNOSTIC PROCEDURES[124,128,132,137,138]

The general consensus is that there is no metabolic abnormality. When performed, skin and muscle biopsies are normal. The mitochondrial cytopathy is exceptional. Other causes of progressive infantile epileptic myoclonic encephalopathies should be excluded.

GENETIC ANALYSIS

Given that no mutations are found in a relatively high percentage of patients with a typical picture of Dravet syndrome, one cannot include genetic analysis in the diagnostic criteria.[139] A severe *SCN1A* gene defect, if present, is strongly supportive but not diagnostic of Dravet syndrome. The diagnosis of Dravet syndrome must remain a clinical one and it is still likely that complex inheritance plays a role even in *de novo* mutations.[154]

BRAIN IMAGING

Brain CT and MRI scans are either normal or show mild cerebral or cerebellar atrophy. Occasionally an increased white matter signal is detected on T2- weighted MRI. Functional brain imaging may be normal or show focal hypoperfusion and hypometabolism even when MRI is normal.[157]

ELECTROENCEPHALOGRAPHY

The EEG shows a similar progression to that of the clinical state, from normal to severely abnormal.[124,128,132,137,138,145]

Inter-ictal EEG

The inter-ictal EEG may initially be normal. The only abnormality at this stage is that approximately 20% of babies show photoparoxysmal discharges of spikes/polyspikes-slow waves. 'Theta pointu alternant pattern' may be seen (page 102).

Within 1 year the EEG becomes very abnormal in two-thirds of cases. The initially normal background becomes progressively slower and slower and is dominated by diffuse theta and delta waves. Paroxysms of polyspikes or spikes-slow waves become frequent and dominate the record. These occur in brief bursts and are usually asymmetrical. Focal and mainly multi-focal abnormalities of sharp or spike-slow waves are frequent. Generalised discharges may not be recorded in 10–15% of the patients.

Drowsiness and sleep are they main facilitators of EEG paroxysmal abnormalities.

Photoparoxysmal discharges occur in 40% of patients and may be the only abnormality in the initial stage of the disease when the EEG is otherwise normal. In series of EEGs, photoparoxysmal abnormalities may only occur once, persisting in less than 5% of patients. Eye closure and pattern stimulation may also induce generalised discharges of polyspikes or spikes and slow waves and myoclonic jerks.

Ictal EEG

The ictal EEG varies according to the type of seizure. Myoclonic jerks are often but not always associated with generalised polyspikes-slow waves. Atypical absences occur with irregular slow GSWD. Focal seizures show focal ictal discharges frequently with localised episodic fast activity and rapid spikes.

DIFFERENTIAL DIAGNOSIS

An early diagnosis of Dravet syndrome can be reliably made on clinical criteria from the second or third seizure in the first year of life.

In the initial pre-seismic period, *febrile seizures* are the most apparent diagnosis to differentiate (Table 7.2).

Difficulties may exist in differentiating Dravet syndrome from *intractable childhood epilepsy with GTCS* (page 155).[153,155]

Lennox–Gastaut syndrome is easy to differentiate because of:

- the absence of repeated febrile mainly clonic seizures in the first year of life
- the predominance of drop attacks, axial tonic seizures and specific EEG patterns
- often pre-existing brain lesions.

Tonic seizures in Dravet syndrome are exceptional and again they are different and never repeated in series.[124,138]

Some difficulties may be imposed by the *'epilepsy with myoclonic astatic seizures'* of Doose (Chapter 10, page 291).[6] However, focal seizures and focal EEG abnormalities do not usually occur in Doose syndrome, which is characterised mainly by myoclonic-atonic seizures.

Benign myoclonic epilepsy in infancy has only brief generalised myoclonic seizures (page 130). If febrile convulsions occur, these are rare and brief. The EEG is markedly different from Dravet syndrome without focal abnormalities.

Progressive myoclonic epilepsies [51] may have similar features, although at this age they may run a different course.[124,138]

PROGNOSIS

Seizure deterioration and mental and neurological decline is relentless and often fatal.

All but a few exceptional cases have a sinister prognosis regarding seizures and psychomotor development, though the progression of the symptoms usually comes to a halt at around the age of 11–12 years in the post-seismic period when the seizures improve but do not cease.[124,128,132,137,138]

In 15% of cases, patients may die either during a seizure or from concomitant diseases.

Neurological deficits persist without worsening and some such as ataxia may improve. Motor coordination is poor, speech is often dysarthric and extrapyramidal rigidity may be present.

All patients show variable but usually severe impairment of cognitive functioning. This usually develops between the second and the sixth years and remains stable later.

Amongst 56 patients of Dravet,[124] only six acquired communicative skills and only one was able to attend school. All 37 patients older than 10 years were dependent or institutionalised. Half had an intelligence quotient lower than 50.

MANAGEMENT

Seizures are intractable. Certain AEDs may reduce them but do not control them and it is doubtful if they can affect the outcome.[124,128,132,137,138] Treatment with valproate, diazepines, melatonin,[158] phenobarbitone (convulsive seizures) and ethosuximide (absence and myoclonic seizures) is partially and temporally beneficial. Adjunctive medication with topiramate[159] and stiripentol had good results in convulsive seizures.[160] Zonisamide and bromides have been found to be useful.[128] Levetiracetam may be the most efficacious of all other AEDs.[161]

Carbamazepine, phenytoin and mainly lamotrigine[162] are contraindicated.[137]

Relatively good results may be obtained with a ketogenic diet starting at the earliest possible stage of Dravet syndrome.[137]

Long, generalised or unilateral seizures should be prevented by early treatment of infectious diseases and hyperthermia, which are their triggering factors.

The treatment of status epilepticus with benzodiazepines such as diazepam, lorazepam, clonazepam, and midazolam is the same as in any other similar condition.

Diagnostic pitfalls in Dravet syndrome

Not all patients develop myoclonic jerks.

Not all patients start with febrile convulsions.

Not all patients develop absence seizures.

Table 7.2 Febrile seizures in Dravet syndrome

Paediatricians should maintain a high index of suspicion for Dravet syndrome if the febrile seizures are:

- prolonged beyond 15 or 30 min
- unilateral
- mainly clonic
- frequent
- precipitated by low fever often below 38°C
- of early onset (before 1 year of age)
- with non-febrile seizures

The diagnosis is nearly certain if intractable myoclonic jerks and mental deterioration appear within 1-2 years from onset.

LENNOX–GASTAUT SYNDROME

Lennox–Gastaut[5,17,163-175] syndrome is a childhood epileptic encephalopathy characterised by the triad of:

1. **Polymorphic intractable seizure that are mainly tonic, atonic and atypical absence seizures**
2. **Cognitive and behavioural abnormalities**
3. **EEG with paroxysms of fast activity and slow (less than 2.5 Hz) generalised spike-wave discharges (GSWD)**

DEMOGRAPHIC DATA

Lennox–Gastaut syndrome starts between 1 and 7 years with a peak at 3–5 years. Boys (60%) are affected slightly more often than girls. The incidence of Lennox–Gastaut syndrome is low at 2.8 per 10,000 live births.[69] However, because of its intractable nature, the prevalence is relatively high at approximately 5–10% of children with seizures.[169,187,189]

CLINICAL MANIFESTATIONS

Lennox–Gastaut syndrome is characterised by polymorphic seizures and neuropsychological decline. The most characteristic seizures are tonic fits, atypical

ILAE definition and considerations of the classification of Lennox–Gastaut syndrome

There is no consensus of what Lennox–Gastaut syndrome is (see Table 7.3 for the inclusion criteria). It is categorised amongst generalised cryptogenic or symptomatic epilepsies (age related) by the ILAE Commission and is defined as follows.[21]

Lennox–Gastaut syndrome manifests itself in children aged 1–8 years, but appears mainly in pre-school age children. The most common seizure types are tonic axial, atonic and absence seizures, but other types such as myoclonic, GTCS or partial are frequently associated with this syndrome. Seizure frequency is high and status epilepticus is frequent (stuporous states with myoclonias and tonic and atonic seizures). The EEG usually has abnormal background activity, slow spikes and waves less than 3 Hz and, often, multi-focal abnormalities. During sleep, bursts of fast rhythms (approximately 10 Hz) appear. In general, there is mental retardation. Seizures are difficult to control and the development is mostly unfavourable. In 60% of cases the syndrome occurs in children suffering from a previous encephalopathy, but it is primary in other cases.

The ILAE Task Force classified Lennox–Gastaut syndrome amongst epileptic encephalopathies.[1]

However, Lennox–Gastaut and other syndromes such as epilepsy with myoclonic astatic seizures (EM-AS) of Doose (page 291) have undefined boundaries resulting in what appears as *'an overlap of syndromes'*.[176,177] There are still significant problems regarding the exact nosological boundaries of Lennox–Gastaut syndrome as emphasised by Aicardi:[51,170,177] "The epilepsies described under the headings of Lennox–Gastaut syndrome and of myoclonic epilepsies raise one of the most controversial problems of childhood epileptology ... There is still considerable confusion surrounding the concept of the Lennox–Gastaut syndrome, so the definition of the syndrome and its relationship to other forms of epilepsy, especially those that feature myoclonic seizures, remains a subject of dispute. Only the more typical syndromes are reasonably well defined, but many patients are impossible to include in a definite category".[170,177]

Doose expressed similar views:[178-180] 'there is hardly another field in paediatric epileptology presenting such terminological uncertainty and confusion as is to be found in the domain of epileptic syndromes with generalised minor seizures of early childhood…'.[178-180]

The so-called "myoclonic variant Lennox-Gastaut syndrome"[181] is another probably artificial situation and by large a mistaken diagnosis of EM-AS.[177,182] Myoclonic seizures are a prominent feature whilst tonic seizures are few and occur only during sleep. Spike and wave complexes may be fast or slow. Most are cryptogenic cases with a similar outcome.

Other myoclonic epilepsies with brief seizures reported[166] as intermediate cases between EM-AS and Lennox–Gastaut syndrome most likely reflect the undefined boundaries of the current definitions.

Focal epilepsies with secondary bilateral synchrony (SBS) has been a major problem of confusion. Sixty percent of the original cases of Gastaut[183-185]when re-evaluated, were suffering from epilepsy with SBS and did not have paroxysms of fast rhythms during sleep.[186]

To emphasise the diversity of opinion regarding what Lennox-Gastaut syndrome is, I take the example of two studies from the same country (*USA*) published in the same journal (*Epilepsia*).[187,188] In one of them[187] the inclusion criteria were (1) the onset of multiple seizure types before age 11 years, (2) at least one seizure type resulting in falls and (3) an EEG demonstrating slow GSWD (less than 2.5 Hz). In the other study[188] the criteria were (1) multiple seizures (two or more) with one being tonic seizures and (2) slow GSWD (at least in one EEG) and (3) age at onset could be at any time. Mental retardation was not used as a diagnostic criterion in either of them.[187,188]

absences and atonic seizures, in that order. Myoclonic jerks occur in 11–28% of patients alone or in combination with other seizures. However, myoclonic jerks do not predominate in the *'pure'* Lennox–Gastaut syndrome.

The onset may be insidious with symptoms appearing *de novo* without conspicuous reason in cryptogenic cases. Previous psychomotor deficits are apparent in symptomatic cases. Cognitive and behavioural abnormalities are present prior to seizure onset in 20–60% of patients.

Half of the cases of West syndrome and other infantile epileptic encephalopathies progress to Lennox–Gastaut syndrome. Conversely, 10–30% of patients with Lennox–Gastaut syndrome develop from West syndrome or other epileptic encephalopathies, though the transition phase is difficult to evaluate. Focal and generalised seizures are also common predecessors.

TONIC SEIZURES

Tonic seizures are the commonest (approximately 80–100%) and probably the most characteristic seizure type in Lennox–Gastaut syndrome (Figures 7.3–7.5). These are usually symmetrical, brief (2–10 s) and of variable severity from inconspicuous to violent. Descriptively, tonic seizures are as follows.[190]

- *Axial* seizures affect the facial, nuchal, trunk, paraspinal, respiratory and abdominal muscles alone or in combination. The symptoms include raising the head from a pillow, elevation of the eyebrows, opening of the eyes, upward deviation of the eyeballs, opening of the mouth and stretching of the lips to a fixed smile. An 'epileptic cry' is common at the onset of attacks.
- *Axo-rhizomelic* seizures, which are axial seizures, also involve the proximal (rhizomelic) muscles of the upper and less often lower limbs. Elevation and abduction or adduction of the upper limbs and shoulders occur together with the other symptoms of axial tonic seizures.
- *Global* seizures, which are axo-rhizomelic seizures, also involve the distal part of the limbs. The arms are forced upwards, abducted and semi-flexed with clenched fists 'like that of a child defending himself from a facial blow'. The lower limbs are forced into triple flexion at the hip, knee and ankle or into extension. Global tonic seizures often cause forceful sudden falls and injuries.

A series of tonic seizures, reminiscent of epileptic spasms but of longer duration, may occur, particularly when Lennox–Gastaut syndrome develops from West syndrome.

Table 7.3 Inclusion criteria for Lennox-Gastaut syndrome

These are not well defined but most authorities demand the following triad:

1. At least two types among tonic, atonic seizures, atypical absences. Some authors demand atypical absences as being one of the mandatory seizure type. Others prefer tonic seizures. Myoclonic seizures are not a prerequisite criterion for inclusion or exclusion.
2. Generalised slow spike wave discharges. Although all agree with this, episodic fast activity is an additional requested EEG abnormality by others.
3. Impaired intellectual functioning. There are recent reports that this is no longer a prerequisite of Lennox-Gastaut syndrome.

Age at onset, abnormal or normal brain imaging and causative factors are usually not considered important. Accordingly, Lennox-Gastaut syndrome may even start in adult life.

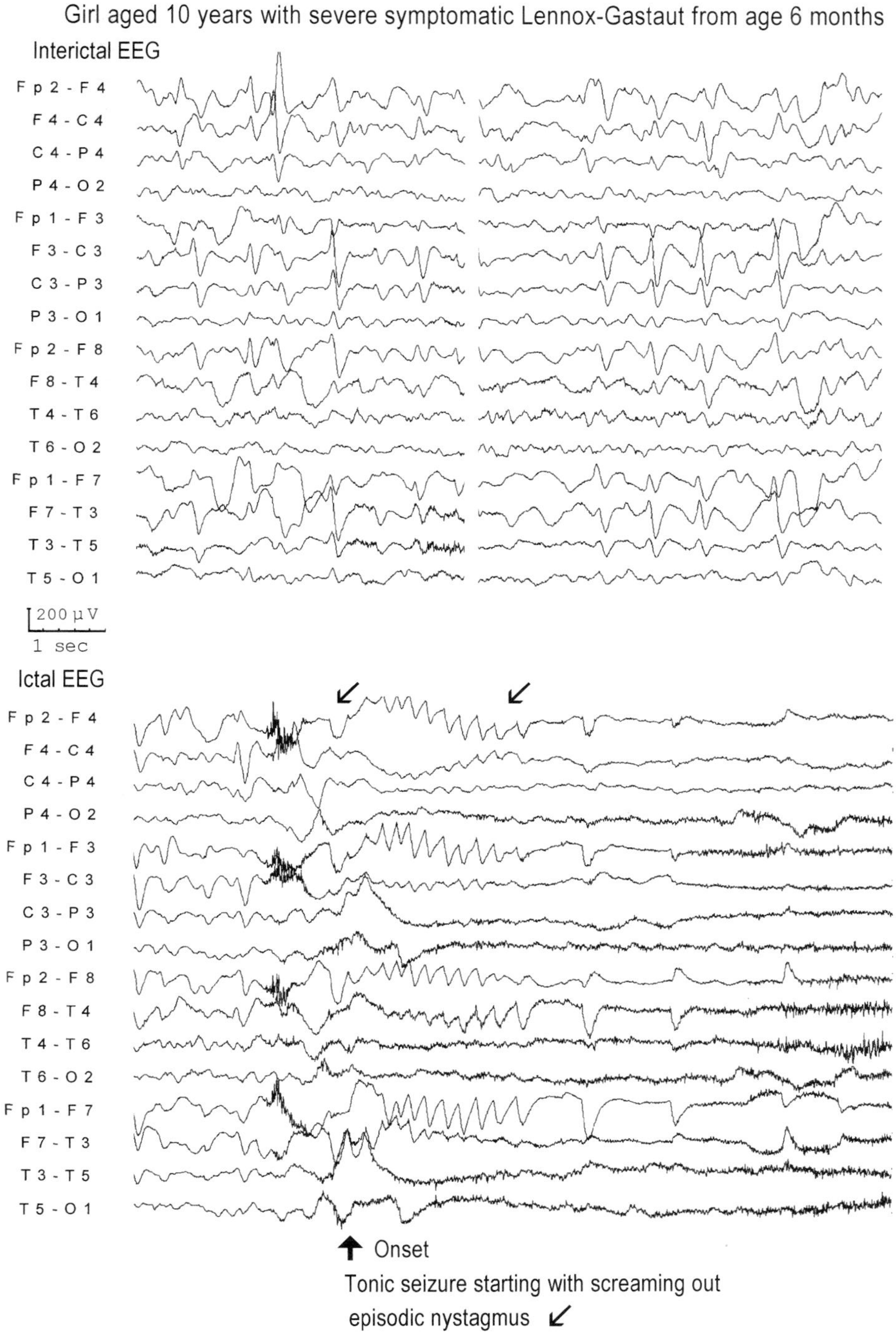

Figure 7.3 Samples from a video-EEG of a 10-year-old girl with severe symptomatic Lennox–Gastaut syndrome from age 6 months.

She had a marked neuronal migration deficit in the right hemisphere and her seizures were multi-form and intractable to any medication. Top: a grossly abnormal inter-ictal EEG with continuous high amplitude sharp-slow waves or spikes-slow waves. These were multi-focal right or left, mainly frontal but also middle line or posterior. Bottom: a tonic seizure started clinically with a scream (vertical arrow) and episodic nystagmus (oblique arrows shows the eye movement artefacts of the nystagmus). The ictal EEG consisted of an abrupt onset of flattening, which lasted for 25 s, followed by high-amplitude generalised sharp and slow waves at approximately 1 Hz. The EEG returned to its pre-ictal state after approximately 1 min from the onset of the seizure. Despite unilateral structural abnormalities, the inter-ictal, ictal and post-ictal EEG abnormalities were not consistently lateralised.

Concurrent autonomic manifestations may occasionally be the prominent symptom of the attacks.

Tonic seizures occur more often during slow wave sleep than states of wakefulness. Some patients may have hundreds of them during sleep. They do not occur during REM sleep. In early onset Lennox–Gastaut syndrome clusters of tonic spasms frequently occur on awakening.

ATYPICAL ABSENCE SEIZURES

Atypical absence seizures (Figures 7.6 and 7.7) occur in approximately two-thirds of patients. There is 'clouding' rather than loss of consciousness with gradual onset and gradual termination. The patients may continue with their activity

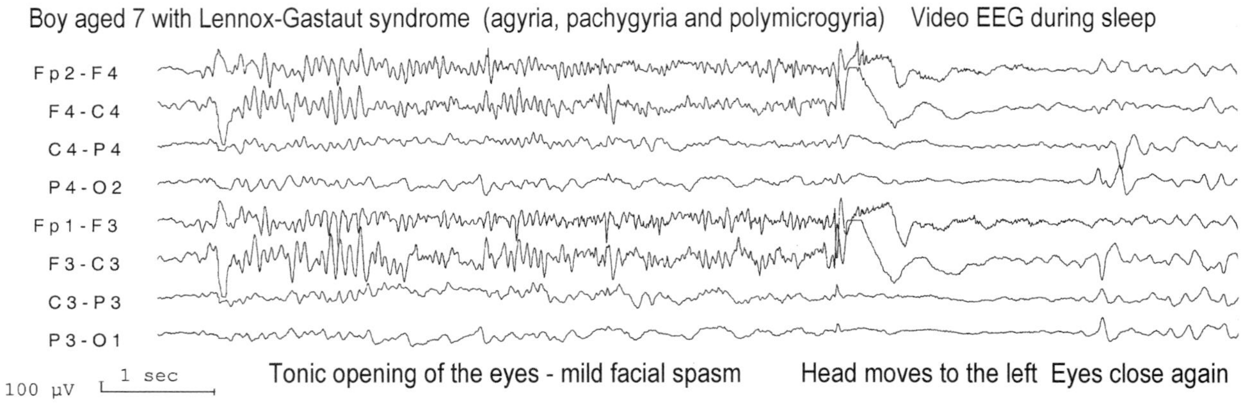

Figure 7.4 From a video–EEG of a child with Lennox–Gastaut syndrome due to malformations of cortical development (his older brother also had the same disease – Figure 3.3, page 48).[191]

EEG fast paroxysms are associated with inconspicuous manifestations of tonic seizures (slight tonic eyelid opening) that would be impossible to detect without video–EEG recording.

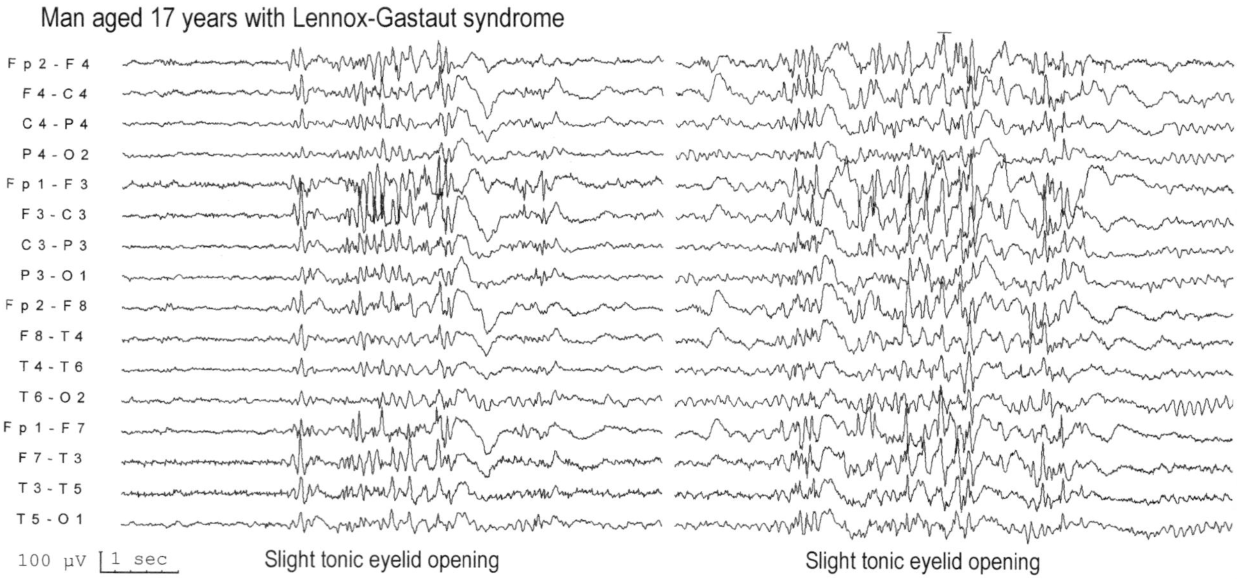

Figure 7.5 From a video–EEG of a man aged 17 years with Lennox–Gastaut syndrome.

A tonic seizure manifesting with mild clinical symptoms occurs during marked paroxysmal fast activity. Turning of the head and symmetrical flattening of the EEG follow this.

though slower and often with mistakes. Impairment of their cognition may be so mild that it can be clinically undetectable. Selective impairment of higher cortical functions with maintained responsiveness may occur.

Changes in tone and myoclonic jerks may be very pronounced. Often, there is loss of trunk or head postural tone, facial muscle or neck muscle stiffening, eyelid or peri-oral myoclonus, random jerks of the head or limbs and head nodding.

Atypical absence seizures, contrary to the typical absences, occur only in the context of mainly severe symptomatic or cryptogenic epilepsies of children with learning difficulties who also suffer from frequent seizures of other types such as atonic, tonic and myoclonic. Other main differences between atypical and typical absence seizures are shown in Table 7.4

ATONIC SEIZURES

Atonic seizures consist of sudden, brief (1–4 s) and severe loss of postural tone. They occur in nearly half of patients. They are frequent and involve the whole body or only the head.

The trunk and head slump forwards and the knees buckle.

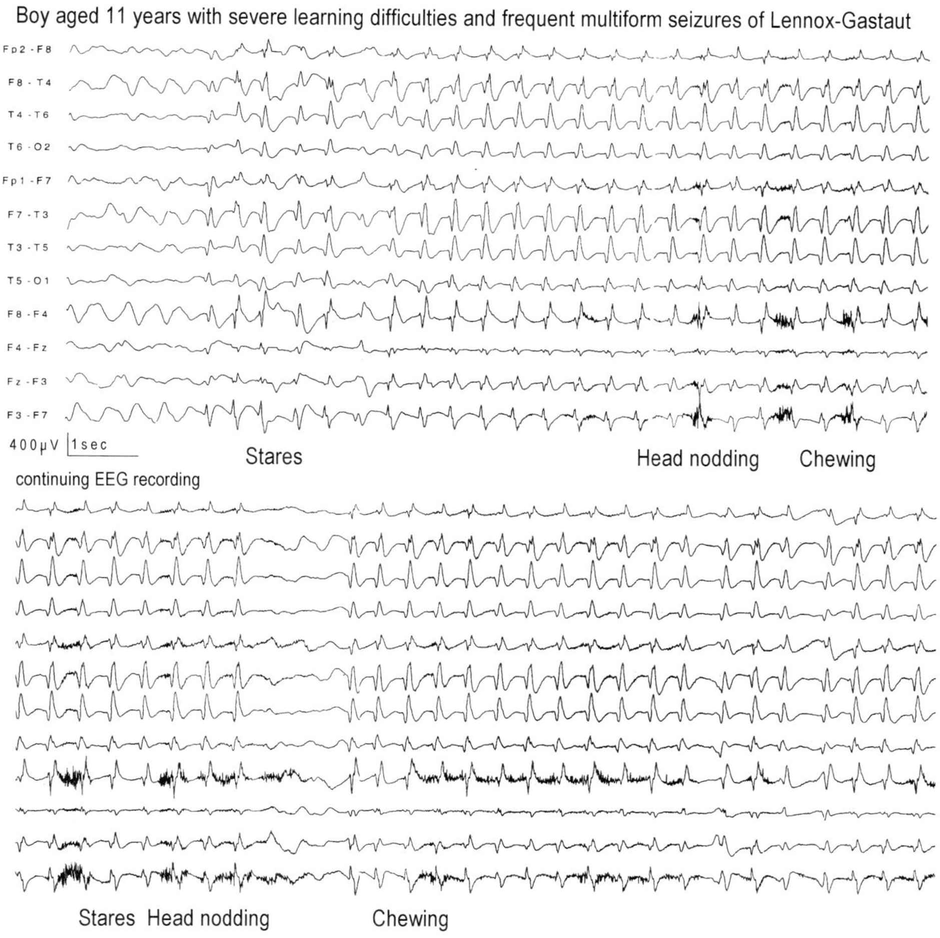

Figure 7.6 A video–EEG sample of a classical and lengthy atypical absence seizure.

The ictal symptoms fluctuated and consisted of staring, head nodding and automatisms. The ictal discharge consisted of slow GSWD at 2–2.5 Hz.

Generalised loss of postural tone causes a lightning-like fall. Atonic seizures are the commonest cause of falls resulting in severe injuries to the nose or teeth.

The patient collapses on the floor irresistibly without impairment of consciousness and then immediately stands up again.

Longer atonic seizures lasting for 30 s up to 1–2 min are rare.

The patient remains on the floor unable to stand up.

In brief and milder attacks there is only head nodding or sagging at the knees.

Atonic seizures always alternate with tonic fits and atypical absences in Lennox–Gastaut syndrome. There may be a predominant tonic component (axial spasm) in these otherwise atonic seizures. In addition, myoclonic jerks may precede or less often intersperse with the atonic manifestations.

Myoclonic jerks

Myoclonic jerks were initially not included amongst the seizures of Lennox–Gastaut syndrome, but they may occur in 11–28% of patients. Myoclonic attacks are very brief shock-like muscle contractions that may be isolated or repeated in a saccadic manner, usually for only a few seconds. The jerks are generally bilateral and symmetrical (massive myoclonus) and preferentially involve the axial flexor muscles and the abductors of the arms. They may cause falls.

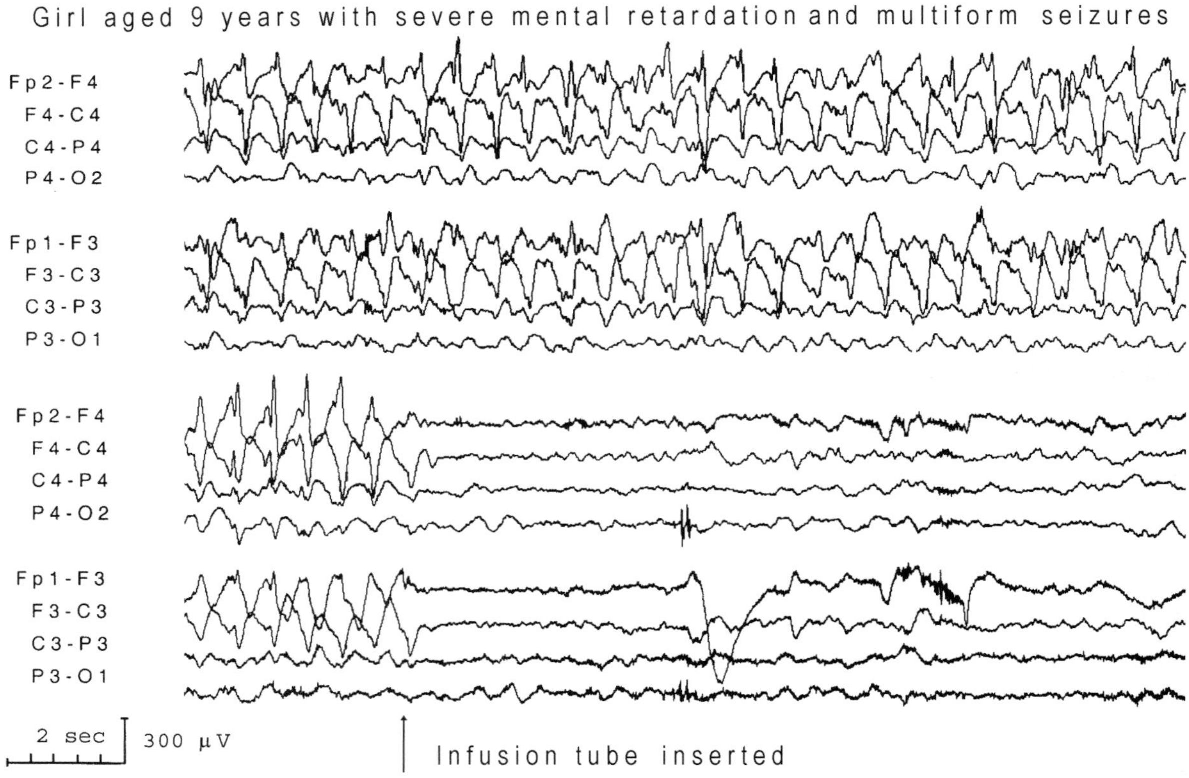

Figure 7.7 A video–EEG sample from a lengthy recording to assess whether this 9-year-old girl with severe symptomatic Lennox–Gastaut syndrome was in atypical status epilepticus.

The EEG consisted of very long slow GSWD at approximately 2 Hz. Because of very severe mental retardation, it was impossible to find any convincing differences in her behaviour and reactivity during or without EEG discharges. The discharge stopped simultaneously when the infusion tube was inserted prior to administering diazepine intravenously.

Epileptic falls

Epileptic falls (drop attacks) may be the result of various types of seizures such as atonic, tonic, myoclonic-atonic and more rarely myoclonic seizures. Tonic seizures are the commonest cause of falls. These are often difficult to differentiate clinically without polygraphic recording.[192] The falls result in recurrent injury.

Non-convulsive status epilepticus

Non-convulsive status epilepticus featuring all types of seizures such as atypical absences, tonic and atonic fits and myoclonic jerks occur in half of patients. It is often of very long duration (days to weeks), exhibits resistance to treatment and is repetitive. Depending on the predominant seizure type, status epilepticus in Lennox–Gastaut syndrome may be one of the following.

- *Absence status epilepticus*, a mild but occasionally severe confusional state that can last for days or weeks.
- *Tonic status epilepticus* is more often seen in adolescents than in children.
- *Myoclonic status epilepticus* is rare, occurring when the myoclonic jerks are the dominant seizure type.
- *Mixed tonic and absence status* is probably the commoner type. It consists of repetitive uninterrupted or discontinuous series of brief tonic seizures alternating with atypical absences. There is usually profound impairment of consciousness or stupor, intermixed with serial tonic attacks and sometimes with myoclonic-atonic falls.

AETIOLOGY

The aetiology is extensive and diverse. Symptomatic Lennox–Gastaut syndrome due to severe and, less often, mild brain disorders of any type is by far the commonest, probably 70% of all cases. The pre-, peri- and postnatal causes are similar to those responsible for West syndrome (Table 7.1), but Aicardi syndrome and lissencephaly, which are common in West syndrome, are rare causes in

Table 7.4 Main differences between atypical and typical absence seizures

Clinical and EEG features	Atypical absences	Typical absences
Onset and termination	Usually gradual	Abrupt
Responsiveness	Decreased but not abolished	Varies from mild to severe
Changes in tone	Usually pronounced	Usually mild
Duration	Usually long sometimes for minutes	Usually brief; never more than 30-40 s
Postictal recovery	Cognitive impairment may persist	Immediately
Inter-ictal EEG	Background often abnormal with frequent discharges of various types and combinations	Background usually normal sometimes with typical IGE discharges
Ictal EEG	Slow (<2.5 Hz) spike-and-wave	Fast (>2.5 Hz) spike-and-slow wave
Normal neurological and mental state	Exceptional	As a rule
Other type of seizures	Commonly atonic and tonic seizures of symptomatic generalised epilepsies	Depend on IGE syndrome (myoclonic jerks, GTCS or both)
Prognosis	Commonly bad	Commonly good

Lennox–Gastaut syndrome. Malformations of cortical development are increasingly identified as a common cause of the Lennox–Gastaut syndrome. Focal cortical dysplasia can produce a typical or an incomplete form of the syndrome.

One-third of Lennox–Gastaut syndrome cases occur without antecedent history or evidence of brain pathology (idiopathic or probably symptomatic cases). There is no evidence of a genetic predisposition.

PATHOPHYSIOLOGY

Lennox-Gastaut syndrome is a non-specific age-dependent diffuse epileptic encephalopathy of unknown pathophysiological mechanisms.[5,12,17,173]

Pathophysiology of the electrical discharges in Lennox-Gastaut syndrome: From the neurophysiological point of view there is no convincing explanation for the electrical interictal or ictal events. They are a severely abnormal response of the maturing brain of early childhood to diffuse, or occasionally localized, brain damage. The response may be similar to that of infants developing West syndrome but at a different age of maturation. The electrographic abnormalities are thought to reflect excessive neocortical excitability and arise from neuronal and synaptic features peculiar to the immature brain. Cortical and subcortical structures are probably involved. Frontal lesions may have a higher responsibility. SBS may be the main pathophysiological mechanism in one-third of cases of typical Lennox-Gastaut syndrome.[193] The response of atypical absence seizures to the same drugs used in typical absence seizures, may indicate similar, but not necessarily the same, pathophysiological mechanisms of an abnormal thalamocortical oscillatory burst-firing circuit (see page).

Pathophysiology of the development cognitive and behavioural abnormalities: Lennox-Gastaut syndrome is considered as an epileptic encephalopathy whereby

A reminder of secondary bilateral synchrony

SBS refers to bilateral and synchronous EEG discharges generated by a unilateral cortical focus.[194-197] The triggering spike of SBS could be at any brain location but mainly in the mesial frontal lobe.

The SBS consists of high amplitude, generalised or diffuse sharp/spike-wave discharges, which appear symmetrical and synchronous. They are usually less than 2.5 Hz but 3 Hz or faster spike/wave is not an uncommon finding. The morphology of each sharp-wave in a series of SBS may vary. Focal spikes/sharp waves immediately preceding most of the GSWD of SBS are apparent and these are of different morphology to those occurring within the discharges of SBS. The lack of focal origin for other GSWD on the EEG does not exclude the presence of SBS. SBS paroxysms may terminate with an enduring focal discharge, which is usually ipsilateral to SBS origin.[196,197]

Contrary to SBS, primary bilateral synchrony manifests with more rapid symmetric and synchronous GSWD caused by a generalised epileptic process independent of any focal hemispheric lesion.

According to Blume,[196,197] identification of SBS requires: (1) the phenomenon to occur at least twice in an EEG, (2) a lead in time of more or equal to 2 s, (3) the morphology of triggering spikes should resemble other focal spikes in the same region and differ from that of the bisynchronous epileptiform paroxysms. This definition was more strict than that of other studies, which required only the coexistence of focal spikes or a lesion and bilaterally synchronous discharges. Magnetoencephalography offers another utility in the evaluation of SBS.[198]

Patients with SBS manifest with seizures that relate (1) directly to SBS itself such as atonic, absence, tonic, myoclonic and GTCS or (2) to epileptogenic leading foci such as focal tonic or clonic seizures and hemi-convulsions.[196,197]

SBS has been implicated in the pathogenesis of epileptic encephalopathies and may be responsible for generalised seizures of certain intractable post-traumatic and other symptomatic or probably symptomatic focal epilepsies.

Focal epilepsies with SBS are often severe and usually of frontal and less often of temporal lobe origin with secondary generalisation of the spike-wave activity. They manifest with a variety of focal and secondarily generalised convulsive and nonconvulsive seizures.[199,200] Sudden falls that resemble the drop attacks[199,200] and myoclonic jerks[201] may occur.[199,200] Tonic seizures are usually missing, and onset is at a later age. Epilepsy with SBS seems to be as severe as Lennox-Gastaut syndrome.[197] This has important therapeutic implications because surgery may be the treatment of choice either by elimination of the driving epileptogenic focus or corpus callosotomy.[173,202]

In comparison with Lennox-Gastaut syndrome, focal epilepsy with SBS begins later (mean age of onset, 10 years and 9 months) with relative infrequent occurence of focal neurological signs, mental retardation, seizure frequency, multiple seizure types in the same patient, astatic seizures and runs of fast paroxysms. Focal seizures are more frequent, atypical absences are not observed, slow GSWD are more often asymmetric and a constant localized epileptic focus is seen in all cases of epilepsy with SBS.[197]

abundant epileptogenic abnormalities of slow GSWD and fast rhythms/rapid spikes play a pivotal role in the development of cognitive and behavioural impairment by altering brain connectivity and neurotransmission of the maturing brain. A reason for this may be that these electrical discharges divert the brain from normal developmental processes toward seizure-preventing mechanisms.[12] AEDs, sleep disruption, and social isolation are significant contributing factors.[12]

DIAGNOSTIC PROCEDURES

A thorough clinical neurodevelopmental assessment, opthalmological and ultraviolent skin examination may reveal the underlying cause particularly in symptomatic cases. The cause may already be known in those who develop from West syndrome. Biochemical, haematological, metabolic and other relevant screening is rarely abnormal depending on the cause.

BRAIN IMAGING

Brain imaging with high-resolution MRI and PET scans is abnormal in nearly all patients.[203-206]

Two-thirds or more of patients with Lennox-Gastaut syndrome have abnormal MRI, which is needed for the detection of subtle focal lesions.

Functional brain imaging is highly sensitive in detecting focal cortical abnormalities in nearly one-third of patients with Lennox-Gastaut syndrome even when MRI is normal.[203-206] FDG-PET usually reveals focal or multi-focal areas of hypometabolism which often correlate with malformations of cortical development and abnormalities of white matter. Diffuse hypometabolism is common. In the studies of Ferrie et al.[204-206] of Lennox-Gastaut syndrome and other childhood epileptic encephalopathies with normal MRI, FDG PET revealed that abnormal cortical up-take (nearly always hypometabolic) occurred in almost two-thirds of patients. Further, in a few patients at least one cortical region showed significantly decreased uptake bilaterally. Also, 90% of patients had evidence of relative thalamic hypometabolism. The abnormalities are stable over time.

ELECTROENCEPHALOGRAPHY[88,207-209]

Inter-ictal EEG

The inter-ictal EEG features at onset may consist of an abnormal background with or without slow GSWD. The background abnormalities are found in almost all cases from the onset of seizures. They consist of a slow and fragmented alpha rhythm, an excess of diffuse slow waves and EEG disorganisation. Focal slow wave abnormalities typically occur in symptomatic cases.

Commonly, EEGs with abnormal background contain paroxysms of fast rhythms characterising tonic seizures and slow (less than 2.5 Hz) GSWD characterising atypical absences (Figures 7.7 and 7.8). These EEG patterns may be clinically silent (inter-ictal) or manifest with inconspicuous or violent seizures (ictal).

Episodic abnormalities are frequent and mainly consist of the following.

- *Slow (less than 2.5 Hz) GSWD.* The slow GSWDs usually at approximately 2 Hz, are considered bilateral, synchronous, symmetrical and of higher amplitude in the anterior regions. However, they are also often asymmetrical, unilateral and less frequently regional.
- *Paroxysms of fast activity or rhythmic rapid spikes* at approximately 10 Hz or much faster. These are the most revealing and characteristic features occurring nearly exclusively during slow wave sleep. Though frequently clinical

manifestations are not apparent, brief and inconspicuous tonic seizures, mainly of the facial muscles, often occur (Figures 7.4 and 7.5), but their detection requires video–EEG monitoring. Fast paroxysms often contain rhythms faster than 10 Hz (Figure 7.9).[5]

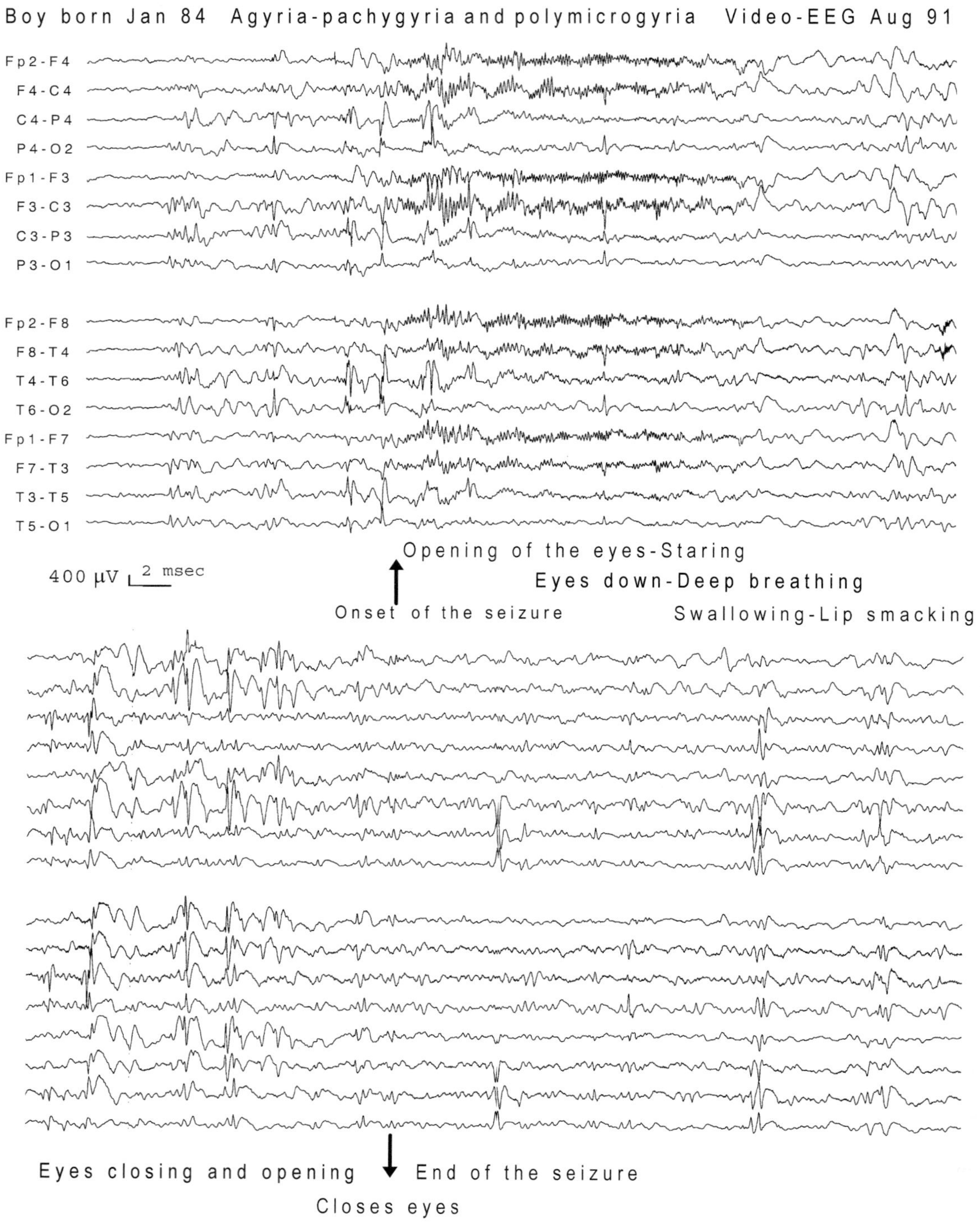

Figure 7.8 A video–EEG-recorded seizure of the same patient depicted in Figure 7.4.

Note that the ictal discharge contains features of tonic (episodic fast activity) and absence (slow spikes and waves) seizure. The clinical manifestations annotated were mild.

- Inter-ictal spikes and multi-focal spike or sharp slow waves are predominant in the frontal and temporal areas in 75% of patients. Multiple independent spike foci mainly occur in the transition from West to Lennox-Gastaut syndrome. The EEG patterns differ among individuals and change from day to day and even moment to moment.

Sleep activates additional spike foci, increases the frequency of GSWD and produces synchronisation of bitemporal and bifrontal spike-wave discharges at 1.5–2.5 Hz.[89]

Useful clarification on the EEG with multi-focal independent spike foci is not a specific diagnostic feature. Though most of the reports emphasise on their association with severe childhood epilepsies and Lennox-Gastaut syndrome [20;210] multiple independent spike foci are a main EEG feature of Panayiotopoulos syndrome.

Ictal EEG

Atypical absences are associated with slow (less than 2.5 Hz) GSWD (Figures 7.6 and 7.7). Tonic seizures have accelerating fast paroxysmal activity, which is bilateral and often predominates in the anterior regions and the vertex (Figures 7.4, 7.5 and 7.9). This may be of two types.[190]

1. Very rapid (20 ± 5 Hz) and initially of low amplitude, progressively increasing to 50–100 mV.
2. A more ample and less rapid rhythmic discharge at 10 Hz, identical to that of the tonic phase of the GTCS (*epileptic recruiting rhythm*) except that it may be of high amplitude from the onset.[66]

Flattening of all EEG activity alone or in combination with fast paroxysms are also common (Figures 7.3 and 7.4). Fast ictal paroxysms may be preceded by generalised spike-slow wave discharges or EEG suppression.

A reminder of multi-focal independent spike foci and their definition

"Patients who have, on a single EEG, epileptiform discharges (spikes, sharp waves, or both) that arise from at least three non-contiguous electrode positions with at least one focus in each hemisphere are considered to have the multiple independent spike foci pattern."[211] Multi-focal independent spike foci have been reported in the EEG of 3.7% of children[210-212] and they are associated with severe and intractable epilepsies.[89,210-212] They have not been described in normal children.[213] Multiple independent spike foci often occur as a transition pattern between hypsarrhythmia and slow GSWD.[89]

The conclusions of Blume and Kaibara (1999)[211] are that multi-focal independent spike foci are:

a. Associated with seizures in more than 90% of patients. Generalized motor seizures are by far more common (80%), with generalized tonic-clonic being the most common single type. Half the patients had more than one type of seizure. Seizures occurred daily in 60% of those who had at least one spike every 10 seconds, but in only 33% of those whose spikes occurred less often.
b. Only one-third of patients are cognitively normal. However, intellect is normal in higher percentages of patients with infrequent spikes (52%), less than 10 spike foci (47%), and normal background activity (39%). Neurological examination is abnormal in about one half of the patients. The incidence of normal intelligence drops from 47% of patients with normal neurological examinations to 16% with abnormal examinations.
c. Presumed aetiologies include the majority of diseases that most commonly afflict the brain in early life, such as perinatal insult, central nervous system infection, neocortical malformations, degenerative conditions, trauma, and anoxia.

According to a recent publication[20] multi-focal independent spikes constitute an "identifiable electroclinical syndrome, which combines intractable motor seizures, mental retardation and multi-focal independent spike discharges" defined as follows:

"Severe epilepsy with multiple independent spike foci is an electroclinical entity with the following characteristics:

1. EEG showing multiple independent spike foci (three or more foci in both hemisphere, i.e., at least one in each hemisphere) and diffuse slowing of the background activity,
2. very frequent multiple types of seizures but mainly generalized minor seizures,
3. frequent association with mental retardation and neurologic abnormalities,
4. underlying causes of various nonspecific prenatal, perinatal, and postnatal cerebral conditions, and
5. poor prognoses for seizures and psychomotor development. It represents a diffuse encephalopathy with mutual transition between other age-dependent epileptic encephalopathies."[20]

However, these conclusions contradict the fact that one-third (30%) of cases of Panayiotopoulos syndrome have EEG with multi-focal spikes in three or many more independent brain locations which by definition are "multiple independent spike foci" (page 243).[214-216] These children are normal, have infrequent or a single seizure, which is focal and not generalised.

Atonic attacks occur with generalised polyspikes, slow GSWD and accelerating fast paroxysms alone or in combination.[190]

Myoclonic attacks have mainly generalised discharges of polyspikes with or without slow waves and fast rhythms.

A combination of clinical manifestations and ictal EEG patterns is common (Figure 7.8).

Massive myoclonus, atonic seizures and myoclonic-atonic seizures mainly consist of a mixture of slow spike-wave, polyspikes and decremental events. Post-ictally, there is diffuse slowing or slow GSWD instead of EEG flattening.

DIFFERENTIAL DIAGNOSIS

There are a number of epileptic and non-epileptic conditions to differentiate from Lennox–Gastaut syndrome (Table 7.5). However, recognising Lennox–Gastaut syndrome in a child is relatively easy because of the characteristic multiple seizure types, pre-existing or developing impairment of cognition and behaviour and EEG features.

The main differential diagnostic problem is between idiopathic Lennox–Gastaut syndrome and EM-AS of Doose syndrome. This is relatively easy in typical presentations (Table 7.6) but many patients present with overlapping features.[166,177]

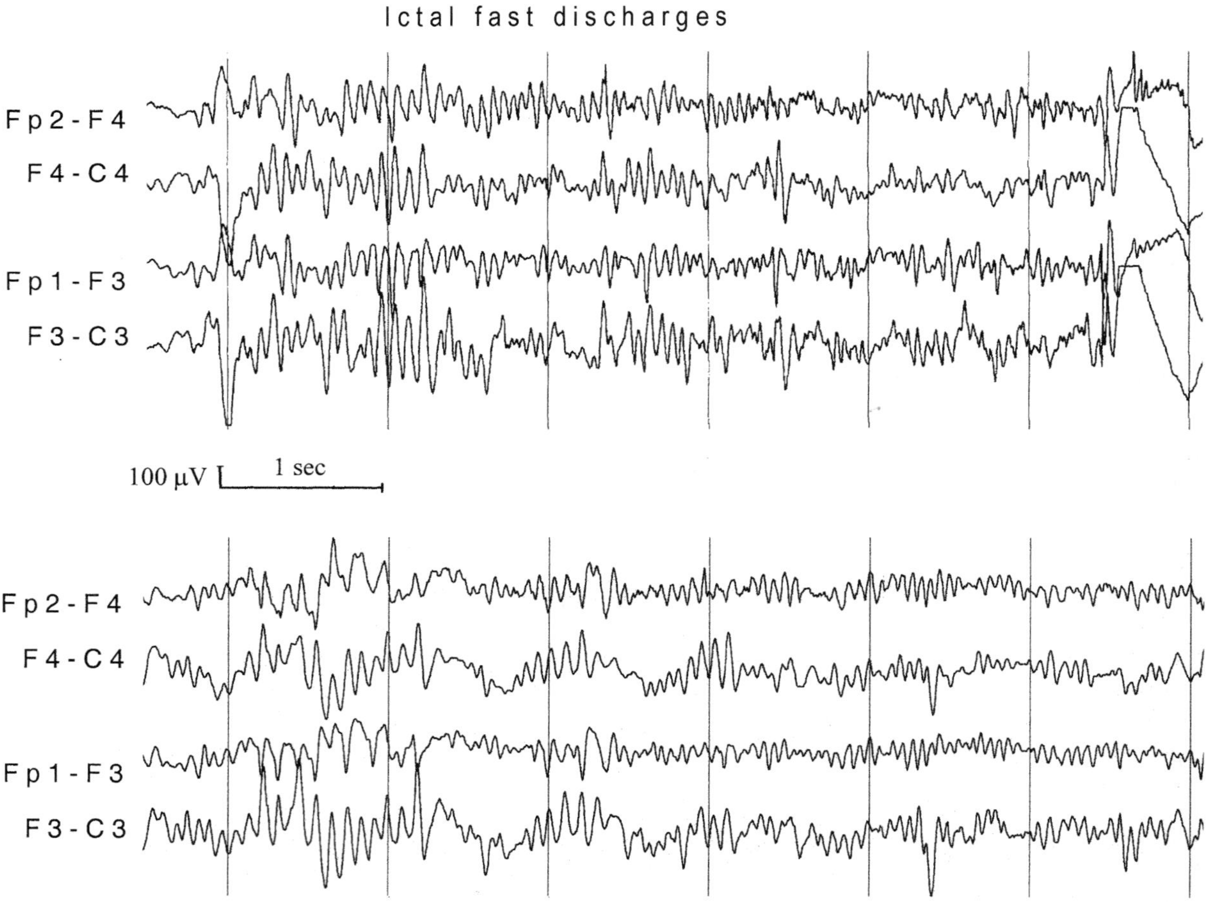

Figure 7.9 Fast ictal paroxysms of various frequencies in Lennox–Gastaut syndrome.

PROGNOSIS

The prognosis is appalling (Table 7.7).[69,168,188,193,217-220] In all, 5% die, 80–90% continue having seizures in adult life and nearly all (85–92%) have severely impaired cognition and behaviour. Many patients are finally institutionalised. A patient achieving normal mental and motor development is a rarity.

Table 7.5 Non-epileptic and epileptic conditions to differentiate from Lennox-Gastaut syndrome

Non-epileptic conditions

- Non-epileptic falls, syncope and cataplexy
- Nocturnal paroxysmal dystonia

Epileptic syndromes

- Late-onset West syndrome
- Myoclonic epilepsies of early childhood
- Dravet syndrome
- Epilepsy with myoclonic absences
- Epilepsy with myoclonic-astatic seizures (Doose syndrome)
- Myoclonic epilepsy of infancy associated with a fixed encephalopathy
- Progressive myoclonic epilepsies and neurodegenerative conditions
- Atypical partial benign epilepsy of childhood
- Epilepsy with electrical status epilepticus during slow-wave sleep
- Focal epilepsies with secondary bilateral synchrony

Table 7.6 Lennox-Gastaut syndrome versus Doose syndrome

	Lennox-Gastaut syndrome	**Doose syndrome**
Main seizures	Tonic, atonic and atypical absences	Myoclonic, atonic and myoclonic-atonic
Tonic seizures	Common and characteristic; diurnal and nocturnal	Probably exclusion criterion (nocturnal tonic seizures are accepted by some authors)
Tonic drop attacks	Common	Incompatible
Atypical absences	Common also occurring independently of other seizures	Uncommon; they usually accompany myoclonic or atonic episodes
Developmental abnormalities before onset of seizures	Common	Exceptional if any
Aetiology	Symptomatic or possibly symptomatic (idiopathic cases are accepted by some authorities)	Idiopathic[1] (although symptomatic or possibly symptomatic cases are included in the ILAE classification of 1989[12])
Genetic predisposition	None	Common
Development from West syndrome	Common	Incompatible
EEG background	Abnormal by rule	Usually normal particularly at onset
EEG episodic fast activity and rapid spikes	Common and often characteristic	Exceptional and mainly in sleep
EEG slow generalised spike wave	Usually <2–2.5 Hz	Usually 2–3 Hz
Prognosis	Commonly bad	Commonly relatively good

Cognitive impairment is more likely to develop in symptomatic or West syndrome-related cases, when the onset is before 3 years of age and when frequent seizures and status epilepticus occur.

Diagnostic tips for Lennox–Gastaut syndrome
Recognising Lennox–Gastaut syndrome is easy due to the characteristics of the multiple seizure types, pre-existing or developing impairment of cognitive functioning and behavioural abnormalities.
Differential diagnosis may be problematic between Lennox–Gastaut syndrome and EM-AS of Doose (Table 7.6).

MANAGEMENT[172-175,221,222]

> My 13-year-old daughter has Lennox–Gastaut syndrome. She is on Sabril, Lamictal and Frisium. It seems multiple drug therapies work best for these children. I have found the best control is when the drug level or types are changed. The initial control is good usually reducing the seizures for a month or so, but they then start up again. Hence, we are always juggling the doses up and down.
>
> From an Internet description by a mother

AED TREATMENT

AED treatments nearly always fail to control seizures completely, although a reduction in seizures, usually temporarily, may be achieved. Lennox–Gastaut syndrome is highly resistant to anti-epileptic medication, often requiring some rational polytherapy that is rarely successful. Tonic attacks that may be numerous during sleep are the most difficult to treat. Atypical absences, myoclonic and atonic seizures are more amicable to treatment. Patients as a rule suffer from sedation and other adverse effects of multiple drugs. Often there is a vicious circle. Sedation increases the incidence of seizures. The severity of the seizures waxes and wanes in time with good and bad days or weeks. More than three AEDs are probably unacceptable. A seizure-free state cannot be achieved.

The beneficial effects of drugs are often transient, lasting for weeks or 2–4 months. AEDs are usually used in combinations according to the predominant seizure type.

Table 7.7 Prognostic factors in Lennox-Gastaut syndrome

Worse prognosis is associated with:

- Symptomatic causes
- Pre-existent West syndrome
- Early onset
- Frequent and intractable seizures
- Repeated episodes of status epilepticus
- Constantly slow EEG background
- Localised and mainly multifocal EEG abnormalities

A better prognosis may be indicated for patients who have:

- Normal development prior to the onset of seizures
- Faster than slower generalized spike-wave activity
- Normal brain imaging
- Normal background EEG
- Activation of generalized spike-wave by hyperventilation

Old anti-epileptic drugs

Valproate is the drug of choice because of its efficacy in all types of seizures seen in Lennox–Gastaut syndrome.[172-175] However, younger children, particularly on polytherapy, are at greater risk of serious hepatotoxic reactions.

Clonazepam and other diazepines such as nitrazepam[172,223] are mainly effective in myoclonic jerks and tonic attacks.

Phenytoin may reduce tonic, vibratory tonic and tonic status epilepticus.

Carbamazepine may be effective in partial seizures, but may exacerbate other types of generalised fits.

Phenobarbital and primidone may control convulsive seizures, but may be prohibited in Lennox–Gastaut syndrome because of cognitive, behavioural and sedative side effects.

Ethosuximide often controls atypical absence seizures and is useful in myoclonic and atonic seizures with falls.[224,225]

New anti-epileptic drugs

In evaluating short-term AED trials in Lennox–Gastaut syndrome it should be remembered that:

- the beneficial effects of AEDs are often transient, lasting for a few weeks
- the Lennox–Gastaut syndrome has a very high percentage of placebo responders
- most trials of Lennox–Gastaut syndrome involve children and adults
- patients have many seizures per day, some of which, such as atypical absences, are difficult to count. Therefore, it is common to use a reduction in drop attacks (tonic or atonic seizures) as the primary outcome variable. This is considered a clinically significant outcome, as drop attacks are one of the most dangerous seizure types, often leading to injuries.[226-229]

Felbamate[230] reduces drop attacks, absences and other seizure types, but because of sometimes fatal side effects it is now only available for specific cases. It should be used with caution and for no longer than 2 months if there is no clear response.[231,232]

Gabapentin is contraindicated because it worsens seizures.[226-229,233]

Lamotrigine appears to be effective in many types of seizure such as drop attacks and absences, but exaggerates myoclonic jerks.[234-236] There is a beneficial pharmakokinetic interaction of lamotrigine with valproate.[237] The major side effect of lamotrigine is skin rash that may be very severe and life threatening.[238] Children on co-medication with valproate are at higher risk for skin rash and for serious hepatotoxic reactions.

Levetiracetam finds an increasingly useful application in the treatment of Lennox–Gastaut syndrome and indeed all other epileptic encephalopathies.[161,239-241] It appears to be effective for all types except tonic seizures, has no adverse effect on alertness and does not interact with other AEDs in polytherapy.

Topiramate significantly reduces the frequency of drop attacks and tonic clonic seizures,[242,243] but many cognitive, behavioural and physical side effects may outweigh any benefits.

Vigabatrin added to monotherapy with valproate had a beneficial effect in 85% of children. They experienced a 50–100% seizure reduction,[244] but the risk of irreversible visual field defects may be too high. In analogy with West syndrome, it may be Lennox–Gastaut syndrome of cortical dysplasia that may benefit most from vigabatrin.

Zonisamide may be useful,[245] although oligohydrosis[246] and other major adverse reactions may be a problem.

Hormonal and other non-AED treatment

Corticosteroids and ACTH may be helpful in idiopathic/cryptogenic Lennox–Gastaut syndrome particularly at onset, in status epilepticus or during periods of marked seizure exaggeration. They should not be tried more than once in the course of the disease.[173]

Intravenous immunoglobulin was found useful in a few case reports.[247]

Amantadine, tryptophan, flumazenil, imipramine and many other treatments have had limited success in some patients.[45]

NON-PHARMACOLOGICAL TREATMENTS

KETOGENIC DIET[248-254]

The ketogenic diet is undergoing a mini-renaissance in epileptic encephalopathies. The ketogenic diet as an effective treatment of intractable epilepsies was introduced in 1921 as a way of duplicating and prolonging the beneficial effects that fasting appeared to have on seizure control. Hence, this diet mimics the changes of starvation.

Indications and efficacy

Although controlled trials are lacking, results from large observational studies, some prospective, are consistent in showing that the ketogenic diet is a relatively safe and effective treatment in infants and children with drug-resistant epilepsies. The diet is particularly effective for epileptic spasms and myoclonic seizures.[255] Overall estimates indicate that complete cessation of all seizures occurs in 16% of patients, a greater than 90% reduction in seizures occurs in 32% and a greater than 50% reduction in seizures occurs in 56%.[249] Half of the children will continue on the diet for at least 1 year, with 40–50% of those starting the diet having a greater than 50% reduction in seizures after 12 months. The majority of parents also report improvements in their child's behaviour and function, particularly with respect to attention/alertness, activity level and socialisation.[255] A concomitant reduction in anti-epileptic medications is often possible. The ketogenic diet is first-line therapy for the treatment of seizures due to rare deficiencies of carbohydrate metabolism. More recently, this diet has also been used for adults.[256]

Mechanism of action

Neurons use ketone bodies rather than glucose as a metabolic substrate. The mechanism of action of the diet remains unknown and it is difficult to assess which biochemical parameters should be monitored as adjustments are made to the diet.[257] It has been suggested that chronic ketosis may control seizures by increasing the cerebral energy reserves in the brain, thus promoting neuronal stability.

The diet

The ketogenic diet is a high-fat, low-carbohydrate and low-protein regimen. The ketogenic ratio (fat:carbohydrate + protein) ranges from 2:1 to a maximum 5:1. The constituents are customised to meet the patient's needs and preferences.

The diet is a radical medical therapy and nutritional well being is a constant concern. The diet is usually commenced for in-patients. It should be initiated, supervised and monitored by a nutrition support team who also instruct family members on the maintenance of the diet at home.

Traditionally, children starting on the ketogenic diet were made to fast for 1–2 days until ketosis was seen. They were then started on one-third of the calories for 24 h and then two-thirds of calories for the next 24 h and finally were advanced to a full diet. This fasting period is often a difficult time for young children and their families, but this is probably not needed.[258]

The Atkins diet

The popular Atkins diet has been recently used in the treatment of epileptic encephalopathies as a less restrictive alternative therapy to the ketogenic diet.[254]

Adverse effects of ketogenic diet

The diet is generally well tolerated and over 94% of patients maintain appropriate growth parameters.[255] Nephrolithiasis is reported in 5–8% of children. Other adverse events include a reduced quantity of bone mass (requiring vitamin D supplementation), gastritis, ulcerative colitis, alteration of mentation and hyperlipidaemia. The altered pharmacokinetics of AEDs may cause toxicity. Carbonic anhydrase inhibitors (acetazolamide, sulthiame, topiramate, zonisamide) should be avoided. When possible, valproate should also be avoided. The diet may be lethal for patients with rare disorders of deranged cerebral energy metabolism such as pyruvate carboxylase deficiency.

VAGUS NERVE STIMULATION

Vagus nerve stimulation in childhood epileptic encephalopathies, though promising in some reports,[259-261] is probably of very limited value in Lennox–Gastaut syndrome.[262,263] There are relatively small changes in the behavioural outcomes, concurrent with the modest effects of vagus nerve stimulation on seizure frequency (an average of 20.6% seizure reduction)[264] and vagus nerve stimulation on seizure did not significantly improve seizure frequency, severity, adaptive behaviour or the EEG during the first year of treatment, although four out of 15 children (27%) had a worthwhile reduction in seizure frequency. There were significant improvements in perceived treatment side effects and general behaviour.[262,263]
See also Chapter 4 page 80.

NEUROSURGERY

Corpus callosotomy [122,265-268] is the only surgical procedure for devastating atonic seizures with traumatic falls (drop attacks) of epileptic encephalopathies (Chapter 4 page 79). Corpus callosotomy may also be considered for intractable tonic and less often GTCS, particularly in cryptogenic cases and provided there is no major diffuse brain malformations.[265] Other seizure types are not benefited. Improvements in behaviour and alertness have been observed in patients with decreased seizure frequency. The adverse side effects of corpus callosotomy are reduced with the anterior two-thirds sections, which may be sufficient in most patients. Despite improvements and modifications of corpus callosotomy with sequential radiofrequency lesions[266] and stereotactic radiosurgery, morbidity is relatively high and there is a tendency for seizures to return after 2 years. More intense focal seizures may occur post-operatively.

Resective neurosurgery is deserved for the few cases with distinctively localised epileptogenic lesions.[173,269]

TREATMENT OF STATUS EPILEPTICUS

In cases of impending status, it is better not to change the treatment dramatically and not to hospitalise the patient in a non-specialised unit. Rectal diazepam or an oral intake of a high dose of clobazam can stop serial attacks. If the status cannot be avoided this should be treated as a medical emergency. Intravenous benzodiazepines (mainly clonazepam) and phenytoin are the most effective drugs, sometimes given with concomitant steroids and with respiratory assistance if necessary. Intravenous diazepam and lorazepam may rarely induce tonic status epilepticus.[270]

ATTENTION TO SEIZURE PRECIPITANTS

Detecting and preventing seizure precipitating factors is part of the appropriate management of Lennox-Gastaut syndrome. A child who is overexcited, for example or lacks sufficient stimulation, may experience more seizures. A stimulating but stable environment can therefore be important in reducing the number of daily seizures. This may include a strict routine of regular meals, sleep and medication.

Triggering factors, such as intercurrent febrile illnessess, a change in drug regimens and psychological stress, may also provoke seizures and status epilepticus. Vomiting and diarrhoea can affect the body's ability to absorb medication.

EDUCATIONAL MANAGEMENT

The control of seizures, which is often unsuccessful, is one aspect of management in Lennox–Gastaut syndrome. However, nearly all patients have equally important educational, behavioural and psychological needs with regard to associated often severe cognitive and behavioural dysfunction. This mandates a multidisciplinary approach to the management of the patient and support for the whole family.

Management tips for Lennox–Gastaut syndrome

With increasing seizures, reducing may be a better option than increasing AEDs.
Evaluate the predominant, severe and disabling seizure type in preparation for selection of the next AED and the elimination of the current drug.
Any AED change, addition or removal, may be temporarily beneficial.

First-line drugs

Valproate: all seizures.
Clonazepam and other diazepines: mainly myoclonic jerks.
Lamotrigine: all (but myoclonic seizures) particularly as an add-on to valproate.
Levetiracetam: all but tonic seizures.
Phenytoin: tonic seizures.
Topiramate: probably all seizures but with many and serious adverse reactions.
Felbamate: probably all seizures but with serious sometimes fatal adverse reactions.

Second-line drugs

Ethosuximide: absences.
Carbamazepine: focal seizures and secondarily GTCS.
Corticosteroids and ACTH if seizures worsen.

Non-pharmacological treatments

The ketogenic diet is undergoing a mini-renaissance.
Neurosurgical resections in selective cases.
Vagus nerve stimulation is an expensive and probably worthless exercise.

LANDAU–KLEFFNER SYNDROME
ACQUIRED EPILEPTIC APHASIA

Landau–Kleffner syndrome[19,28,29,271-283] or acquired epileptic aphasia* is a partly reversible, epileptic encephalopathy of childhood manifesting with acquired verbal auditory agnosia and other predominantly linguistic deficits that often occur together with other cognitive and neuropsychological behavioural abnormalities. Seizures are infrequent and not a prerequisite for Landau-Kleffner syndrome.

DEMOGRAPHIC DATA

The age at onset is 2–8 years with a peak at 5–7 years. Boys are twice as likely as girls to be affected. One or two cases are seen every year in highly specialised centres.

CLINICAL MANIFESTATIONS

> Our son was normal in every way until approximately age 2 years. At first he seemed to be losing his hearing but not for environmental sounds. We thought that he was going deaf, but the hearing test was normal ... When he was 3 years old he didn't say anything for over a month. He improved for a few months and then we saw a very minor seizure.
>
> From the Internet description by a mother.

All children suffer from linguistic abnormalities, but only three-quarters of them also have seizures.

LINGUISTIC ABNORMALITIES

The first symptom is usually auditory verbal agnosia. Children with Landau–Kleffner syndrome become incapable of attributing a semantic value to acoustic signals thus making them appear as hypoacoustic or autistic children. The parents notice a gradual inability of the child to respond to their calls despite raising their voices. Auditory verbal agnosia may later progress to complete word deafness and non-linguistic sound agnosia such as, for example, a doorbell. The diagnosis is often delayed, mistaken for acquired deafness or elective mutism. Many of these children have an audiogram, which is normal.

The language deficit may be initially undermined because of other behavioural or cognitive problems.

---

* Though the language disturbance is described as an acquired aphasia, the main deficit is auditory verbal agnosia occurring in an initially normal child who had achieved developmental milestones at appropriate ages and had already acquired age-appropriate speech.

Considerations on classification of Landau–Kleffner syndrome and epilepsy with CSWS

The 1989 ILAE classification considers Landau–Kleffner syndrome and ECSWS as different epileptic syndromes classified amongst 'epilepsies and syndromes undetermined as to whether they are focal or generalised'.[21]

The ILAE definition is as follows.

Acquired epileptic aphasia (Landau–Kleffner syndrome) is a childhood disorder in which an acquired aphasia, multi-focal spike and spike and wave discharges are associated. Epileptic seizures and behavioural and psychomotor disturbances occur in two-thirds of patients. There is verbal auditory agnosia and a rapid reduction in spontaneous speech. The seizures, usually GTCS or partial motor, are rare and remit before the age of 15 years, as do the EEG abnormalities.

The new ILAE diagnostic scheme also considers them as separate diagnostic entities, which are classified amongst 'epileptic encephalopathies'.[1] Their separation is not universally accepted. Tassinari, a leading authority who has described epilepsy with CSWS, supports the view that Landau–Kleffner syndrome and ECSWS are 'two facets of the same entity', in which the type of neuropsychological dysfunction depends on the location of inter-ictal foci (frontal in ECSWS and temporal in Landau–Kleffner syndrome).[284,285] He considers Landau–Kleffner syndrome as a clinical variant of epileptic encephalopathy with CSWS.[284,285]

The onset may be subacute progressive or stepwise (stuttering) and gradually worsens and affects other linguistic functions with impairment of expressive speech, paraphasias, stereotypes, perseverations and phonological errors. Probably all types of aphasia can occur. The children express themselves in a telegraphic style or in very simple sentences and some cases may develop fluent aphasia or 'jargon'. Finally, the child may become entirely mute also failing to respond to even non-verbal sounds.

One of the most puzzling features of Landau–Kleffner syndrome is the fluctuating course of the linguistic disturbances, characterised by remissions and exacerbations.

COGNITIVE AND BEHAVIOURAL ABNORMALITIES

Cognitive and behavioural abnormalities occur in more than three-quarters of patients with Landau–Kleffner syndrome. Behavioural disorders such as hyperactivity and attention deficit are common and in rare cases there is progression to severe disinhibition and psychosis.

The relative severity of the linguistic, behavioural and cognitive problems can vary over time in the same child and between children. Long-term follow-up studies have shown that Landau–Kleffner syndrome is not always associated with intellectual deterioration.

SEIZURES

Clinically, seizures may also occur in three-quarters of patients, but these are usually infrequent and of good prognosis. Onset is between 4 and 6 years. Only 20% of patients continue having seizures after the age of 10 years and occurrence of seizures after the age of 15 years is exceptional.[286] Seizure symptoms and seizure type are not well described. They may be heterogeneous. GTCS and focal motor seizures (Figure 7.10) are emphasised by the ILAE commission.[21] However, atypical absences, atonic seizures with head drop, minor automatisms and secondarily GTCS are reported. Subtle seizures with minor motor or subjective symptoms may be frequent, but often remain undetected.[277,287] One-third of patients may suffer from a single GTCS or isolated convulsive status epilepticus occurring mainly around 5–10 years. Complex focal seizures of temporal lobe origin are exceptional. Tonic seizures are probably incompatible with Landau–Kleffner syndrome.

Seizures are often nocturnal, infrequent, respond well to treatment and remit before the age of 13–15 years.

The frequency and severity of seizures is not determined by the severity of EEG abnormalities or severity of linguistic and behavioural problems.

AETIOLOGY

This is unknown.

A family history of epilepsy is found in approximately 12% of cases with Landau–Kleffner syndrome who also have seizures.[274] This is reduced to 5% in those cases who do not have seizures.[274] Siblings may be affected.[288,289]

Commonly, there is no detectable underlying structural abnormality and MRI is normal. However, according to some reports 3% of patients have an encephalopathy and a variety of abnormalities were found in brain biopsy specimens of neurosurgical series.[278,282,290]

PATHOPHYSIOLOGY

Landau–Kleffner syndrome is probably the result of an epileptogenic *'functional lesion'* in the speech cortex during a critical period of child development. In other words, focal epileptogenic activity is thought to cause a *functional ablation of eloquent speech areas.*

Landau–Kleffner syndrome and ECSWS are considered to have a common pathophysiological mechanism.[19,29] They are both functional disorders occurring at an age where cortical synaptogenesis with abundant axonal sprouting and elemental functional network is being established in the brain. The number of synapses rapidly increases in excess of the ultimate number needed. Neuronal activity or synaptic use is critical in determining which of these synapses will be established or discarded before the age of 10 years. Aggressive epileptic activity, such as that of CSWS at this active period of brain organisation is detrimental for the establishment of appropriate neuronal connections, normal brain development and functioning.[19] It is likely that epileptic discharges activate and perpetuate synaptic arrangements that are functionally improper.[277] Intense epileptic activity in the dominant temporal region would affect linguistic capabilities, as in Landau–Kleffner syndrome.[277] Conversely, the mainly frontal localisation of CSWS primarily affects higher cognitive and executive functioning.[19,29,282]

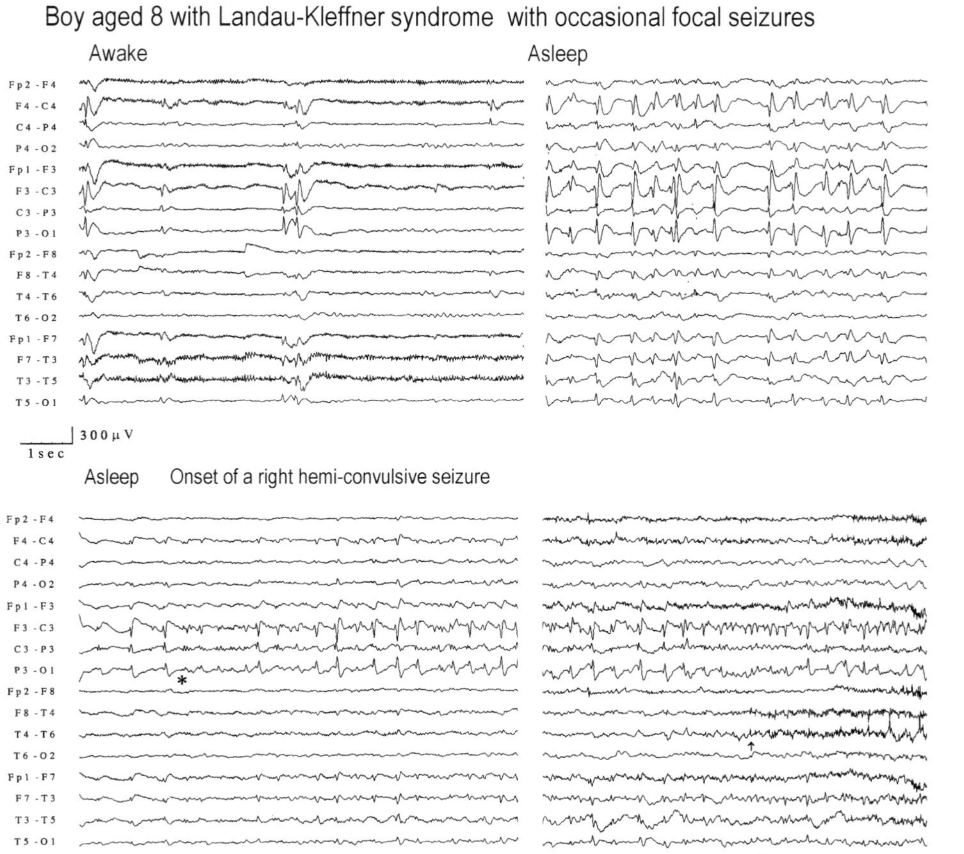

Figure 7.10 From a video–EEG recording of an 8-year-old boy with Landau–Kleffner syndrome prior to a PET scan.

He had infrequent seizures one of which was incidentally captured with video–EEG recording. Top*:* inter-ictally, there were clusters of sharp-slow wave focal discharges maximum around the left Rolandic regions (left). They became continuous during natural sleep (right). Bottom: ictal discharge starts from the left central regions and rapidly spreads to the neighbouring regions. The first clinical signs consisted of right facial spasms (arrow; also note muscle artefacts on the right) progressing to hemi-convulsions.

In my opinion, Landau–Kleffner syndrome and ECSWS is probably an exceptional and extreme part of benign childhood seizure susceptibility syndrome (BCSSS), which is derailed to an epileptic encephalopathy (as detailed in Chapter 9, page 263).[291,292] This extreme deviation results in a more aggressive condition of seizures, neuropsychological manifestations and EEG abnormalities of various combinations and various degrees of severity such as in Landau–Kleffner syndrome, ECSWS and atypical benign partial epilepsy of childhood.[292] The reason for this derailment of such a benign seizure susceptibility is unknown, but may be related to location (temporal spikes in Landau–Kleffner syndrome, frontal spikes in ECSWS) or other intrinsic and external superimposed factors. Additional evidence to support this pathophysiological proposition comes from the atypical evolutions of Rolandic[293] and Panayiotopoulos [214,294,295] syndrome to producing the clinical and EEG features of Landau–Kleffner syndrome, ECSWS and atypical benign partial epilepsy of childhood.

DIAGNOSTIC PROCEDURES

Routine structural brain imaging is often normal but functional brain imaging demonstrates abnormalities in the temporal lobes.[296] MRI volumetric analysis demonstrated volume reduction specifically in planum temporale and superior temporal gyrus (25 to 57%), where receptive language is localized.[297]

ELECTROENCEPHALOGRAPHY

The EEG is characterised by mainly posterior temporal lobe foci of sharp-slow wave complexes that are often multi-focal and bisynchronous, markedly facilitated by NREM sleep (Figure 7.11). CSWS occur at some stage of the illness in nearly all cases, but this is not a prerequisite for diagnosis. This may also persist or deteriorate during REM sleep (a finding that does not happen in ECSWS) (see page 186).

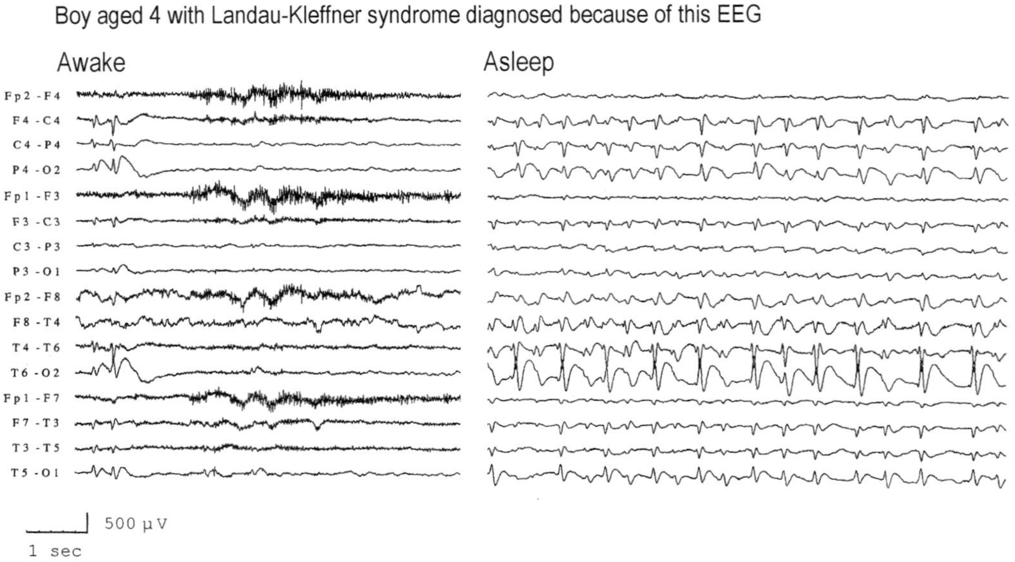

Figure 7.11 From a video–EEG recording of a 4-year-old boy referred for possible 'absence seizures' because of 'frequent episodes of inability to understand commands'.

The EEG showed clusters of sharp-slow wave-focal discharges maximum around the right posterior temporal regions (left). Though this was a request for a routine EEG, the technologist allowed time to proceed with a sleep EEG during which the paroxysms became continuous (right). The possibility of Landau–Kleffner syndrome was raised and this was confirmed with appropriate clinico-psychological testing.

DIFFERENTIAL DIAGNOSIS

Many cases of Landau–Kleffner syndrome are initially investigated for deafness or misdiagnosed as autistic or other psychiatric disorders.

Acute or subacute aphasia in children aged 2–8 years without unilateral acquired paresis or encephalitic symptoms is most probably due to Landau–Kleffner syndrome. This is because receptive or expressive aphasia is unusual in young children unless they have a bitemporal lobe dysfunction.

Although of probably no practical significance, Landau–Kleffner syndrome is often difficult to differentiate from ECSWS because of overlapping clinical and EEG features. The main differences are outlined in Table 7.8.

Linguistic disturbances are a prerequisite for the diagnosis of Landau–Kleffner syndrome, while EEG CSWS is a prerequisite for the diagnosis of ECSWS.[298]

PROGNOSIS

Seizures and EEG abnormalities are age dependent and often remit by the age of 15 years. Language and other neuropsychological disturbances gradually improve at the same age as the disappearance of EEG epileptiform activity. Only half of patients with Landau–Kleffner syndrome may be able to live a relatively normal life with 10–20% achieving complete normalisation. The other half is left with permanent sequelae that may be very severe.

Outcome is not influenced by the frequency and type of epileptic seizures. However, there is a strict correlation between the length of CSWS and persistence of language impairment.[299] Early onset of Landau–Kleffner syndrome is related with the worst prognosis regarding language recovery.

Rarely, spontaneous remissions may occur within weeks or months from onset.

MANAGEMENT

DRUG TREATMENT

Seizures in Landau–Kleffner syndrome are infrequent, age limited and often easily controlled with AEDs. Therefore, the pharmaceutical attempt is to reduce the epileptiform EEG discharges with the assumption that these are responsible for the linguistic, behavioural and other neuropsychological abnormalities. All traditional AEDs, including sleep-modifying drugs such as amitriptyline and amphetamine, have been tried with disappointing results. However, some children responded rather well with high doses of steroids or ACTH.

Table 7.8 Landau-Kleffner syndrome versus ECSWS

EEG aspects	**Landau-Kleffner syndrome**	**ECSWS**
CSWS	80%	100%
Main spike localisation	Temporal	Frontal
Clinical aspects		
Seizures	Three-quarters of patients	All patients
Symptomatic causes	Rare (~10% abnormal MRI)	One third (~33% abnormal MRI)
Primary language impairment	Verbal auditory agnosia	Expressive >receptive aphasia
Psychomotor/behavioural deficits	Common (45%)	Nearly all (95%)
Onset of cognitive impairment	Verbal auditory agnosia	Global
Prognosis	Half reach near-normal life	One-quarter reach near-normal life

The consensus is to first treat Landau–Kleffner syndrome with valproate, ethosuximide and clonazepam or clobazam, alone or in combination. Sulthiame (Ospolot), which is a very old drug, has recently re-emerged as the drug of choice. Phenytoin, phenobarbital and carbamazepine are contraindicated because these drugs may worsen the EEG discharges and neuropsychological deficit.

If AED treatment fails, which is most likely, ACTH or prednisone should be the treatment of choice, particularly in new and younger patients who may respond better, need shorter steroid treatment and are at a high risk of significant residual neuropsychological sequelae. There is an empirical view that the results depend on early treatment with high initial doses of steroids for at least 3 months. Continuation of treatment after this period depends on response and side effects. Some children with a good response may relapse and this may necessitate lengthy continuation of treatment, probably for years. Steroids are usually used with valproate or benzodiazepines and these may remain after steroid weaning.

In isolated cases, intravenous immunoglobulins are successful.

The effect of treatment should be monitored with appropriate neuropsychological evaluation and serial awake and sleep stage EEGs.

However, all these recommendations are empirical and anecdotal from clinical practices using what was available: old AEDs. Treatment now expands to include experience with newer AEDs that may offer more hope for success. In an a case report significant linguistic and seizure improvement was achieved with levetiracetam monotherapy.[300]

NEUROSURGICAL TREATMENT

In medically intractable cases of Landau–Kleffner syndrome subpial intracortical transections (see Chapter 4, page 80) have been used with relatively good success.[277,308] This surgical technique has been designed to eliminate the capacity of cortical tissue for generating seizures while preserving the normal cortical physiological function. Success depends on the selection of cases having severe epileptogenic abnormality that can be demonstrated to be unilateral in origin despite a bilateral electrographic manifestation.

Reminder on sulthiame[301-307]

Sulthiame, a sulphonamide derivative with carbonic anhydrase-inhibiting properties, was first introduced as an AED in the 1950s. Its use was abandoned in the 1970s on the assertion that it had little if any anti-epileptic activity when used alone. Its anti-epileptic action was attributed to raised levels of concomitant medication (phenytoin, phenobarbitone and primidone).[301,302]

Sulthiame appears to have been revitalised recently with reports (including class 1 evidence) that it is probably the most effective drug in benign childhood focal epilepsies with regard to its effect in suppressing seizures and EEG abnormalities.[305-307] It may be very useful and should be tried in epileptic encephalopathies,[303] mainly ECSWS and Landau–Kleffner syndrome. Sulthiame has also re-emerged as an AED in adults.[304]

EPILEPSY WITH CONTINUOUS SPIKE-AND - WAVES DURING SLOW-WAVE SLEEP

EPILEPTIC ENCEPHALOPATHY WITH ELECTRICAL STATUS EPILEPTICUS DURING SLOW-WAVE SLEEP

Epilepsy with continuous spike-and-waves during slow-wave sleep (ECSWS)[28,278,282-285,298,309-311] or encephalopathy with electrical status epilepticus during slow wave sleep (ESES) is a partly reversible, age-related childhood epileptic encephalopathy characterised by the triad of:

1. EEG CSWS (Figure 7.12)
2. seizures
3. neuropsychological and motor impairment.

Continuous spikes and waves during NREM sleep is a prerequisite for the diagnosis of this syndrome.

DEMOGRAPHIC DATA

The syndrome of ECSWS is age dependent, occurring only in children. The onset of seizures is between 2 months and 12 years, with a peak at 4–5 years. The EEG CSWS probably start 1–2 years from the first seizure with a peak at age 8 years and a range of 3–14 years. There may be a male preponderance (62%).[313] The prevalence is no more than 0.5% amongst children with seizures.[310]

CLINICAL MANIFESTATIONS

Half of the affected children are normal prior to the onset of the disease. The other half have pre- or peri-natal illness, neonatal convulsions and neurological abnormalities such as congenital hemiparesis or tetraparesis, ataxia, psychomotor or language deficits.

There are three stages of evolution.

- **The first stage is before the discovery of CSWS.**
- **The second stage is when CSWS is found.**
- **The third stage is after clinical and EEG remission starts.**

FIRST STAGE BEFORE THE DISCOVERY OF CSWS

The first stage is before the discovery of CSWS. The first seizure is usually nocturnal in half of cases and in 40% consists of unilateral convulsions often lasting for more than 30 min and constitutes hemi-clonic status epilepticus. In others, seizures may be focal motor clonic, generalised tonic-clonic, complex focal or myoclonic absence. Seizures are infrequent and mainly nocturnal.

The EEG shows multi-focal spikes and bisynchronous generalised sharp or spike-wave discharges.

Definition and nomenclature of 'ECSWS'

The 1989 ILAE classification classified ECSWS amongst 'epilepsies and syndromes undetermined as to whether they are focal or generalised' and defined it as follows.[21]

"Epilepsy with continuous spike-and-waves during slow-wave sleep results from the association of various seizure types, partial or generalised, occurring during sleep and atypical absences when awake. Tonic seizures do not occur. The characteristic EEG pattern consists of continuous diffuse spikes and waves during slow wave sleep, which is noted after the onset of seizures. The duration varies from months to years. Despite the usually benign evolution of seizures, prognosis is guarded because of the appearance of neuropsychologic disorders."[21]

Tassinari, a leading authority who described ECSWS, prefers the term 'electrical status epilepticus during slow-wave sleep'.[285]

"Slow-wave sleep" in ECSWS refers to all NREM sleep stages I-IV (see page 138). The initial descriptive terminology of "subclinical electrical status epilepticus induced by sleep" [312] was probably more accurate.

SECOND STAGE WITH CSWS

The second stage (with CSWS) commonly starts 1–2 years after the first seizure, with a peak at age 8 years and a range of 4–10 years. The discovery of CSWS is usually due to an increase in seizures and the appearance or deterioration of neuropsychological symptoms that prompt a sleep EEG. The active duration of CSWS is difficult to assess ranging from several months up to 6–7 years.

Seizures during the stage of CSWS[29]

The habitual seizures of the patient become frequent and new types of seizure emerge. Patients may have one or multi-form seizures, which may be frequent or infrequent. All types except tonic seizures occur. These include hemi-facial, hemi-convulsive, GTCS, atypical or typical absences, negative myoclonus, non-convulsive status epilepticus and atonic seizures. Convulsive seizures are predominantly nocturnal.

Tassinari[29] identified the following three groups based on their seizure types.

Group 1. Patients with infrequent motor seizures, which occur during sleep only (11%).

Group 2. Patients with unilateral focal motor seizures or GTCS mainly occurring during sleep. These patients also have typical absence seizures.

Group 3. Patients with rare nocturnal motor seizures who mainly suffer from atypical absences, frequently with atonic or tonic components leading to sudden falls.

Negative myoclonus is a frequent seizure type that may contribute to the development of motor impairment.

The general consensus is that tonic seizures do not occur at any stage and are probably incompatible with the diagnosis of ECSWS.

In the course of the disease over 90% of patients have numerous seizures of sometimes several per day. Infrequent seizure occurrence is unusual (10%).

Neuropsychological state during CSWS

At this second stage of evolution (when CSWS is discovered) the dramatic decline the neuropsychological state is the most disturbing clinical feature. The neuropsychological impairment is usually of insidious onset and progression while sudden commencement is rare. The neuropsychological deficits are largely dependent on spike localisation.

- Frontal or prefrontal CSWS disrupts the higher cognitive and executive functioning before damaging language function and produces a frontal lobe type of mental and behavioural deterioration. These manifest with hyperkinesia, agitation, disinhibition, aggressiveness and inattention often leading to extensive cognitive decline or psychosis described as mental retardation or dementia of frontal lobe syndrome.
- Temporal lobe CSWS produces mainly linguistic disturbances with a tendency towards expressive aphasia rather than verbal or auditory agnosia of Landau-Kleffener syndrome.

Motor disturbances consist of ataxia, hemiparesis and dyspraxia. Some children may develop the clinical features of *'acquired epileptiform opercular syndrome'* with oro-facio-lingual deficits of severe oral motor dysfunction, drooling, dysarthria, speech arrest or weakness of the face and tongue.[282,314,315]

THIRD STAGE OF CLINICAL AND EEG REMISSION

The third stage of clinico-EEG remission starts after a variable period of months to usually 2–7 years from onset.[29] Seizures remit in all patients irrespective of cause and underlying pathology. EEG gradually improves to relative normalisation.[29] The neuropsychological state also improves but children rarely reach average normality. Despite some improvement, many of these children suffer from permanent complex and severe neuropsychological impairment.

AETIOLOGY

The aetiology is unknown. More than one-third of patients with ECSWS have an abnormal pathology such as unilateral or diffuse cortical atrophy, focal porencephaly and malformations of cortical development. Cases of ECSWS evolving from benign childhood focal seizures are well reported.[292,293] There is no evidence of familial epileptic disorders. A family history of epilepsy is very uncommon (approximately 10%).

PATHOPHYSIOLOGY

This is similar to that described in Landau–Kleffner syndrome.

The neuropsychological impairment is attributed to the effect of CSWS as shown by the fact that cognitive and motor impairment in ECSWS is proportional to the duration and severity of CSWS.[19,28,29,282,311]

- The onset and improvement of cognitive and motor impairment coincides with the onset and resolution of CSWS.
- The duration of CSWS is correlated with the final neuropsychological outcome.
- The pattern of neuropsychological derangement depends on the location of the inter-ictal focus. Linguistic impairment relates to epileptogenic abnormalities over one or both temporal lobe regions, whereas mental deterioration and autistic behaviour relates to frontal lobe epileptogenic foci.

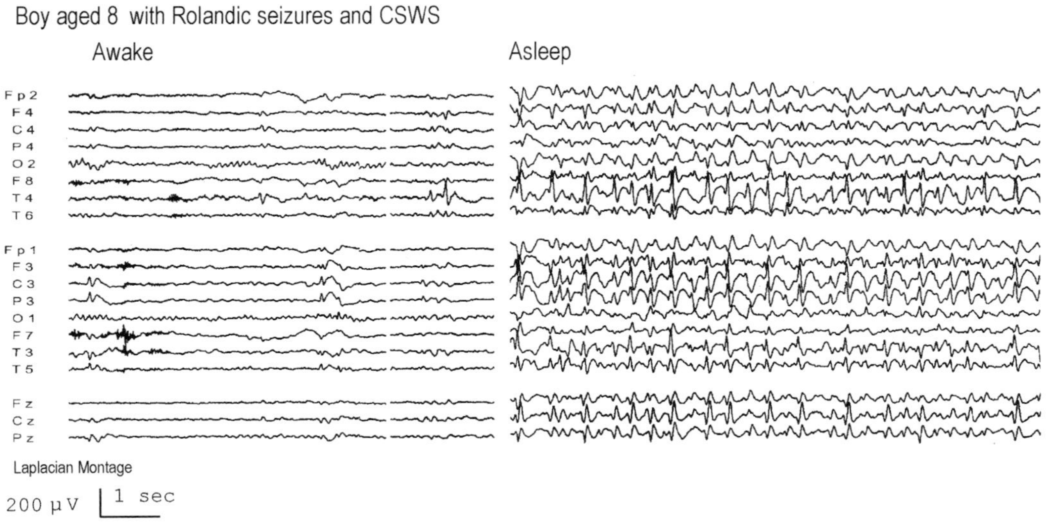

Figure 7.12 This case supports the links between benign neonatal convulsions, Rolandic seizures and ECSWS.

Longitudinal sleep EEG recordings show a progressive improvement over years towards normalisation after an average age of approximately 11 years. The discharges during sleep EEG become shorter, less frequent and more fragmented. Physiological sleep patterns become discernible. Rare focal sharp-slow wave complexes may persist, particularly in sleep EEG, long after clinical improvement. Normalisation, if finally achieved, may take more than 15 years.

In all cases sleep organisation and sleep stages are normal after CSWS remission.

Causative factors for motor impairment such as dyspraxia or dystonia are attributed to the dysfunction of the motor cortex by CSWS and the negative myoclonus during wakefulness.

Based on extensive PET studies Maquet et al.[316] hypothesised that the acquired deterioration of cognitive function with CSWS is caused by an alteration of the maturation of one or several associative cortices, primarily involving local interneurons and cortico-cortical associative neurons.[316]

The mechanism generating CSWS is attributed to secondary bilateral synchrony (page 166). Focal epileptogenic foci rapidly propagate within and between hemispheres to produce diffuse slow GSWD.

DIAGNOSTIC PROCEDURES

BRAIN IMAGING

Brain imaging and particularly MRI are mandatory. More than one-third of patients with ECSWS have abnormal brain imaging such as unilateral or diffuse cortical atrophy, porencephaly and developmental brain malformations. Functional brain imaging (PET or SPECT) is usually abnormal even in patients with normal brain MRI.[316]

In PET with [^{18}F]-fluorodeoxyglucose, the metabolic patterns are variable from one patient to another and in the same patient over time. In the active phase, there is usually a unilateral, focal or regional increase in glucose metabolism of the cortex. Hypermetabolism may occur only during sleep. Decreased regional glucose metabolism may be observed during wakefulness. After recovery, the metabolic pattern is either normal or shows focal or regional, uni- or bilateral hypometabolism.[316]

In SPECT with ^{99m}Tc-HMPAO, focal areas of low cerebral blood flow, when they occur, often correspond with those of the prevalent EEG localisation discharges. The percentage of abnormal SPECT results is significantly higher amongst patients with CSWS for over 1 year.[317]

ELECTROENCEPHALOGRAPHY[29,282]

Epilepsy with continuous spike-and-waves during slow-wave sleep is mainly defined by CSWS. The testing procedures include routine EEG, prolonged video–EEG recording or ambulatory monitoring. The syndrome can be suspected with brief sleep EEG recordings (Figure 7.12), but all-night sleep EEG is usually needed for proper quantification.

EEG findings prior to the development of CSWS[29]

The first EEG is usually obtained after the onset of seizures. It usually shows focal sharp-wave complexes (slow spikes) mainly in the anterior and central regions, while diffuse sharp-waves may occur in 80% of cases. The abnormalities are exaggerated by sleep.

The inter-ictal awake stage routine EEG in more than two-thirds of patients shows focal or multi-focal slow spikes mainly localised in the frontotemporal, centrotemporal and less often in the parieto-occipital electrodes. Often these are morphologically similar to the functional spikes of benign childhood focal seizures (Chapter 9). These are activated by sleep without altering their morphology. In 80% of cases, there are additional diffuse slow GSWD at 1–3 Hz often with an apparent focal driving spike betraying SBS.

Sleep patterns and the cyclic organisation of sleep are normal.

The background EEG varies in accordance with the cause of ECSWS. Focal slow waves, fast spikes and polyspikes may occur in symptomatic cases.

EEG in the second stage of CSWS[29]

The characteristic EEG pattern in this stage occurs during sleep. In wakefulness the EEG is similar to that of the first stage, but the abnormalities are more pronounced.

Continuous spikes and waves during NREM sleep is the defining EEG pattern of ECSWS:

- it consists of mainly bilateral and diffuse slow spikes-waves of 1.5–2 Hz
- it relates to NREM sleep occupying most of its duration.

This pattern is generally found between the ages of 4 and 14 years and seems to develop 1–2 years after the appearance of seizures.

Duration of CSWS

The duration of CSWS is quantitatively expressed as the spike–wave index (SWI) which is the sum of all spike-slow wave complexes in minutes multiplied by 100 and divided by the total duration of NREM sleep in minutes. The SWI is usually more than 85% (sometimes 100%) of the total duration of NREM sleep. Less stringent criteria of a SWI greater than 50% are also accepted providing that the clinical symptomatology resembles that of the classical cases and the dramatic activation of the epileptiform discharges occurs in NREM sleep compared with wakefulness.[28,29,282] Patients with a SWI of less than 85% have better performance tests than those with a higher SWI.[28] The percentage of CSWS is more marked during the first cycle of sleep (95–100%) than in the following cycles (80–70%). An EEG with mainly anterior spikes during wakefulness tends to produce a higher SWI (85–100%) than those with posterior spikes (64%).[28]

> As soon as the patient falls asleep continuous bilateral and diffuse slow spikes and waves appear, mainly at 1.5–2.5 Hz, persisting through all the slow wave sleep stages. An SWI in the range of 85–100%, calculated during all-night sleep EEG recordings, is considered as an essential feature for the diagnosis of ECSWS. This criterion was useful in identifying the tip of the iceberg.[29]

Morphology and distribution of CSWS

The classical CSWS consists of NREM sleep-related, continuous or nearly continuous bilateral and bisynchronous sharp-slow waves, which are morphologically similar to the functional spikes of Rolandic epilepsy with a repetitive rate of 1.5–2 Hz (faster rates of 3–4 Hz may be present). These are of higher amplitude in the anterior or central regions. There are significant variations such that the discharges can be grossly asymmetrical, unilateral or predominantly focal[317] and spikes may be devoid of the slow waves.[29]

The so-called diffuse or generalised spike-wave discharges frequently originate from focal spikes (secondary bilateral synchrony). These focal spikes are often seen in the inter-ictal awake or REM sleep EEG, at the onset of spike and wave stretches or with clearly higher amplitude in relation to the others. They are also discernible during the rare short period of fragmented diffuse spike-wave discharges in NREM sleep.[29]

Polyspikes are rare. Fast episodic activity is exceptional. Focal, frontocentral rhythmic discharges organised as a subclinical seizure were observed at the end of REM sleep in four patients.[313,318]

NREM sleep EEG pattern

The physiological sleep patterns (spindles, K complexes or vertex spikes) are seldom discernible during CSWS. However, these are preserved and become apparent when CSWS is fragmented, in late cycles of sleep and in patients with a low SWI. The cyclic organisation of sleep is grossly preserved, 80% of sleep is NREM and there are no apparent sleep disorders.

REM sleep

In REM sleep the EEG is very similar to that of wakefulness. The electrical status fades away and REM sleep patterns are discernible with superimposed focal, predominantly frontal or frontocentral, sharp slow waves alone or with rare bursts or runs of bilateral paroxysmal discharges.

EEG PROGRESSION TOWARDS RELATIVE NORMALISATION[28,29]

Longitudinal sleep EEG recordings show a progressive improvement over years towards normalisation after an average age of approximately 11 years. The discharges during sleep EEG become shorter, less frequent and more fragmented. Physiological sleep patterns become discernible. Rare focal sharp-slow wave complexes may persist, particularly in sleep EEG, long after clinical improvement. Normalisation, if finally achieved, may take more than 15 years.

In all cases sleep organisation and sleep stages are normal after CSWS remission.

DIFFERENTIAL DIAGNOSIS[19,282,292,311]

The differential diagnosis of ECSWS from Landau–Kleffner syndrome when CSWS occurs in EEG has been detailed on page 181 (Table 7.8). Briefly, in Landau–Kleffner syndrome (1) acquired aphasia is the most predominant linguistic impairment, (2) epileptic seizures may not occur and (3) the inter-ictal EEG foci are mainly temporal while these are mainly frontal in ECSWS.

The differential diagnosis of ECSWS from Rolandic epilepsy and other benign focal seizure susceptibility phenotypes has been emphasised in all recent reviews[19,282,292,311] because of similar EEG features, exaggeration of spikes during sleep, focal motor seizures, mild cognitive impairment and atypical evolutions.

Differentiating ECSWS from Lennox–Gastaut syndrome is easy because tonic seizures and EEG fast paroxysms are prominent in Lennox–Gastaut syndrome while these are practically absent in ECSWS. Furthermore, focal motor seizures and remissions are rare in Lennox–Gastaut syndrome.

PROGNOSIS

Spontaneous resolution of the epileptiform discharges and seizures occurs in the mid-teens and this coincides with stabilisation or improvement of the behavioural and neuropsychological deficits.[28,29,310] The persistence and severity of residual behavioural, cognitive and linguistic deficits depends on the age at onset and the duration of the active phase of electrographic epileptiform activity.

Seizures gradually become less frequent and less severe before they finally remit in all patients, commonly at about the age of 10–15 years. Seizure improvement may be simultaneous with (30%), precede (30%) or follow (40%) the resolution of CSWS. Seizure outcome is independent of aetiology with remission of seizures in symptomatic cases such as multi-lobar polymicrogyria.[319] Delayed resolution of seizures occurs in patients with more severe epilepsy, such as those manifesting with generalised motor, atonic seizures or absences. The total duration of the active seizure period varies from 4 to 17 years.

Cognitive and behavioural abnormalities show a global improvement, which starts after the end of CSWS, but recovery is always slow and often only partial. The majority of affected children never return to normal functioning, particularly in the verbal area and attention.[310,320,321]

Less than one-quarter of patients resume acceptable social and professional levels, but this is more likely amongst those who had a normal pre-morbid neuropsychological state and a shorter active period of CSWS.

MANAGEMENT[19,282,311,322]

Management is similar to that described for Landau–Kleffner syndrome (page 181).

Seizures are not a major problem as their final prognosis is good. Depending on the type of seizures valproate, lamotrigine, levetiracetam[323] and sulthiame may be the most appropriate treatments. Carbamazepine is contraindicated because it exaggerates CSWS.[292]

The treatment of CSWS, which is responsible for the neuropsychological impairment, is entirely empirical and usually of transient efficacy. The following schemes, alone or in combination, have been proposed.[19,29,324]

- Oral benzodiazepines (diazepam, clobazam, clonazepam or lorazepam) combined with valproate.[29] Short cycles (3–4 weeks each) of diazepam (0.5 mg/kg) following a rectal diazepam bolus of 1 mg/kg have been used with some benefit.[324]
- ACTH (80 IU daily with a taper of 3 months) or high-dose prednisone (2–5 mg/kg daily with a taper of 3 months) when CSWS is diagnosed.[19] The earlier the treatment is initiated, the shorter is the duration for which steroids are required and the better is the ultimate outcome.

In cases with severe linguistic impairment, subpial intracortical transections have been used with success.[277,308]

MYOCLONIC STATUS IN NON-PROGRESSIVE ENCEPHALOPATHIES

Myoclonic status in non-progressive (fixed) encephalopathies is considered as a syndrome in development in the new diagnostic scheme of the ILAE.[1,325-328] All patients have a fixed encephalopathy and recurrent episodes of prolonged and erratic atypical myoclonic-absence status epilepticus.

DEMOGRAPHIC DATA

The peak onset is at 12 months (range of 1 day to 5 years). There is a two-fold preponderance in girls. Although its incidence and prevalence are unknown it was found in 0.5–1% of a selected population of children with severe forms of epilepsy.

CLINICAL MANIFESTATIONS

All patients have pre-existing neuropsychological deficits of a fixed encephalopathy characterised by severe axial hypotonia, ataxic gait, continuous abnormal jerky movements tremor and severe cognitive and learning abnormalities.

The defining seizure manifestation is repetitive and long (sometimes for days) episodes of atypical and subtle myoclonic status epilepticus. This consists of myoclonic jerks and discontinuous absences. The myoclonic jerks involving the eyelids, face and limbs are mostly erratic and asynchronous becoming more rhythmic and synchronous during the absences. The myoclonic jerks are often inconspicuous and the babies may appear just apathetic and ataxic. Myoclonic status epilepticus may be the first seizure manifestation. In others onset is with focal motor seizures, myoclonic absences, massive myoclonias and, more rarely, generalised or unilateral clonic convulsions recurring in some cases only during febrile illness. Tonic seizures do not occur.

Many patients also have frequent and sudden spontaneous massive startle attacks of brief and abrupt loss of postural tone and long-lasting episodes of positive/negative myoclonus and tremor.

On electroclinical grounds two main groups are recognised.

- *The first group* shows a mixed pattern of myoclonic-absence seizures, inhibitory phenomena and cortical myoclonus. The myoclonic status is usually sporadic but may also be frequent for years. This pattern mainly occurs in chromosomal abnormalities such as Angelman syndrome.[329,330]
- *The second group* shows a marked predominance of inhibitory phenomena resulting in complete motor inhibition. The status is always permanent throughout the evolution. All patients are females with unknown aetiology.

AETIOLOGY

Half the cases suffer from chromosomal disorders and mainly Angelman and 4p-syndrome. Others have prenatal brain anoxia-ischaemia or malformations of cortical development. The aetiology is unknown in the remaining one-third of cases. One-fifth of cases have a family history of seizure disorders. Metabolic diseases such as non-ketotic hyperglycinaemia may present with similar electroclinical features.

PATHOPHYSIOLOGY

This is uknown but may be multiple. A loss of GABAergic inhibition has been implicated because Angelman syndrome and some patients with 4p-syndrome have a chromosomal deletion eliminating a cluster of $GABA_A$ receptor genes.[327]

DIAGNOSTIC PROCEDURES

Because of different aetiologies these children require brain MRI, chromosomal analysis and metabolic screening. Confirmation of the seizures with video–EEG or polygraphic recordings is needed.

The inter-ictal EEG is diffusely slow with frequent focal or multi-focal abnormalities of slow waves and spikes.

The ictal EEG shows continuous or subcontinuous brief bursts of diffuse slow spikes and waves.

DIFFERENTIAL DIAGNOSIS

Myoclonic status epilepticus is often difficult to recognise without polygraphic or video–EEG recordings because of the severe mental retardation and the continuous abnormal movements of these babies. The diagnosis of non-progressive encephalopathy needs exclusion of progressive diseases manifesting

---

A brief reminder of Angelman syndrome[330,331]

Angelman syndrome is a major cause of childhood mental retardation and epilepsy (6% of all children). Over 70% are due to abnormalities of chromosome 15q11-q13, which encompass a cluster of $GABA_A$ receptor subunit genes. In 20% of patients no genetic abnormality is detected.

Clinical manifestations become apparent just before the first year of life with developmental delay. Other prominent symptoms include impaired expressive language, ataxic gait, tremulousness (tremor-like limb movements), hypermotoric behaviour, and inattention with a happy looking face (happy puppet syndrome). Seizures, microcephaly and scoliosis are common concurrent manifestations in over 80% of patients. All patients even those without seizures have tremulousness which is related to distal cortical myoclonus.[330]

Epileptic seizures are multi-form and include absences, myoclonus and myoclonic status epilepticus. Angelman syndrome may present with symptoms of West or Lennox-Gastaut syndrome.

Inter-ictal EEG is dominated by high amplitude posterior slow waves with or without spikes.

Confirmation of Angelman syndrome is primarily with the methylation test in those with chromosomal deletions or mutations.

with similar seizures/status such as the late infantile form of neuronal ceroid-lipofuscinosis.

PROGNOSIS

Prognosis is poor even for those who initially appear only hypotonic. The initial hypotonic state progressively deteriorates to sometimes-severe neurological and mental deficits. The myoclonic status improves with age but the patients rarely achieve a relatively normal state.

MANAGEMENT

Stopping myoclonic status epilepticus with benzodiazepines is often associated with a global improvement of the patient though commonly this is transient. In some patients with chromosomal abnormalities there may be some beneficial effect of valproate combined with ethosuximide or clobazam, but ACTH treatment is often needed.

ATYPICAL BENIGN PARTIAL EPILEPSY OF CHILDHOOD

Atypical benign partial epilepsy of childhood[51,292,332-335] is rightly not recognised as a syndrome by the ILAE. I present it in this book for two reasons. Firstly because of significant problems in its differentiation from some epileptic encephalopathies (Lennox–Gastaut syndrome, Landau–Kleffner syndrome and ECSWS), EM-AS and atypical evolutions of benign childhood focal seizures.[51,292,332] Secondly because it is of intermediate severity between Landau–Kleffner syndrome and ECSWS versus benign childhood focal seizures.[334]

The main differentiating point is that these children also have nocturnal focal seizures similar to the Rolandic seizures that are often the initial seizure type. In addition, the EEG shows centrotemporal and other functional spikes in various locations.

Some patients may additionally have GTCS, brief absences and occasionally jerks. Focal sensory motor fits are exceptional. Atonic attacks are associated with the slow wave component of spike and wave complexes and the location of the EEG discharges corresponds to that of the atonic episodes.

DEMOGRAPHIC DATA

Atypical benign partial epilepsy of childhood is rare, probably 1 case per 130 patients with Rolandic epilepsy.[337] Onset is between 2 and 6 years of age.

CLINICAL MANIFESTATIONS

Children have normal development and neurological examination before the onset of seizures.

All patients have at least two different seizure types: atonic seizures and nocturnal focal 'Rolandic-like' seizures.

Clarifications on nomenclature

Aicardi and Chevrie[332] used the term *'benign'* for this atypical benign partial epilepsy of childhood, not because of possible similarities with Rolandic seizures, but in order to distinguish it mainly from the Lennox–Gastaut syndrome 'for which it is regularly mistaken'.[332] Others have called it 'pseudo-Lennox syndrome'.[334,336] Retrospectively, Aicardi considered that it now appears that atypical benign partial epilepsy of childhood bears a close relationship to ECSWS. "It may be a mild and intermediate form of ECSWS".[335]

Atonic seizures are the most characteristic of all and occur in clusters lasting for 1 week to several weeks, usually separated by free intervals of several weeks or months. They may involve the whole axial musculature and/or both lower limbs with multiple daily falls that can produce severe injuries. On other occasions, atonic seizures may be subtle and localised manifesting with brief (1–2 s) sudden head or hand drops. Focal atonia of transient dropping of one arm may be very brief (100–150 ms) and is observed when the patients are asked to keep both arms outstretched in front of the body.[338] The brief focal atonia of the arm occasionally progresses to atonic seizures or atonic absence seizures.

Nocturnal focal seizures similar to the Rolandic seizures often occur as a presenting symptom of the disease and are infrequent. Diurnal focal sensory motor fits are exceptional.

Other type of seizures: Some patients may additionally have GTCS, brief absences and occasionally jerks. In some patients, absence seizures may be prominent.

Behavioural and cognitive problems: In the active seizure periods there is some degree of mental slowing or behavioural disturbance, which is often subtle and disappears during seizure-free periods.

DIAGNOSTIC PROCEDURES

All tests except the EEG are normal.

ELECTROENCEPHALOGRAPHY

The awake EEG shows centrotemporal spikes, which are often bilateral. Generalised spikes and waves of 3 Hz are frequent with or without clinical absences.

The sleep EEG is similar or identical to the CSWS. This occurs mainly during the active period of atonic seizures and may disappear in between.

The ictal EEG in unilateral, brief (100–150 ms) focal atonia corresponds exactly with a single sharp-slow wave complex arising from the contralateral centrotemporoparietal region. With progress to atonic or atonic-absence seizures, the localised epileptic discharge spreads into generalised discharges.[338,339]

DIFFERENTIAL DIAGNOSIS

Atypical benign partial epilepsy of childhood, although it 'is regularly mistaken' for Lennox–Gastaut syndrome' has a good outcome with no evidence of residual mental or behavioural deterioration even after some months of evolution. In addition, there are no tonic fits, central spikes occur frequently and the relatively good awake EEG is in marked contrast with the sleep deterioration compatible with CSWS.[51,332,333]

Atypical benign partial epilepsy of childhood may also imitate myoclonic astatic epilepsy because of repeated falls, absences and diffuse slow spike-wave activity mainly in the sleep EEG.[51,292,332] The main differentiating points are as follows.

- Nocturnal focal seizures similar to the Rolandic seizures that are often the initial seizure type.
- EEG centrotemporal and other functional spikes in various locations.

Similar clinico-EEG features may occur in atypical evolutions of Rolandic epilepsy[293,340] and Panayiotopoulos syndrome,[294,295] but these are preceded by typical presentations of these syndromes (see Chapter 9).

A similar but reversible clinico-EEG condition may be induced by carbamazepine in a few children with Rolandic epilepsy.[292,341] This possibility should be considered in children with Rolandic seizures and dramatic deterioration after treatment with carbamazepine or other drugs such as vigabatrin.

PROGNOSIS

The long-term outcome appears to be good with complete remission of seizures, no gross cognitive or behavioural sequelae and children attending mainstream schools.[51,335]

MANAGEMENT

Most of the traditional AEDs are often ineffective against the seizures and the EEG paroxysms. ACTH or corticosteroids were tried unsuccessfully in a few cases. Sulthiame or sulthiame/clobazam has been recommended as an effective treatment.[306,307,342,343] Lamotrigine[344] and phenobarbitone[345] may have a deteriorating effect.

HYPOTHALAMIC (GELASTIC) EPILEPSY

Hypothalamic (gelastic) epilepsy is a rare epileptic disease of hypothalamic hamartomas manifesting with gelastic seizures. This often evolves to a generalised epileptic encephalopathy with severe seizures and cognitive and behaviour decline.[22,346-351] Despite earlier views to the contrary, good evidence now exists that all these clinical features are caused, directly or indirectly, by the hamartoma.[22]

The various aspects of this disorder have been recently authoritatively reviewed by leading experts in a recent issue of *Epileptic Disorders* (December 2003).[352-366]

DEMOGRAPHIC DATA

Onset of habitual seizures typically begins in the neonatal period or early childhood with a peak at 2–3 years. Boys are twice as likely to be affected. Hypothalamic gelastic epilepsy appears to be extremely rare, probably 0.1% amongst patients with seizures. In my experience of a series of 1500 adult and children patients with seizures only two had hypothalamic gelastic epilepsy.

CLINICAL MANIFESTATIONS

Laughter is the defining, inaugural and starting clinical ictal manifestation of hypothalamic gelastic epilepsy. Gelastic seizures may manifest only with laughter, particularly at onset and may not even be recognised as pathological. The laughter may be silent, a facial expression of a smile or loud, with the natural vocalisations at various intensities and combinations. There is no emotional element of pleasure or amusement associated with this: it is a mirthless laughter. The attacks come out of the blue, are out of place and are inappropriate. Although unmotivated as a rule, some of the attacks may be triggered by a pleasant situation.

Classification issues

The association between hypothalamic hamartoma and gelastic seizures, often with a precocious puberty, is now well established thus constituting an epileptic entity (disease) probably amongst epileptic encephalopathies in infancy and early childhood. However, the 1989 ILAE Commission[21] classified hypothalamic gelastic epilepsy amongst' symptomatic generalised epilepsies of specific aetiologies' where epileptic seizures are the presenting or a prominent feature.[21] Similar is the position of the ILAE Task Force, which considers hypothalamic epilepsy amongst 'an example of a classification of diseases frequently associated with epileptic seizures or syndromes' (Table 1.8).[1] Conversely, the new diagnostic scheme correctly recognises gelastic seizures as a seizure type of various aetiologies.[1]

Dacrystic (crying) attacks alone or together with laughter may occur in 13% of patients.[347]

The attacks are usually brief (10–30 s), of sudden onset and termination and occur on a daily basis.[347] Subjectively, patients may be conscious of laughing, but they cannot prevent it or stop it.[347] They feel embarrassed about this, often inventing various excuses to justify it if this occurs at school, church or social meetings.

A few patients report a warning that they cannot describe well.

> A 13-year-old girl had onset of gelastic seizures from age 3 years. The laughter might precede or occur simultaneously with a feeling of her being light as 'if flying in the air'. The ictal laughter is similar to her natural laughter, but her parents can recognise the pathological one. MRI demonstrated a small hypothalamic hamartoma in the right wall of the third ventricle. Despite numerous gelastic seizures, which became longer and more severe with time, she remains highly intelligent with normal behaviour.

Other ictal subjective symptoms concurrent with laughter include disorientation, localised tingling and auditory sensations. The attacks are usually diurnal, but exceptionally they may also occur during sleep.[347,367]

Gelastic seizures may be associated with impairment of consciousness in half of patients.[347] The commoner pattern is that of the gelastic seizures becoming longer with impairment of consciousness and clinical ictal manifestations other than laughter such as automatisms.

Autonomic symptoms associated with the attacks of laughter are common, occurring in one-third of patients.[347,368] These include changes in the respiratory or cardiac rhythm, changes in blood pressure, facial flush or pallor, pupillary dilation, sniffing and urinary incontinence. Gelastic seizures are accompanied by an abrupt sympathetic system activation, probably due to the direct paroxysmal activation of limbic and paralimbic structures or other autonomic centres of the hypothalamus and medulla.[369]

More than half of the patients (66%) also suffer from other types of seizures in addition to gelastic attacks.[347,370,371] These are usually generalised seizures such as tonic, atonic, generalised tonic clonic and absences alone or in combination. Complex focal seizures without laughter are less common. These additional types of seizures may start at the same time as the laughter attacks or usually later within 1 year to a few years.[347]

There are no objective or subjective post-ictal symptoms in non-convulsive seizures of hypothalamic gelastic epilepsy. Pre-ictal activity continues as if nothing had happened.

AETIOLOGY

By definition the aetiology of hypothalamic gelastic epilepsy is due to hypothalamic hamartomas that usually originate in the region of the tuber cinereum and the mamillary bodies (Figure 7.13).[372] Hamartoma is a non-neoplastic, developmental tumour-like nodule that results from aberrant differentiation. Typically, it is a mass composed by disorganised but mature cells, all of which are indigenous to the site of origin (the hypothalamus in cases of hypothalamic gelastic epilepsy).

PATHOPHYSIOLOGY

Hypothalamic hamartomas are directly involved in the pathogenesis of gelastic and dacrystic seizures and they have intrinsic epileptogenicity. There is direct evidence from intracranial recordings that the gelastic seizures of hypothalamic gelastic epilepsy arise from the hamartoma itself.[373] That seizures may also respond to long-acting gonadotrophin-releasing hormone (GnRH) analogue prescribed for precocious puberty, may indicate that the epileptogenic generators reside in the same cells that autonomously produce GnRH.[374]

The acquired cognitive and behavioural symptoms probably result from a direct effect of the seizures.[23] Children with hypothalamic hamartomas and precocious puberty but without seizures do not develop cognitive and behavioural problems.

DIAGNOSTIC PROCEDURES

A clinical diagnosis of hypothalamic gelastic epilepsy would demand confirmation with high-resolution MRI (Figure 7.13). The most modern, detailed and largest study is by Freeman et al. (2004) on 72 patients with hypothalamic hamartoma and refractory epilepsy.[351]

ELECTROENCEPHALOGRAPHY

The inter-ictal EEG is not informative. It may be normal or more commonly show non-specific and non-lateralising episodic abnormalities.

A typical ictal pattern in the surface EEG consists of low-voltage episodic fast rhythms with simultaneous suppression of background activity (Figure 7.14).

DIFFERENTIAL DIAGNOSIS

Hypothalamic gelastic seizures need differentiation from non-epileptic conditions and from seizures arising from other brain locations. Gelastic seizures may initially be so mild and appear so natural that they are understandably unrecognised as pathological. It is only after the appearance of other more traditional seizure manifestations and impairment of consciousness that medical advice is sought.

That gelastic seizures may arise from locations other than the hypothalamus such as temporal (page 374) and frontal lobes (page 398) is well documented.[346,376,377]

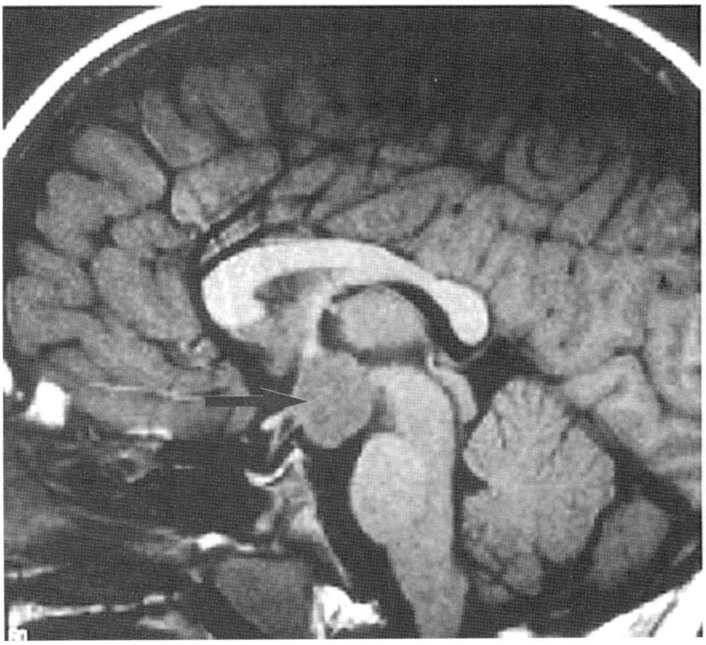

Figure 7.13 MRI showing hypothalamic hamartoma in a child with gelastic seizures.

Figure courtesy of Dr Rod C. Scott, Institute of Child Health, London.

It is difficult to establish exact differential criteria between gelastic seizures of different brain origin. However, gelastic seizures of hypothalamic gelastic epilepsy are unique regarding (1) seizure onset of laughter as the first and often the only ictal manifestation, (2) daily seizure frequency, (3) lack of mirth and (4) awareness of ictal laughter. This clustering of events does not occur in either temporal or frontal gelastic seizures. For example, laughter in the middle of other ictal manifestations, laughter associated with emotions, infrequent seizures of laughter or gelastic seizures starting in adolescence are not features of hypothalamic epilepsy.

PROGNOSIS

Hypothalamic gelastic epilepsy is often a progressive seizure disorder. Typically, neonates or children are normal prior to the onset of seizures. Brief attacks of laughter become more and more frequent with time and longer with associated impairment of consciousness. Later generalised seizures of any type appear as

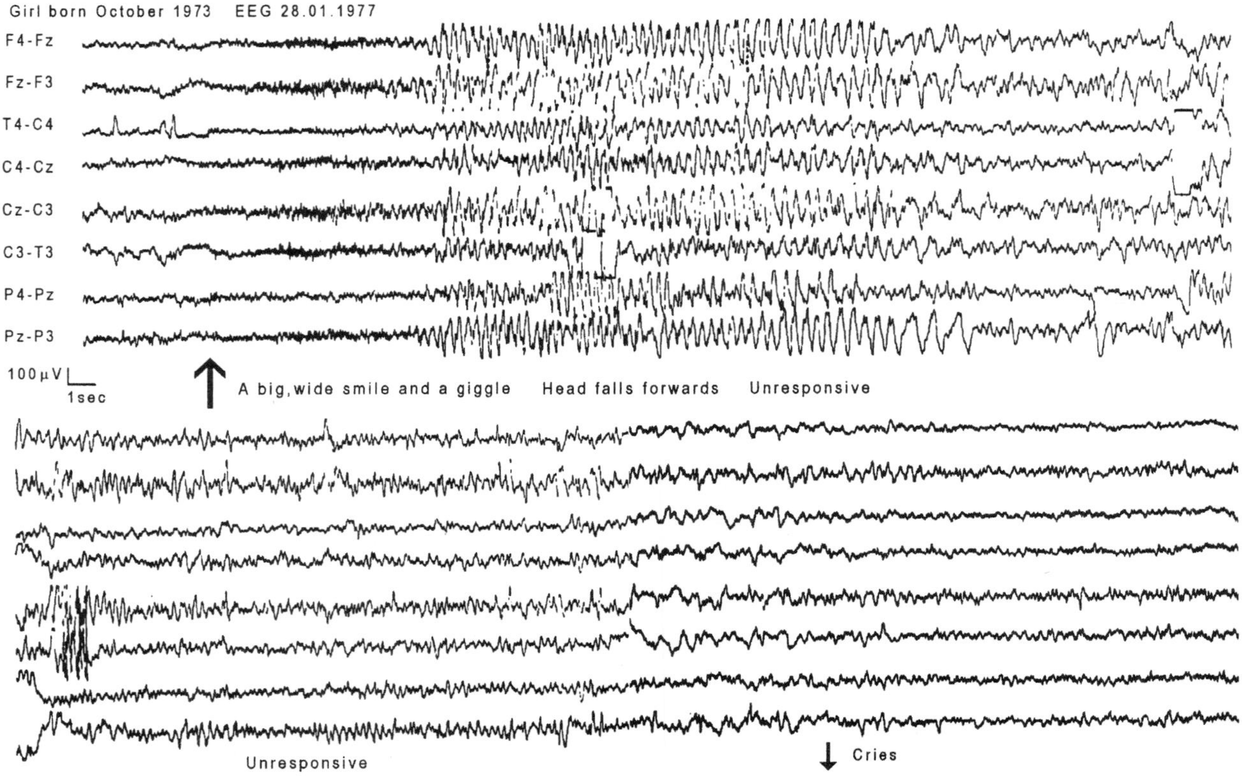

Figure 7.14 Surface ictal EEG of a girl of 3 years and 3 months of age with normal neuropsychological development and frequent daily gelastic seizures.[375]

First noticed at age 2 years when her parents observed that, when told 'how beautiful' she is or 'come and get these candies', she reacted with a 'facial grimace', something like a ' frozen smile', 'a smile that freezes', and 'right-sided deviated lips with a smile'. This initially lasted for only a few seconds, occurred every fortnight and was always provoked as above. Subsequently, within months, this occurred daily, nearly every morning, without precipitating factors, became longer and it was also associated with small giggles. At the first arrow, her mother said'here is her big smile'. The girl suddenly had a big and wide smile, which was associated with a mild giggle. This lasted for only a few seconds followed by the head falling forwards and complete unresponsiveness until the end of the seizure when recovery was manifested by a cry (second arrow). The inter-ictal EEG was normal with a well-organised and symmetrical alpha rhythm. The seizure started (first arrow) with fast episodic activity at approximately 22 Hz which is widely spread with some left-sided emphasis. This was concordant with the gelastic manifestations of the seizure. The rest of the EEG ictal events are self-evident.

symptomatic generalised epilepsies. In addition, progressive cognitive and behavioural impairment develops in most patients. More than half (59%) of them suffer from precocious puberty.[347]

MANAGEMENT

Medical treatment of hypothalamic gelastic epilepsy is often ineffective and polytherapy may cause more harm than good.[347] Two patients treated with GnRH analogue for precocious puberty became free of gelastic seizures.[374] Further trials with GnRH in patients with and without precocious puberty are needed.

Surgical removal of the hamartoma is technically difficult, but it is highly effective if successful. Choices include a transcallosal approach (good for intraventricular lesions), a pterional approach (useful for interpeduncular lesions), a transventricular endoscopic approach or destruction of the lesion with radiofrequency probes or gamma knife radiosurgery.[22] Stereotactic radiofrequency lesioning of the hamartoma may result in seizure remission without surgical complications.[378,379]

Complete lesionectomy results in freedom from seizures and prevents neurobehavioural deterioration.[22] Improvement may occur with incomplete removal.

REFERENCES

1. Engel J, Jr. A proposed diagnostic scheme for people with epileptic seizures and with epilepsy: Report of the ILAE Task Force on Classification and Terminology. *Epilepsia* 2001;**42**:796-803.
2. Dulac OJ, Chiron C. Malignant epileptic encephalopathies in children. *Baillieres Clin Neurol* 1996;**5**:765-81.
3. West Syndrome and other Infantile Epileptic Encephalopathies. Proceedings of an International Symposium. Tokyo, Japan, February 9-11, 2001. *Brain Dev.* 2001;**23**:441-769.
4. Dulac O. Epileptic encephalopathy. *Epilepsia* 2001;**42 Suppl 3**:23-6.
5. Blume WT. Pathogenesis of Lennox-Gastaut syndrome: considerations and hypotheses. *Epileptic Disord.* 2001;**3**:183-96.
6. Guerrini R,Aicardi J. Epileptic encephalopathies with myoclonic seizures in infants and children (severe myoclonic epilepsy and myoclonic-astatic epilepsy). *J Clin Neurophysiol.* 2003;**20**:449-61.
7. Nabbout R,Dulac O. Epileptic encephalopathies: a brief overview. *J Clin Neurophysiol.* 2003;**20**:393-7.
8. Ohtahara S,Yamatogi Y. Epileptic encephalopathies in early infancy with suppression-burst. *J Clin Neurophysiol.* 2003;**20**:398-407.
9. Tharp BR. Epileptic encephalopathies and their relationship to developmental disorders: do spikes cause autism? *Ment Retard Dev Disabil Res Rev* 2004;**10**:132-4.
10. ILAE Task Force. Proposed Diagnostic Scheme for People with Epileptic Seizures and with Epilepsy. http/www.epilepsy.org . 2004.
11. Ohtahara S, Yamatogi Y, Ohtsuka Y. Early epileptic encephalopathies. In Wallace SJ, Farrell K, eds. *Epilepsy in childen*, pp 133-41. London: Arnold, 2004.
12. Blume WT. Lennox-Gastaut syndrome: potential mechanisms of cognitive regression. *Ment Retard Dev Disabil Res Rev* 2004;**10**:150-3.
13. Shields WD. Diagnosis of infantile spasms, Lennox-Gastaut syndrome, and progressive myoclonic epilepsy. *Epilepsia* 2004;**45 Suppl 5**:2-4.
14. Deonna T. Cognitive and behavioral manifestations of epilepsy in children. In Wallace SJ, Farrell K, eds. *Epilepsy in childen*, pp 250-6. London: Arnold, 2004.
15. Swann JW. The effects of seizures on the connectivity and circuitry of the developing brain. *Ment Retard Dev Disabil Res Rev* 2004;**10**:96-100.
16. Holmes GL. Effects of early seizures on later behavior and epileptogenicity. *Ment Retard Dev Disabil Res Rev* 2004;**10**:101-5.
17. Markand ON. Lennox-Gastaut syndrome (childhood epileptic encephalopathy). *J Clin Neurophysiol.* 2003;**20**:426-41.
18. Hrachovy RA, Frost JD, Jr. Infantile epileptic encephalopathy with hypsarrhythmia (infantile spasms/West syndrome). *J Clin Neurophysiol.* 2003;**20**:408-25.
19. Smith MC,Hoeppner TJ. Epileptic encephalopathy of late childhood: Landau-Kleffner syndrome and the syndrome of continuous spikes and waves during slow-wave sleep. *J Clin Neurophysiol.* 2003;**20**:462-72.
20. Yamatogi Y,Ohtahara S. Severe epilepsy with multiple independent spike foci. *J Clin Neurophysiol.* 2003;**20**:442-8.
21. Commission on Classification and Terminology of the International League Against Epilepsy. Proposal for revised classification of epilepsies and epileptic syndromes. *Epilepsia* 1989;**30**:389-99.
22. Berkovic SF, Arzimanoglou A, Kuzniecky R, Harvey AS, Palmini A, Andermann F. Hypothalamic hamartoma and seizures: a treatable epileptic encephalopathy. *Epilepsia* 2003;**44**:969-73.
23. Deonna T,Ziegler AL. Hypothalamic hamartoma, precocious puberty and gelastic seizures: a special model of "epileptic" developmental disorder. *Epileptic Disord.* 2000;**2**:33-7.
24. Shields WD. Catastrophic epilepsy in childhood. *Epilepsia* 2000;**41 Suppl 2**:S2-S6.
25. Conry JA. Pharmacologic treatment of the catastrophic epilepsies. *Epilepsia* 2004;**45 Suppl 5**:12-6.
26. Rho JM. Basic science behind the catastrophic epilepsies. *Epilepsia* 2004;**45 Suppl 5**:5-11.
27. Wheless JW. Nonpharmacologic treatment of the catastrophic epilepsies of childhood. *Epilepsia* 2004;**45 Suppl 5**:17-22.
28. Beaumanoir, A, Bureau, M., Deonna, T., Mira, L., and Tassinari, C. A. eds. *Continuous spike and waves during slow sleep . Electrical status epilepticus during slow sleep.* 1995. London, John Libbey & Company.
29. Tassinari CA, Rubboli G, Volpi L, Billard C, Bureau M. Electrical status epilepticus during slow sleep (ESES or CSWS) including acquired epileptic aphasia (Landau-Kleffner syndrome). In Roger J, Bureau M, Dravet C, Genton P, Tassinari CA, Wolf P, eds. *Epileptic syndromes in infancy, childhood and adolescence (3rd edn)*, pp 265-83. London: John Libbey & Co Ltd, 2002.
30. Blume WT, Luders HO, Mizrahi E, Tassinari C, van Emde BW, Engel J, Jr. Glossary of descriptive terminology for ictal semiology: report of the ILAE task force on classification and terminology. *Epilepsia* 2001;**42**:1212-8.
31. Tassinari CA, Michelucci R, Shigematsu H, Seino M. Atonic and falling seizures. In Engel JJ, Pedley TA, eds. *Epilepsy: A comprehensive Textbook*, pp 605-16. Philadelphia: Lippincott-Raven Publishers, 1997.
32. Plouin P, Jalin C, Dulac O, Chiron C. Ambulatory 24-hour EEG recording in epileptic infantile spasms . *Rev Electroencephalogr Neurophysiol Clin.* 1987;**17**:309-18.
33. Holmes GL, Vigevano F. Infantine spasms. In Engel JJ, Pedley TA, eds. *Epilepsy: A comprehensive Textbook*, pp 627-42. Philadelphia: Lippincott-Raven Publishers, 1997.
34. Oguni H, Fukuyama Y, Tanaka T, Hayashi K, Funatsuka M, Sakauchi M *et al.* Myoclonic-astatic epilepsy of early childhood—clinical and EEG analysis of myoclonic-astatic seizures, and discussions on the nosology of the syndrome. *Brain Dev.* 2001;**23**:757-64.
35. Janz D, Inoue Y, Seino M. Myoclonic seizures. In Engel JJ, Pedley TA, eds. *Epilepsy: A comprehensive Textbook*, pp 591-603. Philadelphia: Lippincott-Raven Publishers, 1997.
36. Guerrini R, Dravet C, Genton P, Bureau M, Roger J, Rubboli G *et al.* Epileptic negative myoclonus. *Neurology* 1993;**43**:1078-83.
37. Tassinari CA, Rubboli G, Parmeggiani L, Valzania F, Plasmati R, Riguzzi P *et al.* Epileptic negative myoclonus. *Adv Neurol* 1995;**67**:181-97.
38. Werhahn KJ, Noachtar S. Epileptic negative myoclonus. In Luders HO, Noachtar S, eds. *Epileptic seizures. Pathophysiology and clinical semiology*, pp 473-83. New York: Churchill Livingstone, 2000.
39. Vigevano F, Fusco L, Yagi K, Seino M. Tonic seizures. In Engel JJ, Pedley TA, eds. *Epilepsy: A comprehensive Textbook*, pp 617-25. Philadelphia: Lippincott-Raven Publishers, 1997.
40. Watanabe K, Iwase K, Hara K. The evolution of EEG features in infantile spasms: a prospective study. *Dev Med Child Neurol* 1973;**15**:584-96.
41. Jeavons PM, Bower BD, Dimitrakoudi M. Long-term prognosis of 150 cases of "West syndrome". *Epilepsia* 1973;**14**:153-64.
42. Negoro T, Matsumoto A, Sugiura M, Iwase K, Watanabe K, Hara K *et al.* Long-term prognosis of 200 cases of infantile spasms. Part II: Electroencephalographic findings at the ages between 5-7. *Folia Psychiatr Neurol Jpn.* 1980;**34**:346-7.
43. Hakamada S, Watanabe K, Hara K, Miyazaki S. Brief atonia associated with electroencephalographic paroxysm in an infant with infantile spasms. *Epilepsia* 1981;**22**:285-8.
44. Matsumoto A, Watanabe K, Negoro T, Sugiura M, Iwase K, Hara K *et al.* Infantile spasms: etiological factors, clinical aspects, and long term prognosis in 200 cases. *Eur J Pediatr.* 1981;**135**:239-44.
45. Matsumoto A, Watanabe K, Negoro T, Sugiura M, Iwase K, Hara K *et al.* Long-term prognosis after infantile spasms: a statistical study of prognostic factors in 200 cases. *Dev Med Child Neurol* 1981;**23**:51-65.
46. Matsumoto A, Watanabe K, Negoro T, Sugiura M, Iwase K, Hara K *et al.* Prognostic factors of infantile spasms from the etiological viewpoint. *Brain Dev.* 1981;**3**:361-4.
47. Donat JF,Wright FS. Clinical imitators of infantile spasms. *J Child Neurol* 1992;**7**:395-9.
48. Jacobi G,Neirich U. Symptomatology and electroencephalography of the 'genuine' type of the West syndrome and its differential diagnosis from the other benign generalized epilepsies of infancy. *Epilepsy Research - Supplement* 1992;**6**:145-51.
49. Cusmai R, Ricci S, Pinard JM, Plouin P, Fariello G, Dulac O. West syndrome due to perinatal insults. *Epilepsia* 1993;**34**:738-42.

60. Vigevano F, Fusco L, Cusmai R, Claps D, Ricci S, Milani L. The idiopathic form of West syndrome. *Epilepsia* 1993;**34**:743-6.

61. Aicardi J. *Epilepsy in Children*. New York: Raven Press, 1994.

62. Baram TZ, Mitchell WG, Brunson K, Haden E. Infantile spasms: hypothesis-driven therapy and pilot human infant experiments using corticotropin-releasing hormone receptor antagonists. *Dev Neurosci.* 1999;**21**:281-9.

63. Chugani HT. Pathophysiology of infantile spasms. *Adv Exp Med Biol.* 2002;**497**:111-21.

64. Chiron C, Dulac O. Drug therapy for West's syndrome. *Adv Exp Med Biol.* 2002;**497**:51-6.

65. Dulac O, Chugani HT, Dalla Bernardina B, eds. *Infantile spasms and West syndrome.* London: W.B.Sanders Company Ltd, 2002.

66. Hoffman HJ. Surgery for West's syndrome. *Adv Exp Med Biol.* 2002;**497**:57-9.

67. Hrachovy RA. West's syndrome (infantile spasms). Clinical description and diagnosis. *Adv Exp Med Biol.* 2002;**497**:33-50.

68. Itomi K, Okumura A, Negoro T, Watanabe K, Natsume J, Takada H *et al.* Prognostic value of positron emission tomography in cryptogenic West syndrome. *Dev Med Child Neurol.* 2002;**44**:107-11.

69. Shields WD. West's syndrome. *J Child Neurol.* 2002;**17 Suppl 1**:S76-S79.

50. Dulac O, Tuxhorn I. Infantile spasms and West syndrome. In Roger J, Bureau M, Dravet C, Genton P, Tassinari CA, Wolf P, eds. *Epileptic syndromes in infancy, childhood and adolescence (3rd edn)*, pp 47-63. London: John Libbey & Co Ltd, 2002.

51. Mackay MT, Weiss SK, Adams-Webber T, Ashwal S, Stephens D, Ballaban-Gill K *et al.* Practice parameter: medical treatment of infantile spasms: report of the American Academy of Neurology and the Child Neurology Society. *Neurology* 2004;**62**:1668-81.

52. Riikonen R. Infantile spasms: therapy and outcome. *J Child Neurol.* 2004;**19**:401-4.

53. Lux AL,Osborne JP. A proposal for case definitions and outcome measures in studies of infantile spasms and west syndrome: consensus statement of the west delphi group. *Epilepsia* 2004;**45**:1416-28.

54. Gibbs, F. A. and Gibbs, E. L. *Atlas of electroencephalography, Vol 2. Epilepsy. (2)*, 214-290. 1952. Reading, MA., Addison-Wesley.

55. Koo B, Hwang P. Localization of focal cortical lesions influences age of onset of infantile spasms. *Epilepsia* 1996;**37**:1068-71.

56. Luthvigsson P, Olafsson E, Sigurthardottir S, Hauser WA. Epidemiologic features of infantile spasms in Iceland. *Epilepsia* 1994;**35**:802-5.

57. Sidenvall R,Eeg-Olofsson O. Epidemiology of infantile spasms in Sweden. *Epilepsia* 1995;**36**:572-4.

58. Trevathan E, Murphy CC, Yeargin-Allsopp M. The descriptive epidemiology of infantile spasms among Atlanta children. *Epilepsia* 1999;**40**:748-51.

59. Rantala H, Putkonen T. Occurrence, outcome, and prognostic factors of infantile spasms and Lennox-Gastaut syndrome. *Epilepsia* 1999;**40**:286-9.

70. West WJ. On a peculiar form of infantile convulsions. *Lancet* 1841;**1**:724-5.

71. Fusco L, Vigevano F. Ictal clinical electroencephalographic findings of spasms in West syndrome. *Epilepsia* 1993;**34**:671-8.

72. Donat JF, Lo WD. Asymmetric hypsarrhythmia and infantile spasms in west syndrome. *J Child Neurol.* 1994;**9**:290-6.

73. Gaily EK, Shewmon DA, Chugani HT, Curran JG. Asymmetric and asynchronous infantile spasms. *Epilepsia* 1995;**36**:873-82.

74. Chugani HT, Conti JR. Etiologic classification of infantile spasms in 140 cases: role of positron emission tomography. *J Child Neurol.* 1996;**11**:44-8.

75. Riikonen R. West syndrome. In Wallace SJ, Farrell K, eds. *Epilepsy in childen*, pp 142-7. London: Arnold, 2004.

76. Vanhatalo S, Riikonen R. Nitric oxide metabolites, nitrates and nitrites in the cerebrospinal fluid in children with west syndrome. *Epilepsy Res.* 2001;**46**:3-13.

77. Riikonen R, Vanhala R. Levels of cerebrospinal fluid nerve-growth factor differ in infantile autism and Rett syndrome. *Dev Med Child Neurol.* 1999;**41**:148-52.

78. Dulac O, Plouin P, Jambaque I. Predicting favorable outcome in idiopathic West syndrome. *Epilepsia* 1993;**34**:747-56.

79. Fleiszar KA, Daniel WL, Imrey PB. Genetic study of infantile spasm with hypsarrhythmia. *Epilepsia* 1977;**18**:55-62.

80. Reiter E, Tiefenthaler M, Freillinger M, Bernert G, Seidl R, Hauser E. Familial idiopathic West syndrome. *J Child Neurol.* 2000;**15**:249-52.

81. Claes S, Devriendt K, Lagae L, Ceulemans B, Dom L, Casaer P *et al.* The X-linked infantile spasms syndrome (MIM 308350) maps to Xp11.4-Xpter in two pedigrees. *Ann Neurol.* 1997;**42**:360-4.

82. Stromme P, Sundet K, Mork C, Cassiman JJ, Fryns JP, Claes S. X linked mental retardation and infantile spasms in a family: new clinical data and linkage to Xp11.4-Xp22.11. *J Med Genet.* 1999;**36**:374-8.

83. Bruyere H, Lewis S, Wood S, MacLeod PJ, Langlois S. Confirmation of linkage in X-linked infantile spasms (West syndrome) and refinement of the disease locus to Xp21.3-Xp22.1. *Clin Genet.* 1999;**55**:173-81.

84. Goodman M, Lamm SH, Bellman MH. Temporal relationship modeling: DTP or DT immunizations and infantile spasms. *Vaccine* 1998;**16**:225-31.

85. Shields MD, Hicks EM, Macgregor DF, Richey S. Infantile spasms associated with theophylline toxicity. *Acta Paediatr.* 1995;**84**:215-7.

86. Yasuhara A, Ochi A, Harada Y, Kobayashi Y. Infantile spasms associated with a histamine H1 antagonist. *Neuropediatrics* 1998;**29**:320-1.

87. Dulac O, Ballaban-Gil K, Moshe SL. West syndrome. In Gilman S, ed. *Medlink Neurology*, San Diego SA: Arbor Publishing Corp, 2004.

88. Niedermeyer, E. and Lopes da Silva, F. eds. *Electroencephalography. Basic principles,clinical applications, and related fields.* Fourth Edition. 1999. Baltimore, Williams & Wilkins.

89. Kotagal P. Multifocal independent Spike syndrome: relationship to hypsarrhythmia and the slow spike-wave (Lennox-Gastaut) syndrome. *Clin Electroencephalogr* 1995;**26**:23-9.

90. Lombroso CT, Fejerman N. Benign myoclonus of early infancy. *Ann Neurol.* 1977;**1**:138-43.

91. Dravet C, Giraud N, Bureau M, Roger J, Gobbi G, Dalla Bernardina B. Benign myoclonus of early infancy or benign non-epileptic infantile spasms. *Neuropediatrics* 1986;**17**:33-8.

92. Maydell BV, Berenson F, Rothner AD, Wyllie E, Kotagal P. Benign myoclonus of early infancy: an imitator of West's syndrome. *J Child Neurol.* 2001;**16**:109-12.

93. Daoust-Roy J, Seshia SS. Benign neonatal sleep myoclonus. A differential diagnosis of neonatal seizures. *Am J Dis Child* 1992;**146**:1236-41.

94. Caraballo R, Yepez I, Cersosimo R, Fejerman N. Benign neonatal sleep myoclonus . *Rev Neurol.* 1998;**26**:540-4.

95. Noone PG, King M, Loftus BG. Benign neonatal sleep myoclonus. *Irish Med J.* 1998;**88**:172-4.

96. Kivity S, Lerman P, Ariel R, Danziger Y, Mimouni M, Shinnar S. Long-term cognitive outcomes of a cohort of children with cryptogenic infantile spasms treated with high-dose adrenocorticotropic hormone. *Epilepsia* 2004;**45**:255-62.

97. Hamano S, Tanaka M, Mochizuki M, Sugiyama N, Eto Y. Long-term follow-up study of West syndrome: Differences of outcome among symptomatic etiologies. *J Pediatr.* 2003;**143**:231-5.

98. Appleton RE. West syndrome: long-term prognosis and social aspects. *Brain Dev.* 2001;**23**:688-91.

99. Glaze DG, Hrachovy RA, Frost JD, Jr., Kellaway P, Zion TE. Prospective study of outcome of infants with infantile spasms treated during controlled studies of ACTH and prednisone. *J Pediatr.* 1988;**112**:389-96.

100. Negoro T, Matsumoto A, Sugiura M, Iwase K, Watanabe K, Hara K *et al.* Long-term prognosis of 200 cases of infantile spasms. Part II: Electroencephalographic findings at the ages between 5-7. *Fol Psychiatr Neurol Jpn.* 1980;**34**:346-7.

101. Matsumoto A, Watanabe K, Negoro T, Sugiura M, Iwase K, Hara K *et al.* Long-term prognosis after infantile spasms: a statistical study of prognostic factors in 200 cases. *Dev Med Child Neurol.* 1981;**23**:51-65.

102. Watanabe K. West syndrome: etiological and prognostic aspects. *Brain Dev.* 1998;**20**:1-8.

103. Hrachovy RA, Glaze DG, Frost JD, Jr. A retrospective study of spontaneous remission and long-term outcome in patients with infantile spasms. *Epilepsia* 1991;**32**:212-4.

104. Sorel L, Dusaucy- Bauloxe A. A propos de 21 cas d'hypsarrthythie de Gibbs. Soutraitement spectaculaire par l'ACTH. Acta Neurol Belg 1958;58:130-41. *Acta Neurol Belg* 1958;**58**:130-41.

105. Hrachovy RA, Frost JD, Jr., Glaze DG. High-dose, long-duration versus low-dose, short-duration corticotropin therapy for infantile spasms. *J Pediatr.* 1994;**124**:803-6.

106. Baram TZ, Mitchell WG, Tournay A, Snead OC, Hanson RA, Horton EJ. High-dose corticotropin (ACTH) versus prednisone for infantile spasms: a prospective, randomized, blinded study. *Pediatrics* 1996;**97**:375-9.

107. Snead OC, III, Benton JW, Jr., Hosey LC, Swann JW, Spink D, Martin D *et al.* Treatment of infantile spasms with high-dose ACTH: efficacy and plasma levels of ACTH and cortisol. *Neurology* 1989;**39**:1027-31.

108. Hrachovy RA, Frost JD, Jr., Kellaway P, Zion TE. Double-blind study of ACTH vs prednisone therapy in infantile spasms. *J Pediatr.* 1983;**103**:641-5.

109. Hancock E, Osborne J, Milner P. Treatment of infantile spasms. *Cochrane Database Syst Rev.* 2003;CD001770.

110. Chiron C, Dumas C, Jambaque I, Mumford J, Dulac O. Randomized trial comparing vigabatrin and hydrocortisone in infantile spasms due to tuberous sclerosis. *Epilepsy Res.* 1997;**26**:389-95.

111. Granstrom ML, Gaily E, Liukkonen E. Treatment of infantile spasms: results of a population-based study with vigabatrin as the first drug for spasms. *Epilepsia* 1999;**40**:950-7.

112. Koo B. Vigabatrin in the treatment of infantile spasms. *Pediatr Neurol.* 1999;**20**:106-10.

113. Appleton RE, Peters AC, Mumford JP, Shaw DE. Randomised, placebo-controlled study of vigabatrin as first-line treatment of infantile spasms. *Epilepsia* 1999;**40**:1627-33.

114. Jambaque I, Chiron C, Dumas C, Mumford J, Dulac O. Mental and behavioural outcome of infantile epilepsy treated by vigabatrin in tuberous sclerosis patients. *Epilepsy Res.* 2000;**38**:151-60.

115. Elterman RD, Shields WD, Mansfield KA, Nakagawa J. Randomized trial of vigabatrin in patients with infantile spasms. *Neurology* 2001;**57**:1416-21.

116. Nabbout R, Melki I, Gerbaka B, Dulac O, Akatcherian C. Infantile spasms in Down syndrome: good response to a short course of vigabatrin. *Epilepsia* 2001;**42**:1580-3.

117. Riikonen RS. Steroids or vigabatrin in the treatment of infantile spasms? *Pediatr Neurol.* 2000;**23**:403-8.

118. Pietz J, Benninger C, Schafer H, Sontheimer D, Mittermaier G, Rating D. Treatment of infantile spasms with high-dosage vitamin B6. *Epilepsia* 1993;**34**:757-63.

119. Mikati MA, Lepejian GA, Holmes GL. Medical treatment of patients with infantile spasms. *Clin Neuropharmacol.* 2002;**25**:61-70.

120. Shields WD, Shewmon DA, Peacock WJ, LoPresti CM, Nakagawa JA, Yudovin S. Surgery for the treatment of medically intractable infantile spasms: a cautionary case. *Epilepsia* 1999;**40**:1305-8.

121. Caplan R, Guthrie D, Komo S, Shields WD, Sigmann M. Infantile spasms: the development of nonverbal communication after epilepsy surgery. *Dev Neurosci.* 1999;**21**:165-73.

122. Pinard JM, Delalande O, Chiron C, Soufflet C, Plouin P, Kim Y *et al.* Callosotomy for epilepsy after West syndrome. *Epilepsia* 1999;**40**:1727-34.

123. Dravet C. Les epilepsies graves de l'enfant. *Vie Med* 1978;**8**:543-8.

124. Dravet C, Bureau M, Guerrini R, Giraud N, Roger J. Severe myoclonic epilepsy in infants. In Roger J, Bureau M, Dravet C, Dreifuss FE, Perret A, Wolf P, eds. *Epileptic syndromes in infancy, childhood and adolescence*, pp 75-8. London: John Libbey & Company, 1992.

125. Wakai S, Ikehata M, Nihira H, Ito N, Sueoka H, Kawamoto Y *et al.* "Obtundation status (Dravet)" caused by complex partial status epilepticus in a patient with severe myoclonic epilepsy in infancy. *Epilepsia* 1996;**37**:1020-2.

126. Guerrini R, Dravet C. Severe epileptic encephalopathies of infancy, other than the West syndrome. In Engel JJr, Pedley TA, eds. *Epilepsy: A Comprehensive Textbook.*, pp 2285-302. Philadelphia: Lippincott-Raven Publishers, 1997.

127. Nieto-Barrera M, Lillo MM, Rodriguez-Collado C, Candau R, Correa A. Severe myoclonic epilepsy in childhood. Epidemiologic analytical study . *Rev Neurol* 2000;**30**:620-4.

128. Oguni H, Hayashi K, Awaya Y, Fukuyama Y, Osawa M. Severe myoclonic epilepsy in infants—a review based on the Tokyo Women's Medical University series of 84 cases. *Brain Dev.* 2001;**23**:736-48.

129. Claes L, Del Favero J, Ceulemans B, Lagae L, Van Broeckhoven C, De Jonghe P. De novo mutations in the sodium-channel gene SCN1A cause severe myoclonic epilepsy of infancy. *Am J Hum Genet.* 2001;**68**:1327-32.

130. Singh R, Andermann E, Whitehouse WP, Harvey AS, Keene DL Seni MH *et al.* Severe myoclonic epilepsy of infancy: extended spectrum of GEFS+? *Epilepsia* 2001;**42**:837-44.

131. Scheffer IE, Wallace R, Mulley JC, Berkovic SF. Clinical and molecular genetics of myoclonic-astatic epilepsy and severe myoclonic epilepsy in infancy (Dravet syndrome). *Brain Dev.* 2001;**23**:732-5.

132. Dravet C, Bureau M, Oguni H, Fukuyama H, Cokar O. Severe myoclonic epilepsy in infancy (Dravet syndrome). In Roger J, Bureau M, Dravet C, Genton P, Tassinari CA, Wolf P, eds. *Epileptic syndromes in infancy, childhood and adolescence (3rd edn)*, pp 81-103. London: John Libbey & Co Ltd, 2002.

133. Herranz JL. Severe myoclonic epilepsy in infancy (Dravet's syndrome). Some genetic aspects . *Rev Neurol.* 2003;**37**:60-3.

134. Nabbout R, Gennaro E, Dalla BB, Dulac O, Madia F, Bertini E *et al.* Spectrum of SCN1A mutations in severe myoclonic epilepsy of infancy. *Neurology* 2003;**60**:1961-7.

135. Sugawara T, Tsurubuchi Y, Fujiwara T, Mazaki-Miyazaki E, Nagata K, Montal M *et al.* Nav1.1 channels with mutations of severe myoclonic epilepsy in infancy display attenuated currents. *Epilepsy Res.* 2003;**54**:201-7.

136. Wallace RH, Hodgson BL, Grinton BE, Gardiner RM, Robinson R, Rodriguez-Casero V *et al.* Sodium channel alpha1-subunit mutations in severe myoclonic epilepsy of infancy and infantile spasms. *Neurology* 2003;**61**:765-9.

137. Fejerman N. Severe myoclonic epilepsy in infancy. In Wallace SJ, Farrell K, eds. *Epilepsy in childen*, pp 157-60. London: Arnold, 2004.

138. Dravet C, Bureau M. Dravet syndrome (severe myoclonic epilepsy in infancy). In Gilman S, ed. *Medlink Neurology*, San Diego SA: Arbor Publishing Corp, 2004.

139. Fukuma G, Oguni H, Shirasaka Y, Watanabe K, Miyajima T, Yasumoto S *et al.* Mutations of neuronal voltage-gated Na+ channel alpha 1 subunit gene SCN1A in core severe myoclonic epilepsy in infancy (SMEI) and in borderline SMEI (SMEB). *Epilepsia* 2004;**45**:140-8.

140. Hurst DL. Epidemiology of severe myoclonic epilepsy of infancy. *Epilepsia* 1990;**31**:397-400.

141. Yakoub M, Dulac O, Jambaque I, Chiron C, Plouin P. Early diagnosis of severe myoclonic epilepsy in infancy. *Brain Dev.* 1992;**14**:299-303.

142. Ogino T, Ohtsuka Y, Yamatogi Y, Oka E, Ohtahara S. The epileptic syndrome sharing common characteristics during early childhood with severe myoclonic epilepsy in infancy. *Jpn J Psychiatry Neurol* 1989;**43**:479-81.

143. Kanazawa O. Refractory grand mal seizures with onset during infancy including severe myoclonic epilepsy in infancy. *Brain Dev.* 2001;**23**:749-56.

144. Hurst DL. Severe myoclonic epilepsy of infancy. *Pediatr Neurol* 1987;**3**:269-72.

145. Ohtsuka Y, Maniwa S, Ogino T, Yamatogi Y, Ohtahara S. Severe myoclonic epilepsy in infancy: a long-term follow-up study. *Jpn J Psychiatry Neurol* 1991;**45**:416-8.

146. Ohtsuka Y, Ohmori I, Ogino T, Ouchida M, Shimizu K, Oka E. Paroxysmal movement disorders in severe myoclonic epilepsy in infancy. *Brain Dev.* 2003;**25**:401-5.

147. Veggiotti P, Cardinali S, Montalenti E, Gatti A, Lanzi G. Generalized Epilepsy with Febrile Seizures plus and Severe Myoclonic Epilepsy in Infancy: a case report of two Italian families. *Epileptic Disord.* 2001;**3**:29-32.

148. Ohmori I, Ouchida M, Ohtsuka Y, Oka E, Shimizu K. Significant correlation of the SCN1A mutations and severe myoclonic epilepsy in infancy. *Biochem Biophys Res Commun.* 2002;**295**:17-23.

149. Sugawara T, Mazaki-Miyazaki E, Fukushima K, Shimomura J, Fujiwara T, Hamano S *et al.* Frequent mutations of SCN1A in severe myoclonic epilepsy in infancy. *Neurology* 2002;**58**:1122-4.

150. Claes L, Ceulemans B, Audenaert D, Smets K, Lofgren A, Del Favero J *et al.* De novo SCN1A mutations are a major cause of severe myoclonic epilepsy of infancy. *Hum Mutat.* 2003;**21**:615-21.

151. Gennaro E, Veggiotti P, Malacarne M, Madia F, Cecconi M, Cardinali S *et al.* Familial severe myoclonic epilepsy of infancy: truncation of Nav1.1 and genetic heterogeneity. *Epileptic Disord.* 2003;**5**:21-5.

152. Ohmori I, Ohtsuka Y, Ouchida M, Ogino T, Maniwa S, Shimizu K *et al.* Is phenotype difference in severe myoclonic epilepsy in infancy related to SCN1A mutations? *Brain Dev.* 2003;**25**:488-93.

153. Fujiwara T, Sugawara T, Mazaki-Miyazaki E, Takahashi Y, Fukushima K, Watanabe M *et al.* Mutations of sodium channel alpha subunit type 1 (SCN1A) in intractable childhood epilepsies with frequent generalized tonic-clonic seizures. *Brain* 2003;**126**:531-46.

154. Scheffer IE. Severe infantile epilepsies: molecular genetics challenge clinical classification. *Brain* 2003;**126**:513-4.

155. Doose H, Lunau H, Castiglione E, Waltz S. Severe idiopathic generalized epilepsy of infancy with generalized tonic-clonic seizures. *Neuropediatrics* 1998;**29**:229-38.

156. Harkin LA, Bowser DN, Dibbens LM, Singh R, Phillips F, Wallace RH *et al.* Truncation of the GABA(A)-receptor gamma2 subunit in a family with generalized epilepsy with febrile seizures plus. *Am J Hum Genet.* 2002;**70**:530-6.

157. Ferrie CD, Robinson RO, Panayiotopoulos CP. Psychotic and severe behavioural reactions with vigabatrin: a review. *Acta Neurol Scandin* 1996;**93**:1-8.

158. Peled N, Shorer Z, Peled E, Pillar G. Melatonin effect on seizures in children with severe neurologic deficit disorders. *Epilepsia* 2001;**42**:1208-10.

159. Coppola G, Capovilla G, Montagnini A, Romeo A, Spano M, Tortorella G *et al.* Topiramate as add-on drug in severe myoclonic epilepsy in infancy: an Italian multicenter open trial. *Epilepsy Res.* 2002;**49**:45-8.

160. Chiron C, Marchand MC, Tran A, Rey E, D'Athis P, Vincent J *et al.* Stiripentol in severe myoclonic epilepsy in infancy: a randomised placebo-controlled syndrome-dedicated trial. STICLO study group. *Lancet* 2000;**356**:1638-42.

161. Crest C, Dupont S, LeGuern E, Adam C, Baulac M. Levetiracetam in progressive myoclonic epilepsy: an exploratory study in 9 patients. *Neurology* 2004;**62**:640-3.

162. Guerrini R, Dravet C, Genton P, Belmonte A, Kaminska A, Dulac O. Lamotrigine and seizure aggravation in severe myoclonic epilepsy. *Epilepsia* 1998;**39**:508-12.

163. Gastaut H. The Lennox-Gastaut syndrome: comments on the syndrome's terminology and nosological position amongst the secondary generalized epilepsies of childhood. *Electroencephalogr Clin Neurophysiol. Suppl* 1982;71-84.

164. Roger J, Remy C, Bureau M, Oller-Daurella L, Beaumanoir A, Favel P *et al.* Lennox-Gastaut syndrome in the adult . *Rev Neurol.* 1987;**143**:401-5.

165. Niedermeyer E, Degen R, eds. *The Lennox-Gastaut syndrome.* New York: Alan R Liss, 1988.

166. Aicardi J, Levy Gomes A. Clinical and electroencephalographic symptomatology of the 'genuine' Lennox-Gastaut syndrome and its differentiation from other forms of epilepsy of early childhood. *Epilepsy Research - Supplement* 1992;**6**:185-93.

167. Beaumanoir A, Dravet C. The Lennox-Gastaut syndrome. In Roger J, Bureau M, Dravet C, Dreifuss FE, Perret A, Wolf P, eds. *Epileptic syndromes in infancy, childhood and adolescence,* pp 115-32. London: John Libbey & Company, 1992.

168. Oguni H, Hayashi K, Osawa M. Long-term prognosis of Lennox-Gastaut syndrome. *Epilepsia* 1996;**37 Suppl 3**:44-7.

169. Genton P, Dravet C. Lennox-Gastaut syndrome and other childhood epileptic encephalopathies. In Engel JJr, Pedley TA, eds. *Epilepsy: A Comprehensive Textbook.,* pp 2355-66. Philadelphia: Lippincott-Raven Publishers, 1997.

170. Aicardi J. Lennox-Gastaut syndrome. In Wallace S, ed. *Epilepsy in Children,* pp 249-61. London: Chapman & Hall, 1996.

171. Niedermeyer E. Lennox-Gastaut syndrome. Clinical description and diagnosis. *Adv Exp Med Biol.* 2002;**497**:61-75.

172. Farrell K. Drug therapy in Lennox-Gastaut syndrome. *Adv Exp Med Biol.* 2002;**497**:77-86.

173. Beaumanoir A, Blume W. The Lennox-Gastaut syndrome. In Roger J, Bureau M, Dravet C, Genton P, Tassinari CA, Wolf P, eds. *Epileptic syndromes in infancy, childhood and adolescence (3rd edn),* pp 113-35. London: John Libbey & Co Ltd, 2002.

174. Crumrine PK. Lennox-Gastaut syndrome. *J Child Neurol.* 2002;**17 Suppl 1**:S70-S75.

175. Aicardi J. Lennox-Gastaut syndrome. In Wallace SJ, Farrell K, eds. *Epilepsy in childen,* pp 169-77. London: Arnold, 2004.

176. Doose H. Myoclonic-astatic epilepsy. *Epilepsy Research - Supplement* 1992;**6**:163-8.

177. Aicardi J. Myoclonic epilepsies difficult to classify either as Lennox-Gastaut syndrome or myoclonic-astatic epilepsy. In Wallace S, ed. *Epilepsy in Children,* pp 271-3. London: Chapman & Hall, 1996.

178. Doose H. Myoclonic-astatic epilepsy. *Epilepsy Res Suppl* 1992;**6**:163-8.

179. Doose H. Myoclonic astatic epilepsy of early childhood. In Roger J, Dravet C, Bureau M, Dreifuss FE, Wolf P, eds. *Epileptic syndromes in infancy, childhood and adolescence,* pp 103-14. London: John Libbey & Company, 1985.

180. Doose H, Baier WK. Epilepsy with primarily generalized myoclonic-astatic seizures: a genetically determined disease. *Eur J Pediatr.* 1987;**146**:550-4.

181. Chevrie JJ, Aicardi J. Childhood epileptic encephalopathy with slow spike-wave. A statistical study of 80 cases. *Epilepsia* 1972;**13**:259-71.

182. Beaumanoir A. History of reflex epilepsy. *Adv Neurol* 1998;**75**:1-4.

183. Gastaut H, Roger J, Soulayrol R, Tassinari CA, Regis H, Dravet C *et al.* Childhood epileptic encephalopathy with diffuse slow spike-waves (otherwise known as "petit mal variant") or Lennox syndrome. *Epilepsia* 1966;**7**:139-79.

184. Gastaut H, Roger J, Soulayrol R, Saint-Jean M, Tassinari CA, Regis H *et al.* Epileptic encephalopathy of children with diffuse slow spikes and waves (alias "petit mal variant") or Lennox syndrome . *AnnPediatr.(Paris)* 1966;**13**:489-99.

185. Bernard R, Pinsard N, Dravet C, Gastaut H, Roger J, Soulayrol R *et al.* Diagnostic and evolutive aspects of epileptic encephalopathy in children with diffuse slow wave spikes (petit mal variant) . *Pediatrie.* 1966;**21**:712-4.

186. Gastaut H, Zifkin BG. Secondary bilateral synchrony and Lennox-Gastaut syndrome. In Niedermeyer E, Degen R, eds. *The Lennox-Gastaut syndrome,* pp 221-42. New York: Alan R Liss, 1988.

187. Trevathan E, Murphy CC, Yeargin-Allsopp M. Prevalence and descriptive epidemiology of Lennox-Gastaut syndrome among Atlanta children. *Epilepsia* 1997;**38**:1283-8.

188. Goldsmith IL, Zupanc ML, Buchhalter JR. Long-term seizure outcome in 74 patients with Lennox-Gastaut syndrome: effects of incorporating MRI head imaging in defining the cryptogenic subgroup. *Epilepsia* 2000;**41**:395-9.

189. Heiskala H. Community-based study of Lennox-Gastaut syndrome. *Epilepsia* 1997;**38**:526-31.

190. Gastaut, H. and Broughton, R. Epileptic seizures.Clinical and electrographic features,diagnosis and treatment. 1972. Illinois, Charles C Thomas.

191. Ferrie CD, Jackson GD, Giannakodimos S, Panayiotopoulos CP. Posterior agyria-pachygyria with polymicrogyria: evidence for an inherited neuronal migration disorder. *Neurology* 1995;**45**:150-3.

192. Ikeno T, Shigematsu H, Miyakoshi M, Ohba A, Yagi K, Seino M. An analytic study of epileptic falls. *Epilepsia* 1985;**26**:612-21.

193. Ohtahara S, Ohtsuka Y, Kobayashi K. Lennox-Gastaut syndrome: a new vista. *Psychiatry Clin Neurosci.* 1995;**49**:S179-S183.

194. Tukel K, Jasper H. The electroencephalogram in parasagittal lesions. *Electroencephalog .Clin Neurophysiol.Suppl* 1952;**4**:481-94.

195. Lombroso CT, Erba G. Primary and secondary bilateral synchrony in epilepsy; a clinical and electroencephalographic study. *Arch Neurol* 1970;**22**:321-34.

196. Blume WT, Pillay N. Electrographic and clinical correlates of secondary bilateral synchrony. *Epilepsia* 1985;**26**:636-41.

197. Blume WT. Lennox-Gastaut syndrome and secondary bilateral synchrony: a comparison. In Wolf P, ed. *Epileptic seizures and syndromes,* pp 285-97. London: John Libbey & Company Ltd, 1994.

198. Smith MC. The utility of magnetoencephalography in the evaluation of secondary bilateral synchrony: a case report. *Epilepsia* 2004;**45 Suppl 4**:57-60.

199. Niedermeyer E, Walker AE, Burton C. The slow spike-wave complex as a correlate of frontal and fronto- temporal post-traumatic epilepsy. *Eur Neurol* 1970;**3**:330-46.

200. Roger J, Dravet C, Bureau M. The Lennox-Gastaut syndrome. *Cleve Clin J Med.* 1989;**56 Suppl Pt 2**:S172-S180.

201. Kobayashi K, Maniwa S, Ogino T, Yoshinaga H, Ohtsuka Y, Oka E. Myoclonic seizures combined with partial seizures and probable pathophysiology of secondary bilateral synchrony. *Clin Neurophysiol.* 2000;**111**:1813-6.

202. Chevrie JJ, Specola N, Aicardi J. Secondary bilateral synchrony in unilateral pial angiomatosis: successful surgical treatment. *J Neurol Neurosurg Psychiatry* 1988;**51**:663-70.

203. Chugani HT, Mazziotta JC, Engel J, Jr., Phelps ME. The Lennox-Gastaut syndrome: metabolic subtypes determined by 2-deoxy-2[18F]fluoro-D-glucose positron emission tomography. *Ann Neurol.* 1987;**21**:4-13.

204. Ferrie CD, Marsden PK, Maisey MN, Robinson RO. Cortical and subcortical glucose metabolism in childhood epileptic encephalopathies. *J Neurol Neurosurg Psychiatry* 1997;**63**:181-7.

205. Ferrie CD, Marsden PK, Maisey MN, Robinson RO. Visual and semiquantitative analysis of cortical FDG-PET scans in childhood epileptic encephalopathies. *J Nucl Med.* 1997;**38**:1891-4.

206. Parker AP, Ferrie CD, Keevil S, Newbold M, Cox T, Maisey M *et al.* Neuroimaging and spectroscopy in children with epileptic encephalopathies. *Arch Dis Child* 1998;**79**:39-43.

207. Fitzgerald LF, Stone JL, Hughes JR, Melyn MA, Lansky LL. The Lennox-Gastaut syndrome: electroencephalographic characteristics, clinical correlates, and follow-up studies. *Clin Electroencephalogr.* 1992;**23**:180-9.

208. Velasco AL, Boleaga B, Santos N, Velasco F, Velasco M. Electroencephalographic and magnetic resonance correlations in children with intractable seizures of Lennox-Gastaut syndrome and epilepsia partialis continua. *Epilepsia* 1993;**34**:262-70.

209. Hughes JR, Patil VK. Long-term electro-clinical changes in the Lennox-Gastaut syndrome before, during, and after the slow spike-wave pattern. *Clin Electroencephalogr.* 2002;**33**:1-7.

210. Blume WT. Clinical and electroencephalographic correlates of the multiple independent spike foci pattern in children. *Ann Neurol.* 1978;**4**:541-7.

211. Blume, W. T. and Kaibara, M. eds. *Atlas of pediatric electroencephalography.* 1999. Philadelphia, Lippincott-Raven.

212. Noriega-Sanchez A, Markand ON. Clinical and electroencephalographic correlation of independent multifocal spike discharges. *Neurology* 1976;**26**:667-72.

213. Petersen I, Eeg-Olofsson O. The development of the electroencephalogram in normal children from the age of 1 through 15 years. Non-paroxysmal activity. *Neuropadiatrie* 1971;**2**:247-304.

214. Panayiotopoulos CP. *Panayiotopoulos syndrome:A common and benign childhood epileptic syndrome.* London: John Libbey & Company, 2002.

215. Ohtsu M, Oguni H, Hayashi K, Funatsuka M, Imai K, Osawa M. EEG in Children with Early-onset Benign Occipital Seizure Susceptibility Syndrome: Panayiotopoulos Syndrome. *Epilepsia* 2003;**44**:435-42.

216. Sanders S, Rowlinson S, Manidakis I, Ferrie CD, Koutroumanidis M. The contribution of the EEG technologists in the diagnosis of Panayiotopoulos syndrome (Susceptibility to early onset benign childhood autonomic seizures). *Seizure* 2004;**13**:565-73.

217. Ogawa K, Kanemoto K, Ishii Y, Koyama M, Shirasaka Y, Kawasaki J *et al.* Long-term follow-up study of Lennox-Gastaut syndrome in patients with severe motor and intellectual disabilities: with special reference to the problem of dysphagia. *Seizure.* 2001;**10**:197-202.

218. Yagi K. Evolution of Lennox-Gastaut syndrome: a long-term longitudinal study. *Epilepsia* 1996;**37 Suppl 3**:48-51.

219. Ohtsuka Y, Amano R, Mizukawa M, Ohtahara S. Long-term prognosis of the Lennox-Gastaut syndrome. *Jpn J Psychiatry Neurol.* 1990;**44**:257-64.

220. Yagi K, Seino M. Lennox-Gastaut syndrome—clinical seizure outcome and social prognosis. *Jpn J Psychiatry Neurol.* 1990;**44**:374-5.

221. Schmidt D, Bourgeois B. A risk-benefit assessment of therapies for Lennox-Gastaut syndrome. *Drug Saf* 2000;**22**:467-77.

222. Hancock E, Cross H. Treatment of Lennox-Gastaut syndrome. *Cochrane Database Syst Rev.* 2003;CD003277.

223. Hosain SA, Green NS, Solomon GE, Chutorian A. Nitrazepam for the treatment of Lennox-Gastaut syndrome. *Pediatr Neurol.* 2003;**28**:16-9.

224. Oguni H, Uehara T, Tanaka T, Sunahara M, Hara M, Osawa M. Dramatic effect of ethosuximide on epileptic negative myoclonus: implications for the neurophysiological mechanism. *Neuropediatrics* 1998;**29**:29-34.

225. Snead OC, III, Hosey LC. Treatment of epileptic falling spells with ethosuximide. *Brain Dev.* 1987;**9**:602-4.

226. French JA, Kanner AM, Bautista J, Abou-Khalil B, Browne T, Harden CL *et al.* Efficacy and tolerability of the new antiepileptic drugs II: treatment of refractory epilepsy: report of the Therapeutics and Technology Assessment Subcommittee and Quality Standards Subcommittee of the American Academy of Neurology and the American Epilepsy Society. *Neurology* 2004;**62**:1261-73.

227. French JA, Kanner AM, Bautista J, Abou-Khalil B, Browne T, Harden CL *et al.* Efficacy and Tolerability of the New Antiepileptic Drugs, II: Treatment of Refractory Epilepsy: Report of the TTA and QSS Subcommittees of the American Academy of Neurology and the American Epilepsy Society. *Epilepsia* 2004;**45**:410-23.

228. French JA, Kanner AM, Bautista J, Abou-Khalil B, Browne T, Harden CL *et al.* Efficacy and tolerability of the new antiepileptic drugs I: treatment of new onset epilepsy: report of the Therapeutics and Technology Assessment Subcommittee and Quality Standards Subcommittee of the American Academy of Neurology and the American Epilepsy Society. *Neurology* 2004;**62**:1252-60.

229. French JA, Kanner AM, Bautista J, Abou-Khalil B, Browne T, Harden CL *et al.* Efficacy and Tolerability of the New Antiepileptic Drugs, I: Treatment of New-Onset Epilepsy: Report of the TTA and QSS Subcommittees of the American Academy of Neurology and the American Epilepsy Society. *Epilepsia* 2004;**45**:401-9.

230. French J, Smith M, Faught E, Brown L. Practice advisory: The use of felbamate in the treatment of patients with intractable epilepsy: report of the Quality Standards Subcommittee of the American Academy of Neurology and the American Epilepsy Society. *Neurology* 1999;**52**:1540-5.

231. Bourgeois BF. Felbamate. *Semin.Pediatr.Neurol.* 1997;**4**:3-8.

232. Siegel H, Kelley K, Stertz B, Reeves-Tyer P, Flamini R, Malow B *et al.* The efficacy of felbamate as add-on therapy to valproic acid in the Lennox-Gastaut syndrome. *Epilepsy Res.* 1999;**34**:91-7.

233. Vossler DG. Exacerbation of seizures in Lennox-Gastaut syndrome by gabapentin. *Neurology* 1996;**46**:852-3.

234. Dulac O, Kaminska A. Use of lamotrigine in Lennox-Gastaut and related epilepsy syndromes. *J Child Neurol* 1997;**12 Suppl 1**:S23-S28.

235. Motte J, Trevathan E, Arvidsson JF, Barrera MN, Mullens EL, Manasco P. Lamotrigine for generalized seizures associated with the Lennox-Gastaut syndrome. Lamictal Lennox-Gastaut Study Group. *N Engl J Med.* 1997;**337**:1807-12.

236. Timmings PL, Richens A. Lamotrigine as an add-on drug in the management of Lennox-Gastaut syndrome. *Eur Neurol* 1992;**32**:305-7.

237. Ferrie CD, Robinson RO, Knott C, Panayiotopoulos CP. Lamotrigine as an add-on drug in typical absence seizures. *Acta Neurol Scand.* 1995;**91**:200-2.

238. Guberman AH, Besag FM, Brodie MJ, Dooley JM, Duchowny MS, Pellock JM *et al.* Lamotrigine-associated rash: risk/benefit considerations in adults and children. *Epilepsia* 1999;**40**:985-91.

239. Huber B, Bommel W, Hauser I, Horstmann V, Liem S, May T *et al.* Efficacy and tolerability of levetiracetam in patients with therapy-resistant epilepsy and learning disabilities. *Seizure* 2004;**13**:168-75.

240. Kadhim H, Nassogne MC, Bonnier C, van Rijckevorsel K. Migrating partial seizures in infancy: first report on a positive response to levetiracetam in youngest patient. *Epilepsia* 2004;**45 (Suppl 3.)**:204.

241. Los Reyes EC, Sharp GB, Williams JP, Hale SE. Levetiracetam in the treatment of Lennox-Gastaut syndrome. *Pediatr Neurol* 2004;**30**:254-6.

242. Glauser TA, Levisohn PM, Ritter F, Sachdeo RC. Topiramate in Lennox-Gastaut syndrome: open-label treatment of patients completing a randomized controlled trial. Topiramate YL Study Group. *Epilepsia* 2000;**41 Suppl 1**:S86-S90.

243. Coppola G, Caliendo G, Veggiotti P, Romeo A, Tortorella G, De Marco P *et al.* Topiramate as add-on drug in children, adolescents and young adults with Lennox-Gastaut syndrome: an Italian multicentric study. *Epilepsy Res.* 2002;**51**:147-53.

244. Feucht M, Brantner-Inthaler S. Gamma-vinyl-GABA (vigabatrin) in the therapy of Lennox-Gastaut syndrome: an open study. *Epilepsia* 1994;**35**:993-8.

245. Glauser TA, Pellock JM. Zonisamide in pediatric epilepsy: review of the Japanese experience. *J Child Neurol.* 2002;**17**:87-96.

246. Knudsen JF, Thambi LR, Kapcala LP, Racoosin JA. Oligohydrosis and fever in pediatric patients treated with zonisamide. *Pediatr Neurol.* 2003;**28**:184-9.

247. van Engelen BG, Renier WO, Weemaes CM, Strengers PF, Bernsen PJ, Notermans SL. High-dose intravenous immunoglobulin treatment in cryptogenic West and Lennox-Gastaut syndrome; an add-on study. *Eur J Pediatr.* 1994;**153**:762-9.

248. Caraballo R, Tripoli J, Escobal L, Cersosimo R, Tenembaum S, Palacios C *et al.* Ketogenic diet: efficacy and tolerability in childhood intractable epilepsy . *Rev Neurol.* 1998;**26**:61-4.

249. Lefevre F, Aronson N. Ketogenic diet for the treatment of refractory epilepsy in children: A systematic review of efficacy. *Pediatrics* 2000;**105**:E46.

250. Vining EP. The ketogenic diet. *Adv Exp.Med Biol.* 2002;**497**:225-31.

251. Nordli D. The ketogenic diet: uses and abuses. *Neurology* 2002;**58**:S21-S24.

252. Levy R, Cooper P. Ketogenic diet for epilepsy. *Cochrane Database Syst Rev.* 2003;CD001903.

253. Thiele EA. Assessing the efficacy of antiepileptic treatments: the ketogenic diet. *Epilepsia* 2003;**44 Suppl 7**:26-9.

254. Kossoff EH. More fat and fewer seizures: dietary therapies for epilepsy. *Lancet Neurol.* 2004;**3**:415-20.

255. Nordli DR, Jr., Kuroda MM, Carroll J, Koenigsberger DY, Hirsch LJ, Bruner HJ *et al.* Experience with the ketogenic diet in infants. *Pediatrics* 2001;**108**:129-33.

256. Mady MA, Kossoff EH, McGregor AL, Wheless JW, Pyzik PL, Freeman JM. The ketogenic diet: adolescents can do it, too. *Epilepsia* 2003;**44**:847-51.

257. Vining EP. Clinical efficacy of the ketogenic diet. *Epilepsy Res.* 1999;**37**:181-90.

258. Wirrell EC, Darwish HZ, Williams-Dyjur C, Blackman M, Lange V. Is a fast necessary when initiating the ketogenic diet? *J Child Neurol* 2002;**17**:179-82.

259. Valencia I, Holder DL, Helmers SL, Madsen JR, Riviello JJ, Jr. Vagus nerve stimulation in pediatric epilepsy: a review. *Pediatr Neurol* 2001;**25**:368-76.

260. Hosain S, Nikalov B, Harden C, Li M, Fraser R, Labar D. Vagus nerve stimulation treatment for Lennox-Gastaut syndrome. *J Child Neurol* 2000;**15**:509-12.

261. Ben Menachem E. Vagus-nerve stimulation for the treatment of epilepsy. *Lancet Neurol.* 2002;**1**:477-82.

262. Parker AP, Polkey CE, Binnie CD, Madigan C, Ferrie CD, Robinson RO. Vagal nerve stimulation in epileptic encephalopathies. *Pediatrics* 1999;**103**:778-82.

263. Parker AP, Polkey CE, Robinson RO. Vagal nerve stimulation in the epileptic encephalopathies: 3-year follow-up. *Pediatrics* 2001;**108**:221.

264. Aldenkamp AP, Majoie HJ, Berfelo MW, Evers SM, Kessels AG, Renier WO *et al.* Long-term effects of 24-month treatment with vagus nerve stimulation on behaviour in children with Lennox-Gastaut syndrome. *Epilepsy Behav.* 2002;**3**:475-9.

265. Rougier A, Claverie B, Pedespan JM, Marchal C, Loiseau P. Callosotomy for intractable epilepsy: overall outcome. *J Neurosurg Sci.* 1997;**41**:51-7.

266. Pendl G, Eder HG, Schroettner O, Leber KA. Corpus callosotomy with radiosurgery. *Neurosurgery* 1999;**45**:303-7.

267. Pressler RM, Binnie CD, Elwes RD, Polkey CE. Return of generalized seizures and discharges after callosotomy. *Adv Neurol* 1999;**81**:171-82.

268. Kwan SY, Wong TT, Chang KP, Yang TF, Lee YC, Guo WY *et al.* Postoperative seizure outcome after corpus callosotomy in reflex epilepsy. *Chung Hua I Hsueh Tsa Chih (Taipei)* 2000;**63**:240-6.

269. Gates JR. Surgery in Lennox-Gastaut syndrome. Corpus callosum division for children. *Adv Exp Med Biol.* 2002;**497**:87-98.

270. Tassinari CA, Dravet C, Roger J, Cano JP, Gastaut H. Tonic status epilepticus precipitated by intravenous benzodiazepine in five patients with Lennox-Gastaut syndrome. *Epilepsia* 1972;**13**:421-35.

271. Landau WM, Kleffner FR. Syndrome of acquired aphasia with convulsive disorder in children. *Neurology* 1957; **7:** 523-530 (reproduced in reference 272).

272. Landau WM, Kleffner FR. Syndrome of acquired aphasia with convulsive disorder in children. 1957 [classical article]. *Neurology* 1998;**51**:1241-9.

273. Worster-Drought C. An usual form of acquired aphasia in children. *Dev Med Child Neurol* 1971;**13**:563-71.

274. Beaumanoir A. The Landau-Kleffner syndrome. In Roger J, Bureau M, Dravet C, Dreifuss FE, Perret A, Wolf P, eds. *Epileptic syndromes in infancy, childhood and adolescence*, pp 231-43. London: John Libbey & Company, 1992.

275. Dugas M, Franc S, Gerard CL, Lecendreux M. Evolution of acquired epileptic aphasia with or without continuous spikes and waves during slow sleep. In Beaumanoir A, Bureau M, Deonna T, Mira L, Tassinari CA, eds. *Continuous spikes and waves during slow sleep. Electrical status epilepticus during slow sleep. Acquired epileptic aphasia and related conditions*, pp 47-55. John Libbey & Company Ltd, 1995.

276. Deonna T, Roulet E. Acquired epileptic aphasia (AEA): definition of the syndrome and current problems. In Beaumanoir A, Bureau M, Deonna T, Mira L, Tassinari CA, eds. *Continuous spikes and waves during slow sleep. Electrical status epilepticus during slow sleep. Acquired epileptic aphasia and related conditions*, pp 37-45. John Libbey & Company Ltd, 1995.

277. Morrell F, Whisler WW, Smith MC, Hoeppner TJ, de Toledo-Morrell L, Pierre-Louis SJ *et al.* Landau-Kleffner syndrome. Treatment with subpial intracortical transection. *Brain* 1995;**118**:1529-46.

278. Smith MC. Landau-Kleffner Syndrome and Continuous Spikes and Waves During Slow Sleep. In Engel JJ, Pedley TA, eds. *Epilepsy: A Comprehensive Textbook*, Philadelphia: Lippincott-Raven Publishers, 1997.

279. Kaga M. Language disorders in Landau-Kleffner syndrome. *J Child Neurol.* 1999;**14**:118-22.

280. Panayiotopoulos CP. Landau-Kleffner syndrome. In Panayiotopoulos CP, ed. *Benign childhood partial seizures and related epileptic syndromes*, pp 337-48. London: John Libbey & Company Ltd, 1999.

281. Metz-Lutz MN, Maquet P, de Saint MA, Rudolf G, Wioland N, Hirsch E *et al.* Pathophysiological aspects of Landau-Kleffner syndrome: from the active epileptic phase to recovery. *Int Rev Neurobiol.* 2001;**45**:505-26.

282. Galanopoulou AS, Bojko A, Lado F, Moshe SL. The spectrum of neuropsychiatric abnormalities associated with electrical status epilepticus in sleep. *Brain Dev.* 2000;**22**:279-95.

283. McVicar KA, Shinnar S. Landau-Kleffner syndrome, electrical status epilepticus in slow wave sleep, and language regression in children. *Ment Retard Dev Disabil Res Rev* 2004;**10**:144-9.

284. Tassinari CA. The problems of 'continuous spikes and waves during slow sleep' or 'electrical status epilepticus during slow sleep' today. In Beaumanoir A, Bureau M, Deonna T, Mira L, Tassinari CA, eds. *Continuous spikes and waves during slow sleep. Electrical status epilepticus during slow sleep. Acquired epileptic aphasia and related conditions*, pp 251-5. John Libbey & Company Ltd, 1995.

285. Tassinari CA, Rubboli G, Volpi L, Meletti S, d'Orsi G, Franca M *et al.* Encephalopathy with electrical status epilepticus during slow sleep or ESES syndrome including the acquired aphasia. *Clin Neurophysiol.* 2000;**111 Suppl 2**:S94-S102.

286. Beaumanoir A, Bureau M, Mira L. Identification of the syndrome. In Beaumanoir A, Bureau M, Deonna T, Mira L, Tassinari CA, eds. *Continuous spikes and waves during slow sleep. Electrical status epilepticus during slow sleep. Acquired epileptic aphasia and related conditions*, pp 243-9. John Libbey & Company Ltd, 1995.

287. Morrell F. Electrophysiology of CSWS in Landau-Kleffner syndrome. In Beaumanoir A, Bureau M, Deonna T, Mira L, Tassinari CA, eds. *Continuous spikes and waves during slow sleep. Electrical status epilepticus during slow sleep. Acquired epileptic aphasia and related conditions*, pp 77-90. John Libbey & Company Ltd, 1995.

288. Mantovani JF, Landau WM. Acquired aphasia with convulsive disorder: course and prognosis. *Neurology* 1980;**30**:524-9.

289. Nakano S, Okuno T, Mikawa H. Landau-Kleffner syndrome. EEG topographic studies. *Brain Dev.* 1989;**11**:43-50.

290. Roulet PE, Seeck M, Mayer E, Despland PA, de Tribolet N, Deonna T. Childhood epilepsy with neuropsychological regression and continuous spike waves during sleep: epilepsy surgery in a young adult. *Eur J Paediatr Neurol.* 1998;**2**:303-11.

291. Panayiotopoulos CP. Benign childhood partial epilepsies: benign childhood seizure susceptibility syndromes [editorial]. *J Neurol Neurosurg Psychiatr* 1993;**56**:2-5.

292. Panayiotopoulos CP. Benign childhood partial seizures and related epileptic syndromes. London: John Libbey & Company Ltd, 1999.

293. Fejerman N, Caraballo R, Tenembaum SN. Atypical evolutions of benign localization-related epilepsies in children: are they predictable? *Epilepsia* 2000;**41**:380-90.

294. Caraballo RH, Astorino F, Cersosimo R, Soprano AM, Fejerman N. Atypical evolution in childhood epilepsy with occipital paroxysms (Panayiotopoulos type). *Epileptic Disord.* 2001;**3**:157-62.

295. Ferrie CD, Koutroumanidis M, Rowlinson S, Sanders S, Panayiotopoulos CP. Atypical evolution of Panayiotopoulos syndrome: a case report [published with video- sequences]. *Epileptic Disord.* 2002;**4**:35-42.

296. da Silva EA, Chugani DC, Muzik O, Chugani HT. Landau-Kleffner syndrome: metabolic abnormalities in temporal lobe are a common feature. *J Child Neurol.* 1997;**12**:489-95.

297. Takeoka M, Riviello JJ, Jr., Duffy FH, Kim F, Kennedy DN, Makris N *et al.* Bilateral volume reduction of the superior temporal areas in Landau-Kleffner syndrome. *Neurology* 2004;**63**:1289-92.

298. Genton P, Guerrini R. What differentiates Landau-Kleffner syndrome from the syndrome of continuous spikes and waves during slow sleep? . *Arch Neurol.* 1993;**50**:1008-9.

299. Robinson RO, Baird G, Robinson G, Simonoff E. Landau-Kleffner syndrome: course and correlates with outcome. *Dev Med Child Neurol.* 2001;**43**:243-7.

300. Kossoff EH, Boatman D, Freeman JM. Landau-Kleffner syndrome responsive to levetiracetam. *Epilepsy Behav.* 2003;**4**:571-5.

301. Green JR, Troupin AS, Halperm LM, Friel P, Kanarek P. Sulthiame: evaluation as an anticonvulsant. *Epilepsia* 1974;**15**:329-49.

302. Houghton GW, Richens A. Phenytoin intoxication induced by sulthiame in epileptic patients. *J Neurol Neurosurg Psychiatry* 1974;**37**:275-81.

303. Lerman P, Nussbaum E. The use of sulthiame- in myoclonic epilepsy of childhood and adolescence. *Acta Neurol Scand. Suppl* 1975;**60**:7-12.

304. Koepp MJ, Patsalos PN, Sander JW. Sulthiame in adults with refractory epilepsy and learning disability: an open trial. *Epilepsy Res.* 2002;**50**:277-82.

305. Kramer U, Shahar E, Zelnik N, Lerman-Sagie T, Watemberg N, Nevo Y *et al.* Carbamazepine versus sulthiame in treating benign childhood epilepsy with centrotemporal spikes. *J Child Neurol.* 2002;**17**:914-6.

306. Bast T, Volp A, Wolf C, Rating D. The influence of sulthiame on EEG in children with benign childhood epilepsy with centrotemporal spikes (BECTS). *Epilepsia* 2003;**44**:215-20.

307. Engler F, Maeder-Ingvar M, Roulet E, Deonna T. Treatment with Sulthiame (Ospolot) in benign partial epilepsy of childhood and related syndromes: an open clinical and EEG study. *Neuropediatrics* 2003;**34**:105-9.

308. Sawhney IM, Robertson IJ, Polkey CE, Binnie CD, Elwes RD. Multiple subpial transection: a review of 21 cases. *J Neurol Neurosurg Psychiatr* 1995;**58**:344-9.

309. Bureau M. 'Continuous spikes and waves during slow sleep'(CSWS): definition of the syndrome. In Beaumanoir A, Bureau M, Deonna T, Mira L, Tassinari CA, eds. *Continuous spikes and waves during slow sleep. Electrical status epilepticus during slow sleep. Acquired epileptic aphasia and related conditions*, pp 17-26. John Libbey & Company Ltd, 1995.

310. Morikawa T, Seino M, Watanabe MD. Long-term outcome of CSWS syndrome. In Beaumanoir A, Bureau M, Deonna T, Mira L, Tassinari CA, eds. *Continuous spikes and waves during slow sleep. Electrical status epilepticus during slow sleep. Acquired epileptic aphasia and related conditions*, pp 27-36. John Libbey & Company Ltd, 1995.

311. Tassinari CA, Volpi L, Michellluchi R. Electrical status epilepticus during slow sleep. In Gilman S, ed. *Medlink Neurology*, San Diego SA: Arbor Publishing Corp, 2004.

312. Patry G, Lyagoubi S, Tassinari CA. Subclinical "electrical status epilepticus" induced by sleep in children. A clinical and electroencephalographic study of six cases. *Arch Neurol* 1971;**24**:242-52.

313. Tassinari CA, Bureau M, Dravet C, Dalla Bernardina B, Roger J. Epilepsy with continuous spikes amd waves during slow sleep-otherwise described as ESES (epilepsy with electrical status epilepticus during slow sleep). In Roger J, Bureau M, Dravet C, Dreifuss FE, Perret A, Wolf P, eds. *Epileptic syndromes in infancy, childhood and adolescence*, pp 245-56. London: John Libbey & Company, 1992.

314. Shafrir Y, Prensky AL. Acquired epileptiform opercular syndrome: a second case report, review of the literature, and comparison to the Landau-Kleffner syndrome. *Epilepsia* 1995;**36**:1050-7.

315. Tachikawa E, Oguni H, Shirakawa S, Funatsuka M, Hayashi K, Osawa M. Acquired epileptiform opercular syndrome: a case report and results of single photon emission computed tomography and computer-assisted electroencephalographic analysis. *Brain Dev.* 2001;**23**:246-50.

316. Maquet P, Hirsch E, Metz-Lutz MN, Motte J, Dive D, Marescaux C *et al.* Regional cerebral glucose metabolism in children with deterioration of one or more cognitive functions and continuous spike-and-wave discharges during sleep. *Brain* 1995;**118**:1497-520.

317. Gaggero R, Caputo M, Fiorio P, Pessagno A, Baglietto MG, Muttini P *et al.* SPECT and epilepsy with continuous spike waves during slow-wave sleep. *Childs Nerv Syst.* 1995;**11**:154-60.

318. Dalla Bernardina B, Tassinari CA, Dravet C, Bureau M, Beghini G, Roger J. Benign focal epilepsy and "electrical status epilepticus" during sleep. *Rev Electroencephal Neurophysiol Clinique* 1978;**8**:350-3.

319. Guerrini R, Genton P, Bureau M, Parmeggiani A, Salas-Puig X, Santucci M *et al.* Multilobar polymicrogyria, intractable drop attack seizures, and sleep-related electrical status epilepticus. *Neurology* 1998;**51**:504-12.

320. Roulet PE, Davidoff V, Despland PA, Deonna T. Mental and behavioural deterioration of children with epilepsy and CSWS: acquired epileptic frontal syndrome. *Dev Med Child Neurol* 1993;**35**:661-74.

321. Roulet PE. Syndromes of acquired epileptic aphasia and epilepsy with continuous spike-waves during sleep: models for prolonged cognitive impairment of epileptic origin. *Semin Pediatr Neurol* 1995;**2**:269-77.

322. Smith MC, Spitz MC. Treatment strategies in Landau-Kleffner syndrome and paraictal psychiatric and cognitive disturbances. *Epilepsy Behav.* 2002;**3**:24-9.

323. Hoppen T, Sandrieser T, Rister M. Successful treatment of pharmacoresistent continuous spike wave activity during slow sleep with levetiracetam. *Eur J Pediatr.* 2003;**162**:59-61.

324. De Negri M. Electrical status epilepticus during sleep (ESES). Different clinical syndromes: towards a unifying view?*Brain Dev.* 1997;**19**:447-51.

325. Chiron C, Plouin P, Dulac O, Mayer M, Ponsot G. Myoclonic epilepsy with non-progressive encephalopathy . *Neurophysiol Clin.* 1988;**18**:513-24.

326. Dalla Bernardina B, Fontana E, Sgro M, Colamaria V, Elia M. Myoclonic epilepsy ('myoclonic status') in non-progressive encephalopathies. In Roger J, Bureau M, Dravet C, Dreifuss FE, Perret A, Wolf P, eds. *Epileptic syndromes in infancy, childhood and adolescence*, pp 89-96. London: John Libbey & Company Ltd, 1992.

327. Dalla Bernardina B, Fontana E, Darra F. Myoclonic status in nonprogressive encephalopathies. In Gilman S, ed. *Medlink Neurology*, San Diego SA: 2004.

328. Dalla Bernardina B, Fontana E, Darra F. Myoclonic status in non-progressive encephalopathies. In Roger J, Bureau M, Dravet C, Genton P, Tassinari CA, Wolf P, eds. *Epileptic syndromes in infancy, childhood and adolescence (3rd edn)*, pp 137-44. London: John Libbey & Co Ltd, 2002.

329. Guerrini R, De Lorey TM, Bonanni P, Moncla A, Dravet C, Suisse G *et al.* Cortical myoclonus in Angelman syndrome. *Ann Neurol.* 1996;**40**:39-48.

330. Guerrini R, Carrozzo R, Rinaldi R, Bonanni P. Angelman syndrome: etiology, clinical features, diagnosis, and management of symptoms. *Paediatr Drugs* 2003;**5**:647-61.

331. Cersosimo R, Caraballo R, Espeche A, Cassar L, Torrado MV, Chertkoff L *et al.* Angelman syndrome: the electroclinical characteristics in 35 patients . *Rev Neurol.* 2003;**37**:14-8.

332. Aicardi J, Chevrie JJ. Atypical benign partial epilepsy of childhood. *Dev Med Child Neurol* 1982;**24**:281-92.

333. Aicardi J. Atypical semiology of rolandic epilepsy in some related syndromes. *Epileptic Disord.* 2000;**2 Suppl 1**:S5-S9.

334. Doose H, Hahn A, Neubauer BA, Pistohl J, Stephani U. Atypical "benign" partial epilepsy of childhood or pseudo-lennox syndrome. Part II: family study. *Neuropediatrics* 2001;**32**:9-13.

335. Arzimanoglou A, Guerrini R, Aicardi J, eds. Aicardi's epilepsy in children. Philadelphia: Lippincott Williams & Wilkins, 2004.

336. Doose H, Baier WK. Benign partial epilepsy and related conditions: multifactorial pathogenesis with hereditary impairment of brain maturation. *Eur J Pediatr* 1989;**149**:152-8.

337. Rodriguez-Barrionuevo AC, Bauzano-Poley E, Delgado-Marques MP, Mora-Ramirez MD, Tosina-Garcia E. Atypical benign partial epilepsy of childhood. Clinical follow-up EEG study of 3 patients . *Rev Neurol* 1998;**26**:197-204.

338. Oguni H, Sato F, Hayashi K, Wang PJ, Fukuyama Y. A study of unilateral brief focal atonia in childhood partial epilepsy. *Epilepsia* 1992;**33**:75-83.

339. Kanazawa O, Kawai I. Status epilepticus characterized by repetitive asymmetrical atonia: two cases accompanied by partial seizures. *Epilepsia* 1990;**31**:536-43.

340. Fejerman N. Atypical evolution of benign partial epilepsy in children. *Rev Neurol* 1996;**24**:1415-20.

341. Caraballo, R, Fontana, E, Michelizza, B, Zullini, B, Sgro, V, Pajno-Ferrara, F, Dalla Bernardina, B, and Espositio, S. Carbamazepina, 'assenze atipiche', 'crisi atoniche', 'crisi atoniche' e stato di PO continua del sonno. *Boll Lega It Epil* 1989; **66/67**: 379-81.

342. Gross-Selbeck G. Treatment of "benign" partial epilepsies of childhood, including atypical forms. *Neuropediatrics* 1995;**26**:45-50.

343. Rating D, Wolf C, Bast T. Sulthiame as monotherapy in children with benign childhood epilepsy with centrotemporal spikes: a 6-month randomized, double-blind, placebo-controlled study. Sulthiame Study Group. *Epilepsia* 2000;**41**:1284-8.

344. Battaglia D, Iuvone L, Stefanini MC, Acquafondata C, Lettori D, Chiricozzi F *et al.* Reversible aphasic disorder induced by lamotrigine in atypical benign childhood epilepsy. *Epileptic Disord.* 2001;**3**:217-22.

345. Hamano S, Mochizuki M, Morikawa T. Phenobarbital-induced atypical absence seizure in benign childhood epilepsy with centrotemporal spikes. *Seizure.* 2002;**11**:201-4.

346. Tassinari CA, Riguzzi P, Rizzi R, Passarelli D, Volpi L. Gelastic seizures. In Tuxhorn I, Holthausen H, Boenigk H, eds. *Paediatric epilepsy syndromes and their surgical treatment*, pp 429-46. London: John Libbey & Comapny Ltd, 1997.

347. Munari C, Quarato P, Kahane P, Tassi L, Minotti L, Hoffman D *et al.* Gelastic and dacrystic seizures. In Luders HO, Noachtar S, eds. *Epileptic seizures. Pathophysiology and clinical semiology*, pp 458-71. New York: Churchill Livingstone, 2000.

348. Striano S, Striano P, Cirillo S, Nocerino C, Bilo L, Meo R *et al.* Small hypothalamic hamartomas and gelastic seizures. [Published with videosequences]. *EpilepticDisord.* 2002;**4**:129-33.

349. Fohlen M, Lellouch A, Delalande O. Hypothalamic hamartoma with refractory epilepsy: surgical procedures and results in 18 patients. *Epileptic Disord.* 2003;**5**:267-73.

350. Brandberg G, Raininko R, Eeg-Olofsson O. Hypothalamic hamartoma with gelastic seizures in Swedish children and adolescents. *Eur.J Paediatr Neurol.* 2004;**8**:35-44.

351. Freeman JL, Coleman LT, Wellard RM, Kean MJ, Rosenfeld JV, Jackson GD *et al.* MR imaging and spectroscopic study of epileptogenic hypothalamic hamartomas: analysis of 72 cases. *Am J Neuroradiol.* 2004;**25**:450-62.

352. Ryvlin P, Ravier C, Bouvard S, Mauguire F, Le Bars D, Arzimanoglou A *et al.* Positron emission tomography in epileptogenic hypothalamic hamartomas. *Epileptic Disord.* 2003;**5**:219-27.

353. Polkey CE. Resective surgery for hypothalamic hamartoma. *Epileptic Disord.* 2003;**5**:281-6.

354. Perez-Jimenez A, Villarejo FJ, Fournier del Castillo MC, Garcia-Penas JJ, Carreno M. Continuous giggling and autistic disorder associated with hypothalamic hamartoma. *Epileptic Disord.* 2003;**5**:31-7.

355. Palmini A, Paglioli-Neto E, Montes J, Farmer JP. The treatment of patients with hypothalamic hamartomas, epilepsy and behavioural abnormalities: facts and hypotheses. *Epileptic Disord.* 2003;**5**:249-55.

356. Mullatti N. Hypothalamic hamartoma in adults. *Epilepti .Disord.* 2003;**5**:201-4.

357. Kuzniecky RI, Guthrie BL. Stereotactic surgical approach to hypothalamic hamartomas. *Epileptic Disord.* 2003;**5**:275-80.

358. Kremer S, Minotti L, Thiriaux A, Grand S, Satre V, Le Bas JF *et al.* Epilepsy and hypothalamic hamartoma: look at the hand Pallister-Hall syndrome. *Epileptic Disord.* 2003;**5**:27-30.

359. Kahane P, Ryvlin P, Hoffmann D, Minotti L, Benabid AL. From hypothalamic hamartoma to cortex: what can be learnt from depth recordings and stimulation? *Epileptic Disord.* 2003;**5**:205-17.

360. Harvey AS, Freeman JL, Berkovic SF, Rosenfeld JV. Transcallosal resection of hypothalamic hamartomas in patients with intractable epilepsy. *Epileptic Disord.* 2003;**5**:257-65.

361. Freeman JL, Zacharin M, Rosenfeld JV, Harvey AS. The endocrinology of hypothalamic hamartoma; surgery for intractable epilepsy. *Epileptic Disord.* 2003;**5**:239-47.

362. Freeman JL. The anatomy and embryology of the hypothalamus in relation to hypothalamic hamartomas. *Epileptic Disord.* 2003;**5**:177-86.

363. Fohlen M, Lellouch A, Delalande O. Hypothalamic hamartoma with refractory epilepsy: surgical procedures and results in 18 patients. *Epileptic Disord.* 2003;**5**:267-73.

364. Biesecker LG. Heritable syndromes with hypothalamic hamartoma and seizures: using rare syndromes to understand more common disorders. *Epileptic Disord.* 2003;**5**:235-8.

365. Arzimanoglou AA, Hirsch E, Aicardi J. Hypothalamic hamartoma and epilepsy in children: illustrative cases of possible evolutions. *Epileptic Disord.* 2003;**5**:187-99.

366. Andermann F, Arzimanoglou A, Berkovic SF. Hypothalamic hamartoma and epilepsy: the pathway of discovery. *Epileptic Disord.* 2003;**5**:173-5.

367. Feeks EF, Murphy GL, Porter HO. Laughter in the cockpit: gelastic seizures—a case report. *Aviat Space Environ Med* 1997;**68**:66-8.

368. Thom M, Gomez-Anson B, Revesz T, Harkness W, O'Brien CJ, Kett-White R *et al.* Spontaneous intralesional haemorrhage in dysembryoplastic neuroepithelial tumours: a series of five cases. *J Neurol Neurosurg Psychiatry* 1999;**67**:97-101.

369. Cerullo A, Tinuper P, Provini F, Contin M, Rosati A, Marini C *et al.* Autonomic and hormonal ictal changes in gelastic seizures from hypothalamic hamartomas. *Electroencephalogr Clin Neurophysiol* 1998;**107**:317-22.

370. Berkovic SF, Andermann F, Melanson D, Ethier RE, Feindel W, Gloor P. Hypothalamic hamartomas and ictal laughter: evolution of a characteristic epileptic syndrome and diagnostic value of magnetic resonance imaging. *Ann Neurol* 1988;**23**: 429-39.

371. Rosenfeld JV, Harvey AS, Wrennall J, Zacharin M, Berkovic SF. Transcallosal resection of hypothalamic hamartomas, with control of seizures, in children with gelastic epilepsy. *Neurosurgery* 2001;**48**:108-18.

372. Berkovic SF, Kuzniecky RI, Andermann F. Human epileptogenesis and hypothalamic hamartomas: new lessons from an experiment of nature [editorial]. *Epilepsia* 1997;**38**:1-3.

373. Munari C, Kahane P, Francione S, Hoffmann D, Tassi L, Cusmai R *et al.* Role of the hypothalamic hamartoma in the genesis of gelastic fits (a video-stereo-EEG study). *Electroencephalogr Clin Neurophysiol* 1995;**95**:154-60.

374. Zaatreh M, Tennison M, Greenwood RS. Successful treatment of hypothalamic seizures and precocious puberty with GnRH analogue. *Neurology* 2000;**55**:1908-10.

375. Panayiotopoulos CP. Gelastic epilepsy. *Materia Medica Greca* 1979;**7**:570-5.

376. Dreyer R, Wehmeyer W. Laughing in complex partial seizure epilepsy. A video tape analysis of 32 patients with laughing as symptom of an attack. *Fortschr Neurol Psychiatr Grenzgeb.* 1978;**46**:61-75.

377. Sartori E, Biraben A, Taussig D, Bernard AM, Scarabin JM. Gelastic seizures: video-EEG and scintigraphic analysis of a case with a frontal focus; review of the literature and pathophysiological hypotheses. *Epileptic Disord.* 1999;**1**:221-8.

378. Kuzniecky R, Guthrie B, Mountz J, Bebin M, Faught E, Gilliam F *et al.* Intrinsic epileptogenesis of hypothalamic hamartomas in gelastic epilepsy. *Ann Neurol* 1997;**42**:60-7.

379. Fukuda M, Kameyama S, Wachi M, Tanaka R. Stereotaxy for hypothalamic hamartoma with intractable gelastic seizures: technical case report. *Neurosurgery* 1999;**44**:1347-50.

SEVERE NEOCORTICAL EPILEPTIC SYNDROMES IN INFANCY AND CHILDHOOD

8

The following are severe neocortical epileptic syndromes with onset in infancy and childhood.[1,2]

- Kozhevnikov-Rasmussen syndrome
- Hemiconvulsion-hemiplegia syndrome
- Migrating partial epilepsy of early childhood*

KOZHEVNIKOV-RASMUSSEN SYNDROME

Kozhevnikov**[3]-Rasmussen[4] syndrome is a severe, probably acquired, neocortical disorder characterised by intractable, mainly focal, motor seizures, epilepsia partialis continua and progressive neuropsychological deterioration with hemiparesis, and cognitive and linguistic deficits.[5-17]

This syndrome should not be equated with *'epilepsia partialis continua'*, which is a form of focal motor status epilepticus with various causes and prognoses as detailed in Table 12.2, page 405. Only 60% of patients with Kozhevnikov-Rasmussen syndrome manifest with epilepsia partialis continua.

DEMOGRAPHIC DATA

Onset is in childhood between 1 and 10 years of age (median 5 years of age).[5] Late onset, in adolescence or adulthood is rare.[21,22] Both sexes are equally affected. Kozhevnikov-Rasmussen syndrome is a very rare disease.[8] Highly specialised tertiary centres may see one case per year: only 48 cases have been seen over 50 years at the Montreal Neurological Hospital, Canada;[5] and similarly, only 10 cases have been seen at the Centre Saint-Paul, Marseilles, France in 10 years.[23]

*Syndrome in development according to the new ILAE diagnostic scheme.[2]

**I use the English spelling of the name Kozhevnikov in this book, as opposed to various other forms such as Kojewnikow[1,18] or Kojevnikov[2] that have appeared in the literature.

Clarifications on the nomenclature for the Kozhevnikov-Rasmussen syndrome and ILAE definitions

The name *'Kozhevnikov-Rasmussen syndrome'* is in compliance with the ILAE nomenclature of 1985[18] and 1989[1] and in respect of medical history.

This syndrome was initially called *'Kozhevnikov type 2 syndrome'*,[18] which was retained in the currently valid classification of 1989[1] where *"Rasmussen syndrome"* was introduced as a sharing synonym after a symposium in the Montreal Neurological Institute (June 1988).[7,19]

The 1985[18] and 1989[1] ILAE classification recognises two syndromes:

'Kozhevnikov type 1 syndrome', which is not a syndrome, but a type of seizure and status epilepticus with many causes and prognoses (see Table 12.2, page405).

'Kozhevnikov type 2 syndrome' described in this chapter and defined as follows:

"Childhood disorder, suspected to be of viral aetiology, has onset between 2 and 10 years (peak, 6 years) with seizures that are motor partial seizures, but are often associated with other types. Fragmentary motor seizures appear early in the course of the illness and are initially localized, but later become erratic and diffuse, and persist during sleep. A progressive motor deficit follows, and mental deterioration occurs. The EEG background activity shows asymmetric and slow diffuse delta waves, with numerous ictal and interictal discharges that are not strictly limited to the Rolandic area."[18]

The recent ILAE diagnostic scheme[2] rightly differentiates these two and classifies:

1. 'Epilepsia partialis continua of Kozhevnikov' among seizure types.[2]
2. 'Rasmussen syndrome' among syndromes of neocortical origin.[2]

The omission of Kozhevnikov's name in this ILAE diagnostic scheme[2] is an historical error based on the misconception that Kozhevnikov described an acute rather than chronic encephalitis (see page 214).[15,19] Kozhevnikov-Rasmussen syndrome is the only proper nomenclature to honour both these great men, who independently described this epileptic syndrome of chronic encephalitis, half a century apart.[20]

CLINICAL MANIFESTATIONS [6,7,9,12,13,24-27]

Typically, affected children are initially normal. Onset is usually with focal motor seizures, epilepsia partialis continua, generalised tonic clonic seizures (GTCS) or complex focal seizures without automatisms. Status epilepticus may be the presenting feature in about 20% of patients. In 50% of cases, there is a history of upper respiratory tract infection, otitis media or tonsillitis, which precedes the seizures by about 6 months.

Initially, the focal motor seizures involve a small group of mainly distal muscles (thumb, fingers, corner of the mouth or the eye), but with time they progress to neighbouring regions, become erratic and more diffuse, and also persist during sleep. Seizures of any type, and usually a combination, gradually become more frequent, longer in duration and are often associated with postictal hemiplegia. Epilepsia partialis continua occurs in 60% of patients and may last for days, often interspersed with hemi-tonic-clonic convulsions that may also become generalised. Hemiplegia is initially postictal and transient, but gradually becomes permanent. Histologically confirmed cases of Kozhevnikov-Rasmussen syndrome without seizures have been reported.[28]

The clinical course follows three stages.[5,6]

First stage

The first stage is characterised mainly by simple motor or somatosensory seizures. Less frequently, onset may comprise epilepsia partialis continua, complex focal seizures without automatisms or secondarily GTCS. A combination of these types of seizures may occur. Gradually, over weeks or months, seizures become more frequent.

Second stage

The second stage is characterised by worsening of the seizures and progressive neurological symptoms with mainly unilateral hemispheric involvement. This stage usually starts about 3 months after seizure onset, but may be delayed for as long as 10 years after the first symptoms of the disease. Seizures become more frequent, more widespread and of longer duration. Permanent psychomotor deficits appear with a progressive intensity. These consist of hemiparesis, hemi-hypoaesthesia, hemianopia with cognitive and linguistic (including dysphasia and dysarthria) impairment. Most of the brain damage occurs during the first 8–12 months.[13]

Progressive deterioration of the neurological and psychological state, either with or without seizure deterioration, is a typical feature of Kozhevnikov-Rasmussen syndrome.

Third stage

In the third stage, the disease appears to abate with regard to seizure frequency and severity, as well as progression of neurological deficits but patients manifest with serious neurocognitive residuals.

AETIOLOGY

The aetiology is unknown,[29] though chronic encephalitis is believed to be the main causative factor, as postulated 100 years ago by Kozhevnikov[3] and later by Rasmussen.[4]

Pathology reveals an inflammatory process, which is initially relatively localised, but later progresses to more extensive unilateral or bilateral, mainly cortical involvement.[30] The lesion appears to extend in a confluent rather than multifocal manner.[29] The pathological abnormalities range from those of active to those of remote disease.[31,32]

Robitaille[31,32] classified the pathological specimens into four groups:

Group 1 consists of an ongoing inflammatory process, with numerous microglial nodules, with or without neuronophagia, perivascular round cells and glial scarring.

Group 2 contains features of 'active and remote disease' with several microglial nodules, cuffs of perivascular round cells, and at least one gyral segment of complete necrosis and cavitation including full-thickness cortex.

Group 3 is of a less active 'remote' disease, with neuronal loss and gliosis, moderately abundant perivascular round cells and only a few microglial nodules.

Group 4 has non-specific changes, with few or no microglial nodules and only mild perivascular inflammation, but with various degrees of neuronal loss and glial scarring.[31,32]

In a more recent report, patterns of pathological changes and stages of cortical abnormalities were studied by histology and immunocytochemistry methods in the cerebral cortex of 45 hemispherectomies.[33] The burden of pathology was quantified in all brain regions of each of the 45 hemispheres. There was significant heterogeneity in the stages of cortical pathology and the multifocal nature of the disease. These stages varied from early inflammation defined by infiltration of T lymphocytes and neuroglial reactions, to more severe stages with extensive neuronal cell death and cavitation of the cerebral cortex. A greater burden of pathology was significantly associated with an early age at onset and longer duration of disease. The burden of pathology was similar in all brain regions except the occipital lobe, where it was significantly lower. The authors concluded that "the multifocal distribution of pathologic changes, as well as the heterogeneity in the stages of cortical damage in each patient, is consistent with an ongoing and progressive immune-mediated process of neuronal damage that involves neuroglial and lymphocytic responses, resembling other autoimmune CNS disorders such as multiple sclerosis".[33]

PATHOPHYSIOLOGY

Converging lines of evidence suggest that an autoimmune process may be important in the pathogenesis of this syndrome. Direct analysis of resected brain tissue for virus by polymerase chain reaction or in situ hybridisation has yielded inconsistent results. This may be a consequence of the variable presence of non-disease-related viral genomes, either in neural cells or in inflammatory cells in the lesions. The precise role played by antibody-mediated mechanisms, T-cell immunity and viral antigens remains unclear.[16]

Proposed causes of the pathological changes are:

- chronic viral infection, but so far no virus has been isolated
- acute viral infection leading to a local immune response
- independent autoimmune process, not linked to infection, but results have been both for and against it.

The viral hypothesis remains controversial and unresolved[15,34]

So far no virus has been isolated.[35] Serological studies to detect antecedent viral infection and direct analysis of resected brain tissue for virus have been inconclusive.[29] Enteroviruses, Epstein-Barr virus, cytomegalovirus, herpes simplex virus (HSV) type 1 and HSV type 2 have been implicated in some cases.[15,34] HSV infection of the brain seems an unlikely direct cause of Kozhevnikov-Rasmussen syndrome.[36]

Immunopathogenetic mechanisms

Immunopathogenetic mechanisms may be important,[10] but results have been both for[37,38] and against it.[39,40]

An attractive proposition is that Kozhevnikov-Rasmussen syndrome is due to an autoimmune process directed against the glutamate/AMPA receptor subunit 3 (GluR3).[41,42] Antibodies appear to activate the receptor and may directly trigger seizures by overstimulating the glutamate receptors.[43] GluR immunoreactivity appeared to correlate with disease activity, but cases without antibody have been described.[44]

Rabbits immunised systemically with fusion proteins containing a portion of GluR3 (amino acids 245–457) developed seizures and changes characteristic of Kozhevnikov-Rasmussen syndrome were demonstrated pathologically.[41] This was further supported by human and animal data.[43]

The proposition is that the initial insult, traumatic or infectious, may cause a breach in the blood-brain barrier.[41,43] In individuals with autoantibodies to GluR3, this 'crack' in the blood-brain barrier allows entry of these antibodies into the brain, causing activation of the receptors and subsequent seizures. The result is a vicious circle in which the seizures result in more rifts in the blood-brain barrier. Alternatively, the GluR3 antibodies may arise as a result of the initial CNS damage, thus leading to further damage.[41,43]

Patients with Kozhevnikov-Rasmussen syndrome may have autoantibodies against several neural molecules, and these autoantibodies may be produced in the CNS as a result of cytotoxic T cell-mediated neuronal damage.[45]

Double pathology

Some patients with typical Kozhevnikov-Rasmussen syndrome may have, in addition to the pathological changes of chronic encephalitis, other pathology such as vascular abnormalities resembling cavernous angiomata, tuberous sclerosis and tumours.[46,47]

Genetics

Reports of Kozhevnikov-Rasmussen syndrome in families are exceptional.[48] Two brothers with epilepsia partialis continua alternately involving both sides of the body have been described.[49] They rapidly developed severe psychomotor regression and cerebral atrophy. Brain biopsy specimens revealed chronic inflammatory changes.[49]

DIAGNOSTIC PROCEDURES

There is no specific diagnostic procedure or abnormality in Kozhevnikov-Rasmussen syndrome. Antibodies to GluR3 are detected in the serum of some, but not all, patients.[14,50] At onset, all methods for functional and structural abnormalities may be normal. It is the progression of symptoms and signs, and their localisation that may be consistent with the diagnosis.

Cerebrospinal fluid[12,15] shows non-specific abnormalities in 50% of patients. Oligoclonal or monoclonal banding may be found.

Brain imaging:[9,13,51] Serial CT brain scans, and preferably MRI, show progressive hemiatrophy (Figure 8.1). This usually starts unilaterally in the temporo-insular region with enlargement of the temporal horn and Sylvian fissure. The abnormalities usually spread from one discrete area to an adjacent region or multifocally, at the same time.[52]

Magnetic resonance spectroscopy (MRS) has been applied in a few cases.[53,54] In the most recent report,[54] following complex focal status epilepticus a T2-weighted

MRI showed transient signal increase in the left superior temporal gyrus and mesial temporal structures. Subsequent scans showed resolution of the swelling and signal normalization, with development of slight focal atrophy. MRS also showed a reduction in N-acetylaspartate, total creatine and trimethylamines. Subsequent scans showed complete resolution of these metabolite abnormalities, followed later by development of further abnormal metabolite values. Lactate and glutamine/glutamate were elevated after status.

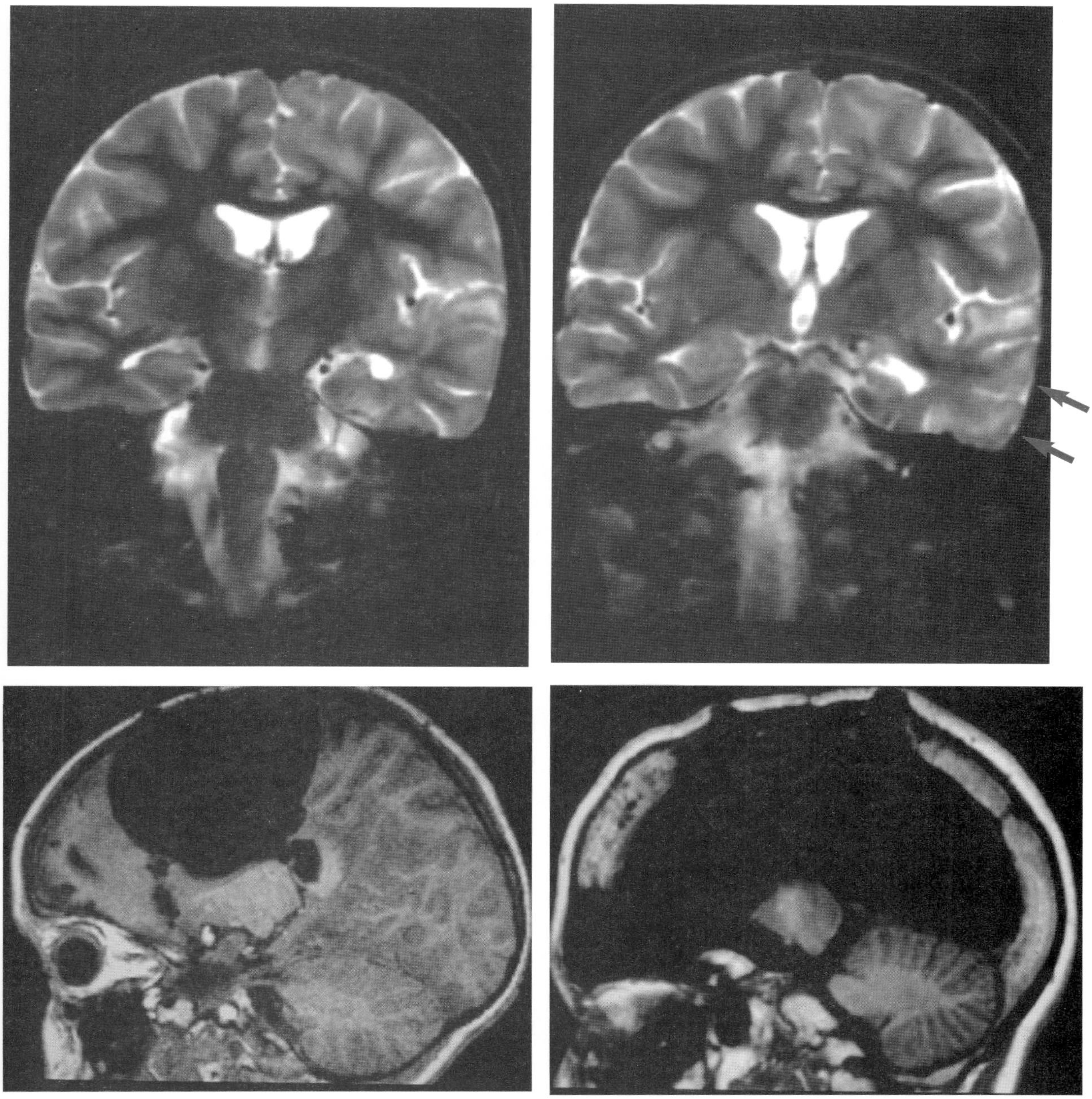

igure 8.1 Brain MRI of a 5-year-old boy with Kozhevnikov-Rasmussen syndrome confirmed by histology.

op: Progression of the disease as documented by brain MRI; the images on the right were obtained 5 months fter those on the left.

Bottom. Further disease progression with severe atrophy is documented even after functional hemispherectomy.

Figure courtesy of Dr Rod C. Scott, Institute of Child Health, London, UK

After surgery, ex vivo high-field (1)H and (31)P MRS confirmed metabolite abnormalities (elevated choline and decreased aspartate, N-acetylaspartate, [(1)H]glutamate together with altered [(31)P]phospholipid ratios. These findings suggested active disease process in the anterior region of the excised superior temporal gyrus. The authors concluded that Kozhevnikov-Rasmussen syndrome "is a combination of progressive encephalitic damage and fluctuating seizure effects, in which neuronal injury and recovery can occur".[54]

Functional brain imaging with single photon emission computed tomography (SPECT) and 5-fluoro-D-glucose positron emission tomography (PET) demonstrates interictal hypoperfusion and hypometabolism in the affected side that is widely distributed, more intense in the Rolandic and temporo-insular regions, worsens with progression of the disease and may be abnormal at a stage when MRI is normal.[55] Ictally, there is regional hyperperfusion corresponding to the epileptogenic locus.[56]

ELECTROENCEPHALOGRAPHY

EEG may be normal initially, but gradually severe multifocal unilateral and later diffuse abnormalities appear.[30,57] Frequency, duration and intensity of clinical seizures are directly correlated with the abundance of interictal epileptiform activity on serial EEG.[50]

Background EEG and interictal spikes

The background EEG may be normal at the onset of the disease. Subsequent abnormalities consist of focal slow, usually high amplitude, delta waves, which gradually dominate in one hemisphere and often become bilateral with lateralised prevalence. Gradual disappearance and poverty of physiological rhythms (alpha, photic following, sleep spindles and drug-induced fast activity) in the affected side is the rule. Focal slow waves may appear prior to MRI abnormalities.[58]

Interictal epileptiform foci and paroxysms: Nearly all the EEGs show interictal spikes or sharp–slow waves. A single focus is rare. Multiple independent foci in the same hemisphere occur in 50% of patients and, in one-third, are bilateral with lateralised emphasis. Also, 50% of cases show bilateral synchronous discharges that are often bi-frontal, but also generalised. Again, they frequently predominate on the affected side.

Ictal EEG

The onset of ictal EEG patterns is variable. Exceptionally, they remain localised. Commonly, seizures have a multifocal onset either confined to one hemisphere or, less frequently, from one or the other side. The discharge appears to have higher amplitude in the secondarily involved hemisphere. Focal motor seizures may occur without concomitant EEG changes. Conversely, ictal EEG paroxysms may frequently occur without discernible clinical manifestations.[27,30,30,57]

Epilepsia partialis continua is notorious with regard to the lack of clinico-EEG correlations. The myoclonic jerks do not have a chronological relation with the interictal spikes.[27,30,30,57] It is exceptional to have jerks associated with EEG discharges.

Similarly, in electrocorticography, interictal epileptiform activity is widespread and the onset of seizures occurs in multiple independent sites.[57] Stereo-EEG correctly identifies the origin of the discharge and the clinico-EEG sequence.[25,59]

Evolution of EEG

As the disease progresses, the abnormalities tend to become bilateral. Background slow activity and poverty of physiological rhythms affect both hemispheres, epileptiform abnormalities become more widespread and multifocal, and also affect the contralateral hemisphere.

DIFFERENTIAL DIAGNOSIS

The diagnosis of Kozhevnikov-Rasmussen syndrome relies on:[60]

- progressive neurological deficit, mainly hemiparesis
- progressive hemispheric atrophy on brain imaging
- presence of oligoclonal or monoclonal banding on examination of CSF
- biopsy evidence of chronic encephalitis, in neurosurgical cases.

In the initial stages, the diagnosis is difficult, particularly in patients without epilepsia partialis continua. High resolution brain imaging is mandatory to exclude other more common causes of focal seizures, such as malformations of cortical development, brain tumours, tuberous sclerosis, vascular anomalies, parasitic diseases (e.g. cysticercosis) and other infectious disorders (see Table 12.2, page 405). An EEG is also mandatory at this stage as it may reveal functional spikes of Rolandic seizures or other ictal and interictal abnormalities that may suggest another epileptic syndrome. These tests are also important as baseline measurements for follow-up comparisons.

Other more serious diseases, such as mitochondrial encephalomyopathy, lactic acidosis and stroke-like episodes (MELAS), are less likely to cause diagnostic difficulties despite the high prevalence of epilepsia partialis continua. Acute encephalitis of any cause that leads to hemiplegia and seizures should also be apparent from the onset. In endemic areas, Russian spring-summer and other tick-borne encephalitides should also be considered in patients with *acute* onset of symptoms.

Despite these difficulties, according to a recent report,[14] the diagnosis was made within 4 months from the onset of the first symptoms and all cases had the following features: (a). refractory focal seizures with a predominant motor component; (b). slow focal activity on EEG contralateral to the motor manifestations; and (c). focal contralateral white matter hyperintensity with insular cortical atrophy on neuroimaging. Less constant or later findings were epilepsia partialis continua, oligoclonal bands and serum anti-GluR3 antibodies.[14]

PROGNOSIS

This is a progressive disorder of increasing seizure frequency and severity with the development of fixed neurological, mainly hemiplegia, and cognitive and language deficits ranging from mild to severe.[13,16]

MANAGEMENT

There is no effective treatment other than dramatic hemispherectomy, which appears to stop progression.[64-70] Focal resections are of no lasting benefit.

A variety of empirical treatments have been tried.[15]

Anti-epileptic medication is usually ineffective, though a reduction of secondarily GTCS may be achieved.[71]

Antiviral treatments, including the use of ganciclovir and zidovudine, produces no definite benefit.[15,72,73]

Corticosteroids (dexamethasone, prednisone) and adrenocorticotropin have no sustained benefit.[71]

High-dose steroids, other immunosuppressive treatments and immunomodulatory trials with immunoglobulins, alone or in combination, may arrest the disease temporarily, but relapse within a few months of the cessation of treatment is probably inevitable.[26,27,38,60,74,75] These treatments may be more effective if given in the early stage of the disease, before permanent neuronal damage and extreme derailment has occurred.

Leach et al. (1999)[76] advocated high-dose, long-term human intravenous immunoglobulin therapy based on their results in two patients with advanced adult-onset Rasmussen's encephalitis, throughout 1 year of treatment.

Plasmapheresis has produced dramatic but transient clinical improvements in some patients.[50] This may be useful in patients with status epilepticus and in the evaluation of patients prior to surgery, when residual function may be unmasked by the reduction in seizure frequency.[50]

Intraventricular alpha-interferon, because of its immunomodulating activity, has also been tried, but improvement is transient.[77,78]

Thalidomide has been recently used with minor improvement.[79]

Immunosuppression: Recently, 7 patients treated with the immunosuppressant tacrolimus had a superior outcome regarding neurological function and progression rate of cerebral hemiatrophy but no better seizure outcome in comparison with 12 untreated patients.[80] None of the treated patients, but 7 of 12 control patients, became eligible for hemispherectomy.

Surgical treatments

The current consensus is that limited focal resection is of little lasting benefit and that only functional hemispherectomy is a reasonable option. Hemispherectomy appears to arrest the disease process in the majority of patients at the expense of the consequent neurological deficits.[25,39,64-67,69,70]

HISTORICAL MISCONCEPTIONS [20]

The following misconceptions are inappropriately perpetuated in nearly all recent reports:

> Russian spring-summer tick-borne encephalitis, described by Kozhevnikov[15]
>
> Epilepsia partialis continua was first described by Kozhevnikov and is still known as Kozhevnikov's epilepsy in francophone countries. Omorokov then showed that it was due to spring-summer encephalitis.[19]

These are all incorrect because:

a. A Kozhevnikov (1894)[3] described a seizure/status *"epilepsia corticalis sive partialis continua"* (epilepsia partialis continua) that he attributed to a syndrome of *"chronic encephalitis"*:[3]

> "In recent years I happened to observe several cases of cortical epilepsy... that it may be called epilepsia corticalis sive partialis continua, in that here the convulsive manifestations were continuous... The question of the nature of the disease process is much more difficult.... in all cases the illness developed little by little and once it had developed persisted for a very long time, so that we can postulate only chronic processes here... Thus, of the chronic processes, encephalitis with transition to secondary hardening of the brain, or sclerosis cerebri, is almost the only possibility...Thus, not knowing precisely what we are dealing with, and proposing the presence of chronic encephalitis..."[3]

b. No one ever showed that Kozhevnikov's four patients had tick-borne encephalitis, an *acute* disease that was described in 1937;[34] 38 years after his death. Furthermore, only one of his four cases had acute illness *"in all cases the illness developed little by little"*.[3] What Omorokov found is that many of his own cases with epilepsia partialis continua (the seizure) in Siberia (Kozhevnikov was practising in Moscow) had acute encephalitis and a few had cysticercosis (see translation of the original report of Omorokov in ref [61]).

c. Kozhevnikov syndrome (type 1 and type 2) was already recognised in the two ILAE Classifications.[1,18] It was well cited around the world, including in the American literature from the beginning of the previous century.[62] Encephalitis as a definite cause of epilepsia partialis continua was confirmed in the Western literature.[24,62] For example, Wilson and Winkelman (1924)[62] described three cases with neuropathological confirmation and Dereux (1955),[24] in his thesis on *Le syndrome de Kojewnikow (epilepsie partialis continue),* described over 100 cases, many of which had chronic encephalitis.

However, it was Theodore Rasmussen,[63] the great neurosurgeon, who through painstaking work over many years established many aspects of what we now know about this devastating disease.[12] In his original article with J Olszewski and D Lloyd-Smith (1958)[4] on *Focal seizures due to chronic localized encephalitis,* he described three children with refractory focal seizures, progressive hemiparesis and cognitive impairment, and the pathological changes of chronic encephalitis. Hemispherectomy was beneficial in two cases, but limited resection was unhelpful. The pathological changes seen included perivascular cuffing, the presence of microglia, spongy degeneration and gliosis, limited to one cerebral hemisphere in the patient undergoing post-mortem examination. The conclusion was that "these three children were suffering from a chronic illness, producing focal seizures and gradually producing severe damage to one cerebral hemisphere. The histological appearance in each instance suggests the lesion is a chronic focal encephalitis. The aetiology is undetermined, but the suggestion is made that it may be viral in nature." The possible role of similar focal encephalitis-like processes in producing certain cases was raised.

Kozhevnikov-Rasmussen syndrome is the only proper nomenclature to honour both these great men, who independently described this epileptic syndrome of chronic encephalitis, half a century apart.

HEMICONVULSION-HEMIPLEGIA EPILEPSY SYNDROME

'Hemiconvulsion-hemiplegia syndrome' is a rare dramatic sequence comprising a sudden and prolonged unilateral clonic seizure, followed by permanent ipsilateral hemiplegia.[81-90] The event occurs suddenly in an otherwise normal child, often during a febrile illness. Subsequently, 80% of patients develop focal epilepsy of the complete *hemiconvulsion-hemiplegia-epilepsy syndrome*.

DEMOGRAPHIC DATA

Peak age onset occurs in the first 2 years of life (range of 5 months–4 years). This may be an extremely rare condition today, with improved emergency care for status epilepticus. There was only one (0.06%) equivocal case in the National Institute of Neurological and Communicative Disorders and Stroke Collaborative Perinatal Project in the USA.[91,92] Though Gastaut initially reported 150 cases,[81] the number of reported cases dramatically decreased in subsequent reports.[83,84,89]

CLINICAL MANIFESTATIONS

Hemiconvulsions occur suddenly out of the blue and consist of unilateral, often

Considerations on classification

The new ILAE diagnostic scheme[2] considers *'hemiconvulsion-hemiplegia epilepsy'* as a syndrome, though rightly it is not recognised as a separate epileptic syndrome in the 1989 ILAE classification.[1]

asynchronous, clonic jerks that last for hours or days if not appropriately treated. If very prolonged, convulsions may spread to the other side or more rarely change sides. Eye and head deviation may occur or may be the first seizure symptom. Consciousness may be intact.

By definition, severe ipsilateral post-convulsive flaccid hemiplegia follows in all cases. It lasts for more than 7 days and is permanent in more than 80% of cases. The face is always involved and aphasia is present if the dominant side is involved. These signs distinguish acquired post convulsive from congenital hemiplegia.[93]

AETIOLOGY

The initial hemiconvulsion-hemiplegia event usually occurs in the course of a febrile illness that is often due to a CNS infection, such as herpes encephalitis. In a few cases, the cause may be traumatic or vascular. Leiden Factor V mutation has been implicated in two cases.[94] Elevation of CSF interleukin-6 to levels seen in patients with encephalitis has been reported 2 hours after seizure onset in a child.[95] However, frequently no cause is found, though the family history may reveal a high incidence of febrile seizures.

DIAGNOSTIC PROCEDURES

Diagnostic procedures should include examination of CSF, which is probably mandatory in children less than 18 months of age in view of the high possibility of a CNS infection. Routine investigation for Leiden Factor V mutation has been suggested.[94] If possible, brain imaging should precede lumbar puncture. In the acute stage, there is usually evidence of oedema in the affected hemisphere. Later,

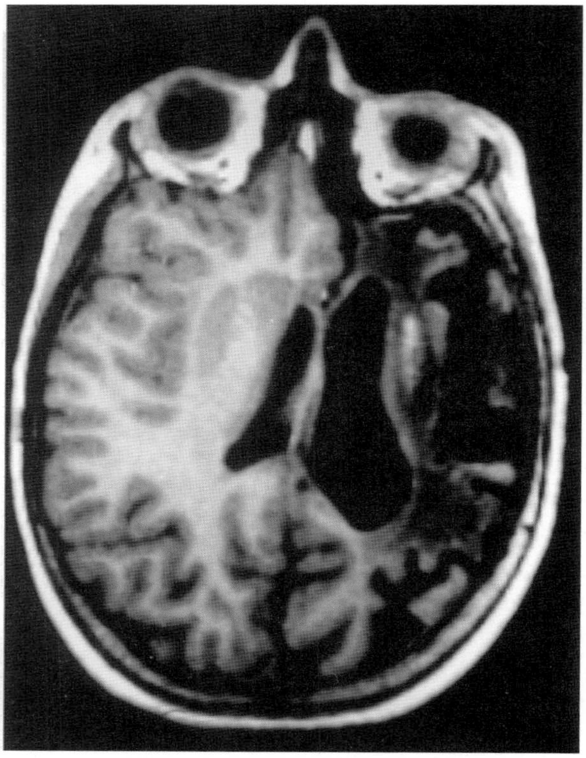

Figure 8.8 Brain MRI showing severe hemiatrophy in a patient with long-standing hemiconvulsion-hemiplegia-epilepsy syndrome.

Figure courtesy of Dr Rod C. Scott, Institute of Child Health, London, UK.

a rather characteristic, uniform hemiatrophy follows prolonged episodes (Figure 8.2). SPECT reveals hyperperfusion during the acute stage, followed later by hypoperfusion.[96]

ELECTROENCEPHALOGRAPHY[90,97]

EEG is not important in the acute stage, because it will simply confirm the clinical situation without offering any specific clues to the underlying cause and development.

Ictal EEG consists of a mixture of high amplitude rhythmical 2–3-Hz slow waves, intermixed with spikes, sharp waves, spike–wave complexes and episodic fast activity of 10–12 Hz. The amplitude is higher and spikes predominate in the affected hemisphere with posterior emphasis. There is no consistent relation between clonic convulsions and EEG discharges.

PROGNOSIS

The prognosis depends on the cause and speed of effective acute management. Focal seizures of temporal, extratemporal or multifocal origin appear within 1–5 years of the acute episode in 80% of patients. Most patients also have secondarily GTCS and often convulsive status epilepticus. Seizures are usually intractable to anti-epileptic medication. Learning difficulties are probably the rule.

MANAGEMENT

Immediate control of the seizure is a medical emergency as in status epilepticus. A benzodiazepine, usually intravenous diazepam or lorazepam, is probably the first choice. Treatment of the fever and the underlying illness is of equal importance. In the few cases with factor V Leiden mutation, careful consideration should be given to therapeutic and prophylactic anticoagulation, as this may improve long-term outcome.[94] Apart from conservative management of the residual neurological deficits, little can be done after the establishment of hemiplegia. Hemispherectomy may be very beneficial.

MIGRATING FOCAL SEIZURES OF INFANCY
MALIGNANT MIGRATING PARTIAL SEIZURES IN INFANCY

Migrating focal seizures of infancy[98-102] (synonym: malignant migrating partial seizures in infancy) is a devastating syndrome in development, with early onset of nearly continuous multifocal seizures arising independently from multiple regions of both hemispheres, and relentless psychomotor deterioration.[98-102]

DEMOGRAPHIC DATA

About 25 cases have been reported. Both sexes are equally affected. Age at onset is between the first day of life to 7 months of age (mean age 3 months).

CLINICAL MANIFESTATIONS

Seizures start without antecedent risk factors, and manifest with motor and autonomic symptoms, alone or combined. Lateral deviation of head and eyes, unilateral eyelid and eye jerking, and unilateral tonic or clonic convulsions of one limb are common motor manifestations that frequently progress to secondarily GTCS. Both sides are alternately affected. Autonomic manifestations of apnoea, cyanosis, flushing, hiccups, sweating and hypersalivation are striking and may not be recognised as seizure symptoms. The same patient has mild or severe, short or prolonged seizures and status epilepticus with a variable clinical expression and a polymorphous combination of ictal manifestations. Epileptic spasms are exceptional (one case).

Within a few weeks of onset, the seizures get relentlessly worse in frequency, duration and symptomatology. They usually occur in clusters, mainly on awakening and during drowsiness, and finally become virtually continuous.

AETIOLOGY

The aetiology is unknown. There is no family history of epilepsies or neurological disorders. In two cases, post-mortem brain pathology showed only severe hippocampal neuronal loss and accompanying gliosis, but this was normal in another case.[101]

DIAGNOSTIC PROCEDURES

CT and MRI brain scans are normal. Electroretinography and evoked potentials are normal.

The interictal EEG shows slow activity from the onset of the seizures, which becomes rapidly worse over time, with alternating side emphasis from one EEG to the next. Spikes are initially sparse, but soon become frequent and multifocal.

Ictal EEG discharges involve multiple independent sites randomly, moving from one cortical area to another in consecutive seizures. Morphologically, they consist of rhythmic alpha or theta activity, spreading to involve an increasing area of the cortical surface. Consecutive seizures overlap and the next seizure starts before the end of the previous one, with the topographical ictal onset markedly shifting from one area to another of the same or the other hemisphere.

PROGNOSIS

All children regress developmentally and develop severe psychomotor abnormalities. They become quadriplegic with major axial hypotonia, pyramidal and extrapyramidal signs, and athetosis.

Death often occurs soon after onset of the disease, within a year or rarely a few years. Control of the seizures and normal development is exceptional.

MANAGEMENT

Anti-epileptic drug treatment and ketogenic diet are ineffective.[103] Potassium bromide,[100] stiripentol combined with clonazepam[104] and, more recently, levetiracetam[85] has had a temporary beneficial effect in individual cases.

REFERENCES

1. Commission on Classification and Terminology of the International League Against Epilepsy. Proposal for revised classification of epilepsies and epileptic syndromes. *Epilepsia* 1989;**30**:389-99.
2. Engel J, Jr. A proposed diagnostic scheme for people with epileptic seizures and with epilepsy: Report of the ILAE Task Force on Classification and Terminology. *Epilepsia* 2001;**42**:796-803.
3. Kozhevnikov A Y. A peculiar type of cortical epilepsy (epilepsia corticalis sive partialis continua). *Miditsinskoe Obozreni* 1894;**42/14**:33-62. *Translated in English by DM Asher* . In Andermann F, ed. *Chronic encephalitis and epilepsy:Rasmussen's syndrome*, pp 245-61. Boston: Butterworth-Heinemann, 1991.
4. Rasmussen T, Olszweski J, Lloyd-Smith DL. Focal seizures due to chronic localized encephalitis. *Neurology* 1958;**8**:435-55.
5. Oguni H, Andermann F, Rasmussen TB. The natural history of the syndrome of chronic encephalitis and epilepsy: A study of the Montreal Neurological Institute series of forty-eight cases. In Andermann F, ed. *Chronic encephalitis and epilepsy:Rasmussen's syndrome*, pp 7-35. Boston: Butterworth-Heinemann, 1991.
6. Oguni H, Andermann F, Rasmussen TB. The syndrome of chronic encephalitis and epilepsy. A study based on the MNI series of 48 cases. *Adv Neurol* 1992;**57**:419-33.
7. Andermann,F. ed. Chronic encephalitis and epilepsy:Rasmussen's syndrome. Boston: Butterworth-Heinemann, 1991.
8. Cockerell OC, Rothwell J, Thompson PD, Marsden CD, Shorvon SD. Clinical and physiological features of epilepsia partialis continua. Cases ascertained in the UK. *Brain* 1996;**119 (Pt 2)**:393-407.
9. Bhatjiwale MG, Polkey C, Cox TC, Dean A, Deasy N. Rasmussen's encephalitis: neuroimaging findings in 21 patients with a closer look at the basal ganglia. *Pediatr Neurosurg.* 1998;**29**:142-8.
10. Aarli JA. Rasmussen's encephalitis: a challenge to neuroimmunology [editorial]. *Curr Opin Neurol* 2000;**13**:297-9.
11. Kaiboriboon K, Cortese C, Hogan RE. Magnetic resonance and positron emission tomography changes during the clinical progression of Rasmussen encephalitis. *J Neuroimaging* 2000;**10**:122-5.
12. Hart Y, Andermann F. Rasmussen's syndrome. In Roger J, Bureau M, Dravet C, Genton P, Tassinari CA, Wolf P, eds. *Epileptic syndromes in infancy, childhood and adolescence (3rd edn)*, pp 495-511. London: John Libbey & Co Ltd, 2002.
13. Bien CG, Widman G, Urbach H, Sassen R, Kuczaty S, Wiestler OD *et al.* The natural history of Rasmussen's encephalitis. *Brain* 2002;**125**:1751-9.
14. Granata T, Gobbi G, Spreafico R, Vigevano F, Capovilla G, Ragona F *et al.* Rasmussen's encephalitis: early characteristics allow diagnosis. *Neurology* 2003;**60**:422-5.
15. Andermann F, Hart Y. Rasmussen's syndrome. In Gilman S, ed. *Medlink Neurology*, San Diego SA: 2004.
16. Hart Y. Rasmussen's encephalitis. *Epilept Disord.* 2004;**6**:133-4.
17. Morse RP. Rasmussen encephalitis. *Arch Neurol.* 2004;**61**:592-4.
18. Commission on Classification and Terminology of the International League Against Epilepsy. Proposal for classification of epilepsy and epileptic syndromes. *Epilepsia* 1985;**26**: 268-78.
19. Andermann F, Rasmussen TB. Chronic encephalitis and epilepsy:an overview. In Andermann F, ed. *Chronic encephalitis and epilepsy:Rasmussen's syndrome*, pp 283-8. Boston: Butterworth-Heinemann, 1991.
20. Panayiotopoulos CP, Andermann F. Kozhevnikov-Rasmussen syndrome and the new proposal on classification. *Epilepsia* 2002;**43**:948-50.
21. Hart YM, Andermann F, Fish DR, Dubeau F, Robitaille Y, Rasmussen T *et al.* Chronic encephalitis and epilepsy in adults and adolescents: a variant of Rasmussen's syndrome? *Neurology* 1997;**48**:418-24.
22. Vadlamudi L, Galton CJ, Jeavons SJ, Tannenberg AE, Boyle RS. Rasmussen's syndrome in a 54 year old female: more support for an adult variant. *J Clin Neurosci.* 2000;**7**:154-6.
23. Dravet C, Genton P, Bureau M, Roger J. Kojewnikow's syndrome. In Wallace S, ed. *Epilepsy in Children*, pp 395-7. London: Chapman & Hall, 1996.
24. Dereux J. Le syndrome de Kojewnikow (epilepsie partialis continue). Paris: Thesis, 1955.
25. Bancaud J. Kojewnikow's syndrome (epilepsia partialis continua) in children. In Roger J, Bureau M, Dravet C, Dreifuss FE, Perret A, Wolf P, eds. *Epileptic syndromes in infancy, childhood and adolescence*, pp 363-74. London: John Libbey, 1992.
26. Chinchilla D, Dulac O, Robain O, Plouin P, Ponsot G, Pinel JF *et al.* Reappraisal of Rasmussen's syndrome with special emphasis on treatment with high doses of steroids. *J Neurol Neurosurg Psychiatry* 1994;**57**:1325-33.
27. Caraballo R, Tenembaum S, Cersosimo R, Pomata H, Medina C, Soprano AM *et al.* Rasmussen syndrome. *Rev Neurol* 1998;**26**:978-83.
28. Korn-Lubetzki I, Bien CG, Bauer J, Gomori M, Wiendl H, Trajo L *et al.* Rasmussen encephalitis with active inflammation and delayed seizures onset. *Neurology* 2004;**62**:984-6.
29. Antel JP,.Rasmussen T. Rasmussen's encephalitis and the new hat [editorial]. *Neurology* 1996;**46**:9-11.
30. Bancaud J. Kojewnikow's syndrome (epilepsia partialis continua) in children :Up-date. In Roger J, Bureau M, Dravet C, Dreifuss FE, Perret A, Wolf P, eds. *Epileptic syndromes in infancy, childhood and adolescence*, pp 374-9. London: John Libbey, 1992.
31. Robitaille Y. Neuropathological aspects of chronic encephalitis. In Andermann F, ed. *Chronic encephalitis and epilepsy:Rasmussen's syndrome*, pp 79-110. Boston: Butterworth-Heinemann, 1991.
32. Robitaille Y, Rasmussen T, Dubeau F, Tampieri D, Kemball K. Histopathology of nonneoplastic lesions in frontal lobe epilepsy. Review of 180 cases with recent MRI and PET correlations. *Adv Neurol* 1992;**57**:499-513.
33. Pardo CA, Vining EP, Guo L, Skolasky RL, Carson BS, Freeman JM. The pathology of Rasmussen syndrome: stages of cortical involvement and neuropathological studies in 45 hemispherectomies. *Epilepsia* 2004;**45**:516-26.
34. Asher DM, Gadjusek.D.C. Virologic studies in chronic encephalitis. In Andermann F, ed. *Chronic encephalitis and epilepsy:Rasmussen's syndrome*, pp 147-58. Boston: Butterworth-Heinemann, 1991.
35. Atkins MR, Terrell W, Hulette CM. Rasmussen's syndrome: a study of potential viral etiology. *Clin Neuropathol.* 1995;**14**:7-12.
36. Vinters HV, Wang R, Wiley CA. Herpesviruses in chronic encephalitis associated with intractable childhood epilepsy. *Hum Pathol.* 1993;**24**:871-9.
37. Andrews JM, Thompson JA, Pysher TJ, Walker ML, Hammond ME. Chronic encephalitis, epilepsy, and cerebrovascular immune complex deposits. *Ann Neurol* 1990;**28**:88-90.
38. Antozzi C, Granata T, Aurisano N, Zardini G, Confalonieri P, Airaghi G *et al.* Long-term selective IgG immuno-adsorption improves Rasmussen's encephalitis. *Neurology* 1998;**51**:302-5.
39. Rasmussen T. Further observations on the syndrome of chronic encephalitis and epilepsy. *Appl Neurophysiol.* 1978;**41**:1-12.
40. Farrell MA, Cheng L, Cornford ME, Grody WW, Vinters HV. Cytomegalovirus and Rasmussen's encephalitis. *Lancet* 1991;**337**:1551-2.
41. Rogers SW, Andrews PI, Gahring LC, Whisenand T, Cauley K, Crain B *et al.* Autoantibodies to glutamate receptor GluR3 in Rasmussen's encephalitis. *Science* 1994;**265**:648-51.
42. McNamara JO, Whitney KD, Andrews PI, He XP, Janumpalli S, Patel MN. Evidence for glutamate receptor autoimmunity in the pathogenesis of Rasmussen encephalitis. *Adv Neurol* 1999;**79**:543-50.
43. Twyman RE, Gahring LC, Spiess J, Rogers SW. Glutamate receptor antibodies activate a subset of receptors and reveal an agonist binding site. *Neuron* 1995;**14**:755-62.
44. Watson R, Jiang Y, Bermudez I, Houlihan L, Clover L, McKnight K *et al.* Absence of antibodies to glutamate receptor type 3 (GluR3) in Rasmussen encephalitis. *Neurology* 2004;**63**:43-50.
45. Whitney KD, Andrews PI, McNamara JO. Immunoglobulin G and complement immunoreactivity in the cerebral cortex of patients with Rasmussen's encephalitis. *Neurology* 1999;**53**:699-708.
46. Hart YM, Andermann F, Robitaille Y, Laxer KD, Rasmussen T, Davis R. Double pathology in Rasmussen's syndrome: a window on the etiology? *Neurology* 1998;**50**:731-5.
47. Yacubian EM, Rosemberg S, Marie SK, Valerio RM, Jorge CL, Cukiert A. Double pathology in Rasmussen's encephalitis: etiologic considerations. *Epilepsia* 1996;**37**:495-500.

48. Andermann E, Oguni H, Guttmann RD, Osterland SK, Antel JP, Eeg-Olofsson O *et al.* Genetic aspects of chronic encephalitis. In Andermann F, ed. *Chronic encephalitis and epilepsy:Rasmussen's syndrome*, pp 167-75. Boston: Butterworth-Heinemann, 1991.

49. Silver K, Andermann F, Meagher-Villemure K. Familial alternating epilepsia partialis continua with chronic encephalitis: another variant of Rasmussen syndrome? *Arch Neurol.* 1998;**55**:733-6.

50. Andrews PI, McNamara JO, Lewis DV. Clinical and electroencephalographic correlates in Rasmussen's encephalitis. *Epilepsia* 1997;**38**:189-94.

51. Geller E, Faerber EN, Legido A, Melvin JJ, Hunter JV, Wang Z *et al.* Rasmussen encephalitis: complementary role of multitechnique neuroimaging. *AJNR Am J Neuroradiol.* 1998;**19**:445-9.

52. Maeda Y, Oguni H, Saitou Y, Mutoh A, Imai K, Osawa M *et al.* Rasmussen syndrome: multifocal spread of inflammation suggested from MRI and PET findings. *Epilepsia* 2003;**44**:1118-21.

53. Turkdogan-Sozuer D, Ozek MM, Sav A, Dincer A, Pamir MN. Serial MRI and MRS studies with unusual findings in Rasmussen's encephalitis. *Eur Radiol.* 2000;**10**:962-6.

54. Wellard RM, Briellmann RS, Wilson JC, Kalnins RM, Anderson DP, Federico P *et al.* Longitudinal study of MRS metabolites in Rasmussen encephalitis. *Brain* 2004.

55. Lee JS, Juhasz C, Kaddurah AK, Chugani HT. Patterns of cerebral glucose metabolism in early and late stages of Rasmussen's syndrome. *J Child Neurol* 2001;**16**:798-805.

56. Paladin F, Capovilla G, Bonazza A, Mameli R. Utility of Tc 99m HMPAO SPECT in the early diagnosis of Rasmussen's syndrome. *Ital J Neurol Sci.* 1998;**19**:217-20.

57. So NK, Gloor P. Electroencephalographic and electrocorticographic findings in chronic encephalitis of Rasmussen type. In Andermann F, ed. *Chronic encephalitis and epilepsy:Rasmussen's syndrome*, pp 37-45. Boston: Butterworth-Heinemann, 1991.

58. Capovilla G, Paladin F, Bernardina BD. Rasmussen's syndrome: longitudinal EEG study from the first seizure to epilepsia partialis continua. *Epilepsia* 1997;**38**:483-8.

59. Chauvel P, Liegeois-Chauvel C, Marquis P, Bancaud J. Distinction between the myoclonus-related potential and the epileptic spike in epilepsia partialis continua. *Electroencephalogr Clin Neurophysiol.* 1986;**64**:304-7.

60. Hart YM, Cortez M, Andermann F, Hwang P, Fish DR, Dulac O *et al.* Medical treatment of Rasmussen's syndrome (chronic encephalitis and epilepsy): effect of high-dose steroids or immunoglobulins in 19 patients. *Neurology* 1994;**44**:1030-6.

61. Omorokov LI. Kozhevnikov's epilepsy in Siberia (1927) Translation in English by DM Asher. In Andermann F, ed. *Chronic encephalitis and epilepsy:Rasmussen's syndrome*, pp 263-9. Boston: Butterworth-Heinemann, 1991.

62. Wilson G, Winkelman NW. Partial continuous epilepsy with special reference to that produced by microscopic cortical lesions. *Arch Neurol Psychiat* 1924;**11**: 530-42.

63. Feindel W. Theodore Brown Rasmussen (1910-2002): epilepsy surgeon, scientist, and teacher. *J.Neurosurg.* 2003;**98**:631-7.

64. Villemure JG, Rasmussen T. Functional hemispherectomy in children. *Neuropediatrics* 1993;**24**:53-5.

65. Caplan R, Curtiss S, Chugani HT, Vinters HV. Pediatric Rasmussen encephalitis: social communication, language, PET and pathology before and after hemispherectomy. *Brain Cogn* 1996;**32**:45-66.

66. Vining EPG, Freeman JM, Pillas DJ, Uematsu S, Carson BS, Brandt J *et al.* Why Would You Remove Half a Brain? The Outcome of 58 Children After Hemispherectomy-The Johns Hopkins Experience: 1968 to 1996. *Pediatrics* 1997;**100**:163-71.

67. Devlin AM, Cross JH, Harkness W, Chong WK, Harding B, Vargha-Khadem F *et al.* Clinical outcomes of hemispherectomy for epilepsy in childhood and adolescence. *Brain* 2003;**126**:556-66.

68. Thomas P, Zifkin B, Ghetau G, Delalande O. Persistence of ictal activity after functional hemispherectomy in Rasmussen syndrome. *Neurology* 2003;**60**:140-2.

69. Cook SW, Nguyen ST, Hu B, Yudovin S, Shields WD, Vinters HV *et al.* Cerebral hemispherectomy in pediatric patients with epilepsy: comparison of three techniques by pathological substrate in 115 patients. *J.Neurosurg.* 2004;**100**:125-41.

70. Pulsifer MB, Brandt J, Salorio CF, Vining EP, Carson BS, Freeman JM. The cognitive outcome of hemispherectomy in 71 children. *Epilepsia* 2004;**45**:243-54.

71. Dubeau F, Sherwin A. Pharmacologic principles in the management of chronic focal encephalitis. In Andermann F, ed. *Chronic encephalitis and epilepsy:Rasmussen's syndrome*, pp 179-92. Boston: Butterworth-Heinemann, 1991.

72. McLachlan RS, Levin S, Blume WT. Treatment of Rasmussen's syndrome with ganciclovir. *Neurology* 1996;**47**:925-8.

73. DeToledo JC, Smith DB. Partially successful treatment of Rasmussen's encephalitis with zidovudine: symptomatic improvement followed by involvement of the contralateral hemisphere. *Epilepsia* 1994;**35**:352-5.

74. Dulac O. Rasmussen's syndrome. *Curr Opin Neurol* 1996;**9**:75-7.

75. Dulac O, Robain O, Chiron K, Plouin P, Pinnel JF, Vigevano F *et al.* High-dose steroid treatment of epilepsia partialis continua due to chronic focal encephalitis. In Andermann F, ed. *Chronic encephalitis and epilepsy:Rasmussen's syndrome*, pp 193-9. Boston: Butterworth-Heinemann, 1991.

76. Leach JP, Chadwick DW, Miles JB, Hart IK. Improvement in adult-onset Rasmussen's encephalitis with long- term immunomodulatory therapy. *Neurology* 1999;**52**:738-42.

77. Dabbagh O, Gascon G, Crowell J, Bamoggadam F. Intraventricular interferon-alpha stops seizures in Rasmussen's encephalitis: a case report. *Epilepsia* 1997;**38**:1045-9.

78. Maria BL, Ringdahl DM, Mickle JP, Smith LJ, Reuman PD, Gilmore RL *et al.* Intraventricular alpha interferon therapy for Rasmussen's syndrome. *Can J Neurol Sci.* 1993;**20**:333-6.

79. Marjanovic BD, Stojanov LM, Zdravkovic DS, Kravljanac RM, Djordjevic MS. Rasmussen syndrome and long-term response to thalidomide. *Pediat Neurol* 2003;**29**:151-6.

80. Bien CG, Gleissner U, Sassen R, Widman G, Urbach H, Elger CE. An open study of tacrolimus therapy in Rasmussen encephalitis. *Neurology* 2004;**62**:2106-9.

81. Gastaut H, BroughtonR. Epileptic seizures.Clinical and electrographic features,diagnosis and treatment. 1972. Illinois, Charles C Thomas.

82. Mori Y. Anatomopathology and pathogeny of the hemiconvulsion-hemiplegia-epilepsy syndrome. Part II. *J Neurosurg Sci.* 1979;**23**:1-22.

83. Salih MA, Kabiraj M, Al Jarallah AS, El Desouki M, Othman S, Palkar VA. Hemiconvulsion-hemiplegia-epilepsy syndrome. A clinical, electroencephalographic and neuroradiological study. *Childs Nerv Syst.* 1997;**13**:257-63.

84. Roger J, Dravet C, Bureau M. Unilateral seizures: hemiconvulsions-hemiplegia syndrome (HH) and hemiconvulsions-hemiplegia-epilepsy syndrome (HHE). *Electroencephalogr Clin Neurophysiol.Suppl* 1982;211-21.

85. Kadhim H, Nassogne MC, Bonnier C, van Rijckevorsel K. Migrating partial seizures in infancy: first report on a positive response to levetiracetam in youngest patient. *Epilepsia* 2004;**45 (Suppl 3)**:204.

86. Kataoka K, Okuno T, Mikawa H, Hojo H. Cranial computed tomographic and electroencephalographic abnormalities in children with post-hemiconvulsive hemiplegia. *Eur Neurol* 1988;**28**:279-84.

87. Blume WT, Luders HO, Mizrahi E, Tassinari C, van Emde BW, Engel J, Jr. Glossary of descriptive terminology for ictal semiology: report of the ILAE task force on classification and terminology. *Epilepsia* 2001;**42**:1212-8.

88. Freeman JL, Coleman LT, Smith LJ, Shield LK. Hemiconvulsion-hemiplegia-epilepsy syndrome: characteristic early magnetic resonance imaging findings. *J Child Neurol.* 2002;**17**:10-6.

89. Herbst F, Heckmann M, Reiss I, Hugens-Penzel M, Gortner L, Neubauer B. Hemiconvulsion-Hemiplegia-Epilepsy-Syndrome (HHE). *Klin Padiatr.* 2002;**214**:126-7.

90. Arzimanoglou A, Dravet C. Hemiconvulsion-hemiplegia syndrome. In Gilman S, ed. *Medlink Neurology*, San Diego SA: Arbor Publishing Corp, 2004

91. Nelson KB, Ellenberg JH. Predictors of epilepsy in children who have experienced febrile seizures. *NEJM* 1976;**295**:1029-33.

92. Nelson KB, Ellenberg JH. Prognosis in children with febrile seizures. *Pediatrics* 1978;**61**:720-7.

93. Aicardi J. Epilepsy in Children. New York: Raven Press, 1994.
94. Scantlebury MH, David M, Carmant L. Association between factor V Leiden mutation and the hemiconvulsion, hemiplegia, and epilepsy syndrome: report of two cases. *J Child Neurol* 2002;**17**:713-7.
95. Kimura M, Tasaka M, Sejima H, Takusa Y, Ichiyama T, Yamaguchi S. Hemiconvulsion-hemiplegia syndrome and elevated interleukin-6: case report. *J Child Neurol* 2002;**17**:705-7.
96. Tanaka Y, Nakanishi Y, Hamano S, Nara T, Aihara T. Brain perfusion in acute infantile hemiplegia studied with single photon emission computed tomography. *No To Hattatsu* 1994;**26**:68-73.
97. Vigouroux M. EEG study of hemiconvulsions followed by hemiplegia (the hemiconvulsion-hemiplegia syndrome) & its epileptic sequelae (the hemiconvulsion-hemiplegiaepilepsy syndrome). *Rev.Neurol (Paris)* 1958;**99**:39-53.
98. Coppola G, Plouin P, Chiron C, Robain O, Dulac O. Migrating partial seizures in infancy: a malignant disorder with developmental arrest. *Epilepsia* 1995;**36**:1017-24.
99. Guerrini R, Dravet C. Severe epileptic encephalopathies of infancy, other than the West syndrome. In Engel JJr, Pedley TA, eds. *Epilepsy: A Comprehensive Textbook.*, pp 2285-302. Philadelphia: Lippincott-Raven Publishers, 1997.
100. Okuda K, Yasuhara A, Kamei A, Araki A, Kitamura N, Kobayashi Y. Successful control with bromide of two patients with malignant migrating partial seizures in infancy. *Brain Dev.* 2000;**22**:56-9.
101. Wilmshurst JM, Appleton DB, Grattan-Smith PJ. Migrating partial seizures in infancy: two new cases. *J Child Neurol* 2000;**15**:717-22.
102. Dulac O. Malignant migrating partial seizures in infancy. In Roger J, Bureau M, Dravet C, Genton P, Tassinari CA, Wolf P, eds. *Epileptic syndromes in infancy, childhood and adolescence (3rd edn)*, pp 65-8. London: John Libbey & Co Ltd, 2002.
103. Francois LL, Manel V, Rousselle C, David M. Ketogenic regime as anti-epileptic treatment: its use in 29 epileptic children. *Arch Pediatr.* 2003;**10**:300-6.
104. Perez J, Chiron C, Musial C, Rey E, Blehaut H, D'Athis P *et al.* Stiripentol: efficacy and tolerability in children with epilepsy. *Epilepsia* 1999;**40**:1618-26.

BENIGN CHILDHOOD FOCAL SEIZURES AND RELATED EPILEPTIC SYNDROMES

BENIGN CHILDHOOD SEIZURE SUSCEPTIBILITY SYNDROME

Benign childhood focal seizures and related epileptic syndromes are the commonest and probably the most fascinating and rewarding topic in paediatric epileptology.[1] They affect 25% of children with non-febrile seizures and form a significant part of the everyday practice of paediatricians, neurologists and clinical neurophysiologists who care for children with seizures. Rolandic seizures (RS) are widely recognised and are associated with an excellent prognosis thanks to appropriate research and publications. Paediatricians have been receptive to and have made excellent use of this knowledge. Panayiotopoulos syndrome (PS), a common disorder with dramatic clinical and EEG manifestations, eluded us until recently. PS has now been formally recognised in the new ILAE diagnostic scheme and is becoming more readily diagnosed by physicians. Less common phenotypes, such as the

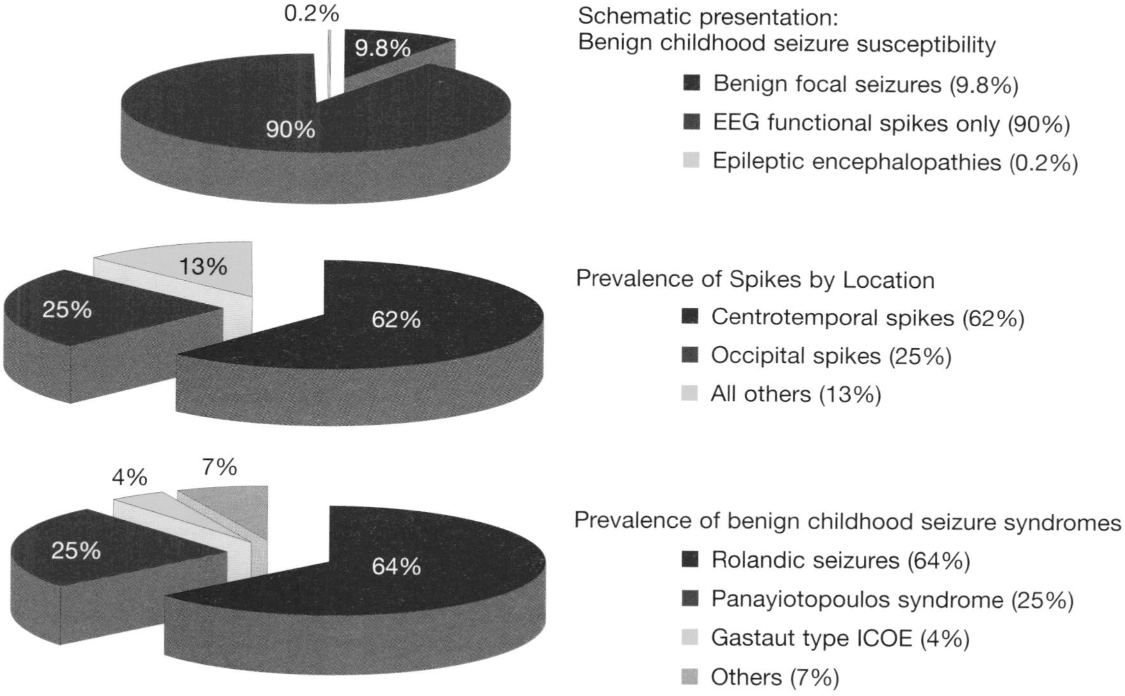

Figure 9.1 Schematic presentation of benign childhood seizure susceptibility syndrome.*

Top: Over 90% of functional spikes are clinically silent.
Middle: Prevalence of functional spikes by location. Centrotemporal spikes predominate followed by occipital spikes.
Bottom: Rolandic seizures (64%) are 2.5 times more common than PS (25%), but this figure may change with increasing awareness of PS and the inclusion of less typical cases.
*The percentages are approximate estimations from available relevant clinical and EEG data on the prevalence of clinical phenotypes of benign childhood focal seizures and functional spikes in childhood.[1;4]

Considerations on nomenclature

These are detailed in the individual description of each of these benign childhood focal syndromes. Overall, benign childhood focal syndromes and their main representatives, BCECTS and PS, do not fulfil the diagnostic criteria of *'epilepsy'* defined as *"chronic neurological condition characterised by recurrent epileptic seizures"*.[3] BCECTS and PS are age-limited (not *"chronic"*) and at least one-third of patients have a single (not *"recurrent"*) seizure. They should be classified among *"Conditions with epileptic seizures that do not require a diagnosis of epilepsy"*, which is a new concept in the ILAE diagnostic scheme to incorporate "febrile, benign neonatal, single seizures or isolated clusters of seizures and rarely repeated seizures (oligoepilepsy)" (Table 1.7).[2]

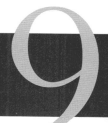

Gastaut type-idiopathic childhood occipital epilepsy (G-ICOE) and idiopathic photosensitive occipital lobe epilepsy have also been recognised and defined. Furthermore, there are also children who manifest with seizures of predominantly affective symptoms, and there are claims of other benign childhood seizures associated with certain interictal EEG foci, such as frontal, midline or parietal, with or without extreme somatosensory evoked spikes.

It should also be emphasised that functional spikes of whatever location occur in 2–4% of children with or without seizures including apparently normal children without seizures and even more often children with non-epileptic neurological or medical disorders. (Figure 9.1).[1]

All these conditions may be linked together in a broad age-related and age-limited benign childhood seizure susceptibility syndrome (BCSSS), which may also constitute a biological continuum with febrile seizures and benign infantile and neonatal seizures. It is my thesis that the clinical, EEG, pathophysiological and management aspects of BCSSS should be properly re-examined and redefined.
The 1989 ILAE classification recognised three "age-related and localization-related (focal, local, partial) epilepsies and syndromes" (Table 1.5):

- **Benign childhood epilepsy with centrotemporal spikes (BCECTS)**
- **Childhood epilepsy with occipital paroxysms (Gastaut type)**
- **Primary reading epilepsy**

The new diagnostic scheme rightly reclassified "reading epilepsy" as a reflex epileptic syndrome (Table 1.7) and recognised three syndromes of "idiopathic childhood focal epilepsy":[2]

- **Benign childhood epilepsy with centrotemporal spikes**
- **Early onset benign childhood occipital epilepsy (Panayiotopoulos type)**
- **Late onset childhood occipital epilepsy (Gastaut type)**

BENIGN CHILDHOOD EPILEPSY WITH CENTROTEMPORAL SPIKES

ROLANDIC SEIZURES

Benign childhood epilepsy with centrotemporal spikes [1;5-12] or Rolandic seizures/epilepsy is the commonest manifestation of a childhood seizure susceptibility syndrome that is age related and genetically determined.

This chapter is based on an exhaustive review of the literature regarding all aspects of Rolandic seizures and their EEG manifestations.[1] The history of the 'discovery of benign Rolandic epilepsy' has been vividly described by the main French protagonists Marc Beaussart and Pierre Loiseau.[9]

DEMOGRAPHIC DATA

Onset of RS is between 1 and 14 years; in 75% of patients, onset is between 7 and 10 years, and there is a peak at 8–9 years.[1;7] There is a 1.5 male predominance. Prevalence is around 15% in children with seizures aged 1–15 years. Incidence is 10–20/100,000 children aged 0–15 years.[1]

CLINICAL MANIFESTATIONS

The cardinal features of RS are infrequent, often single, focal seizures consisting of unilateral facial sensorimotor symptoms, oro-pharyngo-laryngeal (OPL) manifestations, speech arrest and hypersalivation.[1]

Hemifacial sensorimotor seizures occur in approximately one-third of patients. These are mainly motor seizures, which may be entirely localised in the lower lip manifesting with sudden, continuous or bursts of clonic contractions, usually lasting from a few seconds to 1 minute. Ipsilateral tonic deviation of the mouth is also common. More rarely, hemifacial convulsions may appear nearly simultaneously or spread to the ipsilateral upper extremity. Involvement of the leg is rare.

Hemifacial sensory seizures are less common and consist of numbness in the corner of the mouth.

Consciousness is usually preserved.

Hemifacial sensorimotor symptoms may be the only ictal manifestations, but are often associated with an inability to speak and hypersalivation.

> The left side of my mouth felt numb and started jerking and pulling to the left, and I could not speak to say what was happening to me.

Oro-pharyngo-laryngeal ictal manifestations, which occur in more than half of seizures (53%), are the most characteristic of all other ictal symptoms of RS. They consist of unilateral sensory and motor manifestations inside the mouth, tongue, inner cheek, gums, teeth and pharyngo-laryngeal regions. Sensory symptoms manifest with unilateral numbness and more commonly paraesthesias (tingling, prickling, freezing and their variations), and are usually diffuse on one side or, exceptionally, may be highly localised to even one tooth. Motor OPL symptoms produce strange sounds, such as death rattle, gargling, grunting, guttural sounds and their combinations.

> In his sleep, he was making guttural noises, with his mouth pulled to the right, "as if he was chewing his tongue".

> We heard her making strange noises "like roaring" and found her unresponsive, head raised from the pillow, eyes wide open, rivers of saliva coming out of her mouth, rigid.

Arrest of speech is another common ictal symptom that occurs in more than 40% of RS. The child is inarticulate and attempts to communicate with gestures. A few mainly laryngeal sounds, not words, may be uttered, particularly at the beginning.

LAE classification and considerations on omenclature

enign childhood epilepsy with centrotemporal spikes (best nown among paediatricians as Rolandic epilepsy) is defined by he ILAE as follows:[13]

Benign childhood epilepsy with centrotemporal spikes is a yndrome of brief, simple, partial, hemifacial motor seizures, equently having associated somatosensory symptoms which ave a tendency to evolve into generalised tonic clonic eizures. Both seizure types are often related to sleep. Onset ccurs between the ages of 3 and 13 years (peak 9–10 years) nd recovery occurs before the age of 15–16 years. Genetic redisposition is common, and there is a male predominance. he EEG has blunt high-voltage centrotemporal spikes, often ollowed by slow waves that are activated by sleep and tend to hift or spread from side to side." [13]

he following should be considered in future revisions of the lassification of BCECTS:

a). Most of centrotemporal spikes are, in fact, Rolandic spikes; hey are rarely located in the temporal electrodes

b). The word 'temporal' is misleading because these children o not have symptoms from the temporal lobes

c). BCECTS may occur without centrotemporal spikes and onversely centrotemporal spikes may occur in children without seizures or other clinical phenotypes of benign childhood seizure susceptibility syndrome

(d). Similar clinical features may appear in patients with spikes in other than centrotemporal locations

(e). Children with centrotemporal spikes may manifest with symptoms typical of PS.[14]

Rolandic seizures/epilepsy may be the most appropriate nomenclature. Rolandic epilepsy is very well established and well identified by neurologists, neurophysiologists and paediatricians with this form of benign childhood focal seizures. They all understand it as a benign seizure syndrome of children with ictal symptoms, originating from a well-known anatomical region of the brain, the inferior part of the pre-and post-central gyrus.

Rolandic fissure (or central fissure) is a well-established anatomical name that can not change, though the central (or Rolandic) sulcus was probably first described by the French anatomist Vicq d'Azy and not by the Italian anatomist Luigi Rolando.[15] Also, epileptic symptoms do not come from the Rolandic (central) fissure, but from the pre- and post-central gyrus.[15]

In this book I use BCECTS, Rolandic seizures or Rolandic epilepsy synomymously though I would prefer the term Rolandic seizures.

There is no impairment of the cortical language mechanisms. The child is perfectly able to understand what is being said, but unable to utter a single intelligible word. Some authors call this *aphemia* or *aphonia*. However, *aphemia* means motor aphasia or pure word mutism and does not appear to be correct, and *aphonia* is an inability to produce sounds by laryngeal mechanisms, which also does not appear to be the case in RS. The arrest of speech in RS is more of an *anarthria,* that is loss of the power and coordination for the articulation of words, which also explains why this is equally common in left or right sided RS.

> My right hand was numb and stiff. My mouth opened and I could not speak. I wanted to say I can not speak. At the same time, it was as if somebody was strangling me.

> She was trying to speak but only noises came out of her mouth as if her tongue was tied up in her mouth.

Some RS patients are dysarthric rather than anarthic that is they were able to pronounce some words but with difficulty as:

> if there are stones in my mouth.

Hypersalivation is one of the most characteristic ictal symptoms of RS and probably occurs in as many as one-third of cases. It is often associated with OPL symptoms, but is also associated with pure hemifacial seizures and may be the most pronounced ictal manifestation. Hypersalivation is not just frothing:

> Suddenly my mouth is full of saliva, it runs out like a river and I can not speak.

Ictal syncope may occur probably as a concurrent symptom of PS (page 237).

> She lies there, unconscious with no movements, no convulsions, like a wax work, no life.

Consciousness is fully retained in more than half (58%) of RS and the patient is able to describe the events after the end of the fits well.

> I felt that air was forced into my mouth, I could not speak and I could not close my mouth. I could understand well everything said to me. Other times I feel that there is food in my mouth and there is also a lot of salivation. I can not speak.

Secondarily GTCS are reported in between one- and two-thirds of children with RS. Primarily GTCS are not part of the syndrome of RS.

Duration of RS is usually brief, lasting for 1–2 min, but may become longer if seizures progress to convulsions.

Circadian distribution. Three-quarters of seizures occur during non-REM sleep, mainly at sleep onset or just before awakening. Seizures during sleep are usually longer and may progress to GTCS, which rarely occurs during wakefulness.

STATUS EPILEPTICUS

Generalised convulsive status epilepticus is exceptional. Though rare, focal motor status epilepticus[16] and hemiconvulsive status epilepticus are more likely to occur.

> While skating, he felt that the left side of his tongue was numb and that he could not see well. This was followed within seconds by repetitive and continuous left-sided clonic hemifacial spasms, involving the mouth and eye that ended 40 min later with left hemiconvulsions. There was postictal Todd's paralysis.

Hemiconvulsive status epilepticus may be more common in children aged 2–5 years; this is often associated with postictal Todd's paralysis, which generally does not include the face.[12;16]

Opercular status epilepticus usually occurs in atypical evolutions of BCECTS.[12;17-21] or exceptionally it may be carbamazepine-induced.[22;23] These are often associated with EEG continuous spikes and waves during slow-wave sleep (page 183). The status may last for hours to months and consists of continuous unilateral or bilateral contractions of the mouth, tongue or eyelids, positive or negative subtle perioral or other myoclonia, dysarthria, anarthria or speech arrest, difficulties in swallowing, buccofacial apraxia and hypersalivation.

AETIOLOGY

Benign childhood epilepsy with centrotemporal spikes is genetically determined and there is evidence of linkage with chromosome 15q14[24]. The mode of inheritance is unknown. Autosomal dominant inheritance with age-dependent penetrance refers to the EEG centrotemporal spikes, and not to the clinical syndrome of BCECTS (see review in ref [1]).[25;26] A multifactorial pathogenesis with hereditary impairment of brain maturation has been proposed by Doose and associates.[27] However, according to a recent study conventional genetic influences may be less important than other mechanisms, which need to be explored.[28] This study compared the concordance of twins with Rolandic epilepsy with the concordance of a twin sample of IGEs. All eight twins (six monozygous and two dizygous) with RS were discordant.[28] Monozygous pairwise concordance was 0 (95% confidence interval, 0-0.4) for Rolandic epilepsy compared with 0.7 (95% confidence interval, 0.5-0.9) for 26 IGE monozygous pairs.[28]

Siblings or parents of patients with BCECTS may rarely have the same type of seizures or other phenotypes of BCSSS, such as PS (page 240). Febrile seizures are common (10–20%) prior to RS.

My view that RS are part of a BCSSS is detailed on page 262.[1;29] All these benign childhood conditions are linked together through a common, genetically determined, mild and reversible, functional derangement of the brain cortical maturational process.[1;29]

PATHOPHYSIOLOGY

The ictal manifestations of RS agree well with the symptoms elicited by electrical stimulation of the lower part of the precentral and postcentral gyrus in man.[30]

Hypersalivation, like other autonomic manifestations in childhood focal seizures, is difficult to explain; it is extremely rare in adults.

DIAGNOSTIC PROCEDURES

Apart from the EEG, all tests are normal.

Brain imaging is not needed when the diagnosis of RS is certain though 15% of patients with RS may have abnormal findings because of static or other brain diseases unrelated to the pathophysiology of RS[31]. Further, hippocampal abnormalities have been detected in some children with RS on MRI and proton magnetic resonance spectroscopy [32] which may be incompatible with such an age-related and benign seizure disorder.

The presence of brain lesions has no influence on the prognosis of RS.[31.]

INTERICTAL EEG

Centrotemporal spikes are the hallmark of the syndrome of BCECTS (Figures 9.2, 9.3, 9.4 and 9.5). They are characterised by their morphology, amplitude and duration, location and field distribution, frequency and pattern of occurrence, reactivity to external stimuli and the sleep-wake cycle, as well as age-dependence and evolution.

Although called centrotemporal spikes, these are mainly high amplitude sharp and slow wave complexes localised in the C3/C4 (central) or C5/C6 (midway between central and temporal) electrodes (Figure 9.3).[35] The main spike (sharp wave) component is diphasic with a maximum surface, negative, rounded peak that is followed by a smaller positive peak (Figure 9.2). This is followed by a negative or negative-positive slow wave. A relatively minute positive spike often precedes this spike–slow wave complex (Figure 9.2). The amplitude of the main spike (or sharp wave) component often exceeds 200 μV, though it may be much smaller or much higher. The negative phase is larger than the positive phase of the spike, as well as the preceding or following components of the spike–slow wave complex. CTS may be unilateral, but are more often bilateral, independently right or left. They are abundant (4–20/min) and usually occur in clusters.

CTS increase during stages I-IV of sleep by a factor of 2-5 times without disturbing the sleep organisation (Figure 9.2).

Rarely, children with RS may have a normal EEG, the spikes may be very small or CTS appear only during sleep stages (3-35%).[1] In serial EEG, CTS may appear right or left, infrequent or abundant, small or giant, alone or with functional spikes in other locations.

In this book, I comply with the nomenclature "centrotemporal spikes", though they are rarely temporal; "Rolandic spikes" or simply "central spikes" would be a more accurate name (see Figure 9.3).

Dipoles of centrotemporal spikes

The main negative spike component of CTS can usually be modelled by a single and stable tangential dipole source along the Rolandic region, with the negative pole maximum in the centrotemporal region and the positive pole maximum in the frontal regions (Figure 9.3).[36-39] The tangential dipole and the location of CTS have been confirmed with magnetoencephalography.[40;41]

Concurrent spikes in locations other than the centrotemporal region

CTS may occur simultaneously in the same EEG with morphologically similar sharp and slow waves in other locations, such as the midline, parietal, frontal and occipital regions.[1] These multifocal sharp waves are more frequently seen in serial EEGs. Occipital spikes are usually the first to appear.

The frequency, location and persistence of CTS do not determine the clinical manifestations, severity and frequency of seizures or the prognosis.

Centrotemporal spikes in normal and children without Rolandic seizures

CTS occur in 2–3% of normal school-age children, of whom less than 10% develop RS.[1;42-45] CTS are age-dependent, appearing at a peak age of 7–10 years, often persisting despite clinical remission, and usually disappearing before the age of 16 years. They are common among relatives of children with RS. Age-dependent CTS frequently occur in a variety of organic brain diseases with or without seizures, such as cerebral tumours, Rett syndrome, fragile X syndrome and focal cortical dysplasia. Furthermore, CTS may incidentally be found in non-epileptic children with various symptoms, such as headache (Figure 9.4), speech, behavioural and learning difficulties.

Definitions[33]

Sharp wave: A transient, clearly distinguished from background activity, with pointed peak at conventional paper speeds and duration of 70-200 ms i.e. over 1/14-1/5 s approximately. The main component is generally negative relative to other areas. Amplitude is variable. [33]

Spike: A transient, clearly distinguished from background activity, with pointed peak at conventional paper speeds and duration of 20 to under 70 ms i.e. over 1/50-1/14 s approximately. The main component is generally negative relative to other areas. Amplitude is variable. [33]

According to the above definition what we call centrotemporal spikes are centrotemporal sharp waves because their duration is usually more than 70 ms.

Niedermeyer explained: "EEG spikes should be differentiated from sharp waves (i.e. transients having similar characteristics but longer duration). However, it is well to keep in mind that that this distinction is largely arbitrary and serves primarily descriptive purposes. It is certainly not incorrect to use the term 'spike' and 'sharp wave' synonymously when a local paroxysmal event is discussed, although purists of nomenclature would regard this as a breach of etiquette."[34]

Extreme somatosensory evoked potentials/spikes

After sleep, the most common form of activation of CTS (10%–20%) is somatosensory stimulation mainly of the fingers or toes (Figures 9.2 and 9.4).[1;46-53] These are called extreme somatosensory evoked spikes (ESES), extreme somatosensory evoked potentials or giant somatosensory evoked spikes. Like normal somatosensory evoked potentials, their location depends on the site and side of stimulation (Figures 9.2 and 9.4), but their size and morphology is identical to that of CTS. ESES correspond to mid- or long-latency somatosensory evoked potentials with peaks at 35–80 ms depending on the height of the individual and the site of the stimulation (Figure 9.2). ESES persist during sleep. ESES, like

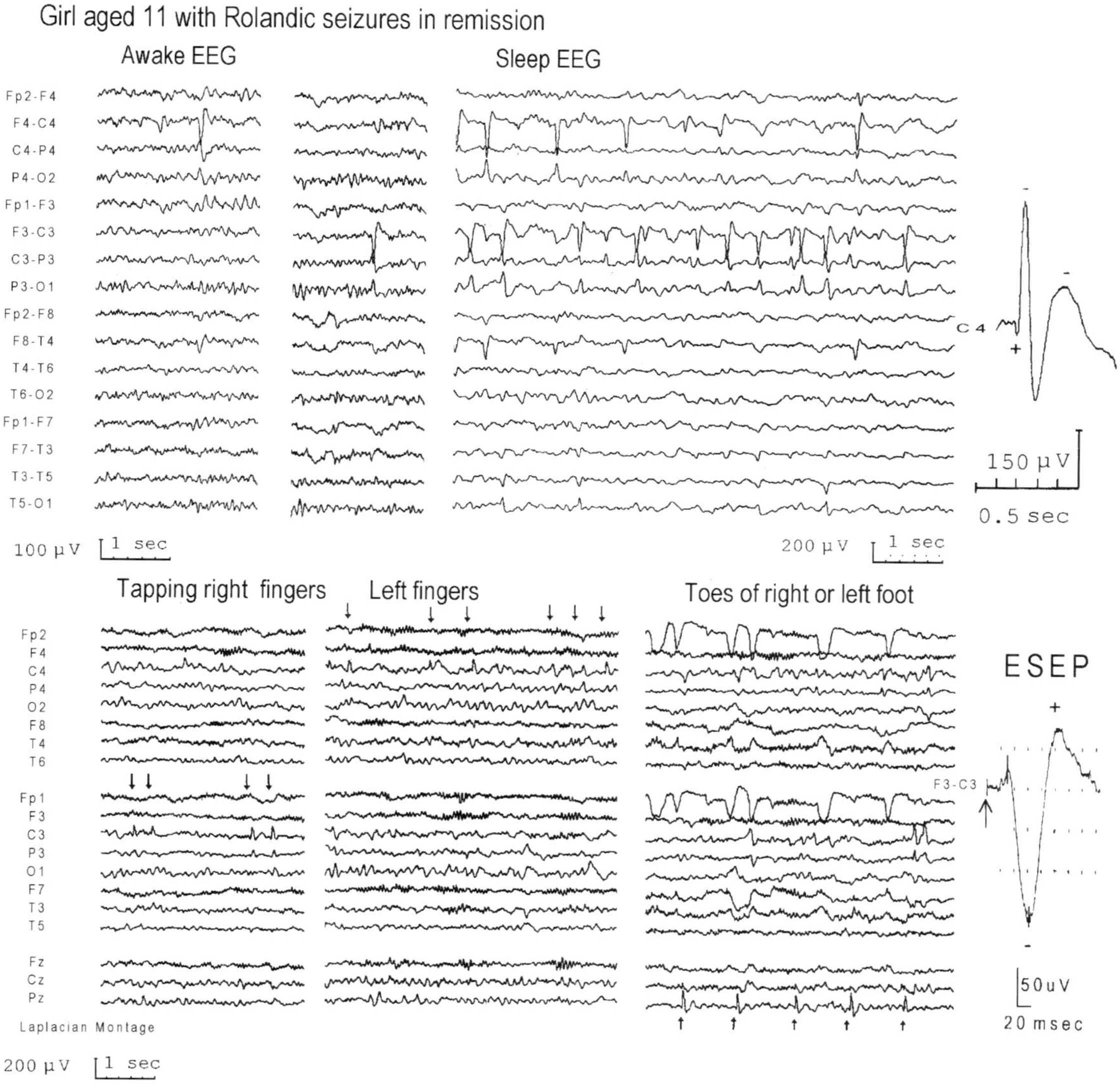

Figure 9.2 Video EEG of an 11-year-old girl with Rolandic seizures who has been in remission since the age of 8 years.

Top: High amplitude centrotemporal spikes (in fact these are central spikes) occur independently on the right or left, and are markedly exaggerated during natural sleep.
Top extreme right: Typical morphology and polarity of CTS in Laplacian montage.
Bottom: ESES, which are evoked by tapping fingers or toes. Note that their location corresponds to the location of the activating stimulus.
Bottom extreme right: ESES from another patient, which were evoked by electrical stimulation of the right thumb (onset at arrow). Peak latency of the somatosensory spike is 58 ms.

spontaneous CTS, occur in children with or without seizures and disappear with age. They may be detected in EEGs with or without spontaneous CTS or other functional spikes of childhood.

Techniques to elicit extreme somatosensory evoked spikes

Any type of mechanical or electrical stimulus can elicit ESES in susceptible children providing that it is properly applied. It must be abrupt and strong enough (without being uncomfortable), and delivered to the appropriate sensitive body region. Percussion of the distal parts of the legs (toes and heels) or arms (palms and mainly tips of fingers) with a reflex hammer or with the plantar tips of the examiner's fingers is very effective in eliciting ESES (Figure 9.2). A hammer can also be connected to a channel of the EEG in order to mark the exact timing of the stimulus and measure the latency of the evoked spike. Electrical stimulation with digital electrodes as in orthodromic sensory nerve testing, or electrical stimulation of the nerve as in antidromic sensory nerve testing, is equally effective for eliciting ESES, but this is used only for research purposes (Figure 9.2).[49;50] It may not be necessary for routine EEG, because it is no more efficient than the mechanical stimulation described above, which is a more child-friendly method.

In clinical EEG practice, asking the child to tap together the palmar surface of the tips of his/her fingers of both hands is an easy method of testing for ESES (Figure 9.4). The child should be instructed to strike them with sufficient strength and at random intervals of varying frequency. This may elicit either bilateral or unilateral ESES (Figure 9.4).

Generalised discharges

The reported prevalence of generalised discharges in RS varies from as low as 0% to as high as 54%.[1] In my studies, generalised discharges occurred in about 4% of patients with RS and consisted of brief 1–3 s generalised bursts of 3–5 Hz slow waves intermixed with small spikes.[1] These brief generalised discharges are identical to those seen in PS (Figure 9.6, page 242).

The combination of a normal child with infrequent seizures and an EEG showing disproportionately severe focal epileptogenic activity is highly suggestive of benign childhood seizure susceptibility syndrome.[1]

ICTAL EEG

There are very few reports of ictal EEG of RS. One example captured with video EEG is shown in Figure 9.5.[1] There is an initial paucity of spontaneous CTS prior to the onset of the ictal discharge, which appears in the ipsilateral Rolandic regions and consists of slow waves intermixed with fast rhythms and spikes.

EVOLUTION AND PROGNOSIS

Remission occurs within 2–4 years of onset and before the age 16 years. The total number of seizures is low. The majority of patients have less than 10 seizures; 10-20% have a single seizure only. Around 10–20% may have frequent seizures, but these also remit with age.

Figure 9.3 Centrotemporal spikes are mainly Rolandic not temporal spikes.[1;35] Facing page

Top, middle and bottom: The same EEG sample is shown in 3 different montages.

This is from an 8-year-old boy referred for an EEG because of "recent GTCS and a 2-year history of unilateral facial spasms. Previously, the EEG and CT brain scan were normal. No medication. Focal seizures with secondarily generalised convulsions?"

The EEG showed frequent clusters of repetitive centrotemporal spikes on the left. Because the spikes appeared to be of higher amplitude in the temporal electrode (T3) (black arrows), the technologist rightly applied additional electrodes at C5 and C6 (Rolandic localisation). This showed that the spike is of higher amplitude in the left Rolandic region (C5) (open arrows).

Another EEG 16 months later, showed a few small spikes in the right frontal and central midline electrodes.

Boy aged 8 with Rolandic seizures- Spikes are Rolandic not Centrotemporal

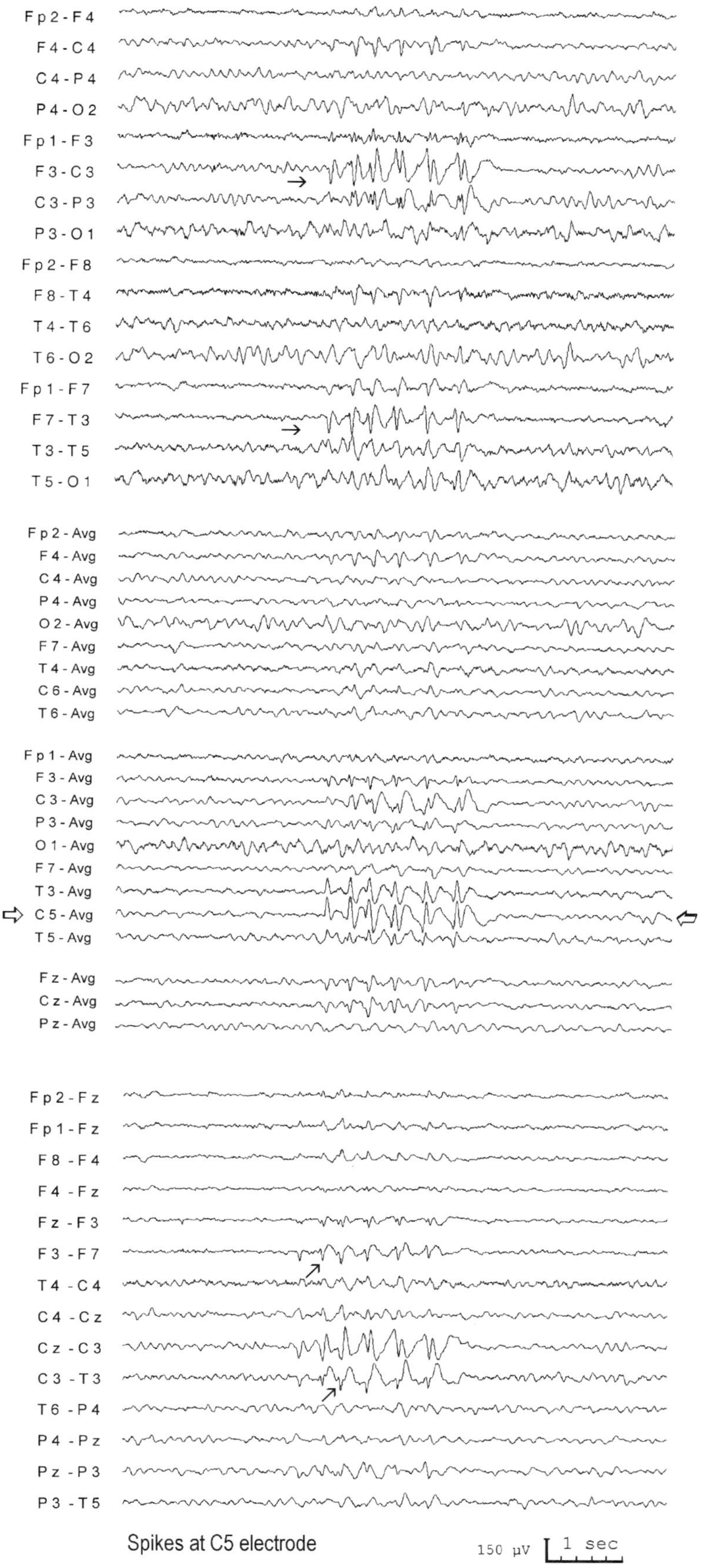

Children with RS may develop reversible linguistic abnormalities during the active phase of their disease.[1;54-56] Hospital-based studies emphasise learning or behavioural problems that require intervention.[56-58] A few patients (< 1%) may progress to atypical evolutions of more severe syndromes of linguistic, behavioural and neuropsychological deficits, such as Landau-Kleffner syndrome, atypical focal epilepsy of childhood, or epilepsy with continuous spikes and waves during slow wave sleep.[20;21]

The prognosis of RS is invariably excellent, with a less than 2% risk of developing infrequent generalised seizures in adult life; absence seizures may be more common than GTCS.[1;59-62]

Development, social adaptation and occupation of adults with a previous history of RS is normal. [1;61;62]

> The only problem was with five patients who had difficulties in obtaining their driving licences and one patient who despite a 15-year seizure-free period was still on phenytoin because of concerns of her physician regarding her driving licence. [61]

> For unknown reasons social levels of patients with Rolandic epilepsy seem to be even higher than for non-epileptic controls.[62]

MANAGEMENT

Children with RS may not need antiepileptic medication, particularly if the seizures are infrequent, mild or nocturnal, or the onset is close to the age of natural remission of this age-limited disorder. Patients with frequent seizures and secondarily GTCS or with comorbid conditions (tics, attention-deficit hyperactivity disorder, learning disability) may need medication.[63] In a recent study, AEDs significantly reduced GTCS, but did not reduce focal seizures.[64] On an empirical basis, carbamazepine is the preferred AED. However, some children might experience particular learning difficulties and exaggeration and new types of seizures while receiving carbamazepine.[1;22;23;65]

> Within days after re-introduction of carbamazepine, she suffered nearly continuous, brief atonic attacks of head and arm drop and also absences (case 17.3 in ref [1])

Lamotrigine may be contraindicated in RS, because of case reports with exacerbation of the condition and new types of seizures.[66-68]

See details in “Management of benign childhood focal seizures” (page 257).

Figure 9.4 Activation of functional centrotemporal and occipital spikes. Facing page

Top: Video EEG of a 6-year-old girl with headaches and abdominal pains of recent onset (case 16.2 in ref [1]). Neurological examination and MRI were normal. Symptoms improved over the following year. She never had seizures and her development was normal.
EEG showed normal background with the following abnormalities:
(a). Spontaneously central spikes, occurring independently on the right or left.
(b). High amplitude central spikes elicited by somatosensory stimulation of the contralateral side. Simultaneous stimulation of the fingers of the hands by the patient herself elicited simultaneous bilateral central spikes.
(c). Brief, mainly anterior, bursts of polyspikes.
(d). Brief and high amplitude generalised discharges of 3–5 Hz slow waves interspersed with small spikes or small polyspikes.
Note that the ESES are bilateral and synchronous when the stimulus is also bilateral and synchronous (tapping together and simultaneously the palmar tips of her fingers). Unilateral tapping evoked contralateral ESES.
Middle: ESES of a patient with PS (case 17 in ref [4]). At the age of 8 years, this boy had a single nocturnal seizure, which started with repetitive vomiting and “he was lost”. He then clenched his teeth and became rigid, but there were no clonic convulsions. The last follow-up, at the age of 14 years, disclosed no further seizures and normal development, though school performance was moderate. Three EEGs showed right CTS that were also evoked by somatosensory stimuli. Occipital spikes were never observed.
Bottom: Sample EEG from a patient with PS and occipital paroxysms (case 6 in ref [4]). Occipital paroxysms are bilateral and synchronous, because they are activated in the hyperexcitable occipital cortices by the elimination of central vision and fixation.

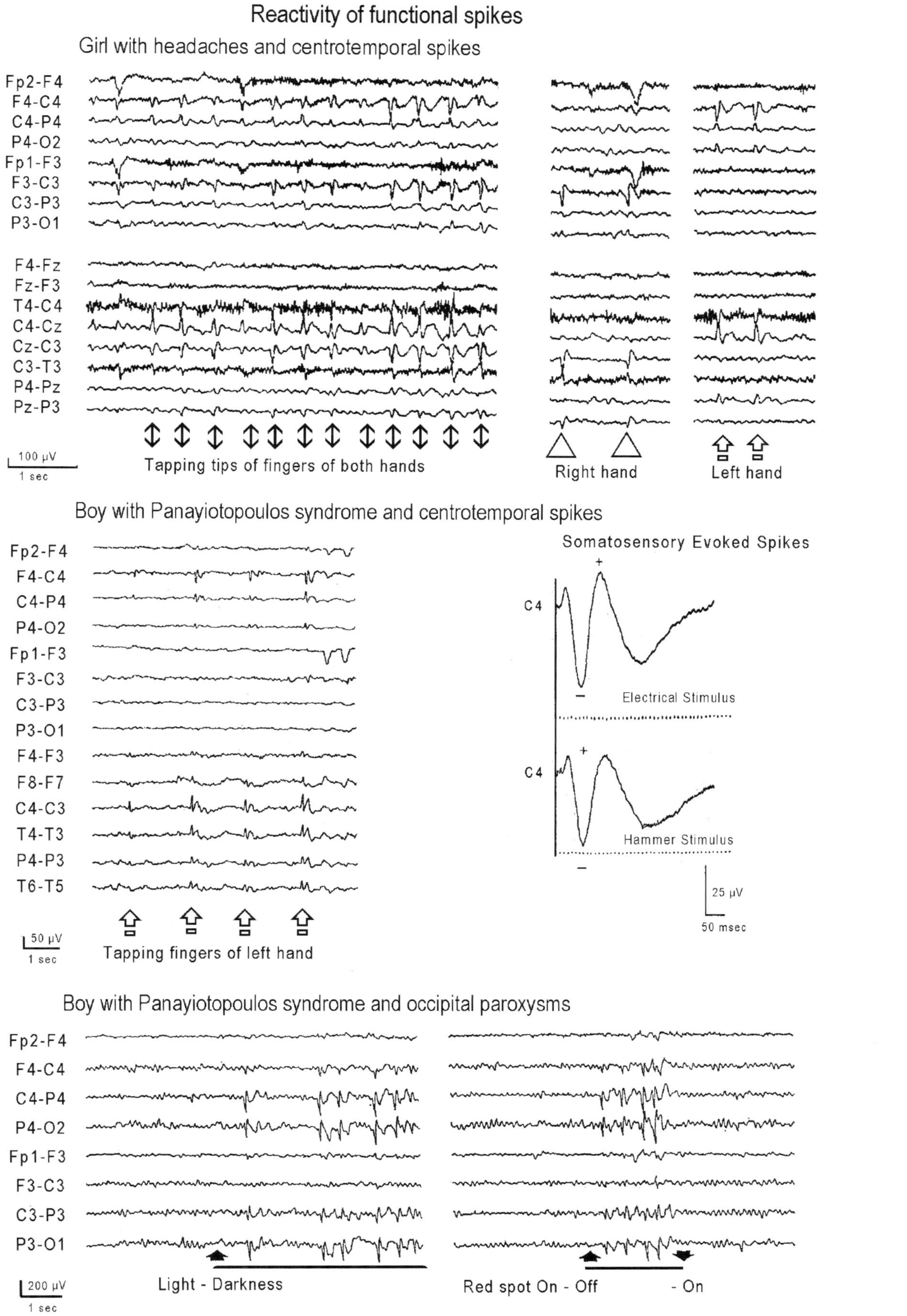
Reactivity of functional spikes
Girl with headaches and centrotemporal spikes
Fp2-F4
F4-C4
C4-P4
P4-O2
Fp1-F3
F3-C3
C3-P3
P3-O1
F4-Fz
Fz-F3
T4-C4
C4-Cz
Cz-C3
C3-T3
P4-Pz
Pz-P3
100 µV
1 sec
Tapping tips of fingers of both hands
Right hand
Left hand
Boy with Panayiotopoulos syndrome and centrotemporal spikes
Fp2-F4
F4-C4
C4-P4
P4-O2
Fp1-F3
F3-C3
C3-P3
P3-O1
F4-F3
F8-F7
C4-C3
T4-T3
P4-P3
T6-T5
50 µV
1 sec
Tapping fingers of left hand
Somatosensory Evoked Spikes
C4
+
−
Electrical Stimulus
C4
+
−
Hammer Stimulus
25 µV
50 msec
Boy with Panayiotopoulos syndrome and occipital paroxysms
Fp2-F4
F4-C4
C4-P4
P4-O2
Fp1-F3
F3-C3
C3-P3
P3-O1
200 µV
1 sec
Light - Darkness
Red spot On - Off
- On

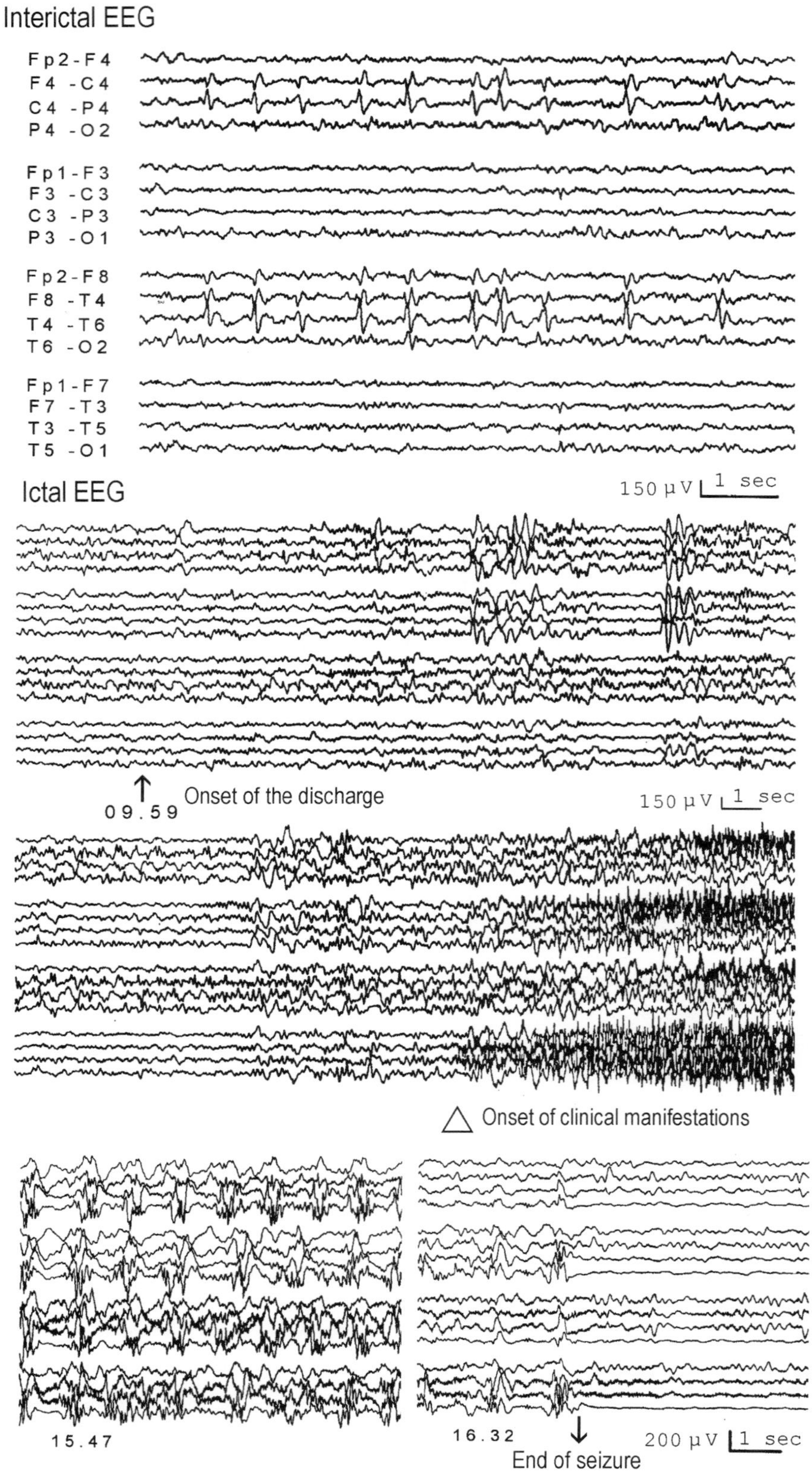

Figure 9.5 Video EEG of a 10-year-old girl with Rolandic seizures (case 5.1 in ref [1]).

Top: High amplitude right-sided centrotemporal spikes (C5 and C6 electrodes were not applied).
Bottom: Onset of ictal discharge in the right centrotemporal regions during sleep. Arrow shows onset of clinical manifestations that started with contractions of the left facial muscles (note muscle artefacts on the left), progressing to a prolonged generalised clonic seizure, which lasted for 5 min.

PANAYIOTOPOULOS SYNDROME

Panayiotopoulos syndrome (PS) is a childhood-related idiopathic benign susceptibility to focal, mainly autonomic, seizures and autonomic status epilepticus.[4;14;69-82] Affected children have normal physical and neuropsychological development. Autonomic manifestations are the cardinal seizure symptoms in PS, and have immense pathophysiological, clinical and treatment implications. All functions of the autonomic system may be affected during the ictus. Nearly half of these seizures last between 30 min and 7 hours, and constitute autonomic status epilepticus.

DEMOGRAPHIC DATA

Age at onset is 1–14 years with a peak at 4–5 years; in 76% of cases, onset occurs at 3–6 years of age. Boys and girls are equally affected.[4] Children of all races are vulnerable. Prevalence is around 13% in children 3–6 years old with one or more non-febrile seizures and 6% in the 1–15-year age group. In the general population, 2–3/1000 children may be affected. These figures may be higher if cases that are currently considered to have atypical features are included.[4]

CLINICAL MANIFESTATIONS

Seizures comprise an unusual constellation of autonomic, mainly emetic, symptoms, behavioural changes, unilateral deviation of the eyes and other more conventional ictal manifestations.[4;14;70;74;78-80;82] Consciousness and speech, as a rule, are preserved at seizure onset. The seizure commonly starts with autonomic manifestations (81%), which are mainly emetic (72%). In a typical presentation, the child is fully conscious, able to speak and understand, complains "I feel sick", looks pale and vomits.

> He complained of nausea and he looked pale. Five min later he vomited while still standing... He gradually became disorientated, but was still able to walk. However, 10 min from onset his eyes turned to the right and he became unresponsive.

ICTUS EMETICUS

The full emetic triad (nausea, retching, vomiting) culminates in vomiting in 74% of seizures; in others, only nausea or retching occur and, in a few cases, emesis may

---

Considerations on classification and nomenclature of Panayiotopoulos syndrome

Panayiotopoulos syndrome has been recognised in the new diagnostic scheme[2] as: "Early onset benign childhood occipital epilepsy (Panayiotopoulos type)". However, PS is not "occipital" epilepsy: [4;83]

(a). Onset is with autonomic manifestations, which are unlikely to be of occipital origin. Of all the other seizure symptoms, only eye deviation, which is often not the first ictal symptom, may originate from the occipital lobes.
(b). Interictal occipital spikes may never occur.
(c). Even ictal EEG has documented anterior or posterior origin.

Currently, most authors prefer the eponymic nomenclature "Panayiotopoulos syndrome" to include all patients with this syndrome irrespective of EEG spikes or topographic terminology [4;14;76;77;79-82;84] as in the original study of Panayiotopoulos.[70]

In that study of 900 seizure-patients of all ages, only 24 had ictal vomiting and all of these were children. [70] Of these 24 children with ictal vomiting:
(a). 21 had normal development with EEG occipital spikes (12 patients), extra-occipital spikes (5 patients), brief generalised discharges (1 patient) or normal EEG (3 patients)
(b). 3 had an abnormal neurological state (symptomatic childhood autonomic epilepsy).

Of the 21 idiopathic patients (which constitutes what is now known as Panayiotopoulos syndrome), attention was directed towards the predominant group of occipital spikes and occipital paroxysms (hence the name *"occipital epilepsy"* or *"epilepsy with occipital paroxysms"*).[85] The fact that the other 9 patients without occipital spikes had the same disorder with those of occipital spikes was documented much later.[86]

The terms "early onset" and "late onset" have been used adjunctively with "childhood occipital epilepsy" or "epilepsy with occipital paroxysms" in order to discriminate between PS (with median age of onset in early childhood) and G-ICOE (with median age of onset in late childhood). It should be clarified that these terms ("early onset" and "late onset") were first introduced at a time that G-ICOE was the only recognised syndrome associated with "occipital paroxysms"[85] and prior to the documentation that PS manifests with multi-focal EEG spikes with one-third not having occipital spikes.

For those few that they may disapprove *certain* eponyms (see for example reference [87]) the most precise descriptive term I can propose for PS is "benign childhood autonomic seizures and autonomic status epilepticus" and not "early onset benign childhood epilepsy with occipital spikes".

not be apparent. Emesis is usually the first apparent ictal symptom, but may also occur long after the onset of other manifestations.

Typically, nausea is the first complaint of a child who suffers a seizure (while awake or who wakes from sleep) prior to vomiting and other ictal manifestations. This initial stage does not suggest an epileptic seizure; the child simply complains of feeling sick and being unwell, and looks pale. The patient may be quiet or agitated, vacant or restless but fully conscious and able to understand and answer questions. Ictus emeticus at this stage is no different from any other disease that causes emesis – just a child who feels sick or wants to be sick.

> On returning home from school, she looked tired and had a nap. After half an hour, she woke up looking pale and complained of feeling sick. She ran to the toilet and vomited repeatedly. Then her eyes deviated to one side and she became unresponsive and flaccid for 10 min. Soon after, she started recovering, answering simple questions and 1 hour later she was playing again as if nothing had happened.

Timing of the vomiting. When vomiting occurs, it commonly starts 1–5 min after the onset of nausea, while the child is still conscious and otherwise well. Less often, vomiting may occur later during other more conventional seizure symptoms.

Intensity and duration of vomiting. This varies considerably from mild to often severe and repetitive. Usually, the child vomits 3–5 times; however, some children may repeatedly vomit for hours leading to dehydration, while others may vomit only once.

OTHER AUTONOMIC MANIFESTATIONS

Autonomic manifestations other than ictus emeticus may occur concurrently or appear later in the course of the ictus. These include pallor and less often flushing or cyanosis, mydriasis and less often miosis, cardiorespiratory and thermoregulatory alterations, coughing, incontinence of urine and/or faeces, and modifications of intestinal motility. Hypersalivation (probably a concurrent Rolandic symptom) may occur. Headache and more often cephalic auras may occur particularly at onset.

Pallor is one of the commonest ictal manifestations. It mainly occurs at onset, usually with emetic symptoms. Exceptionally, pallor may be among the first symptoms without apparent emesis.

Cyanosis is less common than pallor. It principally occurs during the evolution of the seizures, often while the child is unresponsive.

Incontinence of urine and faeces occur when consciousness is impaired prior to, or without, convulsions: "became unresponsive and incontinent of urine" is a common association. These symptoms do not occur at onset.

Mydriasis is sometimes so prominent that it may be reported spontaneously.

> Her pupils were as big as her eyes.

Definitions of autonomic seizures and autonomic status epilepticus

Autonomic auras consist of a subjective awareness of a change in the activity of autonomic nervous system function.[88]
Autonomic seizures consist of episodic altered autonomic function of any type at onset or as the sole manifestation of an epileptic event. These may be objective, subjective or both. They must be distinguished from secondary (indirect effects) on the autonomic system by other seizure symptoms.[89]
Pure autonomic seizures are those that consist solely of episodic altered autonomic function from onset to the end.
In the absence of a definition for autonomic status epilepticus, the terms I propose are:
Autonomic status epilepticus: is an autonomic seizure that lasts for more than 30 minutes.[4;90]
Pure autonomic status epilepticus is a pure autonomic seizure that lasts for more than 30 minutes.[4;90]

Terminology of the emetic components

The emetic process consists of the triad of nausea, retching and vomiting, which are three separate functional entities occurring independently of each other and in any combination.
Vomiting refers to the forcible oral expulsion of gastric contents and is usually preceded by symptoms (e.g. pallor, salivation, sweating) attributed to autonomic nervous system discharges, which are not, however, essential for the act of vomiting.
Ictus emeticus: emetic manifestations (nausea, retching, vomiting alone or in combination) caused by seizure discharges.
Ictal vomiting: forcible oral expulsion of gastric contents due to seizure discharges.

Mydriasis occurs concurrently with other marked autonomic manifestations. Dilated pupils may not be reactive to light.

Miosis is rare and occurs with other severe autonomic manifestations while the child is unresponsive.

Hypersalivation is also rare in PS, in contrast to its common occurrence in RS. Combined speech arrest and hypersalivation, as in RS, is even rarer.

Cephalic auras, though rare, are of interest, because they are considered to be autonomic manifestations and because of the diagnostic confusion they may cause with migraine if not properly evaluated. Cephalic auras commonly occur with other autonomic symptoms, mainly nausea, at seizure onset. Occasionally, the child may also complain of "headache" but whether the complaint of "headache" is a true perception of pain, discomfort or some odd sensation in the head is uncertain.

"funny feeling in my head", "warm sensation", "pressure", "headache"

Coughing may occur as an initial ictal symptom either with or without ictus emeticus. It is described as "strange coughing" or "cough as if about to vomit".

Thermoregulatory changes. Raised temperature may be subjectively or objectively documented during the seizure or immediately post-ictally. Whether this is a coincidental finding, a precipitating factor or an ictal abnormality is uncertain. It could be any of these. However, pyrexia recorded immediately after seizure onset is probably an ictal autonomic manifestation.

Abnormalities of intestinal motility. Diarrhoea (3%) is occasionally reported during the progression of seizures.

Breathing and cardiac irregularities are rarely reported, but may be much more common in a mild form. Breathing changes prior to convulsions include descriptions of "heavy, irregular, abnormal breathing" or "brief cessation of breathing for a few seconds". Tachycardia is a consistent finding, sometimes at the onset, of ictal EEG (Figures 9.8 and 9.9).

Cardiorespiratory arrest is exceptional, but is potentially fatal without immediate medical intervention (case 37 in ref [4]).

At the age of 3 years, while dozing in his mother's car, his head went back, eyes were "rolling", colour clay-like grey, pupils dilated, unresponsive and incontinent of urine. Arms were initially rigid, but then he became floppy. At this stage, 5–10 min from onset, a Swiss paediatrician who happened to be present diagnosed cardiopulmonary arrest and resuscitated him: "Lips blue and then white. No respiration. No heart beat and wide pupils without reaction to light. External heart massage and mouth-to-nose resuscitation, less than 1 minute. Total time of asystole reckoned to be 2 min. Unconsciousness went on for 20 min then he started to cry and he recognised his mother". He was well after a few hours' sleep.[4]

I have been made aware of three other children with PS and cardiorespiratory arrest. Sadly, one of them died. Though tragic and exceptional, this should be expected to happen in view of the frequent occurrence of autonomic status epilepticus in children (page 239).

Ictal syncope

Ictal syncope is an intriguing and important ictal feature of PS.[4] It is a common and dramatic occurrence. In at least one-fifth of seizures, the child becomes *'completely unresponsive and flaccid like a rag doll'* before and often without convulsions or in isolation.

Terminology of the cephalic auras

Cephalic auras are ictal symptoms of non-specific sensory perceptions involving or limited to the head.[91]

While talking to her teacher, suddenly and without warning, she fell on the floor pale, flaccid and unresponsive for 2 min. She had a complete recovery, but 10 min later she complained of feeling sick, vomited repeatedly and again became unresponsive and flaccid with pupils widely dilated for 1 hour. She had an unremarkable recovery and was normal after a few hours' sleep.

She complained of 'dizziness' and then her eyes deviated to the left, she fell on the floor and she became totally flaccid and unresponsive for 5 min.

I proposed the descriptive term *'ictal syncope'*[4;90] to describe this state, because *'unresponsiveness with loss of postural tone'* are the defining clinical symptoms of syncope.[92;93] Other authors prefer *'syncope-like symptoms'*.[94]

ICTAL BEHAVIOURAL CHANGES

Ictal behavioural changes usually consist of restlessness, agitation, terror or quietness, which appear at the onset of seizures, often concurrently with emetic or other autonomic manifestations. These symptoms are often similar to those occurring in 'benign childhood epilepsy with affective symptoms' (page 255).

He was happily playing and asking questions when he started complaining that he was feeling sick, and became very pale and quiet. He did not want to drink or eat. Gradually, he was getting paler and paler, and kept complaining that he felt sick. He then became restless and frightened. Ten min from the onset, his head and eyes slowly turned to the left. The eyes were opened, but fixed to the left upper corner. We called his name, but he was unresponsive. He had completely gone. We tried to move his head, but this was fixed to the left. There were no convulsions. This lasted for another 15 min when his head and eyes returned to normal and he looked better, although he was droopy and really not there. At this stage he vomited once.

At age 9 years, on return from school, he looked tired and pale. He said that his head was killing him "something that would cause me to be sick". In 10 min, he started screaming and banging his head on the wall. Within the next 20 min, he gradually became disorientated and floppy 'like a rag doll'. He was staring.

CONVENTIONAL SEIZURE-SYMPTOMS

In PS, pure autonomic seizures and pure autonomic status epilepticus occur in 10% of patients. They start and end solely with autonomic symptoms. In all others, autonomic manifestations are followed by conventional seizure-symptoms and these in order of prevalence are:

- Impairment of consciousness (94%)
- Deviation of the eyes (60-80%)
- Hemiconvulsions (26%)
- Generalised convulsions (20%)
- Speech arrest (8%)
- Visual hallucinations (6%)
- Other manifestations occur less than 3% each.

Impairment of consciousness: Though initially fully conscious, the child gradually or suddenly becomes confused and unresponsive. Impairment of consciousness may be mild or moderate, with the child retaining some ability to respond to verbal commands, but often talking out of context. Complete unresponsiveness is probably exceptional at the beginning of the seizure. In diurnal seizures observed from

Definition of ictal syncope

'Ictal syncope' denotes transient loss of consciousness and postural tone that occurs in a seizure before or without convulsions.[4;90] *'Transient loss of consciousness and postural tone'* are the defining symptoms of syncope irrespective of underlying cause.[92] Ictal syncope is purely a name for a cluster of seizure symptoms that, until now, have lacked a descriptive term. Ictal syncope does not occur or may be very rare in other types of seizures, except in postictal states after GTCS.

onset, clouding of consciousness usually starts after the appearance of autonomic and behavioural symptoms, becoming progressively worse until complete unresponsiveness is reached. Good awareness may be preserved throughout the ictus in around 6% of seizures.

Deviation of the eyes: Unilateral deviation of the eyes with, or rarely without, ictal vomiting is a common ictal manifestation, which seldom occurs at onset. The eyes shift to the extreme of one side and the head may also turn ipsilaterally. This pursuit-like deviation of the eyes may be brief (for min) or prolonged (for hours). It may be continuous or less often intermittent, with eyes returning to the midline and shifting again towards the same side. The eyelids remain open, but may be half open or open wide and, at this stage, consciousness is often, but not invariably, impaired.

Deviation of the eyes may occur without vomiting in 10–20% of patients and, in some children, the eyes may be open wide and remain in the midline before other convulsions occur.

Other ictal symptoms in order of prevalence are speech arrest (8%), hemifacial spasms (6%), visual hallucinations (6%), OPL movements (3%), unilateral drooping of the mouth (3%), eyelid jerks (1%), myoclonic jerks (1%), ictal nystagmus and automatisms (1%). These probably reflect the primary area of seizure discharge generation. The seizures may end with hemiconvulsions often with Jacksonian march (19%) or generalised convulsions (21%).

Ictal visual symptoms, such as elementary visual hallucinations, illusions or blindness, occur after more typical seizure symptoms of PS.

Hemiconvulsive (2%) or generalised convulsive status (2%) is exceptional.

The same child may have seizures with marked autonomic manifestations and seizures in which autonomic manifestations may be inconspicuous or absent. Seizures without autonomic manifestations are rare (7%).[4]

The clinical seizure manifestations are roughly the same irrespective of EEG localisations though there may be slightly less autonomic and slightly more focal motor features at onset in children without occipital spikes.[4]

SEIZURES WITHOUT AUTONOMIC MANIFESTATIONS

Such seizures are rare (7%) and occur in patients who may also have additional autonomic seizures.

Case 3 of ref [4] had three seizures with ictus emeticus. An additional lengthy diurnal seizure manifested only with deviation of the eyes and mild impairment of consciousness prior to generalised convulsions.

DURATION OF SEIZURES AND AUTONOMIC STATUS EPILEPTICUS

Nearly half (44%) of the seizures last for more than 30 min and can persist for up to 7 hours (mean about 2 hours), constituting autonomic status epilepticus. The rest of the seizures (54%) last from 1–30 min with a mean of 9 min. Lengthy seizures are equally common in sleep and wakefulness. Even after the most severe seizures and status, the patient is normal after a few hours' sleep. There is no record of residual neurological or mental abnormalities. The same child may have brief and lengthy seizures. Hemi-convulsive or convulsive status epilepticus is exceptional (4%).

Despite the high incidence of autonomic status epilepticus, convulsive status epilepticus is exceptional in PS.

CIRCADIAN DISTRIBUTION

Two-thirds of seizures start in sleep; the child may wake up with similar complaints while still conscious or else may be found vomiting, conscious, confused or unresponsive.

Clinically, while asleep, "he suddenly got up with both eyes open, vomited several times and then showed a prolonged atonic state with cyanosis and irregular respiration for 3 min" (from ictal EEG documentation by Oguni and associates).[72]

The same child may suffer seizures while asleep or awake.

A 10-year-old boy of normal development suffered an episode of autonomic status epilepticus at 5 years of age. Half an hour after he had gone to sleep, he woke up looking pale and then complained that he felt sick before vomiting repeatedly. Within min his eyes deviated and fixed laterally, and soon after he became flaccid 'like a rag doll', unresponsive, and incontinent of urine and faeces. His breathing was short and shallow, and stopped for a few seconds before he started vomiting again. Two hours after onset, he had brief hemiconvulsions with Jacksonian marching for 5 min. On arrival at hospital, he was recovering and his temperature was mildly raised to 37.4^{0} C. A CT brain scan, CSF examination and relevant blood tests were normal. Triple treatment for encephalitis was started, though he was entirely normal and apyrexial after a few hours of sleep. EEG the next day showed a few scattered occipital and central spikes. Treatment was stopped 4 days later.

A similar autonomic status epilepticus occurred 6 months later on a ferryboat while on holiday. He said that he felt sick and looked pale. He vomited a couple of times, and then his eyes turned to one side and he talked out of context and vomited again. "Then I knew that he was having another fit" his mother said. "He was as if drifting in and out of sleep. He did not become unconscious, but he was continuously vomiting for several hours." On arrival at hospital 3 hours later, he was improving and able to talk and walk. He was diagnosed and treated for dehydration. He was normal the next morning. A new EEG showed repetitive multifocal spike-wave complexes.

No further seizures occurred in the next 5 years, and his development and EEG were normal.

PRECIPITATING FACTORS

There are no apparent precipitating factors other than sleep. Fixation off sensitivity is an EEG phenomenon, which may not be clinically important.

Many seizures have been witnessed while a child is travelling in a car, boat or aeroplane. There are two explanations for this: (a) the seizures are more likely to be witnessed during travelling; or (b), children are more vulnerable because travelling also precipitates motion sickness which is particularly common in children.

AETIOLOGY

PS, like RS, is probably genetically determined. Usually, no family history of similar seizures exists, though siblings with PS or PS and Rolandic epilepsy have been reported.[14;71;74;79] There is a high prevalence of febrile seizures (about 17%). Also, there may be a high incidence of abnormal birth deliveries, but these all need re-evaluation.[4]

Considerations on the classification of autonomic status epilepticus

Childhood autonomic status epilepticus, though common and specific in childhood, is ignored in all classifications even now, long after its first description by Panayiotopoulos.[4;70;90] The new ILAE diagnostic scheme[2] recognises four forms of focal status epilepticus (Table 1.4):[2;95]

(a). Epilepsia partialis continua of Kozhevnikov
(b). Aura continua[95]
(c). Limbic status epilepticus (psychomotor status)
(d). Hemiconvulsive status with hemi-paresis

From a clinical point of view aura continua is classified into:[95]
(1) somatosensory, i.e. dysaesthesia phenomena that involve the trunk, head and extremities,
(2) aura continua that involve the special senses (visual, auditory, vertiginous, gustatory and olfactory).
(3) aura continua with predominantly autonomic symptoms, and with psychic symptoms.[95]

It is anticipated that future revisions of the ILAE classifications will recognise this type of age-related autonomic status epilepticus. This is mandated by its high prevalence and its high rate of misdiagnosis and mismanagement.[4;90;96] Four-fifths of childhood autonomic status epilepticus occur in PS and the remaining one-fifth occurs in symptomatic childhood epileptic disorders.[4;90;96] Ignoring these facts, as indeed happens even now, results in avoidable morbidity and probably mortality.[4;90]

PS, Rolandic epilepsy and all other benign childhood focal seizures are probably linked together by a common, genetically determined, mild and reversible functional derangement of the brain cortical maturational process that I proposed to call 'benign childhood seizure susceptibility syndrome' (see Figure 9.1 and pages 223).

PATHOPHYSIOLOGY

Autonomic symptoms of any type are often encountered in seizures, focal or generalised, in adults or children and they are implicated in occurrences of sudden death.[89;97] However, autonomic seizures and autonomic status with ictus emeticus and ictal syncope, with the symptomatology and the sequence as detailed in this chapter, are specific in childhood.[90] This clinical picture does not occur in adults: only about 30 cases of ictal vomiting have been reported, but not in the same sequence as in children – adult patients usually have amnesia about the vomiting, which often occurs after the seizure has started with other symptoms (see page 373).[88;97-99] An explanation for this is that children are vulnerable to emetic disturbances as exemplified by the 'cyclic vomiting syndrome', a non-seizure disorder of unknown aetiology that is also specific to childhood.[100] Ictal syncope is even more difficult to explain.

Symptoms at the onset of seizures are important, because they indicate the possible location of the epileptic focus. However, autonomic and emetic disturbances are of uncertain value with regard to localisation in PS and may occur in seizures starting from the anterior or posterior regions. The localisation of ictal vomiting in adults does not appear to apply in children (page 373).

Clinical and EEG findings indicate that, in PS, there is a diffuse cortical hyperexcitability, which is maturation-related. This diffuse epileptogenicity may be unequally distributed, predominating in one area, which is often posterior. The preferential involvement of emetic and other autonomic manifestations may be attributed to epileptic discharges triggering low-threshold emetic centres and hypothalamus of vulnerable children .[4;90] In other words, it is likely that in vulnerable children a "weak" epileptic electrical discharge (irrespective of localisation) activates at its onset susceptible autonomic centres to autonomic seizures and autonomic status epilepticus. This is prior to the generation of clinical manifestations from brain regions that are topographically related to the ictal electrical discharge (occipital, frontal, central, parietal and less often temporal) with seizure thresholds higher than those of the autonomic centers.

DIAGNOSTIC PROCEDURES

By definition, in an idiopathic syndrome, neurological and mental states and high resolution MRI are normal. The most useful laboratory test is the EEG (Figure 9.6). The most important determinant of the neurodiagnostic procedures is the state of the child at the time of first medical attendance.[4]

- *The child has a typical brief or lengthy seizure of PS, but has fully recovered before arriving at the accident and emergency department or being seen by a physician.* A child with the distinctive clinical features of PS, particularly ictus emeticus and lengthy seizures, may not need any investigations other than EEG. However, because approximately 10–20% of children with similar seizures may have brain pathology, an MRI may be indicated.
- *The child with a typical lengthy seizure of PS has partially recovered, though is still in a postictal stage, tired, mildly confused and drowsy on arrival at the accident and emergency department or when seen by a physician.* The child should be kept under medical supervision until full recovery, which is the rule after a few hours of sleep. Then guidelines are the same as above

- *The child is brought to the accident and emergency department or is seen by a physician while ictal symptoms continue.* This is the most difficult and challenging situation. Symptoms may dramatically accumulate in succession, and demand rigorous and experienced evaluation. A history of a previous similar seizure is reassuring and may help to avoid unnecessary investigation.

ELECTROENCEPHALOGRAPHY

In about 90% of cases, the EEG reveals functional, mainly multi-focal, high amplitude sharp-slow wave complexes (Figure 9.6).[4;14;79;80;82;84;94;101] Spikes may

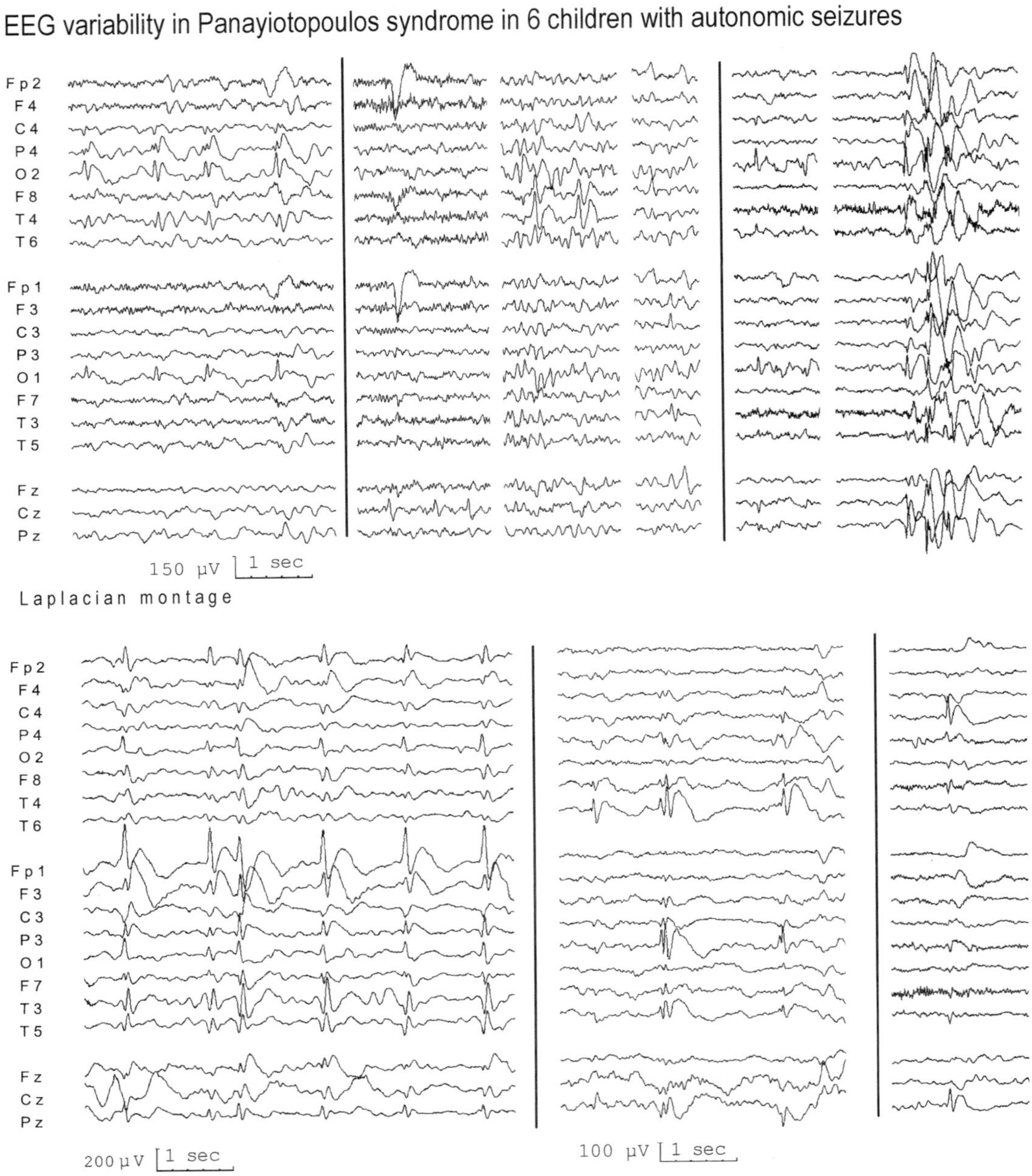

Figure 9.6 EEG variability in Panayiotopoulos syndrome.

Samples from EEGs of six children with typical clinical manifestations of PS. Spikes may occur in all electrode locations, and they are usually of high amplitude and frequent or repetitive (cloned-like repetitive multifocal spike wave complexes). but may also be small and sparse. Brief generalised discharges of small spikes and slow waves may be present.

appear anywhere. They are often independent, and occur at various posterior locations and, less often anterior locations, in the same or the contralateral hemisphere, and may appear as cloned-like, repetitive, multifocal spike-wave complexes. In order of prevalence, the complexes most commonly occur in occipital, frontal and centrotemporal regions; right and left regions are equally involved. Midline spikes occur in 17% of cases.

The EEG shows great variability in functional focal spikes at various electrode locations. All brain regions are involved, though posterior areas predominate (Figures 9.6 and 9.7).

Two-thirds of patients (68%) have at least one EEG with occipital paroxysms or, more commonly, occipital spikes, which are often (64%) concurrent with extra-occipital spikes in at least one EEG.[4] The other third (32%) never show occipital spikes (Figures 9.4 and 9.6). Instead, they have extra-occipital spikes (21%) only, a consistently normal EEG (9%) or brief generalised discharges only (2%). An EEG with multifocal spikes in more than two, and often many, brain locations occurs in one-third of patients; single spike foci are rare (9%). Cloned-like, repetitive, multifocal spike-wave complexes may be characteristic features when they occur (19%).[4] They have never been studied or reported before in idiopathic epilepsies. On the contrary, multifocal repetitive spikes are considered to be suggestive of a bad prognosis and indicative of symptomatic epilepsies (page 169). Cloned-like, repetitive, multifocal spike-wave complexes do not determine the prognosis, because they occur equally in children with single or multiple seizures.

Spikes are usually of high amplitude and morphologically similar to CTS. They often show stable dipoles in the occipital regions.[84]

Small and even inconspicuous spikes may appear in the same or a previous EEG of children with giant spikes. Though rare, positive spikes or other unusual EEG spike conFigurations may occur.[4]

Brief generalised discharges of slow waves intermixed with small spikes may occur either alone (4%) or more often with focal spikes (15%).

The EEG spikes may be stimulus sensitive; occipital paroxysms are commonly (47%) activated by the elimination of central vision and fixation, while CTS may be elicited by somatosensory stimuli (Figure 9.4).[4] EEG occipital photosensitivity is an exceptional finding.[4]

Functional spikes in whatever location are accentuated by sleep. If a routine EEG is normal, a sleep EEG should be performed. There is no particular relationship between the likehood of an abnormal EEG and the interval since the last seizure. EEGs recorded a short or long time after a seizure are equally likely to manifest with functional spikes, which may occur only once in serial routine and sleep EEGs.

The background EEG is usually normal, but diffuse or localised slow wave abnormalities may also occur in at least one EEG in 20% of cases, particularly postictally.

Definition of cloned-like, repetitive, multifocal spike-wave complexes[4]

Cloned-like repetitive multifocal spike wave complexes are repetitive spike or sharp and slow wave complexes that appear concurrently in different brain locations of one or both hemispheres. There may be just two discrete foci unilaterally or contralaterally, but the complexes are usually multifocal and often give the impression of generalised discharges or secondary bilateral synchrony. They are stereotypically and identically repetitive in the same and often subsequent EEGs from the same patient, which is the reason that I coined the name 'cloned-like'. On the surface, in routine EEG recordings, they appear synchronous but usually one spike focus leads the others by a few milliseconds. The leading focus commonly occurs alone without spikes in other locations. Cloned-like repetitive multifocal spike-wave complexes can occur without the primary spike and can be so abundant that they dominate the EEG and obscure its background, which is otherwise normal. On other occasions, they are scarce and appear in a well-organised EEG with normal background.

EEG abnormalities, particularly functional spikes, may persist for many years after clinical remission; they disappear when the patient reaches the mid-teens. Conversely, spikes may appear only once in one of a series of EEGs.

Frequency, location and persistence of functional spikes do not determine clinical manifestations, duration, severity and frequency of seizures, or prognosis.

ICTAL EEG

Typical autonomic seizures and autonomic status epilepticus of PS have been documented by ictal EEG (Figures 9.8 and 9.9).[72;81;90;102;103] The seizure discharge consists mainly of rhythmic theta or delta activity, usually intermixed with small spikes. Onset is unilateral, often posterior, but may also be anterior and not strictly localised to one electrode. Figure 9.8 shows autonomic status epilepticus captured from the onset on video EEG. Ictal clinical manifestations may start minutes after the onset of the electrical seizure discharge (Figure 9.8).

DIFFERENTIAL DIAGNOSIS

PS is easy to diagnose, because of the characteristic clustering of clinical seizure semiology, which is often supported by interictal EEG findings. However, despite sound clinical EEG manifestations, PS escaped recognition for many years for a number of reasons. Ictus emeticus is rarely considered a seizure event. When it is associated with a deteriorating level of consciousness, followed by convulsions,

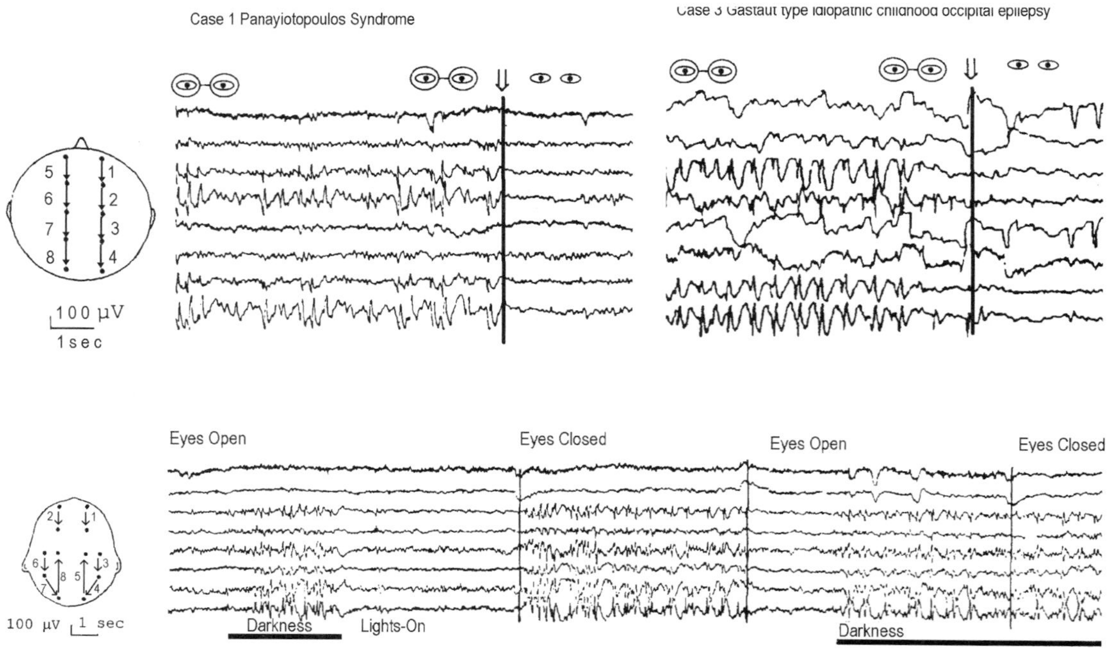

Figure 9.7 Occipital paroxysms in their classical form with fixation-off sensitivity from the initial study of Panayiotopoulos (1981).[69]

Top: EEGs from two patients with PS and G-ICOE. In routine EEG, repetitive, high amplitude, occipital sharp and slow wave complexes (occipital paroxysms) occur immediately after the eyes are closed and persist for as long as the eyes remain closed. The EEG normalises immediately after the eyes are opened and for as long as the eyes remain open. The activation of the occipital paroxysms is due to the elimination of central vision and fixation (left of the vertical bar, symbol of eyes with glasses) and inhibition by fixation (right of the vertical bar, symbol of eyes without glasses).

Bottom: Effect of darkness on occipital paroxysms:

(a). Complete darkness activates the occipital paroxysms even when eyes are open.

(b). The occipital paroxysms become continuous in darkness irrespective of whether the eyes are open or closed.

Modified from Panayiotopoulos (1981)[69] and reproduced with the permission of the Editor of *Neurology*

encephalitis or other acute cerebral insults are the prevailing diagnoses in the acute stage. If the child is seen after complete recovery, atypical migraine, gastroenteritis, motion sickness or a first seizure are likely diagnoses. Similarly, ictal syncope has only recently been recognised as an important clinical

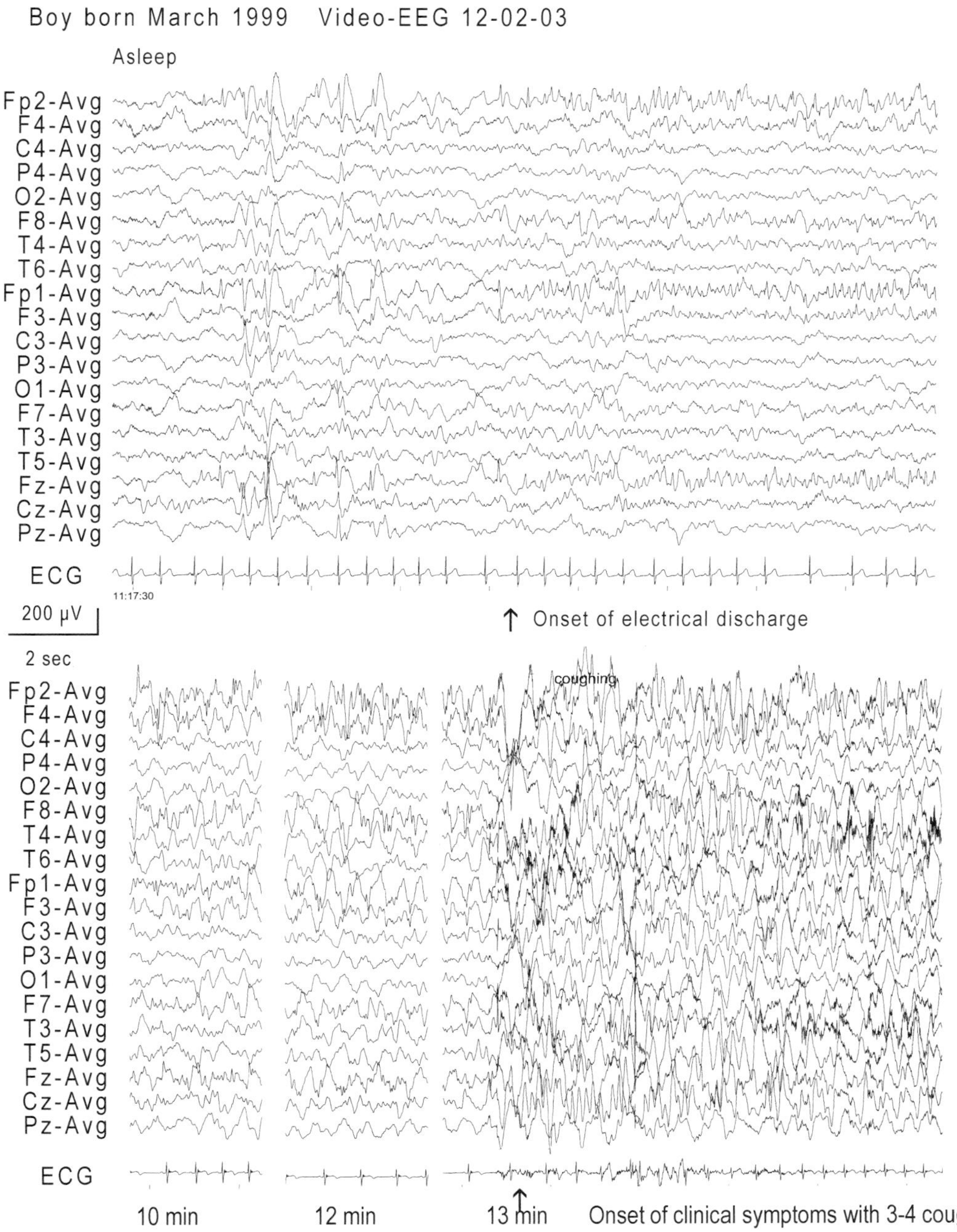

Figure 9.8 EEG of a 4-year-old boy with autonomic status epilepticus recorded from onset to termination.

Top: High amplitude spikes and slow waves are recorded from the bifrontal regions prior to the onset of the electrical discharge, which is also purely bifrontal (arrow). *Bottom:* First clinical symptoms with three or four coughs and marked tachycardia appeared 13 min after the onset of the electrical discharge, when this had become bilaterally diffuse. Subsequent clinical symptoms were tachycardia, ictus emeticus (without vomiting) and impairment of consciousness. No other ictal manifestations occurred until termination of the seizure with diazepines 70 min after onset.

Another lengthy autonomic seizure was recorded on video EEG 1 year later. The onset of symptoms was different with mainly tachycardia and agitation.

From Panayiotopoulos (2004)[90] with the permission of the Editor of *Epilepsy and Behaviour*.
Figure courtesy of Dr Michael Koutroumanidis, MD from the Department of Clinical Neurophysiology and Epilepsies, Guy's & St. Thomas' NHS Trust, UK.

manifestation of PS; ictal syncope may be misdiagnosed as cardiogenic syncope, pseudoseizure or a more severe encephalopathic state.[4]

The main problem is to recognise emetic and other autonomic manifestations as seizure events, and not to dismiss them or erroneously consider them as unrelated to the ictus and as a feature of encephalitis, migraine, syncope or gastroenteritis.

Similarly, 10–20% of autonomic seizures and autonomic status epilepticus with a similar presentation to PS are due to heterogeneous cerebral pathology, such as focal or diffuse brain lesions of diverse aetiology. These autonomic seizures are also restricted to childhood. In these symptomatic cases, there is often abnormal neurological or mental symptomatology, abnormal brain imaging, and

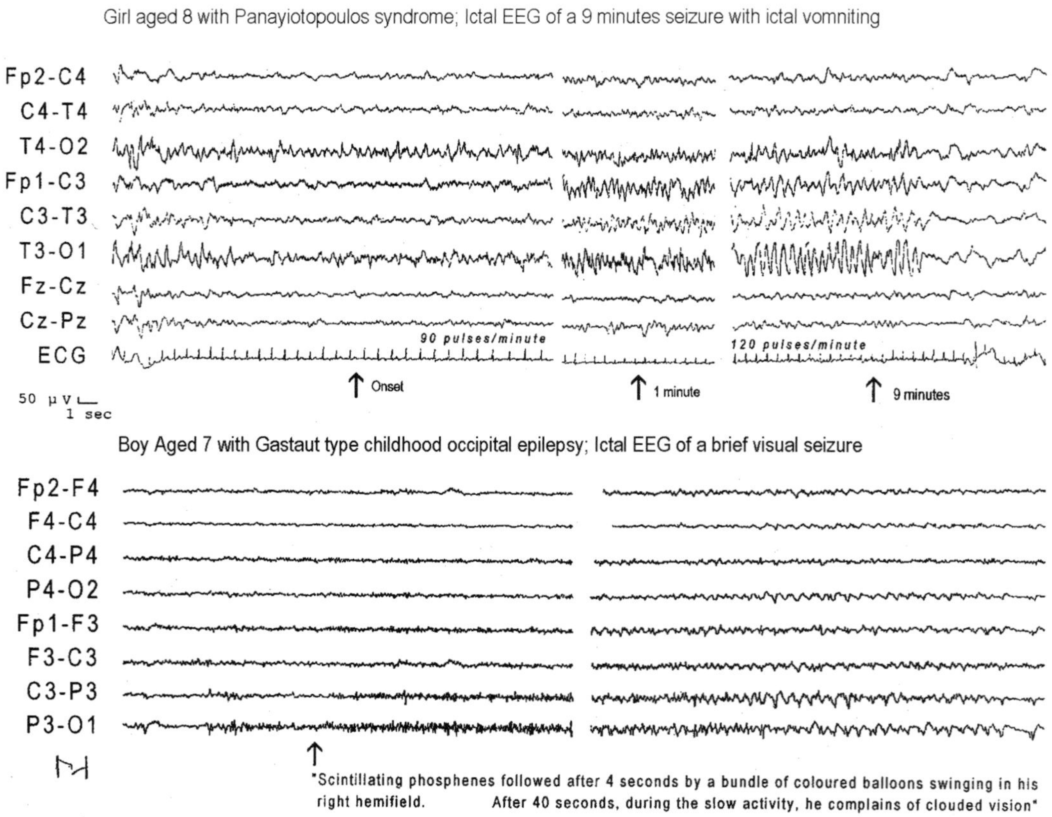

Figure 9.9 Ictal EEGs in Panayiotopoulos syndrome (top) and Gastaut-type childhood occipital epilepsy (bottom).

Top: Samples of continuous EEG recording from the onset to the end of a 9-minute seizure during sleep stage II in an 8-year-old girl. Clinically, the seizure manifested with awakening, eyes opening, frequent vomiting efforts and complaints of frontal headache.[102] The ictal EEG started with remission of the interictal occipital paroxysms and the appearance of occipital sharp rhythms progressing to monomorphic rhythmic theta activity in the bi-occipital regions, but mainly involving the right hemisphere in a wider posterior distribution. The slow activity slowed down with the progress of the seizure and ended without postictal abnormalities. The ECG showed significant tachycardia during the ictus.[102] *Bottom:* Ictal EEG during a visual seizure in a boy with Gastaut-type childhood occipital epilepsy. The seizure starts in the left occipital region with fast rhythms associated with visual symptoms. This spreads, 4 s later, to the parietal regions and the child sees a bundle of coloured balloons swinging in his right hemifield. This lasted for 40 s and was followed by slow waves that progressively became slower and diffuse over the whole brain. At this stage, he complained of clouded vision. This boy was normal physically and intellectually, and also had a normal CT brain scan. At the age of 3 years, he had a nocturnal, left hemiconvulsion. His first EEG showed occipital paroxysms with fixation-off sensitivity. Since the age of 4 years, he had started having frequent, brief visual seizures (simple, coloured, visual hallucinations) provoked by sudden darkness.

From Beaumanoir (1993)[102] and reproduced with the kind permission of the author and the publisher John Libbey

background EEG abnormalities (Figure 9.10). Also, patients commonly have additional types of seizures without autonomic symptoms that continue in adult life. Management and treatment is similar to any other form of lesional epilepsy.

- *Gastaut-type idiopathic childhood occipital epilepsy* has entirely different clinical manifestations, despite common interictal EEG features when occipital paroxysms occur in PS. Visual seizures are predominant in G-ICOE. Visual symptoms in PS, when present, occur with other typical clinical, mainly autonomic, vomiting and behavioural manifestations. They are not the predominant seizure symptom. They are never the sole symptom of a seizure and do not occur alone. Usually, they develop after the seizure has started. Their presence signifies spreading of the discharge to the occipital regions of the brain. Exceptionally (in 1% of cases), visual symptoms occur at onset suggesting an occipital origin for the epileptic discharge in these patients.

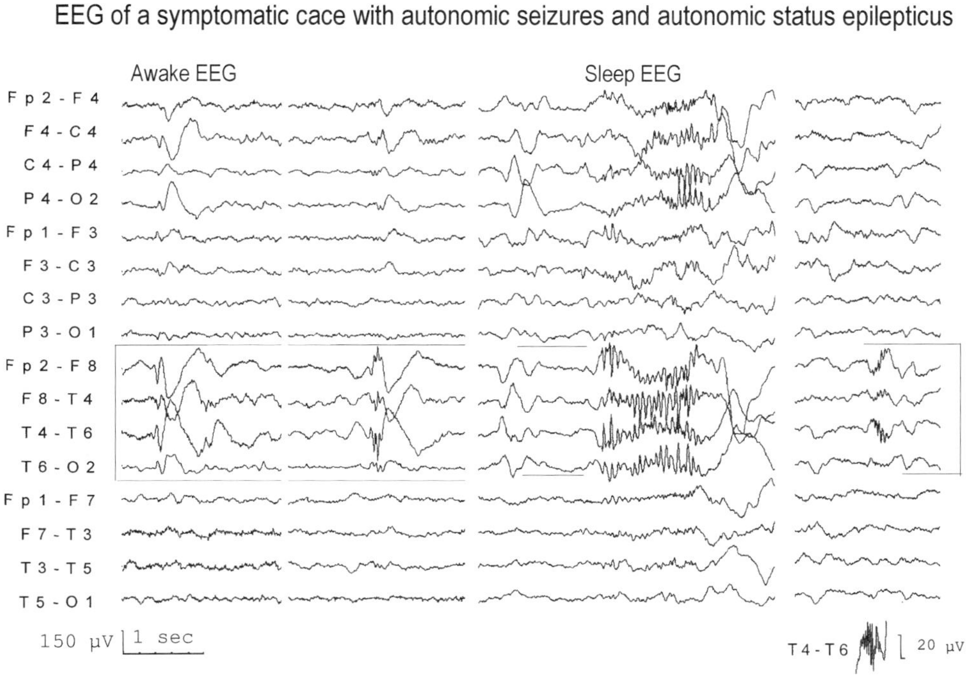

Figure 9.10 EEG of a 10-year-old girl with autonomic seizures and autonomic status epilepticus identical to those of PS (case 60 in ref [4]). The neurological findings and development were normal. However, the EEG had features that were markedly different to the idiopathic cases (rectangle). This prompted an MRI examination, which showed an extensive dysembryoblastic neuroepithelial tumour in the right temporo-parieto-occipital regions, corresponding to severe EEG abnormalities in the same areas.

Since 7 years of age, she had experienced about 10 brief nocturnal seizures lasting 5-10 min each. During these episodes, she jumps out of bed, calls her parents, and complains of feeling sick and of headache. She screams and vomits, her eyes stare and roll, her eyelids blink, her pupils are dilated and she sweats profusely.

A dramatic diurnal autonomic status epilepticus occurred at school. She complained of frontal headache and she had gone out for fresh air when she started feeling "funny". She screamed that she was hot, and she was sweating and vomiting. Subsequently, she became vacant, her speech slurred slightly, her eyes twitched and she dribbled a lot. She asked for water, but did not drink. She talked "gobbledegook" and gradually got worse. Her head deviated to the left and she became unresponsive. This was followed by a series of left hemiconvulsions lasting 5–10 min each. Convulsions were stopped with intravenous diazepam. She gradually recovered. The neurological examination was normal. She was amnesic of the events the next morning and she looked well, complaining only of photophobia.

The CT brain scan was normal. CSF and other relevant investigations were normal. She received triple therapy for encephalitis for 4 days after which she was discharged home.

- *Rolandic seizures* have different clinical manifestations. Emesis, when it occurs, is a concomitant symptom of PS.[14] Conversely, in some cases of PS, there are concurrent Rolandic symptoms. This should not be a problem as the management and the prognosis of both syndromes is the same.
- Cases of PS with seizures occurring when the child is febrile may be diagnosed as *febrile seizures*, but this again is of no prognostic significance.

An EEG demonstrating multifocal spikes may be indispensable in the diagnosis of patients with PS if clinical information is inadequate or emetic manifestations are inconspicuous.

PROGNOSIS

PS is a remarkably benign condition despite the high incidence of autonomic status epilepticus. One-third of patients (27%) have only a single seizure, half (47%) have 2–5 seizures and only 5% have more than 10 seizures, which can sometimes be very frequent, but again the outcome is favourable. Furthermore, the active seizure period is very brief and remission commonly occurs within 1–2 years from onset. The risk of developing epilepsy in adult life is probably no more than that in the general population. However, one-fifth of patients (21%) may develop another type of infrequent, usually Rolandic (13%), seizures during their childhood and early teens. These seizures are also age-related and remit before the age of 16 years. Atypical evolutions with absences and drop attacks, such as those occurring in Rolandic epilepsy, are exceptional.[104;105]

However, despite its benign course, some seizures of PS may occasionally manifest with potentially fatal autonomic symptoms, such as cardiorespiratory arrest.[4]

MANAGEMENT

Current guidelines for febrile seizures, if appropriately modified, may provide the basis for similar guidelines for PS. Based on the risks and benefits of the effective therapies, continuous anticonvulsant therapy is not recommended for children with one or brief seizures. Most clinicians treat recurrent seizures with carbamazepine. Lengthy seizures are a medical emergency and rectal diazepam is prescribed for home administration.

See details in "Management of benign childhood focal seizures" (page 257).

Diagnostic tips

Paediatricians should be alerted by lengthy autonomic seizures and electroencephalographers by frequent multifocal spikes in a normal child with one or a few seizures.

In terms of the EEG, it is important to remember that frequent epileptogenic foci in a normal child with infrequent seizures should raise the possibility of the benign childhood focal seizures.

GASTAUT-TYPE IDIOPATHIC CHILDHOOD OCCIPITAL EPILEPSY

IDIOPATHIC CHILDHOOD OCCIPITAL EPILEPSY

Gastaut type-idiopathic childhood occipital epilepsy (G-ICOE) or idiopathic childhood occipital epilepsy of late onset [1;106-109] is a rare manifestation of a childhood seizure susceptibility syndrome that has an age-related onset, is often age limited and may be genetically determined. It is a pure form of idiopathic occipital epilepsy.

DEMOGRAPHIC DATA

Age at onset is 3–15 years with a mean around 8 years of age. Girls and boys are equally affected. The disorder accounts for about 2–7% of benign childhood focal seizures.

CLINICAL MANIFESTATIONS

Seizures are purely occipital and primarily manifest with elementary visual hallucinations, blindness or both (see also detailed symptomatology of occipital lobe epilepsy, page 417). They are usually frequent and diurnal. They develop rapidly within seconds and are brief, lasting from a few seconds to 1–3 min, rarely longer.

Elementary visual hallucinations are the commonest and most characteristic ictal symptom, and are most likely to be the first and often the only clinical manifestation. Ictal elementary visual hallucinations mainly consist of small multicoloured circular patterns that often appear in the periphery of a visual field, becoming larger and multiplying during the course of the seizure, frequently moving horizontally towards the other side (page 250 and Figure 9.11).

> I see millions of small, very bright, mainly blue and green coloured, circular spots of light, which appear on the left side and sometimes move to the right

Other occipital symptoms, such as sensory illusions of ocular movements and ocular pain, tonic deviation of the eyes, eyelid fluttering or repetitive eye closures, may occur at the onset of the seizures or appear after the elementary visual hallucinations.

Deviation of the eyes, often associated with ipsilateral turning of the head, is the most common (in around 70% of cases) non-visual symptom. It is often associated with ipsilateral turning of the head and usually starts after visual hallucinations, but may also occur while the hallucinations still persist. It may be mild, but more often it is severe and progresses to hemiconvulsions and GTCS. It has been well established that children with benign occipital seizures may have motor focal seizures of eye deviation ab initio without visual hallucination. It is likely that these cases have a better prognosis and shorter seizure life span than those with

---

ILAE definition

The 1989 ILAE Commission named this syndrome "childhood epilepsy with occipital paroxysms" and defined it as follows:[13] "The syndrome of childhood epilepsy with occipital paroxysms is, in general respects, similar to that of benign childhood epilepsy with centrotemporal spikes. The seizures start with visual symptoms (amaurosis, phosphenes, illusions, or hallucinations) and are often followed by a hemiclonic seizure or automatisms. In 25% of cases, the seizures are immediately followed by migrainous headache. The EEG has paroxysms of high-amplitude spike waves or sharp waves recurring rhythmically on the occipital and posterior temporal areas of one or both hemispheres, but only when the eyes are closed. During seizures the occipital discharge may spread to the central or temporal region. At present, no definite statement on prognosis is possible."

This purely *'idiopathic'* and purely *'occipital'* epilepsy has been recognised in the new diagnostic scheme[2] as: "Late onset childhood occipital epilepsy (Gastaut type)".[2]

Uncertainty in regard to prognosis is reflected by the fact that the term 'benign' (used in all other benign childhood focal seizures) is not included in the ILAE descriptive terminology of this syndrome.[2;13]

G-ICOE, but this has not yet been properly investigated.[109]

Forced eyelid closure and eyelid blinking are interesting ictal clinical symptoms of occipital seizures that occur in approximately 10% of patients, usually at a stage in which consciousness is impaired. They signal impending secondary GTCS.

Ictal blindness, appearing ab initio or less commonly after other manifestations of occipital seizures, usually lasts for 3–5 min. It can occur alone and can be the only ictal event in patients who may, at other times, have visual hallucinations without blindness.

> Everything went suddenly black, I could not see and I had to ask other swimmers to show me the direction to the beach.

Complex visual hallucinations, without the emotional and complicated character of temporal lobe seizures, visual illusions and other symptoms resulting from more anterior ictal spreading, may rarely occur ab initio or as a result of seizure progress that may terminate in hemiconvulsions or generalised convulsions.

Ictal headache, or mainly orbital pain, may occur and often precedes the visual or other ictal occipital symptoms in a small number of patients.[1;110]

Consciousness in not impaired during the elementary or complex visual hallucinations, blindness and other occipital seizure symptoms (simple focal seizures), but may be disturbed or lost in the course of the seizure, usually prior to eye deviation or convulsions.

Ictal syncope is rare.[4]

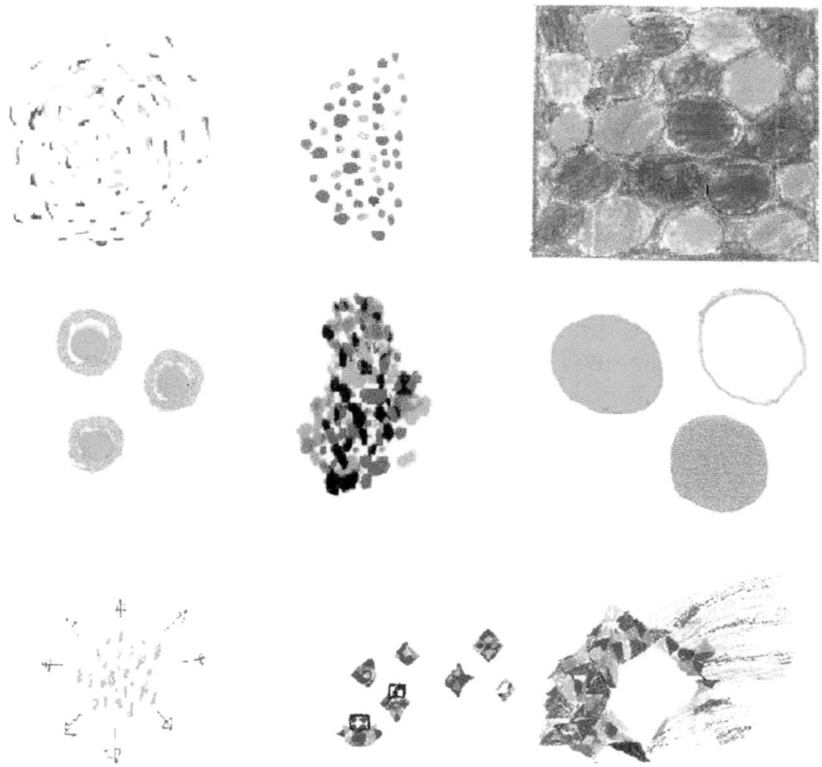

Figure 9.11 Elementary visual hallucinations as perceived and drawn by patients with visual seizures.

From Panayiotopoulos 1999[110] and reproduced with the permission of the Editor of the *Journal of Neurology, Neurosurgery and Psychiatry*.

A 10-year-old child had frequent visual seizures of elementary hallucinations and blindness. He also had 4 episodes of ictal syncope in its most pure and challenging form: brief (1-2 minutes), transient loss of consciousness and postural tone with pallor of sudden onset and sudden recovery. They occurred whilst sitting or standing. He falls down and becomes unresponsive. One episode witnessed by a physician was described "clumsiness, vacant, unresponsive for a minute or so. No convulsions". Another one was witnessed by his parents: "he was next to us in a shop. We heard a bang and saw him on the ground. Colour white not blue. He was out for a few seconds." He never had anything like this in the next 9 years of follow-up. This is case 26 in ref.[1]

Occipital seizures of Gastaut-type childhood occipital epilepsy may rarely progress to extra-occipital manifestations, such as hemiparaesthesia. Spreading to produce symptoms of temporal lobe involvement is exceptional and may indicate a symptomatic cause.

Postictal headache, mainly diffuse, but also severe, unilateral and pulsating, or indistinguishable from migraine headache occurs in half of the patients and, in 10% of these cases, it may be associated with nausea and vomiting.[1;110]

I then have a left-sided severe throbbing headache for an hour or so.

CIRCADIAN DISTRIBUTION

Visual seizures are predominantly diurnal and occur at any time of the day. Longer seizures, with or without secondary hemi- or generalised convulsions, tend to occur either during sleep, causing the patient to wake, or after awakening. Thus, some children may have numerous diurnal visual seizures and only a few seizures that are exclusively nocturnal or that occur on awakening secondary to GTCS.

FREQUENCY OF SEIZURES

In untreated, patients experience brief visual seizures frequently (often several each day or weekly). However, propagation to other seizure manifestations, such as focal or generalised convulsions, is much less frequent (monthly, yearly or exceptionally).

AETIOLOGY

There may be an increased family history of epilepsies (37% of cases) or migraine (16% of cases),[107] but a family history of similar seizures is exeptional.[111]
G-ICOE is considered to be a late onset phenotype of BCSSS (see page 262).

PATHOPHYSIOLOGY

The seizures are purely of cortical occipital origin.[109]

The mechanisms of postictal headache, which is common even after minor idiopathic or symptomatic visual seizures, with or without a predisposition to migraine, are unknown. It is likely that the occipital seizure discharge triggers a genuine migraine headache through trigeminovascular or brain-stem mechanisms.[110;112]

The occipital paroxysms are bilateral and synchronous when they occur, because they are activated in the bi-occipital regions by the elimination of fixation and central vision (Figures 9.4;9.12).[4;113] They are not due to a thalamocortical mechanism, driven by a thalamic pacemaker, as proposed by Gastaut and Zifkin.[107]

DIAGNOSTIC PROCEDURES

By definition, all tests other than the EEG are normal. However, high resolution MRI is probably mandatory, because of the high incidence of symptomatic occipital epilepsies with the same clinical EEG manifestations.

ELECTROENCEPHALOGRAPHY

The interictal EEG shows occipital paroxysms often demonstrating fixation-off sensitivity (Figure 9.12). However, some patients may have only random occipital spikes, while others may have occipital spikes in only the sleep EEG and a few may have a consistently normal EEG. Centrotemporal, frontal and giant somatosensory spikes may occur, but less often than in PS. Whether occipital photosensitivity is part of this syndrome or not is debated (page 469).

Ictal EEG, preceded by regression of occipital paroxysms, is characterised by the sudden appearance of an occipital discharge that consists of fast rhythms, fast spikes or both (Figures 9.9 and 9.13).[102;106;107;116-120] This is of much lower amplitude than the occipital paroxysms. Elementary visual hallucinations are related to the fast spike activity that may spread to the other hemisphere. Complex visual hallucinations may occur when the discharge is slower. In oculoclonic seizures, spikes and spike and waves are slower and a localised ictal fast spike rhythm may occur prior to the deviation of the eyes. Ictal EEG during blindness is characterised by pseudoperiodic slow waves and spikes, which differs from that seen in ictal visual hallucinations.

There are usually no postictal abnormalities.

DIFFERENTIAL DIAGNOSIS

The differential diagnosis of G-ICOE is mainly from probably symptomatic (cryptogenic) or symptomatic occipital epilepsy, coeliac disease, migraine with aura, and basilar or acephalgic migraine where misdiagnosis is high.[1;110]

The differential diagnosis from migraine should be easy if all clinical elements are properly assessed and synthesised as described in Table 12.3, page 427.

Basilar migraine with occipital spikes does not exist; the relevant reports described cases with genuine G-ICOE (see page 427) imitating basilar migraine.[110;121]

In a typical case of G-ICOE, an 8-year-old child started complaining of elementary visual hallucinations that consisted of unilateral multicoloured small circles lasting for a few seconds. Their frequency and duration increased over the next few months and these symptoms were followed by diffuse headache. A diagnosis of migraine with aura was made and relevant treatment was initiated without success. On the contrary, the child had two seizures in which the same visual hallucinations became so intense as to obscure his vision, followed by deviation of the eyes and head. An EEG showed bilateral occipital paroxysms with fixation-off sensitivity. MRI was normal. The child had two

Definition of occipital paroxysms

Occipital paroxysms are by far more common in G-ICOE than PS (Figures 9.7 and 9.12) They are defined as 'long runs of repetitive, high amplitude sharp and slow wave complexes in the occipital regions, which are morphologically similar to the CTS'.[113] The word 'paroxysm' in EEG terminology is a 'Group of waves that appears and disappears abruptly, which is clearly distinguishable from background activity by its different frequency, morphology or amplitude'. The individual complexes of the occipital paroxysms show a diphasic spike component with a main surface negative peak in the occipital electrodes and an amplitude often exceeding 200 µV. This is followed by a smaller positive peak and a high amplitude, negative slow wave. Occipital paroxysms are often bilateral and synchronous, but may also be unilateral and predominantly right sided. Occipital paroxysms appear and persist only when the eyes are closed and may not be recorded in children who keep their eyes open during the EEG. This is because occipital paroxysms are activated by the elimination of fixation and central vision (fixation-off sensitivity, Figure 9.12).[69]

Occipital paroxysms may persist long after remission of clinical seizures, but also may not be detected interictally during the active seizure phase.

Random occipital spikes that do not have the repetitive character of occipital paroxysms are more common than occipital paroxysms.

Reminder about occipital spikes

Occipital spikes are not pathognomonic of a particular syndrome, because they also occur in a variety of organic brain diseases with or without seizures, in children with congenital or early onset visual and ocular deficits, and even in 0.5–1.2 % of normal preschool-age children.[42;113-115] They are common in young children with a peak age at first discovery of 4–5 years and "tend to disappear in adult life, and the subsidence of the EEG abnormality is usually accompanied by a cessation of seizures".[42;114]

episodes of complete blindness without convulsions. The diagnosis of basilar migraine was suspected, but visual hallucinations continued, one of them ending with GTCS. No more seizures of any other type occurred after treatment with carbamazepine, which continued for 3 years. By 20 years of age, the patient was attending university, was well, free of seizures with no treatment and had a normal EEG.

Symptomatic occipital epilepsy often imitates G-ICOE; neuro-ophthalmological examination and brain imaging may be normal, and high resolution MRI may be required to detect subtle lesions.[122] Occipital seizures of mitochondrial disorders, Lafora disease and coeliac disease[123] should be considered (see details on pages 422–3).[1]

PROGNOSIS

The prognosis is unclear, though available data indicate that remission occurs in 50–60% of patients within 2–4 years from onset. Seizures show a dramatically good response to carbamazepine in more than 90% of patients. However, 40–50% of patients may continue to have visual seizures and infrequent secondary GTCS, particularly if they have not been appropriately treated with carbamazepine. Rarely, atypical evolutions to epilepsy with continuous spike waves during slow wave sleep with cognitive deterioration have been reported.[124]

Although no significant differences were found in basic neurophysiological functions between patients with G-ICOE and control groups, patients' performance scores for in attention, memory and intellectual functioning were lower.[125]

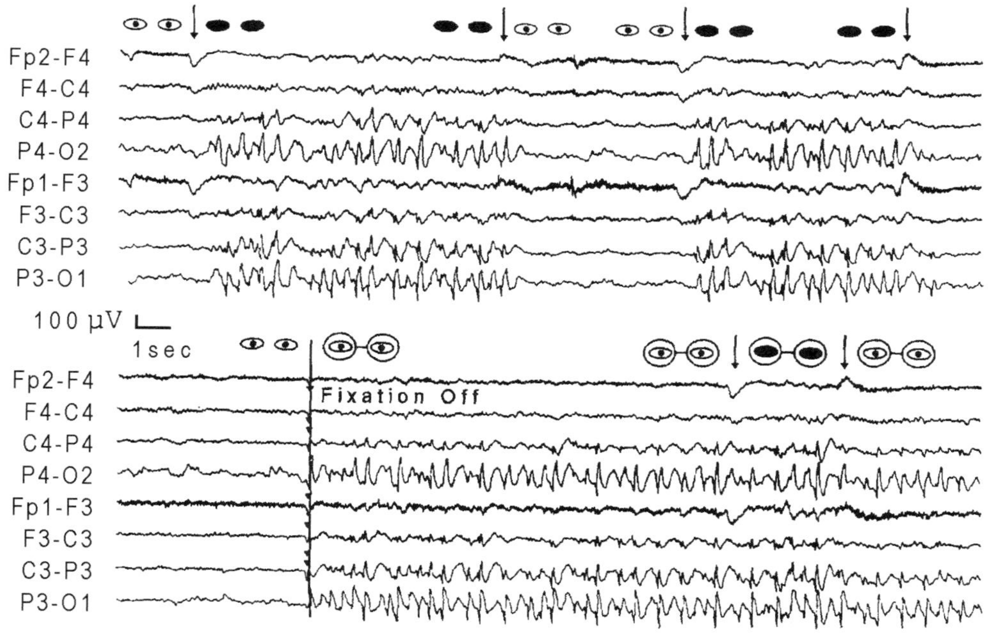

Figure 9.12 Occipital paroxysms in their classical form with fixation-off sensitivity in a 10-year-old boy with Gastaut-type childhood occipital epilepsy (case 26 in ref [1]).

Occipital paroxysms occur as long as fixation and central vision are eliminated by any means (eyes closed, darkness, +10 spherical lenses, Ganzfeld stimulation). Under these conditions, eye opening is not capable of inhibiting the spikes.

Symbols of the eyes open or closed without glasses denote that the recording was made with the lights on and whenever fixation was possible.

Symbols of the eyes open or closed with glasses denote that the recording was made when fixation and central vision were eliminated by any of the above means.

MANAGEMENT

In contrast to other phenotypes of the BCSSS, patients with Gastaut-type childhood occipital epilepsy often suffer from frequent seizures and therefore medical treatment, mainly with carbamazepine, is probably mandatory.[1;110] Secondary GTCS are probably unavoidable without medication.

A slow reduction in the dose of medication 2–3 years after the last visual or other minor or major seizure may be advised, but if visual seizures reappear, treatment should be restored.

OTHER PHENOTYPES OF BENIGN CHILDHOOD SEIZURE SUSCEPTIBILITY SYNDROME[1]

There are well-documented reports of children suffering from benign childhood focal seizures with clinical EEG manifestations that can not be classified as typical cases of Rolandic epilepsy, PS or Gastaut-type childhood occipital epilepsy. Their existence verifies the unified concept of BCSSS. They may represent atypical presentations of the recognised syndromes within the BCSSS.

BENIGN CHILDHOOD SEIZURES WITH AFFECTIVE SYMPTOMS

Benign childhood seizures with affective symptoms[12;126] are a rare clinical phenotype of the BCSSS. This disorder has features in common with both PS

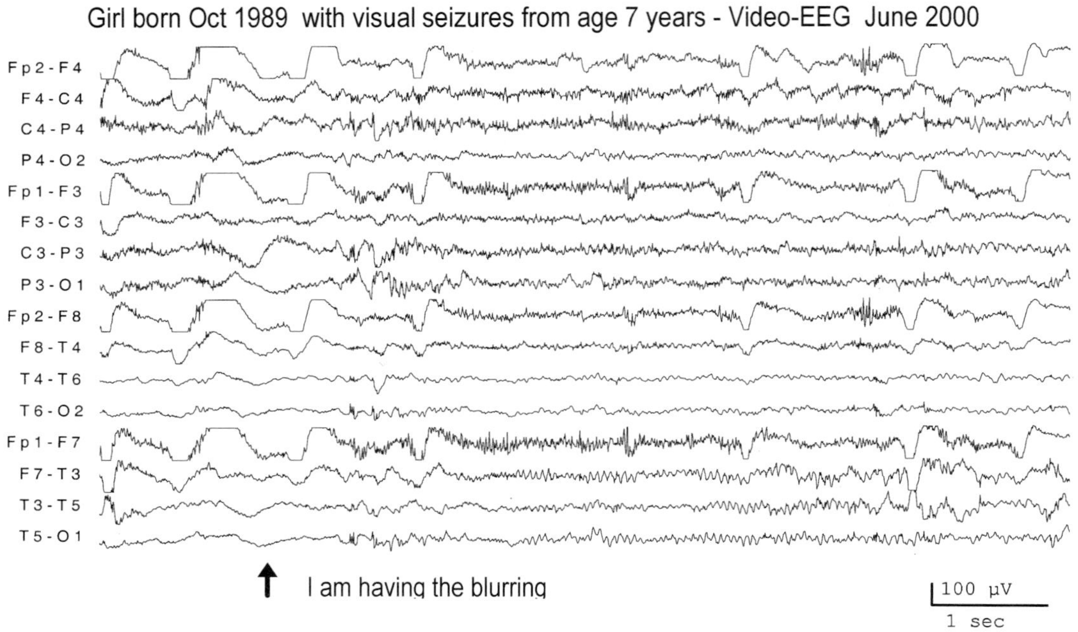

Figure 9.13

Ictal video EEG telemetry of an 11-year-old girl with frequent daily visual seizures since 7 years of age. The seizures were intractable to any appropriate medication. The child had learning difficulties, but all appropriate tests, including high resolution brain MRI, were normal. This may be a case of probable symptomatic occipital epilepsy rather than G-ICOE.

Note that the first ictal symptom is blurring of vision. The ictal EEG starts with small bi-occipital spikes followed by symmetrical, episodic, fast activity in the posterior regions.

(behavioural and autonomic symptoms) and Rolandic epilepsy (arrest of speech and hypersalivation). Dalla Bernandina et al.[126] consider 'benign partial epilepsy with affective symptoms' a relatively rare variant of RS.

DEMOGRAPHIC DATA

The onset of afebrile seizures occurs at 2–9 years of age and both sexes are equally affected. One-fifth of patients have febrile seizures and family history of epilepsy is common (36%).

CLINICAL MANIFESTATIONS

Seizures are brief, but multiple, diurnal and nocturnal, and manifest with terror and screaming, autonomic disturbances (pallor, sweating, abdominal pain, salivation), chewing and other automatisms, arrest of speech and mild impairment of consciousness.

The predominant seizure symptom is sudden fear or terror:

> "This terror was expressed by the child starting to scream, to yell or to call his mother; he clung to her or to anyone nearby or went to a corner of the room hiding his face in his hands. His terrorised expression was sometimes associated with either chewing or swallowing movements, distressed laughter, arrest of speech with glottal noises, moans and salivation, or some kind of autonomic manifestation, such as pallor, sweating or abdominal pain, that the child expressed by bringing his hands onto his abdomen and saying 'It hurts me, it hurts me'. These phenomena were associated with changes in awareness (loss of contact) that did not amount to complete unconsciousness."[126]

The seizures are brief, lasting between 1–2 min and a maximum of 10 min.

Half of the children have frequent (several times a day) seizures from the onset, which may occur with the same semiology whether awake or asleep. Some children may have brief and infrequent nocturnal RS at the same time as the affective attacks. Generalised seizures do not occur.

DIAGNOSTIC PROCEDURES

All tests, apart from the EEG, are normal.

The interictal EEG shows high amplitude sharp and slow wave complexes, which are morphologically similar to Rolandic spikes and are located around the fronto-temporal and parieto-temporal electrodes. In common with the other benign childhood focal seizures, EEG abnormalities are exaggerated by sleep and may be associated with generalised discharges.

Ictal EEG discharges are localized to the fronto-temporal, centrotemporal or parietal areas or may be diffuse. They are stereotypical in each individual patient.

PROGNOSIS

The response to treatment is excellent and remission is reported to occur within 1–2 years. At the active stage of the disease, behavioural problems may be prominent, but subside with the seizures.

TREATMENT

In the active phase of the disease and because of frequent seizures antiepileptic medication, mainly with carbamazepine, may be needed.

BENIGN CHILDHOOD EPILEPSY WITH PARIETAL SPIKES AND FREQUENT GIANT SOMATOSENSORY EVOKED POTENTIALS[46;51;127]

Benign childhood epilepsy with parietal spikes and frequent giant somatosensory evoked potentials may be another phenotype of BCSSS. The defining features are

EEG spikes in the parietal regions, which are often elicited by tactile stimulation. However, somatosensory evoked giant potentials/spikes (page 229)[1;4;46-48;51;52] are not specific for any syndrome as they also occur in 10–20% of children with RS,[51] in a few patients with PS (Figure 9.4)[1;4] and in children without seizures (Figure 9.4).[128]

Clinically, patients suffer from versive seizures of the head and body, often without impairment of consciousness. These are mainly diurnal and infrequent. Multiple daily seizures and focal status epilepticus are exceptional.

Remission usually occurs within 1 year from seizure onset, but EEG abnormalities may persist for longer.

BENIGN CHILDHOOD FOCAL SEIZURES ASSOCIATED WITH FRONTAL SPIKES OR MIDLINES SPIKES

Benign childhood focal seizures associated with frontal spikes[1;129;130] or midline spikes[1;131] have been described and long follow-up reports have confirmed a benign course, but no systematic studies have been published. However, it should be remembered that EEG spike foci of various locations are also seen in Rolandic epilepsy and more commonly in PS. Midline spikes are more common in children than in adults and they are not specific for any type of epilepsy.[132;133] Of six children with at least one EEG having midline spikes only, five had normal development with febrile seizures (one case), Rolandic epilepsy (one case), PS (one case), a single occipital complex partial seizure (one case) and brief seizures with loss of consciousness only (one case). The only symptomatic case had generalised convulsions.[133]

BENIGN FOCAL EPILEPSY IN INFANTS WITH CENTRAL AND VERTEX SPIKES AND WAVES DURING SLEEP

Benign focal epilepsy in infants with central and vertex spikes and waves during sleep has been recently described as a new BCSSS.[134;135] In terms of age, this is on the borderline between benign infantile seizures (page 124) and BCSSS. Age at onset is in the first 2 years of life with both sexes equally affected. Infants are normal and all tests other than EEG are normal. Seizures consist mainly of staring, motion arrest, facial cyanosis, loss of consciousness and stiffening of the arms. Clonic convulsions and automatisms are rare. Duration is from 1–5 min. Seizures are mainly diurnal (but may also occur during sleep) and may occur in clusters, but are generally infrequent (1–3 seizures/year).

Interictal EEG abnormalities are seen only in non-REM sleep and consist of small, mostly singular, spikes and waves localised in the vertex and central electrodes.

There is a strong family history of epilepsy with benign epilepsies prevailing.

The prognosis is excellent with remission of seizures, normal development and normalisation of the EEG before the age of 4 years.

MANAGEMENT OF BENIGN CHILDHOOD FOCAL SEIZURES

Short- and long-term treatment strategies of benign childhood focal seizures are empirical and there is no consensus regarding their management.[1;4] However, current practice parameter guidelines for febrile seizures,[136;137] if appropriately modified, may be the basis for similar guidelines in benign childhood focal seizures and, particularly, Rolandic epilepsy[1] and PS.[4] Based on the risks and benefits of the effective therapies, continuous antiepileptic medication is not recommended for children who have had only one or brief seizures. Most clinicians treat recurrent seizures with carbamazepine, but in exceptional cases this may worsen seizures. Lengthy seizures are a medical emergency; rectal diazepam is prescribed for home administration. Recurrent and lengthy seizures create anxiety in parents and patients, and, as such, appropriate education and emotional support should be provided.

ACUTE MANAGEMENT OF A CHILD WITH PROLONGED SEIZURES

Control of the seizure is paramount. On the rare occasions that the child is febrile, treatment of possible fever and the underlying illness is also important.

Long-lasting seizures (> 10 min) or status epilepticus (> 30 min–hours) is a feature in two-thirds of children (70%) with PS. This is a genuine paediatric emergency that demands appropriate and vigorous treatment as for status epilepticus.[138;139] Early, usually parental administration of appropriate AEDs is more effective than late emergency treatment.[139]

The treatment of prolonged febrile seizures and febrile status epilepticus is described on pages 123.

PROPHYLACTIC MANAGEMENT OF BENIGN CHILDHOOD FOCAL SEIZURES

Continuous anticonvulsant treatment is usually not recommended. Although there are effective therapies that could prevent the occurrence of additional seizures, the potential adverse effects of such therapy are not commensurate with the benefit. The great majority of children with benign focal seizures do not need anticonvulsant treatment even if they suffer lengthy seizures or have more than two recurrences. The risks are small and the potential side effects of drugs appear to outweigh the benefits.

In patients with recurrent seizures and/or when parental anxiety associated with seizures is severe, small doses of antiepileptic medication may be effective in preventing recurrence. There is no convincing evidence, however, that any therapy will alleviate the possibility of recurrences. In deciding management for a child with benign childhood focal seizures the following should be considered:

- Most children have an excellent prognosis: 10–30% of patients may have only a single seizure and seizures may be infrequent (usually 2–10) in 60–70%. However, 10–20% of patients may have frequent seizures, which are sometimes resistant to treatment.
- Remission of benign childhood focal seizures is expected in all patients by 15–16 years of age at the latest.
- The possibility of future epilepsy is a most unlikely event and probably not higher than that in the general population.
- There is no evidence that the long-term prognosis is worse in untreated children, though they may not be protected against seizure recurrences.

- Some children become frightened even by simple focal seizures and some parents are unable to cope with the possibility of another fit despite firm reassurances.
- Persistence and frequency of EEG functional spikes are not predictive of clinical severity, frequency and degree of liability to seizures.

Continuous prophylaxis consists of daily monotherapy using any antiepileptic drug with proven efficacy in focal seizures, usually carbamazepine. However, carbamazepine may exaggerate seizures in a minority of children with RS. Recently, sulthiame has been revived as an excellent drug for the treatment of benign childhood epilepsy with centrotemporal spikes.[140-142] Sulthiame may be the drug of choice in children with BCSSS and cognitive impairment, because it often normalises the EEG.[140-142] Of the newer drugs, levetiracetam has been reported as therapeutic in the few children in whom it has been tried.[143] Lamotrigine may be associated with significant seizure and cognitive derioration.[66-68]

STOPPING MEDICATION

Methods of withdrawing medication differ between experts, though all agree that there is no need to continue medication 1–3 years after the last seizure and certainly not after 14 years of age when most benign childhood focal seizures remit or 16 years of age when they are practically non-existent. My practice is to start gradual withdrawal of medication 2 years after the last seizure, making sure that the child does not have any minor seizures. However, I do not adhere to fixed rules and may continue medication until the age of 13–15 years depending on the severity, frequency and age at onset of seizures. Thus, in a child that had frequent, severe and difficult to control fits in early childhood, I would not stop medication if the child had a seizure-free period of 2–3 years by the age 7 years. Conversely, for a child who had three or four nocturnal seizures at age 11 and 12 years, I would certainly slowly discontinue medication after a 2-year seizure-free period. I advise very slow withdrawal, reducing the dose in monthly steps so that the drug is completely discontinued approximately 6 months later. The reason for this is that I expect that any possible seizure recurrence during the process of very slow drug withdrawal would manifest with mild, brief and simple focal without secondary generalised convulsions. In the case of barbiturates and diazepines, slow withdrawal of medication is mandatory in order to avoid risking a possible withdrawal seizure.

PARENTAL ATTITUDE, REACTION AND EDUCATION IN BENIGN CHILDHOOD FOCAL SEIZURES*

By Thalia Valeta

The traditional goal of care for children with epilepsies has been optimal seizure control. This has now been widely broadened to include optimal health-related quality of life outcomes.[144] These outcomes assess the physical, mental and psychological functioning of the epileptic child within his/her family, educational and social environment, and reflect the impact of seizures and their treatments on patients and their parents. Parents are integral to the functioning and quality of life of their children and, therefore, the health-related quality of life of a child largely depends on the parents' attitudes, reactions, education and adjustment.

***Author's note:** Searching through appropriate sources of information, I found no work or reference to the reactions and needs of parents with children of benign focal seizures. The on-going study of Thalia Valeta is the first of this kind.

Thus, it is crucial that parents are given sufficient time and opportunity to discuss their concerns with the specialists, who should provide the following:

- an accurate diagnosis of the child's condition including precise cause, risk of recurrence, prognosis, and type and length of management, as well as possible hereditary factors and adverse reactions of treatments
- an assessment of the immediate and future effects on the physical, mental, behavioural, educational, family, social and vocational aspects of their life
- information about the parental role in preventing (leisure and other activities) or early detection of an epileptic attack including means of terminating a seizure, particularly if this is lengthy and life threatening.

The adjustment and other problems experienced by children with a diagnosis of epilepsy and their parents have always been a concern to clinicians and health-care providers. It is understandable that this has been primarily focused on parents of children with severe and intractable epilepsy, who face profound challenges in dealing with their child's frequent and severe seizures, the additional physical, social and psychological problems, and ongoing quest of seizure control through a variety of drugs, diet and surgery.[145] However, the significant burden of anxieties placed on the parents of children with benign epileptic conditions has been less emphasised because, comparatively, they are more fortunate with regard to prognosis, management, current and future prospects, and responsibilities. The only exception to this is in relation to febrile seizures where parental reactions and concerns have been well documented[146-152] and properly addressed.[136;137] These reactions are often severe and contrast with the physician's perception of febrile seizures as a uncomplicated and benign condition. In one such study,[146] 52 parents of a child with febrile seizures were interviewed about their immediate and long-term reactions. Most parents knew little about febrile convulsions before the fit and most of them thought the child was dying (77%), was suffocating or had meningitis (15%). Afterwards, parental behaviour altered: 60% experienced restless sleep, 29% had dyspepsia, and 6% watched over their child at night and 8% when feverish. Parents with previous knowledge of febrile seizures took more appropriate measures, but only 21% positioned the child correctly during the seizure.[146]

It is now part of good clinical practice to provide the parents of children with febrile seizures specific information about fever and febrile seizures, and comprehensive instructions about what to do if a seizure happens again. [136;137;153] The parents of children with recurrent febrile seizures should be advised on what to do if a seizure recurs since early treatment provided by parents is more effective than late treatment in an emergency facility. The guidelines also provide room for starting anti-epileptic drug treatment in "the unlikely event of parental insistence" or "situations in which parental anxiety associated with seizures is severe". [136;137]

Talking extensively to parents of children with benign childhood focal seizures I realised that, despite the fact that these seizures are of excellent prognosis, they are a dramatic experience for patients and their parents. Consequently, I have initiated an on-going study aiming to define and analyse the psychosocial effects of benign childhood focal seizures on parents and children. I have designed a questionnaire in order to identify the main concerns of parents about the seizure itself and its impact on the child's development and future. The questionnaire includes questions on beliefs and attitudes about epilepsy, as well as concerns about the prognosis, necessity of evaluation and information on daily care. I hope that the results of my study will assist the patient and parents, inform the physician and, consequently, help to improve the treatment outcome.

QUESTIONAIRE ON PARENTAL ATTITUDE AND REACTIONS TO BENIGN CHILDHOOD FOCAL SEIZURES

I. Parental reaction during and after the seizure prior to medical attention

a. What did you think was happening to your child?

b. What was your reaction and how did you help your child?

c. How did you feel?

II. Parental reaction after the child had recovered

a. How did you feel?

b. What do you think about the future?

c. Did you think that this was a one-off event?

d. Did you take any further actions?

III. Parental reaction after consultation with the attending physician

a. Was this useful?

b. How did you feel? (1) re-assured, (2) uncertain or (3) anxious.

IV. Short- and long-term effects of the event on you as parents, other members of the family and the child

a. Did you discuss the event with the child and what did you say?

b. Did your attitude change towards the child?

c. If yes, in what way did it change?

d. How did the event affect you over the following weeks/months/years (fears, sleep, appetite, work, relation with the child and other members of your family)?

e. Did the event change the child's behaviour and attitude?

f. Did the event affect the family?

V. When the diagnosis of your child was established and explained to you did this affect your state of mind and your reactions?

VI. Any questions and comments that you may still have?

The commonest fears and expressions were:

> I thought he/she was dying, choking, asphyxiated, electrocuted never to come around again
>
> I thought he had a stroke
>
> I was terrified, petrified
>
> The doctor told me that because the seizure was longer than half an hour this may affect the brain and that time will tell.
>
> We sleep with our daughter in between us on a large bed, and we keep an eye on her as she enters and exits sleep.

The most dominant points emerging from this study are:

- *Uncertainty of what this event was.*

The majority of parents felt uncertain about what this event was and that they were not given sufficient information or reassurance, and some were told that the child had not had a seizure. Initially, some children were diagnosed as having encephalitis, atypical migraine, fainting, gastroenteritis or motion sickness.

- *Anxiety of what the cause of the event was.*

This was often associated with a feeling of guilt, either of parental acts directly associated with the event (child relatively unattended, preceding parental arguments, child involved in leisure activity that may have caused the attack), heredity or with previous events in the child's development (birth, trauma, illness, family history of illness).

- *The effect of the seizure on the child's development.* "Is this going to affect his/her brain?"

Most parents were reassured that one brief seizure would not affect the child's development. However, some parents of children with lengthy seizures were left with the impression that, because the seizure was prolonged, it may have had some adverse effect on the child and only "time will tell".

- *No specific advice was provided about the possibility of relapses and what the parents should do if such a seizure recurred.*

These results indicate that there is a need for supportive family management, education and specific instructions about emergency procedures in possible subsequent seizures. Demonstrations of first aid practices for seizures are necessary. Parents of young children should be given general information about benign childhood focal seizures and, in particular, Panayiotopoulos syndrome in which seizures may last for many hours, compounded by physicians' uncertainty regarding diagnoses, management and prognosis. Parents who have watched their child during a fit need specific information and psychological support to overcome anxiety and panic. Anxiety may result in overprotection, which interferes with parent-child separation and independence. Educating parents about the epilepsies and different types of seizure through seminars, courses and lectures will help to alleviate the social stigma surrounding these conditions, which parents often pass on to their children who are the patients. Parents must be offered training to remain calm and confident about their children's condition in order to improve the quality of life of both the child and the family. Medicine can now profit from a holistic approach to care through counselling and helping people with epilepsies and their families. Practice parameter guidelines regarding parental management and education of children with benign seizures should be updated.

UNIFIED CONCEPT FOR THE BENIGN CHILDHOOD FOCAL SEIZURES

BENIGN CHILDHOOD SEIZURE SUSCEPTIBILITY SYNDROME[1;4;154]

Benign childhood focal seizures with focal EEG sharp slow wave complexes are a group of syndromes of probably one disease, which, in my opinion, share common clinical and EEG characteristics. Seizures are infrequent, usually nocturnal and remit within 1–3 years from onset. Brief or prolonged seizures, even status epilepticus, may be the only clinical event of the patient's lifetime. Ictal autonomic manifestations, such as hypersalivation, vomiting, headache, pallor or sweating, and ictal syncope, which is unusual in other epileptic syndromes, are frequent and may occasionally appear in isolation. The clinical and EEG characteristics of one syndrome may evolve into another or a child may simultaneously develop features of another form of benign childhood focal seizures. Febrile seizures are common. Neurological examination and intellect are normal, but some children may experience mild and reversible neuropsychological problems during the active stage of the disorder. Brain imaging is normal. There are usually severe EEG abnormalities, which are disproportionate to the frequency of seizures. Epileptogenic foci, irrespective of their location, manifest as abundant, high amplitude, sharp, slow wave complexes that occur mainly in clusters. They are often bilateral, independent or synchronous, frequently combined with foci from other cortical areas or brief generalised discharges, and are exaggerated in sleep stages I–IV. A normal EEG is rare and should provoke a sleep EEG study. Similar EEG features resolving with age are frequently found in normal school-age children (2–4%) and children having an EEG for reasons other than seizures.

There is no reason to suggest that all these syndromes differ from each other merely because an 'epileptogenic' focus is a little anterior or posterior, lateral or

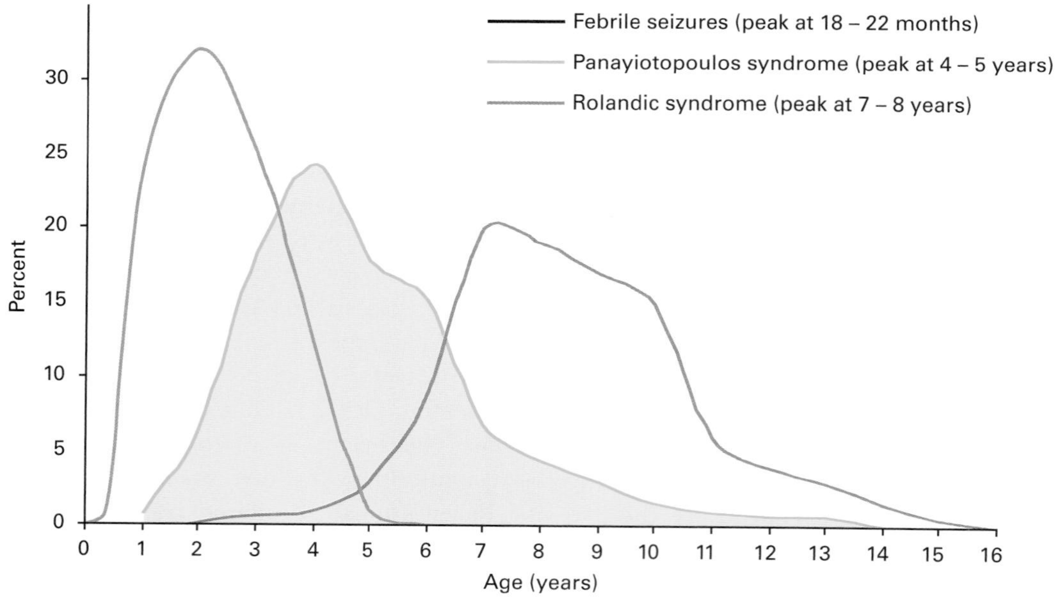

Figure 9.14 Diagramatic age-related presentation of febrile, Rolandic and Panayiotopoulos syndromes.

medial to the centrotemporal regions. A unified concept of benign childhood focal seizures is also suggested by the frequency of more than one type of benign childhood focal seizures in an affected child, siblings or both.

It is likely and I have proposed that all these conditions are linked together by a common, genetically determined, mild and reversible, functional derangement of the brain cortical maturational process.[1;29] This is often clinically silent and manifests in more than 90% with EEG sharp and slow waves with an age-related localisation (Figure 9.1). The remaining minority have infrequent focal seizures with symptoms that are also localisation- and age-related and -dependent. It is possible that a few of these children, with or without seizures, also have usually minor and fully reversible neuropsychological symptoms that are rarely clinically overt and that can only be detected by formal neuropsychological testing. Finally, there may be a very small number of patients (< 1%) in whom this derangement of the brain maturation process may be further derailed in a more aggressive condition with seizures, neuropsychological manifestations and EEG abnormalities of various combinations and various degrees of severity, such as in atypical benign focal epilepsy of childhood, Landau-Kleffner syndrome, and epilepsy with continuous spikes and slow waves during sleep.

My overall impression is that benign childhood focal seizures, their clinical and EEG manifestations and evolutions, need appropriate prospective studies, such as those performed for febrile seizures.

FEBRILE SEIZURES AND BENIGN CHILDHOOD SEIZURE SUSCEPTIBILITY SYNDROME

One of the most interesting aspects of benign childhood seizures is their striking age-related sequence. Common benign seizure disorders are specific to children and do not occur in adults. The fact that children are particularly susceptible to seizures is well documented.

There are three main periods of age-related childhood susceptibility to seizures. Febrile mainly *generalised* convulsions first appear in early childhood at a peak age of 18–22 months. Rolandic *focal* seizures occur in late childhood at a peak age of 7–10 years. Panayiotopoulos syndrome covers the intermediate period, occurring at a peak of 4–5 years, and manifests with mainly autonomic seizures (Figure 9.14). Let me analyse this further as this is likely to be highly significant in our understanding of the disordered age-related maturational processes.

In the first, early period (febrile seizures), the brain is vulnerable to seizures that are triggered by fever and mainly manifest with *convulsions* that are commonly *generalised*. The second intermediate period (Panayiotopoulos syndrome) consists of spontaneous seizures that are often *prolonged* for hours and manifest principally with *autonomic* and mainly *emetic* symptoms. The third late period (Rolandic syndrome) consists of spontaneous focal, motor or sensorimotor seizures.

These three periods of clinical seizure susceptibility also have peculiar EEG accompaniments. The EEG is practically normal in the first period of febrile seizures, shows mainly posterior and multifocal spikes in the intermediate period of Panayiotopoulos syndrome and Rolandic spikes in the late period of the Rolandic syndrome.

All these indicate that the brain in early childhood has a low threshold to generalised convulsions provoked by fever with a relatively silent EEG spike capacity. Subsequently, the autonomic system and particularly the emetic centres become vulnerable, the seizure discharges may be self-sustained and the cortex exhibits a diffuse epileptogenicity, which is unequally distributed and mainly affects the posterior regions. Finally, in the third period of late childhood, brain epileptogenicity shrinks to around the Rolandic regions to produce the distinctive clinical and EEG manifestations of the Rolandic syndrome.

These are incontrovertible facts that tell us something very important about the developing brain that we have not yet explored. We should also consider the neonatal and the early infantile periods, because they also have their own peculiarities as indicated by the benign familial and non-familial neonatal seizures that occur around the first few days of life, and the benign infantile focal seizures of the Watanabe-Vigevano syndrome. This point is exemplified by reports of children with neonatal seizures who later developed Rolandic[155] or PS.[79] Maihara et al.[155] described a family with benign familial neonatal seizures in which two siblings later developed RS and EEG centrotemporal spikes. Lada et al.[79] reported an otherwise normal boy who first had benign neonatal seizures, then two febrile seizures at the age of 18 months and 3 years. This was followed by a brief autonomic seizure of PS with ictal vomiting and deviation of the eyes occurred during sleep at 6 years of age; the EEG showed occipital paroxysms. I have also described a boy who, at 8 weeks old, had three focal seizures of right-sided convulsions involving the face and upper limbs (benign neonatal non-familial seizures of Watanabe-Vigevano syndrome). Subsequent EEGs were normal and treatment stopped at age 10 months. He was well until the age of 7 years when he started having RS seizures and later developed epilepsy with continuous spikes and waves during slow wave sleep (see Figures 6.1 and 7.12). The brain MRI was normal (case 17.2 of Panayiotopoulos[1]).

BENIGN (ISOLATED) FOCAL SEIZURES OF ADOLESCENCE

Benign (isolated) focal seizures of adolescence[156-163] constitute an idiopathic, short-lived and transient period of seizure susceptibility during the second decade of life.

DEMOGRAPHIC DATA

This is a seizure susceptibility of the second decade of life with a peak at 13–15 years of age. There is a 71.2% male preponderance. According to Loiseau and Louiset (1992)[157] a quarter of focal seizures with an onset between 12 and 18 years of age have a benign course (i.e. they are single or occur in a cluster of up to five seizures during 36 hours, never to occur again). The disorder may account for between 7.5%[158] and 22%[160] of patients having simple focal seizures in the second decade of life. Around 200 cases have been described.[157;160-162;164;165]

CLINICAL MANIFESTATIONS

The syndrome manifests with a single or a cluster of 2–5 focal, mainly motor and sensory, seizures, which progress to secondary generalized tonic-clonic convulsions in 50% of cases. There are no epileptic events preceding or following this limited seizure period, which lasts for no more than 36 hours. The physical and mental states of the patients are normal.

Consideration on classification

Benign (isolated) focal seizures of adolescence are not a recognised syndrome in the new diagnostic scheme.[2] Loiseau and Jallon (2002)[162] consider that this is a syndrome of "isolated focal seizures of adolescence", which is in accordance with my proposition to classify them among "Conditions with epileptic seizures that do not require a diagnosis of epilepsy".[2]

The seizures are, by definition, focal, but the temporal lobes are rarely involved. Most of the seizures are diurnal (87%). The commonest ictal clinical manifestations are motor, usually without Jacksonian marching, and somatosensory. Visual, vertiginous and autonomic symptoms are reported in one-fifth of cases. Experiential phenomena, such as those seen in temporal lobe seizures, practically never occur. The teenager is fully aware and can give a reliable account of the onset of the clinical manifestations (simple focal seizures) in the majority of episodes (88%). However, consciousness rarely remains intact throughout the whole event; the seizures usually evolve to impaired cognition, and/or to secondary GTCS, which occur in 50% of cases.

DIAGNOSTIC PROCEDURES

Laboratory tests and brain imaging are normal. The EEG may show some minor, non-specific, abnormalities without spikes or focal slowing. In a recent report, 9 of 37 cases had functional spikes,[161] which is incompatible with this syndrome; these patients probably suffered from benign childhood focal seizures as described earlier in this chapter.

DIFFERENTIAL DIAGNOSIS

These patients are difficult to diagnose, as there are no specific features at onset to differentiate them from others with similar clinical manifestations, but of different aetiology, such as symptomatic or cryptogenic focal epilepsies. My practice is to investigate all adolescents with onset of focal seizures with MRI and EEG, which, if normal, would make the diagnosis of benign focal seizures of adolescence more likely. A definitive diagnosis cannot be made until the patient has been free of seizures for 1–5 years.[157;160]

PROGNOSIS

The prognosis is excellent; in 80% of patients, there is a single, isolated seizure event and, in the remaining 20%, a cluster of 2–5 seizures all occurring within 36 hours.

MANAGEMENT

No drug treatment is needed because only one or a cluster of 2–5 focal seizures (which can not be predicted) occurs within 36 hours.

REFERENCES

1. Panayiotopoulos CP. Benign childhood partial seizures and related epileptic syndromes. London: John Libbey & Company Ltd, 1999.
2. Engel J, Jr. A proposed diagnostic scheme for people with epileptic seizures and with epilepsy: Report of the ILAE Task Force on Classification and Terminology. *Epilepsia* 2001;**42**:796-803.
3. Blume WT, Luders HO, Mizrahi E, Tassinari C, van Emde BW, Engel J, Jr. Glossary of descriptive terminology for ictal semiology: report of the ILAE task force on classification and terminology. *Epilepsia* 2001;**42**:1212-8.
4. Panayiotopoulos CP. Panayiotopoulos syndrome:A common and benign childhood epileptic syndrome. London: John Libbey & Company, 2002.
5. Loiseau P,.Beaussart M. The seizures of benign childhood epilepsy with Rolandic paroxysmal discharges. *Epilepsia* 1973;**14**:381-9.
6. Loiseau P, Duche B. Benign rolandic epilepsy. *Adv Neurol* 1992;**57**:411-7.
7. Bouma PA, Bovenkerk AC, Westendorp RG, Brouwer OF. The course of benign partial epilepsy of childhood with centrotemporal spikes: a meta-analysis. *Neurology* 1997;**48**:430-7.
8. Lerman P. Benign childhood epilepsy with centrotemporal spikes. In Engel JJr, Pedley TA, eds. *Epilepsy: A comprehensive textbook*, pp 2307-14. Philadelphia: Lippincott-Raven Publishers, 1997.
9. Beaussart M, Loiseau P, Roger H. The discovery of "benign rolandic epilepsy". In Berkovic SF, Genton P, Hirsch E, Picard F, eds. *Genetics of focal epilepsies*, pp 3-6. London: John Libbey & Company, 1999.
10. Stephani U, ed. Spectrum of rolandic epilepsy: Agreements, disagreements and open questions. *Epilep Disord.* 2000;**2 (Suppl 1)**.
11. Loiseau P. Idiopathic and benign partial epilepsies. In Wyllie E, ed. *The treatment of epilepsy: Principles and practices*, pp 475-84. Philadelphia: Lippincott Williams & Wilkins, 2001.
12. Dalla Bernardina B, Sgro M, Fejerman N. Epilepsy with centro-temporal spikes and related syndromes. In Roger J, Bureau M, Dravet C, Genton P, Tassinari CA, Wolf P, eds. *Epileptic syndromes in infancy, childhood and adolescence (3rd edn)*, pp 181-202. London: John Libbey & Co Ltd, 2002.
13. Commission on Classification and Terminology of the International League Against Epilepsy. Proposal for revised classification of epilepsies and epileptic syndromes. *Epilepsia* 1989;**30**:389-99.
14. Covanis A, Lada C, Skiadas K. Children with rolandic spikes and ictus emeticus: Rolandic epilepsy or Panayiotopoulos syndrome? *Epilep Dis.* 2003;**5**:139-43.
15. Van Huffelen AC. A tribute to Martinus Rulandus. A 16th-century description of benign focal epilepsy of childhood. *Arch Neurol* 1989;**46**:445-7.
16. Gregory DL, Farrell K, Wong PK. Partial status epilepticus in benign childhood epilepsy with centrotemporal spikes: are independent right and left seizures a risk factor? *Epilepsia* 2002;**43**:936-40.
17. Fejerman N, Di Blasi AM. Status epilepticus of benign partial epilepsies in children: report of two cases. *Epilepsia* 1987;**28**:351-5.
18. Colamaria V, Sgro V, Caraballo R, Simeone M, Zullini E, Fontana E *et al.* Status epilepticus in benign rolandic epilepsy manifesting as anterior operculum syndrome. *Epilepsia* 1991;**32**:329-34.
19. Deonna TW, Roulet E, Fontan D, Marcoz JP. Speech and oromotor deficits of epileptic origin in benign partial epilepsy of childhood with rolandic spikes. Relationship to the acquired aphasia-epilepsy syndrome. *Neuropediatrics* 1993;**24**:83-7.
20. Fejerman N, Caraballo R, Tenembaum SN. Atypical evolutions of benign partial epilepsy of infancy with centro- temporal spikes. *Rev Neurol* 2000;**31**:389-96.
21. Fejerman N, Caraballo R, Tenembaum SN. Atypical evolutions of benign localization-related epilepsies in children: are they predictable? *Epilepsia* 2000;**41**:380-90.
22. Caraballo R, Fontana E, Michelizza B, Zullini B, Sgro V, Pajno-Ferrara F, Dalla Bernardina B, Espositio S. Carbamazepina, 'assenze atipiche', 'crisi atoniche', 'crisi atoniche' e stato di PO continua del sonno. *Boll Lega It Epil* 1989;**66/67**:379-81.
23. Parmeggiani L, Seri S, Bonanni P, Guerrini R. Electrophysiological characterization of spontaneous and carbamazepine-induced epileptic negative myoclonus in benign childhood epilepsy with centro-temporal spikes. *Clin Neurophysiol.* 2004;**115**:50-8.
24. Neubauer BA, Fiedler B, Himmelein B, Kampfer F, Lassker U, Schwabe G *et al.* Centrotemporal spikes in families with rolandic epilepsy: linkage to chromosome 15q14. *Neurology* 1998;**51**:1608-12.
25. Bray PF, Wiser WC. Evidence for a genetic etiology of temporal-central abnormalities in focal epilepsy. *NEJM* 1964;**271**:926-33.
26. Bray PF, Wiser WC. Hereditary characteristics of familial temporal-central focal epilepsy. *Pediatrics* 1965;**36**:207-21.
27. Doose H, Brigger-Heuer B, Neubauer B. Children with focal sharp waves: clinical and genetic aspects. *Epilepsia* 1997;**38**:788-96.
28. Vadlamudi L, Harvey AS, Connellan MM, Milne RL, Hopper JL, Scheffer IE *et al.* Is benign rolandic epilepsy genetically determined? *Ann Neurol.* 2004;**56**:129-32.
29. Panayiotopoulos CP. Benign childhood partial epilepsies: benign childhood seizure susceptibility syndromes [editorial]. *J Neurol Neurosurg Psychiatr* 1993;**56**:2-5.
30. Penfield W, Rasmussen T. The cerebral cortex of man:A clinical study of localisation of function. New York: The Macmillan Company, 1957.
31. Gelisse P, Corda D, Raybaud C, Dravet C, Bureau M, Genton P. Abnormal neuroimaging in patients with benign epilepsy with centrotemporal spikes. *Epilepsia* 2003;**44**:372-8.
32. Lundberg S, Weis J, Eeg-Olofsson O, Raininko R. Hippocampal region asymmetry assessed by 1H-MRS in rolandic epilepsy. *Epilepsia* 2003;**44**:205-10.
33. International Federation of Societies for Electroencephalography and Clinical Neurophysiology. A glossary of terms most commonly used by clinical electroencephalographers. *Electroencephal Clin Neurophysiol* 1974;**37:** 538-48.
34. Niedermeyer, E. and Lopes da Silva, F. Electroencephalography. Basic principles,clinical applications, and related fields. Baltimore:Williams & Wilkins, 1999
35. Legarda S, Jayakar P, Duchowny M, Alvarez L, Resnick T. Benign rolandic epilepsy: high central and low central subgroups. *Epilepsia* 1994;**35**:1125-9.
36. Gregory DL, Wong PK. Clinical relevance of a dipole field in rolandic spikes. *Epilepsia* 1992;**33**:36-44.
37. Yoshinaga H, Sato M, Oka E, Ohtahara S. Spike dipole analysis using SEP dipole as a marker. *Brain Topography* 1995;**8**:7-11.
38. Tsai ML, Hung KL. Topographic mapping and clinical analysis of benign childhood epilepsy with centrotemporal spikes. *Brain Dev.* 1998;**20**:27-32.
39. Jung KY, Kim JM, Kim DW. Patterns of interictal spike propagation across the central sulcus in benign rolandic epilepsy. *Clin.Electroencephalogr.* 2003;**34**:153-7.
40. Minami T, Gondo K, Yamamoto T, Yanai S, Tasaki K, Ueda K. Magnetoencephalographic analysis of rolandic discharges in benign childhood epilepsy. *Ann Neurol* 1996;**39**:326-34.
41. Huiskamp G, Van der MW, Van Huffelen A, Van Nieuwenhuizen O. High resolution spatio-temporal EEG-MEG analysis of rolandic spikes. *J Clin Neurophysiol.* 2004;**21**:84-95.
42. Gibbs FA, Gibbs EL. Medical Electroencephalography.Reading, Massachusetts: Addison-Wesley Publishing Company, 1967.
43. Petersen I, Eeg-Olofsson O. The development of the electroencephalogram in normal children from the age of 1 through 15 years. Non-paroxysmal activity. *Neuropadiatrie* 1971;**2**:247-304.
44. Cavazzuti GB, Cappella L, Nalin A. Longitudinal study of epileptiform EEG patterns in normal children. *Epilepsia* 1980;**21**:43-55.
45. Okubo Y, Matsuura M, Asai T, Asai K, Kato M, Kojima T *et al.* Epileptiform EEG discharges in healthy children: prevalence, emotional and behavioral correlates, and genetic influences. *Epilepsia* 1994;**35**:832-41.
46. De Marco P, Tassinari CA. Extreme somatosensory evoked potential: an EEG sign forecasting the possible occurrence of seizures in children. *Epilepsia* 1981;**22**:569-75.
47. Tassinari CA, De Marco P, Plasmati R, Pantieri R, Blanco M, Michelucci R. Extreme somatosensory evoked potentials (ESEPs) elicited by tapping of hands or feet in children: a somatosensory cerebral evoked potentials study. *Neurophysiol Clinique* 1988;**18**:123-8.
48. Minami T, Gondo K, Yanai S, Yamamoto T, Tasaki K, Ueda K. Rolandic discharges and somatosensory evoked potentials in

benign childhood partial epilepsy: magnetoencephalographical study. *Psychiatr Clinic Neurosci* 1995;**49**:S227-8.
49. Manganotti P, Miniussi C, Santorum E, Tinazzi M, Bonato C, Polo A *et al.* Scalp topography and source analysis of interictal spontaneous spikes and evoked spikes by digital stimulation in benign rolandic epilepsy. *Electroencephalogr Clin Neurophysiol.* 1998;**107**:18-26.
50. Manganotti P, Miniussi C, Santorum E, Tinazzi M, Bonato C, Marzi CA *et al.* Influence of somatosensory input on paroxysmal activity in benign rolandic epilepsy with 'extreme somatosensory evoked potentials'. *Brain* 1998;**121**:647-58.
51. Fonseca LC, Tedrus GM. Somatosensory evoked spikes and epileptic seizures: a study of 385 cases. *Clin Electroencephalogr* 2000;**31**:71-5.
52. Kubota M, Takeshita K, Sakakihara Y, Yanagisawa M. Magnetoencephalographic study of giant somatosensory evoked responses in patients with rolandic epilepsy. *J Child Neurol* 2000;**15**:370-9.
53. Langill L,.Wong PK. Tactile-evoked rolandic discharges: a benign finding? *Epilepsia* 2003;**44**:221-7.
54. D'Alessandro P, Piccirilli M, Tiacci C, Ibba A, Maiotti M, Sciarma T *et al.* Neuropsychological features of benign partial epilepsy in children. *Italian J Neurol Scienc* 1990;**11**:265-9.
55. Piccirilli M, D'Alessandro P, Sciarma T, Cantoni C, Dioguardi MS, Giuglietti M *et al.* Attention problems in epilepsy: possible significance of the epileptogenic focus. *Epilepsia* 1994;**35**:1091-6.
56. Baglietto MG, Battaglia FM, Nobili L, Tortorelli S, De Negri E, Calevo MG *et al.* Neuropsychological disorders related to interictal epileptic discharges during sleep in benign epilepsy of childhood with centrotemporal or Rolandic spikes. *Dev Med Child Neurol* 2001;**43**:407-12.
57. Staden U, Isaacs E, Boyd SG, Brandl U, Neville BG. Language dysfunction in children with Rolandic epilepsy. *Neuropediatrics* 1998;**29**:242-8.
58. Yung AW, Park YD, Cohen MJ, Garrison TN. Cognitive and behavioral problems in children with centrotemporal spikes. *Pediatr Neurol* 2000;**23**:391-5.
59. Beaumanoir A, Ballis T, Varfis G, Ansari K. Benign epilepsy of childhood with Rolandic spikes. A clinical, electroencephalographic, and telencephalographic study. *Epilepsia* 1974;**15**:301-15.
60. Lerman P,.Kivity S. Benign focal epilepsy of childhood. A follow-up study of 100 recovered patients. *Arch Neurol* 1975;**32**:261-4.
61. Blom S, Heijbel J. Benign epilepsy of children with centrotemporal EEG foci: a follow-up study in adulthood of patients initially studied as children. *Epilepsia* 1982;**23**:629-32.
62. Loiseau P, Pestre M, Dartigues JF, Commenges D, Barberger-Gateau C, Cohadon S. Long-term prognosis in two forms of childhood epilepsy: typical absence seizures and epilepsy with rolandic (centrotemporal) EEG foci. *Ann Neurol* 1983;**13**:642-8.
63. Al Twajri WA, Shevell MI. Atypical benign epilepsy of childhood with rolandic spikes: features of a subset requiring more than one medication for seizure control. *J Child Neurol.* 2002;**17**:901-4.
64. Peters JM, Camfield CS, Camfield PR. Population study of benign rolandic epilepsy:Is treatment needed? *Neurology* 2001;**57**:537-9.
65. Seidel WT, Mitchell WG. Cognitive and behavioral effects of carbamazepine in children: data from benign rolandic epilepsy. *J Child Neurol* 1999;**14**:716-23.
66. Catania S, Cross H, De Sousa C, Boyd S. Paradoxic reaction to lamotrigine in a child with benign focal epilepsy of childhood with centrotemporal spikes. *Epilepsia* 1999;**40**:1657-60.
67. Battaglia D, Iuvone L, Stefanini MC, Acquafondata C, Lettori D, Chiricozzi F *et al.* Reversible aphasic disorder induced by lamotrigine in atypical benign childhood epilepsy. *Epilep Disord.* 2001;**3**:217-22.
68. Cerminara C, Montanaro ML, Curatolo P, Seri S. Lamotrigine-induced seizure aggravation and negative myoclonus in idiopathic rolandic epilepsy. *Neurology* 2004;**63**:373-5.
69. Panayiotopoulos CP. Inhibitory effect of central vision on occipital lobe seizures. *Neurology* 1981;**31**:1330-3.
70. Panayiotopoulos CP. Vomiting as an ictal manifestation of epileptic seizures and syndromes. *J Neurol Neurosurg Psychiatr* 1988;**51**:1448-51.
71. Ferrie CD, Beaumanoir A, Guerrini R, Kivity S, Vigevano F, Takaishi *et al.* Early-onset benign occipital seizure susceptibility syndrome. *Epilepsia* 1997;**38**:285-93.
72. Oguni H, Hayashi K, Imai K, Hirano Y, Mutoh A, Osawa M. Study on the early-onset variant of benign childhood epilepsy with occipital paroxysms otherwise described as early-onset benign occipital seizure susceptibility syndrome. *Epilepsia* 1999;**40**:1020-30.
73. Kivity S, Ephraim T, Weitz R, Tamir A. Childhood epilepsy with occipital paroxysms:Clinical variants in 134 patients. *Epilepsia* 2000;**41**:1522-3.
74. Caraballo R, Cersosimo R, Medina C, Fejerman N. Panayiotopoulos-type benign childhood occipital epilepsy: a prospective study. *Neurology* 2000;**55**:1096-100.
75. Berg AT, Panayiotopoulos CP. Diversity in epilepsy and a newly recognized benign childhood syndrome [Editorial]. *Neurology* 2000;**55**:1073-4.
76. Ferrie CD, Grunewald RA. Panayiotopoulos syndrome: a common and benign childhood epilepsy [Commentary]. *Lancet* 2001;**357**:821-3.
77. Koutroumanidis M. Panayiotopoulos syndrome: a common benign but underdiagnosed and unexplored early childhood seizure syndrome [Editorial]. *BMJ* 2002;**324**:1228-9.
78. Panayiotopoulos CP. Benign childhood occipital seizures (Panayiotopoulos syndrome). In Gilman S, ed. *Medlink Neurology*, San Diego, USA: Arbor Publishing Corporation, 2004.
79. Lada C, Skiadas K, Theodorou V, Covanis A. A study of 43 patients with Panayiotopoulos syndrome: A common and benign childhood seizure suceptibility. *Epilepsia* 2003;**44**:81-8.
80. Ohtsu M, Oguni H, Hayashi K, Funatsuka M, Imai K, Osawa M. EEG in Children with Early-onset Benign Occipital Seizure Susceptibility Syndrome: Panayiotopoulos Syndrome. *Epilepsia* 2003;**44**:435-42.
81. Demirbilek V, Dervent A. Panayiotopoulos syndrome: video-EEG illustration of a typical seizure. *Epilep Disord.* 2004;**6**:121-4.
82. Sanders S, Rowlinson S, Manidakis I, Ferrie CD, Koutroumanidis M. The contribution of the EEG technologists in the diagnosis of Panayiotopoulos syndrome (Susceptibility to early onset benign childhood autonomic seizures). *Seizure* 2004;**13**:565-73.
83. Martinovic Z. Panayiotopoulos Syndrome or Early-onset Benign Childhood Occipital Epilepsy. *Epilepsia* 2002;**43**:1268-72.
84. Yoshinaga H, Koutroumanidis M, Shirasawa A, Kikumoto K, Ohtsuka Y, Oka A. Dipole analysis in Panayiotopoulos syndrome. *Brain Develop* 2004;*(in press).*
85. Panayiotopoulos CP. Benign childhood epilepsy with occipital paroxysms: a 15-year prospective study. *Ann Neurol* 1989;**26**:51-6.
86. Panayiotopoulos CP. Extraoccipital benign childhood partial seizures with ictal vomiting and excellent prognosis. *J Neurol Neurosurg Psychiatry* 1999;**66**:82-5.
87. Krauss GL, Sinha SR. Book review: A clinical guide to epileptic syndromes and their treatment. *Ann Neurol* 2003;**54**:280.
88. Luders HO, Noachtar S, Burgess RC. Semiologic classification of epileptic seizures. In Luders HO, Noachtar S, eds. *Epileptic seizures. Pathophysiology and clinical semiology*, pp 263-85. New York: Churchill Livingstone, 2000.
89. Burgess RC. Autonomic signs associated with seizures. In Luders HO, Noachtar S, eds. *Epileptic seizures. Pathophysiology and clinical semiology*, pp 631-41. New York: Churchill Livingstone, 2000.
90. Panayiotopoulos CP. Autonomic seizures and autonomic status epilepticus peculiar to childhood: diagnosis and management. *Epilepsy Behav.* 2004;**5**:286-95.
91. Nair DR, Luders HO. Cephalic and whole-body auras. In Luders HO, Noachtar S, eds. *Epileptic seizures. Pathophysiology and clinical semiology*, pp 355-60. New York: Churchill Livingstone, 2000.
92. Schnipper JL, Kapoor WN. Diagnostic evaluation and management of patients with syncope. *Med Clin North Am* 2001;**85**:423-56, xi.
93. Lempert T. Recognizing syncope: pitfalls and surprises. *J R Soc Med* 1996;**89**:372-5.
94. Manidakis I, Sanders S, Rowlinson S, Akanuma N, Ferrie CD, Koutroumanidis M. The electroclinical spectrum of Panayiotopoulos syndrome. *Epilepsia* 2004;**45 (Suppl.3)**:70.
95. Wieser HG. Aura Continua. In Gilman S, ed. *Medlink Neurology*, San Diego, USA: Arbor Publishing Corporation, 2004.
96. Panayiotopoulos CP. Panayiotopoulos syndrome. *Lancet* 2001;**358**:68-9.
97. Baumgartner C, Lurger S, Leutmezer F. Autonomic symptoms during epileptic seizures. *Epileptic Disord.* 2001;**3**:103-16.
98. Schauble B, Britton JW, Mullan BP, Watson J, Sharbrough FW, Marsh WR. Ictal vomiting in association with left temporal lobe seizures in a left hemisphere language-dominant patient. *Epilepsia* 2002;**43**:1432-5.

99. Koutroumanidis M. Ictal Vomiting in Association with Left Temporal Lobe Seizures in a Left Hemisphere Language-Dominant Patient. *Epilepsia* 2003;**44**:1259.
100. Li BU, Issenman RM, Sarna SK. Consensus statement—2nd International Scientific Symposium on CVS. The Faculty of The 2nd International Scientific Symposium on Cyclic Vomiting Syndrome. *Dig Dis Sci.* 1999;**44**:9S-11S.
101. Ferrie CD, Sanders S, Rowlinson S, Valeta T. Panayiotopoulos syndrome - a benign childhood susceptibility to autonomic rather than occipital seizures. *Epilepsia* 2003;**44 (Suppl 9)**:306.
102. Beaumanoir A. Semiology of occipital seizures in infants and children. In Andermann F, Beaumanoir A, Mira L, Roger J, Tassinari CA, eds. *Occipital seizures and epilepsies in children*, pp 71-86. London: John Libbey and Company Ltd, 1993.
103. Vigevano F, Lispi ML, Ricci S. Early onset benign occipital susceptibility syndrome: video-EEG documentation of an illustrative case. *Clin Neurophysiol* 2000;**111 Suppl 2**:S81-S86.
104. Caraballo RH, Astorino F, Cersosimo R, Soprano AM, Fejerman N. Atypical evolution in childhood epilepsy with occipital paroxysms (Panayiotopoulos type). *Epileptic Disord.* 2001;**3**:157-62.
105. Ferrie CD, Koutroumanidis M, Rowlinson S, Sanders S, Panayiotopoulos CP. Atypical evolution of Panayiotopoulos syndrome: a case report [published with video- sequences]. *Epileptic Disord.* 2002;**4**:35-42.
106. Gastaut H. A new type of epilepsy: benign partial epilepsy of childhood with occipital spike-waves. *Clin Electroencephalogr* 1982;**13**:13-22.
107. Gastaut H, Zifkin BG. Benign epilepsy of childhood with occipital spike and wave complexes. In Andermann F, Lugaresi E, eds. *Migraine and epilepsy*, pp 47-81. Boston: Butterworths, 1987.
108. Gastaut H, Roger J, Bureau M. Benign epilepsy of childhood with occipital paroxysms. Up-date. In Roger J, Bureau M, Dravet C, Dreifuss FE, Perret A, Wolf P, eds. *Epileptic syndromes in infancy, childhood and adolescence*, pp 201-17. London: John Libbey & Company Ltd, 1992.
109. Panayiotopoulos CP. Idiopathic childhood occipital epilepsies. In Roger J, Bureau M, Dravet C, Genton P, Tassinari CA, Wolf P, eds. *Epileptic syndromes in infancy, childhood and adolescence (3rd edn)*, pp 203-27. London: John Libbey & Co Ltd, 2002.
110. Panayiotopoulos CP. Elementary visual hallucinations, blindness, and headache in idiopathic occipital epilepsy: differentiation from migraine. *J Neurol Neurosurg Psychiatry* 1999;**66**:536-40.
111. Nagendran K, Prior PF, Rossiter MA. Benign occipital epilepsy of childhood: a family study. *J R Soc Med* 1990;**83**:804-5.
112. Panayiotopoulos CP. Visual phenomena and headache in occipital epilepsy: a review, a systematic study and differentiation from migraine. *Epilept Disord.* 1999;**1**:205-16.
113. Panayiotopoulos CP. Occipital spikes, occipital paroxysms and other electroencephalographic findings in children with benign childhood occipital seizures . Occipital spikes in normal children and those without seizures. In Panayiotopoulos CP, ed. *Benign childhood partial seizures and related epileptic syndromes*, pp 173-202. London: John Libbey & Company Ltd, 1999.
114. Gibbs FA, Gibbs EL. Atlas of electroencephalography, Vol 2. Epilepsy. (2), pp: 214-290. Reading, MA: Addison-Wesley, 1952.
115. Kellaway P. The incidence, significance and natural history of spike foci in children. In Henry CE, ed. *Current clinical neurophysiology. Update on EEG and Evoked Potentials.*, pp 151-75. New York: Elsevier/North Holland, 1980.
116. Aso K, Watanabe K, Negoro T, Takaesu E, Furune A, Takahashi I *et al.* Visual seizures in children. *Epilepsy Research* 1987;**1**:246-53.
117. De Romanis F, Feliciani M, Cerbo R. Migraine and other clinical syndromes in children affected by EEG occipital spike-wave complexes. *Functional Neurology* 1988;**3**:187-203.
118. De Romanis F, Buzzi MG, Cerbo R, Feliciani M, Assenza S, Agnoli A. Migraine and epilepsy with infantile onset and electroencephalographic findings of occipital spike-wave complexes. *Headache* 1991;**31**:378-83.
119. De Romanis F, Buzzi MG, Assenza S, Brusa L, Cerbo R. Basilar migraine with electroencephalographic findings of occipital spike-wave complexes: a long-term study in seven children. *Cephalalgia* 1993;**13**:192-6; discussion 150.
120. Beaumanoir A. An EEG contribution to the study of migraine and of the association between migraine and epilepsy in childhood. In Andermann F, Beaumanoir A, Mira L, Roger J, Tassinari CA, eds. *Occipital seizures and epilepsy in children*, pp 101-10. London: John Libbey & company Ltd, 1993.
121. Panayiotopoulos CP. Basilar migraine: a review. In Panayiotopoulos CP, ed. *Benign childhood partial seizures and related epileptic syndromes*, pp 303-8. London: John Libbey & Company Ltd, 1999.
122. Kuzniecky R, Gilliam F, Morawetz R, Faught E, Palmer C, Black L. Occipital lobe developmental malformations and epilepsy: clinical spectrum, treatment, and outcome. *Epilepsia* 1997;**38**:175-81.
123. Gobbi G, Bertani G, Italian Working Group on Coeliac Disease and Epilepsy. Coeliac disease and epilepsy. In Gobbi G, Andermann F, Naccarato S, Banchini G, eds. *Epilepsy and other neurological disorders in coeliac disease*, pp 65-79. London: John Libbey & Company Ltd, 1997.
124. Tenembaum S, Deonna T, Fejerman N, Medina C, Ingvar-Maeder M, Gubser-Mercati D. Continuous spike-waves and dementia in childhood epilepsy with occipital paroxysms. *J Epilepsy* 1997;**10**:139-45.
125. Gulgonen S, Demirbilek V, Korkmaz B, Dervent A, Townes BD. Neuropsychological functions in idiopathic occipital lobe epilepsy. *Epilepsia* 2000;**41**:405-11.
126. Dalla Bernardina B, Colamaria V, Chiamenti C, Capovilla G, Trevisan E, Tassinari CA. Benign partial epilepsy with affective symptoms ('benign psychomotor epilepsy'). In Roger J, Bureau M, Dravet C, Dreifuss FE, Perret A, Wolf P, eds. *Epileptic syndromes in infancy, childhood and adolescence*, pp 219-23. London: John Libbey & Company Ltd, 1992.
127. Tassinari CA, De Marco P. Benign partial epilepsy with extreme somato-sensory evoked potentials. In Roger J, Bureau M, Dravet C, Dreifuss FE, Wolf P, Perret A, eds. *Epileptic syndromes in infancy, childhood and adolescense*, pp 225-9. London: John Libbey, 1992.
128. Negrin P,.De Marco P. Parietal focal spikes evoked by tactile somatotopic stimulation in sixty non-epileptic children: the nocturnal sleep and clinical and EEG evolution. *Electroencephalogr Clin Neurophysiol* 1977;**43**:312-6.
129. Beaumanoir A, Nahory A. Benign partial epilepsies: 11 cases of frontal partial epilepsy with favorable prognosis. *Rev Electroencephalograph Neurophysiolog Clinique* 1983;**13**:207-11.
130. Martin-Santidrian MA, Garaizar C, Prats-Vinas JM. Frontal lobe epilepsy in infancy: is there a benign partial frontal lobe epilepsy? *Rev Neurol* 1998;**26**:919-23.
131. Bagdorf R, Lee SI. Midline spikes: is it another benign EEG pattern of childhood? *Epilepsia* 1993;**34**:271-4.
132. Kutluay E, Passaro EA, Gomez-Hassan D, Beydoun A. Seizure semiology and neuroimaging findings in patients with midline spikes. *Epilepsia* 2001;**42**:1563-8.
133. Sanders S, Rowlinson S, Koutroumanidis M, Ferrie CD, Panayiotopoulos CP. Midline spikes in children and clinical correlations. *Epilepsia* 2002;**43**:1436-9.
134. Bureau M, Cokar O, Maton B, Genton P, Dravet C. Sleep-related, low voltage Rolandic and vertex spikes: an EEG marker of benignity in infancy-onset focal epilepsies. *Epilept Disord.* 2002;**4**:15-22.
135. Capovilla G, Beccaria F. Benign partial epilepsy in infancy and early childhood with vertex spikes and waves during sleep: a new epileptic form. *Brain Dev.* 2000;**22**:93-8.
136. American Academy of Pediatrics. Practice parameter: long-term treatment of the child with simple febrile seizures. American Academy of Pediatrics. Committee on Quality Improvement, Subcommittee on Febrile Seizures. *Pediatrics* 1999;**103**:1307-9.
137. Baumann RJ. Technical report: treatment of the child with simple febrile seizures. *Pediatrics* 1999;**103**:e86.
138. Mitchell WG. Status epilepticus and acute repetitive seizures in children, adolescents, and young adults: etiology, outcome, and treatment. *Epilepsia* 1996;**37 Suppl 1**:S74-S80.
139. Knudsen FU. Febrile seizures: treatment and prognosis. *Epilepsia* 2000;**41**:2-9.
140. Engler F, Maeder-Ingvar M, Roulet E, Deonna T. Treatment with Sulthiame (Ospolot) in benign partial epilepsy of childhood and related syndromes: an open clinical and EEG study. *Neuropediatrics* 2003;**34**:105-9.
141. Rating D, Wolf C, Bast T. Sulthiame as monotherapy in children with benign childhood epilepsy with centrotemporal spikes: a 6-month randomized, double-blind, placebo-controlled study. Sulthiame Study Group. *Epilepsia* 2000;**41**:1284-8.
142. Bast T, Volp A, Wolf C, Rating D. The influence of sulthiame on EEG in children with benign childhood epilepsy with centrotemporal spikes. *Epilepsia* 2003;**44**:215-20.
143. Bello-Espinosa LE, Roberts SL. Levetiracetam for benign epilepsy of childhood with centrotemporal spikes-three cases. *Seizure.* 2003;**12**:157-9.

144. Austin EJ, Santilli N. Quality of life in children with epilepsy. In Pellock JM, Dodson WE, Bourgeois BFD, eds. *Pediatric epilepsy*, pp 601-11. New York: Demos, 2001.
145. Farnalls SL, Rennick J. Parents' caregiving approaches: facing a new treatment alternative in severe intractable childhood epilepsy. *Seizure.* 2003;**12**:1-10.
146. Balslev T. Parental reactions to a child's first febrile convulsion. A follow-up investigation. *Acta Paediatr Scand* 1991;**80**:466-9.
147. Kurugol NZ, Tutuncuoglu S, Tekgul H. The family attitudes towards febrile convulsions. *Indian J Pediatr* 1995;**62**:69-75.
148. Deng CT, Zulkifli HI, Azizi BH. Parental reactions to febrile seizures in Malaysian children. *Med J Malaysia* 1996;**51**:462-8.
149. Miller R. The effect on parents of febrile convulsions. *Paediatr Nurs.* 1996;**8**:28-31.
150. Shuper A, Gabbay U, Mimouni M. Parental anxiety in febrile convulsions. *Isr J Med Sci.* 1996;**32**:1282-5.
151. van Stuijvenberg M, de Vos S, Tjiang GC, Steyerberg EW, Derksen-Lubsen G, Moll HA. Parents' fear regarding fever and febrile seizures. *Acta Paediatr.* 1999;**88**:618-22.
152. Rasmussen NH, Noiesen E. Parents of children with febrile convulsions. Multidisciplinary quality development of information and documentation. *Ugeskr Laeger* 2001;**163**:1103-6.
153. Baram TZ, Shinnar S. Febrile Seizures. San Diego, California: Academic Press, 2002.
154. Panayiotopoulos CP. Benign childhood partial epilepsies: benign childhood seizure susceptibility syndromes [editorial]. *J Neurol Neurosurg Psychiatry* 1993;**56**:2-5.
155. Maihara T, Tsuji M, Higuchi Y, Hattori H. Benign familial neonatal convulsions followed by benign epilepsy with centrotemporal spikes in two siblings. *Epilepsia* 1999;**40**:110-3.
156. Loiseau P, Orgogozo JM. An unrecognized syndrome of benign focal epileptic seizures in teenagers? *Lancet* 1978;**2**:1070-1.
157. Loiseau P, Louiset P. Benign partial seizures of adolescence. In Roger J, Bureau M, Dravet C, Dreifuss FE, Perret A, Wolf P, eds. *Epileptic syndromes in infancy, childhood and adolescence*, pp 343-5. London: John Libbey & Company, 1992.
158. Panayiotopoulos CP. Benign partial seizures of adolescence. In Wallace S, ed. *Epilepsy in Children*, pp 377-8. London: Chapman & Hall, 1996.
159. Caraballo R, Galicchio S, Granana N, Cersosimo R, Fejerman N. Benign partial convulsions in adolescence. *Rev Neurol* 1999;**28**:669-71.
160. King MA, Newton MR, Berkovic SF. Benign partial seizures of adolescence. *Epilepsia* 1999;**40**:1244-7.
161. Capovilla G, Gambardella A, Romeo A, Beccaria F, Montagnini A, Labate A *et al.* Benign partial epilepsies of adolescence: a report of 37 new cases. *Epilepsia* 2001;**42**:1549-52.
162. Loiseau P, Jallon P. Isolated partial seizures of adolescence. In Roger J, Bureau M, Dravet C, Genton P, Tassinari CA, Wolf P, eds. *Epileptic syndromes in infancy, childhood and adolescence (3rd edn)*, London: John Libbey & Co Ltd, 2002.
163. Horacio CR, Cersosimo RO, Fejerman N. Benign focal seizures of adolescence: a prospective study. *Epilepsia* 2004;**45**:1600-3.
164. Mauri JA, Iniguez C, Jerico I, Morales F. Benign partial seizures of adolescence. *Epilepsia* 1996;**37 (Suppl 4)**:102.
165. Jallon P, Loiseau J, Loiseau P, de Zelicourt M, Motte J, Vallee L *et al.* The risk of recurrence after a first unprovoked seizure in adolescence. *Epilepsia* 1999;**40 (Suppl 7)**:87-8.

10

IDIOPATHIC GENERALISED EPILEPSIES

Idiopathic generalised epilepsies (IGEs) constitute one-third of all epilepsies.[1-6] They are genetically determined and affect otherwise normal people of both sexes and all races. IGEs manifest with typical absences, myoclonic jerks and generalised tonic clonic seizures (GTCS), alone or in varying combinations and severity. Absence status epilepticus (ASE) is common. Most syndromes of IGE start in childhood or adolescence, but some have an adult onset. They are usually life long, though a few are age related. The EEG is the most sensitive test in the diagnosis and confirmation of IGE. EEG shows generalised discharges of spikes, polyspikes or spike/polyspike-wave either ictally or inter-ictally. These discharges are often precipitated by hyperventilation, sleep deprivation and intermittent photic stimulation. Inconspicuous clinical manifestations become apparent on video EEG and with breath counting during hyperventilation. The EEG is unlikely to be normal in untreated patients. In suspected cases with normal routine awake EEG, an EEG during sleep and awakening should be obtained. Molecular genetic analyses have led to important breakthroughs in the identification of candidate genes and loci;[7,8] genetic heterogeneity is common.[8-11] Genetic mutations found in γ-aminobutyric acid ($GABA_A$) receptor subunits strongly implicate the $GABA_A$ receptor in IGEs.[12] Treatment of IGEs is demanding for two main reasons. Firstly, anti-epileptic drugs (AEDs) beneficial in focal epilepsies may be deleterious in IGEs.[4,13] Secondly, efficacy of AEDs differs even within IGE seizures. This is because the generation of absences, for example, is due to a predominance of inhibitory activity, in contrast to generalised convulsive seizures in which an excess of excitatory activity is present.[13] Most IGEs respond well to appropriate AEDs, but treatment is often life long. The fact that nearly 50% of patients with IGE are currently taking *"ill-advised AED"* medication[14] is a grave problem that needs to be addressed.

SEIZURES OF IDIOPATHIC GENERALISED EPILEPSIES

The syndromes of IGEs manifest with three main types of seizures alone or in combination. These are:

1. **Typical absence seizures**
2. **Myoclonic seizures**
3. **Generalised tonic clonic seizures**

ILAE definition of idiopathic generalised epilepsies

The ILAE Commission[1] defined IGE as follows:

"Idiopathic generalised epilepsies are forms of generalised epilepsies in which all seizures are initially generalised (absences, myoclonic jerks and generalised tonic clonic seizures), with an EEG expression that is a generalised bilateral, synchronous, symmetrical discharge (such as is described in the seizure classification of the corresponding type). The patient usually has a normal interictal state, without neurological or neuroradiologic signs. In general, interictal EEGs show normal background activity and generalised discharges, such as spikes, polyspike spike-waves, and polyspike-waves ≥ 3 Hz. The discharges are increased by slow sleep. The various syndromes of idiopathic generalised epilepsies differ mainly in age of onset. No aetiology can be found other than a genetic predisposition towards these disorders."[1]

TYPICAL ABSENCE SEIZURES*

Typical absences (previously known as petit mal) are brief (lasting seconds) generalised epileptic seizures of abrupt onset and abrupt termination (Table 10.1). They have two essential components:

1. a clinical component manifesting with impairment of consciousness (absence)
2. an EEG component manifesting with generalised spike-slow wave discharges of 3–4 Hz (> 2.5 Hz).[1-4,15,16]

The absence seizures are fundamentally different and pharmacologically unique compared with any other type of seizure, which also makes their treatment different.[4,16,17]

The clinical and EEG manifestations of typical absences are extensive and syndrome-related.[1-4,15,16,18]

Clinical manifestations: Impairment of consciousness may be severe, moderate, mild or inconspicuous (and special cognitive testing may be required to detect it). It is often associated with other concomitant symptoms, such as myoclonia, automatisms and autonomic disturbances. Myoclonia may be rhythmic or random, mild or severe, regional (mouth or eyes) or widespread (head, limbs and trunk).

Typical absences are predominantly spontaneous, though they are precipitated by hyperventilation in around 90% of untreated patients. Other specific modes of precipitation include photic, pattern, video games and thinking (reflex absences).

Ictal EEG: The ictal EEG consists of generalised discharges with repetitive and rhythmic 3–4 Hz single or multiple spike-slow wave complexes (Figure 10.1).

These generalised spike-wave discharges (GSWD) may be brief (sometimes less than 3 s) or long (≥ 30 s), and continuous or fragmented. The intradischarge frequency of the spike-wave may be relatively constant or may vary.

Typical absence seizures in IGE syndromes. Typical absences are severe in childhood absence epilepsy (CAE) and juvenile absence epilepsy (JAE), but mild or inconspicuous in other syndromes, such as juvenile myoclonic epilepsy (JME).

They may occur alone or in combination with other types of generalised seizures. IGE with absences may remit with age or be lifelong.

Typical ASE occurs in approximately one-third of patients who suffer from typical absence seizures.[19]

CLINICAL MANIFESTATIONS OF TYPICAL ABSENCE SEIZURES

The clinical manifestations of typical absence seizures vary significantly between patients.[3,4,15,18,20-26] Impairment of consciousness may be the only clinical symptom, but it is often combined with other manifestations (Table 10.1).

Typical absences are categorised as:

- *simple absences* with impairment of consciousness <u>only</u>
- *complex absences* when impairment of consciousness combines with other ictal motor manifestations.

Complex absences are far commoner than simple absences in children. Simple absences are commoner in adults. The same patient may have both simple and complex absences.

---

*The term *'typical'* is used not to characterise them as *'classical'*, but to differentiate them from *'atypical'* absence seizures.

Absence with impairment of consciousness only[1]

The classical[27] and ILAE[1] descriptions refer to absence seizures with severe impairment of consciousness as in CAE and JAE.

> "Transient loss of consciousness without conspicuous convulsions. A patient stops for a moment whatever he or she is doing, very often turns pale, may drop whatever is in the hand.....There may be a slight stoop forward, or a slight quivering of the eyelids...The attack usually lasts only a few seconds. The return of the consciousness may be sudden and the patient after the momentary lapse, may be in just the same state as before the attack, may even continue a sentence or action which was commenced before it came on, and suspended during the occurrence." *W.R.Gowers (1885)* [27]

The hallmark of severe absence seizures is a sudden onset and interruption of ongoing activities, often with a blank stare. If the patient is speaking, speech is slowed or interrupted; if walking, he/she stands transfixed. Usually the patient will be unresponsive when spoken to. Attacks are often aborted by auditory or sensory stimulation.

In less severe absences, the patient may not stop his/her activities, though reaction time and speech may slow down. In their mildest form, absences may be inconspicuous to the patient and imperceptible to the observer *(phantom absences)*, as disclosed by video EEG recordings showing errors and delays during breath counting or other cognitive tests during hyperventilation.

Absence with clonic components[1]

During the absence, as described above, clonic motor manifestations, rhythmic or arrhythmic and singular or repetitive, are particularly frequent at the onset. They

Table 10.1 Clinical and EEG manifestations of typical absence seizures[21]

Typical absence seizures: clinical manifestations

The hallmark of the absence attack is a sudden onset, interruption of ongoing activities, a blank stare, possibly a brief upward rotation of the eyes. If the patient is speaking, speech is slowed or interrupted, if walking, he stands transfixed; if eating, the food will stop on his way to the mouth. Usually the patient will be unresponsive when spoken to. In some, attacks are aborted when the patient is spoken to. The attack lasts from a few seconds to half a minute and evaporates as rapidly as it commenced.

Clinical seizure type

- *Absence with impairment of consciousness only.* The above description fits the description of absence simple in which no other activities take place during the attack.
- *Absence with mild clonic components.* Here the onset of the attack is indistinguishable from the above, but clonic components may occur in the eyelids, at the corner of the mouth, or in other muscle groups, which may vary in severity from almost imperceptible movements to generalised myoclonic jerks. Objects held in the hand may be dropped.
- *Absence with atonic components.* Here there may be a diminution in tone of muscles subserving posture as well as in the limbs leading to drooping of the head, occasionally slumping of the trunk, dropping of the arms, and relaxation of the grip. Rarely tone is sufficiently diminished to cause this person to fall.
- *Absence with tonic components.* Here during the attack tonic muscular contraction may occur, leading to increase in muscle tone, which may affect the extensor muscles or the flexor muscles symmetrically or asymmetrically. If the patient is standing the head may be drawn backward and the trunk may arch. This may lead to retropulsion. The head may tonically draw to one or another side.
- *Absence with automatisms.* Purposeful or quasipurposeful movements occurring in the absence of awareness during an absence attack are frequent and may range from lip licking and swallowing to clothes fumbling or aimless walking. If spoken to, the patient may grunt or to the spoken voice and when touched or tickled may rub the site. Automatisms are quite elaborate and may consist of combinations of the above described movements or may be so simple as to be missed by causal observation.
- *Absence with autonomic components.* These may be pallor and less frequently flushing, sweating, dilatation of pupils and incontinence of urine.

Mixed forms of absence frequently occur.

Absence EEG manifestations

Ictal EEG

- Usually regular and symmetrical 3Hz but may be 2-4 Hz spike-and-slow wave complexes and may have multiple spike-and-slow wave complexes. Abnormalities are bilateral.

EEG interictal expression

- Background activity usually normal although paroxysmal activity (such as spikes or spike-and-slow wave complexes) may occur. This activity is usually regular and symmetrical.

From the Commission on Classification and Terminology of the ILAE[21] with the permission of the Commission and the editor of Epilepsia

may be continuous. They may also occur at any other stage of the seizure. The most common manifestations are clonic jerking of the eyelids, eyebrows and eyeballs, together or independently, as well as random or repetitive eye closures. Fast flickering of the eyelids is probably the most common ictal clinical manifestation, and may occur during brief GSWD without discernible impairment of consciousness. Myoclonias at the corner of the mouth and jerking of the jaw are less common. Myoclonic jerks of the head, body and limbs may be singular or rhythmical and repetitive, and they may be mild or violent. In some patients with absence seizures, single myoclonic jerks of the head and less often of the limbs may occur during the progression of ictus; in my opinion, these are indicative of a bad prognosis and may constitute an epileptic syndrome, but this needs further documentation.[15,16]

Absence with atonic components

Diminution of muscle tone is usual when absences are severe. This manifests with drooping of the head and, occasionally, slumping of the trunk, dropping of the arms and relaxation of the grip. Rarely, tone is sufficiently diminished to cause falls.

Absence with tonic components

Tonic seizures alone do not occur in IGEs. However, tonic muscular contractions are common concomitant manifestations during typical absence seizures. They mainly affect facial and neck muscles symmetrically or asymmetrically. The eyes and head may be drawn backwards (retropulsion) or to one side, and the trunk may arch. Tonic manifestations are prominent in myoclonic absence seizures.

Absence with automatisms

Automatisms are common in typical absences when consciousness is sufficiently impaired, and they are more likely to occur 4–6 s after the onset of GSWD. They do not occur in mild absence seizures irrespective of duration as for example in ASE. Automatisms of typical absence seizures are simple and void of behavioural changes (see definitions in Chapter 12). They vary in location and character from seizure to seizure. Perioral automatisms, such as lip licking, smacking, swallowing or 'mute' speech movements, are the most common. Scratching, fumbling with clothes and other limb automatisms are also common. Automatisms can be evoked; passive movements, postural repositioning or other stimuli can change their pattern and distribution.[24]

Absence with autonomic components

Autonomic components consist of pallor and, less frequently, flushing, sweating, dilatation of the pupils and incontinence of urine. During absence seizures, pronounced changes in cerebral oxygenation occur with a decrease in oxygenated and an increase in deoxygenated haemoglobin. Oxygenation changes start several seconds after the EEG-defined onset of the absence and outlast the clinically defined event by 20–30 s.[28]

Absences with focal motor components, hallucinations and other manifestations of neocortical or limbic symptomatology

During a typical absence seizure, patients frequently manifest with concomitant focal motor components (tonic or clonic) imitating focal motor seizures. Hallucinations and other manifestations such as concurrent epigastric sensations[29] may occur; these are particularly more apparent during ASE.[16]

> I was in that state of confused mind. The surroundings were vertical and flat and I lost depth perception. People around me appeared as be wearing wigs in pastel shades.[30]

ELECTROENCEPHALOGRAPHY

The ictal EEG is characteristic with regular and symmetrical 3-4 Hz GSWD (Figure 10.1). The intradischarge spike-wave frequency varies from onset to termination (Figure 10.2). It is usually faster and unstable in the *opening phase* (first second), becomes more regular and stable in the *initial phase* (first 3 s),

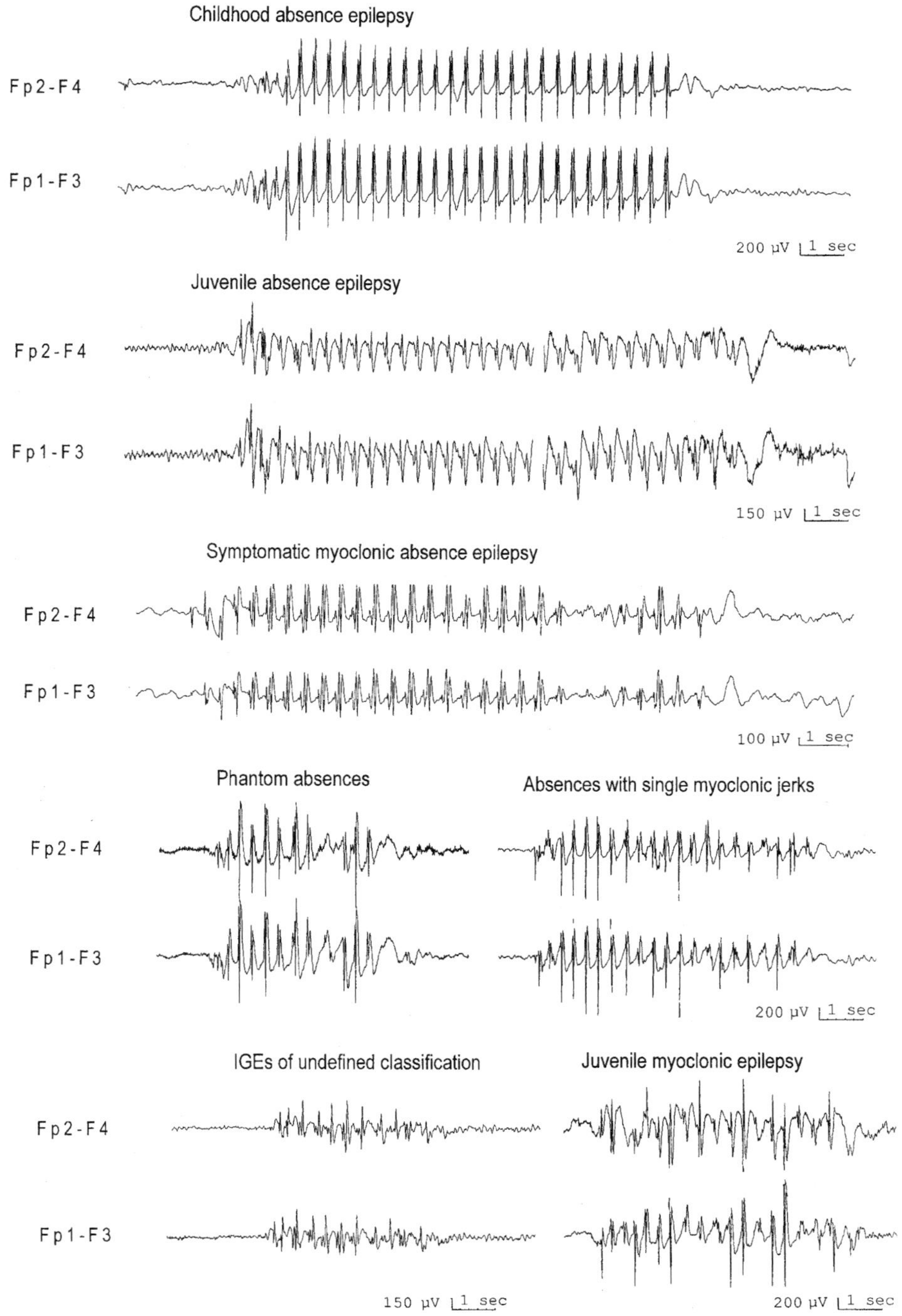

Figure 10.1

Examples from video EEG recorded generalised discharges of 3 Hz spikes or multiple spikes-waves of typical absence seizures. These seven patients had different syndromes of idiopathic and symptomatic absence epilepsies. Note that the GSWD may be brief or prolonged, with or without polyspikes and of regular or irregular sequence. Also, note that the intradischarge frequency of the spike–wave complexes may show significant diversity. Though there are significant variations between different syndromes, the GSWD is not itself pathognomonic of any syndrome. The syndromic diagnosis requires homogeneous clustering of symptoms and signs.

and slows down towards the *terminal phase* (last 3 s).[24] The intradischarge relationship between spike or multiple spike and slow wave frequently varies. The GSWD is often of higher amplitude in the anterior regions. A generalised discharge with an onset or a higher amplitude in the posterior regions may indicate a bad prognosis.[31]

Duration of the discharges commonly varies from 3 to 30 s (Figure 10.1).

The background interictal EEG is usually normal, though some paroxysmal activity (such as spikes or spike–wave complexes) may occur. Focal abnormalities or other asymmetries are common.[32,33]

Sleep EEG patterns are normal. GSWD are more likely to increase, but decrease during sleep. The discharges are often shorter and usually devoid of discernible clinical manifestations in sleep, even in those patients who have numerous clinical seizures with motor manifestations during the alert state.

Important note

Though the EEG GSWD of typical absences is defined as symmetrical and synchronous, this is rarely the case at its onset. Commonly, the discharge starts with single or multiple spikes-slow waves that are asymmetrical and usually have a regional onset, mainly frontal (Figures 10.1 and 10.2). Often (but not always), there is an alternating side emphasis. Unilateral onset of the GSWD may be confused with secondary bilateral synchrony. The end of the discharge may be abrupt or consists of brief rhythmic or irregular slow waves (Figure 10.2). Sometimes more focal or fragmentary spikes occur, representing a 'forme fruste' of GSWD. These are more often recorded from the anterior regions, but other locations are also common.

GENETICS

IGEs with typical absences are genetically determined, as indicated by the high incidence of similar disorders among families. However, the precise mode of inheritance and the genes involved remain largely unknown.[7] Currently, various

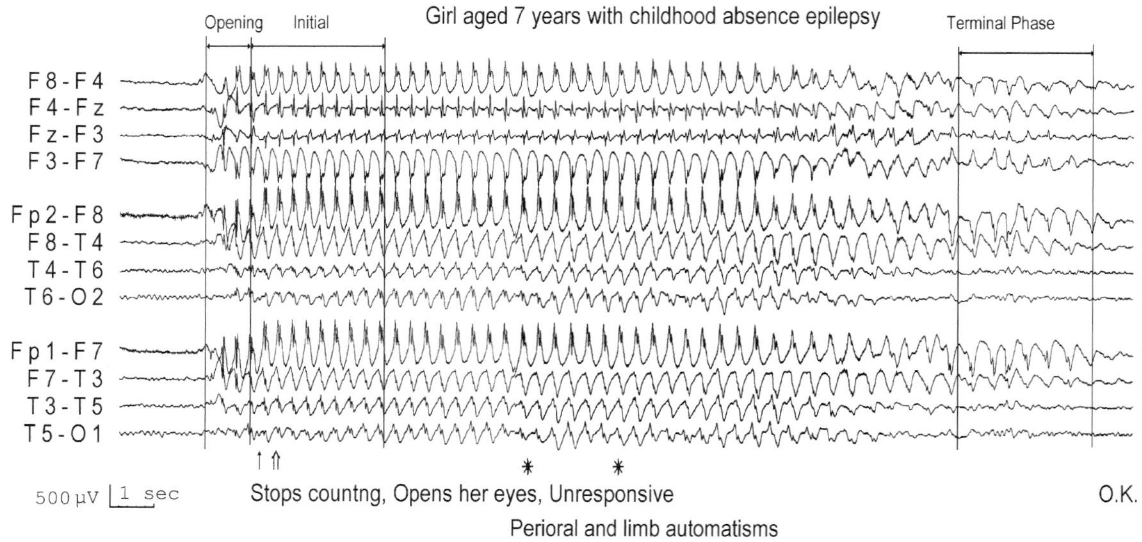

Figure 10.2 Girl, aged 7 years, with childhood absence epilepsy.

The seizure occurred during hyperventilation with breath counting. She stopped counting (black arrow), opened her eyes (open arrow) and became unresponsive. Marked perioral automatisms occurred later (*). She abruptly recovered at the end of the discharge (O.K.).
The GSWD is artificially divided into the opening phase (first 1 s of the GSWD), the initial phase of stabilisation (following 3 s) and terminal phase (last 3 s).[24] Note that the frequency of the regular spike–wave complexes gradually slows down from 3 Hz in the initial phase to 2 Hz in the terminal phase. The opening phase is asymmetrical and asynchronous with faster or irregular spike wave frequencies.
See also Figures 2.3 and 10.1.

chromosomal loci have been identified for IGEs, as detailed in the description of individual syndromes. Furthermore, there is now evidence available to suggest that mutations in genes encoding GABA receptors[34-36] or brain expressed voltage-dependent calcium channels[37] may underlie CAE.

Genetic heterogeneity of the GSWD phenotype in animal models of absences favours a similar, and probably much wider, genetic heterogeneity in humans.[7,13,17]

PATHOPHYSIOLOGY OF ABSENCE SEIZURES

The pathophysiological mechanisms of absence seizures have been studied in various animal models with GSWD associated with behavioural arrest.[7,13,17,38,39] It appears that the GSWD are generated and sustained by highly synchronised abnormal oscillatory rhythms in thalamocortical networks that mainly involve neocortical pyramidal cells, the reticular thalamic nucleus and the relay nuclei of the thalamus. Neither the cortex nor the thalamus alone can sustain these discharges, indicating that both structures are involved in their generation.

The involvement of thalamus as the generator of GSWD is documented by the fact that:

- stimulation of the medial thalamus induces a cortical GSWD without leading to self-sustained activity
- thalamic neurons can intrinsically generate action potentials in both a tonic and a burst firing mode[7,13,17,40]
- magnetic resonance spectroscopy (MRS) and neuroimaging in vivo provides evidence of progressive thalamic neuronal dysfunction in patients with IGE.[41,42]

The relative importance of the cortex in the initiation and synchronisation of GSWD is mainly documented by the finding that, following thalamectomy, instigation of GSWD persists though the thalamus is required to maintain rhythmicity once the GSWD is established. More recently, in a rat model of absence, Meeren et al.[43] showed that, during GSWD, cortical and thalamic interactions lag behind an initial burst of activity in the perioral region of the primary somatosensory cortex (S1po) during the first 500 ms of GSWD activity. These findings suggest that, in this animal model, a cortical focus within S1po is the dominant factor in initiating the paroxysmal oscillation within the corticothalamic loops, and that the large scale synchronisation is mediated by an extremely fast intracortical spread of seizure activity.[43] This is also supported by experiments whereby microinfusion of ethosuximide into S1po produces an immediate cessation of GSWD.[44]

The basic intrinsic neuronal mechanisms involve low threshold T-type calcium currents elicited by activating the low threshold calcium channels. These channels are present in high densities in thalamic neurons and trigger regenerative burst firing that drive normal and pathological thalamocortical rhythms, including the GSWD of absence seizures. Ethosuximide exerts its anti-absence effect by either reducing thalamic low threshold calcium currents, probably by a direct channel blocking action that is voltage dependent,[45] or through a potent inhibitory effect in the perioral region of the primary somatosensory cortex.[13,44]

It is likely that the generation of absence seizures is due to a predominance of inhibitory activity, in contrast to generalised or focal convulsive seizures in which an excess of excitatory activity is present.[13]

Both inhibitory and excitatory neurotransmissions are involved in the genesis and control of absence seizures. This may be the result of excessive cortical excitability due to an imbalance between inhibition and excitation, or excessive thalamic oscillations due to abnormal intrinsic neuronal properties under the control of inhibitory GABAergic mechanisms. $GABA_B$ receptors play the most prominent role by eliciting long-standing hyperpolarisation required to drive low threshold calcium channels for the initiation of sustained burst firing. Typical absences are aggravated by $GABA_B$ agonists, such as baclofen, and suppressed by $GABA_B$ antagonists. GABAergic drugs (e.g. vigabatrin, tiagabine) are pro-absence substances; they interfere with the degradation of, and the re-uptake of, GABA.[4,13] The only exception to GABAergic activation inhibiting absences is the reticular thalamic nucleus, which has exclusively $GABA_A$ receptors; it functions as a pacemaker to synchronise thalamocortical oscillations.[46,47] Enhanced activation of $GABA_A$ receptors in this nucleus decreases the pacemaking capacity of these cells, thereby decreasing the likelihood of generating absence seizures.

Functional imaging using positron emission tomography (PET) demonstrates normal cerebral glucose metabolism and benzodiazepine receptor density in absence epilepsies, with diffuse hypermetabolism during 3 Hz GSWD.[48,49] There is no evidence of any overall interictal abnormality of opioid receptors in IGE, but typical absences have been found to displace 11C-diprenorphine from the association areas of the neocortex. In contrast, binding of 11C-flumazenil to central benzodiazepine receptors has been shown to be unaffected by serial absences.[49]

Ictal single photon emission computed tomography (SPECT) shows an overall increase in cerebral blood flow[50,51] and may be useful in detecting cases of frontal or other secondarily generalised absences.[52] Interictally, relative hypoperfusion occurs in the frontal lobes, and may involve neighbouring parietal and temporal regions.[51] Ictally, there is relative hyperperfusion in the same brain regions that are hypoperfused in the baseline study.[51]

Microdysgenesis and other cerebral structural changes were reported in some patients with CAE and JAE at autopsy[53] and MRI[54] studies. These results were not replicated in a more recent, blinded study.[55] Microdysgenesis may be inconceivable for a benign, age-dependent and age-limited epileptic syndrome, such as CAE, though the current ion channel hypothesis for the pathogenesis of IGE does not preclude microscopic or ultramicroscopic abnormalities. Furthermore, recent quantitative MRI, PET and MRS studies have challenged the belief that IGEs are not associated with tissue pathology.[42]

DIAGNOSING ABSENCES AND DIFFERENTIAL DIAGNOSIS

The brief duration of absence seizures with abrupt onset and abrupt termination of ictal symptoms, daily frequency and nearly invariable provocation by hyperventilation makes the diagnosis easy.[4,16,18]

The differential diagnosis of typical absence seizures with severe impairment of consciousness in children is relatively straightforward. The absences may be missed if mild or void of myoclonic components. Automatisms, such as lip smacking or licking, swallowing, fumbling or aimless walking, are common and should not be taken as evidence of complex partial (focal) seizures, which require entirely different management.

The EEG or, ideally, video EEG can confirm the diagnosis of typical absence seizures in more than 90% of untreated patients, mainly during hyperventilation.[16] If not, the diagnosis of absences should be questioned.

In practical terms, a child with suspected typical absences should be asked to overbreathe for 3 minutes, counting his or her breaths while standing with hands extended in front. Hyperventilation will provoke an absence in more than 90% of those with typical absences. This procedure should preferably be videotaped to document the clinical manifestations. It may reveal features favouring a specific epileptic syndrome and, therefore, may determine the long-term prognosis and management. Video EEG documentation may be particularly useful if absences prove resistant to treatment, if other seizures develop, or for future genetic counselling. Focal spike abnormalities and asymmetrical onset of the ictal GSWD are common and may be a cause of misdiagnosis, particularly in resistant cases.[15] If video EEG is not available, documentation of absences using a camcorder or modern digital means of recording is recommended.

The differentiation of typical from atypical absence seizures is shown in Table 7.4. Briefly, atypical absences differ from typical absences in the following ways:

- Atypical absences occur only in the context of mainly severe symptomatic or cryptogenic epilepsies of children with learning difficulties, who also suffer from frequent seizures of other types, such as atonic, tonic and myoclonic seizures.
- In atypical absences, onset and termination is not as abrupt as in typical absences, and changes in tone are more pronounced.
- The ictal EEG of atypical absence has slow (< 2.5 Hz) GSWD. These are heterogeneous, often asymmetrical, and may include irregular spike–wave complexes and other paroxysmal activity. Background interictal EEG is usually abnormal.

The differentiation of typical absences from complex focal seizures, detailed in Table 10.2, may be more difficult when the motor components of the absence are unilateral and in adults in whom absences are often misdiagnosed as temporal lobe seizures.[56-58] Absences occur in 10% of adult patients with epileptic seizures.[56-58]

Misconceptions

Petit mal is seen almost exclusively in children, more rarely in adolescents and is a real curiosity in adults and the elderly.[59]

Contrary to the dominant view above, typical absence seizures occur in approximately 10% of adults with epilepsy.[56,57] The alarming problem is that these are underdiagnosed or misinterpreted as focal seizures.

Table 10.2 Differential diagnosis of typical absences from complex focal seizures

Clinical criteria	**Typical absences**	**Complex focal seizures**
Duration for less than 30 seconds	As a rule	Exceptional
Duration for more than 1 minute	Exceptional	As a rule
Non-convulsive status epilepticus	Frequent	Rare
Daily frequency	As a rule	Rare
Simple automatisms	Frequent	Frequent
Complex behavioural automatisms	Exceptional	Frequent
Simple and complex hallucinations or illusions	Exceptional	Frequent
Bilateral facial myoclonic jerks or eyelid closures	Frequent	Exceptional
Evolving to other focal seizure manifestations	Never	Frequent
Sudden onset and termination	As a rule	Frequent
Postictal symptoms	Never	Frequent
Reproduced by hyperventilation	As a rule	Exceptional
Elicited by photic stimulation	Frequent	Exceptional
EEG criteria		
Ictal generalised 3–4 Hz spike and wave	Exclusive	Never
Interictal generalised discharges	Frequent	Exceptional
Interictal focal abnormalities of slow waves	Exceptional	Frequent
Normal EEG in untreated state	Exceptional	Frequent

The primary differences are shown in red.

From Panayiotopoulos (2002)[16] with the permission of the Editor of *Medlink*.

MYOCLONIC JERKS

Myoclonic jerks are shock-like, irregular and often arrhythmic, clonic-twitching movements that are singular or repetitive.[21,60,61] They are of variable amplitude and force, ranging from mild and inconspicuous to sufficiently violent to make the patient fall on the ground, drop or throw things, or kick. Commonly, the same patients experience mild and violent jerks. Myoclonic jerks predominantly affect the eyelids, facial and neck muscles, the upper limbs more than the lower limbs and the body. Myoclonic jerks of IGE mainly occur on awakening. Precipitating factors are sleep deprivation, fatigue, excitement or distress and often photic stimulation. The patient is fully aware of myoclonic jerks unless they occur during impairment of consciousness in absence seizures. The location and extent of myoclonic jerks varies between IGE syndromes.

Polyspikes are the EEG accompaniment of myoclonic jerks (Figures 10.2, 10.3 and 10.5).

DIAGNOSING MYOCLONIC JERKS

Elicitation of the characteristic history of myoclonic jerks is something of an art. It is often necessary to physically demonstrate mild myoclonic jerks of the fingers and hands, and to inquire about morning clumsiness and tremors.[62] Questions like 'do you spill your morning tea?' and 'do you drop things in the morning?', together with a simultaneous demonstration of how myoclonic jerks produce this effect, may be answered positively by patients who denied experiencing myoclonic jerks on direct questioning. Further elaboration is required to confirm that clumsiness was due to genuine myoclonic jerks. If the patient reports normal hypnagogic jactitations, it is reassuring that the concept of myoclonic jerks has been understood. Diagnostic yield may be improved by emphasising the close relationship between jerks and fatigue, alcohol and sleep deprivation. Some patients do not report their jerks, erroneously assuming that this is a self-inflicted normal phenomenon related to excess of alcohol and lack of sleep.

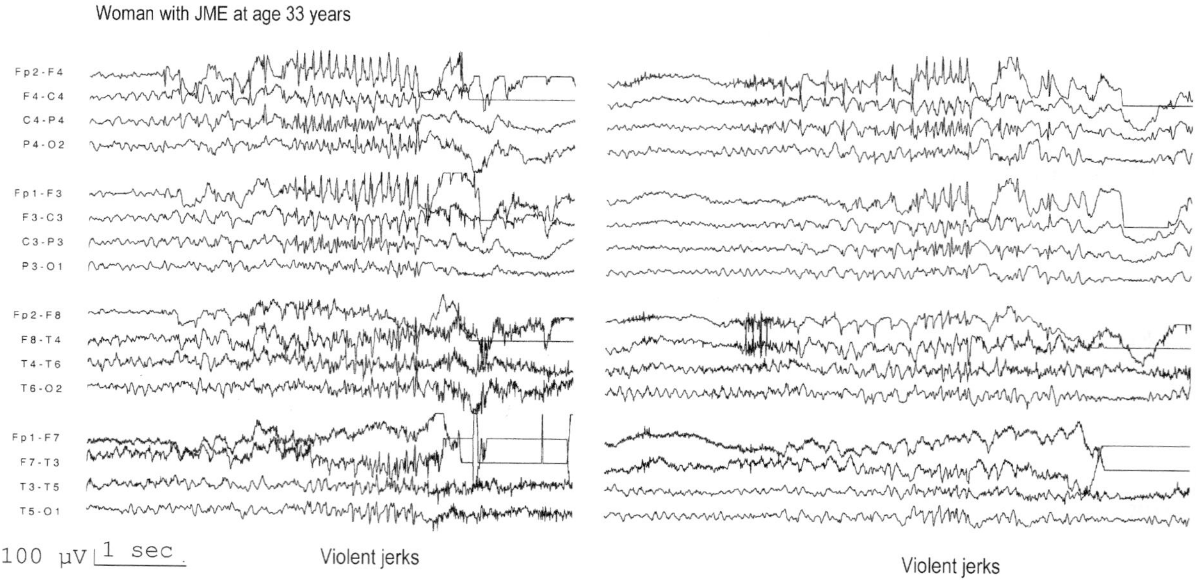

Figure 10.3

Samples from the video EEG of a woman with JME on carbamazepine. Violent myoclonic jerks occur with generalised multiple spike discharges (see also Figure 10.14 of the same patient).

GENERALISED TONIC CLONIC SEIZURES IN IGES

In IGEs, GTCS are primary (primarily) in the sense that they are generalised from onset without preceding auras or objective ictal focal symptoms, though they are often heralded by a series of myoclonic jerks or absences. This contrasts with secondarily GTCS of focal epilepsies that are often preceded by an aura or motor-sensory focal symptoms. Overall, primarily GTCS occur on awakening (17–53% of patients), diffusely while awake (23–36%) or during sleep (27–44%), or randomly (13–26%).[63] The proportion of these patients who also have other generalised seizures, such as jerks or absences, is undetermined.

DIFFERENTIAL DIAGNOSIS OF PRIMARILY FROM SECONDARILY GENERALISED TONIC CLONIC SEIZURES*

GTCS are dramatic in their presentation, which is the main reason for referral for medical consultation. This firstly demands careful exclusion of syncopal and other non-epileptic events. Once an unequivocal diagnosis of genuine epileptic GTCS has been established, the main differential diagnosis is between primarily and secondarily GTCS.

GTCS whether primarily (IGEs) or secondarily (focal epilepsies) are identical in their clinical presentation. Their differentiation, which is of immense clinical importance regarding overall management and AED treatment, is often easy (Table 10.3) based on:

- clinical history regarding other types of coexisting seizures, precipitating factors, circadian distribution and family history

* The terminological differences between primarily as opposed to primary and secondarily as opposed to secondary have been detailed in Chapter 1.

Table 10.3 Differentiation of primarily versus secondarily GTCS

	Primarily GTCS	Secondarily GTCS
GTCS with other clinically evident seizures	About 90%	About 90%
Typical absences	About 40%	None
Myoclonic jerks	About 60%	None
Focal seizures	None	About 90%
GTCS without other clinically evident seizures	About 10%**	About 10%**
Precipitating factors	> 60%	< 10%
Consistently on awakening	Common	Uncommon
Family history of similar epilepsies	Common	Uncommon
EEG in untreated patients		
Generalised discharges	About 80%	Exceptional
Focal abnormalities alone	About 10%	About 60%
Generalised discharges and focal abnormalities	About 30%	Exceptional
High resolution brain imaging		
Focal abnormalities	Exceptional	About 60%
Normal	By definition	About 40%

**It is these patients, who make up about 10% of each category, without clinically apparent other types of seizures that constitute the main problem in the differential diagnosis between primarily and secondarily GTCS. However, other features, such as precipitating factors, circadian distribution, EEG and brain imaging, are often of diagnostic significance.

- EEG manifestations
- brain imaging.

SPECT studies have shown activation of selective frontal, parietal and temporal networks after both spontaneous and induced primarily or secondarily GTCS, but thalamic cerebral blood flow is only increased after primarily GTCS.[42]

STATUS EPILEPTICUS IN IDIOPATHIC GENERALISED EPILEPSIES

IGEs manifest with all types of generalised status epilepticus. ASE is probably the most common of all and the most likely to escape diagnosis or be misdiagnosed as focal status epilepticus or non-epileptic confusion, psychogenic or behavioural disorder.[1,15,19,64-66]

The new ILAE diagnostic scheme[5] considers status epilepticus as a "continuous seizure" with two main categories (Table 1.2):

I. Generalised status epilepticus

II. Focal status epilepticus

The subcategories of generalised status epilepticus are relevant to this chapter:*

- Generalised tonic-clonic status epilepticus
- Clonic status epilepticus
- Absence status epilepticus
- Tonic status epilepticus
- Myoclonic status epilepticus

CLASSIFICATION OF ABSENCE STATUS EPILEPTICUS

Absence status epilepticus is divided into:

a. typical ASE occurring in patients with IGEs who also have absence seizures

* Non-convulsive status epilepticus is a term that has been rightly discarded in the new diagnostic scheme,[5] because it encompasses heterogeneous conditions which may be focal, such as limbic status epilepticus, or generalised, such as ASE.[71,72] Convulsive elements and particularly myoclonic jerks are common in generalised non-convulsive status epilepticus as, for example, in eyelid or perioral status epilepticus. Non-convulsive status epilepticus is not synonymous with ASE. If this term is used, the distinction between 'focal non-convulsive' and 'generalised non-convulsive' should be made for clinical and management purposes.

Definition of status epilepticus

There is no satisfactory definition of status epilepticus.[64] Its definition is mainly influenced by the convulsive status epilepticus, because of its high morbidity, mortality and the need for early detection and early treatment.

The World Health Organization defines status epilepticus as "a condition characterised by epileptic seizures that are sufficiently prolonged or repeated at sufficiently brief intervals so as to produce an unvarying and enduring epileptic condition".[67] By consensus, "sufficient length of time" was defined as being more than 30 minutes' duration[68] although more recent opinions argue for shorter periods of 5-10 minutes in defining convulsive status epilepticus.[69] These short periods may not be applicable in other than convulsive types of status epilepticus.

The recent ILAE glossary makes no significant contribution in defining status epilepticus as "A seizure that shows no clinical signs of arresting after a duration encompassing the great majority of seizures of that type in most patients or recurrent seizures without interictal resumption of baseline central nervous system function".[70] Also, etymologically, status epilepticus is not a 'continuous seizure' as the ILAE Task Force proposed;[5] it is a prolonged, enduring or rapidly repeated seizure which may also be 'discontinuous' and often stops without medical intervention.

Shorvons' operational definition is more appealing "status epilepticus is condition in which epileptic activity persists for 30 minutes or more, causing a wide spectrum of clinical symptoms, and with a highly variable pathophysiological, anatomical and aetiological basis".[64] This definition implies that status is not simply a prolonged seizure or rapid repetition of seizures (in fact the word 'seizure' is no longer retained), but a condition (or group of conditions) in its own right with distinctive pathophysiological features.

b. atypical ASE occurring in patients with symptomatic epilepsies and epileptic encephalopathies (Figure 7.7)

c. de novo or situation related absence status epilepticus occurring mainly in adults without a history of previous epileptic seizures commonly as the result of benzodiazepine or other drug discontinuation. [73,74] The most well-documented example is diazepine withdrawal. De novo ASE is often misdiagnosed as a psychotic state or dementia.[66,73,74]

TYPICAL ABSENCE STATUS EPILEPTICUS IN IGE

Typical (idiopathic) absence status epilepticus in IGEs is defined as a prolonged (> 30 minutes), generalised non-convulsive seizure of impairment of the content of consciousness (absence) and EEG generalised spike/polyspike-wave discharges.[19,65,66,75,76]

It should be emphasised that typical ASE, like absence seizures, is of many types with impairment of cognition as a shared common symptom. Impairment of consciousness may be mild or severe. It may occur alone (Figure 10.18) or more frequently be associated with other symptoms such as those listed in Table 10.1 for complex absence seizures. Motor manifestations such as myoclonic jerks, eyelid or perioral myoclonia, may predominate and be syndrome related (Figures 10.6 and 13.7).

Accordingly, typical (idiopathic) absence status epilepticus may be subdivided to:

- typical absence status epilepticus with impairment of consciousness only (Figure 10.18)
- myoclonic-atonic status epilepticus (Figure 10.6)
- myoclonic-absence status epilepticus (Figure 10.14)
- perioral myoclonic status epilepticus (Figure 10.16)
- eyelid myoclonic status epilepticus (Figure 13.8).

The ictal EEG is characteristic with usually regular and symmetrical 3 Hz (range 1–4 Hz) GSWD, which is continuous or repetitive (Figures 10.6, 10.14, 10.16, 10.18 and 13.7).

With the possible exception of CAE, all IGEs with typical absences may manifest with typical ASE, either as a spontaneous expression of their natural course or provoked by external factors or inappropriate treatment manoeuvres.

Impairment of consciousness, memory and higher cognitive functions

The cardinal symptom shared by all cases of typical ASE is altered content of consciousness in a usually fully alert patient. Memory and higher cognitive intellectual functions, such as abstract thinking, computation and personal awareness, are the main areas of disturbance, which varies from very mild to very severe with intermediate states of severity occurring more often.

Mild disturbance is experienced as a state of slow reaction, behaviour and mental functioning:

> My mind slows down and I am able to understand, but it takes longer to formulate answers.
>
> I become slow, but can communicate verbally with others.
>
> My behaviour slows down and I muddle up words.
>
> It's like being in a trance and missing pieces of conversation.

Moderate and severe impairment of consciousness manifest with varying degrees of confusion, global disorientation and inappropriate behaviour:

> Confused, cannot recognise people other than close relatives, disorientated in time and place, very quiet.
>
> Disturbed, vague, uncooperative, confused.
>
> Markedly confused, goes into a dreamy state, able to formulate some single word answers to simple questions, puts trousers on over pyjamas.
>
> Confused, makes coffee twice, fades away mentally and physically, disoriented in time and place.

Usually, the patient is alert, attentive and cooperative. Verbal functioning is relatively well preserved, but is often slow with stereotypic and usually monosyllabic or monolectic answers. Movement and coordination are intact. Complete unresponsive is rare.

Behavioural abnormalities and experiential phenomena

Though the most common behavioural changes refer to daily activities disturbed by the impairment of consciousness, some patients become depressed, agitated and, occasionally, hostile and aggressive. Experiential and sensational phenomena are more common than is usually appreciated and may include:

> Sensation of viewing the world through a different medium and a feeling of not being in the same world as everyone else. Uncontrollable rush of thoughts. A feeling of fear of losing control of my mind.
>
> A feeling of closeness.
>
> A funny feeling that I can not elaborate.
>
> A strange feeling of not being myself.
>
> Edgy, worry and uncomfortable.
>
> My character changes completely, I become extremely snappy, have a severe headache.
>
> Weird.

Simple gestural and ambulatory automatisms, and automatic behavioural and fugue-like states may occur in the 20% of patients who also have severe impairment of consciousness:

> Replies yes to any question and fumbles with his clothes.

Myoclonic jerks in absence status epilepticus

Segmental myoclonic jerks, usually involving the eyelids or perioral region and less often the limbs, frequently occur during typical ASE, and vary in degree and severity. They are most likely to occur in syndromes that manifest with similar myoclonic phenomena during brief absences (see descriptions in the relevant sections of individual IGE syndromes).

GTCS associated with typical absence status epilepticus

ASE ending with a GTCS is probably the rule irrespective of the syndrome. However, in one-third of patients, ASE always ends with GTCS. In the remaining two-thirds, it may also terminate spontaneously without GTCS. It is exceptional for GTCS to precede or be interspersed with ASE. It is also exceptional for more than one GTCS to occur following ASE.

Duration and frequency of typical absence status epilepticus

ASE usually lasts for an average of 3–4 hours, rarely as little as half an hour, often exceeds 6–10 hours and occasionally lasts for 2–10 days. Frequency also varies from once in a lifetime to an average of 10–20 episodes/year, or be consistently catamenial. The duration and frequency depend on treatment strategies and syndromic classification.

Postictal state

Amnesia of the event is exceptional. Commonly patients are aware of what happens during the ASE and some are able to write down their experiences even when in status. Other patients have a patchy recollection of events and usually miss the last part prior to the GTCS. After a GTCS, the patient feels tired, has a headache and is confused for a varying duration of time.

Age at onset and sex

Mean age at onset of ASE is 29 years, with a range of 9–56 years. It is rare for ASE in IGE to start before the first decade of life. Other types of seizures, such as absences, myoclonic jerks and GTCS, may predate the first ASE by many years. ASE rarely is the first overt type of seizure.[77]

Precipitating factors

Inappropriate use of AEDs, such as tiagabine,[78,79] vigabatrin,[66] carbamazepine and phenytoin,[80] as well as discontinuation of proper anti-absence medication are the commonest precipitants of ASE. Sleep deprivation, stress and excess alcohol consumption, alone or usually in combination are common precipitating factors. Some women may have consistent catamenial precipitation.[81-83]

DIFFERENTIAL DIAGNOSIS

A confusional state lasting for hours and ending with GTCS creates significant diagnostic difficulties regarding its nature and cause. Causes to consider are intoxication, and psychogenic, metabolic or systemic diseases. If these are excluded, the differential diagnosis is between focal (complex, partial) or ASE.

Idiopathic ASE is commonly unrecognised or misdiagnosed. It is surprising how often physicians are deceived by the general good appearance, alertness and cooperation of the patient.[66] Basic testing of memory and higher cognitive functions, essential for diagnosis, are rarely carried out. It is important to remember that more than half of patients are aware of the situation when entering or during ASE, which is of great practical significance with regard to termination of the ASE and prevention of the impending GTCS by self-administered appropriate medication.

Idiopathic ASE is easy to diagnose on the basis of proper identification of the IGE syndrome.

Differentiation of generalised ASE from complex focal status epilepticus

Complex focal status epilepticus (including limbic status epilepticus) is rarer than generalised ASE. Patients frequently have recurring complex focal seizures with incomplete recovery between attacks, or a continuous 'epileptic twilight state' with cycling between unresponsiveness and partial responsiveness. The ictal EEG reveals recurrent epileptiform patterns consistent with those encountered in isolated complex focal seizures. The interictal EEG usually shows a unilateral or bilateral cortical focus. In complex focal status epilepticus, conscious levels fluctuate during the attack and patients experience postictal confusion and amnesia of the episode. Although automatisms may occur in both forms of status epilepticus, they are more complex and prolonged in complex focal status epilepticus.

The commonest reason for misdiagnosis between the two conditions is because absences are not recognised or misdiagnosed as complex focal seizures

(Table 10.2). A previous or new EEG invariably shows generalised discharges in IGE. It may be normal or show specific focal spikes in focal epilepsies, mainly temporal lobe epilepsy. Ictal EEG with GSWD is diagnostic of IGE. Coexisting focal abnormalities should not be interpreted as evidence of focal epilepsy.

The differentiation of typical (idiopathic) ASE from atypical (usually symptomatic or probably symptomatic) ASE is also easy

The major distinguishing feature of atypical ASE is that it occurs mainly in children with symptomatic or cryptogenic generalised epilepsies, who also have a plethora of other types of frequent seizures, such as atypical absences, tonic and atonic seizures, myoclonic jerks and GTCS. Most of these patients also have moderate or severe learning and physical handicaps. In addition, the interictal EEG is often very abnormal with slow background activity and frequent, brief or long runs of slow generalised spike–wave complexes, paroxysmal fast activity and paroxysms of polyspikes. It is often difficult to define the boundaries, onset and termination of atypical ASE, because these children frequently have alterations of behaviour and alertness as well as long interictal slow GSWD.

Atypical ASE is clinically characterised by fluctuating impairment of consciousness often with other ictal symptoms, such as repeated series of tonic or atonic seizures and segmental or generalised jerks. The ictal EEG pattern is of slow (< 2.5 Hz) GSWD. Both the clinical patterns and the EEG abnormalities are more variable than of the typical ASE.

Additional discriminating features of atypical ASE are:

- gradual onset and offset
- level of consciousness and other coexisting types of seizures tend to fluctuate sometimes for weeks, with little distinction between ictal and interictal phases
- initiation or termination with a GTCS is exceptional
- incontinence is common.

EPILEPTIC SYNDROMES OF IDIOPATHIC GENERALISED EPILEPSIES

The recognised syndromes of IGEs are shown in Table 1.5 (1989 ILAE classification)[1] and Table 1.6 (new ILAE classification scheme).[5] Listed according to the age at onset, these are:

- **Benign myoclonic epilepsy in infancy** (Chapter 6)
- **Generalised epilepsy with febrile seizures plus*** (Chapter 6)
- **Epilepsy with myoclonic absences**
- **Epilepsy with myoclonic-astatic seizures**
- **Childhood absence epilepsy**
- **Idiopathic generalised epilepsies with variable phenotypes**
  - **Juvenile absence epilepsy**
  - **Juvenile myoclonic epilepsy**
  - **Epilepsy with generalised tonic-clonic seizures only**

Other possible syndromes of IGE for consideration, which are not yet recognised by the ILAE Committees, are:[1,5]

- IGE with absences of early childhood
- Perioral myoclonia with absences
- Idiopathic generalised epilepsy with phantom absences
- Jeavons syndrome (eyelid myoclonia with absences)
- Benign adult familial myoclonic epilepsy
- Autosomal dominant cortical myoclonus and epilepsy

*Syndrome in development

Considerations on the classification of idiopathic generalised epilepsies:

The classification of IGE is probably one of the most significant and debated issues. There are two schools of thought, with diversely opposing views:[2] (a). IGE is one disease, (b). IGE comprises a large group of many distinct syndromes. The evidence so far is not conclusive in favour of one or the other, and any new classification should not take sides unreasonably. In practical terms, the view that 'IGE is one disease' would, overall, be an easy clinical diagnostic approach, but it would discourage the diagnostic precision required for genetic studies, prognosis and management decisions. The view that 'IGE comprises a large group of many distinct syndromes' would be more demanding diagnostically and occasionally require exhaustive clinical and video EEG data. However, this is often the price that we, as physicians, have to pay in pursuing an accurate diagnosis, which is is the golden rule in medicine. This view also satisfies: (a). "maximum practical application to differential diagnosis,"[84] which is the main reason for reorganising the classification of epileptic syndromes in the forthcoming revisions; and (b). takes advantage of "significant advances in our understanding"[85] of IGEs, which constitute one-third of cases of 'epilepsy'. Similarly, there is no justification for the unification of 'IGEs with onset in adolescence' in a single syndrome as has been recently proposed.[86] The major conceptual problem with this proposition is that it takes 'onset in adolescence' as the most significant almost defining factor, which is at variance with the definition of a syndrome.[1] Further, the same IGE syndromes may start in childhood, adolescence and occasionally adult life.[1] On the surface, syndromes of IGE may look alike if their clinical EEG manifestations are not properly analysed and synthesised. For example, JME and JAE both manifest with absences, myoclonic jerks and GTCS. However, severe absences are the main and most disturbing type of seizure in JAE, and myoclonic jerks may not occur or be randomly distributed.[16] Conversely, myoclonic jerks on awakening is the defining symptom of JME; absences are mild and occur in only one-third of patients. The clinical-EEG features of typical absence seizures that may be syndrome-related are well described in video EEG studies.[16,18] Unifying all typical absence seizures as a single type is of no benefit to any cause. Animal genetic studies have documented numerous syndromes of IGE[17] and this is likely to be the case in humans.[2]

Recognised syndromes of IGEs in the ILAE classification of 1989 versus the newly proposed diagnostic scheme

The new ILAE diagnostic scheme[5] has some significant differences in relation to the ILAE classification of 1989[1] regarding IGE of childhood and adolescence. These are:
(1). The syndromes of JAE, JME and IGE with GTCS only are considered as phenotypical variants of IGE of adolescence
(2). A new syndrome of 'IGE with GTCS only' has been proposed to replace 'epilepsy with GTCS on awakening'
(3). 'Epilepsy with myoclonic-astatic seizures' and 'epilepsy with myoclonic absences' are included among *idiopathic* generalised epilepsies; these were previously categorised as *symptomatic or cryptogenic* generalised epilepsies.
(4). 'Generalised epilepsy with febrile seizures plus' is proposed as a new syndrome in development

EPILEPSY WITH MYOCLONIC ABSENCES

Epilepsy with myoclonic absences (MAE) is a rare syndrome of childhood, which demands scrupulous exclusion of other forms of symptomatic or probably symptomatic cases manifesting with the same seizure (myoclonic absences).[173-177]

DEMOGRAPHIC DATA

Age at onset varies from the first months of life to early teens with a median of 7 years. Boys (69%) predominate. MAE is a very rare disorder with an approximate prevalence of 0.5–1% among selected patients with epileptic disorders.[173,177,178] I have seen only three cases (two of which were idiopathic MAE) over a period of 15 years out of nearly 200 patients with video EEG-recorded typical absence seizures.[4,24,177]

CLINICAL MANIFESTATIONS

MYOCLONIC ABSENCES

The myoclonic absences are the hallmark of MAE.[173,178] They consist of impairment of consciousness, which varies from mild to severe and rhythmic myoclonic jerks, mainly of the shoulders, arms and legs with a concomitant tonic contraction. Eyelid twitching is practically absent, but perioral myoclonias are frequent. The jerks and the tonic contraction may be unilateral or asymmetrical, and head/body deviation may be a constant feature in some patients. The tonic contraction mainly affects the shoulder and deltoid muscles, and may cause elevation of the arms. Some patients maintain awareness of the jerks.

The duration of the absences varies from 8 to 60 s. Myoclonic absences occur many times a day.

OTHER TYPES OF SEIZURE

Other types of seizure also occur in two-thirds of patients.[173,174,179] These are infrequent GTCS and atonic seizures, which may precede or occur concurrently with the myoclonic absences. ASE is rare.

PRECIPITATING FACTORS

Hyperventilation is the main precipitating factor.[173,178] Photosensitivity is uncommon (14%).[178] Non-photosensitive myoclonic absences precipitated by eye-closure or eye-opening have been described.[173,178] Seizures induced by emotionally gratifying stimuli, such as cheek-kissing or after viewing pleasant or funny events have been reported in a child with inverted chromosomal 15 duplications.[24]

NEUROLOGICAL AND MENTAL STATE

Neurological examination is usually normal, but nearly half of patients (45%) have impaired cognitive functioning prior to the onset of absences.[175,178]

Considerations on the classification of epilepsy with myoclonic absences

Myoclonic absences (the seizures) may feature either in normal or children with neurocognitive impairment.[16,176]
The 1989 ILAE Commission, discounting the idiopathic form, classified 'epilepsy with myoclonic absences' among 'cryptogenic/symptomatic' generalised epilepsies, that is in the same group of disorders as the Lennox-Gastaut syndrome and EM-AS.[1] "The syndrome of epilepsy with myoclonic absences is clinically characterised by absences accompanied by severe bilateral rhythmical clonic jerks, often associated with a tonic contraction. On the EEG, these clinical features are always accompanied by bilateral, synchronous, and symmetrical discharge of rhythmical spike–waves at 3 Hz, similar to childhood absence. Seizures occur many times a day. Awareness of the jerks may be maintained. Associated seizures are rare. Age of onset is ~7 years, and there is a male preponderance. Prognosis is less favourable than in pyknolepsy owing to resistance to therapy of the seizures, mental deterioration, and possible evolution to other types of epilepsy such as Lennox-Gastaut syndrome or JME."[1]
Contrary to this, the new ILAE diagnostic scheme considers only the idiopathic form (Table 1.7),[5] which probably represents around one-third of the whole spectrum of epileptic disorders manifesting with myoclonic absences. The others are symptomatic or probably symptomatic cases.[1]

AETIOLOGY

Only one-third of patients with myoclonic absences are idiopathic cases and only these belong to this syndrome of MAE. The other two-thirds with myoclonic absences (the seizures, not the syndrome) are due to symptomatic causes including chromosomal abnormalities, such as trisomy 12p, Angelman syndrome, inverted chromosomal 15 duplications[179,180] and malformations of brain development.[176,177,181]

DIAGNOSTIC PROCEDURES

By definition, in idiopathic MAE, all tests but the EEG should be normal. Brain MRI and chromosomal testing[179] are needed to detect symptomatic cases.

ELECTROENCEPHALOGRAPHY

Background EEG is usually normal at onset, but may deteriorate later or be abnormal in symptomatic cases. Interictal EEG shows brief generalised, focal or multifocal spike and slow waves in 50% of cases.[173,177]

Ictal EEG shows 3 Hz GSWD, even in those with unilateral or asymmetrical clinical manifestations. Polygraphic studies have revealed that each myoclonic jerk coincides with the spike component of the discharge.[173,177]

DIFFERENTIAL DIAGNOSIS

The differential diagnosis of MAE from other types of syndromes with absences is easy because of the characteristic type of myoclonic absences. The difficulty is between idiopathic and symptomatic/cryptogenic cases that manifest with the same seizure type (myoclonic absences). Symptomatic patients often have an abnormal neurological state, abnormal background EEG and abnormal brain MRI. Chromosomal abnormalities are common.[179] Additionally, absences with rhythmic myoclonic jerking, but less than 2.5 Hz spike/polyspike–wave complexes and other characteristics of atypical absences may occur in epileptic encephalopathies[173,178,182] and include some of the cases with chromosomal abnormalities.[179]

PROGNOSIS

Myoclonic absences remit after an average of 5 years in one-third of patients.[176,177] In the remaining (perhaps symptomatic) patients, absences continue into adult life together with other types of seizures, such as GTCS and atonic seizures, or they develop features of other types of epilepsy, such as Lennox-Gastaut syndrome or JME.

Nearly half of the children with MAE have impaired cognitive functioning prior to the onset of absences, but these are probably symptomatic cases. However, half of those who were normal prior to the onset of absences develop cognitive and behavioural impairment. This may mean that the EEG discharges have a deteriorating effect on cognition unless eliminated early with treatment.

MANAGEMENT

The aim is to stop myoclonic absence seizures as early as possible. Early control of absences may prevent subsequent cognitive deterioration and secure normal development.[178]

Myoclonic absences are often resistant to treatment. Treatment frequently requires high doses of valproate often combined with ethosuximide or lamotrigine.[177] Interestingly, Tassinari et al.[173] had a few cases that responded only to phenobarbitone alone or in combination with anti-absence drugs. Newer drugs, such as levetiracetam,[183] or old drugs, such as clonazepam and acetazolamide, may be tried in resistant cases.

Baclofen a $GABA_B$ agonist used for the treatment of spasticity in neurologically impaired patients is contraindicated because of significant provocation of absence seizures.

See also AEDs contraidicated in IGEs (page 337).

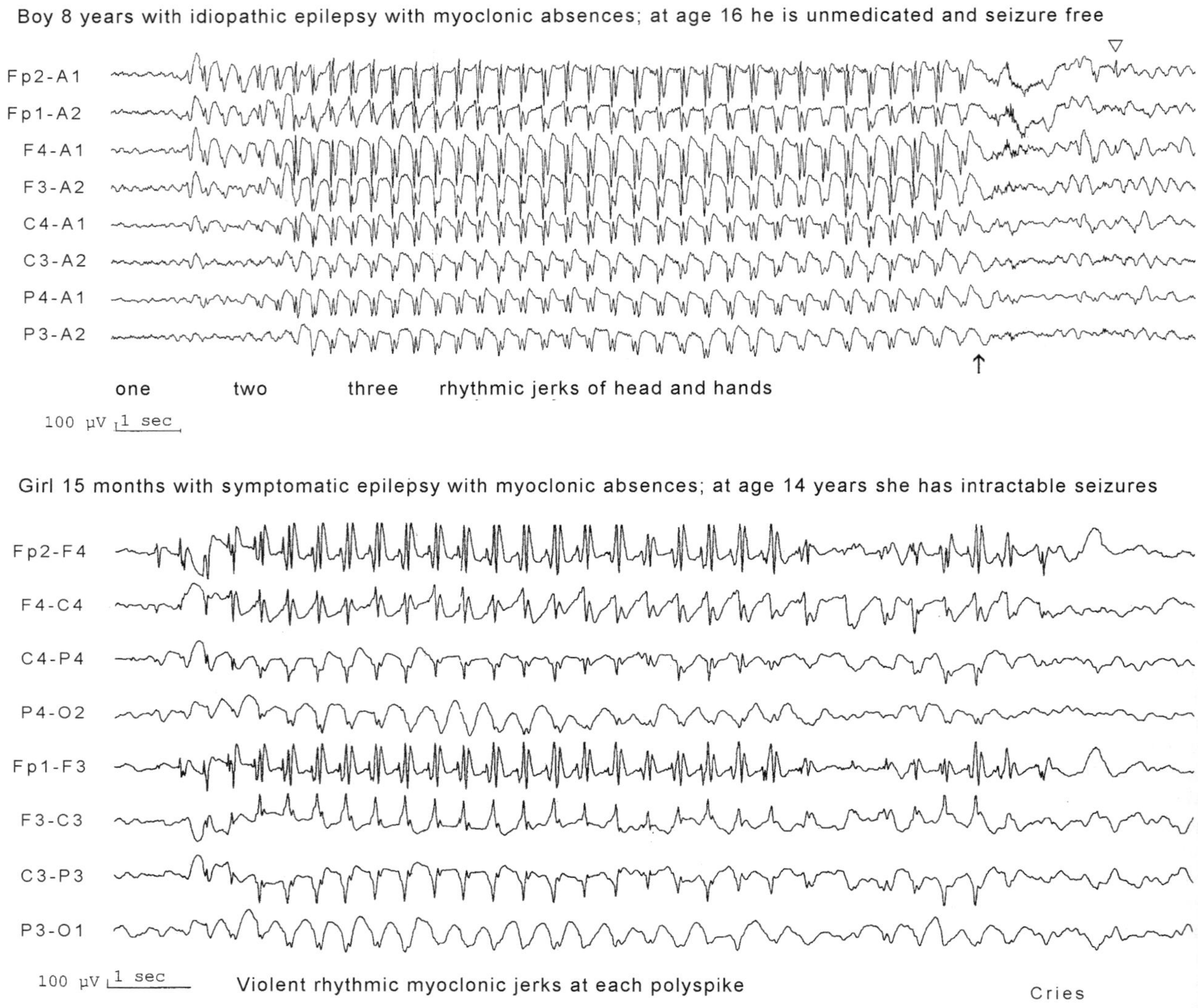

Figure 10.4 Samples from a video EEG showing idiopathic and symptomatic myoclonic absence seizures. The EEG GSWD are similar with no apparent differentiating features or asymmetry in the symptomatic patient.

Top: Video EEG of a boy aged 8 years with myoclonic absences from the age of 6 years. These were frequent, hundreds per day, and manifested with rhythmic myoclonic jerks and unresponsiveness. Valproate failed to achieve control, but absences ceased completely when ethosuximide was added at the age of 8 years. Medication was withdrawn at 11 years of age. No further seizures occurred in the next 8 years of follow-up and he is academically successful.
The absence is terminated by somatosensory stimulation (tapping his shoulder).

Bottom: Video EEG of a girl aged 15 months with myoclonic absences due to birth anoxia. Myoclonic absences started at 15 months of age, occurred many times a day, lasted for 8–10 s and were characterised by synchronous and bilateral myoclonic jerks of the limbs and head with apparent loss of consciousness. Subsequently, she developed frequent, mainly nocturnal GTCS while myoclonic absences continued. These were intractable to any appropriate medication. At 8 years of age, she had severe learning difficulties and spastic quadraparesis.

EPILEPSY WITH MYOCLONIC-ASTATIC SEIZURES

DOOSE SYNDROME

Epilepsy with myoclonic-astatic seizures (EM-AS)* or Doose syndrome**[87-97] is considered as an IGE in the new ILAE diagnostic sceme.[5] Diagnosis of this syndrome requires careful application of inclusion and exclusion criteria. Its characteristic symptom, myoclonic-astatic seizures, is shared by many other childhood syndromes and particularly epileptic encephalopathies.

DEMOGRAPHIC DATA

Onset occurs between 7 months and 6 years, and peaks at 2–4 years. Two-thirds are boys. EM-AS accounts for about 1–2% of all childhood epilepsies.

CLINICAL MANIFESTATIONS

Doose syndrome is characterised by myoclonic-astatic seizures that often occur together with atonic, myoclonic and absence seizures; myoclonic-astatic status epilepticus is common.

Children are normal prior to the onset of seizures. In two-thirds of children, febrile and afebrile generalised tonic clonic seizures appear first, several months prior to the onset of myoclonic-astatic seizures.

**Astatic* is not synonymous with *atonic* seizures. The term astatic seizures is abandoned in the new ILAE diagnostic scheme, which uses only the term '*atonic*' or '*myoclonic-atonic*' seizures.[5]

**I use the eponymic nomenclature '*Doose syndrome*' only for the pure form of '*idiopathic epilepsy with myoclonic-astatic seizures*' to exclude cases of symptomatic cause manifesting with myoclonic-astatic seizures.

Considerations on the classification of EM-AS

The 1989 ILAE Commission classifies EM-AS among 'cryptogenic/symptomatic' generalised epilepsies, that is in the same group of disorders as Lennox-Gastaut syndrome.[1] It is defined as follows:

"Manifestations of myoclonic-astatic seizures begin between the ages of 7 months and 6 years (mostly between the ages of 2 and 5 years), with (except if seizures begin in the first year) twice as many boys affected. There is frequently hereditary predisposition and usually a normal developmental background. The seizures are myoclonic, astatic, myoclonic-astatic, absence with clonic and tonic components, and tonic-clonic. Status frequently occurs. Tonic seizures develop late in the course of unfavorable cases. The EEG, initially often normal except for 4–7 Hz rhythms, may have irregular fast spike-wave or polyspike wave. Course and outcome are variable."[1]

Contrary to this, the ILAE Task Force considers EM-AS as IGE,[5] a view which is similar to that of Doose (Table 10.4):[98]

"Myoclonic-astatic epilepsy belongs to the epilepsies with primarily generalized seizures and thus stands in one line with absence epilepsies, JME, as well as the infantile and juvenile idiopathic epilepsy with generalized tonic clonic seizures. Like these types of epilepsy, myoclonic-astatic epilepsy is polygenically determined with little nongenetic variability. The disease is characterized by the following criteria: genetic predisposition (high incidence of seizures and/or genetic EEG patterns in relatives); mostly normal development and no neurological deficits before onset; primarily generalized myoclonic, astatic or myoclonic-astatic seizures, short absences and mostly generalized tonic clonic seizures; no tonic seizures or tonic drop attacks during daytime (except for some rare cases with a most unfavourable course); generalized EEG patterns (spikes and waves, photosensitivity, 4–7 Hz rhythms), no multifocal EEG-abnormalities (but often pseudofoci)."[98]

The problem may reflect lack of specific diagnostic criteria and undefined boundaries of certain epileptic syndromes and particularly epileptic encephalopathies, which may manifest with myoclonic-astatic seizures. This particularly refers to Dravet, Lennox-Gastaut syndrome and atypical benign epilepsy of childhood. Cases of benign and severe myoclonic epilepsy in infants may have been included in EM-AS.[89] Other myoclonic epilepsies with brief seizures reported as intermediate cases between EM-AS and Lennox-Gastaut syndrome probably prove this point.[99]

However, it is generally accepted that some children with myoclonic-astatic seizures are otherwise normal with no discernible causes other than a strong genetic epileptic background and probably represent the genuine 'Doose syndrome' of 'idiopathic epilepsy with myoclonic-astatic seizures'. This point is exemplified in the study of Kaminska *et al.*,[100] who found evidence that EM-AS is distinct from Lennox-Gastaut syndrome, and the distinction appears from the first year of the disorder.

A further exciting development is that myoclonic-astatic seizures frequently occur in patients with 'generalised epilepsy with febrile seizures plus'[101], a syndrome that also has strong genetic links with Dravet syndrome.

Myoclonic-astatic (in fact myoclonic-atonic) seizures are the defining symptoms (100% of cases).[89] These manifest with symmetrical myoclonic jerks immediately followed by loss of muscle tone (post-myoclonic atonia) (Figure 10.5).

Atonic seizures of sudden, brief and severe loss of postural tone may involve the whole body or only the head. Attacks are brief, lasting 1–4 s and frequent. Generalised loss of postural tone causes a lightning-like fall. The patient collapses on the floor irresistibly. In brief and milder attacks, there is only head nodding or bending of the knees.

Myoclonic jerks may precede or less often intersperse with the atonic manifestations (Figures 10.5 and 10.6).

Brief absence seizures happen in more than 50% of cases. These often occur together with myoclonic jerks, facial myoclonias and atonic manifestations. Atonic and absence seizures may occur frequently, sometimes many times a day in the active period of the disease. Absence seizures alone are exceptional.

Tonic seizures are an exclusion criterion.

Myoclonic-atonic status epilepticus lasting for hours or even days (Figure 10.6) is common affecting one-third of patients. It manifests with varying degrees of usually severe cognitive impairment or cloudiness of consciousness interspersed with repetitive myoclonic and atonic fits. Facial myoclonus of eyelids and mouth may be continuous together with irregular jerks of the limbs and atonic seizures of head nodding or falls. Myoclonic-atonic status epilepticus may occur several times during a period of 1–2 years.

AETIOLOGY

Doose syndrome may be genetically determined in a multifactorial polygenic fashion with variable penetrance.[87-89] One-third of patients have familial seizure disorders and mainly IGEs.[87-89] Of significant interest are the clinical and molecular studies in 'generalised epilepsy with febrile seizures plus' in which myoclonic-atonic seizures are common in some families.[101] 'Generalised epilepsy with febrile seizures plus' also has strong genetic links with Dravet syndrome.

DIAGNOSTIC PROCEDURES

By definition, all tests other than the EEG are normal.

Electroencephalography

Interictal EEG may be normal at the stage of febrile or afebrile GTCS. Rhythmic theta activity in the parasagittal regions may be the only significant abnormality. Subsequently, when myoclonic-atonic seizures appear, there are frequent clusters of 2–3 Hz GSWD interrupted by high amplitude slow waves in cases with predominant atonic or myoclonic-atonic seizures. In children with predominantly myoclonic seizures, paroxysms of irregular spikes or polyspike–wave complexes prevail.

The ictal EEG of myoclonic and atonic seizures manifests with discharges of irregular spike–wave or polyspike–wave complexes at a frequency of 2.5–3 Hz or more (Figures 10.5 and 10.6). Atonia is usually concurrent with the slow wave of a single or multiple spike–wave complex and the intensity of the atonia is proportional to the amplitude of the slow wave. Drop attacks are associated with diffuse EMG paucity indicating their true atonic nature.[91] The myoclonus of Doose syndrome appears to be a primary generalised epileptic phenomenon, which differs from that of Lennox-Gastaut syndrome.[102]

In myoclonic-atonic status epilepticus, the EEG shows continuous or discontinuous and repetitive 2–3 Hz spike-wave complexes (Figure 10.6).

DIFFERENTIAL DIAGNOSIS

Differentiation of EM-AS is mainly between:

- benign myoclonic epilepsy in infancy
- Dravet syndrome
- Lennox-Gastaut syndrome
- late onset West syndrome.

In general, children with the Doose syndrome are normal prior to the development of seizures, have a strong family history of IGE, and the background EEG and brain imaging are normal.

Progressive myoclonic epilepsies, such as myoclonic epilepsy with ragged-red fibres, Lafora and Unverricht-Lundborg disease, may initially imitate Doose syndrome. However, the associated relevant neurological abnormalities and, sometimes, the relentless progression and deterioration will establish the diagnosis.

Table 10.4 Diagnostic criteria for Doose syndrome (idiopathic EM-AS)[91]

Inclusion criteria

1. Normal development prior to the onset of seizures and normal MRI
2. Onset of myoclonic, myoclonic-atonic or atonic seizures between 7 months and 6 years of age
3. Normal background EEG with 2–3 Hz GSWD without consistent focal spikes

Exclusion criteria

1. Dravet syndrome, Lennox-Gastaut syndrome, benign myoclonic epilepsy in infancy or other epileptic syndromes manifesting with myoclonic-astatic seizures
2. Tonic seizures

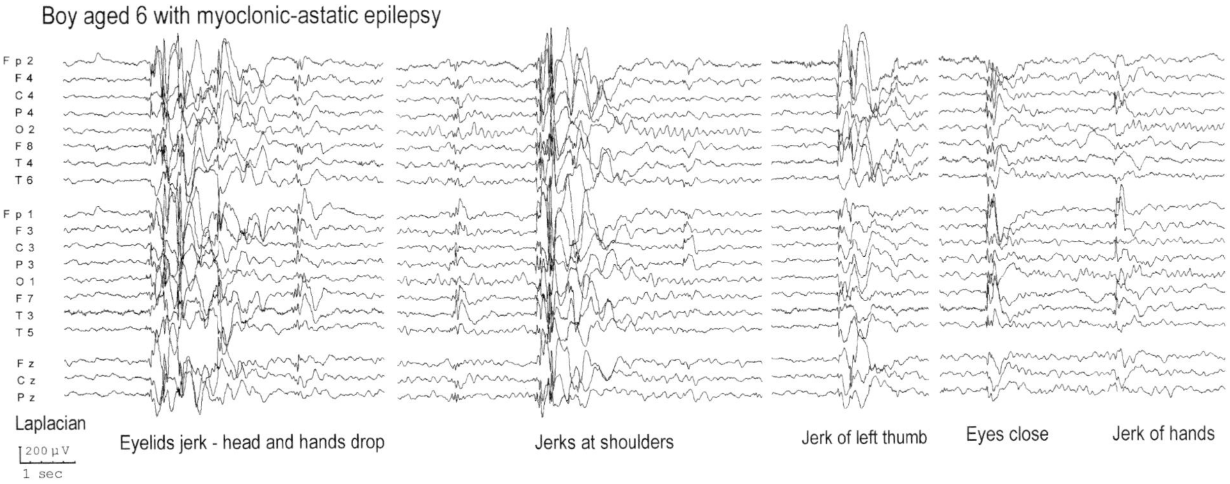

Figure 10.5 Samples from a video EEG of a 6-year-old normal boy with Doose syndrome

The background activity was normal, but there were frequent (at least every 10 s) generalised discharges of high-voltage spike/polyspike–wave complexes at 3-6 Hz with an anterior maximum. They were brief lasting 1–4 s and were frequently associated with single jerks of mainly the shoulders, but occasionally of the hands, thumbs, eyelids or elsewhere. The jerks occurred simultaneously with the first or the second polyspike–wave complex of the GSWD. Some jerks were followed by atonic attacks. The EEG also showed brief (< 0.5 s) abortive generalised discharges of polyspikes at around 15 Hz with anterior maximum and alternating, but not consistent, side emphasis. There were no clinical manifestations.

The paroxysmal discharges occurred with the eyes open and closed, spontaneously and during overbreathing. Intermittent photic stimulation (IPS) did not evoke photoparoxysmal responses.

Atypical benign partial epilepsy of childhood may also imitate Doose syndrome, because of repeated falls, absences and diffuse slow spike–wave activity mainly in the sleep EEG.[31,103-105] The main differentiating point is that these children also have nocturnal focal seizures similar to the Rolandic seizures (RS) that are often the presenting seizure symptom. Also, the EEG shows centrotemporal and other functional spikes in various locations.

Atypical evolutions of RS[106,107] and Panayiotopoulos syndrome[108,109] may have clinico-EEG features similar to those of Doose syndrome, but they are preceded by typical presentations of these syndromes (see Chapter 9). A similar, but reversible, clinico-EEG condition may be induced by carbamazepine,[31] oxcarbazepine[110] and lamotrigine[111] in a few children with RS. This possibility should be considered in children with RS and dramatic deterioration after treatment with these AEDs.

Children with 'epilepsy with continuous spike–wave complexes during slow-wave sleep' may also have drop attacks due to atypical absences or negative epileptic myoclonus.

Non-epileptic myoclonus of many neurological disorders rarely raises a diagnostic problem with Doose syndrome, unless it is a symptom of a degenerative disease with associated epileptic features.[90]

Diagnostic tips

The diagnosis of Doose syndrome is probably safe if myoclonic-atonic seizures start in a previously normal child with pre-existing febrile or afebrile GTCS and familial seizure disorders.

Differential diagnostic problems from Lennox-Gastaut syndrome probably reflect ill-defined inclusion and exclusion criteria.

PROGNOSIS

The prognosis is unclear probably because of different selection criteria.

Half of the patients may achieve a seizure-free state and normal or near normal development.[95] Myoclonic-atonic seizures remit within 1–3 years from onset despite initial resistance to treatment, but GTCS or clonic seizures tend to continue.[95] These patients who have a good prognosis may correspond to the genuine Doose syndrome of the idiopathic form of EM-AS. Spontaneous remission with normal development has been observed in a few untreated cases, but these may belong to benign myoclonic epilepsy in infancy.

The others, probably belonging to symptomatic or probably symptomatic cases or other syndromes, may continue with seizures, severe impairment of cognitive functions and behavioural abnormalities. Ataxia, poor motor function, dysarthria and poor language development may emerge.

MANAGEMENT

Drug therapy is dictated by seizure type. Valproate, which is effective in myoclonic jerks, atonic seizures and absences, is the most efficacious. Add-on small doses of lamotrigine have a beneficial pharmacodynamic interaction with valproate. Topiramate reduces the frequency of atonic seizures.[112] Levetiracetam may be an effective substitute AED for valproate.

In resistant cases, ketogenic diet, followed by adrenocorticotropin hormone (ACTH) and ethosuximide, have been found to be highly beneficial.[95] Benzodiazepines, acetazolamide, sulthiame and even bromides are also used.

Carbamazepine, phenytoin, and vigabatrin are contraindicated.

In myoclonic-atonic status epilepticus, intravenous benzodiazepines are often efficacious, but rarely may precipitate tonic status.

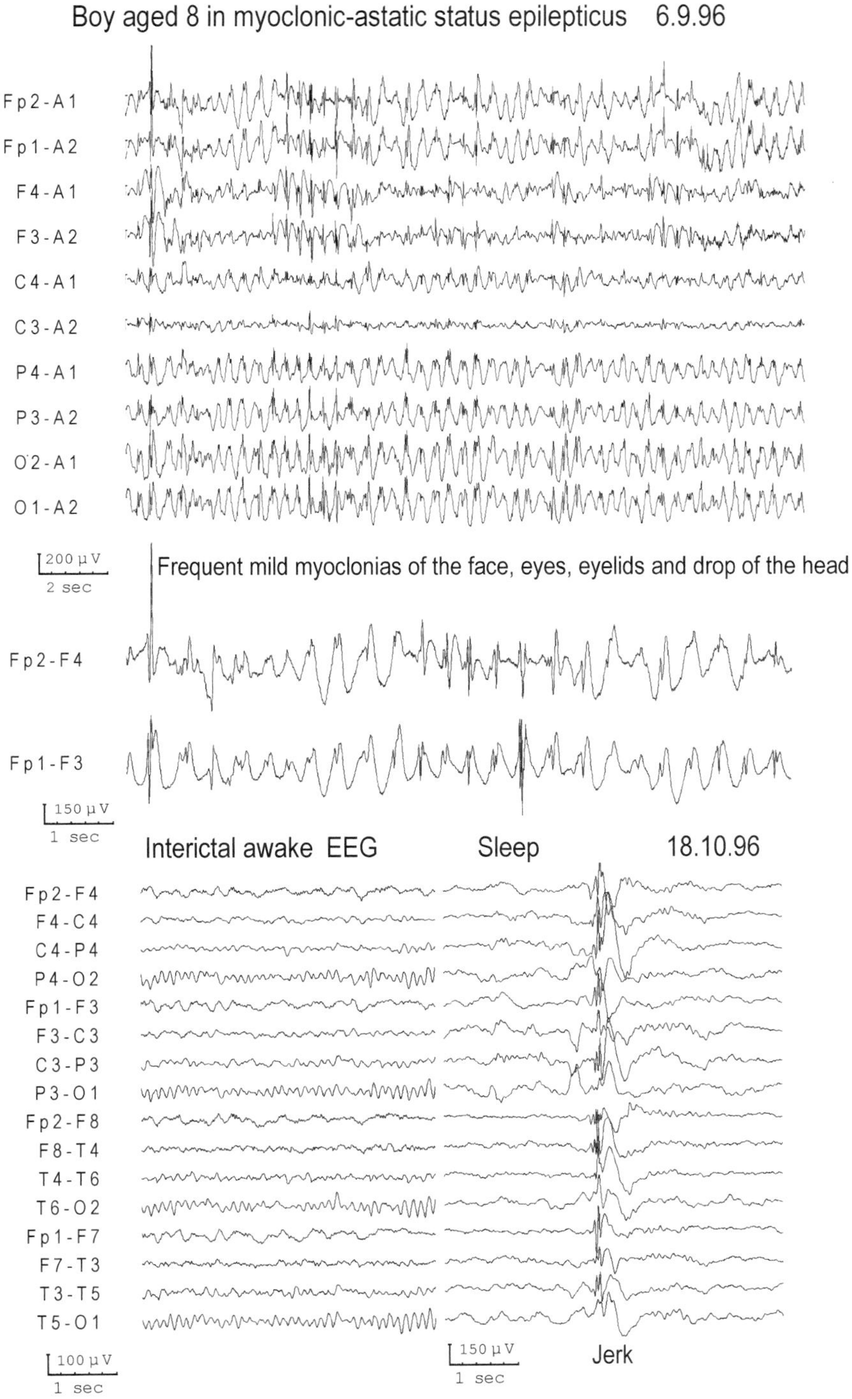

Figure 10.6 Samples of a video EEG of a boy in myoclonic-atonic status epilepticus

Top: The EEG showed electrical status epilepticus during wakefulness and sleep. This consisted of nearly continuous generalised discharges of spikes (or double spikes) and slow wave complexes at 2.5-3Hz. This pattern occasionally alternated with relatively normal background activity lasting less than 30 s.

The main clinical manifestations were frequent facial subtle myoclonias (eyelid fluttering, upwards deviation of the eyes with spontaneous eye opening associated with fast eyelid fluttering, subtle facial twitches) and a few massive myoclonic jerks occasionally with some atonic components. Clinically, there was no apparent impairment of consciousness.

Middle: Details of the EEG in the top of the Figure. Magnified frontal EEG channels and increased time scale.

Bottom: The video EEG 1 month later was normal during wakefulness with a few myoclonic jerks only during sleep.

CHILDHOOD ABSENCE EPILEPSY

"...a disease with an explosive onset between the ages of 4 and 12 years, of frequent short, very slight, monotonous minor epileptiform seizures of uniform severity, which recur almost daily for weeks, months, or years, are uninfluenced by anti-epileptic remedies, do not impede normal and psychical development, and ultimately cease spontaneously never to return. At most, the eyeballs may roll upwards, the lids may flicker, and the arms may be raised by a feeble tonic spasm. Clonic movements, however slight, obvious vasomotor disturbances, palpitations, and lassitude or confusion after the attacks are equivocal symptoms strongly suggestive of oncoming grave epilepsy, and for the present they should be considered as foreign to the more favourable disease." [113]

W. J. Adie (1924) [113] defining CAE as an epileptic syndrome

CAE is the prototype IGE of typical absence seizures.[7,15,16,18,114] It is genetically determined, age related and affects otherwise normal children.

DEMOGRAPHIC DATA

Onset is between 4 and 10 years of age, with a peak at 5–6 years.[15,114-117] The onset of typical absence seizures in CAE before 4 years of age [118-121] and after 10 years of age[118-121] is uncertain or at least exceptional.

Comments and debate on the ILAE definition of CAE

The ILAE Commission of 1989 [1] largely defined CAE by age at onset and frequency of absences:

"Childhood absence epilepsy (pyknolepsy) occurs in children of school age (peak manifestation age 6–7 years), with a strong genetic predisposition in otherwise normal children. It appears more frequently in girls than in boys. It is characterised by very frequent (several to many per day) absences. The EEG reveals bilateral, synchronous symmetrical spike–waves, usually 3 Hz, on a normal background activity. During adolescence, GTCS often develop. Otherwise, absences may remit or more rarely, persist as the only seizure type."[1]

The new ILAE diagnostic scheme also classifies CAE as IGE.[5]

The ILAE definition is a very broad and requires revision. Otherwise, any type of frequent absence seizures occurring in childhood would be erroneously equated with CAE. Because of this ambiguity, the epidemiology, genetics, age at onset, clinical manifestations, other types of seizures, long-term prognosis and treatment of CAE reviewed in this chapter may not accurately reflect the syndrome of CAE. It is also because of this ambiguity that some authors: (a.) have divided patients with childhood onset absence seizures into 'subsyndromes' including those who remit, those who persist into adolescence and develop GTCS, and those who develop both GTCS and myoclonic seizures during adolescence;[138] and (b.) consider that patients with CAE 'evolve' into JAE or JME.[139,140]

The inclusion and exclusion criteria of Table 10.5 proposed by Loiseau and Panayiotopoulos[114] for CAE should not be taken as an extreme position. They do not differ significantly from the ILAE (1989)[1] criteria of CAE with:

a. age at onset in childhood
b. very frequent (several to many per day) absences presumably with severe impairment of consciousness
c. ictal EEG with bilateral, synchronous and symmetrical 3 Hz GSWD, on a normal background activity (that presumably excludes fragmented, asymmetrical and asynchronous 3–5 Hz GSWD with intradischarge variations)
d. GTCS accepted only if they develop later in adolescence.

Also, the Commission (1989)[1] by accepting 'epilepsy with myoclonic absences' as a separate syndrome differentiates myoclonic absences from typical absences of CAE. It is along this line that Loiseau and Panayiotopoulos[114] also considered eyelid myoclonia (which is a predominantly myoclonic and less of an absence syndrome) as an exclusion criterion. Whether, perioral myoclonia or single violent jerks during the ictus of an absence seizure is an exclusion criterion may be debatable. However, their presence indicates a worse prognosis.[15,16,141] The same applies to multiple spikes (more than three spikes/wave), which also indicate a bad prognosis,[138,142] and coexistent myoclonic jerks or GTCS.[24] Further, the Commission (1989),[1] by accepting 'typical absence seizures consistently provoked by specific stimuli' as a specific type of reflex seizures, indicates that these may be a separate group from CAE.[16,114,136,143]

Age at onset of absences does not determine syndromic classification of CAE

We have studied 39 adults with IGE with typical absences starting before 10 years of age.[144] All were older than 18 years (31.5±10.5; range 18-56) at the last follow-up and all had EEG (15 with video-EEG) recorded typical absence seizures. Typical absences had onset at 6.2±1.9 years (range 2-9) that persisted into adulthhood in 28 (71.8%) cases. GTCS occurred in 87.2% (onset 13±7.2 years; range 2-36). Myoclonic jerks occurred in 38.5% (onset 2.6±4.1 years; range 7-18). Women (82%) and photosensitivity (56.4%) markedly predominated. Eight patients have EMA, 5 JAE, 4 perioral myoclonia with absences, 3 JME, 3 absences with single myoclonic jerk, 1 CAE, 3 predominantly reflex absences. Twelve patients (8 with photosensitivity) could not be classified. Only 6 patients were free from all type of seizures (1 CAE, 2 JAE, 2 unclassified IGE with reflex absences). [144]

Synonyms

Pyknolepsy. Many European clinicians use the word 'pyknolepsy' (from the Greek words pyknos = dense and epilepsy) either to define a high daily frequency of absences or as a synonym to CAE.

Two-thirds of patients are girls[115,116,122,123] despite some studies indicating that boys and girls are equally affected.[124,125]

The prevalence is about 10%[126-128] and the annual incidence is about 7/100,000[129-131] in children with epileptic seizures who are less than 15–16 years of age. Recruitment bias explains the wide range in the reported incidence (1.9–8/100,000 of children < 16 years) and prevalence (2–37% of children with epileptic disorders) of CAE.[124,129,130,132-137]

CLINICAL MANIFESTATIONS

TYPICAL ABSENCE SEIZURES

CAE manifests with the most characteristic and classical example of typical absence seizures, which are characterised by:

- short duration
- abrupt onset and abrupt termination
- severe impairment of consciousness
- high daily frequency.

Probably any other types of seizure are incompatible with this diagnosis.
Mild impairment of consciousness in untreated patients is an exclusion criterion.[114]

Absences are severe and frequent, with from ten to hundreds per day, for which reason CAE is also known as pyknolepsy.[113] They are of abrupt onset and abrupt termination (Figures 10.2, 10.7 and 10.8). Their duration varies from 4–20 s, though most last around 10 s. Clinically, the hallmark of the absence is abrupt, brief and severe impairment of consciousness with unresponsiveness and interruption of the ongoing voluntary activity, which is not restored during the ictus. The eyes open spontaneously, overbreathing, and speech and other voluntary activity stop within the first 3 s from the onset of the discharge. Simple automatisms occur in two-thirds of seizures, but are not stereotyped. The eyes stare or move slowly. Mild myoclonic elements of the eyes, eyebrows and eyelids may feature in CAE, but are usually mild and occur at the onset of the GSWD. However, more severe and sustained myoclonic jerks of the facial muscles may indicate other IGEs with absences.

The attack ends as abruptly as it commenced with sudden resumption of the pre-absence activity as if it was not interrupted.

Typical absence seizures are nearly invariably provoked by hyperventilation.

OTHER TYPES OF SEIZURES

Seizures other than typical absences are not compatible with CAE. The only exceptions are (a). febrile seizures that may precede the onset of CAE and (b). solitary or infrequent GTCS that occur long after the onset of absence seizures and usually in adolescence after absences have remitted.

GTCS or myoclonic jerks preceding the onset of typical absences or concomitant with the stage of active absence seizures do not occur in CAE.[15,114,143,145,146] However, about 10% of patients may later develop a few, solitary or infrequent GTCS in adolescence or adult life.[145,146] This contrasts with the fact that focal seizures, myoclonic jerks, GTCS and other more bizarre fits have been described with CAE but these are probably other epileptic syndromes starting with absences in childhood.[134]

Status epilepticus, whether convulsive or non-convulsive, is incompatible with CAE. If this occurs, the diagnosis of CAE should be seriously challenged. Also, though absence status epilepticus may occur in 5–16% of patients with typical absence seizures starting before the age of 10 years,[117,140,147] this is probably incompatible with CAE.[15,19,77]

Atonic falls do not occur in CAE.[136]

SEIZURE-PRECIPITATING FACTORS

Typical absence seizures occur spontaneously, but they are also influenced by various other factors, mainly hyperventilation (Figures 10.2, and 10.6). Hyperventilation is the most potent precipitating factor that induces absences in more than 90% of the trials,[148,149] ranging from 75%[150] or 80%[151] to 100%.[143] A diagnosis of CAE should be seriously questioned in an untreated child who does not have an attack on hyperventilation.

Other precipitating or facilitating factors are emotional (anger, sorrow, fear, surprise, embarrassment), intellectual (lack of interest, release of attention, mealtimes for some children and school-time for others) and metabolic (hypoglycaemia).[114] Typical absence seizures generally do not occur when the

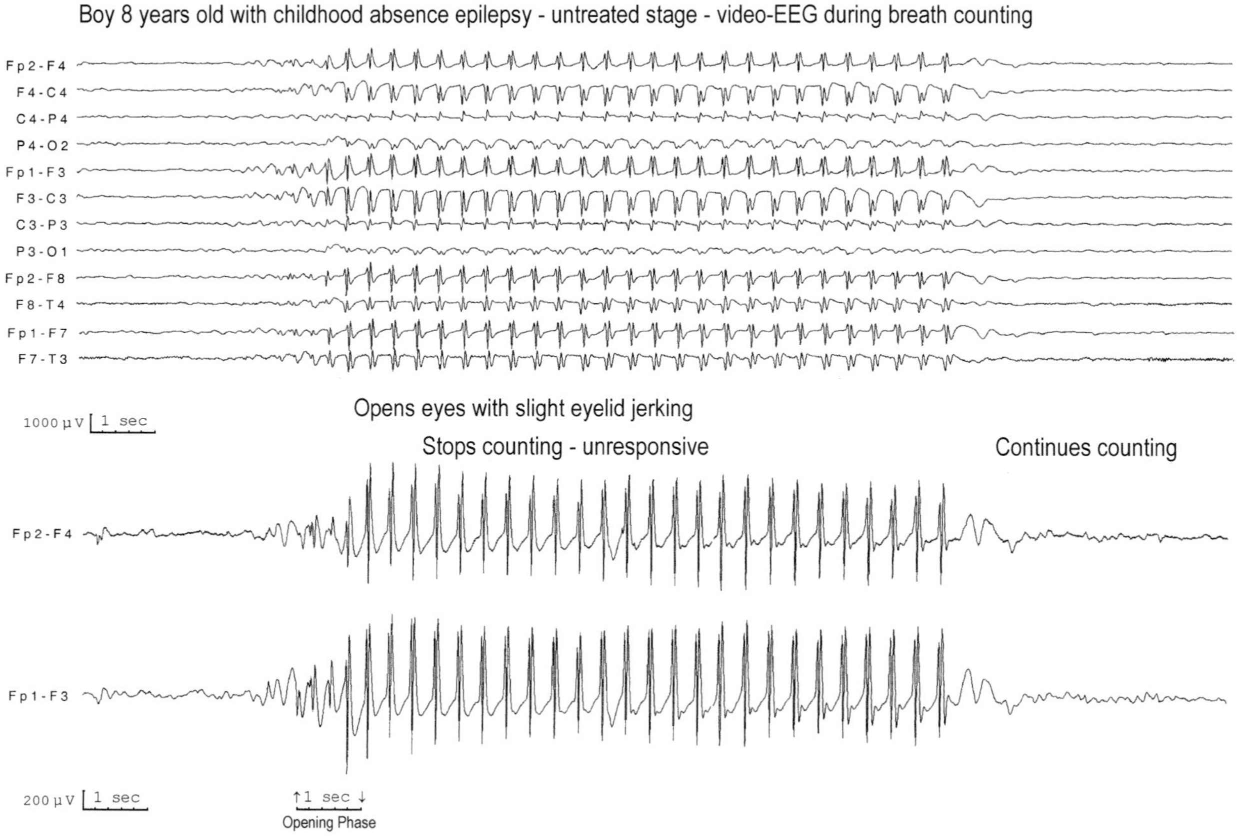

Figure 10.7 Video EEG of an 8-year-old boy with classical CAE.

He was referred for EEG because of "blanks and day dreaming"; the diagnosis had been overlooked despite frequent absences for 2 years, which also interfered with his scholastic performance.

The seizure had all the characteristic features of typical absences in CAE. Initially there was some brief eyelid flickering in the opening phase of the GWSD followed by opening of the eyes, eyes and head deviating upwards and to the right, and simultaneous cessation of breath counting. He remained unresponsive during the rest of the GSWD. Counting was restored immediately after the end of the GSWD.

Note the fast and asymmetrical onset of the GSWD in the opening phase during the first second. Subsequently, the GSWD is entirely rhythmical and regular with abrupt termination to clinical and EEG normality.[24]

child is busy and stimulated by physical or mental activity, or has sustained attention.[136] Emotional or conflicting situations, such as reading difficulties, may provoke absences.[152] In a given patient, typical absence seizures are often triggered by the same factor.

There are no other precipitating factors in CAE, which is at variance with nearly all other forms of IGE. In particular, though photosensitivity is accepted according to the ILAE Commission's definition,[1] most other authors consider clinical photosensitivity as a significant exclusion criterion.[15,136,143] Mild EEG photosensitivity or facilitation (not consistent provocation) of photoparoxysmal responses and absences may occur.

AETIOLOGY

Although CAE is genetically determined, the precise mode of inheritance and the genes involved remain largely unidentified.[7]

In monozygotic twins, 84% had 3 Hz GSWD and only 75 % of pairs had clinical absence seizures. These events occurred 16 times less often in dizygotic twins.[115] Currently, various chromosomal loci have been identified in families with absences of childhood onset (not necessarily equated with CAE). Linkage to chromosome 1 was found in families with absences starting in childhood and the later development of myoclonic jerks and GTCS, as in JME.[9] Linkage analysis in five generations of a family in which affected patients had childhood absences and GTCS provided evidence of a locus on chromosome 8q24.[9,138] The candidate region for this locus, designated ECA 1, has been refined, but a gene remains to be identified. According to the criteria proposed in this chapter, neither of these groups is CAE. There are also reports implicating chromosome 5q31.1 and 19p13.2 (see ref [7] for an excellent recent review).

Furthermore, there is now evidence available to suggest that mutations in genes encoding GABA receptors[34-36] or brain-expressed voltage-dependent calcium channels[37] may underlie CAE. Feucht et al.[34] found a significant association between a polymorphism in $GABA_A$ receptor gamma 3 subunit in chromosome 15q11 in 50 families with CAE. Marini et al.[36] found $GABA_A$ receptor gamma 2 subunit gene mutations on chromosome 5 in a large family with CAE and febrile seizures (including febrile seizures plus and other seizure phenotypes). This gene mutation segregated with febrile seizures and CAE, and also occurred in individuals with the other phenotypes. The clinical and molecular data suggested that the $GABA_A$ receptor subunit mutation alone could account for the febrile seizure phenotype, but an interaction of this gene with another gene or genes was required for the childhood absence phenotype in this family. Linkage analysis for a putative second gene contributing to the childhood absence phenotype suggested possible loci on chromosomes 10, 13, 14 and 15.[36] Chen et al.[37] found 68 variations, including 12 missense mutations in the calcium channel *CACNA1H* gene in CAE patients. The identified missense mutations occurred in the highly conserved residues of the T-type calcium channel gene.[37] However, another study of 33 nuclear families, each with two or more individuals with CAE each provided conclusive evidence that the genes encoding $GABA_A$ and $GABA_B$ receptors, voltage-dependent calcium channels and the ECA1 region on chromosome 8q do not account independently for the childhood absence trait in a majority of the families.[153]

Acquired factors may play a facilitating role.

DIAGNOSTIC PROCEDURES

In typical cases nothing but an EEG is needed.

INTERICTAL EEG

The interictal EEG in CAE has normal background activity, with frequent rhythmic posterior delta activity (Figure 10.8). Benign functional spikes (mainly centrotemporal and less frequently occipital or frontal) may be seen and do not alter the prognosis.

Posterior rhythmic slow activity is considered a characteristic finding in CAE. This consists of long runs of bilateral rhythmic and fusiform, high amplitude slow waves at 3 Hz in the distribution regions of alpha rhythm. It is bilateral, often of higher amplitude on the right, but occasionally may be lateralised to one side or fluctuate from side to side in emphasis. It occurs in less than half of patients at a peak age of 6–10 years. Patients with this EEG finding tend to have longer absence seizures, a better prognosis and less often develop GTCS.[154,155]

Sleep EEG has not been studied systematically in pure forms of CAE. Generally, in IGE, GSWD are more likely to increase, but a reduction is also observed during sleep. The discharges are shorter and usually devoid of discernible clinical manifestations, even in those patients who have numerous clinical seizures during the alert state. However, clinical absence seizures that may awake the patient have been recorded during sleep. Sleep EEG patterns are normal.

Photic stimulation: Clinical photosensitivity or consistent provocation of typical absences by IPS is an exclusion criterion for CAE. However, IPS may act as a facilitatory factor in that these children may have more typical absences during IPS than in the resting EEG, but these are far less common than during hyperventilation.

ICTAL EEG

Ictal EEG consists of high amplitude 3 Hz GSWD which are of higher voltage in the anterior regions. They are rhythmic at around 3 Hz (2.5–4 Hz) with a gradual and regular slowing down of the frequency by 0.5–1 Hz from the initial to the terminal phase of the discharge. The opening phase of the discharge, 1–2 s from

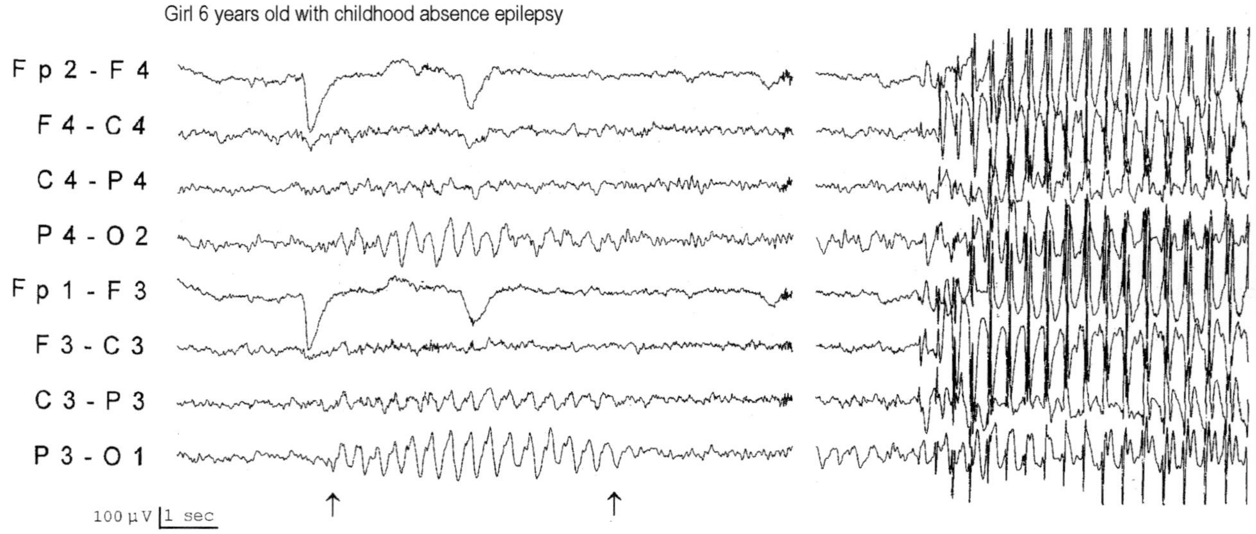

Figure 10.8 Girl aged 6 years with untreated childhood absence epilepsy

Left: Long runs of bilateral, rhythmic and fusiform, high amplitude 3 Hz slow waves appear in the posterior regions (between arrows).
Right: Onset of a typical absence seizure.

the onset, is usually fast and unreliable for these measurements. There are no marked variations in the relationship of the spike to the slow wave, no fluctuations in the intradischarge frequency and certainly no fragmentations of the ictal discharges (Figure 10.7).

Diagnostic tips

Typical absence seizures of CAE are easy to diagnose and reproduce by hyperventilation.

Any child with sudden, brief and frequent cessation of physical and mental activity should be tested clinically for absences. This is easily performed with the hyperventilation test.

Ask the child to overbreathe for 3 minutes while counting his/her breaths and holding his/her hands in front. This will evoke an absence in more than 90% of children with childhood absence epilepsy.

It is essential that a video EEG is performed prior to initiating treatment for appropriate confirmation and documentation of the clinical EEG characteristics of the absences. If this is not possible, the clinical manifestations should be documented with home camcorders or modern digital recorders.

DIFFERENTIAL DIAGNOSIS

CAE should be the easiest type of epileptic syndrome to diagnose, because seizures have an abrupt onset and termination, high daily frequency and are nearly invariably provoked by hyperventilation. In practical terms, a child with suspected typical absences should be asked to overbreathe for 3 minutes while standing, counting his/her breaths and with the hands extended in front. This will provoke an absence in as many as 90% of those affected.

Clarification

CAE is not synonymous with any type of absence seizures starting in childhood. Therefore, other epilepsy syndromes with absence seizures that may be life-long and have a worse prognosis should be meticulously differentiated from CAE.

Table 10.5 Criteria for childhood absence epilepsy

Inclusion criteria

1. Age at onset between 4 and 10 years and a peak at 5–7 years.
2. Normal neurological state and development.
3. Brief (4–20 seconds, exceptionally longer) and frequent (tens per day) absence seizures with abrupt and severe impairment (loss) of consciousness. Automatisms are frequent but have no significance in the diagnosis.
4. EEG ictal discharges of generalised high-amplitude spike and double (maximum occasional three spikes are allowed) spike and slow wave complexes. Spike-wave is rhythmic at around 3 Hz with a gradual and regular slowdown from the initial to the terminal phase of the discharge. The duration of the discharges varies from 4 to 20 seconds.

Exclusion criteria

The following may be incompatible with childhood absence epilepsy:

1. Other than typical absence seizures such as GTCS, or myoclonic jerks before or during the active stage of absences.
2. Eyelid myoclonia, perioral myoclonia, rhythmic massive limb jerking, and single or arrhythmic myoclonic jerks of the head, trunk or limbs. However, mild myoclonic elements of the eyes, eyebrows, and eyelids may be featured – particularly in the first 3 seconds of the absence seizure.
3. Mild or no impairment of consciousness during the 3–4 Hz discharges.
4. Brief EEG 3–4 Hz spike wave paroxysms of <4 seconds, multiple spikes (>3) or ictal discharge fragmentations.
5. Visual (photic) and other sensory precipitation of clinical seizures.

Diagnosis should improve with heightened awareness and video EEG studies. Exclusion criteria for CAE are as important as inclusion criteria (Table 10.5). Automatisms have no significance in the diagnosis. They should not be taken as evidence of complex focal seizures (see Table 10.2), which require entirely different management.

PROGNOSIS

> "For myself I shall be well satisfied if I have made it appear probable to you that there does exist a form of epilepsy in children which is distinguishable by its clinical features and in which the prognosis is always good." Adie (1924)[113]

Most of the studies on the prognosis of CAE are based on the seizure/symptom itself and not on the relevant syndrome. Absences and therefore their prognosis are syndrome related.[15,24,141]

Studies on the prognosis of typical absences with onset in childhood (which are not necessarily CAE) [115-117,145,147,151,154,156-169] give an overall rate of remission from 30-80%. Thus, 20-70 % of patients continue having typical absences in adult life and of these 90% will develop other generalised seizures such as GTCS and myoclonic jerks. Absences become less frequent and less severe with age. The diagnostic confusion is further indicated by the finding that some cases develop motor or versive seizures of frontal lobe epilepsies. If CAE is defined by age at onset alone, half of the patients develop GTCS later.[168]

The factors indicating a worse prognosis in these studies were:

- mental retardation, neurological and EEG background abnormalities (which by definition are against IGE)
- GTCS or other type of seizures preceding or coinciding with the onset of typical absences (an exclusion criterion for CAE)
- photosensitivity (exclusion criterion)
- onset in late childhood or adolescence (are these JAE? or JME?) or very early childhood (are these MAE? or EMA?).

Note on the prognosis of childhood absence epilepsy

In my opinion, based on prospective studies of children fulfilling the strict criteria of CAE (see Table 10.5) and retrospective evaluation of adults with absences[15,56,57] the long-term prognosis of CAE is excellent. This implies complete remission of absences 2–6 years after onset and no more than 3% of patients developing infrequent GTCS in adult life. There is indirect, but not definite, evidence for this. In our series of 85 adult patients (> 16 years of age with mean age 32 years) with absences and syndromes of IGEs, none had CAE, though in 37 patients absences had started in childhood, before the age of 10 years.[57] Most patients had JME (30 patients), but others had JAE (10 patients), IGE with phantom absences (12 patients), eyelid myoclonia with absences (11 patients), perioral myoclonia with absences (PMA; 7 patients), photosensitive absence syndromes (4 patients), absences with single myoclonic jerks (1 patient), and 10 patients were unclassified. Half of these patients would have been classified as CAE continuing in adult life, if the only criteria for diagnosis were age at onset and frequency of absences.

This optimistic view of mine is also supported by the results of long-term studies in which the remission rate for absences starting in childhood increased with the application of exclusion criteria.[114,145,154]

Loiseau and associates[145,146] studied 53 patients over the age of 20 years at last follow-up. Inclusion criteria were age at onset (3–10 years) of daily and EEG-recorded typical absences as a presenting symptom of normal children, with no history of preceding seizures other than febrile convulsions. Patients with EEG multiple or irregular spike–wave complexes and/or photosensitivity were excluded. Absences persisted in five children (< 10%) and were the only type of seizure in two of them. GTCS occurred in 14 patients (26%), but were isolated or rare in 11 cases. GTCS were more common among patients with onset of absences at 9–10 years and without posterior delta rhythms. Response to treatment varied. Control was achieved in 12 patients within weeks, but in most cases absences persisted for years. In this scholarly study, the prognosis could probably have been improved if video EEG had been used to exclude patients who perhaps had other types of IGE with frequent absences from childhood. In other words, patients who did not remit may have had other epileptic syndromes, particularly JAE, which may start before the age of 10 years.

- prominent ictal myoclonic components (are these absences with perioral or single myoclonic jerks?
- poor response to treatment.

All the above studies involve long-term follow-up of patients with onset of absences in childhood or adolescence. Most were based on clinico-EEG documented 'absences', probably with severe impairment of consciousness, without reference to syndromic classification and without the help of video-EEG recordings. Myoclonic jerks or GTCS occurring independently of absences, severity of impairment of consciousness during the absence ictus, syndromic criteria of epilepsies and video-EEG documentation have not been utilised in these studies.

By applying strict diagnostic criteria, an excellent prognosis may be anticipated for CAE. At a time when no anti-absence drugs existed, Adie[113] concluded that even if absence seizures in CAE (he called it pyknolepsy) persisted for a long time, they ultimately ceased, never to return. Adie considered only the pure form of CAE with severe pyknoleptic absences while with the advent of EEG this group was broaden to include any type absences starting in childhood.

A good prognosis is consistent with recent findings that absences of CAE, even if they persist for several years, they finally disappear with age in more than 90% of cases.[18,154] In a Swedish population-based study, a 91% remission rate was found when patients with absence epilepsy had only absence seizures.[162]

Remission occurs before the age of 12 years. Less than 10% of patients develop infrequent or solitary GTCS in adolescence or adult life. It is exceptional for patients to continue having absence seizures when adults. Poor social adjustment has been reported in one-third of patients.[122,147,154,160] This may be due to frequent absence seizures, particularly if they were not treated early at their onset, the attitudes of school mates and parents, or medication.

MANAGEMENT

Monotherapy either with valproate or ethosuximide controls absences in 80% of patients.[4] Another option is lamotrigine monotherapy, though this is less effective and only nearly half of patients become seizure free.[4,170,171]

If monotherapy fails or unacceptable adverse reactions appear, replacement of one drug with the other is the alternative. Adding small doses of lamotrigine to valproate may be the best combination in resistant cases.

There are anecdotal reports that children may not respond to syrup of valproate despite adequate levels, but seizures stop if this is replaced with tablets of valproate. It is also anecdotal experience that, once seizure cessation has been achieved, valproate may be safely reduced to more moderate doses without relapses.[4]

Contraindicated drugs, which make seizures worse and may induce status epilepticus are: carbamazepine, gabapentin, oxcarbazepine, phenytoin, phenobarbitone, vigabatrin and tiagabine.

Withdrawing anti-epileptic medication: In the pure form of CAE, drug therapy can be gradually withdrawn (within 3–6 months) after 2–3 years free of seizures.

Note of practical significance

In evaluating the efficacy of therapy or anticipating AED withdrawal, it should be remembered that:

a. the true frequency of typical absence seizures is difficult to assess without prolonged video EEG monitoring, because the clinical manifestations can be easily missed.

b. parents' assessment is often an underestimate.[4,172]

JUVENILE ABSENCE EPILEPSY

JAE is an IGE syndrome[1,5,15] mainly manifesting with severe typical absence seizures; nearly all patients (80%) also suffer from GTCS and one-fifth from sporadic myoclonic jerks.[15,16,24,184,185]

DEMOGRAPHIC DATA

Usual age at onset is 9–13 years (70% of patients), but can range from 5 to 20 years.[15,185] Myoclonic jerks and GTCS usually begin 1–10 years after the onset of absences. Rarely, GTCS may precede the onset of absences.[15,184] Both sexes are equally affected.

The exact prevalence of JAE is unknown because of variable criteria. In adults over 20 years of age, the prevalence of JAE may be around 2–3% of all epilepsies and around 8–10% of IGEs.[57,186]

CLINICAL MANIFESTATIONS

JAE manifests with severe typical absences.[15,184,185] Nearly all patients also develop GTCS and one-fifth also suffer from mild myoclonic jerks.

TYPICAL ABSENCE SEIZURES

Frequent and severe typical absences are the defining seizure type of JAE.[15,184,185] The seizures are similar to those of CAE, though they may be milder. The usual frequency of absences is approximately 1–10/day, but this may be much higher for some patients. The hallmark of the absence is abrupt, brief and severe impairment of consciousness with total or partial unresponsiveness. Mild or inconspicuous impairment of consciousness is not compatible with JAE. The ongoing voluntary activity usually stops at onset, but may be partly restored during the ictus. Automatisms are frequent, usually occurring 6–10 s after the onset of the EEG discharge (Figure 10.9). In JAE, mild myoclonic elements of the eyelids are common during the absence. However, more severe and sustained myoclonic jerks of the facial muscles may indicate other IGE with absences. Severe eyelid or

Considerations on classification

The 1989 ILAE classification broadly defined JAE as follows:[1] "The absences of JAE are the same as in pyknolepsy, but absences with retropulsive movements are less common. Manifestation occurs around puberty. Seizure frequency is lower than in pyknolepsy, with absences occurring less frequently than every day, mostly sporadically. Association with GTCS is frequent, and GTCS precede the absence manifestations more often than in childhood absence epilepsy, often occurring on awakening. Not infrequently, the patients also have myoclonic seizures. Sex distribution is equal. The spike-waves are often >3 Hz. Response to therapy is excellent."

Age at onset (around puberty) and frequency of seizures (less frequent than CAE) are insufficient criteria for the categorisation of any syndrome.[15] Thus, epidemiology, genetics, age at onset, clinical manifestations, other types of seizure, long-term prognosis and treatment may not accurately reflect the syndrome of JAE. Recently, JAE has been redefined based on a cluster of clinical and EEG manifestations studied in video EEG recordings (Table10.6).[15,24]

The ILAE Task Force has not yet reached definite conclusions regarding the definition of JAE, though there is a tendency to consider JAE as part of a broader syndrome of IGE in adolescence.[5,86]

Age at onset of absences does not determine syndromic classification of JAE

We have studied 71 adults with onset of typical absences after the age of 10 years (median 13 years). All were over 18 years of age and all had experienced typical absences, verified by EEG or video EEG. Two-thirds were women (43 patients). Mean age at last follow-up was 36 years.

In 65 patients (92%), absences continued during adulthood. All but two patients had GTCS with a mean age at onset of 19 years. A total of 33 patients (47%) also had myoclonic jerks with a mean age at onset of 16 years. One-third of patients (26 patients were clinically or EEG photosensitive.

In terms of epileptic syndromes, 21 had JME, 13 phantom absences with GTCS, 11 JAE, 5 eyelid myoclonia with absences, 3 perioral myoclonia with absences, 2 purely photosensitive IGE, 2 GTCS on awakening and 1 absences with single myoclonic jerks; 13 patients could not be classified.

Patients with briefer, milder and later onset absence seizures had a worse prognosis.

perioral myoclonus, rhythmic limb jerking and single or arrhythmic myoclonic jerks of the head, trunk or limbs during the absence ictus are probably incompatible with JAE.

Duration of the absences varies from 4–30 s, but it is usually long (about 16 s).

GENERALISED TONIC CLONIC SEIZURES

GTCS are probably unavoidable in untreated patients. They occur in 80% of patients, mainly after awakening, though nocturnal or diurnal GTCS may also be experienced.[15,57,168,184,185,187] GTCS are usually infrequent, but may also become severe and intractable.

MYOCLONIC JERKS

Myoclonic jerks occur in 15–25% of patients and are infrequent, mild and of random distribution. They usually occur in the afternoon when the patient is more tired than in the morning after awakening.[15,66]

ABSENCE STATUS EPILEPTICUS

ASE is truly generalised non-convulsive (without any type of jerks) and occurs in one-fifth of patients.[19,66]

SEIZURE-PRECIPITATING FACTORS

Mental and psychological arousal is the main precipitating factor for absences. Conversely, sleep deprivation, fatigue, alcohol, excitement and lights, either alone or more usually in combination, are the main precipitating factors for GTCS.

Some authors have reported that 8% of JAE patients suffer from photosensitivity clinically or on the EEG.[184] However, clinical photosensitivity that is consistent with provocation of seizures (absences, GTCS or jerks) may be incompatible with JAE. These patients may have another IGE syndrome.[15] EEG photosensitivity (i.e. facilitation of absences by IPS) may not be uncommon.

AETIOLOGY

JAE is determined by genetic factors, but mode of transmission and its relation to other forms of IGE, particularly CAE and JME, has not yet been established. A single Mendelian mode appears to be unlikely.

There is an increased incidence of epileptic disorders in families of patients with JAE and there are reports of monozygotic twins with JAE.[24,185,188] A proband with JAE was found in 3 of 37 families selected, because at least three members were affected by IGE in one or more generations.[189] However, only one sibling also had JAE, while other members mainly had GTCS.[189]

In various reports JAE has been linked to chromosome 8,[190] 21,[191] 18[10] and probably 5.[10] Heterogeneity may be common. Autopsy[192] and MRI studies[54] found microdysgenesis and other cerebral changes in patients with JAE.

DIAGNOSTIC PROCEDURES

All tests apart from the EEG are normal.

ELECTROENCEPHALOGRAPHY

In untreated patients, absences are easily elicited by hyperventilation (Figure 10.9), if not the diagnosis of JAE should be questioned.

The interictal EEG is normal or with mild abnormalities only. Focal epileptiform abnormalities and abortive asymmetrical bursts of spike/multiple spikes are common.

The ictal EEG shows 3–4 Hz GSWD. The frequency at the initial phase of the discharge is usually fast (3–5 Hz). There is a gradual and smooth decline in frequency from the initial to the terminal phase. The discharge is regular, with well-formed spikes and polyspikes, which retain a constant relation with the slow waves (Figure 10.9).

DIFFERENTIAL DIAGNOSIS

In general, and particularly in adults, absences are often misdiagnosed as complex focal seizures, though they are easy to differentiate (Table 10.2).[56,57]

The differentiation of JAE from other IGE with absences may be more difficult without appropriate video EEG evaluation.[4,15,24] In children, it is often difficult to distinguish between CAE and JAE, because their features often overlap and manifestations are similar. In JAE, absences start later, usually they are less frequent and impairment of cognition is less severe.[24] Automatisms are equally prominent in both. Limb myoclonic jerks (not during the absences) and/or GTCS in the presence of severe absences indicate JAE.

JAE is distinctly different from the Jeavons syndrome of very brief seizures marked with rapid eyelid myoclonia, PMA with rhythmic perioral myoclonia during the absence, and MAE with rhythmic myoclonic jerks during the absence. In adolescents, the differential diagnosis between JAE and JME should not be difficult. Severe absences are the major problem in JAE while myoclonic jerks are the main seizure type in JME (Table 10.7). Absences in JME are mild and often inconspicuous.

PROGNOSIS

JAE is a lifelong disorder, though seizures can be controlled in 70–80% of patients. However, there is a tendency for the absences to become less severe, in terms of

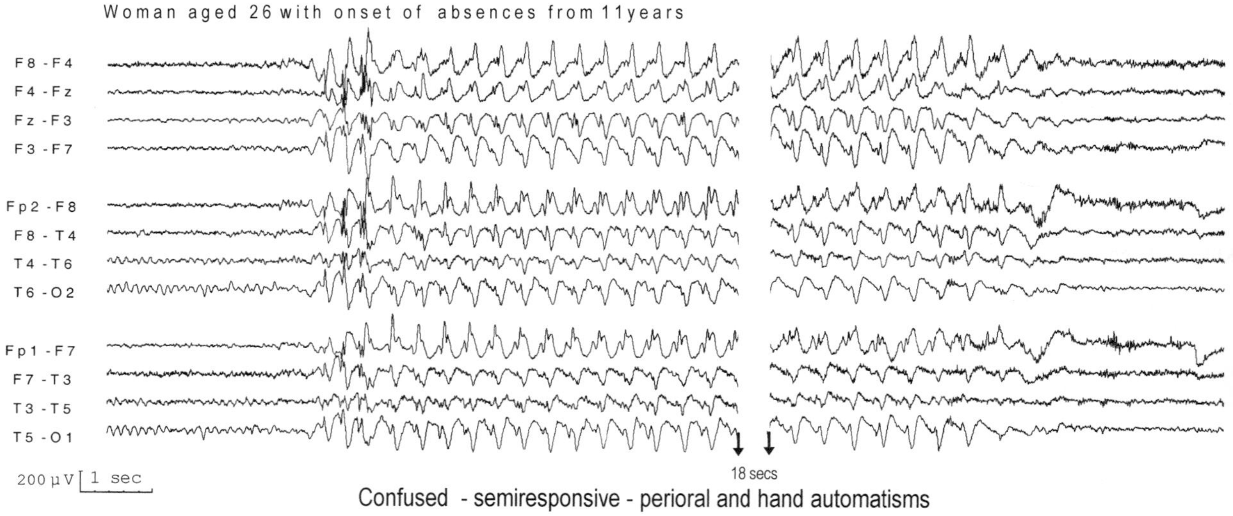

Figure 10.9 Video EEG of a 26-year-old normal woman.

She started having frequent typical absence seizures (tens of seizures each day) with severe impairment of consciousness at the age of 11 years, but medical attendance was sought only after her first GTCS at the age of 14 years. Severe and lengthy absences of 20–30 s occur 5–10 times/day. Also she has had 3–5 GTCS every year, mostly after awakening and mainly premenstrually. GTCS are preceded by clusters of absences. Occasionally, she also has random, infrequent and mild limb myoclonic jerks, which started at the age of 20 years. Treatment with various appropriate anti-absence drugs resulted in minor improvement, but compliance varies.

From Panayiotopoulos (2004)[16] with the permission of the Editor of *Medlink.*

impairment of cognition, duration and frequency, with age and particularly after the fourth decade of life.[168,184] GTCS are usually infrequent and are often precipitated by sleep deprivation, fatigue and alcohol consumption. Myoclonic jerks, if present, are not troublesome to the patient. However, one-fifth of patients may have frequent and sometimes intractable absences and GTCS, and this figure may be higher if appropriate treatment is not initiated in the early stages of JAE.

MANAGEMENT

In JAE, the consensus is that because of the frequent combination of absences and GTCS, the drug of choice is valproate, which controls all seizures in 70–80% of patients.[4] Lamotrigine, though less effective than valproate, probably controls absences and GTCS in half of patients and may be a monotherapy option, particularly in women of childbearing age.[193,194]

If seizure control with valproate monotherapy is inadequate, add-on treatment with lamotrigine or ethosuximide (if absences persist) may control the situation. If patients are unwilling to receive treatment with valproate, combining lamotrigine with levetiracetam may prove a potent efficacious option based on their different seizure efficacy and mode of action. In one study of 5 patients with JAE all became seizure free with levetiracetam alone or as add-on therapy.[183]

Control of absences is usually associated with good control of GTCS (90% of cases).

Patients should be warned about the factors precipitating GTCS.

Treatment may be lifelong, because attempts to withdraw medication nearly invariably leads to relapses even after many years free of seizures.

Table 10.6 Main inclusion and exclusion criteria for juvenile absence epilepsy (JAE)

Inclusion criteria

1. Unequivocal clinical evidence of absence seizures with severe impairment of consciousness. Nearly all patients may have GTCS. More than half have myoclonic jerks but these are mild and do not show the circadian distribution of JME.
2. Documentation of ictal 3–4 Hz generalised discharges of spike or multiple spike and slow wave discharges longer than 4 seconds that are associated with severe impairment of consciousness and often with automatisms. Normal EEGs in treated patients are common.

Exclusion criteria

The following may be incompatible with juvenile absence epilepsy:

Clinical exclusion criteria

1. Absences with marked eyelid or perioral myoclonus or marked single or rhythmic limb and trunk myoclonic jerks.
2. Absences with exclusively mild or clinically undetectable impairment of consciousness.
3. Consistent visual, photosensitive and other sensory precipitation of clinical absences is probably against the diagnosis of JAE. However, on EEG, intermittent photic stimulation often facilitates generalised discharges and absences.

EEG exclusion criteria

1. Irregular, arrhythmic spike/multiple spike and slow wave discharges with marked variations of the intra-discharge frequency.
2. Significant variations between the spike/multiple spike and slow wave relations.
3. Predominantly brief discharges (<4 seconds).

JUVENILE MYOCLONIC EPILEPSY
JANZ SYNDROME

Juvenile myoclonic epilepsy (JME) is one of the most important syndromes of IGE and is genetically determined.[1,60,195-201]

DEMOGRAPHIC DATA

The triad of absences, jerks and GTCS shows a characteristic age-related onset (Figure 10.10). Absences, when a feature, begin between the ages of 5 and 16 years. Myoclonic jerks follow between 1 and 9 years later, usually around the age of 14–15 years. GTCS usually appear a few months after, occasionally earlier, the myoclonic jerks. Exceptionally, JME may start or become clinically identifiable in adult life as *'adult myoclonic epilepsy'*.[202] Both sexes are equally affected. The reported prevalence of JME in hospital-based clinics has increased since the syndrome was first described, from 2.7%,[201] 5.7%,[203,204] 8.7%,[205] to 10.2%.[60] In community-based studies,[206,207] the reported prevalence is lower and probably reflects underdiagnosis, which may improve with heightened medical awareness.

CLINICAL MANIFESTATIONS

Juvenile myoclonic epilepsy is characterised by the triad of:

1. Myoclonic jerks on awakening (all patients)
2. Generalised tonic clonic seizures (> 90% of patients)
3. Typical absences (about one-third of patients).

Seizures have an age-related onset.
Myoclonic status epilepticus is common.

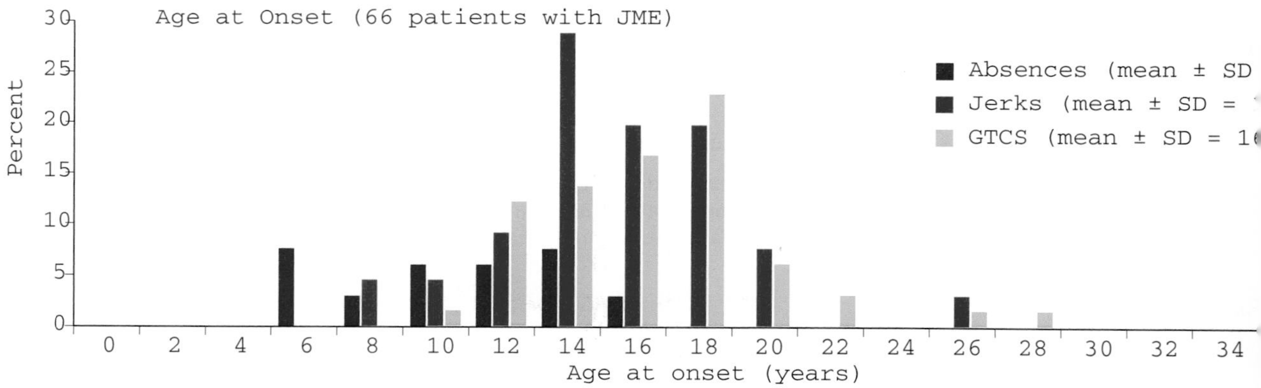

Figure 10.10 Age at onset of absences, myoclonic jerks and GTCS in 66 consecutive patients with JME.

Modified from Panayiotopoulos et al[60] with the permission of the Editor of *Epilepsia*

Classification and definition of juvenile myoclonic epilepsy

The 1989 ILAE Commission classified JME as a distinct syndrome of IGE and defined it as follows:[1] "Juvenile myoclonic epilepsy (impulsive petit mal) appears around puberty and is characterised by seizures with bilateral, single or repetitive, arrhythmic, irregular myoclonic jerks, predominantly in the arms. Jerks may cause some patients to fall suddenly. No disturbance of consciousness is noticeable. The disorder may be inherited, and sex distribution is equal. Often, there are GTCS and, less often, infrequent absences. The seizures usually occur shortly after awakening and are often precipitated by sleep deprivation. Interictal and ictal EEG have rapid, generalized, often irregular spike–waves and polyspike–waves; there is no close phase correlation between EEG spikes and jerks. Frequently, the patients are photosensitive. Response to appropriate drugs is good."

The ILAE Task Force has not yet reached definite conclusions regarding the definition of JME though there is a tendency to consider JME as part of a broader syndrome of IGE in adolescence.[5,86]

Lots of blanks and jerks; then I had a grand mal...I usually have fits when rushing after getting up; usually does not happen later in the day [198]

MYOCLONIC JERKS

Myoclonic jerks occurring after awakening are the most prominent and characteristic seizure type (Figures 10.3 and 10.11). They are shock-like, irregular and arrhythmic, clonic movements of proximal and distal muscles mainly of the upper extremities. They are often inconspicuous, restricted to the fingers, making the patient prone to drop things or look clumsy. They may be violent enough to cause falls. One-fifth of patients describe their jerks as unilateral, but video EEG shows that the jerks affect both sides (Figure 10.3).[199,208]

Some patients (< 10%) with mild forms of JME have myoclonic jerks only without developing GTCS.[60,209]

TYPICAL ABSENCE SEIZURES

One-third of patients have typical absences, which are brief with subtle impairment of consciousness. They are different from the absence seizures of childhood or JAE.[24,25,60]

Absences appearing before the age of 10 years may be more severe. They become less frequent and less severe with age.[24,25,60]

One-tenth of patients, do not perceive absences despite GSWD lasting more than 3 s.[25,60] However, the GSWD seen on video EEG with breath counting during hyperventilation often manifest with mild impairment of cognition, eyelid flickering or both (Figures 10.12, and 10.13).[4]

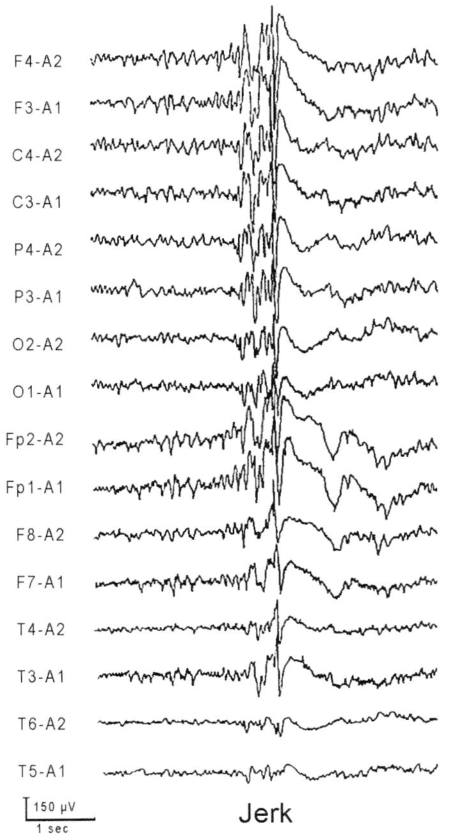

Figure 10.11 Violent myoclonic jerks of the hands associated with typical EEG manifestations.

From Panayiotopoulos et al. (1994)[60] with the permission of the Editor of *Epilepsia*.

GENERALISED TONIC CLONIC SEIZURES

GTCS usually follow the onset of myoclonic jerks. Myoclonic jerks, which usually occur in clusters and often with an accelerating frequency and severity, may precede GTCS, a so-called clonic-tonic-clonic generalised seizure.[199]

STATUS EPILEPTICUS

Myoclonic status epilepticus is probably more common than appreciated.[60,210] It almost invariably starts on awakening and is associated with precipitating factors, such as sleep deprivation or missing medication. Consciousness may not be impaired, though in some patients absences are often interspersed with myoclonic jerks (myoclonic-absence status epilepticus) (Figure 6.10).

Pure ASE with impairment of consciousness only is exceptional.[19] Convulsive generalised tonic clonic status epilepticus is relatively rare.

CIRCADIAN DISTRIBUTION

Seizures, principally myoclonic jerks, occurring within 30 min to 1 hour of awakening are characteristic of JME. Myoclonic jerks rarely occur at other times unless the patient is tired.

GTCS occur mainly on awakening, but may also be purely nocturnal or random. Absence seizures occur during any time of the day while the patient is awake.

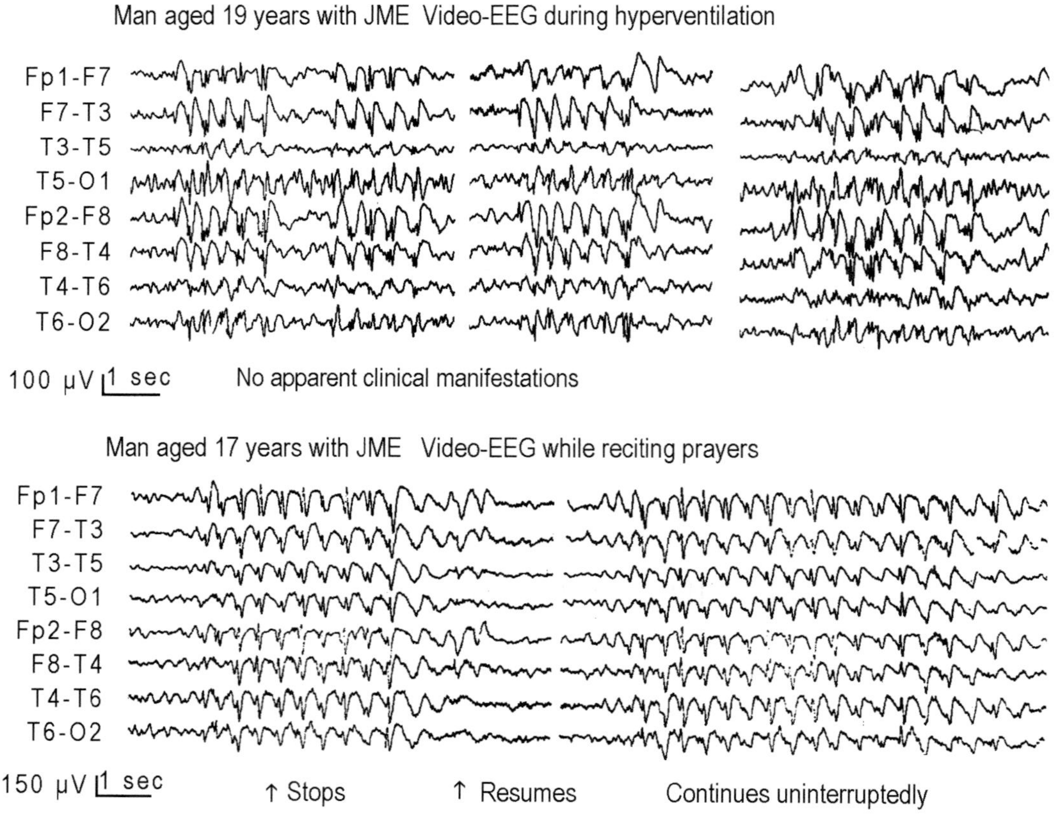

Figure 10.12 Video EEG of two patients with JME.

Top: GSWD are not associated with apparent clinical manifestations (but these may have been revealed if breath counting was performed during hyperventilation).

Bottom: GSWD are associated with mild impairment of cognition.

Modified from Panayiotopoulos et al[60] with the permission of the Editor of *Epilepsia*

SEIZURE-PRECIPITATING FACTORS

Sleep deprivation and fatigue, particularly after excessive alcohol intake, are the most powerful precipitants of jerks and GTCS in JME.

Sleep deprivation means a late night followed by a brief sleep suddenly interrupted by either compulsory early awakening in order to go to work or on a trip. An unscheduled telephone call early next morning may frequently have disastrous effects.

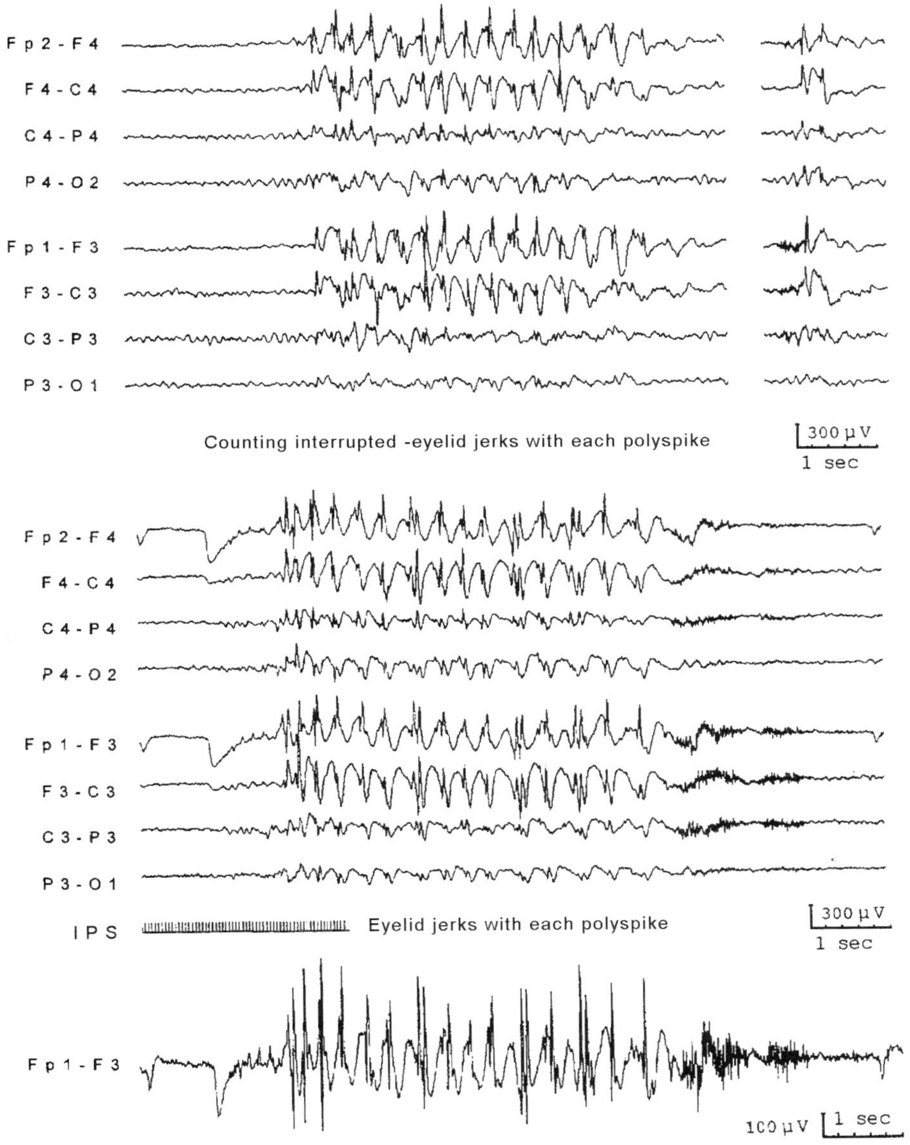

Figure 10.13 Sample from a video EEG of a woman aged 28 years who had suffered from JME since the age of 9 years.

This woman was referred for a routine EEG because she had experienced "probable IGE-absences from age 9 until age 18 years. Myoclonus as a teenager when sleep deprived. Recently suffered her first ever GTCS following sleep deprivation. No absence or myoclonus for 10 years. Treatment with valproate was withdrawn at age 18 years despite continuing myoclonic jerks and absences."
The video EEG documented that she still had brief absences, which manifest with mild impairment of cognition and eyelid jerks. These were spontaneous, or induced by hyperventilation (top) and intermittent photic stimulation (bottom).
Note the multiple spike–wave of the discharges and the irregular intradischarge frequency (magnification on the bottom). Also note the bifrontal spike-slow wave discharges (upper right).

Photosensitivity is confirmed by the EEG in one-third of patients, but probably less than one-tenth of patients with JME have clinical seizures induced by photic stimulation in daily life (Figure 10.13).

Other common and prominent precipitants of seizures are mental stress, emotion and, in particular, excitement, concentration, mental and psychological arousal, failed expectations and frustration.[60,211,212] Video games may precipitate seizures because of the photic/pattern effect, mental and psychological excitement, or both.[60]

Reading,[213] writing[214] and proprioceptive stimuli[56] are exceptional precipitants of seizures in patients with typical features of JME.

Women often have their seizures premenstrually, particularly if other precipitating factors are also present.[60]

Hyperventilation is an effective precipitant of EEG generalised discharges, which may often be the only abnormality in a routine EEG.[60]

Frequently, patients with JME have seizures when these precipitating factors cluster together, such as during exams, trips or vacations.

AETIOLOGY

JME is genetically determined.[61,199,215,216] Between 50% and 60% of families of probands with JME report seizures in first- or second-degree relatives.[216,217] Inheritance is probably complex.[9,203,218,219] Families with autosomal recessive[215] or dominant[215,218] Mendelian inheritance have been described.

Susceptibility loci for JME have been found in chromosome 6p11-12 (EJM1)[9] and 15q14 (EJM2).[220,221] Genes *C6orf33*[222] or *BRD2* (*RING3*)[223] in the EJM1 region have been recently identified.

An association reported between JME and an HLA-DR allele[224,225] has not been replicated.[226]

Genetic heterogeneity of JME is a possible explanation for such discordant observations.

Families with phenotypic overlap between JME and idiopathic photosensitive occipital epilepsy have been described.[227]

Magnetic resonance spectroscopy studies found reductions of N-acetyl aspartate (NAA) in the prefrontal and frontal brain regions of JME patients, but not in other forms of IGE.[42] JME patients with reduced frontal NAA concentrations showed poor performance on neuropsychological tests of executive functions, but not JME patients with normal frontal NAA levels. Frontal glutamate plus glutamine concentrations were elevated, which suggests possible increased neuronal excitability.[42]

DIAGNOSTIC PROCEDURES

All tests other than the EEG are normal. Using new MRI technologies, abnormalities of cerebral structure in some patients with JME involving mesiofrontal cortical structures have been reported.[42,228]

ELECTROENCEPHALOGRAPHY[25,32,60,198,229]

Interictal EEG

A normal EEG in a patient suspected of having JME should prompt an EEG on sleep and awakening.

The EEG in untreated patients is usually abnormal, with generalised discharges of an irregular mixture of 3–6 Hz spike/polyspikes-slow waves, with intradischarge fragmentations and unstable intradischarge frequency (Figures 2..1, 10.12 and 10.13). One-third of patients have photoparoxysmal responses.

Focal abnormalities are recorded in approximately one-third of patients.[32] These consist of focal single spikes, spike–wave complexes or focal slow waves.

Ictal EEG

The typical EEG discharge of a myoclonic jerk is a generalised burst of multiple spikes of 0.5–2 s duration (Figures 10.3, and 10.11).

The ictal discharges of absences in JME are distinctly different from those in CAE and JAE.[24,25] They consist of single, double, treble or multiple spikes usually preceding or superimposed on a slow wave. Multiple spikes consist of up to 8–10 spikes with a characteristic *'worm-like'* or *"compressed capital W"* appearance (*'Ws'*). The number and amplitude of the spikes shows considerable inter- and intradischarge variation. The intradischarge frequency of the GSWD varies from 2–10 Hz and is mainly 3–5 Hz. The frequency is often higher in the first second of onset. Fragmentations of the discharge are common and characteristic. Ws and fragmentation of discharges are observed in all patients, but vary quantitatively between patients and between discharges (Figures 2..1, 10.12, and 10.13).

Brief GSWD are far more common than long ones and most of them last for 1–4 s.

Photoparoxysmal discharges are evoked in 27% of patients (Figure 10.12).

DIFFERENTIAL DIAGNOSIS

JME is a typical example of a frequently misdiagnosed common epileptic syndrome resulting in avoidable morbidity.[205,230] Failure to diagnose JME is a

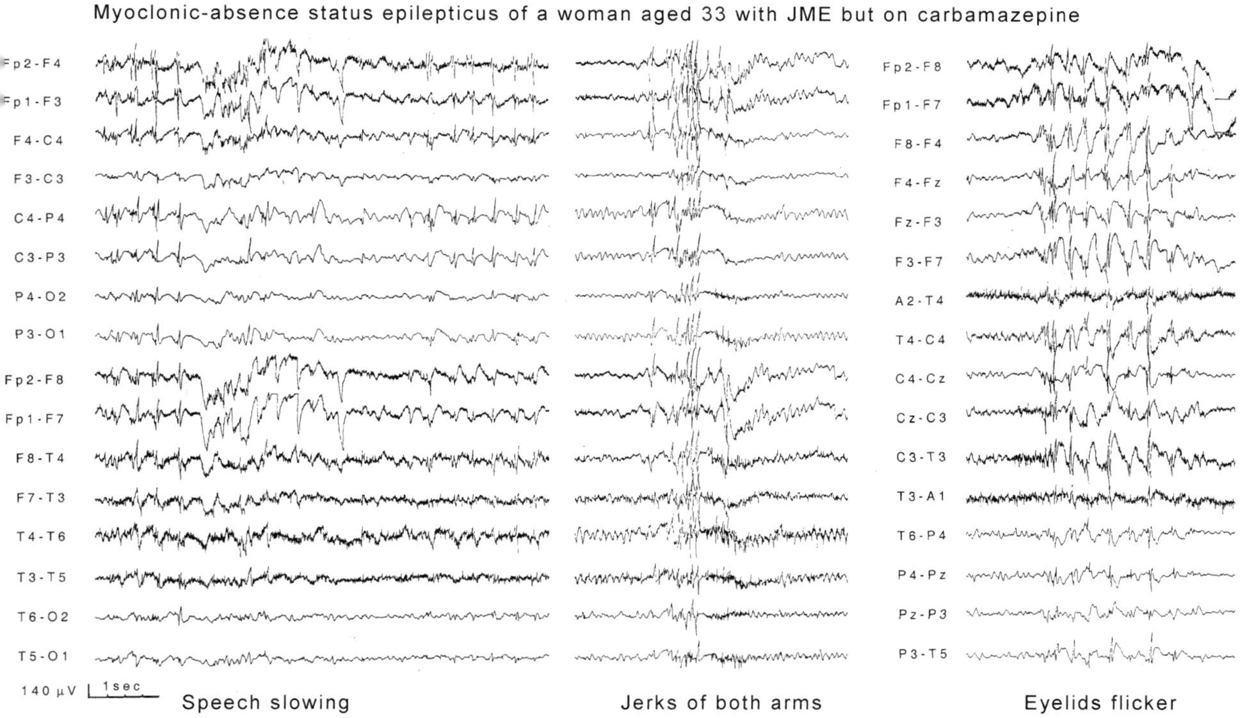

Figure 10.14 Myoclonic-absence status epilepticus in JME.

Video EEG of a woman with classical JME, but on carbamazepine at the time of this recording (see also Figure 10.3 from the same patient). The patient was mildly confused with continuous jerking of the hands (middle) and rarely the eyelids. The ictal EEG consisted of repetitive and discontinuous frequent GSWD interrupted by brief intervals of relative normality. Each GSWD consisted of varying numbers of polyspikes/spikes-wave in various combinations and morphologies.

serious medical error, because JME defies all aspects of general advice regarding 'epilepsy'. Diagnosis should improve with heightened medical awareness. Physicians should be ever alert to the possibility of JME, which is common.

High rate of misdiagnosis

The rate of misdiagnosis of JME is as high as 90%.[205,230] Factors responsible include lack of familiarity with JME, failure to elicit a history of myoclonic jerks, misinterpretation of absences as complex focal seizures, misinterpretation of jerks as focal motor seizures, and a high prevalence of focal EEG abnormalities.

JME is easy to diagnose because of the characteristic clustering of myoclonic and other generalised seizures of IGEs, the circadian distribution, precipitating factors and EEG manifestations. Patients are otherwise normal and there is no mental or physical deterioration if properly diagnosed and treated early.

Of the other IGEs, JAE is more difficult to differentiate, because this syndrome may also manifest with similar clinical and EEG manifestations (Table 10.7). The main differentiating factor is that absences with severe impairment of consciousness, not the myoclonic jerks, are the main seizure type in JAE. Myoclonic jerks, if they occur, are mild and random often lacking the circadian distribution of JME.

Another formidable situation is when JME starts with absences in childhood prior to the development of myoclonic jerks. There are no prospective video EEG studies of these patients. Examining the EEG and clinical manifestations of these patients retrospectively, I am of the opinion that their absences are distinct from CAE or JAE in that they are usually shorter, milder and the ictal EEG often contains multiple spike–slow waves. Certainly, this situation is not CAE progressing to JME as some authors have reported:[140] it is JME starting with absences prior to the development of myoclonic jerks.

Diagnostic tips for juvenile myoclonic epilepsy

GTCS, usually preceded by myoclonic jerks, are nearly pathognomonic of JME if they occur in the morning after:

a. a party to celebrate a birthday, end of school term or New Year's eve
b. waking up early in the morning to travel on a vacation, particularly after a late night
c. replacement of valproate with carbamazepine in women wishing to start a family
d. withdrawal of appropriate medication after many seizure-free years.

Table 10.7 Main differences between JME and JAE

	JME	JAE
Main type of seizures	Myoclonic jerks	Typical absences
Circadian distribution	Mainly on awakening	Any time during the day
Typical absences	Mild and often imperceptible; they occur in one-third of patients	Defining seizure type; they are very severe and occur in all patients
Myoclonic jerks	Defining seizure type; they occur in all patients and mainly on awakening	Mild; they occur in one-third of patients and are random
GTCS	They mainly occur after a series of myoclonic jerks on awakening	They mainly occur independently or less commonly after a series of absence seizures
EEG	Brief (1–3 s) 3-6 Hz GSWD which are usually asymptomatic	Lengthy (8–30 s) 3-4 Hz GSWD, which are usually associated with severe impairment of consciousness.

PROGNOSIS

All seizures are probably lifelong, though improve after the fourth decade of life. JME may vary in severity from mild myoclonic jerks to frequent and severe falls and GTCS if not appropriately diagnosed and treated.

Seizures are generally well controlled with appropriate medication in up to 90% of patients.[60,198,199,231] Patients with all three types of seizures are more likely to be resistant to treatment.[232]

Accepted practice for the management of 'epilepsy' is often inappropriate in JME

a. "Treatment of epilepsy should not start after a first GTCS."
Withholding treatment in JME is an erroneous medical decision. A JME patient may have his/her first GTCS long after many myoclonic jerks on awakening, absences or both.

b. "Treatment for epilepsy may be withdrawn after 2–3 years freedom of seizures."
Withdrawing treatment in JME is often an erroneous medical decision. More than 80% of patients will relapse.

MANAGEMENT

LIFESTYLE AND AVOIDANCE OF SEIZURE PRECIPITANTS

Advice regarding circadian distribution, lifestyle and seizure precipitants may be as important as drug treatment. Avoidance of precipitating factors and adherence to long-term medication is essential to avoid seizures.

Some patients experience GTCS or myoclonic jerks only after encountering precipitating factors. Patients may have myoclonic jerks despite treatment only after excessively violating these factors and others may have seizures exclusively after awakening that may not affect their daily duties.

Advice on the risk of sleep deprivation and alcohol is mandatory; avoidance of alcohol indulgence and compensating for sleep deprivation is essential.

A young person can not probably do without late night entertainment. It is natural and understandable. However, sleeping longer the next morning may well compensate for staying up late at night. A glass of wine is acceptable providing that this is not followed by another five or more. Patients with JME are often intelligent. They understand these simple rules. There are some restrictions, but they do not deprive patients from their rights in life. Sometimes, they experiment against these rules. They find what is right or wrong for them by trial and error.

ANTI-EPILEPTIC MEDICATION

The current state of knowledge of the drug treatment of JME is mainly based on clinical experience of prospective and retrospective studies with little evidence from randomised control trials (RCTs). There are no head-to-head comparisons between old and new AEDs.[233] Thus, the assessment of new AED monotherapy or polytherapy in JME and, indeed all IGEs, is notoriously problematic. My evaluation of the AED treatment of JME is based on a thorough review of the literature including abstracts, exchanging views with eminent colleagues in the field and my own clinical research over the last 25 years. The following are the most pragmatic recommendations that I could reach. Briefly these are as follows:

Monotherapy: Valproate is unquestionably the most effective AED in JME but is humbled by serious adverse reactions in women. Other options include levetiracetam and lamotrigine. When cost is of concern, phenobarbitone is effective in around 60% of patients. In mild JME with *myoclonic jerks only*, clonazepam alone may be recommended.

Polytherapy: Valproate with small doses of clonazepam or small doses of lamotrigine is the most effective combination. When valproate is undesirable, combining levetiracetam with lamotrigine or lamotrigine with clonazepam (to counteract the pro-myoclonic effect of lamotrigine) may be the best option. Persisting absences are practically never a problem so ethosuximide may not have a place in the polytherapy of JME. Combination regimens with levetiracetam have the advantage that other comedications may be gradually withdrawn without seizure deterioration.[234-236]

Contraindicated or ineffective AEDs should be excluded and these are: carbamazepine, gabapentin, oxcarbazepine, phenytoin, tiagabine and vigabatrin.

Old anti-epileptic drugs in JME

The indications and contraindications of old AEDs in JME have been established through numerous prospective and retrospective studies, and clinical experience over many years of use.

Valproate has been recognised as the most effective drug with full control of seizures in about 80% of patients with JME.[4,237] Valproate monotherapy controls absence seizures in around 75%, GTCS in 70% and myoclonic jerks in 75%.[4] The valproate dosage depends on the severity of JME. In a RCT, no difference in control of various types of JME could be demonstrated between 1000 mg and 2000 mg of valproate. [238]

The usual dose is 500 mg twice daily. Resistant cases require higher doses of up to 1500 mg twice daily. Mild cases may be well controlled with smaller doses of 300 mg twice daily. The best way to find the most appropriate dose in individual patients is to start with a low dose and increase in small increments until all seizures stop. Similarly, any attempt at withdrawal should be tested with small decrements of approximately 200 mg daily every 3 months. Relapses may be heralded by myoclonic jerks indicating the need to reinstate drug treatment.

The major problem is that valproate is undesirable in women because of its teratogenic effects[239-244] and its tendency to cause weight gain and polycystic ovary syndrome.[245] Women exposed to valproate during pregnancy have a relatively small, but statistically significant increased risk of having a child with a major malformation (spina bifida, cardiac and kidney abnormalities, extra fingers and clubfoot) compared with mothers not exposed to AEDs. This risk with valproate was found to be 5% against a background risk of 1.62%[243] or 5.9% versus 2.4%.[244]

Currently, media, internet and various other campaigns make it nearly impossible to prescribe valproate to women. There are increasing numbers of litigations against physicians and health authorities by parents of children with foetal valproate syndrome (even if the risks were appropriately explained to them) on a scale characterised as 'bigger than thalidomide'.

Phenobarbitone is extensively used as a very effective form of monotherapy in JME by European neurologists.[61,201,216] It is effective in controlling GTCS and

Teratogenicity and AEDs [246,247]

The FDA categorization of drug risks to the foetus runs from "Category A" (safest) to "Category X" (known danger—do not use).

Valproate is a category D drug that is: there is positive evidence of human foetal risk, but the benefits from use in pregnant women may be acceptable despite the risk (e.g., if the drug is needed in a life-threatening situation or for a serious disease for which safer drugs cannot be used or are ineffective).

All newer AEDs are classified as Category C that is: either studies in animals have revealed adverse effects on the foetus (teratogenic or embryocidal or other) and there are no controlled studies in women, or studies in women and animals are not available. Drugs should be given only if the potential benefit justifies the potential risk to the foetus.

On preliminary basis from humans, gabapentin,[248] lamotrigine[249] and levetiracetam[250] may be relatively safe but certainly their use in women of child-bearing age should be extremely cautious and their use should be based on the risk-benefit ratio.

See also Chapter 14, on pregnancy registries as a new method for assessing the foetal risks from exposures in pregnancy.[251,252] Overall, the results are generally encouraging, in that of the total groups of all pregnancies, over 95% of offspring do *not* have a *major* congenital malformation.

myoclonic jerks, but may exacerbate absences. It is the AED of choice when cost is of concern. One dose of 100-200 mg of phenobarbitone prior to going to sleep is often sufficient. Some patients may be controlled with 60-90 mg nocte.

Clonazepam is predominantly used as adjunctive treatment. It is one of the most effective anti-myoclonic drugs, but clonazepam alone may not suppress and may even precipitate GTCS. [253] Furthermore, clonazepam may deprive patients of the warning of an impending GTCS provided by the myoclonic jerks.[60,253-255]

Clonazepam should be given in small add-on doses (0.5–2 mg at night) when myoclonic jerks persist and are troublesome despite adequate monotherapy with another broad-spectrum AED. Monotherapy with clonazepam may be considered for mild cases of JME with myoclonic jerks only.

Clobazam has not been evaluated in JME, but it may be effective in some cases.[233,256] Clobazam is a very useful AED in focal epilepsies as I described on pages 432. However, in IGEs, I found clobazam to be far inferior to clonazepam in controlling myoclonic jerks, and to valproate and ethosuximide in controlling absences.

Acetazolamide has been used for treating GTCS in cases resistant to conventional treatment, though its use may induce nephrolithiasis.[257]

New anti-epileptic drugs in JME

The adverse effects of valproate and its lack of efficacy in 20% of patients with JME have prompted the search for alternatives. Of the new AEDs, only lamotrigine,[4,193,258,259] levetiracetam,[234,260-265]topiramate[266,267] and possibly zonisamide[268] appear to be therapeutic agents in JME. Levetiracetam, because of its efficacy in all seizure types[234,260-265,269] and safer adverse reactions profile,[270,271] appears to be the most promising substitute for valproate (Table 10.8).

Levetiracetam

Levetiracetam fulfils all expectations as probably the best new AED in the treatment of JME and it is the likely candidate to replace valproate in the treatment of this disorder, because of its high and sustained efficacy, fast action, good safety profile and lack of clinically meaningful interactions with other drugs.

Table 10.8 Efficacy and safety of new AEDs in the JME triad of seizures and photosensitivity in comparison with valproate

	Myoclonic jerks	GTCS	Absences	Photosensitivity	Serious adverse reactions[194;271]	Titration	Drug-drug interactions
Patients (%)	100%	90%	30%	30%			
Valproate	Very effective	Very effective	Very effective	Very effective	Yes	Optional (1–2 weeks)	Mainly with lamotrigine
Levetiracetam	Very effective	Very effective	Effective	Very effective	No	Optional (1–2 weeks)	None
Lamotrigine	Exaggerates in 50%	Very effective	Very effective	Probably effective	Yes	Mandatory (6–8 weeks)	Many
Topiramate	Probably effective	Very effective	Weakly effective	Undetermined	Yes	Mandatory (6–8 weeks)	Many

The results of treatment with levetiracetam in JME are very impressive.[234-236,272,273] In three independent studies, 62%,[234] 67%[235] and 63%[236] of patients with intractable JME became seizure free with levetiracetam monotherapy or polytherapy.

In a USA study, levetiracetam monotherapy was assessed in 24 patients with JME and GTCS.[235]

> "Sixteen (66.7%) had been free of GTCS; 3 of them had a single convulsive seizure after either stopping levetiracetam for 24 hours or reducing the dose to 500 mg per day but subsequently have remained free of convulsive seizures. Myoclonic seizures were effectively controlled in 22 of 24 patients."[235]

In a UK case-note review of more than 30 patients with resistant JME, 62% became seizure free with levetiracetam.[234]

In a Dutch study of 16 intractable JME patients, levetiracetam had excellent effects achieving freedom from seizures in 10 (63%) and a greater than 50% seizure reduction in 2 patients (12%). No clinically meaningful change was seen in two patients (12%); one patient experienced an increase in myoclonic jerks (6%).[236]

A controlled study compared 12-week baseline and levetiracetam treatment periods in 55 patients with idiopathic generalised seizures (myoclonic, GTCS and absence seizures), in whom other anticonvulsants had failed. Three-quarters (76%) of patients had a greater than 50% seizure reduction with levetiracetam therapy and 40% became seizure free; 15% discontinued levetiracetam because of adverse events, mostly sedation.[264]

The high efficacy of levetiracetam in JME is consistent with its effectiveness against all types of epileptic seizure, epileptic and non-epileptic myoclonus and photosensitivity.

Levetiracetam has a potent antimyoclonic effect,[254,255,274,275] even in severe myoclonic epilepsies, such as post-anoxic myoclonus and Unverricht-Lundborg disease,[276] as well as non-epileptic myoclonus.[262,277-279] This may be explained by its structural similarity to piracetam.

The prevalence of photosensitivity in IGE is high,[280,281] with 30% of patients having EEG photoparoxysmal responses.[60] Levetiracetam is the only new AED with well-established efficacy in EEG and clinical photosensitivity.[263,282,283] Levetiracetam reduces or eliminates both the photoparoxysmal responses and the myoclonic jerks elicited by IPS.[282]

> "Long-term use of levetiracetam in some visually sensitive patients has shown a remarkably good suppressive effect for > 4 years; discontinuation of the drug before becoming pregnant resulted in a return of myoclonic jerks and an increase of IPS sensitivity."[283]

Levetiracetam monotherapy was also studied in 18 patients aged 6–22 years with well-documented IGEs.[261] The majority of patients (14) had the typical JME seizure triad (absences, myoclonic jerks and GTCS) and most were photosensitive. Eight patients (44.5%), five of whom were photosensitive, became clinically seizure free and the EEG normalised in seven patients. All but one of the other six patients improved with levetiracetam alone or in combination with valproate. One patient with absences and myoclonic jerks worsened with levetiracetam, but responded well to valproate.[261]

In a case series of highly refractory IGE (absence seizures, myoclonic jerks and GTCS), three patients in whom treatment with at least three AEDs had failed became seizure free when treated with levetiracetam monotherapy.[260]

Further evidence for the efficacy of levetiracetam in IGEs is that it reduces the density and duration of GSWD, which is documented with continuous EEG monitoring.[265]

In view of some conflicting evidence in regard to behavioural adverse reactions particularly in children treated with levetiracetam [284-287]it is advisable to apply the rule 'start slow and go slow'. Thus, the starting dose of levetiracetam should be lower (250 mg) and titration should be slower (250 mg daily per week) than recommended by the manufacturers. Control of seizures is usually achieved at a maintenance dose of 1000–1500 mg in two divided doses daily. Higher doses may be unnecessary.

Lamotrigine

Lamotrigine is a very useful AED in IGEs, because of its efficacy in controlling GTCS and absence seizures. However, lamotrigine is often a pro-myoclonic AED that exaggerates myoclonic jerks in around 50% of patients. Cases with severe deterioration of JME are well reported.[288,289] In view of the fact that JME is predominantly a myoclonic epileptic syndrome, it is unlikely that lamotrigine will be the successor to valproate, because of its weaker efficacy and the deterioration of myoclonic syndromes (Table 10.8). Lamotrigine monotherapy in JME is debatable and probably not recommended.[4,290-292] Lamotrigine was the first of the new AEDs that appeared to be effective in JME.[4,258,259] However, in most reports, the efficacy of lamotrigine in JME was evaluated not as monotherapy, but in polytherapy with valproate.[4,258,259] Withdrawal of valproate often resulted in relapses.

Lamotrigine added to valproate is very effective in resistant cases,[4,258] because of beneficial pharmacokinetic interactions.[4,293] I should emphasise that *small doses* of lamotrigine (25–50 mg) added to adequate dosage of valproate are sufficient. This is clinically important for two reasons. Firstly, the combination of these drugs has an additive effect on adverse reactions associated with one or both of them.[294] Secondly, on anecdotal evidence the beneficial pharmacodynamic interaction with valproate may be lost with increasing dosage of lamotrigine.[295]

With regard to photosensitivity, lamotrigine also appears to be effective;[193] suppression of EEG photoparoxysmal discharges with lamotrigine has been reported in five patients, of whom four were also taking valproate.[296]

Small doses of lamotrigine added to valproate are very effective in resistant cases,[4,258] because of pharmacokinetic interactions.[4,293] Withdrawal of valproate often results in relapses even when lamotrigine dosage is increased. Regarding photosensitivity, lamotrigine was reported to have a beneficial effect in a small number of patients who were also on valproate.[296]

In a recent report of 962 patients with various IGE syndromes (including JME), a 1-year period of remission was achieved mainly with valproate monotherapy (52.1%) with lower rates for lamotrigine (16.7%) and topiramate (34.6%).[297] The combination of valproate and lamotrigine achieved a remission rate of 15.3%.[297] In another report of JME patients who had also received phenytoin and carbamazepine often as initial treatment, poor outcome was more likely with lamotrigine than valproate; worsening of seizures occurred in 6% of patients with lamotrigine.[291,292]

Topiramate

Topiramate[266,267,291,298]is another broad-spectrum AED that is effective in primarily GTCS,[299-302] but with a weak anti-absence[303] and anti-myoclonic action. Irrespective of efficacy, the major problem with topiramate is the high incidence of adverse reactions, some of which are very serious and include significant cognitive disturbances.[304,305] Also, topiramate imposes severe drug–drug interactions, including with hormonal contraception.[306]

In IGE, including JME, topiramate appears to be much less effective than valproate, but more effective than lamotrigine;[297] a 1-year period of remission was achieved in 34.6% of patients treated with topiramate compared with 52.1% with valproate.[297] In one study, a poor outcome was less likely with valproate than topiramate, which worsened seizures in 5% of patients. Furthermore, tolerability of topiramate was low and worse than valproate.[291]

Topiramate polytherapy may be a remote option for the few patients in whom treatment with valproate, levetiracetam and lamotrigine treatment alone or in combination fails.[291] Topiramate, which is less effective and has a worse safety profile than valproate, is unlikely to be useful as monotherapy in JME.

Zonisamide [307-309] is also a broad-spectrum AED, but its role in JME is largely unknown and probably weak.[310]

AEDs contraindicated in JME

Carbamazepine is contraindicated in JME as 68% of patients suffer an increase in seizures,[195,196,200,311,312] though it may improve control of GTCS in a few patients.[313]

Oxcarbazepine like carbamazepine is also contraindicated in JME.[314]

Phenytoin is often ineffective and may worsen seizures of JME. [312] In the original studies of Janz, it was significantly inferior to phenobarbitone.[201]

Gabapentin, tiagabine and vigabatrin are detailed on pages 337.

PREVENTION OF GTCS AND TERMINATION OF MYOCLONIC-ABSENCE STATUS EPILEPTICUS

It is important to remember that patients with JME often experience myoclonic jerks or myoclonic-absence status epilepticus long before terminating to a GTCS, which can be prevented by home administration of an appropriate benzodiazepine preparation. Rectal absorption of liquid diazepam is very rapid, reaches the brain within minutes and has a near-intravenous efficacy. Rectal tubes containing liquid diazepam are the most widely used formulation (Stesolid). Diazepam rectal gel is now available (Diastad). Buccal or nasal application of midazolam is another alternative.

DURATION OF AED TREATMENT AND WITHDRAWAL OF MEDICATION IN JME

Lifelong AED treatment is usually considered necessary in patients with JME. Withdrawal of medication results in relapses, even in patients who have been seizure free for many years with an appropriate AED.[60] In mild forms of JME, it may be safe to reduce the dose of medication slowly over months or years, especially after the fourth decade of life. Persistence or recrudescence of myoclonic jerks necessitates continuation of medication.

IDIOPATHIC GENERALISED EPILEPSY WITH GENERALISED TONIC CLONIC SEIZURES ONLY

'Idiopathic generalised epilepsy with GTCS only' is a newly proposed IGE syndrome of undetermined definition and boundaries.[5] All patients suffer from primarily GTCS occurring at any time in wakefulness, sleep or awakening. Thus, this syndrome is to include 'epilepsy with GTCS on awakening' (EGTCSA) which has been extensively studied by Janz. [315-317]

DEMOGRAPHIC DATA

Age at onset varies from 6 to 47 years with a peak at 16–17 years; 80% of patients have their first GTCS in the second decade of life. Men (55%) predominate slightly, probably because of differences in alcohol exposure and sleep habits to women.

The prevalence of 'IGE with GTCS only' is unknown. In my experience, it is very rare if strict criteria are applied (*GTCS only*). Of 1000 patients with one or more afebrile seizures, 356 patients (35.6%) had various syndromes of IGEs, but only 9 patients (0.9%) had GTCS *only*, though this was often the reason for referral. The low yield of 'IGE with GTCS only' in this sample reflects both the fact that we methodically question patients and witnesses regarding the occurrence of minor seizures and that we make long video EEG recordings, including video EEG during sleep and on awakening. As a result of this approach, for example, we found that 14 patients mainly referred for late onset GTCS had 'IGE with phantom absences'.[58,319]

In the experience of other authors, the prevalence of 'IGE with GTCS only' varies from 10–15%[314,320-322] to as high as 62%[14] among IGEs. Of 253 patients with IGEs, 30 (12%) had EGTCSA and 39 (15%) had "a mild form of IGE characterised by infrequent GTCS and generalised interictal EEG discharges of spike wave".[320] Of 1033 patients with IGEs, 138 (13%) had GTCS only with onset between 3 and 18 years of age.[321] Of 101 patients with IGE beginning in adolescence, 10 had *GTCS only*, but neither on awakening nor in the evening period of relaxation.[322]

The reported prevalence of epilepsy with GTCS on awakening also varies from 0%[207] to as high as 17%[315] in patients with epileptic seizures.

CLINICAL MANIFESTATIONS

GTCS are the defining clinical manifestations. [63,316,317,319]

[I]LAE definition and considerations on [c]lassification

[T]he 1989 ILAE Commission[1] recognised a syndrome of [']epilepsy with GTCS on awakening' among IGEs and defined [it] as follows:

[“]Epilepsy with GTCS on awakening is a syndrome with onset [o]ccurring mostly in the second decade of life. The GTCS [o]ccur exclusively or predominantly (> 90% of the time) [s]hortly after awakening regardless of the time of day or in a [s]econd seizure peak in the evening period of relaxation. If [o]ther seizures occur, they are mostly absence or myoclonic, as [i]n JME. Seizures may be precipitated by sleep deprivation and [o]ther external factors. Genetic predisposition is relatively [f]requent. The EEG shows one of the patterns of idiopathic [g]eneralised epilepsy. There is a significant correlation with [p]hotosensitivity."[1]

[T]he new ILAE diagnostic scheme [5,86] broadens this to a [s]yndrome of 'IGE -GTCS only' in which 'epilepsy with GTCS [o]n awakening (EGTCSA)' is incorporated though there is some evidence that this is genetically different.[318]

'IGE with GTCS only' has not been defined by the ILAE Task Force.[5] Its name implies that it includes only those patients with GTCS alone (i.e. without absences and/or jerks) and that these may occur at any time. However, it is more likely that it is a broader category (rather than a syndrome) of 'IGE with predominantly GTCS' (which also includes patients with mild absences, myoclonic jerks or both). If this is so, it is undetermined what proportion of patients also has other generalised seizures (jerks or absences) and there may be significant overlap with other syndromes of IGEs.

GTCS commonly feature in IGEs and occur predominantly on awakening.[319] GTCS are the most severe form of epileptic seizures, while absences and myoclonic jerks may be mild and sometimes inconspicuous to the patient and imperceptible to the observer.[58] They are often detected only by taking a meticulous history or video EEG. A patient with a first GTCS has often suffered from minor seizures (absences, myoclonic jerks or both), sometimes for many years prior to a GTCS.

In EGTCSA, GTCS occur within 1–2 hours of awakening from either nocturnal or diurnal sleep. The seizure may occur while the patient is still in bed, having his breakfast or on arriving at work. Seizures may also occur during relaxation or leisure.

However, GTCS in the syndrome of 'IGE with GTCS only' may also occur at any other time during sleep, wakefulness or awakening. Overall, GTCS are reported to occur on awakening in 17–53% of patients, diffusely while awake in 23–36%, during sleep in 27–44% or randomly in 13–26%.[63]

With age, GTCS tend to increase in frequency and become more unpredictable. Janz described patients with EGTCSA as unreliable, unstable and prone to neglect.[315,316] Their sleep patterns are particularly unstable and modifiable by external factors (i.e. AEDs), and patients may suffer from chronic sleep deficit.[63,316,317]

PRECIPITATING FACTORS

Sleep deprivation, fatigue and excessive alcohol consumption are the main precipitants of seizures. Shift work, changes in sleep habits, particularly during holidays and celebrations, predispose to GTCS on awakening. A few patients may be clinically photosensitive.

AETIOLOGY

There is a high incidence of epileptic disorders in other family members.[63,316] Recently, a link to the EJM-1 locus has been reported in EGTCSA while no such link was found in adolescent-onset idiopathic epilepsy with GTCS at any time while awake.[318] Microdysgenesis has been reported in pathological specimens of EGTCSA.[323]

DIAGNOSTIC PROCEDURES

By definition, all tests apart from the EEG are normal.

ELECTROENCEPHALOGRAPHY

The EEG shows generalised discharges of 3-4 Hz spike/multiple spike–wave complexes (GSWD) in 50% of patients with pure EGTCSA (Figure 10.15) and 70% of those with additional absences or myoclonic jerks.

A normal routine EEG should prompt a video EEG during sleep and on awakening. Myoclonic jerks or, more frequently, brief absences will often be revealed.

Focal EEG abnormalities occur in one-third of patients but these are exceptional in the absence of GSWD. Photoparoxysmal responses are reported in 17% of females and 9% of males with EGTCSA.[63]

DIFFERENTIAL DIAGNOSIS

The differential diagnosis is mainly from other IGEs that share with EGTCSA the same propensity to seizures after awakening and the same precipitating factors. JME, JAE and eyelid myoclonia with absences are examples of IGE syndromes that may cause diagnostic difficulties (see Chapter 14). Symptomatic and focal epileptic seizures with secondary generalisation may also occur, predominantly on awakening.

PROGNOSIS

As in all other types of IGEs with onset in the mid-teens, EGTCSA is probably a lifelong disease with a high incidence of relapse (83%) on withdrawal of treatment.[316] Characteristically, the intervals between seizures become shorter with time, the precipitating factors less obvious and GTCS may become more random (diurnal and nocturnal), either as a result of the evolution of the disease or drug-induced modifications.[63,316,317]

MANAGEMENT

Patients should be warned of the common seizure precipitants, namely sleep deprivation with early awakening and alcohol consumption, and when possible should avoid occupational night shifts. Patients, after adjusting their lifestyles, may become seizure free.

Treatment is with AEDs that control primarily GTCS, such as valproate, phenobarbitone, lamotrigine, levetiracetam and topiramate. In the pure forms of 'GTCS only', carbamazepine, oxcarbazepine and phenytoin may be used, but require exclusion of other types of seizures that may be exacerbated by these AEDS.

Primarily GTCS in AED RCT

Results of RCTs of AEDs in primarily GTCS present significant difficulties in interpretation:

a. secondarily GTCS may contaminate the selected populations for the active AED and the comparator agent (established AED or placebo)
b. patients with primarily GTCS and absences or myoclonic jerks are often included though these seizures respond differently to AEDs
c. inappropriate AEDs for IGEs, such as carbamazepine, have been used in one-quarter of IGE patients as a comparator agent.

The results of such studies are of uncertain value and should be interpreted with caution.

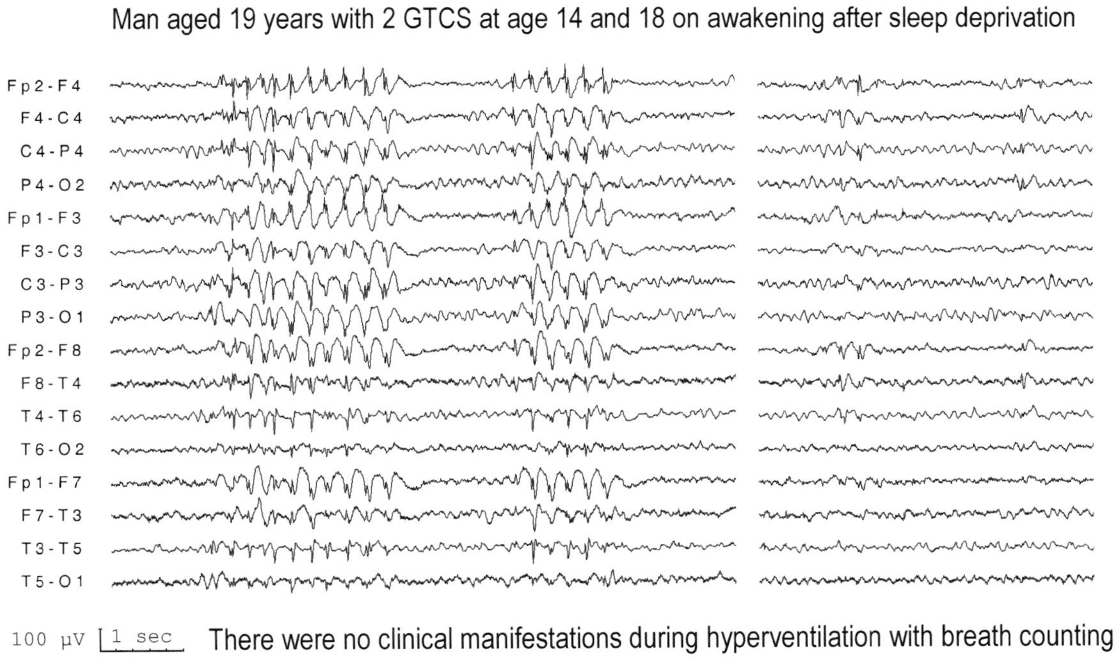

Figure 10.15

Asymptomatic GSWD on video EEG of a 19-year-old university student who had two GTCS at 14 and 18 years of age. They both occurred half an hour after awakening from a brief sleep during exam periods. There was no clinical history of any other type of seizures and there were no other symptoms preceding either of the GTCS.

Note that the discharges may start from right or left. Also note focal spikes at various locations.

IGE WITH ABSENCES OF EARLY CHILDHOOD

Typical absence seizures starting in early childhood (between a few months and 4 years of age)[187,324-327] are not a specific expression of a distinct syndrome. This may be the first manifestation of various syndromes of IGEs with absences or more severe forms of generalised epilepsies. By excluding all these conditions, it is realistic to accept that there is a syndrome of IGE that starts in early childhood primarily manifesting with absences, often combined with GTCS and possibly with myoclonic jerks.

Doose,[325,326] having studied 140 cases with onset of absences in early childhood, rightly concluded that:
"this is an heterogeneous subgroup within IGE. There is a distinct overlap with early childhood epilepsy with GTCS and myoclonic-astatic epilepsy on the one side and with childhood absence epilepsy on the other. Thus it should not be regarded as a special syndrome". [325,326]

I am in complete agreement with this statement. Age at onset of absence seizures alone can not define an epileptic syndrome. However, with improved diagnostic skills, applying inclusion (e.g. including absences and GTCS) and exclusion criteria (e.g. excluding CAE and symptomatic cases), it appears that there is a rare IGE, which needs a precise definition.

This is an IGE syndrome (occurring in otherwise normal children). [325,326]

- Onset of absences occurs between 1–5 years of age. Absences are markedly different from CAE. Clinically, they are less severe and less frequent. Ictal EEG 2.5–4 Hz GSWD is very irregular and termination is not abrupt, but often fades with spike–wave complexes.
- GTCS are common (affecting two-thirds of patients) and are often the first seizure type. Boys are more likely to suffer GTCS than girls.
- Myoclonic jerks and myoclonic-astatic seizures occur in 40% of patients.
- Absence status epilepticus may lead to cognitive impairment.
- Background EEG shows a moderate excess of slow waves.
- Long-term prognosis is worse than in CAE.
- There is a strong family history of IGE and GSWD in the EEG of unaffected members, particularly mothers.

PERIORAL MYOCLONIA WITH ABSENCES

Typical absences with ictal motor symptoms of perioral myoclonia is a type of seizure.[16,26,328-331] However, this is often combined with a clustering of other clinical and EEG features probably constituting an interesting IGE syndrome of perioral myoclonia with absences (PMA).[16,18,328,331]

DEMOGRAPHIC DATA

Age at onset covers a wide range from 2–13 years (median 10 years). Girls are far more frequently affected than boys.

The syndrome is uncommon in children (< 1% with typical absences) but, because it fails to remit, is relatively common in adults (9.3%) with typical absence seizures.[16,328,331]

CLINICAL MANIFESTATIONS

Typical absence seizures with perioral myoclonia are the defining symptom. The characteristic feature is perioral myoclonia, which consists of rhythmic contractions of the orbicularis oris muscle that cause protrusion of the lips, contractions of the depressor anguli oris resulting in twitching of the corners of the mouth or, rarely, more widespread involvement, including the muscles of mastication producing jaw jerking (Figure 10.16). Impairment of consciousness varies from severe to mild. Most patients are usually aware of the perioral myoclonia. Duration is usually brief, lasting a mean of 4 s (range 2–9 s). Absences with perioral myoclonia may be very frequent and occur many times a day or 1–2 times a week, or they are rare.

Generalised tonic clonic seizures occur in all patients. GTCS often start before or soon after the onset of clinically apparent absences. Exceptionally, GTCS may start many years after the onset of absences. GTCS are usually infrequent (ranging from once in a lifetime to 12/year) and are often heralded by clusters of absences or ASE.

Absence status epilepticus is very common in PMA (57%) and frequently ends with GTCS (Figure 10.16). It is more common than in any other syndrome of IGE with typical absences.[19] Perioral myoclonia may be more apparent than impairment of consciousness or vice versa.

AETIOLOGY

Half of patients with PMA have first degree relatives and mainly siblings with IGE and absences.[141]

DIAGNOSTIC PROCEDURES

All tests apart from the EEG are normal.

ELECTROENCEPHALOGRAPHY

Interictal EEG frequently shows: (a). abortive bursts or brief less than 1 s generalised discharges of 4–7 Hz spikes/multiple spikes-waves, which are usually asymmetrical and may give the impression of a localised focus; and (b). focal abnormalities, including single spikes, spike–wave complexes and theta waves with variable side emphasis.

Ictal EEG consists of 3–4 Hz GSWD with frequent irregularities in terms of the number of spikes in the spike–wave complex, the fluctuations in spike amplitude and the occurrence of fragmentations (Figure 10.16).

There is no photosensitivity.

DIFFERENTIAL DIAGNOSIS

Patients with PMA are frequently erroneously diagnosed as having focal motor seizures because: (a). the prominent motor features of the absences, which are often reported or sometimes recorded as unilateral; and (b). the presence of interictal focal EEG abnormalities.

However, this error is unlikely to happen if EEG is properly recorded and interpreted. Also, patients with focal motor seizures are unlikely to suffer ASE, which is common in PMA.

Considerations on classification

Absences with perioral myoclonia despite unequivocal documentation with video EEG[16,328,331] have not been recognised by the ILAE as a seizure type.[1,5] Perioral myoclonia may occur in typical and atypical absence seizures of idiopathic and symptomatic epilepsies. Therefore, absences with perioral myoclonia alone can not be taken as evidence of any syndrome. However, they often occur together with other symptoms that cluster in a non-fortuitous manner thus constituting the main manifestation of a syndrome within the broad spectrum of IGE, which we proposed to call perioral myoclonia with absences. [16,328] Other manifestations of this syndrome include GTCS, which often start early prior or together with the absences, frequent occurrence of ASE, resistance to treatment and persistence in adult life.[16,328,331]

The main differential diagnosis is from other syndromes of IGEs such as CAE, JAE and MAE depends on the age at onset. Video EEG invariably reveals perioral myoclonia that sometimes, and particularly in treated patients, may be subtle. Onset of GTCS before or at the same age as typical absences, the relatively brief duration of the absences with the concurrent perioral myoclonia and the frequent occurrence of ASE are useful clinical indicators in favour of PMA and against childhood, juvenile or other forms of IGE. PMA may be difficult to differentiate from MAE, particularly if the latter presents with mild myoclonic jerks localised

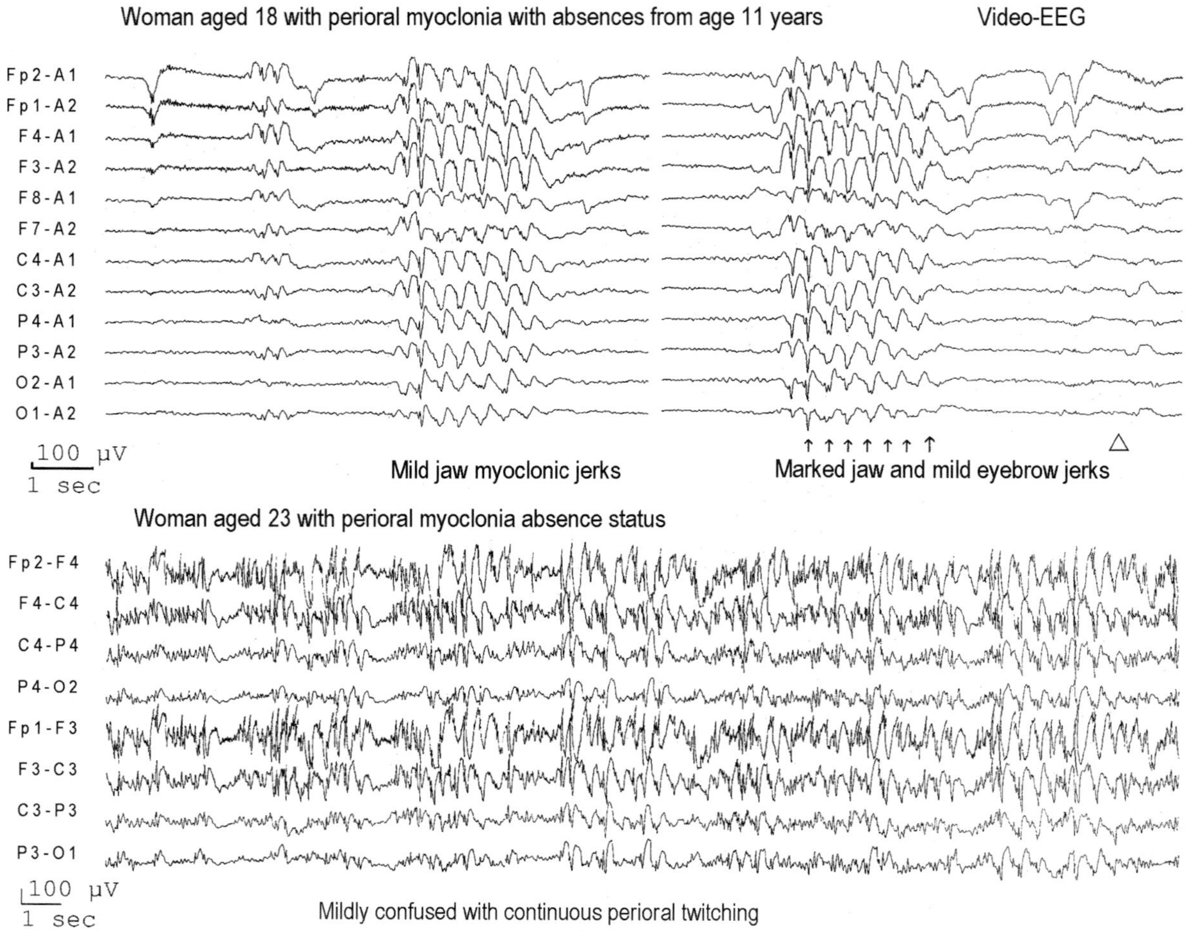

Figure 10.16 Diagnostic errors in PMA

Top: Video EEG recording of an 18-year-old woman with perioral myoclonia with absences (case 6 in ref [328]). She was referred because of 'focal motor seizures and secondarily GTCS'. She had onset of GTCS and absences at 11 years of age, which continued despite treatment with various combinations of valproate, ethosuximide, clonazepam, lamotrigine and acetazolamide. Absences were frequent, often in daily clusters and consisted of brief (about 5 s) moderate impairment of consciousness with violent rhythmic jerking of the jaw. GTCS occurred 1–10 times a year, usually after awakening, preceded by clusters of absences with the jaw myoclonus spreading to limb jerks prior to generalised convulsions. She was more concerned about the absences because they interfered with her daily life "everyone notices the jerks of my jaw" and less about the GTCS, which usually occurred at home. The initial misdiagnosis of 'focal motor seizures' was because the jaw jerking was perceived and described by her mother as unilateral.

Bottom: EEG of 23-year-old woman while in perioral status epilepticus (case 2 in ref [328]). She was mildly confused with continuous perioral twitching. This ended with a GTCS. Initial presentation at 11 years of age was with GTCS. PMA was noted at the same time and was diagnosed as focal motor seizures. Despite medication with valproate, she continues having infrequent episodes of ASE terminated with self-administered benzodiazepines.

in the face.[26] However, MAE is often symptomatic and is rarely associated with generalised non-convulsive status epilepticus.[177]

PROGNOSIS

Absences and GTCS may be resistant to medication, unremitting and possibly lifelong.[16,328,331]

MANAGEMENT

Treatment is with valproate alone or combined with ethosuximide, small doses of lamotrigine or clonazepam. Levetiracetam may be effective, because of the myoclonic elements of the absences.

ASE with perioral myoclonia, of which most patients are aware, should be terminated with immediate self-administered medication of oral midazolam or rectal diazepam.

IDIOPATHIC GENERALISED EPILEPSY WITH PHANTOM ABSENCES

The syndrome of IGE with phantom absences[58] is characterised by the triad of:

1. phantom absences that are inconspicuous or never appreciated prior to the onset of GTCS
2. GTCS, which are commonly the first overt clinical manifestations, usually start in adulthood and are infrequent
3. ASE, which occurs in 50% of patients.

DEMOGRAPHIC DATA

The first overt clinical manifestations of GTCS appear in adult life, though absences may have started much earlier. ASE as the first overt symptom in childhood is rare.[77] Men and women are equally affected. The prevalence was estimated to be 15% among IGE with typical absences, 10% of IGE and 3% of 410

Definition of phantom absences

'Phantom absences' denote typical absence seizures, which are so mild that they are inconspicuous to the patient and imperceptible to the observer.[16,58]

Why the name phantom absences? Is this synonymous with 'subclinical or larval absences'.

We use the term 'phantom absences' because of their clinically elusive and inconspicuous character.[58] Cognitive impairment during 'subclinical, larval' GSWD are well documented[332,333] and phantom absences may be a good example of them. However, it should be emphasised that patients with phantom absences have, by definition,[1,15] active, clinical absence seizures that manifest with mild impairment of cognition, as demonstrated by errors and discontinuation during breath counting on video EEG (Figure 10.17).[334] It should also be emphasised that phantom absences in these adults do not represent aborted past childhood or juvenile absences modified by age or medical treatment.[58]

Furthemore, phantom absences is not synonymous with the EEG pattern of abortive *"phantom 4-6 Hz spike and slow wave"*, which is a non-specific EEG abnormality of no clinical significance.[335-337]

Considerations on classification

Phantom absences, or mild absence seizures, have not been categorised as such by the ILAE.[1,5] The absences are simple, brief (usually 2–4 s) causing only inconspicuous impairment of cognition, which is not clinically disturbing to the patient. Though not classical, they fulfil the criteria of typical absences with more than 2.5 Hz GSWD.[58]

There is reasonable evidence to suggest that phantom absences are not only discrete seizures, but may also constitute the main symptom of a syndrome within the broad spectrum of IGE. There is non-fortuitous clustering of other symptoms, such as GTCS of usually late onset, frequent occurrence of ASE and persistence in adult life.[58] That these patients have IGE is beyond any doubt, as they all are of normal intelligence and physical state, high resolution MRI is normal, the EEG shows GSWD, and the seizures are generalised.

The syndrome of IGE with phantom absences has not been recognized by the ILAE.[1,5] Accordingly, these cases are probably orphaned or probably categorised among undefined IGE or other syndromes of IGE.

consecutive patients over 16 years of age with epileptic seizures.[58] Genton et al.[338] reported that, among 253 consecutive cases of IGE, 32 (15.4%) patients had rare GTCS with GSWD in the interictal EEG. It is possible that these patients suffered from IGE with GTCS only and/or IGE with phantom absences.

CLINICAL MANIFESTATIONS

Phantom absences are the defining and consistent symptom in these patients.[58] Phantom absences manifest with mild, but definite, impairment of cognition documented by video EEG (Figure 10.17). There are no other clinical symptoms except eyelid flickering that consistently occurs in some patients. However, patients are not usually aware, even retrospectively, that absences interfere with their daily life, even when driving or in demanding professions, such as computer programming, civil engineering, major business and administration.[58]

Patients may retrospectively admit to momentary lack of concentration and forgetfulness, which in their opinion was of no practical significance.[58] Rarely patients or witnesses also become aware of some minor motor manifestations during the absence:

occasional, very brief episodes of quick flickering of the eyeballs upwards accompanied by a brief lack of concentration

Phantom absences are common in patients with IGEs, but are often unrecognised. These absences are impossible to detect without breath counting and video EEG.

Generalised tonic clonic seizures occur in all adult patients that seek medical attention. They are usually the first overt clinical manifestation.[58] They are of late onset, infrequent and without consistent circadian distribution or specific precipitating factors.

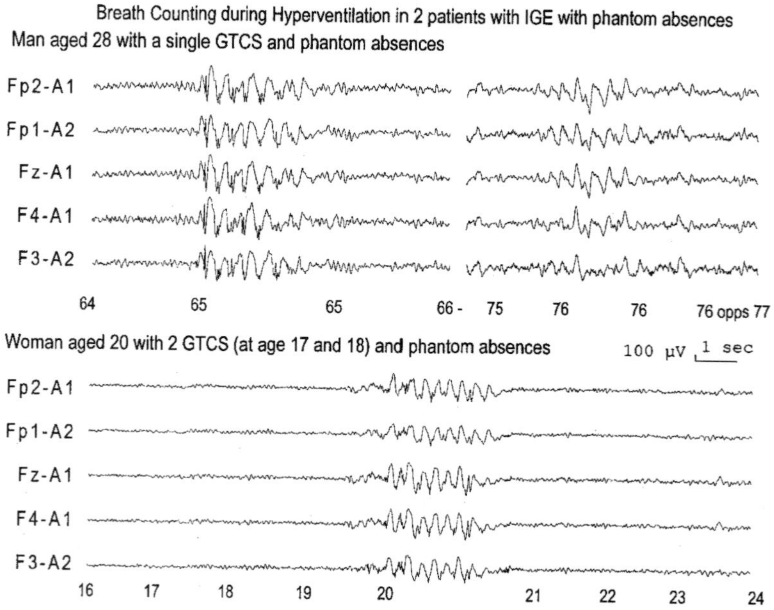

Figure 10.17 Video EEG of two patients suffering from IGE with phantom absences.

The numbers denote the actual breath counting during hyperventilation. Note that errors, when they occur, are only related to these brief GSWD. Errors consist of hesitation in pronouncing the next consecutive number, repetitions and erroneous counting sequence.

Absence status epilepticus occurs in 50% of patients. This often lasts for many hours alone or prior to GTCS (Figure 10.18).[58,76] It manifests with cognitive impairment, which is usually of mild or moderate severity.

At the age of 28, this patient was able to drive for 2–3 hours while in ASE. This was on Christmas Eve with no precipitating factors. For the whole day he was feeling unwell, "tired, unable to compute conversations, clouded mind, missing words, as if sleep waking, slow mind". Despite this, he had his haircut and then drove alone on a 1-hour trip through busy roads to relatives, offering the wrong Christmas gifts to the wrong persons. He then drove back home for another hour, picked up his wife and drove again towards a friend's house. His wife noticed that he appeared "slow and very quiet during the drive, but I though he was just tired. I was not alerted because he was driving very well, not making any errors". She did not notice any abnormal movements, including gestural automatisms or jerking. He became completely silent for 1–2 minutes prior to a GTCS, which occurred while parking; his wife managed to stop the car and avoid an accident. No further seizures occurred in the next 5 years while on valproate 1000 mg daily.

Impaired cognition during ASE varies. Most patients often communicate poorly and slowly, feel strange and confused, make errors at work and look depressed, but do not become unresponsive (Figures 10.17, and 10.18). Experiential, mental and sensational symptoms are more common than is usually appreciated.[30] Frequently, they have a good recollection of the ictal events and may be able to write down their experiences while in ASE.[30,58]

Neuropsychological examination under video EEG monitoring during ASE in 2 patients revealed only mild attentional and executive disturbances.[339] GSWD were associated with selective impairment in the initiation of response and self-generated action, whereas short-term storage of external information was fully preserved.[339]

Patients with recurrent ASE are often aware of the impeding GTCS and try to find a safe place to have it.

AETIOLOGY

IGE with phantom absences is probably genetically determined.[58] It is difficult to explain the high frequency of ASE in these patients, with such brief and mild absences and infrequent GTCS. It is possible that, under the influence of precipitating factors that are not fully understood, phantom absences might cluster and evolve into ASE facilitated either by lack of or inappropriate treatment. Vuilleumier et al.[339] proposed that a predominant involvement of frontomesial thalamocortical circuitry may underlie an 'inconspicuous' disorder of consciousness, as seen in phantom absences with selective loss of initiation and goal-oriented behaviour, whereas involvement of more lateral frontal areas in typical absences may also disrupt working memory processes.[339]

DIAGNOSTIC PROCEDURES

All tests apart from the EEG are normal.

Interictal EEG: The background activity is normal, 50% of patients have EEG focal paroxysmal abnormalities consisting of short transients of localised slow, sharp waves or spikes, or both, occurring either independently or in association with brief GSWD. [58,340] EEG photosensitivity is exceptional.

Ictal EEG consists of 3-4 Hz GSWD with occasional fragmentations (Figure 10.17). They are typically brief lasting of no more than 5 s. Mild cognitive impairment manifested with hesitation, discontinuation and errors in breath counting is the only clinical ictal symptom during GSWD. A few may also have mild ictal eyelid fluttering.[58,340] Hyperventilation is a major provocative factor.

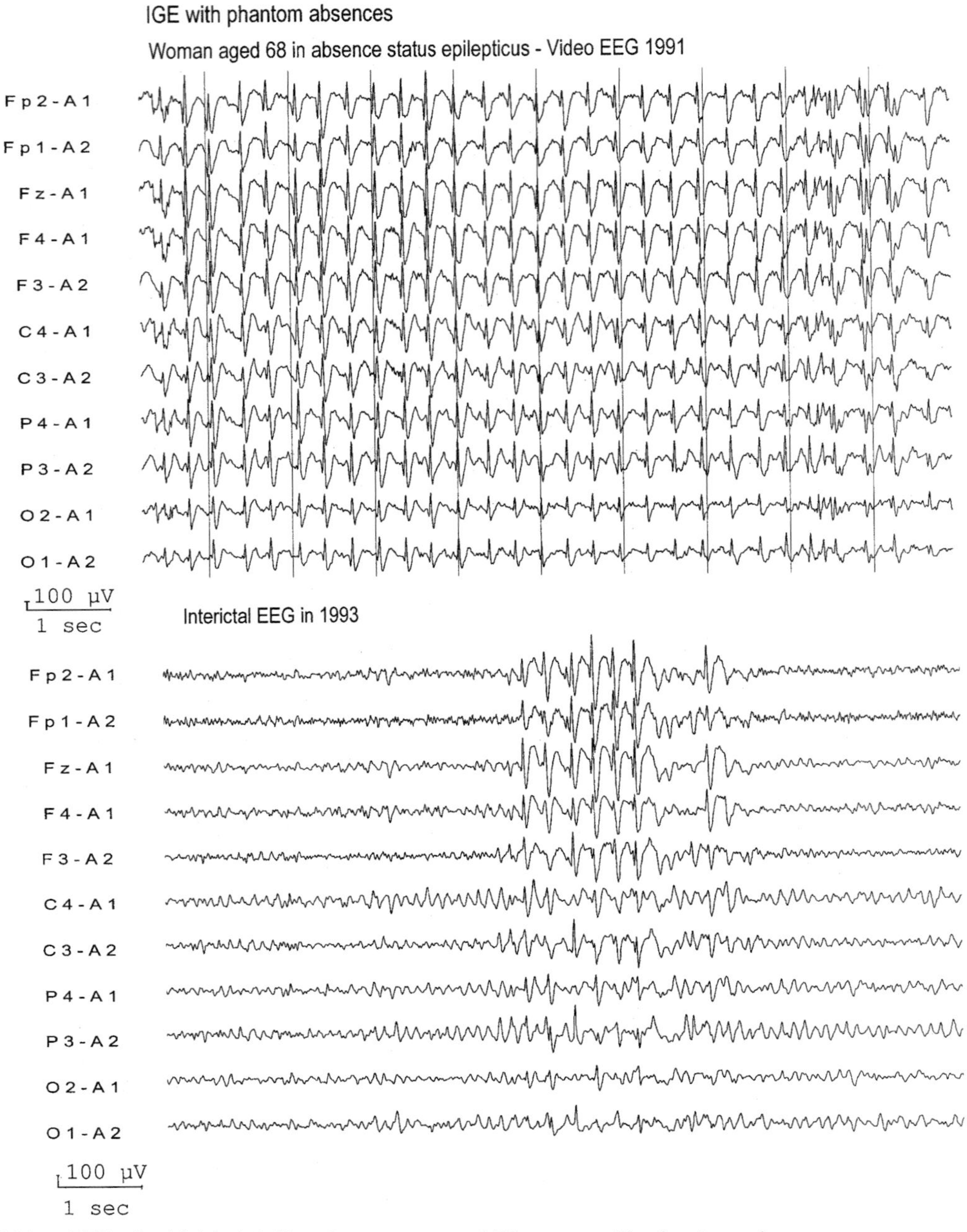

Figure 10.18 Video EEG of a highly intelligent woman, aged 79 years, with phantom absences.

ASE and GTCS (case 1 in ref [58]). She had her first overt seizure at the age of 30 years. She was moderately confused for 12 hours prior to a GTCS. Since then she had 1–3 similar episodes of ASE every year. She was misdiagnosed as temporal lobe epilepsy and was on primidone and sulthiame for nearly 40 years. Retrospectively, she admits brief episodes of mild impairment of cognition: "The absences lasted a couple of seconds; the other state (ASE) lasts much longer, for 24 hours or more. They may be linked I suppose." No further seizures of any type occurred in the next 11 years of follow-up on monotherapy with valproate 1000 mg daily
Upper: ASE with continuous spike and occasional polyspike-slow wave activity mainly at 3 Hz. Note also slower or faster components and some topographic variability of the discharge. The patient was fully alert, attentive and cooperative. Movements and speech were normal. There were no abnormal ictal symptoms other than severe global memory deficit and global diminution of content of consciousness. She was unable to remember her name, how many children she had, the date and her location. She could not perform simple calculations, but could repeat up to five numbers given to her. She could read text correctly and she correctly wrote her address, though she could not remember it on verbal questioning. She did not know where she was, but given the choice between various locations, she correctly recognised that she was in a hospital. This ASE was successfully interrupted with intravenous administration of diazepam.
Bottom: Interictal video-EEG showing brief 3 Hz GSWD lasting 2–3 s without apparent clinical manifestations.

During ASE, the EEG shows continuous, generalised, mainly 3 Hz spike/multiple spike slow wave activity (Figure 10.4 **??????????????????**).

DIFFERENTIAL DIAGNOSIS

The diagnostic and management errors involved in adult patients with IGE and typical absence seizures have been well reported.[56,58] The magnitude of the problem is worse in IGE with phantom absences, in which the absences are very mild, ASE is confused with non-epileptic events or temporal lobe epilepsy, and GTCS are of late onset. This is compounded by frequent EEG focal abnormalities and the current practice of most EEG departments to not test cognition appropriately during brief GSWD.

The main problems to consider in IGE with phantom absences are:

- the first overt unprovoked GTCS appears in adult life
- absence status epilepticus
- differentiation from other syndromes of IGE.

It is essential to take a careful clinical history and to interpret symptoms correctly, which may be suggestive of typical absences and ASE. A history of altered consciousness preceding GTCS should not be taken as evidence of complex focal seizures, depression or an unspecified seizure prodrome.

Other forms of the so-called 'adult onset IGE' may be otherwise typical examples of JME, JAE or other IGE syndromes that start or become clinically identifiable after the age of 20 years.[202,341-344] Some of the patients described may suffer from IGE with phantom absences.

PROGNOSIS

IGE with phantom absences may be a lifelong propensity to seizures, which is of undetermined onset and remission. Patients are of normal intelligence, which does not show any signs of deterioration. Further, phantom absences, though frequent, do not appear to affect daily activity.

MANAGEMENT

There are many unanswered questions as to whether patients with phantom absences need treatment. All patients with IGE with phantom absences had a normal life without medication until their first GTCS, probably many years after the onset of frequent daily mild absence seizures. We do not know how many people there are in the general population with the same problem but without GTCS or conspicuous ASE. If treatment is considered necessary (driving a car is a significant factor), valproate, levetiracetam and lamotrigine are AEDs to consider.

A reminder of "adult onset idiopathic generalised epilepsies"

Recently, there has been increasing interest in the so-called adult-onset IGE.[202,341-344] Seizures consist of GTCS, myoclonic jerks and absences, alone or in combination, which first become clinically detectable after the age of 20 years. I emphasise clinically detectable, because these patients may have had minor seizures (as is the case with phantom absences) long before seeking medical advice, which is usually prompted by a GTCS. Thus, adult onset IGE appears to consist of classical syndromes of IGE, but with delayed onset or delayed identification. Other than age at the time of the first overt seizure, all other clinical and EEG manifestations are typical of JME, JAE or IGE with GTCS only. For example, 'adult myoclonic epilepsy' is identical to JME.[202] When grouped together on the basis of age at onset, clinical manifestations, EEG and family history of epilepsies, there is a similarity between 'adult onset IGE' and 'IGE of classical late childhood or adolescence onset'.[342-344] However, an exemption exists with 'benign familial adult myoclonic epilepsy',[345] which is a distinct autosomal epileptic syndrome with seizures first appearing in adult life.

FAMILIAL (AUTOSOMAL DOMINANT) GENERALISED EPILEPTIC SYNDROMES

There is an increasing number of reports of familial idiopathic generalised epilepsies which have not been recognised by the ILAE yet. These include:

1. Benign adult familial myoclonic epilepsy[345-353]
2. Autosomal dominant cortical myoclonus and epilepsy[354]

BENIGN FAMILIAL ADULT MYOCLONIC EPILEPSY

Benign familial adult myoclonic epilepsy (FAME)[345] is probably the most common of the autosomal epileptic syndromes not yet recognised by the ILAE. FAME has been initially identified in Japanese[346,347,352,355] and more recently in European families.[351,353] FAME is a relatively benign non-progressive autosomal dominant idiopathic epileptic syndrome with high penetrance.

Clinically, FAME is characterised by adult-onset cortical myoclonus and tremor of the fingers; 80% of patients also have infrequent GTCS in periods of worsening myoclonus. Movement and emotional stress intensify the myoclonus. Age at onset varies from 30 to 60 years (mean 40 years). Families with members having concurrent migraine or blindness have been reported.

The EEG shows generalised polyspikes and waves, photosensitivity and giant somatosensory evoked potentials. Consistent with cortical myoclonus, long-loop C reflexes are enhanced and there is a preceding wave on jerk-locked back EEG averaging.

The genes for FAME have been mapped to 8q24 in Japanese families[346,347,352,355] and 2p11.1-q12.2 in European[351,353] families. There may be allelism with 'autosomal dominant cortical myoclonus and epilepsy syndrome'.

AUTOSOMAL DOMINANT CORTICAL MYOCLONUS AND EPILEPSY

Autosomal dominant cortical myoclonus and epilepsy (ADCME) with complex focal and generalised seizures is based on a study by Guerrini et al[354] of a pedigree, in which eight individuals presented with a non-progressive disorder with onset between the ages of 12 and 50 years.[354] It was characterised by predominantly distal, semicontinuous rhythmic myoclonus (all patients), GTCS (all patients) and complex focal seizures (three patients). Most patients had suffered infrequent seizures and had a normal cognitive level, but three patients with intractable seizures had mild mental retardation. The pattern of inheritance was autosomal dominant with high penetrance. All patients had frontotemporal as well as generalised interictal EEG abnormalities. Back-averaging analysis and other neurophysiological studies of the myoclonus suggested a cortical origin. The C-reflex at rest was enhanced and somatosensory, and visual evoked potentials were of high amplitude. The resting motor threshold intensity in response to transcranial magnetic stimulation was significantly reduced and the post-motor evoked potential silent period was significantly shortened compared with the controls. These clinical and neurophysiological characteristics suggest diffuse cortical hyperexcitability and a high propensity for intra-hemispheric and inter-hemispheric cortical spread, as well as rhythmic myoclonic activity. The disease has been linked to chromosome 2p11.1-q12.2.[354]

Syndromes of autosomal recessive inheritance such as 'familial infantile myoclonic epilepsy'[356,357] have also been described and may be considered in ILAE revisions.

TREATMENT OF IDIOPATHIC GENERALISED EPILEPSIES

Consider the following facts:

> "A majority (48%) of patients with idiopathic generalised epilepsy initially receive ill-advised AED, which cause IGE to appear intractable." Benbadis et al.[14]

> "Carbamazepine is still being inappropriately prescribed to children (47%) with typical absence syndromes to their detriment." Parker et al.[358]

> "In a class 1 control AED study, one quarter (27%) of patients with IGE, including JME, were treated with carbamazepine (a contra-indicated drug in IGE) which was the comparator drug on the basis of the physicians' 'intention to treat'." Privitera et al.[301]

These are striking, recent examples of commonly occurring and disturbing inappropriate medications in patients with IGEs. The most important of the multiple reasons for this continuing error are:

- diagnostic misclassification of IGEs as focal epilepsies[233]
- sparse or methodologically ambiguous AED RCTs [233]
- official guidelines and publications paying scant attention to important management aspects of IGEs [359]
- a *'one size fits all'* policy with regard to *'how to treat epilepsy'*. RCTs studying *'epilepsy'* and its treatment in its *'universe'* [301,302] are of no benefit and should be discouraged.[359] As Faught said, even for IGEs "we can not lump them all together in clinical trials".[233]
- Formal national formularies are conspicuously void of warning against established pro-epileptic action of certain AEDs in certain types of seizures and syndromes of IGEs.

I take some examples from the *British National Formulary (BNF)*, which are more or less the same everywhere:

> "Indications for carbamazepine: partial and secondary generalised tonic-clonic seizures and some primary generalised seizures."

Thus, physicians may reasonably prescribe carbamazepine for absences and myoclonic jerks (which are primary generalised seizures as also defined in the *BNF*) with disastrous effects.

> "Indications for tiagabine or vigabatrin: adjunctive treatment for partial seizures with or without secondary generalisation."

There is no warning that these AEDs are deleterious for IGEs, which are often misdiagnosed as partial epilepsies.

IGEs demand different treatment strategies to focal epilepsies.[4,14,310,360-363] Ignoring this fact results in avoidable morbidity and sometimes mortality. There is an urgent need for clear and unequivocal guidelines in the use of old and new AEDs in IGEs and its various types of seizures. Practising physicians have a colossal task in not only properly diagnosing IGE, but also in deciding which of the many old and new AEDs is the most suitable and which is contraindicated for the seizures and preferably the syndromes of IGEs.

The methodology followed in this book regarding treatment recommendations for AEDs is detailed in Chapter 4. The treatment of each individual IGE syndrome has been detailed in the appropriate chapter. Recent reviews and publications on the AED treatment of IGEs are recommended reading.[14,233,310,314,360,362,363]

Important established documentation to remember is that:

1. **Certain AEDs that are beneficial in focal epilepsies are ineffective or even contraindicated in IGE.**[4,276,292,364,365]
   - Tiagabine and vigabatrin are major pro-absence agents.
   - Carbamazepine, oxcarbazepine and phenytoin exacerbate absences and myoclonic jerks.
   - Gabapentin is ineffective in all types of idiopathic epileptic seizures and may exacerbate some of them.
2. **A drug efficacious in one type of generalised seizure may be ineffective or exaggerate another type of generalised seizure.**
   - Clonazepam is the best choice of drug for myoclonic jerks, but is ineffective in GTCS. Ethosuximide is highly efficacious only for absence seizures and negative epileptic myoclonus, but is ineffective or may exaggerate GTCS.
   - Carbamazepine and oxcarbazepine are effective in primarily GTCS, but often aggravate myoclonic jerks and absences.
   - Lamotrigine is effective in primarily GTCS and absences, but may exacerbate myoclonic jerks.
3. **If a drug is found to be efficacious in 'generalised' childhood epileptic encephalopathies, it does not mean that this is also the case in IGEs.**
   - Vigabatrin is the drug of first choice in West syndrome, but it is contraindicated in IGE.
4. **A drug found to be efficacious in secondarily GTCS, may be ineffective in primarily GTCS or deleterious in IGEs.**
   - Gabapentin, an AED licensed for the treatment of focal and secondarily GTCS is ineffective in primarily GTCS and may aggravate other types of IGE seizures.
   - Tiagabine, an AED licensed for the treatment of focal and secondarily GTCS, is a potent pro-absence agent that induces absence seizures and provokes ASE often ending with GTCS in IGE.
5. **IGEs are often easily treatable which means that a *small dose* of an appropriate AED is as good as a *large dose*.** [233]
   - No difference in control of various types of JME could be demonstrated between 1000 mg and 2000 mg of valproate. [238]

DIAGNOSIS AND TREATMENT OF NEWLY IDENTIFIED IGES

Diagnosis should first establish that the patient suffers from genuine epileptic seizures and then define:

- this is IGE and not focal epilepsy
- the types of seizures that the patient suffers
- if possible, the IGE syndrome.

In choosing the first AED to be recommended from Table 10.8 efficacy and adverse reactions have to be carefully balanced, because treatment is often lifelong.

Old anti-epileptic drugs in IGEs

Briefly, prior to the introduction of new AEDs, the position was as follows.

Valproate has superior efficacy in all seizures and syndromes of IGEs but its use in certain populations and particularly in women of reproductive age is highly problematic and sometimes impossible.

Clonazepam, even in small doses of 0.5 –1 mg, is probably the most potent antimyoclonic drug with some anti-absence effect;[4] it may deteriorate GTCS or deprive patients from the warning symptoms of an impeding GTCS in JME (see page 317).[253-255]

Ethosuximide is a potent drug against absences. It may improve myoclonic seizures (particularly negative epileptic myoclonus), but is ineffective and may worsen GTCS.[4]

Phenytoin is effective in primarily GTCS, but deteriorates absences and possibly myoclonic jerks; it is often ineffective or worsens JME.[312]

Carbamazepine is effective in primarily GTCS, but aggravates absences and myoclonic jerks.

Phenobarbitone was historically the preferred drug in JME and is still used in Europe and developing countries; it worsens absences.[61,201]

Evolving treatment of IGE in the era of new anti-epileptic drugs

The adverse effects of valproate and its lack of efficacy in 20% of patients has prompted the search for alternatives. Half of the new AEDs appear to be either ineffective or contraindicated (vigabatrin, tiagabine, oxcarbazepine, gabapentin)[366] in IGE (Table 4.1). Of the other four new AEDs, lamotrigine,[4,258,259] levetiracetam,[234,260-265] topiramate[266,267,298] and zonisamide[268] appear to be therapeutic agents. Levetiracetam, because of its efficacy in all types of seizure[234,260-265] and safer adverse reactions profile,[270,271] appears to be the most promising substitute for valproate. Lamotrigine is effective in GTCS and absence seizures, but often aggravates myoclonic jerks. It has important beneficial synergistic interactions with valproate. Topiramate is mainly effective in GTCS, but its adverse effect profile and drug–drug interactions are possibly worse than those of valproate. Zonisamide may have a weak therapeutic effect.

Prescribing errors in IGEs

The error of prescribing tiagabine or vigabatrin in patients with absence seizures may be of the same magnitude as prescribing a gluten-rich diet in the treatment of coeliac disease.[4] Prescribing carbamazepine in patients with JME is a similar situation.

New anti-epileptic drugs useful in IGEs

These have been detailed on pages 315-18 in the treatment of JME. Briefly, in order of preference:

Levetiracetam,[4,367] so far fulfils all expectations as probably the best new AED in the treatment of IGEs and is the likely candidate to replace valproate in at least JME, with its high and sustained efficacy, fast action, excellent safety profile, lack of clinically meaningful interactions with other drugs and no need for laboratory tests. Its role in syndromes with predominant absence seizures (CAE and JAE) is yet unclear though it has a unique mode of action in animal models of absence seizures.[368] In a recent report 3 of 4 patients with CAE and 5 of 5 patients with JAE became seizure free with levetiracetam alone or in combination with other AEDs. [183]

Lamotrigine has proven efficacy in controlling GTCS and absence seizures in at least 50% of patients, but may exaggerate myoclonic jerks. It is inferior to valproate in terms of efficacy, but superior with respect to adverse reactions despite a high incidence of idiosyncratic reactions that can occasionally be fatal. Efficacy and adverse reactions have to be carefully balanced in these cases, because treatment is often lifelong.

Lamotrigine is recommended in the treatment of CAE and JAE either alone[170,171] or in combination with other anti-absence AEDs.[4,170,171,194,246,247,271]

However, lamotrigine monotherapy in JME is probably not recommended but small doses of lamotrigine added to valproate are probably the most effective combination treatment for resistant cases.

Topiramate[266,298,369] is another broad-spectrum AED that is effective in primary GTCS[299-302] with a weak anti-absence[303] and anti-myoclonic action.[291,297] In IGEs, including JME, it appears to be much less effective than valproate, but more effective than lamotrigine.[297]

In a well-cited class 1 study, topiramate has been found to be effective in primarily GTCS.[299,301,302] Methodological drawbacks of these studies included: (a). patients with symptomatic generalised seizures were enrolled; (b). one fourth (27%) of patients with IGEs were assigned to carbamazepine as a comparator AED; and (c). carbamazepine was statistically decreased in the topiramate group thus favouring the results in this group for at least the 'subtypes of generalised seizures', such as absences and myoclonic jerks that deteriorate with carbamazepine.

Topiramate is unlikely to achieve monotherapy status in the long-term treatment of IGEs mainly because of its many short and long term adverse effects and drug-drug interactions.

Zonisamide[307-310] is also a broad-spectrum AED, but its role in IGEs is largely unknown and probably weak. In the long experience of eminent Japanese colleagues that I consulted, zonisamide is effective in the treatment of focal seizures, secondarily GTCS, epileptic encephalopathies (West syndrome responds much better than Lennox-Gastaut syndrome) and progressive myoclonic epilepsies. Zonisamide appears to be much less effective in IGE, primarily GTCS, absences and jerks, though a few patients may have an excellent response. In children, cognitive adverse reactions may be troublesome. Currently in Japan, zonisamide is a second-line AED for focal epilepsies after carbamazepine and for symptomatic generalised epilepsy after valproate, clonazepam and clobazam.

POLYTHERAPY

For patients in whom monotherapy with valproate fails, the combination of valproate with small doses of lamotrigine (25–50 mg) appears to be the most effective.[4] In those with persistent myoclonic jerks, clonazepam is the best add-on drug to valproate.[4] Ethosuximide should be added only for uncontrolled absence seizures. However, in all these scenarios, valproate is the principal AED. The situation is likely to change dramatically with use of levetiracetam instead of valproate but this needs RCTs.

The consensus is that IGEs have a better prognosis with, and a more favourable response to, appropriate AEDs than symptomatic and focal epilepsies. "Most patients with IGE are easily controlled with appropriate medication, refractory patients are rare."[246,247] However, there is no reliable Figure regarding the prevalence of intractable IGE, which may be in the order of 10–30%.[370] A factor contributing to this uncertainty and probably high incidence of intractable IGEs is that IGEs are often inappropriately treated with AEDs that are either ineffective or contraindicated. Table 4.1 lists AEDs that are indicated and contraindicated in IGE seizures.

Management of patients with intractable IGEs, providing that they truly suffer from epileptic seizures, should take the following steps:

1. Based on clinical and EEG evidence, establish the type or types of seizures (absences, myoclonic jerks and GTCS alone or in combination), and make sure that these are primarily and not secondarily generalised. Previous EEGs particularly, in untreated stages, are invaluable.
2. Establish precipitating factors and circadian distribution as well as their effect regarding intractability.

3. List in chronological order, all AEDs used, and in what doses and combinations. Establish which drugs were beneficial and which made the situation worse.
4. Consider thoroughly the current situation regarding: (a). seizures – which are the more predominant and more disturbing; and (b). AEDs – which are definitely or possibly effective, ineffective or contraindicated with respect to seizures and adverse reactions.
5. Consider thoroughly all the above, including compliance, in making a definite plan (Tables 1.3) of which AEDs with adverse effects (seizure efficacy and patient tolerability) should be withdrawn and which of the indicated AEDs should be increased in dosage or added to the scheme.
6. Of the new AEDs, those which are likely to be effective as monotherapy (Table 4.1 and Table 10.8) are also the most likely to be suitable in polytherapy. The order of priority as determined by efficacy, safety, drug–drug interactions and other parameters are levetiracetam, lamotrigine, topiramate and zonisamide. All other new AEDs –tiagabine, oxcarbazepine and gabapentin –are unsuitable.

New AEDs contraindicated in IGEs

Gabapentin: all relevant studies have shown that gabapentin is, at least, ineffective in IGEs including primary GTCS, and it may exacerbate absences and myoclonic jerks.[194,246,247,271,371-373]

Oxcarbazepine appears to have a similar seizure profile to carbamazepine. In IGEs, like carbamazepine, oxcarbazepine mainly aggravates absences and myoclonic jerks; GTCS may also worsen.[365] In a case series, all six IGE patients showed significant deterioration in terms of absences and myoclonic jerks related to oxcarbazepine treatment; GTCS also worsened in three patients.[365]

Vigabatrin and tiagabine are contraindicated. These are pro-absence AEDs, because of their GABAergic action, which explains the high incidence of drug-induced ASE and the appearance of new types of seizures.[4]

DRUG WITHDRAWAL

In CAE, treatment may be slowly withdrawn 1–3 years after controlling all absences.[4] All other IGE syndromes are probably lifelong and confront the usual textbook advice of withdrawal of medication after 2–3 years from the last seizure. Relapses are probably unavoidable. However, if seizures are mild and infrequent, drug withdrawal may be attempted. This should be done in small decrements, probably over years, warning the patient that re-emergence of even minor seizures, such as absences or myoclonic jerks, mandates continuation of treatment. EEG confirmation of the seizure-free state is needed during the withdrawal period.[4]

First-line drugs
Valproate (the most effective of all but often unsuitable for women)
Levetiracetam (but needs RCTs)
Lamotrigine (may exaggerate myoclonic jerks)
Ethosuximide (only for absences and negative myoclonus; may exaggerate GTCS)
Clonazepam (only for pure myoclonic syndromes; may exaggerate GTCS)

Second-line or adjunctive drugs
Topiramate (but with serious adverse reactions and drug–drug interactions)
Zonisamide (needs further documentation regarding efficacy and adverse reactions)
Phenobarbitone (may be first line AED for those without absence seizures if cost is a major issue)
Acetazolamide (only for absences)

Contraindicated drugs
Carbamazepine, oxcarbazepine and phenytoin (though they may control primarily GTCS if added to first-line drugs)
Gabapentin (ineffective in primarily GTCS and may exacerbate absences and myoclonic jerks)
Tiagabine and vigabatrin (pro-absence drugs with a high incidence of induced ASE)

TREATMENT OF STATUS EPILEPTICUS IN IDIOPATHIC GENERALISED EPILEPSY

Idiopathic generalised ASE with all its variations (generalised non-convulsive status epilepticus) has a high prevalence in IGE, though it is often unrecognised, because symptoms may be mild. Generalised tonic clonic status epilepticus is less common in IGE than symptomatic and probably symptomatic focal or generalised epilepsies.

The emergency treatment of convulsive or non-convulsive status epilepticus is the same irrespective of causes, idiopathic or symptomatic, in focal or generalised epilepsies. There are recent major publications and reviews for more extensive reading.[363,371,374-379,379-388]

CONVULSIVE STATUS EPILEPTICUS

Convulsive status epilepticus (CSE) is a medical emergency and should be managed urgently and properly according to established and well-publicised protocols.[371,374-379] Following any of these protocols results in appropriate and rapid management of CSE, which reduces morbidity and mortality.[377] The mortality of CSE is around 10%. The commonest cause of CSE is withdrawal of anti-epileptic medication, which should be reintroduced as soon as possible after the onset of CSE. The longer CSE lasts, the harder it is to treat and the greater the morbidity and mortality.

The aim of treatment is early termination of CSE in order to prevent neuronal damage caused by systemic and metabolic disturbances and by the direct excitotoxic effect of electrical seizure discharges. Control of overt and electrical seizures is imperative. The risk of brain damage increases progressively if continuous CSE persists for more than 30 minutes and particularly after 1–2 hours. This is because compensatory mechanisms to prevent brain damage are relatively satisfactory during the first 30 minutes. Subsequently, compensatory mechanisms break down with increasing speed if the seizures are not stopped during the first 30 minutes. Neuronal damage leads to transient or permanent neurological, epileptic and cognitive sequelae or even death.

DRUG TREATMENT OF CSE CAN BE DIVIDED INTO THREE STAGES.

1. *In the early stage (first 30 minutes),* treatment comprises intravenous administration of a fast-acting benzodiazepine of which diazepam, lorazepam or midazolam are the most effective agents. Diazepam is the traditional drug, then lorazepam came to prominence as the drug of first choice[377] and, recently, midazolam infusion has become increasingly popular as an effective and well-tolerated therapeutic agent.[389] Most cases are controlled with this approach. If CSE is not controlled at this stage, the patient enters into the second stage of established status epilepticus, which carries an appreciable morbidity.

2. *In the stage of established CSE,* first-line drug options are intravenous phenytoin or fosphenytoin. If these are ineffective, subanaesthetic doses of phenobarbitone are used. If seizures are not controlled at this stage the patient enters refractory status epilepticus.

3. *The last stage of refractory status epilepticus* requires general anaesthesia and a continuous infusion of AEDs, such as pentobarbital, midazolam or propofol, and concomitant EEG monitoring of seizure or EEG background suppression.[381] Despite these measures, the mortality of refractory CSE is more than 20%.[381]

ABSENCE (GENERALISED NON-CONVULSIVE) STATUS EPILEPTICUS

Absence status epilepticus[19,66,390] occurs in 10–20% of cases of IGE and in as many as 50% of cases of some syndromes of IGE such as those manifesting with phantom absences or perioral myoclonia. Additionally, nearly all patients are fully aware of this epileptic status and know that it may inevitably lead to a GTCS, though it is avoidable:

> It is the same feeling of: "slowing down", "uncontrollable rush of thoughts", "losing control of my mind", "taking me much longer to formulate my response which occasionally is inappropriate and bumbled. Then I know that I will have the fit. If I can, I just go to a private place and wait for it."

This stage is unlikely to be considered as a genuine status epilepticus by the physicians in accident and emergency departments. Therefore, advice to the patient regarding therapeutic options for self-administration of drugs is imperative. Benzodiazepines and, mainly, diazepam, lorazepam or midazolam are the most effective agents.

Self-administration: Rectal diazepam (10–20 mg for adults and 0.5 mg/kg for children) as soon as the first symptoms appear may stop ASE and prevent an impending GTCS. Rectal absorption of liquid diazepam is very rapid, reaches the brain within minutes and has a near-intravenous efficacy. Proprietary rectal tubes (Stesolid) containing ready-made liquid diazepam are the most widely used formulation. Suppositories of diazepam are not useful, because of their slow absorption. Diazepam rectal gel is now available in the USA and some other countries.[391] However, adult patients, either because of embarrassment or inconvenience, rarely use rectal preparations. An oral bolus dose of valproate (usually twice the daily prophylactic dose) from onset of symptoms is often effective in terminating the ASE and preventing GTCS (most patients prefer this to rectal preparations of drugs).

Buccal[392,393] or intranasal[394] application of midazolam may be the best practical and effective therapeutic option. Midazolam buccal administration has equal efficacy and rapidity of action to rectal diazepam. It is more convenient and less traumatising than rectal preparations of diazepam. Midazolam (0.3 mg/kg for children and 10–20 mg for adults) drawn up from an ampoule is dissolved with peppermint (otherwise it smells and tastes terrible) and should be swirled around the mouth for 4–5 min and then spat out.

Clonazepam (1–4 mg) may be given orally at the onset of generalised non-convulsive status epilepticus and is the preferred option in patients with mainly myoclonic jerks.

> This helps me to go to sleep and when I wake up I am fine.

Hospital management: With intravenous administration of any type of the benzodiazepines discussed above, generalised non-convulsive status epilepticus usually stops abruptly. The problem is that this condition is not recognised and the patients are not believed when they seek such treatment even when they produce a relevant letter from their treating physician, which clearly explains their situation and the need for urgent attention.

> She started doing the same silly things. I recognised it. The doctor told me that she is OK. No, no I said, she is going to have a fit.

REFERENCES

1. Commission on Classification and Terminology of the International League Against Epilepsy. Proposal for revised classification of epilepsies and epileptic syndromes. *Epilepsia* 1989;**30**:389-99.
2. Malafosse A, Genton P, Hirsch E, Marescaux C, Broglin D, Bernasconi R, eds. Idiopathic generalised epilepsies. London: John Libbey & Company Ltd, 1994.
3. Duncan JS, Panayiotopoulos CP, eds. Typical absences and related epileptic syndromes. London: Churchill Communications Europe, 1995.
4. Panayiotopoulos CP. Treatment of typical absence seizures and related epileptic syndromes. *Paediatr Drugs* 2001;**3**:379-403.
5. Engel J, Jr. A proposed diagnostic scheme for people with epileptic seizures and with epilepsy: Report of the ILAE Task Force on Classification and Terminology. *Epilepsia* 2001;**42**:796-803.
6. Panayiotopoulos CP, ed. Idiopathic generalised epilepsies:A review and modern approach. *Epilepsia* 2005;**Suppl** (in press).
7. Crunelli V, Leresche N. Childhood absence epilepsy: genes, channels, neurons and networks. *Nat Rev Neurosci.* 2002; **3**:371-82.
8. Gourfinkel-An I, Baulac S, Nabbout R, Ruberg M, Baulac M, Brice A *et al.* Monogenic idiopathic epilepsies. *Lancet Neurol.* 2004;**3**:209-18.
9. Delgado-Escueta AV, Medina MT, Serratosa JM, Castroviejo IP, Gee MN, Weissbecker K *et al.* Mapping and positional cloning of common idiopathic generalized epilepsies: juvenile myoclonus epilepsy and childhood absence epilepsy. *Adv Neurol* 1999;**79**:351-74.
10. Durner M, Keddache MA, Tomasini L, Shinnar S, Resor SR, Cohen J *et al.* Genome scan of idiopathic generalized epilepsy: evidence for major susceptibility gene and modifying genes influencing the seizure type. *Ann Neurol* 2001;**49**:328-35.
11. Noebels JL. Exploring new gene discoveries in idiopathic generalized epilepsy. *Epilepsia* 2003;**44 Suppl 2**:16-21.
12. Jones-Davis DM, Macdonald RL. GABA(A) receptor function and pharmacology in epilepsy and status epilepticus. *Curr Opin Pharmacol.* 2003;**3**:12-8.
13. Manning JP, Richards DA, Bowery NG. Pharmacology of absence epilepsy. *Trends Pharmacol Sci.* 2003;**24**:542-9.
14. Benbadis SR, Tatum WO, Gieron M. Idiopathic generalized epilepsy and choice of antiepileptic drugs. *Neurology* 2003;**61**:1793-5.
15. Panayiotopoulos CP. Absence epilepsies. In Engel JJ, Pedley TA, eds. *Epilepsy: A comprehensive Textbook*, pp 2327-46. Philadelphia: Lippincott-Raven Publishers, 1997.
16. Panayiotopoulos CP. Typical absence seizures. In Gilman S, ed. *Medlink Neurology*, San Diego SA: Arbor Publishing Corp, 2004.
17. Snead OC, III, Depaulis A, Vergnes M, Marescaux C. Absence epilepsy: advances in experimental animal models. *Adv Neurol* 1999;**79**:253-78.
18. Loiseau P, Panayiotopoulos CP, Hirsch E. Childhood absence epilepsy and related syndromes. In Roger J, Bureau M, Dravet C, Genton P, Tassinari CA, Wolf P, eds. *Epileptic syndromes in infancy, childhood and adolescence (3rd edn)*, pp 285-304. London: John Libbey & Co Ltd, 2002.
19. Agathonikou A, Panayiotopoulos CP, Giannakodimos S, Koutroumanidis M. Typical absence status in adults: diagnostic and syndromic considerations. *Epilepsia* 1998;**39**:1265-76.
20. Penry JK, Porter RJ, Dreifuss RE. Simultaneous recording of absence seizures with video tape and electroencephalography. A study of 374 seizures in 48 patients. *Brain* 1975;**98**:427-40.
21. Commission of Classification and Terminology of the International League Against Epilepsy. Proposal for revised clinical and electroencephalographic classification of epileptic seizures. *Epilepsia* 1981;**22**:489-501.
22. Stefan H. Epileptic absences. Studies on the structure, pathophysiology and clinical course of the seizure. *Fortschr Med* 1983;**101**:996-8.
23. Stefan H, Snead OC, III. Absence seizures. In Engel JJ, Pedley TA, eds. *Epilepsy:A comprehensive textbook*, pp 579-90. Philadelphia: Lippincott-Raven Publishers, 1997.
24. Panayiotopoulos CP, Obeid T, Waheed G. Differentiation of typical absence seizures in epileptic syndromes. A video EEG study of 224 seizures in 20 patients. *Brain* 1989;**112**:1039-56.
25. Panayiotopoulos CP, Obeid T, Waheed G. Absences in juvenile myoclonic epilepsy: a clinical and video- electroencephalographic study. *Ann Neurol* 1989;**25**:391-7.
26. Capovilla G, Rubboli G, Beccaria F, Lorenzetti ME, Montagnini A, Resi C *et al.* A clinical spectrum of the myoclonic manifestations associated with typical absences in childhood absence epilepsy. A video-polygraphic study. *Epileptic Disord.* 2001;**3**:57-62.
27. Gowers WR. Epilepsies and other chronic convulsive diseases. Their causes, symptoms and treatment. London: Churchill,J.A, 1881.
28. Buchheim K, Obrig H, Pannwitz W, Muller A, Heekeren H, Villringer A *et al.* Decrease in haemoglobin oxygenation during absence seizures in adult humans. *Neurosci.Lett.* 2004;**354**:119-22.
29. Wiest R, Schindler K, Kollar M, Donati F. Epigastric sensations as an unusual manifestation of adult absence epilepsy. *Epileptic Disord.* 2001;**3**:13-6.
30. Ferner RE, Panayiotopoulos CP. 'Phantom' typical absences, absence status and experiential phenomena. *Seizure* 1993;**2**:253-6.
31. Panayiotopoulos CP. Benign childhood partial seizures and related epileptic syndromes. London: John Libbey & Company Ltd, 1999.
32. Aliberti V, Grunewald RA, Panayiotopoulos CP, Chroni E. Focal electroencephalographic abnormalities in juvenile myoclonic epilepsy. *Epilepsia* 1994;**35**:297-301.
33. Lombroso CT. Consistent EEG focalities detected in subjects with primary generalized epilepsies monitored for two decades. *Epilepsia* 1997;**38**:797-812.
34. Feucht M, Fuchs K, Pichlbauer E, Hornik K, Scharfetter J, Goessler R *et al.* Possible association between childhood absence epilepsy and the gene encoding GABRB3. *Biol Psychiatry* 1999;**46**:997-1002.
35. Wallace RH, Marini C, Petrou S, Harkin LA, Bowser DN, Panchal RG *et al.* Mutant GABA(A) receptor gamma2-subunit in childhood absence epilepsy and febrile seizures. *Nat Genet.* 2001;**28**:49-52.
36. Marini C, Harkin LA, Wallace RH, Mulley JC, Scheffer IE, Berkovic SF. Childhood absence epilepsy and febrile seizures: a family with a GABA(A) receptor mutation. *Brain* 2003;**126**:230-40.
37. Chen Y, Lu J, Pan H, Zhang Y, Wu H, Xu K *et al.* Association between genetic variation of CACNA1H and childhood absence epilepsy. *Ann Neurol.* 2003;**54**:239-43.
38. Danober L, Deransart C, Depaulis A, Vergnes M, Marescaux C. Pathophysiological mechanisms of genetic absence epilepsy in the rat. *Prog Neurobiol.* 1998;**55**:27-57.
39. Futatsugi Y, Riviello JJ, Jr. Mechanisms of generalized absence epilepsy. *Brain Devel.* 1998;**20**:75-9.
40. Blumenfeld H. From molecules to networks: cortical/subcortical interactions in the pathophysiology of idiopathic generalized epilepsy. *Epilepsia* 2003;**44 Suppl 2**:7-15.
41. Bernasconi A, Bernasconi N, Natsume J, Antel SB, Andermann F, Arnold DL. Magnetic resonance spectroscopy and imaging of the thalamus in idiopathic generalized epilepsy. *Brain* 2003;**126**:2447-54.
42. Koepp MJ, Duncan JS. Epilepsy. *Curr Opin Neurol* 2004;**17**:467-74.
43. Meeren HK, Pijn JP, van Luijtelaar EL, Coenen AM, Lopes da Silva FH. Cortical focus drives widespread corticothalamic networks during spontaneous absence seizures in rats. *J Neurosci.* 2002;**22**:1480-95.
44. Manning JP, Richards DA, Leresche N, Crunelli V, Bowery NG. Cortical-area specific block of genetically determined absence seizures by ethosuximide. *Neuroscience* 2004;**123**:5-9.
45. Coulter DA. Antiepileptic drug cellular mechanisms of action: where does lamotrigine fit in? *J Child Neurol.* 1997;**12 Suppl 1**:S2-9.
46. Gibbs JW3, Schroder GB, Coulter DA. GABAA receptor function in developing rat thalamic reticular neurons: whole cell recordings of GABA-mediated currents and modulation by clonazepam. *J Neurophysiol* 1996;**76**:2568-79.
47. Hosford DA, Lin FH, Wang Y, Caddick SJ, Rees M, Parkinson NJ *et al.* Studies of the lethargic (lh/lh) mouse model of absence seizures: regulatory mechanisms and identification of the lh gene. *Adv Neurol* 1999;**79**:239-52.

48. Ryvlin P, Mauguiere F. Functional imaging in idiopathic generalized epilepsy. *Rev Neurol (Paris)* 1998;**154**:691-3.

49. Duncan JS. Positron emission tomography receptor studies. *Adv Neurol* 1999;**79**:893-9.

50. Yeni SN, Kabasakal L, Yalcinkaya C, Nisli C, Dervent A. Ictal and interictal SPECT findings in childhood absence epilepsy. *Seizure* 2000;**9**:265-9.

51. Kapucu LO, Serdaroglu A, Okuyaz C, Kose G, Gucuyener K. Brain single photon emission computed tomographic evaluation of patients with childhood absence epilepsy. *J Child Neurol.* 2003;**18**:542-8.

52. Iannetti P, Spalice A, De Luca PF, Boemi S, Festa A, Maini CL. Ictal single photon emission computed tomography in absence seizures: apparent implication of different neuronal mechanisms. *J Child Neurol* 2001;**16**:339-44.

53. Meencke HJ. Pathological findings in childhood absence epilepsy. In Duncan JS, Panayiotopoulos CP, eds. *Typical absences and related epileptic syndromes*, pp 122-32. London: Churchill Communications Europe, 1995.

54. Woermann FG, Sisodiya SM, Free SL, Duncan JS. Quantitative MRI in patients with idiopathic generalized epilepsy. Evidence of widespread cerebral structural changes. *Brain* 1998;**121**:1661-7.

55. Opeskin K, Kalnins RM, Halliday G, Cartwright H, Berkovic SF. Idiopathic generalized epilepsy: lack of significant microdysgenesis. *Neurology* 2000;**55**:1101-6.

56. Panayiotopoulos CP, Chroni E, Daskalopoulos C, Baker A, Rowlinson S, Walsh P. Typical absence seizures in adults: clinical, EEG, video-EEG findings and diagnostic/syndromic considerations. *J Neurol Neurosurg Psychiatr* 1992;**55**:1002-8.

57. Panayiotopoulos CP, Giannakodimos S, Chroni E. Typical absences in adults. In Duncan JS, Panayiotopoulos CP, eds. *Typical absences and related epileptic syndromes*, pp 289-99. London: Churchill Communications Europe, 1995.

58. Panayiotopoulos CP, Koutroumanidis M, Giannakodimos S, Agathonikou A. Idiopathic generalised epilepsy in adults manifested by phantom absences, generalised tonic-clonic seizures, and frequent absence status. *J Neurol Neurosurg Psychiatr* 1997;**63**:622-7.

59. Gastaut, H. The epilepsies:Electro-clinical correlations. Springfield,Illinois, CC Thomas, 1954.

60. Panayiotopoulos CP, Obeid T, Tahan AR. Juvenile myoclonic epilepsy: a 5-year prospective study. *Epilepsia* 1994;**35**:285-96.

61. Janz D, Durner M. Juvenile myoclonic epilepsy. In Engel JJ, Pedley TA, eds. *Epilepsy: A comprehensive Textbook*, pp 2389-400. Philadelphia: Lippincott-Raven Publishers, 1997.

62. Diagnosing juvenile myoclonic epilepsy [editorial]. *Lancet* 1992;**340**:759-60.

63. Wolf P. Epilepsy with grand mal on awakening. In Roger J, Bureau M, Dravet C, Dreifuss FE, Perret A, Wolf P, eds. *Epileptic syndromes in infancy, childhood and adolescence*, pp 329-41. London: John Libbey & Company, 1992.

64. Shorvon, S. D. Status epilepticus:its clinical features and treatment in children and adults. Cambridge, Cambridge University Press, 1994.

65. Shorvon S. Absence status epilepticus. In Duncan JS, Panayiotopoulos CP, eds. *Typical absences and related epileptic syndromes*, pp 263-74. London: Churchill Communications Europe, 1995.

66. Panayiotopoulos CP. Absence status epilepticus. In Gilman S, ed. *Medlink Neurology*, San Diego SA: Arbor Publishing Corp, 2004.

67. Gastaut H. Dictionary of epilepsies. Part I:Definitions. Geneva: World Health Organisation, 1973.

68. Treatment of convulsive status epilepticus. Recommendations of the Epilepsy Foundation of America's Working Group on Status Epilepticus. *JAMA* 1993;**270**:854-9.

69. Bleck TP. Management approaches to prolonged seizures and status epilepticus. *Epilepsia* 1999;**40 Suppl 1**:S59-S63.

70. Blume WT, Luders HO, Mizrahi E, Tassinari C, van Emde BW, Engel J, Jr. Glossary of descriptive terminology for ictal semiology: report of the ILAE task force on classification and terminology. *Epilepsia* 2001;**42**:1212-8.

71. Kaplan PW. Assessing the outcomes in patients with nonconvulsive status epilepticus: nonconvulsive status epilepticus is underdiagnosed, potentially overtreated, and confounded by comorbidity. *J Clin Neurophysiol.* 1999;**16**:341-52.

72. Kaplan PW. Behavioral Manifestations of Nonconvulsive Status Epilepticus. *Epilepsy Behav.* 2002;**3**:122-39.

73. Thomas P, Andermann F. Late-onset absence status epilepticus is most often situation- related. In Malafosse A, Genton P, Hirsch E, Marescaux C, Broglin D, Bernasconi R, eds. *Idiopathic generalized epilepsies*, pp 95-109. London: John Libbey & Company Ltd, 1994.

74. Thomas P. Absence status epilepsy. *Rev Neurol (Paris)* 1999;**155**:1023-38.

75. Snead OC, III, Dean JC, Penry JK. Absence status epilepticus. In Engel JJ, Pedley TA, eds. *Epilepsy:a comprehensive textbook*, pp 701-7. Philadelphia: Lippincott-Raven Publishers, 1997.

76. Baykan B, Gokyigit A, Gurses C, Eraksoy M. Recurrent absence status epilepticus: clinical and EEG characteristics. *Seizure* 2002;**11**:310-9.

77. Panayiotopoulos CP, Ferrie CD, Koutroumanidis M, Rowlinson S, Sanders S. Idiopathic generalised epilepsy with phantom absences and absence status in a child. *Epileptic Disord.* 2001;**3**:63-6.

78. Skardoutsou A, Voudris KA, Vagiakou EA. Non-convulsive status epilepticus associated with tiagabine therapy in children. *Seizure.* 2003;**12**:599-601.

79. Schapel G, Chadwick D. Tiagabine and non-convulsive status epilepticus. *Seizure* 1996;**5**:153-6.

80. Osorio I, Reed RC, Peltzer JN. Refractory idiopathic absence status epilepticus: A probable paradoxical effect of phenytoin and carbamazepine. *Epilepsia* 2000;**41**:887-94.

81. Agathonikou A, Koutroumanidis M, Panayiotopoulos CP. Fixation-off-sensitive epilepsy with absences and absence status: video- EEG documentation. *Neurology* 1997;**48**:231-4.

82. Ming X, Kaplan PW. Fixation-off and eyes closed catamenial generalized nonconvulsive status epilepticus with eyelid myoclonic jerks. *Epilepsia* 1998;**39**:664-8.

83. Foldvary-Schaefer N, Falcone T. Catamenial epilepsy: pathophysiology, diagnosis, and management. *Neurology* 2003;**61**:S2-15.

84. Engel J, Jr. Classifications of the International League Against Epilepsy: time for reappraisal. *Epilepsia* 1998;**39**:1014-7.

85. Engel J, Jr. Classification of Epileptic Disorders. *Epilepsia* 2001;**42**:316.

86. Andermann F, Berkovic SF. Idiopathic generalized epilepsy with generalised and other seizures in adolescence. *Epilepsia* 2001;**42**:317-20.

87. Doose H. Das akinetische petit mal. *Arch Psychiatr Nervenkr* 1965;**205**:638-54.

88. Doose H, Gerken H, Leonhardt T, Volz E, Volz C. Centrencephalic myoclonic-astatic petit mal. Clinical and genetic investigation. *Neuropadiatrie* 1970;**2**:59-78.

89. Doose H. Myoclonic-astatic epilepsy. *Epilepsy Research - Supplement* 1992;**6**:163-8.

90. Aicardi J. Myoclonic-astatic epilepsy. In Wallace S, ed. *Epilepsy in Children*, pp 263-70. London: Chapman & Hall, 1996.

91. Oguni H, Fukuyama Y, Tanaka T, Hayashi K, Funatsuka M, Sakauchi M *et al.* Myoclonic-astatic epilepsy of early childhood—clinical and EEG analysis of myoclonic-astatic seizures, and discussions on the nosology of the syndrome. *Brain Dev.* 2001;**23**:757-64.

92. Dulac O, Dreifuss F. Myoclonic-astatic epilepsy of childhood. In Gilman S, ed. *Medlink Neurology*, San Diego SA: Arbor Publishing Corp, 2004.

93. Weber P, Tillmann B, Minet JC, Blauenstein U. Myoclonic-astatic epilepsy in early childhood: review of clinical signs, EEG features, etiology, and therapy. *Klin Padiatr.* 2002;**214**:279-84.

94. Guerrini R, Parmeggiani A, Kaminska A, Dulac O. Myoclonic astatic epilepsy. In Roger J, Bureau M, Dravet C, Genton P, Tassinari CA, Wolf P, eds. *Epileptic syndromes in infancy, childhood and adolescence (3rd edn)*, pp 105-12. London: John Libbey & Co Ltd, 2002.

95. Oguni H, Tanaka T, Hayashi K, Funatsuka M, Sakauchi M, Shirakawa S *et al.* Treatment and long-term prognosis of myoclonic-astatic epilepsy of early childhood. *Neuropediatrics* 2002;**33**:122-32.

96. Guerrini R, Aicardi J. Epileptic encephalopathies with myoclonic seizures in infants and children (severe myoclonic epilepsy and myoclonic-astatic epilepsy). *J Clin Neurophysiol.* 2003;**20**:449-61.

97. Aicardi J. Myoclonic-astatic epilepsy. In Wallace SJ, Farrell K, eds. *Epilepsy in childen*, pp 163-8. London: Arnold, 2004.

98. Doose H. Myoclonic-astatic epilepsy. *Epilepsy Res Suppl* 1992;**6**:163-8.

99. Aicardi J, Levy Gomes A. Clinical and electroencephalographic symptomatology of the 'genuine' Lennox-Gastaut syndrome and its differentiation from other forms of epilepsy of early childhood. *Epilepsy Res- Suppl* 1992;**6**:185-93.

100. Kaminska A, Ickowicz A, Plouin P, Bru MF, Dellatolas G, Dulac O. Delineation of cryptogenic Lennox-Gastaut syndrome and myoclonic astatic epilepsy using multiple correspondence analysis. *Epilepsy Res.* 1999;**36**:15-29.

101. Scheffer IE, Wallace R, Mulley JC, Berkovic SF. Clinical and molecular genetics of myoclonic-astatic epilepsy and severe myoclonic epilepsy in infancy (Dravet syndrome). *Brain Dev.* 2001;**23**:732-5.

102. Bonanni P, Parmeggiani L, Guerrini R. Different neurophysiologic patterns of myoclonus characterize Lennox-Gastaut syndrome and myoclonic astatic epilepsy. *Epilepsia* 2002;**43**:609-15.

103. Aicardi J. Epilepsy in Children. New York: Raven Press, 1994.

104. Aicardi J, Chevrie JJ. Atypical benign partial epilepsy of childhood. *Devel Med Child Neurol* 1982;**24**:281-92.

105. Arzimanoglou A, Guerrini R, Aicardi J. Aicardi's epilepsy in children. Philadelphia: Lippincott Williams & Wilkins, 2004.

106. Fejerman N, Caraballo R, Tenembaum SN. Atypical evolutions of benign localization-related epilepsies in children: are they predictable? *Epilepsia* 2000;**41**:380-90.

107. Fejerman N. Atypical evolution of benign partial epilepsy in children. *Rev Neurol* 1996;**24**:1415-20.

108. Ferrie CD, Panayiotopoulos CP. Idiopathic generalised epilepsy with generalised tonic clonic seizures on awakening. In Wallace SJ, Farrell K, eds. *Epilepsy in Children (2nd edition)*, London: Edward Arnold (Publishers) Limited, 2002.

109. Caraballo RH, Astorino F, Cersosimo R, Soprano AM, Fejerman N. Atypical evolution in childhood epilepsy with occipital paroxysms (Panayiotopoulos type). *Epileptic Disord.* 2001;**3**:157-62.

110. Chapman K, Holland K, Erenberg G. Seizure exacerbation associated with oxcarbazepine in idiopathic focal epilepsy of childhood. *Neurology* 2003;**61**:1012.

111. Catania S, Cross H, De Sousa C, Boyd S. Paradoxic reaction to lamotrigine in a child with benign focal epilepsy of childhood with centrotemporal spikes. *Epilepsia* 1999;**40**:1657-60.

112. Jayawant S, Libretto SE. Topiramate in the treatment of myoclonic-astatic epilepsy in children: A retrospective hospital audit. *J.Postgrad Med.* 2003;**49**:202-6.

113. Adie WJ. Pyknolepsy:a form of epilepsy occurring in children with a good prognosis. *Brain* 1924;**47**:96-102.

114. Loiseau P, Panayiotopoulos CP. Childhood absence epilepsy. In Gilman S, ed. *Medlink Neurology*, San Diego SA: Arbor Publishing Corp, 2004.

115. Lennox WG, Lennox MA. Epilepsy and related disorders. Boston: Little,Brown & Co.1960.

116. Currier RD, Kooi KA, Saidman, J. Prognosis of pure petit mal:a follow-up study. *Neurology* 1963;**13**: 959-67.

117. Livingston S, Torres J, Pauli LL, Rider RV. Petit mal epilepsy: results of a prolonged follow-up study of 117 patients. *JAMA* 1965;**194**, 227-32.

118. Beaumanoir A. Les épilepsies infantiles. Problèmes de diagnostic et de traitement. Bâle, Editions Roche, 1976.

119. Cavazzuti GB, Ferrari F, Galli V, Benatti A. Epilepsy with typical absence seizures with onset during the first year of life. *Epilepsia* 1989;**30**:802-6.

120. Darra F, Fontana E, Scaramuzzi V, Santorum E, Zoccante L, Zulumi E *et al.* Typical absence seizures in the first three years of life: electroclinical study of 31 cases. *Epilepsia* 1996;**37 Suppl 4** :95.

121. Aicardi J. Typical absences in the first two years of life. In Duncan JS, Panayiotopoulos CP, eds. *Typical absences and related epileptic syndromes*, pp 284-8. London: Churchill Communications Europe, 1995.

122. Hertoft P. The clinical, electroencephalographic and social prognosis in petit mal epilepsy. *Epilepsia* 1963;**4**:298-314.

123. Bergamini L, Bram S, Broglia S, Riccio A. L'insorgenza tardiva di crisi Grande Male nel Piccolo Male puro. Studio catamnestico di 78 casi. *Arch Suisses Neurol Neurochir Psychiatr* 1965;**96**:306-17.

124. Rocca WA, Sharbrough FW, Hauser WA, Annegers JF, Schoenberg BS. Risk factors for absence seizures: a population-based case- control study in Rochester, Minnesota. *Neurology* 1987;**37**:1309-14.

125. Hollowack J, Thurston DL, O'Leary J L. Petit mal epilepsy. *Pediatrics* 1962;**60**: 893-901.

126. Callenbach PM, Geerts AT, Arts WF, van Donselaar CA, Peters AC, Stroink H *et al.* Familial occurrence of epilepsy in children with newly diagnosed multiple seizures: Dutch Study of Epilepsy in Childhood. *Epilepsia* 1998;**39**:331-6.

127. Berg AT, Levy SR, Testa FM, Shinnar S. Classification of childhood epilepsy syndromes in newly diagnosed epilepsy: interrater agreement and reasons for disagreement. *Epilepsia* 1999;**40**:439-44.

128. Berg AT, Shinnar S, Levy SR, Testa FM, Smith-Rapaport S, Beckerman B. How well can epilepsy syndromes be identified at diagnosis? A reassessment 2 years after initial diagnosis. *Epilepsia* 2000;**41**:1269-75.

129. Olsson I. Epidemiology of absence epilepsy. I. Concept and incidence. *Acta Paediatr Scand* 1988;**77**:860-6.

130. Loiseau J, Loiseau P, Guyot M, Duche B, Dartigues JF, Aublet B. Survey of seizure disorders in the French southwest. I. Incidence of epileptic syndromes. *Epilepsia* 1990;**31**:391-6.

131. Blom S, Heijbel J, Bergfors PG. Incidence of epilepsy in children: a follow-up study three years after the first seizure. *Epilepsia* 1978;**19**:343-50.

132. Olsson I, Hagberg G. Epidemiology of absence epilepsy. III. Clinical aspects. *Acta Paediatr Scand* 1991;**80**:1066-72.

133. Olsson I, Hedstrom A. Epidemiology of absence epilepsy. II. Typical absences in children with encephalopathies. *Acta Paediatr Scand* 1991;**80**:235-42.

134. Berkovic SF. Childhood absence epilepsy and juvenile absence epilepsy. In Wyllie E, ed. *The treatment of epilepsy:Principles and practice*, pp 547-51. Philadelphia: Lea & Febiger, 1993.

135. Berkovic SF. Generalised absence seizures. In Wyllie E, ed. *The treatment of epilepsy:Principles and practice*, pp 401-10. Philadelphia: Lea & Febiger, 1993.

136. Loiseau P. Childhood absence epilepsy. In Roger J, Bureau M, Dravet C, Dreifuss FE, Perret A, Wolf P, eds. *Epileptic syndromes in infancy, childhood and adolescence*, pp 135-50. London: John Libbey & Company, 1992.

137. Sander JWAS. The epidemiology and prognosis of typical absence seizures. In Duncan JS, Panayiotopoulos CP, eds. *Typical absences and related epileptic syndromes*, pp 135-44. London: Churchill Communications Europe, 1995.

138. Fong GC, Shah PU, Gee MN, Serratosa JM, Castroviejo IP, Khan S *et al.* Childhood absence epilepsy with tonic-clonic seizures and electroencephalogram 3-4-Hz spike and multispike-slow wave complexes: linkage to chromosome 8q24. *Am J Hum Genet.* 1998;**63**:1117-29.

139. Wirrell EC. Natural history of absence epilepsy in children. *Can J Neurol Sci.* 2003;**30**:184-8.

140. Wirrell EC, Camfield CS, Camfield PR, Gordon KE, Dooley JM. Long-term prognosis of typical childhood absence epilepsy: remission or progression to juvenile myoclonic epilepsy. *Neurology* 1996;**47**:912-8.

141. Panayiotopoulos CP. Typical absences are syndrome related. In Duncan JS, Panayiotopoulos CP, eds. *Typical absences and related epileptic syndromes*, pp 304-10. London: Churchill Communications Europe, 1995.

142. Fakhoury T, Abou-Khalil B. Generalized absence seizures with 10-15 Hz fast discharges. *Clin Neurophysiol* 1999;**110**:1029-35.

143. Hirsch E, Marescaux C. What are the relevant criteria for a better classification of epileptic syndromes with typical absences? In Malafosse A, Genton P, Hirsch E, Marescaux C, Broglin D, Bernasconi R, eds. *Idiopathic generalised epilepsies*, pp 87-93. London: John Libbey & Company Ltd, 1994.

144. Agathonikou A, Giannakodimos S, Koutroumanidis M, Parker APJ, Ahmed Sharoqi I, Rowlinson S *et al.* Idiopathic GeneralisedEpilepsies in Adults with Onset of Typical Absences before the Age of 10 Years. *Epilepsia* 1997;**38 Suppl 3**:213.

145. Loiseau P, Duche B, Pedespan JM. Absence epilepsies. *Epilepsia* 1995;**36**:1182-6.

146. Loiseau P, Duche B. Childhood absence epilepsy. In Duncan JS, Panayiotopoulos CP, eds. *Typical absences and related epileptic syndromes*, pp 152-60. London: Churchill Communications Europe, 1995.

147. Dieterich E, Baier WK, Doose H, Tuxhorn I, Fichsel H. Longterm follow-up of childhood epilepsy with absences. I. Epilepsy with absences at onset. *Neuropediatrics* 1985;**16**:149-54.

148. Panayiotopoulos CP. Lamictal (lamotrigine) monotherapy for typical absence seizures in children. *Epilepsia* 2000;**41**:357-9.

149. Panayiotopoulos CP. Typical absence seizures and their treatment. *Arch Dis Child* 1999;**81**:351-5.

150. Wirrell EC, Camfield PR, Gordon KE, Camfield CS, Dooley JM, Hanna BD. Will a critical level of hyperventilation-induced hypocapnia always induce an absence seizure? *Epilepsia* 1996;**37**:459-62.

151. Dalby MA. Epilepsy and 3 per second spike and wave rhythms. A clinical,electroencephalographic and prognostic analysis of 346 patients. Acta Neurol Scand 1969;**40 Suppl** , 1-183.

152. Bureau M, Guey J, Dravet C, Roger J. Etude de la répartition des absences chez l'enfant en fonction de ses activités. *Rev Neurol* 1968;**118**:493-4.

153. Robinson R, Taske N, Sander T, Heils A, Whitehouse W, Goutieres F *et al.* Linkage analysis between childhood absence epilepsy and genes encoding GABAA and GABAB receptors, voltage-dependent calcium channels, and the ECA1 region on chromosome 8q. *Epilepsy Res.* 2002;**48**:169-79.

154. Loiseau P, Pestre M, Dartigues JF, Commenges D, Barberger-Gateau C, Cohadon S. Long-term prognosis in two forms of childhood epilepsy: typical absence seizures and epilepsy with rolandic (centrotemporal) EEG foci. *Ann Neurol* 1983;**13**:642-8.

155. Niedermeyer E, Lopes da Silva F, eds. Electroencephalography. Basic principles,clinical applications, and related fields. Fourth Edition. 1999. Baltimore, Williams & Wilkins.

156. Lees F, Liversedge LA. The prognosis of petit mal and minor epilepsy. Lancet 1962;**i**: 797-82.

157. Charlton MH, Yahr M D. Long term follow up of patients with petit mal. Arch Neurol 1967;**16**: 595-8.

158. Gibberd FB. The prognosis of petit mal. Brain 1966;**89**:531-8.

159. Gibberd F B. The prognosis of petit mal in adults. Epilepsia 1972; **3**, 171-5.

160. Lugaresi E, Pazzaglia PP, Franck L, Roger J, Bureau-Paillas M, Ambrosetto G *et al.* Evolution and prognosis of primary generalised epilepsy of petit mal absence type. In Lugaressi E, Pazzaglia PP, Tassinari CA, eds. *Evolution and prognosis of epilepsy*, pp 3-22. Bologna: Auto Gaggi, 1973.

161. Gastaut H, Zifkin BG, Mariani E, Puig JS. The long-term course of primary generalized epilepsy with persisting absences. *Neurology* 1986;**36**:1021-8.

162. Hedstrom A, Olsson I. Epidemiology of absence epilepsy: EEG findings and their predictive value. *Pediat Neurol* 1991;**7**:100-4.

163. Sato S, Dreifuss FE, Penry JK. Prognostic factors in absence seizures. *Neurology* 1976;**26**:788-96.

164. Sato S, Dreifuss FE, Penry JK, Kirby DD, Palesch Y. Long-term follow-up of absence seizures. *Neurology* 1983;**33**:1590-5.

165. Covanis A, Skiadas K, Loli N, Lada C, Theodorou V. Absence epilepsy: early prognostic signs. *Seizure* 1992;**1**:281-9.

166. Dieterich E, Doose H, Baier WK, Fichsel H. Longterm follow-up of childhood epilepsy with absences. II. Absence-epilepsy with initial grand mal. *Neuropediatrics* 1985;**16**:155-8.

167. Bartolomei F, Roger J, Bureau M, Genton P, Dravet C, Viallat D *et al.* Prognostic factors for childhood and juvenile absence epilepsies. *Eur Neurol* 1997;**37**:169-75.

168. Oller L. Prospective study of the differences between the syndromes of infantile absence epilepsy and syndromes of juvenile absence epilepsy. *Rev Neurol* 1996;**24**:930-6.

169. Trinka E, Baumgartner S, Unterberger I, Unterrainer J, Luef G, Haberlandt E *et al.* Long-term prognosis for childhood and juvenile absence epilepsy. *J Neurol.* 2004;**251**:1235-41.

170. Frank LM, Enlow T, Holmes GL, Manasco P, Concannon S, Chen C *et al.* Lamictal (lamotrigine) monotherapy for typical absence seizures in children. *Epilepsia* 1999;**40**:973-9.

171. Coppola G, Licciardi F, Sciscio N, Russo F, Carotenuto M, Pascotto A. Lamotrigine as first-line drug in childhood absence epilepsy: a clinical and neurophysiological study. *Brain Dev.* 2004;**26**:26-9.

172. Browne TR, Dreifuss FE, Penry JK, Porter RJ, White BG. Clinical and EEG estimates of absence seizure frequency. *Arch Neurol.* 1983;**40**:469-72.

173. Tassinari CA, Bureau M, Thomas P. Epilepsy with myoclonic absences. In Roger J, Bureau M, Dravet C, Dreifuss FE, Perret A, Wolf P, eds. *Epileptic syndromes in infancy, childhood and adolescence*, pp 151-60. London: John Libbey & Company, 1992.

174. Manonmani V, Wallace SJ. Epilepsy with myoclonic absences. *Arch Dis Child* 1994;**70**:288-90.

175. Verrotti A, Greco R, Chiarelli F, Domizio S, Sabatino G, Morgese G. Epilepsy with myoclonic absences with early onset: a follow-up study. *J Child Neurol* 1999;**14**:746-9.

176. Tassinari CA, Rubboli G, Michellluchi R. Epilepsy with myoclonic absences. In Gilman S, ed. *Medlink Neurology*, San Diego SA: Arbor Publishing Corp, 2004.

177. Tassinari CA, Rubboli G, Gardella E, Michellluchi R. Epilepsy with myoclonic absences. In Wallace SJ, Farrell K, eds. *Epilepsy in childen*, pp 189-94. London: Arnold, 2004.

178. Tassinari CA, Michelucci R, Rubboli G, Passarelli D, Riguzzi P, Parmeggiani L *et al.* Myoclonic absence epilepsy. In Duncan JS, Panayiotopoulos CP, eds. *Typical absences and related epileptic syndromes*, pp 187-95. London: Churchill Communications Europe, 1995.

179. Elia M, Guerrini R, Musumeci SA, Bonanni P, Gambardella A, Aguglia U. Myoclonic absence-like seizures and chromosome abnormality syndromes. *Epilepsia* 1998;**39**:660-3.

180. Aguglia U, Le Piane E, Gambardella A, Messina D, Russo C, Sirchia SM *et al.* Emotion-induced myoclonic absence-like seizures in a patient with inv- dup(15) syndrome: a clinical, EEG, and molecular genetic study. *Epilepsia* 1999;**40**:1316-9.

181. Kimura S, Adachi K. Localization-related epilepsy mimicking epilepsy with myoclonic absence in a patient with pachygyria. *Pediatr.Int.* 2002;**44**:171-3.

182. Ferrie CD, Giannakodimos S, Robinson RO, Panayiotopoulos CP. Symptomatic typical absence seizures. In Duncan JS, Panayiotopoulos CP, eds. *Typical absences and related epileptic syndromes*, pp 241-52. London: Churchill Communications Europe, 1995.

183. Fattouch J, Di Bonaventura C, Mari F, Egeo G, Vaudano AE, Mascia A *et al.* Role of levetiracetam in the treatment of primary generalised epilepsy. *Epilepsia* 2004;**45 Suppl 3**:142.

184. Wolf P. Juvenile absence epilepsy. In Roger J, Bureau M, Dravet C, Dreifuss FE, Perret A, Wolf P, eds. *Epileptic syndromes in infancy, childhood and adolescence*, pp 307-12. London: John Libbey & Company, 1992.

185. Obeid T. Clinical and genetic aspects of juvenile absence epilepsy. *J Neurol* 1994;**241**:487-91.

186. Osservatorio Regionale per L'Epilessia (OREp), Lombardy. Osservatorio Regionale per L'Epilessia (OREp) L. ILAE classification of epilepsies: its applicability and practical value of different diagnostic categories. *Epilepsia* 1996;**37**:1051-9.

187. Doose H, Volzke E, Scheffner D. Verlaufsformen kindlicher epilepsien mit spike wave-absencen. *Arch Psychiatr Nervenkr* 1965;**207**:394-415.

188. Berkovic SF, Howell RA, Hay DA, Hopper JL. Epilepsies in twins. In Wolf P, ed. *Epileptic seizures and syndromes*, pp 157-64. London: John Libbey & Company Ltd, 1994.

189. Bianchi A, and the Italian LAE Collaborative Group. Study of concordance of symptoms in families with absence epilepsies. In Duncan JS, Panayiotopoulos CP, eds. *Typical absences and related epileptic syndromes*, pp 328-37. London: Churchill Communications Europe, 1995.

190. Durner M, Zhou G, Fu D, Abreu P, Shinnar S, Resor SR *et al.* Evidence for linkage of adolescent-onset idiopathic generalized epilepsies to chromosome 8-and genetic heterogeneity. *Am J Hum Genet.* 1999;**64**:1411-9.

191. Sander T, Hildmann T, Kretz R, Furst R, Sailer U, Bauer G *et al.* Allelic association of juvenile absence epilepsy with a GluR5 kainate receptor gene (GRIK1) polymorphism. *Am J Med Genet.* 1997;**74**:416-21.

192. Meencke HJ, Janz D. The significance of microdysgenesia in primary generalized epilepsy: an answer to the considerations of Lyon and Gastaut. *Epilepsia* 1985;**26**:368-71.

193. Gericke CA, Picard F, Saint-Martin A, Strumia S, Marescaux C, Hirsch E. Efficacy of lamotrigine in idiopathic generalized epilepsy syndromes: a video-EEG-controlled, open study. *Epileptic Disord.* 1999;**1**:159-65.

194. French JA, Kanner AM, Bautista J, Abou-Khalil B, Browne T, Harden CL *et al.* Efficacy and tolerability of the new antiepileptic drugs I: treatment of new onset epilepsy: report of the

Therapeutics and Technology Assessment Subcommittee and Quality Standards Subcommittee of the American Academy of Neurology and the American Epilepsy Society. *Neurology* 2004;**62**:1252-60.

195. Thomas P, Genton P, Wolf P. Juvenile myoclonic epilepsy. In Roger J, Bureau M, Dravet C, Genton P, Tassinari CA, Wolf P, eds. *Epileptic syndromes in infancy, childhood and adolescence (3rd edn)*, pp 335-56. London: John Libbey & Co Ltd, 2002.
196. Genton P, Gelisse P. Juvenile myoclonic epilepsy. *Arch Neurol* 2001;**58**:1487-90.
197. Panayiotopoulos CP. Juvenile myoclonic epilepsy: an uderdiagnosed syndrome. In Wolf P, ed. *Epileptic seizures and syndromes*, pp 221-30. London: John Libbey & Company Ltd, 1994.
198. Grunewald RA, Panayiotopoulos CP. Juvenile myoclonic epilepsy. A review. *Arch Neurol* 1993;**50**:594-8.
199. Delgado-Escueta AV, Enrile-Bacsal F. Juvenile myoclonic epilepsy of Janz. *Neurology* 1984;**34**:285-94.
200. Schmitz B, Sander T. Juvenile myoclonic epilepsy: the Janz syndrome. Petersfield, UK.: Wrightson Biomedical Publishing Ltd, 2000.
201. Janz D, Christian W. Impulsiv-Petit mal. Zeitschrift f Nervenheilkunde.1957;176:346-386. (Translated in English by Genton,P.). In Malafosse A, Genton P, Hirsch E, Marescaux C, Broglin D, Bernasconi R, eds. *Idiopathic generalised epilepsies*, pp 229-51. London: John Libbey & Company Ltd, 1957.
202. Gilliam F, Steinhoff BJ, Bittermann HJ, Kuzniecky R, Faught E, Abou-Khalil B. Adult myoclonic epilepsy: a distinct syndrome of idiopathic generalized epilepsy. *Neurology* 2000;**55**:1030-3.
203. Tsuboi T, Christian W. On the genetics of the primary generalised epilepsy with sporadic myoclonus of impulsive petit mal type. *Humangenetik 1973;***19**, 155-82.
204. Tsuboi T, Christian W. Epilepsy:A clinical, electroencephalographic and statistical study of 466 patients. 1976. Berlin, Springer.
205. Grunewald RA, Chroni E, Panayiotopoulos CP. Delayed diagnosis of juvenile myoclonic epilepsy. *J.Neurol Neurosurg Psychiatry* 1992;**55**:497-9.
206. Sander JW, Hart YM, Johnson AL, Shorvon SD. National General Practice Study of Epilepsy: newly diagnosed epileptic seizures in a general population. *Lancet* 1990;**336**:1267-71.
207. Manford M, Hart YM, Sander JW, Shorvon SD. The National General Practice Study of Epilepsy. The syndromic classification of the International League Against Epilepsy applied to epilepsy in a general population. *Arch Neurol.* 1992;**49**:801-8.
208. Oguni H, Mukahira K, Oguni M, Uehara T, Su YH, Izumi T *et al.* Video-polygraphic analysis of myoclonic seizures in juvenile myoclonic epilepsy. *Epilepsia* 1994;**35**:307-16.
209. Jain S, Padma MV, Maheshwari MC. Occurrence of only myoclonic jerks in juvenile myoclonic epilepsy. *Acta Neurol Scand* 1997;**95**:263-7.
210. Salas Puig J, Tunon A, Vidal JA, Mateos V, Guisasola LM, Lahoz CH. Janz's juvenile myoclonic epilepsy: a little-known frequent syndrome. A study of 85 patients. *Med.Clin.(Barc).* 1994;**103**:684-9.
211. Matsuoka H. A clinical and electroencephalographic study of juvenile myoclonic epilepsy: its pathophysiological considerations based on the findings obtained from neuropsychological EEG activation. *Seishin Shinkeigaku Zasshi.* 1989;**91**:318-46.
212. Matsuoka H, Takahashi T, Sasaki M, Yoshida S, Numachi Y, Sato M. The long-term course of seizure susceptibility in two patients with juvenile myoclonic epilepsy. *Seizure* 2002;**11**:126-30.
213. Mayer T, Wolf P. Reading epilepsy: clinical and genetic background. In Berkovic SF, Genton P, Hirsch E, Picard F, eds. *Genetics of focal epilepsies*, pp 159-68. London: John Libbey and Company Ltd, 1999.
214. Chifari R, Piazzini A, Turner K, Canger R, Canevini MP, Wolf P. Reflex writing seizures in two siblings with juvenile myoclonic epilepsy. *Acta Neurol Scand.* 2004;**109**:232-5.
215. Panayiotopoulos CP, Obeid T. Juvenile myoclonic epilepsy: an autosomal recessive disease. *Ann Neurol.* 1989;**25**:440-3.
216. Canevini MP, Mai R, Di Marco C, Bertin C, Minotti L, Pontrelli V *et al.* Juvenile myoclonic epilepsy of Janz: clinical observations in 60 patients. *Seizure* 1992;**1**:291-8.
217. Janz D. Juvenile myoclonic epilepsy. Epilepsy with impulsive petit mal. *Cleve Clin J Med.* 1989;**56 Suppl Pt 1**::S23-33; discussion S40-2.
218. Serratosa JM, Delgado-Escueta AV, Medina MT, Zhang Q, Iranmanesh R, Sparkes RS. Clinical and genetic analysis of a large pedigree with juvenile myoclonic epilepsy. *Ann Neurol* 1996;**39**:187-95.
219. Delgado-Escueta AV, Greenberg D, Weissbecker K, Liu A, Treiman L, Sparkes R *et al.* Gene mapping in the idiopathic generalized epilepsies: juvenile myoclonic epilepsy, childhood absence epilepsy, epilepsy with grand mal seizures, and early childhood myoclonic epilepsy. *Epilepsia* 1990;**31 Suppl 3**:S19-29.
220. Elmslie FV, Rees M, Williamson MP, Kerr M, Kjeldsen MJ, Pang KA *et al.* Genetic mapping of a major susceptibility locus for juvenile myoclonic epilepsy on chromosome 15q. *Hum Mol Genet.* 1997;**6**:1329-34.
221. Taske NL, Williamson MP, Makoff A, Bate L, Curtis D, Kerr M *et al.* Evaluation of the positional candidate gene CHRNA7 at the juvenile myoclonic epilepsy locus (EJM2) on chromosome 15q13-14. *Epilepsy Res.* 2002;**49**:157-72.
222. Suzuki T, Ganesh S, Agarwala KL, Morita R, Sugimoto Y, Inazawa J *et al.* A novel gene in the chromosomal region for juvenile myoclonic epilepsy on 6p12 encodes a brain-specific lysosomal membrane protein. *Biochem Biophys Res Commun.* 2001;**288**:626-36.
223. Pal DK, Evgrafov OV, Tabares P, Zhang F, Durner M, Greenberg DA. BRD2 (RING3) is a probable major susceptibility gene for common juvenile myoclonic epilepsy. *Am J Hum Genet.* 2003;**73**:261-70.
224. Greenberg DA, Durner M, Shinnar S, Resor S, Rosenbaum D, Klotz I *et al.* Association of HLA class II alleles in patients with juvenile myoclonic epilepsy compared with patients with other forms of adolescent-onset generalized epilepsy. *Neurology* 1996;**47**:750-5.
225. Obeid T, el Rab MO, Daif AK, Panayiotopoulos CP, Halim K, Bahakim H *et al.* Is HLA-DRW13 (W6) associated with juvenile myoclonic epilepsy in Arab patients? *Epilepsia* 1994;**35**:319-21.
226. Le Hellard S, Neidhart E, Thomas P, Feingold J, Malafosse A, Tafti M. Lack of association between juvenile myoclonic epilepsy and HLA- DR13. *Epilepsia* 1999;**40**:117-9.
227. Taylor I, Marini C, Johnson MR, Turner S, Berkovic SF, Scheffer IE. Juvenile myoclonic epilepsy and idiopathic photosensitive occipital lobe epilepsy: is there overlap? *Brain* 2004;**127**:1878-86.
228. Woermann FG, Free SL, Koepp MJ, Sisodiya SM, Duncan JS. Abnormal cerebral structure in juvenile myoclonic epilepsy demonstrated with voxel-based analysis of MRI. *Brain* 1999;**122**:2101-8.
229. Montalenti E, Imperiale D, Rovera A, Bergamasco B, Benna P. Clinical features, EEG findings and diagnostic pitfalls in juvenile myoclonic epilepsy: a series of 63 patients. *J Neurol Sci.* 2001;**184**:65-70.
230. Panayiotopoulos CP, Tahan R, Obeid T. Juvenile myoclonic epilepsy: factors of error involved in the diagnosis and treatment. *Epilepsia* 1991;**32**:672-6.
231. Penry JK, Dean JC, Riela AR. Juvenile myoclonic epilepsy: long-term response to therapy. *Epilepsia* 1989;**30 Suppl 4**:S19-23; discussion S24-7.
232. Gelisse P, Genton P, Thomas P, Rey M, Samuelian JC, Dravet C. Clinical factors of drug resistance in juvenile myoclonic epilepsy. *J Neurol Neurosurg Psychiatry* 2001;**70**:240-3.
233. Faught E. Clinical trials for treatment of primary generalized epilepsies. *Epilepsia* 2003;**44 Suppl 7**:44-50.
234. Greenhill L, Betts T, Smith K. Effect of levetiracetam on resistant juvenile myoclonic epilepsy. *Epilepsia* 2002;**43 Suppl 7**:179.
235. Resor, S. R. and Resor, L. D. Levetiracetam monotherapy in the treatment of convulsive seizures in juvenile myoclonic epilepsy. American Academy Neurology, 54th annual meeting, April 2002
236. Jongsma M, Janssen G, Engelsman M, Haan D. Promising results of levetiracetam in juvenile myoclonic epilepsy. *Epilepsia* 2002;**43 Suppl 8S**:153.
237. Calleja S, Salas-Puig J, Ribacoba R, Lahoz CH. Evolution of juvenile myoclonic epilepsy treated from the outset with sodium valproate. *Seizure* 2001;**10**:424-7.
238. Sundqvist A, Nilsson BY, Tomson T. Valproate monotherapy in juvenile myoclonic epilepsy: dose- related effects on

electroencephalographic and other neurophysiologic tests. *Ther Drug Monit.* 1999;**21**:91-6.

239. Morrell MJ. Guidelines for the care of women with epilepsy. *Neurology* 1998;**51**:S21-S27.
240. Crawford P, Appleton R, Betts T, Duncan J, Guthrie E, Morrow J. Best practice guidelines for the management of women with epilepsy. The Women with Epilepsy Guidelines Development Group. *Seizure* 1999;**8**:201-17.
241. Yerby MS. Management issues for women with epilepsy: neural tube defects and folic acid supplementation. *Neurology* 2003;**61**:S23-S26.
242. Tatum WO, Liporace J, Benbadis SR, Kaplan PW. Updates on the treatment of epilepsy in women. *Arch Intern Med.* 2004;**164**:137-45.
243. Wyszynski DF, Holmes LB. The AED (antiepileptic drug) pregnancy registry: a six year experience. *Epilepsia* 2004;**45 Suppl 3**:56.
244. Morrow JI, Russell AJC, Irwin B, Guthrie E, Morrison P *et al.* The safety of antiepileptic drugs in pregancy: results of the UK epilepsy and pregnancy register. Epilepsia 2004; **45 Suppl 3**:57.
245. Isojarvi JI, Tauboll E, Tapanainen JS, Pakarinen AJ, Laatikainen TJ, Knip M *et al.* On the association between valproate and poycystic ovary syndrome:A response and an alternative view. *Epilepsia* 2001;**42**:305-10.
246. French JA, Kanner AM, Bautista J, Abou-Khalil B, Browne T, Harden CL *et al.* Efficacy and tolerability of the new antiepileptic drugs II: treatment of refractory epilepsy: report of the Therapeutics and Technology Assessment Subcommittee and Quality Standards Subcommittee of the American Academy of Neurology and the American Epilepsy Society. *Neurology* 2004;**62**:1261-73.
247. French JA, Kanner AM, Bautista J, Abou-Khalil B, Browne T, Harden CL *et al.* Efficacy and Tolerability of the New Antiepileptic Drugs, II: Treatment of Refractory Epilepsy: Report of the TTA and QSS Subcommittees of the American Academy of Neurology and the American Epilepsy Society. *Epilepsia* 2004;**45**:410-23.
248. Montouris G. Gabapentin exposure in human pregnancy: results from the Gabapentin Pregnancy Registry. *Epilepsy Behav.* 2003;**4**:310-7.
249. Tennis P, Eldridge RR. Preliminary results on pregnancy outcomes in women using lamotrigine. *Epilepsia* 2002;**43**:1161-7.
250. Long L. Levetiracetam monotherapy during pregnancy: a case series. *Epilepsy Behav.* 2003;**4**:447-8.
251. Tomson T, Perucca E, Battino D. Navigating toward fetal and maternal health: the challenge of treating epilepsy in pregnancy. *Epilepsia* 2004;**45**:1171-5.
252. Cunnington MC. The international lamotrigine pregnancy registry update for the epilepsy foundation. *Epilepsia* 2004;**45**:1468.
253. Obeid T, Panayiotopoulos CP. Clonazepam in juvenile myoclonic epilepsy. *Epilepsia* 1989;**30**:603-6.
254. Van Zandijcke M. Treatment of myoclonus. *Acta Neurol Belg* 2003;**103**:66-70.
255. Wheless JW, Sankar R. Treatment Strategies for Myoclonic Seizures and Epilepsy Syndromes with Myoclonic Seizures. *Epilepsia* 2003;**44 Suppl 11**:27-37.
256. Canadian Study Group for Childhood Epilepsy. Clobazam has equivalent efficacy to carbamazepine and phenytoin as monotherapy for childhood epilepsy. *Epilepsia* 1998;**39**:952-9.
257. Resor SR, Jr., Resor LD. Chronic acetazolamide monotherapy in the treatment of juvenile myoclonic epilepsy. *Neurology* 1990;**40**:1677-81.
258. Buchanan N. The use of lamotrigine in juvenile myoclonic epilepsy. *Seizure* 1996;**5**:149-51.
259. Isojarvi JI, Rattya J, Myllyla VV, Knip M, Koivunen R, Pakarinen AJ *et al.* Valproate, lamotrigine, and insulin-mediated risks in women with epilepsy. *Ann Neurol.* 1998;**43**:446-51.
260. Cohen J. Levetiracetam monotherapy for primary generalised epilepsy. *Seizure* 2003;**12**:150-3.
261. Covanis A, Katsalouli M. Levetiracetam monotherapy in generalised epilepsy and photosensitivity. *Epilepsia* 2003;**44 Suppl 8**:80.
262. Gelisse P, Crespel A, Genton P, Baldy-Moulinier M. Dramatic effect of levetiracetam on epileptic negative myoclonus. *Acta Neurol Scand.* 2003;**107**:302-3.
263. Kasteleijn-Nolst Trenite DG, Hirsch E. Levetiracetam: preliminary efficacy in generalized seizures. *Epileptic Disord.* 2003;**5 Suppl 1**:S39-S44.
264. Krauss GL, Betts T, Abou-Khalil B, Bergey G, Yarrow H, Miller A. Levetiracetam treatment of idiopathic generalised epilepsy. *Seizure* 2003;**12**:617-20.
265. Gallagher MJ, Eisenman LN, Brown KM, Erbayat-Altay E, Hecimovic H, Fessler AJ *et al.* Levetiracetam Reduces Spike-Wave Density and Duration during Continuous EEG Monitoring in Patients with Idiopathic Generalized Epilepsy. *Epilepsia* 2004;**45**:90-1.
266. Nieto BM. Characteristics and indications of topiramate. *Rev Neurol.* 2002;**35 Suppl 1**:S88-S95.
267. Prasad A, Knowlton RC, Mendez M, Martin R, Kuzniecky R, Faught E. A comparison of lamotrigine and topiramate in juvenile myoclonic epilepsy. *Epilepsia* 2002;**43 Suppl 7**:198-9.
268. Wallace SJ. Myoclonus and epilepsy in childhood: a review of treatment with valproate, ethosuximide, lamotrigine and zonisamide. *Epilepsy Res.* 1998;**29**:147-54.
269. Fattouch J, Di Bonaventura C, Mari F, Egeo, G, Vaudano, A E, Mascia, A, Giallonardo AT, Manfredi M. Role of levetiracetam in the treatment of primary generalised epilepsy. Epilepsia 2004; **45 Suppl 3**:142.
270. Arroyo S, Crawford P. Safety profile of levetiracetam. *Epileptic Disord.* 2003;**5 Suppl 1**:S57-S63.
271. French JA, Kanner AM, Bautista J, Abou-Khalil B, Browne T, Harden CL *et al.* Efficacy and Tolerability of the New Antiepileptic Drugs, I: Treatment of New-Onset Epilepsy: Report of the TTA and QSS Subcommittees of the American Academy of Neurology and the American Epilepsy Society. *Epilepsia* 2004;**45**:401-9.
272. Czapinski, P. P. and Czapinska, E. M. The effectiveness of levetiracetam in drug-resistant juvenile myoclonic epilepsy. *Epilepsia* 2004;**45 Suppl 3**:141.
273. La Neve A, Boero G, Specchio N, Santasabato M, De Paolo A *et al.* Levetiracetam is effective in juvenile myoclonic epilepsy. Epilepsia 2004;**45 Suppl 3**: 141.
274. Agarwal P, Frucht SJ. Myoclonus. *Curr Opin Neurol.* 2003;**16**:515-21.
275. Crest C, Dupont S, LeGuern E, Adam C, Baulac M. Levetiracetam in progressive myoclonic epilepsy: an exploratory study in 9 patients. *Neurology* 2004;**62**:640-3.
276. Genton P, Gelisse P. Antimyoclonic effect of levetiracetam. *Epileptic Disord.* 2000;**2**:209-12.
277. Frucht SJ, Louis ED, Chuang C, Fahn S. A pilot tolerability and efficacy study of levetiracetam in patients with chronic myoclonus. *Neurology* 2001;**57**:1112-4.
278. Krauss GL, Bergin A, Kramer RE, Cho YW, Reich SG. Suppression of post-hypoxic and post-encephalitic myoclonus with levetiracetam. *Neurology* 2001;**56**:411-2.
279. Schauer R, Singer M, Saltuari L, Kofler M. Suppression of cortical myoclonus by levetiracetam. *Mov Disord.* 2002;**17**:411-5.
280. Guerrini R, Genton P. Epileptic syndromes and visually induced seizures. *Epilepsia* 2004;**45 Suppl 1**:14-8.
281. De Bittencourt PR. Photosensitivity: the magnitude of the problem. *Epilepsia* 2004;**45 Suppl 1**:30-4.
282. Kasteleijn-Nolst Trenite DG, Marescaux C, Stodieck S, Edelbroek PM, Oosting J. Photosensitive epilepsy: a model to study the effects of antiepileptic drugs. Evaluation of the piracetam analogue, levetiracetam. *Epilepsy Res.* 1996;**25**:225-30.
283. Covanis A, Stodieck SR, Wilkins AJ. Treatment of photosensitivity. *Epilepsia* 2004;**45 Suppl 1**:40-5.
284. Cramer JA, De Rue K, Devinsky O, Edrich P, Trimble MR. A systematic review of the behavioral effects of levetiracetam in adults with epilepsy, cognitive disorders, or an anxiety disorder during clinical trials. *Epilepsy Behav.* 2003;**4**:124-32.
285. Huber B, Bommel W, Hauser I, Horstmann V, Liem S, May T *et al.* Efficacy and tolerability of levetiracetam in patients with therapy-resistant epilepsy and learning disabilities. *Seizure* 2004;**13**:168-75.
286. Mula M, Trimble MR, Sander JW. Psychiatric adverse events in patients with epilepsy and learning disabilities taking levetiracetam. *Seizure* 2004;**13**:55-7.
287. Besag FM. Behavioral aspects of pediatric epilepsy syndromes. *Epilepsy Behav.* 2004;**5 Suppl 1**:S3-13.

288. Biraben A, Allain H, Scarabin JM, Schuck S, Edan G. Exacerbation of juvenile myoclonic epilepsy with lamotrigine. *Neurology* 2000;**55**:1758.

289. Carrazana EJ, Wheeler SD. Exacerbation of juvenile myoclonic epilepsy with lamotrigine. *Neurology* 2001;**56**:1424-5.

290. Genton P, Bauer J, Duncan S, Taylor AE, Balen AH, Eberle A *et al.* On the association between valproate and poycystic ovary syndrome. *Epilepsia* 2001;**42**:295-304.

291. Prasad A, Kuzniecky RI, Knowlton RC, Welty TE, Martin RC, Mendez M *et al.* Evolving antiepileptic drug treatment in juvenile myoclonic epilepsy. *Arch Neurol.* 2003;**60**:1100-5.

292. Grunewald RA, Genton P, Salas Puig J, Panayiotopoulos CP. Evolving antiepileptic drug treatment in juvenile myoclonic epilepsy. *Arch Neurol.* 2004;**61**:1328-9

293. Ferrie CD, Robinson RO, Knott C, Panayiotopoulos CP. Lamotrigine as an add-on drug in typical absence seizures. *Acta Neurol Scand.* 1995;**91**:200-2.

294. Reutens DC, Duncan JS, Patsalos PN. Disabling tremor after lamotrigine with sodium valproate. *Lancet* 1993;**342**:185-6.

295. Panayiotopoulos CP. Beneficial effect of relatively small doses of lamotrigine. *Epilepsia* 1999;**40**:1171-2.

296. Binnie CD, van Emde BW, Kasteleijn-Nolste-Trenite DG, de Korte RA, Meijer JW, Meinardi H *et al.* Acute effects of lamotrigine (BW430C) in persons with epilepsy. *Epilepsia* 1986;**27**:248-54.

297. Nicolson A, Appleton RE, Chadwick DW, Smith DF. The relationship between treatment with valproate, lamotrigine, and topiramate and the prognosis of the idiopathic generalised epilepsies. *J Neurol Neurosurg Psychiatry* 2004;**75**:75-9.

298. Salas PX, Calleja S, Jimenez L, Gonzalez DM. Juvenile myoclonic epilepsy. *Rev Neurol* 2001;**32**:957-61.

299. Biton V, Montouris GD, Ritter F, Riviello JJ, Reife R, Lim P *et al.* A randomized, placebo-controlled study of topiramate in primary generalized tonic-clonic seizures. Topiramate YTC Study Group. *Neurology* 1999;**52**:1330-7.

300. Waugh J, Goa KL. Topiramate: as monotherapy in newly diagnosed epilepsy. *CNS Drugs* 2003;**17**:985-92.

301. Privitera MD, Brodie MJ, Mattson RH, Chadwick DW, Neto W, Wang S. Topiramate, carbamazepine and valproate monotherapy: double-blind comparison in newly diagnosed epilepsy. *Acta Neurol Scand.* 2003;**107**:165-75.

302. Wheless JW, Neto W, Wang S. Topiramate, carbamazepine, and valproate monotherapy: double-blind comparison in children with newly diagnosed epilepsy. *J Child Neurol* 2004;**19**:135-41.

303. Cross JH. Topiramate monotherapy for childhood absence seizures: an open label pilot study. *Seizure* 2002;**11**:406-10.

304. Aldenkamp AP, Baker G, Mulder OG, Chadwick D, Cooper P, Doelman J *et al.* A multicenter, randomized clinical study to evaluate the effect on cognitive function of topiramate compared with valproate as add-on therapy to carbamazepine in patients with partial-onset seizures. *Epilepsia* 2000;**41**:1167-78.

305. Kockelmann E, Elger CE, Helmstaedter C. Significant improvement in frontal lobe associated neuropsychological functions after withdrawal of topiramate in epilepsy patients. *Epilepsy Res.* 2003;**54**:171-8.

306. Patsalos PN, Perucca E. Clinically important drug interactions in epilepsy: interactions between antiepileptic drugs and other drugs. *Lancet Neurol.* 2003;**2**:473-81.

307. Jain KK. An assessment of zonisamide as an anti-epileptic drug. *Expert Opin Pharmacother.* 2000;**1**:1245-60.

308. Glauser TA, Pellock JM. Zonisamide in pediatric epilepsy: review of the Japanese experience. *J Child Neurol.* 2002;**17**:87-96.

309. Newmark ME, Dubinsky S. Zonisamide monotherapy in a multi-group clinic. *Seizure* 2004;**13**:223-5.

310. Sullivan JE, Dlugos DJ. Idiopathic Generalized Epilepsy. *Curr Treat Options Neurol.* 2004;**6**:231-42.

311. Panayiotopoulos CP. Juvenile myoclonic epilepsy. In Panayiotopoulos CP, ed. *A clinical guide to epileptic syndromes and their treatment*, pp 139-45. Oxford: Bladon Medical Publishing, 2002.

312. Genton P, Gelisse P, Thomas P, Dravet C. Do carbamazepine and phenytoin aggravate juvenile myoclonic epilepsy? *Neurology* 2000;**55**:1106-9.

313. Knott C, Panayiotopoulos CP. Carbamazepine in the treatment of generalised tonic clonic seizures in juvenile myoclonic epilepsy. *J Neurol Neurosurg Psychiatr* 1994;**57**:503.

314. Gelisse P, Genton P, Kuate D, Pesenti A, Baldy-Moulinier M, Crespel A. Worsening of seizures by oxcarbazepine in juvenile idiopathic generalized epilepsies. *Epilepsia* 2004;**45**:1282-8.

315. Janz D. Die epilepsien:Spezielle pathologie and therapie. Stuttgart: Georg Thieme, 1969.

316. Janz D. Pitfalls in the diagnosis of grand mal on awakening. In Wolf P, ed. *Epileptic seizures and syndromes*, pp 213-20. London: John Libbey & Company Ltd, 1994.

317. Janz D. Epilepsy with grand mal on awakening and sleep-waking cycle. *Clin Neurophysiol* 2000;**111 Suppl 2**:S103-S110.

318. Greenberg DA, Durner M, Resor S, Rosenbaum D, Shinnar S. The genetics of idiopathic generalized epilepsies of adolescent onset: differences between juvenile myoclonic epilepsy and epilepsy with random grand mal and with awakening grand mal. *Neurology* 1995;**45**:942-6.

319. Ferrie CD, Panayiotopoulos CP. Idiopathic generalised epilepsy with generalised tonic clonic seizures on awakening. In Wallace SJ, Farrell K, eds. *Epilepsy in Children (2nd edition)*, pp 219-30. London: Edward Arnold (Publishers) Limited, 2004.

320. Roger J, Bureau M, Oller Ferrer-Vidal L, Oller-Daurella L, Saltarelli A, Genton P. Clinical and electroencephalographic characteristics of idiopathic generalised epilepsies. In Malafosse A, Genton P, Hirsch E, Marescaux C, Broglin D, Bernasconi R, eds. *Idiopathic generalised epilepsies*, pp 7-18. London: John Libbey & Company Ltd, 1994.

321. Oller-Daurella LF-V,Oller L. 5000 epilepticos. Clinica y evolucion. Barcelona, Ciba-Geigy. 1994.

322. Reutens DC, Berkovic SF. Idiopathic generalized epilepsy of adolescence: are the syndromes clinically distinct? *Neurology* 1995;**45**:1469-76.

323. Meencke HJ, Janz D, Cervos-Navarro J. Neuropathology of primary generalized epilepsies with awakening grand mal. *Acta Neuropathol.Suppl (Berl)* 1981;**7**:378-80.

324. Baier WK, Doose H. Petit mal-absences of childhood onset: familial prevalences of migraine and seizures. *Neuropediatrics* 1985;**16**:80-3.

325. Doose H. Absence epilepsy of early childhood—genetic aspects. *Eur J Pediatr.* 1994;**153**:372-7.

326. Doose H. Absence epilepsy of early childhood. In Wolf P, ed. *Epileptic seizures and syndromes*, pp 133-5. London: John Libbey & Company Ltd, 1994.

327. Chaix Y, Daquin G, Monteiro F, Villeneuve N, Laguitton V, Genton P. Absence epilepsy with onset before age three years: a heterogeneous and often severe condition. *Epilepsia* 2003;**44**:944-9.

328. Panayiotopoulos CP, Ferrie CD, Giannakodimos S, Robinson RO. Perioral myoclonia with absences: a new syndrome. In Wolf P, ed. *Epileptic seizures and syndromes*, pp 143-53. London: John Libbey & Company Ltd, 1994.

329. Hirsch E. Perioral myoclonia with absences. In Duncan JS, Panayiotopoulos CP, eds. *Typical absences and related epileptic syndromes*, p 230. London: Churchill Communications Europe, 1995.

330. Clemens B. Perioral myoclonia with absences? A case report with EEG and voltage mapping analysis. *Brain Dev.* 1997;**19**:353-8.

331. Bilgic B, Baykan B, Gurses C, Gokyigit A. Perioral myoclonia with absence seizures: a rare epileptic syndrome. *Epileptic Disord.* 2001;**3**:23-7.

332. Aarts JH, Binnie CD, Smit AM, Wilkins AJ. Selective cognitive impairment during focal and generalized epileptiform EEG activity. *Brain* 1984;**107**:293-308.

333. Kasteleijn-Nolst Trenite DG. Transient cognitive impairment during subclinical epileptiform electroencephalographic discharges. *Semin Pediatr Neurol* 1995;**2**:246-53.

334. Giannakodimos S, Ferrie CD, Panayiotopoulos CP. Qualitative and quantitative abnormalities of breath counting during brief generalized 3 Hz spike and slow wave 'subclinical' discharges. *Clin Electroencephalogr* 1995;**26**:200-3.

335. Marsall C. Some clinical correlates of the wave and spike phantom. *Electroencephalogr Clin Neurophysiol* 1955;**7**:633-6.

336. Tharp BR. The 6-per-second spike and wave complex. The wave and spike phantom. *Arch Neurol* 1966;**15**:533-7.

337. Silverman, D. Phantom spike-waves and the fourteen and six per second positive spike pattern: a consideration of their relation. *Electroencephalograph Clin Neurophysiol* 1967; *23*: 207-13.

338. Genton P. Epilepsy with 3Hz spike-and-waves without clinically evideent absences. In Duncan JS, Panayiotopoulos CP, eds. *Typical absences and related epileptic syndromes*, pp 231-8. London: Churchill Communications Europe, 1995.

339. Vuilleumier P, Assal F, Blanke O, Jallon P. Distinct behavioral and EEG topographic correlates of loss of consciousness in absences. *Epilepsia* 2000;**41**:687-93.

340. Panayiotopoulos CP. Epilepsy with generalised tonic-clonic seizures on awakening. In Wallace S, ed. *Epilepsy in Children*, pp 349-53. London: Chapman & Hall, 1996.

341. Cutting S, Lauchheimer A, Barr W, Devinsky O. Adult-onset idiopathic generalized epilepsy: clinical and behavioral features. *Epilepsia* 2001;**42**:1395-8.

342. Marini C, King MA, Archer JS, Newton MR, Berkovic SF. Idiopathic generalised epilepsy of adult onset: clinical syndromes and genetics. *J Neurol Neurosurg Psychiatry* 2003;**74**:192-6.

343. Yenjun S, Harvey AS, Marini C, Newton MR, King MA, Berkovic SF. EEG in adult-onset idiopathic generalized epilepsy. *Epilepsia* 2003;**44**:252-6.

344. Nicolson A, Chadwick DW, Smith DF. A comparison of adult onset and "classical" idiopathic generalised epilepsy. *J Neurol Neurosurg Psychiatry* 2004;**75**:72-4.

345. Okino S. Familial benign myoclonus epilepsy of adult onset: a previously unrecognized myoclonic disorder. *J Neurol Sc* 1997;**145**:113-8.

346. Mikami M, Yasuda T, Terao A, Nakamura M, Ueno S, Tanabe H *et al.* Localization of a gene for benign adult familial myoclonic epilepsy to chromosome 8q23.3-q24.1. *Am J Hum Genet.* 1999;**65**:745-51.

347. Plaster NM, Uyama E, Uchino M, Ikeda T, Flanigan KM, Kondo I *et al.* Genetic localization of the familial adult myoclonic epilepsy (FAME) gene to chromosome 8q24. *Neurology* 1999;**53**:1180-3.

348. Saka E, Saygi S. Familial adult onset myoclonic epilepsy associated with migraine. *Seizure* 2000;**9**:344-6.

349. Labauge P, Amer LO, Simonetta-Moreau M, Attane F, Tannier C, Clanet M *et al.* Absence of linkage to 8q24 in a European family with familial adult myoclonic epilepsy (FAME). *Neurology* 2002;**58**:941-4.

350. Manabe Y, Narai H, Warita H, Hayashi T, Shiro Y, Sakai K *et al.* Benign adult familial myoclonic epilepsy (BAFME) with night blindness. *Seizure* 2002;**11**:266-8.

351. de Falco FA, Striano P, de Falco A, Striano S, Santangelo R, Perretti A *et al.* Benign adult familial myoclonic epilepsy: genetic heterogeneity and allelism with ADCME. *Neurology* 2003;**60**:1381-5.

352. Shimizu A, Asakawa S, Sasaki T, Yamazaki S, Yamagata H, Kudoh J *et al.* A novel giant gene CSMD3 encoding a protein with CUB and sushi multiple domains: a candidate gene for benign adult familial myoclonic epilepsy on human chromosome 8q23.3-q24.1. *Biochem Biophys Res Commun.* 2003;**309**:143-54.

353. Striano P, Chifari R, Striano S, De Fusco M, Elia M, Guerrini R *et al.* A New Benign Adult Familial Myoclonic Epilepsy (BAFME) Pedigree Suggesting Linkage to Chromosome 2p11.1-q12.2. *Epilepsia* 2004;**45**:190-2.

354. Guerrini R, Bonanni P, Patrignani A, Brown P, Parmeggiani L, Grosse P *et al.* Autosomal dominant cortical myoclonus and epilepsy (ADCME) with complex partial and generalized seizures: A newly recognized epilepsy syndrome with linkage to chromosome 2p11.1-q12.2. *Brain* 2001;**124**:2459-75.

355. Sano A, Mikami M, Nakamura M, Ueno S, Tanabe H, Kaneko S. Positional candidate approach for the gene responsible for benign adult familial myoclonic epilepsy. *Epilepsia* 2002;**43 Suppl 9**:26-31.

356. Zara F, Gennaro E, Stabile M, Carbone I, Malacarne M, Majello L *et al.* Mapping of a locus for a familial autosomal recessive idiopathic myoclonic epilepsy of infancy to chromosome 16p13. *Am J Hum Genet.* 2000;**66**:1552-7.

357. de Falco FA, Majello L, Santangelo R, Stabile M, Bricarelli FD, Zara F. Familial infantile myoclonic epilepsy: clinical features in a large kindred with autosomal recessive inheritance. *Epilepsia* 2001;**42**:1541-8.

358. Parker AP, Agathonikou A, Robinson RO, Panayiotopoulos CP. Inappropriate use of carbamazepine and vigabatrin in typical absence seizures. *Dev Med Child Neurol.* 1998;**40**:517-9.

359. Panayiotopoulos CP, Benbadis SR, Covanis A, Dulac O, Duncan JS, Eeg-Olofsson O *et al.* Efficacy and tolerability of the new antiepileptic drugs; commentary on the recently published practice parameters. *Epilepsia* 2004;**45**:1646-9.

360. Bourgeois BF. Chronic management of seizures in the syndromes of idiopathic generalized epilepsy. *Epilepsia* 2003;**44 Suppl 2**:27-32.

361. Posner EB, Mohamed K, Marson AG. Ethosuximide, sodium valproate or lamotrigine for absence seizures in children and adolescents. *Cochrane Database Syst Rev.* 2003;CD003032.

362. Mattson RH. Overview: idiopathic generalized epilepsies. *Epilepsia* 2003;**44 Suppl 2**:2-6.

363. Wheless JW. Acute management of seizures in the syndromes of idiopathic generalized epilepsies. *Epilepsia* 2003;**44 Suppl 2**:22-6.

364. Hirsch E, Genton P. Antiepileptic drug-induced pharmacodynamic aggravation of seizures: does valproate have a lower potential? *CNS Drugs* 2003;**17**:633-40.

365. Gelisse P, Genton P, Kuate D, Pesenti A, Baldy-Moulinier M, Crespel A. Worsening of seizures by oxcarbazepine in juvenile idiopathic generalised epilepsies. *Epilepsia* 2004;**45**:1282-8.

366. Genton P. When antiepileptic drugs aggravate epilepsy. *Brain Dev.* 2000;**22**:75-80.

367. Kasteleijn-Nolst Trenite DG, Marescaux C, Stodieck S, Edelbroek PM, Oosting J. Photosensitive epilepsy: a model to study the effects of antiepileptic drugs. Evaluation of the piracetam analogue, levetiracetam. *Epilepsy Res* 1996;**25**:225-30.

368. Klitgaard H, Matagne A, Gobert J, Wulfert E. Evidence for a unique profile of levetiracetam in rodent models of seizures and epilepsy. *Eur.J.Pharmacol.* 1998;**353**:191-206.

369. Montouris G, Biton V, Rosenfeld W, and the Topiramate YTC/YTCE study group. Nonfocal generalized tonic-clonic seizures:Response during long-trem topiramate treatment. *Epilepsia* 2000;**41 Suppl 1**:S77-S81.

370. Siren A, Eriksson K, Jalava H, Kilpinen-Loisa P, Koivikko M. Idiopathic generalised epilepsies with 3 Hz and faster spike wave discharges: a population-based study with evaluation and long-term follow-up in 71 patients. *Epileptic Disord.* 2002;**4**:209-16.

371. Shorvon, S. Handbook of epilepsy treatment. Oxford, Blackwell Science.2000.

372. Chadwick D, Leiderman DB, Sauermann W, Alexander J, Garofalo E. Gabapentin in generalized seizures. *Epilepsy Res* 1996;**25**:191-7.

373. Trudeau V, Myers S, LaMoreaux L, Anhut H, Garofalo E, Ebersole J. Gabapentin in naive childhood absence epilepsy: results from two double-blind, placebo-controlled, multicenter studies. *J Child Neurol* 1996;**11**:470-5.

374. Scott RC, Neville BG. Pharmacological management of convulsive status epilepticus in children. *Dev Med Child Neurol* 1999;**41**:207-10.

375. Smith BJ. Treatment of status epilepticus. *Neurol Clin.* 2001;**19**:347-69.

376. Lowenstein DH, Alldredge BK, Allen F, Neuhaus J, Corry M, Gottwald M *et al.* The prehospital treatment of status epilepticus (PHTSE) study: design and methodology. *Control Clin Trials* 2001;**22**:290-309.

377. Shorvon S. The management of status epilepticus. *J Neurol Neurosurg Psychiatry* 2001;**70 Suppl 2**:II22-II27.

378. Alldredge BK, Gelb AM, Isaacs SM, Corry MD, Allen F, Ulrich S *et al.* A comparison of lorazepam, diazepam, and placebo for the treatment of out-of-hospital status epilepticus. *NEJM* 2001;**345**:631-7.

379. Hirsch LJ, Claassen J. The current state of treatment of status epilepticus. *Curr Neurol Neurosci Rep.* 2002;**2**:345-56.

380. Appleton R, Martland T, Phillips B. Drug management for acute tonic-clonic convulsions including convulsive status epilepticus in children. *Cochrane Database Syst Rev.* 2002;CD001905.

381. Claassen J, Hirsch LJ, Emerson RG, Mayer SA. Treatment of refractory status epilepticus with pentobarbital, propofol, or midazolam: a systematic review. *Epilepsia* 2002;**43**:146-53.

382. Claassen J, Hirsch LJ, Mayer SA. Treatment of status epilepticus: a survey of neurologists. *J.Neurol Sci.* 2003;**211**:37-41.

383. Gaitanis JN, Drislane FW. Status epilepticus: a review of different syndromes, their current evaluation, and treatment. *Neurolog.* 2003;**9**:61-76.

384. Manno EM. New management strategies in the treatment of status epilepticus. *Mayo Clin.Proc.* 2003;**78**:508-18.

385. Ruegg SJ, Dichter MA. Diagnosis and Treatment of Nonconvulsive Status Epilepticus in an Intensive Care Unit Setting. *Curr Treat Options Neurol.* 2003;**5**:93-110.

386. Sirven JI, Waterhouse E. Management of status epilepticus. *Am Fam Physician* 2003;**68**:469-76.

387. Walker MC. Status epilepticus on the intensive care unit. *J Neurol.* 2003;**250**:401-6.

388. Lowenstein DH. Treatment options for status epilepticus. *Curr Opin Pharmacol.* 2003;**3**:6-11.

389. De Negri M, Baglietto MG. Treatment of status epilepticus in children. *Paediatr Drugs* 2001;**3**:411-20.

390. Walker MC. Diagnosis and treatment of nonconvulsive status epilepticus. *CNS Drugs* 2001;**15**:931-9.

391. Fitzgerald BJ, Okos AJ, Miller JW. Treatment of out-of-hospital status epilepticus with diazepam rectal gel. *Seizure* 2003;**12**:52-5.

392. Scott RC, Besag FM, Neville BG. Buccal midazolam and rectal diazepam for treatment of prolonged seizures in childhood and adolescence: a randomised trial . *Lancet* 1999;**353**:623-6.

393. Kutlu NO, Dogrul M, Yakinci C, Soylu H. Buccal midazolam for treatment of prolonged seizures in children. *Brain Dev.* 2003;**25**:275-8.

394. Lahat E, Goldman M, Barr J, Bistritzer T, Berkovitch M. Comparison of intranasal midazolam with intravenous diazepam for treating febrile seizures in children: prospective randomised study. *BMJ* 2000;**321**:83-6.

11

FAMILIAL (AUTOSOMAL DOMINANT) FOCAL EPILEPSIES

In the past two decades, significant progress in molecular and statistical genetics have led to breakthroughs in the mapping and identification of gene variants of genetic diseases that follow Mendelian patterns of inheritance in humans. Of the more than 500 genetic loci associated with Mendelian genetic diseases that have been mapped to specific chromosomal locations, almost 100 gene variants have been cloned, based on their position. The cloning and sequencing of these gene variants has elucidated the function and cellular biology of the gene products encoded by these gene variants.

However, one of the most difficult problems is to find out how genes contribute to diseases that have a complex pattern of inheritance. In all these cases, no one gene determines whether a person has a disease or not. It is likely that more than one mutation is required before the disease is manifest, a number of genes may each make a subtle contribution to the disease and genes may determine how a person reacts to environmental factors contributing to the disease.

Similar advances have been made in identifying the genetic and molecular basis of certain epilepsies.[1-18] Direct molecular diagnosis is now possible in several inherited diseases with progressive symptomatic epileptic seizures. Success has been achieved mainly in identifying many mutations in rare monogenic epilepsy syndromes using linkage analysis. These findings concern only a few families but their potential importance is immense, because the discovered genes are implicated in a wide range of common epileptic disorders, which are more complex, and probably influenced by variation in several susceptibility genes. [19]

"Functional studies of these mutations, while leading to further progress in the neurobiology of the epilepsies will help to refine genotype-phenotype relations and increase our understanding of responses to antiepileptic drugs."[17]

It has been known for a long time that genetic factors play a major role in the aetiology of idiopathic and symptomatic epilepsies.[20] Oligogenic or polygenic inheritance has been suspected in most of these disorders and a few are monogenic. These conditions came to light through the genetic contributions of familial aggregation and twin studies, positional cloning of specific genes that raise risk, and clinical descriptions of families. Linkage analysis to determine candidate genes depends on large families, while association studies in the search for susceptibility genes involve large numbers of sporadic cases to determine if there is significant association of epilepsy with a particular polymorphism within a gene.[19]

Conspicuous features emerging from these discoveries are the marked phenotypic variability of epileptic conditions associated with the known gene mutations and the genetic heterogeneity that underlies all known monogenic syndromes.

"The heterogeneity of mutations described to date has precluded the development of simple diagnostic tests, but advances in the next few years are likely to have an impact on both the clinical diagnosis and the treatment of epilepsies."[15]

Familial (autosomal dominant) focal epilepsies are monogenic (single gene) forms of epilepsy identified in large families with an epileptic trait segregating in the absence of environmental factors.[3;17;21-23] In these families, phenotypes are determined by mutations in susceptibility genes, some of which have been localised and some of which have been identified. Most of the genes discovered code for either voltage-gated or ligand-gated ion channel subunits, which indicates that, at least in part, familial (autosomal dominant) focal epilepsies are a family of channelopathies.[24] Lateral familial temporal lobe epilepsy was the first non-ion channel disease in this group to be described.

The following familial (autosomal dominant) focal epilepsy syndromes have been recognised:

- **Benign familial neonatal seizures** (see page 98)
- **Benign familial infantile seizures** (see page 124)
- **Autosomal dominant nocturnal frontal lobe epilepsy**
- **Familial temporal lobe epilepsy**
  - **Mesial familial temporal lobe epilepsy**
  - **Lateral familial temporal lobe epilepsy**
- **Familial focal epilepsy with variable foci** (syndrome in development)

Useful glossary

Definitions and details on genetics can be found through appropriate Web sites of which the most important are those provided by the National Human Genome Research Institute (www.nhgri.nih.gov), the National Center for Biotechnology Information (www.ncbi.nlm.nih.gov), and the Online Mendelian Inheritance in Man™ (OMIM™) database hosted by Johns Hopkins University.

Autosomal dominant: A gene on one of the non-sex chromosomes that is always expressed, even if only one copy is present. The chance of passing the gene to offspring is 50% for each pregnancy.

Chromosome: The self-replicating genetic structure of cells containing the cellular DNA that bears in its nucleotide sequence the linear array of genes. In prokaryotes, chromosomal DNA is circular, and the entire genome is carried on one chromosome. Eukaryotic genomes consist of a number of chromosomes whose DNA is associated with different kinds of proteins.

Chromosome region p: A designation for the short arm of a chromosome.

Chromosome region q: A designation for the long arm of a chromosome.

Gene: The fundamental physical and functional unit of heredity. A gene is an ordered sequence of nucleotides located in a particular position on a particular chromosome that encodes a specific functional product (i.e., a protein or RNA molecule).

Gene mapping: Determination of the relative positions of genes on a DNA molecule (chromosome or plasmid) and of the distance, in linkage units or physical units, between them.

Genetic screening: Testing a group of people to identify individuals at high risk of having or passing on a specific genetic disorder.

Genetic testing: Analysing an individual's genetic material to determine predisposition to a particular health condition or to confirm a diagnosis of genetic disease.

Genome: All the genetic material in the chromosomes of a particular organism; its size is generally given as its total number of base pairs.

Genotype: The genetic constitution of an organism, as distinguished from its physical appearance (its phenotype).

Insertion: A chromosome abnormality in which a piece of DNA is incorporated into a gene and thereby disrupts the gene's normal function.

Linkage: The proximity of two or more markers (e.g., genes, RFLP markers) on a chromosome; the closer the markers, the lower the probability that they will be separated during DNA repair or replication processes (binary fission in prokaryotes, mitosis or meiosis in eukaryotes), and hence the greater the probability that they will be inherited together.

Linkage map: A map of the relative positions of genetic loci on a chromosome, determined on the basis of how often the loci are inherited together. Distance is measured in centimorgans (cM).

Locus (pl. loci): The position on a chromosome of a gene or other chromosome marker; also, the DNA at that position. The use of locus is sometimes restricted to mean expressed DNA regions.

Mendelian inheritance: Inheritance pattern based on a single affected gene.
The inheritance pattern of a Mendelian disease depends on whether it is autosomal dominant, autosomal recessive, X-linked dominant, X-linked recessive, or Y-linked. Also related but not truly Mendelian are some of the rarer inheritance patterns (e.g. mosaicism, anticipation, triplet repeat).

Monogenic disorder: A disorder caused by mutation of a single gene.

Mutation: Any heritable change in DNA sequence.

Penetrance: The probability of a gene or genetic trait being expressed. "Complete" penetrance means the gene or genes for a trait are expressed in all the population who have the genes. "Incomplete" penetrance means the genetic trait is expressed in only part of the population. The percentage penetrance also may change with the age range of the population.

Phenocopy: A trait not caused by inheritance of a gene but appears to be identical to a genetic trait.

Phenotype: The physical characteristics of an organism or the presence of a disease that may or may not be genetic.

Polygenic disorder: Genetic disorder resulting from the combined action of alleles of more than one gene (e.g., heart disease, diabetes, and some cancers). Although such disorders are inherited, they depend on the simultaneous presence of several alleles; thus the hereditary patterns usually are more complex than those of single-gene disorders.

Recessive gene: A gene which will be expressed only if there are 2 identical copies or, for a male, if one copy is present on the X chromosome.

Sequencing: Determination of the order of nucleotides (base sequences) in a DNA or RNA molecule or the order of amino acids in a protein.

Single-gene disorder: Hereditary disorder caused by a mutant allele of a single gene (e.g., Duchenne muscular dystrophy, retinoblastoma, sickle cell disease).

AUTOSOMAL DOMINANT NOCTURNAL FRONTAL LOBE EPILEPSY

Autosomal dominant nocturnal frontal lobe epilepsy (ADNFLE) [21;25-3637;38] is the first distinctive syndrome of focal epilepsy with single gene inheritance to be described.[39]

DEMOGRAPHIC DATA

Onset is mainly in late childhood at 7–12 years of age (mean 11 years), though it ranges from infancy (2 months) to adulthood (56 years). Overall, 90% of patients have their first seizure before the age of 20 years. Men and women are equally affected. The prevalence is unknown, but the increasing number of publications from 1994 indicates that ADNFLE may not be an uncommon disease.

CLINICAL MANIFESTATIONS

ADNFLE manifests with frequent (nearly every night) clusters of brief (20–50 s) nocturnal motor seizures, with hyperkinetic/dystonic features or tonic manifestations . These hypermotor seizures of ADNFLE are identical to those of the supplementary sensorimotor area as detailed in Chapter 12.

Seizures are of sudden onset and their termination is void of postictal symptoms. Motor symptoms consist of thrashing hyperkinetic movements and dystonic posturing (shoulder or pelvic thrashing movements, bipedal and fencing postures) or tonic stiffening of the limbs and the body, often with superimposed clonic components. Patients may be thrown out of bed or find themselves prone in a crawling position. Injuries may occur. Paroxysmal arousals or awakening during non-rapid eye movement sleep may also represent mild seizures that may or may not be associated with transient dystonic posturing. Two-thirds of patients experience a non-specific aura of somatosensory, sensory, psychic and autonomic symptoms. Consciousness is usually preserved. Sleep is abruptly interrupted, but immediately resumes with the end of the seizure. The postictal state is entirely normal.

Secondarily generalised tonic clonic seizures (GTCS), which occur in two-thirds of patients, are also very infrequent during sleep and are mainly seen in untreated patients or after withdrawal of medication.

There is marked intra- and inter-family variability in severity. Affected family members usually have clusters of seizures with a weekly or monthly frequency, but some patients have attacks every night; a few individuals have mild and rare attacks that are identified only during systematic study of their family.

CIRCADIAN DISTRIBUTION

Seizures are most likely to occur in the hypnagogic state of sleep or shortly before awakening. Diurnal attacks are rare.

PRECIPITATING FACTORS

Stress, fatigue and alcohol increase the frequency of fits. Seizures in children provoked by movement and sound stimulation are reported.[31]

AETIOLOGY

ADNFLE segregates with an autosomal dominant mode of inheritance and incomplete penetrance (about 70%), though it can be much lower in some families.

ADNFLE has been linked to chromosome 20q13.2 and 15q24, but not in many other families, thus demonstrating genetic heterogeneity. ADNFLE is associated with mutations of the alpha 4 or the beta 2 subunit of the neuronal nicotinic acetylcholine receptor (nAChR). At least three mutations have been described in the M2 domain of the nAChR alpha 4 subunit (*CHRNA4*) gene. The nAChR beta 2 subunit (*CHRNB2*) is a second acetylcholine receptor subunit associated with ADNFLE in chromosome 1.[40]

Despite this genetic heterogeneity, the clinical phenotypes appear markedly homogeneous in all families and difficult to separate on clinical grounds, irrespective of chromosomal linkage and mutations.[36]

DIAGNOSTIC PROCEDURES

Brain imaging is normal. Interictal and often ictal EEG are usually normal and unhelpful. On video-polysomnographic EEG, ictal epileptiform abnormalities occur predominantly over frontal areas in 32% of patients, and the EEG showed ictal, rhythmic, slow wave activity over anterior areas in another 47% of patients.[41]

PROGNOSIS

Seizures are lifelong, though in mild cases they may appear only for a brief period. Spontaneous remissions and relapses occur. Some patients have frequent attacks that are refractory to medication. Attacks may become milder in the fifth or sixth decade of life and be described as fragments of previous seizures.

DIFFERENTIAL DIAGNOSIS

Misdiagnosis of seizures as benign nocturnal parasomnias, night terrors, nightmares, or psychiatric and medical disorders is common (around 80% of patients).[41] *'Nocturnal paroxysmal dystonia'*[42] and *'Hypnic tonic postural seizures of frontal lobe origin'*[43] are certainly frontal lobe seizures and most patients probably have ADNFLE.

Some clinical features, such as awakenings with the feeling of choking, abnormal motor activity during sleep and excessive daytime sleepiness are relatively common in both obstructive sleep apnoea syndrome and nocturnal frontal lobe epilepsy. All-night video-polysomnographic monitoring is needed to provide a firm diagnosis.[41]

On clinical and EEG grounds ADNFLE may be identical to symptomatic forms of frontal lobe epilepsy from the supplementary sensorimotor area. The differential diagnosis depends on family history of ADNFLE and MRI abnormalities in epilepsy from the supplementary sensorimotor area.

MANAGEMENT

The management is the same as that described for focal symptomatic epilepsies. Carbamazepine monotherapy is frequently effective, but one-third of patients is resistant to treatment. In refractory cases, multiple anti-epileptic drugs (AEDs) are often ineffective. Add-on clobazam may be useful. Newer drugs, such as levetiracetam, lamotrigine and topiramate, may be effective. Cognitive impairment due to topiramate appears to be easily overlooked and underestimated in patients treated with this drug.[44]

Nicotine patches in conjunction with appropriate AEDs may be of benefit in some individuals with ADNFLE.[45]

FAMILIAL TEMPORAL LOBE EPILEPSY

Temporal lobe epilepsy was considered as an acquired condition secondary to lesions, such as hippocampal sclerosis, tumours, trauma, vascular malformations and malformations of cortical development. The extent of the genetic involvement in some forms of temporal lobe epilepsy only recently has been elucidated. Familial temporal lobe epilepsy is of autosomal dominant inheritance and has two types:[14]

1. **Mesial familial temporal lobe epilepsy** (MFTLE)
2. **Lateral familial temporal lobe epilepsy** (LFTLE), which is also described as partial epilepsy with auditory symptoms.[46]

Both these forms of epilepsy begin in adolescence or adult life and are usually benign epilepsy syndromes. MFTLE is characterised by seizure symptomatology of any type of mesial temporal lobe epilepsy such as déjà vu or autonomic phenomena. LFTLE manifests with subjective ictal symptoms such as auditory hallucinations of lateral temporal lobe origin.

MESIAL FAMILIAL TEMPORAL LOBE EPILEPSY

MFTLE is an autosomal dominant epileptic disease.[21;47-53]

DEMOGRAPHIC DATA

Onset is typically in teenage or early adult life with a median in the middle of the third decade of life. No children under the age of 10 years have been identified with this disorder. Women (58%) may be affected more than men. Epidemiology is unknown. Berkovic proposes that this may be a common condition.[47;48;51]

CLINICAL MANIFESTATIONS

Seizures are generally mild, infrequent and well controlled with AEDs. Simple focal seizures (90%) are far more common than complex focal seizures (66%) and may be the only seizure type (18%). The main ictal manifestations consist of déjà vu, other experiential phenomena and hallucinations (nearly all) alone or together with autonomic disturbances. Emotional symptoms of fear and panic, visual and auditory illusions of distortions of light and sound, and somatosensory sensations of diffuse, not localised, numbness and tingling are other common ictal symptoms.

Rising epigastric sensation does not exist.

GTCS occur in only two-thirds of patients with MFTLE and, in 50% of cases, they occur prior to initiation of appropriate treatment. GTCS are again infrequent with the worse possible scenario of one GTCS per year.

Patients are neurologically and mentally normal, and the condition does not appear to affect their otherwise normal life, particularly when on medication.

AETIOLOGY

Autosomal dominant inheritance with reduced penetrance (60%) is the most likely mode of inheritance.[48;50] The gene responsible for MFTLE has not yet been identified.

DIAGNOSTIC PROCEDURES

All relevant investigations are normal apart from the EEG. MRI is often normal,[47;48] but in severe cases hippocampal atrophy is found, including some rare examples of familial hippocampal sclerosis.[47;54] Minor and non-specific abnormalities manifest as diffuse, small, high signal areas on T2-weighted images may be seen. Interictal FDG-PET may show ipsilateral temporal hypometabolism in patients with active seizures.

The interictal EEG is usually normal (50% of cases), shows mild, focal, slow waves (28%), or sparse, usually unilateral (22%) sharp and slow wave complexes localised to the temporal region.[1;48] Sleep may occasionally activate epileptiform abnormalities.

Only three seizures have been recorded.[51] In one seizure, a right temporal ictal discharge appeared during the attack, which began with fear and was followed by loss of awareness, staring, swallowing and left hand automatisms. The two other seizures occurred in the same patient. No definitive epileptiform changes were recorded in one seizure, which comprised an aura of buzzing in the ears, followed by oral automatisms and impaired awareness. No lateralised EEG changes occurred in the other seizure, which started with an aura and early left-sided dystonia that rapidly progressed to secondarily generalised convulsions.

DIFFERENTIAL DIAGNOSIS

The main difficulty is probably in differentiating patients with very mild and infrequent seizures of predominantly déjà vu from normal phenomena. This may be impossible in individual cases without other overt seizure symptoms or other family members having temporal lobe epilepsy.

Familial temporal lobe epilepsy should be mainly differentiated from hippocampal epilepsy. The main differentiating features in favour of familial temporal lobe epilepsy are:

- onset in the teens or early adult life
- no febrile convulsions or other antecedent factors of epilepsy
- no ictal symptoms of rising epigastric aura
- mild and infrequent seizures that may remit
- usually normal MRI.

PROGNOSIS

The prognosis is commonly good. One-sixth of cases with mild simple partial seizures alone (16%) would never know that they have an epileptic disorder if other family members were not affected. Of the cases with more overt seizure manifestations, only 66% have complex focal seizures and GTCS that are again rather infrequent and respond well to AEDs. It is rare for seizures to continue after drug treatment (10–20% of cases). The cross-sectional nature of the study of Berkovic et al.[47;48;51] precluded accurate determination of remission rates, but the histories of affected individuals suggested that long remissions, with or without therapy, were common. Conversely, in the Montreal series, drawn largely from patients considering surgical treatment for epilepsy, a more severe clinical spectrum was observed.[50;55]

MANAGEMENT

Seizures are usually easily controlled with carbamazepine or phenytoin.[47;48;51] Patients with refractory MFTLE have a good surgical outcome when unilateral or clearly asymmetric hippocampal atrophy is identified.[55] Preoperative investigation should be the same as that in patients with sporadic refractory MFTLE.[55]

LATERAL FAMILIAL (AUTOSOMAL DOMINANT) TEMPORAL LOBE EPILEPSY [56-63]

'Lateral (autosomal dominant) familial temporal lobe epilepsy' is the same disease as 'autosomal dominant focal epilepsy with auditory features', as they are both due to defects in the same gene. It is the first non-ion channel familial epilepsy to have been discovered.[60;62] All the genes for idiopathic epilepsies that were discovered previously have been associated with ion channels.[64]

DEMOGRAPHIC DATA

Onset of LFTLE is typically in teenage or early adult life, but may be earlier (5–10 years of age), or later.

CLINICAL MANIFESTATIONS

LFTLE is characterised by:[49]

- mild seizures with mainly auditory hallucinations
- mainly nocturnal and infrequent GTCS
- excellent response to treatment.

Seizures are generally mild, infrequent and well controlled with AEDs. Simple focal seizures, which are the most common of all, mainly consist of simple auditory hallucinations such as ringing, humming, clicking or unspecified noises. Other sensory symptoms, such as visual (lights, colours, and simple figures), olfactory, vertiginous or cephalic features, are frequent in simple focal seizures, while autonomic, experiential and motor symptoms are less common. Infrequently, simple focal seizures may progress to complex focal seizures. LFTLE with mainly brief aphasic seizures has been described.[65]

Secondarily GTCS are rare and predominantly nocturnal.

AETIOLOGY

LFTLE has autosomal dominant inheritance with high penetrance (about 80%). Genetic analysis showed linkage to chromosome 10q and localised a gene in a common overlapping region of 3-cM at 10q24 (the leucine-rich, glioma-inactivated 1 [LGI1]/Epitempin gene).[60;62;6366]

LGI1 was first described in glial tumours in which it may be deleted or rearranged, but glial tumours do not occur with increased frequency in LFTLE.[14] LGI1 may influence neuronal migration or cortical organisation. Given that the majority of LGI1 mutations cause protein truncation, loss of function is the likely underlying mechanism.[14]

LGI1 mutations are specific for LFTLE but do not occur in all families. LFTLE is genetically heterogeneous, but mutations in LGI2, LGI3, or LGI4 do not account for families without LGI1 mutations.[66]

DIAGNOSTIC PROCEDURES

EEG and MRI are often normal or show usually mild and non-specific abnormalities. Interictal EEG epileptiform abnormalities rarely occur.

PROGNOSIS

The prognosis is excellent. Patients are neurologically and mentally normal, and the condition does not appear to affect their otherwise normal life particularly when on medication.

DIFFERENTIAL DIAGNOSIS

LFTLE should be mainly differentiated from other structural causes of lateral temporal lobe epilepsy, which lack a similar family history. LFTLE is markedly different from hippocampal and other types of MFTLE though their differential diagnosis may sometimes be difficult in cases that overlap. Auditory hallucinations are the main ictal symptom of LFTLE, but may not occur in some patients. Conversely, déjà vu and other experiential phenomena are the predominant seizure manifestations of MFTLE.

MANAGEMENT

The response to carbamazepine is excellent.

FAMILIAL FOCAL EPILEPSY WITH VARIABLE FOCI

Familial partial epilepsy with variable foci is an autosomal dominant syndrome characterised by focal seizures originating from different brain regions in different family members in the absence of detectable structural abnormalities. [67-72]

DEMOGRAPHIC DATA

Age at onset varies markedly (range months to 43 years), though the mean age at onset of seizures is 13 years. To date, the disorder has been reported in eight unrelated families.

CLINICAL MANIFESTATIONS

The defining feature of this syndrome is that different family members have focal seizures emanating from different cortical locations that include temporal, frontal, centroparietal or occipital regions. Each individual patient has the same electroclinical pattern of single location focal epilepsy. Seizures are often nocturnal. There is great intrafamilial variability. Severity varies among family members; some are asymptomatic manifesting with only an EEG spike-focus, and most are easily controlled with AEDs; but a few others may be intractable to medication.

Identification of the various forms of familial focal epilepsy is difficult, particularly in small families, in which insufficient individuals exist to identify a specific pattern. Berkovic et al. have recently provided clinical guidelines for this task, 'which will eventually be supplanted by specific molecular diagnosis'.[72]

AETIOLOGY

Familial focal epilepsy with variable foci is a rare inherited syndrome with autosomal dominant inheritance and penetrance of about 60%. In two families, the disease has been mapped to a locus in a 3.8-cM interval on chromosome 22q11-q12, between markers D22S1144 and D22S685.[69,71,72] However, in the original Australian family, the disorder was not found to be linked to chromosome 22, indicating genetic heterogeneity. In this family, a genome-wide search failed to demonstrate definitive linkage, but a suggestion of linkage was found on chromosome 2q.[67]

DIAGNOSTIC PROCEDURES

Neuroimaging is usually normal.

ELECTROENCEPHALOGRAPHY

Interictal focal epileptiform abnormalities occur in most patients. Their locations vary between family members and may occur in the temporal, frontal, centroparietal or occipital regions, but for each individual a single focus remains constant over time. These abnormalities are facilitated or brought on by sleep. Clinical seizures are concordant with EEG localisation. EEG severity varies significantly in different individuals and does not correlate with seizure frequency. Normal family members may also have an EEG spike focus, which indicates that this is likely to be a marker for the familial partial epilepsy with variable foci trait.

PROGNOSIS

Development is usually normal.

MANAGEMENT

The effects of new AEDs have not been evaluated directly, but carbamazepine and phenytoin appear to be effective.

OTHER POSSIBLE FAMILIAL (AUTOSOMAL DOMINANT) FOCAL EPILEPSIES NOT YET RECOGNISED

Of those syndromes not yet recognised by the ILAE Task Force, the most important and well documented are:

- autosomal dominant rolandic epilepsy and speech dyspraxia[73;74]
- partial epilepsy with pericentral spikes with evidence for linkage to chromosome 4p15.[75]

AUTOSOMAL DOMINANT ROLANDIC EPILEPSY AND SPEECH DYSPRAXIA[73;74]

'Autosomal dominant rolandic epilepsy and speech dyspraxia: a new syndrome with anticipation' appears to be a rare hereditary condition described by the Australian team of Berkovic, Scheffer and associates.[73] They extensively studied a family of nine affected individuals in three generations with nocturnal oro-facio-brachial focal seizures, secondarily GTCS, and centrotemporal epileptiform discharges, associated with oral and speech dyspraxia and cognitive impairment. The speech disorder was prominent, but differed from that of Landau-Kleffner syndrome and of epilepsy with continuous spike and wave during slow-wave sleep. Patients in previous generations were not so severely affected, but they also had neurological deficits, mainly of oral and speech dyspraxia without evidence of dysarthria.

The authors assessed that: "The electroclinical features of this new syndrome of autosomal dominant rolandic epilepsy resemble those of benign rolandic epilepsy, a common inherited epilepsy of childhood. This family shows clinical anticipation of the seizure disorder, the oral and speech dyspraxia, and cognitive dysfunction, suggesting that the genetic mechanism could be expansion of an unstable triplet repeat. Molecular studies on this syndrome, where the inheritance pattern is clear, could also be relevant to identifying a gene for benign rolandic epilepsy where anticipation does not occur and the mode of inheritance is uncertain."

However, the clinical presentation of these patients with a permanent neurological deficit, sometimes preceding the seizures, can hardly be considered as 'resembling benign Rolandic epilepsy' or 'epitomising the archetypal benign rolandic epileptic attack'.

FOCAL EPILEPSY WITH PERICENTRAL SPIKES[75]

Focal epilepsy with pericentral spikes was based on the study of a family in which affected family members manifested a variety of seizure types, including hemiclonic, hemitonic, GTCS, simple focal (stereotyped episodes of epigastric pain) and complex focal seizures consistent with temporal lobe semiology. The syndrome is benign, either requiring no treatment or responding to a single AED. Seizure onset is in the first or second decades of life, with seizures persisting up to 71 years of age and documented EEG changes up to the age of 30 years. A key feature of this syndrome is a characteristic EEG abnormality of spikes or sharp waves in the pericentral region (centroparietal, centrofrontal or centrotemporal). The syndrome may be overlooked, because of the variability in penetrance and seizure types among affected family members. There is evidence for linkage to chromosome 4p15.

Syndromes of focal epilepsy with autosomal recessive inheritance, such as 'autosomal recessive rolandic epilepsy with paroxysmal exercise-induced dystonia and writer's cramp',[76] have not been yet recognised.

REFERENCES

1. Berkovic SF, Steinlein OK. Genetics of partial epilepsies. *Adv Neurol* 1999;**79**:375-81.
2. Steinlein OK. Idiopathic epilepsies with a monogenic mode of inheritance. *Epilepsia* 1999;**40 Suppl 3**:9-11.
3. Ottman R. Progress in the genetics of the partial epilepsies. *Epilepsia* 2001;**42 Suppl 5**:24-30.
4. Hirose S, Okada M, Kaneko S, Mitsudome A. Molecular genetics of human familial epilepsy syndromes. *Epilepsia* 2002;**43 Suppl 9**:21-5.
5. Kaneko S, Okada M, Iwasa H, Yamakawa K, Hirose S. Genetics of epilepsy: current status and perspectives. *Neurosci Res.* 2002;**44**:11-30.
6. Hirose S, Mohney RP, Okada M, Kaneko S, Mitsudome A. The genetics of febrile seizures and related epilepsy syndromes. *Brain Dev.* 2003;**25**:304-12.
7. Scheffer IE. Severe infantile epilepsies: molecular genetics challenge clinical classification. *Brain* 2003;**126**:513-4.
8. Anderson E, Berkovic S, Dulac O, Gardiner M, Jain S, Laue FM *et al.* ILAE genetics commission conference report: molecular analysis of complex genetic epilepsies. *Epilepsia* 2002;**43**:1262-7.
9. Delgado-Escueta AV, Medina MT, Bai DS, Fong CY, Tanaka M, Alonso ME. Genetics of idiopathic myoclonic epilepsies: an overview. *Adv Neurol.* 2002;**89**:161-84.
10. Winawer MR. Epilepsy genetics. *Neurology* 2002;**8**:133-51.
11. Willmore LJ,.Ueda Y. Molecular biology and genetics of epilepsy. *Acta Med Okayama* 2002;**56**:57-68.
12. Iwasaki N, Nakayama J, Hamano K, Matsui A, Arinami T. Molecular genetics of febrile seizures. *Epilepsia* 2002;**43 Suppl 9**:32-5.
13. Kullmann DM. Epilepsy genetics. *Drugs Today (Barc.)* 2003;**39**:725-32.
14. Vadlamudi L, Scheffer IE, Berkovic SF. Genetics of temporal lobe epilepsy. *J Neurol Neurosurg Psychiatry* 2003;**74**:1359-61.
15. Scheffer IE, Berkovic SF. The genetics of human epilepsy. *Trends Pharmacol Sci.* 2003;**24**:428-33.
16. Stephani U, Tauer U, Koeleman B, Pinto D, Neubauer BA, Lindhout D. Genetics of Photosensitivity (Photoparoxysmal Response): A Review. *Epilepsia* 2004;**45 Suppl 1**:19-23.
17. Gourfinkel-An I, Baulac S, Nabbout R, Ruberg M, Baulac M, Brice A *et al.* Monogenic idiopathic epilepsies. *Lancet Neurol.* 2004;**3**:209-18.
18. Gutierrez-Delicado E, Serratosa JM. Genetics of the epilepsies. *Curr Opin Neurol.* 2004;**17**:147-53.
19. Tan NC, Mulley JC, Berkovic SF. Genetic association studies in epilepsy: "the truth is out there". *Epilepsia* 2004;**45**:1429-42.
20. Vadlamudi L, Andermann E, Lombroso CT, Schachter SC, Milne RL, Hopper JL *et al.* Epilepsy in twins: insights from unique historical data of William Lennox. *Neurology* 2004;**62**:1127-33.
21. Genetics of focal epilepsies. Berkovic S F, Genton P, Hirsch E, Picard F, eds. London: John Libbey & Company Ltd, 1999.
22. Berkovic SF, Ottman R. Molecular genetics of the idiopathic epilepsies: the next steps. *Epileptic Disord.* 2000;**2**:179-81.
23. Scheffer IE, Berkovic SF. Genetics of the epilepsies. *Curr Opin Pediatr* 2000;**12**:536-42.
24. Celesia GG. Disorders of membrane channels or channelopathies. *Clin Neurophysiol.* 2001;**112**:2-18.
25. Scheffer IE. Autosomal dominant nocturnal frontal lobe epilepsy. In Berkovic SF, Genton P, Hirsch E, Picard F, eds. *Genetics of focal epilepsies*, pp 81-4. London: John Libbey & Company Ltd, 1999.
26. Bertrand D. Neuronal nicotinic acetylcholine receptors: their properties and alterations in autosomal dominant nocturnal frontal lobe epilepsy. *Rev Neurol (Paris)* 1999;**155**:457-62.
27. Hirose S, Iwata H, Akiyoshi H, Kobayashi K, Ito M, Wada K *et al.* A novel mutation of CHRNA4 responsible for autosomal dominant nocturnal frontal lobe epilepsy. *Neurology* 1999;**53**:1749-53.
28. Provini F, Plazzi G, Tinuper P, Vandi S, Lugaresi E, Montagna P. Nocturnal frontal lobe epilepsy. A clinical and polygraphic overview of 100 consecutive cases. *Brain* 1999;**122**:1017-31.
29. Nakken KO, Magnusson A, Steinlein OK. Autosomal dominant nocturnal frontal lobe epilepsy: an electroclinical study of a Norwegian family with ten affected members. *Epilepsia* 1999;**40**:88-92.
30. Picard F, Chauvel P. Autosomal dominant nocturnal frontal lobe epilepsy: the syndrome. *Rev Neurol (Paris)* 1999;**155**:445-9.
31. Ito M, Kobayashi K, Fujii T, Okuno T, Hirose S, Iwata H *et al.* Electroclinical picture of autosomal dominant nocturnal frontal lobe epilepsy in a Japanese family. *Epilepsia* 2000;**41**:52-8.
32. Steinlein OK, Stoodt J, Mulley J, Berkovic S, Scheffer IE, Brodtkorb E. Independent occurrence of the CHRNA4 Ser248Phe mutation in a Norwegian family with nocturnal frontal lobe epilepsy. *Epilepsia* 2000;**41**:529-35.
33. Duga S, Asselta R, Bonati MT, Malcovati M, Dalpra L, Oldani A *et al.* Mutational analysis of nicotinic acetylcholine receptor beta2 subunit gene (CHRNB2) in a representative cohort of Italian probands affected by autosomal dominant nocturnal frontal lobe epilepsy. *Epilepsia* 2002;**43**:362-4.
34. Motamedi GK, Lesser RP. Autosomal dominant nocturnal frontal lobe epilepsy. *Adv Neurol.* 2002;**89**:463-73.
35. Rozycka A,.Trzeciak WH. Genetic basis of autosomal dominant nocturnal frontal lobe epilepsy. *J Appl Genet.* 2003;**44**:197-207.
36. McLellan A, Phillips HA, Rittey C, Kirkpatrick M, Mulley JC, Goudie D *et al.* Phenotypic comparison of two Scottish families with mutations in different genes causing autosomal dominant nocturnal frontal lobe epilepsy. *Epilepsia* 2003;**44**:613-7.
37. Combi R, Dalpra L, Malcovati M, Oldani A, Tenchini ML, Ferini-Strambi L. Evidence for a fourth locus for autosomal dominant nocturnal frontal lobe epilepsy. *Brain Res Bull.* 2004;**63**:353-9.
38. Combi R, Dalpra L, Tenchini ML, Ferini-Strambi L. Autosomal dominant nocturnal frontal lobe epilepsy—a critical overview. *J Neurol.* 2004;**251**:923-34.
39. Scheffer IE, Bhatia KP, Lopes-Cendes I, Fish DR, Marsden CD, Andermann F *et al.* Autosomal dominant frontal epilepsy misdiagnosed as sleep disorder. *Lancet* 1994;**343**:515-7.
40. Phillips HA, Favre I, Kirkpatrick M, Zuberi SM, Goudie D, Heron SE *et al.* CHRNB2 is the second acetylcholine receptor subunit associated with autosomal dominant nocturnal frontal lobe epilepsy. *Am J Hum Genet.* 2001;**68**:225-31.
41. Oldani A, Zucconi M, Asselta R, Modugno M, Bonati MT, Dalpra L *et al.* Autosomal dominant nocturnal frontal lobe epilepsy. A video- polysomnographic and genetic appraisal of 40 patients and delineation of the epileptic syndrome. *Brain* 1998;**121**:205-23.
42. Lugaresi E, Cirignotta F, Montagna P. Nocturnal paroxysmal dystonia. *Epilepsy Res Suppl* 1991;**2**:137-40.
43. Vigevano F, Fusco L. Hypnic tonic postural seizures in healthy children provide evidence for a partial epileptic syndrome of frontal lobe origin. *Epilepsia* 1993;**34**:110-9.
44. Kockelmann E, Elger CE, Helmstaedter C. Significant improvement in frontal lobe associated neuropsychological functions after withdrawal of topiramate in epilepsy patients. *Epilepsy Res.* 2003;**54**:171-8.
45. Willoughby JO, Pope KJ, Eaton V. Nicotine as an antiepileptic agent in ADNFLE: an N-of-one study. *Epilepsia* 2003;**44**:1238-40.
46. Berkovic SF, Scheffer IE. Genetics of the epilepsies. *Epilepsia* 2001;**42 Suppl 5**:16-23.
47. Berkovic SF, Howell RA, Hopper JL. Familial temporal lobe epilepsy:a new syndrome with adolescent/adult onset and a benign course. In Wolf P, ed. *Epileptic seizures and syndromes*, pp 257-63. London: John Libbey & Company Ltd, 1994.
48. Berkovic SF, McIntosh A, Howell RA, Mitchell A, Sheffield LJ, Hopper *et al.* Familial temporal lobe epilepsy: a common disorder identified in twins. *Ann Neurol* 1996;**40**:227-35.
49. Tassinari CA, Michelucci R. Familial frontal and temporal lobe epilepsies. In Engel JJ, Pedley TA, eds. *Epilepsy: A comprehensive Textbook*, pp 2427-31. Philadelphia: Lippincott-Raven Publishers, 1997.
50. Cendes F, Lopes-Cendes I, Andermann E, Andermann F. Familial temporal lobe epilepsy: a clinically heterogeneous syndrome. *Neurology* 1998;**50**:554-7.
51. Berkovic SF. Familial temporal lobe epilepsy. In Berkovic SF, Genton P, Hirsch E, Picard F, eds. *Genetics of focal epilepsies*, pp 85-93. London: John Libbey & Company Ltd, 1999.
52. Gordon N. Familial temporal-lobe epilepsy. *Dev Med Child Neurol* 1999;**41**:501-2.

53. Gambardella A, Messina D, Le Piane E, Oliveri RL, Annesi G, Zappia M *et al.* Familial temporal lobe epilepsy autosomal dominant inheritance in a large pedigree from southern Italy. *Epilepsy Res* 2000;**38**:127-32.

54. Kobayashi E, D'Agostino MD, Lopes-Cendes I, Berkovic SF, Li ML, Andermann E *et al.* Hippocampal atrophy and T2-weighted signal changes in familial mesial temporal lobe epilepsy. *Neurology* 2003;**60**:405-9.

55. Kobayashi E, D'Agostino MD, Lopes-Cendes I, Andermann E, Dubeau F, Guerreiro CA *et al.* Outcome of surgical treatment in familial mesial temporal lobe epilepsy. *Epilepsia* 2003;**44**:1080-4.

56. Ottman R, Barker-Cummings C, Lee JH, Ranta S. Genetics of autosomal dominant partial epilepsy with auditory features. In Berkovic SF, Genton P, Hirsch E, Picard F, eds. *Genetics of focal epilepsies,* pp 95-102. London: John Libbey & Company Ltd, 1999.

57. Winawer MR, Ottman R, Hauser WA, Pedley TA. Autosomal dominant partial epilepsy with auditory features: defining the phenotype. *Neurology* 2000;**54**:2173-6.

58. Ikeda A, Kunieda T, Miyamoto S, Fukuyama H, Shibasaki H. Autosomal dominant temporal lobe epilepsy in a Japanese family. *J Neurol Sci.* 2000;**176**:162-5.

59. Michelucci R, Passarelli D, Pitzalis S, Dal Corso G, Tassinari CA, Nobile C. Autosomal dominant partial epilepsy with auditory features: description of a new family. *Epilepsia* 2000;**41**:967-70.

60. Kalachikov S, Evgrafov O, Ross B, Winawer M, Barker-Cummings C, Boneschi FM *et al.* Mutations in LGI1 cause autosomal-dominant partial epilepsy with auditory features. *Nat Genet.* 2002;**30**:335-41.

61. Winawer MR, Boneschi FM, Barker-Cummings C, Lee JH, Liu J, Mekios C *et al.* Four new families with autosomal dominant partial epilepsy with auditory features: clinical description and linkage to chromosome 10q24. *Epilepsia* 2002;**43**:60-7.

62. Morante-Redolat JM, Gorostidi-Pagola A, Piquer-Sirerol S, Saenz A, Poza JJ, Galan J *et al.* Mutations in the LGI1/Epitempin gene on 10q24 cause autosomal dominant lateral temporal epilepsy. *Hum Mol Genet.* 2002;**11**:1119-28.

63. Michelucci R, Poza JJ, Sofia V, de Feo MR, Binelli S, Bisulli F *et al.* Autosomal dominant lateral temporal epilepsy: clinical spectrum, new epitempin mutations, and genetic heterogeneity in seven European families. *Epilepsia* 2003;**44**:1289-97.

64. Kullmann DM. Genetics of epilepsy. *J Neurol Neurosurg Psychiatry* 2002;**73 Suppl 2**:II32-II35.

65. Brodtkorb E, Gu W, Nakken KO, Fischer C, Steinlein OK. Familial temporal lobe epilepsy with aphasic seizures and linkage to chromosome 10q22-q24. *Epilepsia* 2002;**43**:228-35.

66. Berkovic SF, Izzillo P, McMahon JM, Harkin LA, McIntosh AM, Phillips HA *et al.* LGI1 mutations in temporal lobe epilepsies. *Neurology* 2004;**62**:1115-9.

67. Scheffer IE, Phillips HA, O'Brien CE, Saling MM, Wrennall JA, Wallace RH *et al.* Familial partial epilepsy with variable foci: a new partial epilepsy syndrome with suggestion of linkage to chromosome 2. *Ann.Neurol.* 1998;**44**:890-9.

68. Scheffer IE. Familial partial epilepsy with variable foci. In Berkovic SF, Genton P, Hirsch E, Picard F, eds. *Genetics of focal epilepsies,* pp 103-8. London: John Libbey & Company Ltd, 1999.

69. Xiong L, Labuda M, Li DS, Hudson TJ, Desbiens R, Patry G *et al.* Mapping of a gene determining familial partial epilepsy with variable foci to chromosome 22q11-q12. *Am J Hum Genet.* 1999;**65**:1698-710.

70. Picard F, Baulac S, Kahane P, Hirsch E, Sebastianelli R, Thomas P *et al.* Dominant partial epilepsies. A clinical, electrophysiological and genetic study of 19 European families. *Brain* 2000;**123**:1247-62.

71. Callenbach PM, van den Maagdenberg AM, Hottenga JJ, van den Boogerd EH, de Coo RF, Lindhout D *et al.* Familial partial epilepsy with variable foci in a Dutch family: clinical characteristics and confirmation of linkage to chromosome 22q. *Epilepsia* 2003;**44**:1298-305.

72. Berkovic SF, Serratosa JM, Phillips HA, Xiong L, Andermann E, Diaz-Otero F *et al.* Familial partial epilepsy with variable foci: clinical features and linkage to chromosome 22q12. *Epilepsia* 2004;**45**:1054-60.

73. Scheffer IE, Jones L, Pozzebon M, Howell RA, Saling MM, Berkovic SF. Autosomal dominant rolandic epilepsy and speech dyspraxia: a new syndrome with anticipation. *Ann Neurol* 1995;**38**:633-42.

74. Scheffer IE. Autosomal dominant rolandic epilepsy with speech dyspraxia. *Epileptic Disord.* 2000;**2 Suppl 1**:S19-S22.

75. Kinton L, Johnson MR, Smith SJM, Farrell F, Stevens J, Rance JB *et al.* Partial epilepsy with pericentral spikes: A new familial epilepsy syndrome with evidence for linkage to chromosome 4p15. *Ann Neurol* 2002;**51**:740-9.

76. Guerrini R, Bonanni P, Nardocci N, Parmeggiani L, Piccirilli M, De Fusco M *et al.* Autosomal recessive rolandic epilepsy with paroxysmal exercise-induced dystonia and writer's cramp: delineation of the syndrome and gene mapping to chromosome 16p12-11.2. *Ann Neurol.* 1999;**45**:344-52.

12 SYMPTOMATIC AND PROBABLY SYMPTOMATIC FOCAL EPILEPSIES

TOPOGRAPHICAL SYMPTOMATOLOGY AND CLASSIFICATION

Focal (anatomical, topographical or localisation related) epilepsies* are defined as seizures that emanate from an epileptogenic focus anywhere within the brain.[1] Ictal symptoms, particularly at onset, are determined by localisation and not by aetiology. However, it is difficult to assign some epilepsies to specific anatomical localisations or lobes, as is often the case with seizures originating from clinically silent epileptogenic regions.

The ILAE Commission (1989) classifies focal epilepsies according to their topographical/anatomical origin as:[1]

- **Temporal lobe epilepsies**
- **Frontal lobe epilepsies**
- **Parietal lobe epilepsies**
- **Occipital lobe epilepsies**

These epilepsies may be idiopathic, cryptogenic or symptomatic. The new diagnostic scheme considers 'symptomatic (or probably symptomatic) focal epilepsies' as a separate group from 'idiopathic focal epilepsies'.[2] This is because of the significant progress made in recent years through the investigation of neurosurgical cases, technological advances in brain imaging methodologies and genetics. This distinction is important in practice, because the prognosis and treatment of idiopathic focal epilepsies differ significantly from those of symptomatic epilepsies. There is now concrete evidence to accept, diagnose and treat certain focal epilepsies on the basis of aetiology rather than simply localisation. Mesial temporal lobe epilepsy (MTLE) with hippocampal sclerosis, which is one of the commoner and most distinct epileptic syndromes, is a striking example of this.

The new ILAE diagnostic scheme further classifies focal epilepsies according to whether they are limbic or neocortical:[2]

LIMBIC EPILEPSIES

Mesial temporal lobe epilepsy with hippocampal sclerosis

Mesial temporal lobe epilepsy defined by specific aetiologies

Other types defined by location and aetiology

NEOCORTICAL EPILEPSIES (see pages 207–221)

Rasmussen syndrome (page 207)

Hemiconvulsion-hemiplegia syndrome (page 215)

Lateral temporal lobe epilepsy

Migrating focal seizures of early childhood (page 217)

Other types defined by location and aetiology

Simple and complex focal seizures may account for 60–70 % of all epilepsies and nearly half originate from temporal lobe structures.[3-5] There are numerous causes of focal symptomatic and probably symptomatic focal epilepsies, such as benign or malignant tumours, viral and other infectious and parasitic diseases,

---

*The terms focal and partial seizures are synonymous and are interchangeable. Focal seizures or focal epilepsies are the preferred term.

cerebrovascular disorders, malformations of cortical development, genetically determined brain and metabolic disorders, trauma and other injuries. The exact prevalence of these aetiological factors in various types of focal epilepsies has not been estimated precisely, and certainly varies significantly between developed and developing countries. For example, cysticercosis and tuberculomas are among the commonest causes of epilepsies in developing countries, but have a minimal prevalence in Western industrialised countries. Malformations of cortical development, which are a significant cause of focal epilepsies, are often revealed only by high resolution MRI.[6]

The other idiopathic and hereditary forms of focal epilepsies have been detailed mainly in Chapters 10 and 11.

TEMPORAL LOBE EPILEPSIES

Temporal lobe epilepsies comprise a heterogeneous group of disorders sharing the same topographical seizure onset (the temporal lobe), but often of diverse aetiology, age at onset, prognosis, and response to medical or surgical management. Anatomically they are broadly divided into those originating from the lateral or mesial regions of the temporal lobe (Figures 12.1 and 12.2). Mesial (or medial) is far more common (accounting for two-thirds of cases) than lateral temporal lobe epilepsy (LTLE). The most common of all is hippocampal epilepsy, which probably constitutes a disease with known pathology rather than a syndrome. Other causes of temporal lobe epilepsy, mesial or lateral, are benign or malignant tumours, viral and other infectious and parasitic diseases, cerebrovascular disorders, malformations of cortical development, trauma and other injuries.[7] The other idiopathic and hereditary forms of temporal lobe epilepsy have been detailed in Chapters 10 and 11. Onset, progress and response to treatment largely depend on causative factors. Ictal manifestations distinguishing lateral from MTLE are often, but not always, pathognomonic. Seizures from other anatomical brain locations may present with similar semiology, mainly because of spread to temporal lobe structures.

Classification and definition

According to the ILAE Commission (1989)[1]

"Temporal lobe syndromes are characterized by simple focal seizures, complex focal seizures, and secondarily generalized seizures, or combinations of these. Frequently, there is a history of febrile seizures, and a family history of seizures is common. Memory deficits may occur. On metabolic imaging studies, hypometabolism is frequently observed [e.g., positron emission tomography]. Unilateral or bilateral temporal lobe spikes are common on EEG. Onset is frequently in childhood or young adulthood. Seizures occur in clusters at intervals or randomly.

General characteristics

Features strongly suggestive of the diagnosis when present include:

1.*Simple focal seizures* typically characterized by autonomic and/or psychic symptoms and certain sensory phenomena such as olfactory and auditory (including illusions). Most common is an epigastric, often rising, sensation.

2.*Complex focal seizures* often but not always begin with motor arrest typically followed by oroalimentary automatisms. Other automatisms frequently follow. The duration is typically >1 min. Postictal confusion usually occurs. The attacks are followed by amnesia. Recovery is gradual.

Electroencephalographic characteristics

In temporal lobe epilepsies the interictal scalp EEG may show the following:

1.No abnormality.

2.Slight or marked asymmetry of the background activity.

3.Temporal spikes, sharp waves and/or slow waves, unilateral or bilateral, synchronous but also asynchronous. These findings are not always confined to the temporal region.

4.In addition to scalp EEG findings, intracranial recordings may allow better definition of the intracranial distribution of the interictal abnormalities.

In temporal lobe epilepsies various EEG patterns may accompany the initial clinical ictal symptomatology, including (a) a unilateral or bilateral interruption of background activity; and (b) temporal or multilobar low-amplitude fast activity, rhythmic spikes, or rhythmic slow waves. The onset of the EEG may not correlate with the clinical onset depending on methodology. Intracranial recordings may provide additional information regarding the chronological and spatial evolution of the discharges." [1]

DEMOGRAPHIC DATA

Temporal lobe epilepsy may comprise 30–35% of all epilepsies. Two-thirds of these epilepsies originate from the mesial and the other third from the lateral temporal lobe regions. The commonest cause, in neurosurgical series, is hippocampal sclerosis, which accounts for 65% of cases.[8-11] Men and women are equally affected. Age at onset largely depends on aetiology.

CLASSIFICATION

The ILAE Task Force classifies temporal lobe epilepsies as:[2]

LIMBIC EPILEPSY

- Mesial temporal lobe epilepsy with hippocampal sclerosis
- Mesial temporal lobe epilepsy defined by specific aetiologies

NEOCORTICAL EPILEPSY

- Lateral temporal lobe epilepsy

CLINICAL MANIFESTATIONS OF TEMPORAL LOBE SEIZURES

Temporal lobe epilepsy manifests with:

- Simple focal seizures
- Complex focal seizures
- Secondarily generalised tonic clonic seizures (GTCS)
- Focal non-convulsive status epilepticus (limbic or neocortical)
- Secondarily convulsive status epilepticus

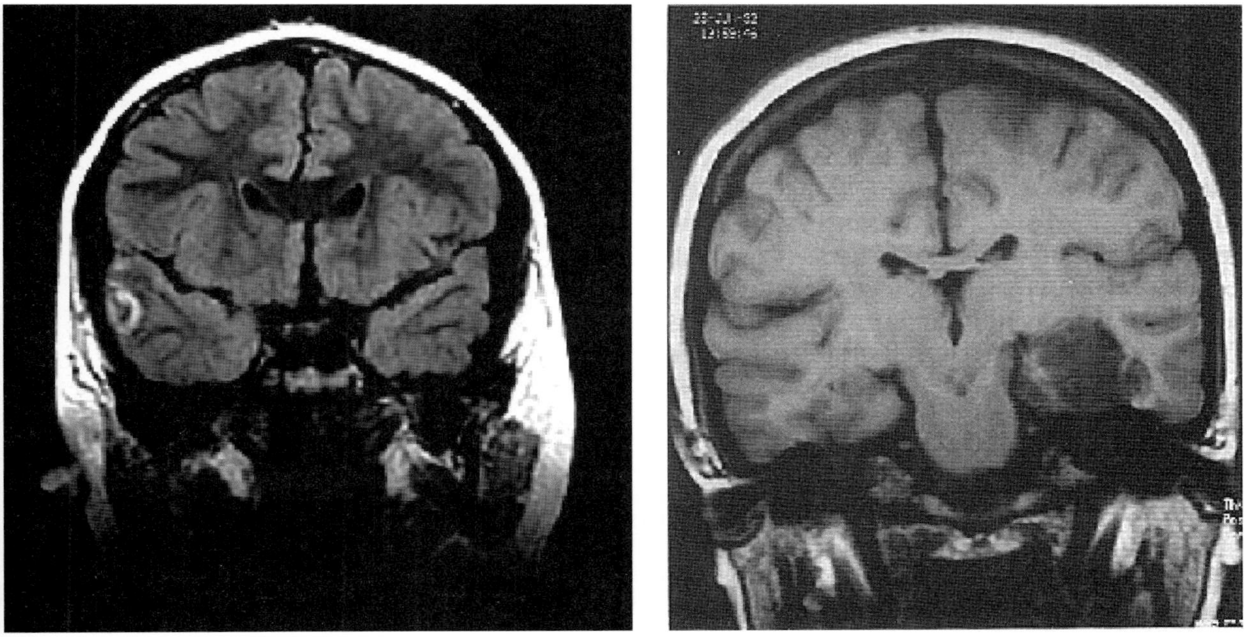

Figure 12.1 MRIs of two patients with mesial (right) and lateral (left) temporal lobe epilepsy due to dysembryoplastic neuroepithelial tumours (DNET).

Left: Coronal FLAIR MRI showing a discrete ring-like lesion in the lateral aspects of the right middle temporal gyrus consistent with a small neoplasm. Pathology revealed a DNET.

Figure courtesy of Dr Ruben Kuzniecky, NYU epilepsy center, New York, USA

Right: Coronal T1-weighted MRI showing a large DNET occupying the left hippocampal areas and adjacent mesial temporal lobe gyri and white matter.

Figure courtesy of Dr Rod C. Scott, Institute of Child Health, London

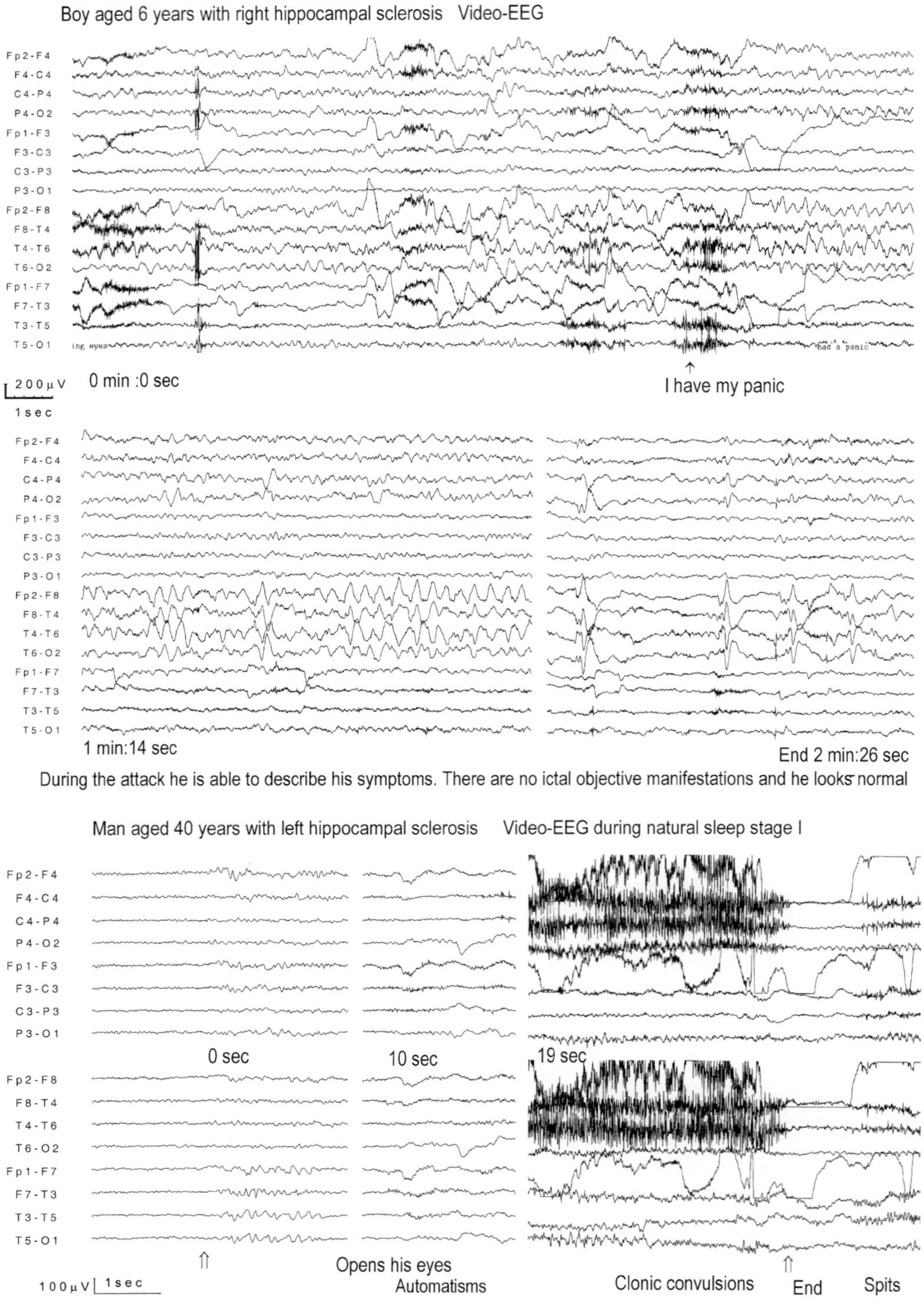

Figure 12.2 Ictal EEG of 2 patients with hippocampal epilepsy.

Top and middle: This was the first EEG of a boy aged 6 referred for episodes of panic attacks and a recent GTCS. The resting EEG was entirely normal but one of his seizures was recorded from onset (0 min:0 s) and lasted for 2 min and 26 s. The child looked disturbed, complaining, "I have my panic". He was able to communicate well during the whole seizure. Speech and cognition were normal. Brain MRI documented right hippocampal sclerosis.

Bottom: Sample of video EEG during a brief seizure of a man aged 40 years with increasing numbers of complex focal seizures typical of hippocampal epilepsy. MRI documented left hippocampal sclerosis. Note that towards the end of the attack the patient had mild clonic convulsions though he never had GTCS. Also note that he immediately spits after the cessation of the seizure.

Ictal clinical symptoms of temporal lobe epilepsy can be subjective, objective or both. They have been accurately localised and studied in neurosurgical series of patients. Simple focal seizures manifest with subjective symptoms of illusions, hallucinations or both (also called auras). These last from a few seconds to 1–2 min. They may be the only seizure type, but commonly progress to complex focal seizures during which objective symptoms, such as automatisms and motor manifestations, appear. Autonomic disturbances are common at any stage of the ictus. Secondarily GTCS may be frequent or rare and one-tenth of patients may never experience GTCS. Postictal fatigue and drowsiness are common.

The clinical manifestations of temporal lobe epilepsy are well described in relevant textbooks. Excellent descriptions can be found in old[12-27] and relatively newer reports[28-34] and reviews[35-39] devoted to this vast subject.

SUBJECTIVE ICTAL CLINICAL MANIFESTATIONS

Subjective ictal clinical manifestations constitute a galaxy of various simple or complex sensations of illusions, hallucinations or both. They are also called auras because they are the first subjective symptom of an epileptic seizure prior to the impairment of consciousness. These symptoms are experienced by nearly all patients (> 90%) with temporal lobe epilepsy.[28,31,35,37,39-41] They can be the only ictal symptom of a focal seizure, but frequently progress to other manifestations of complex focal seizures.[42,43]

Epigastric aura and fear are the commonest and often the initial manifestations of mesial temporal lobe seizures. Simple or complex auditory hallucinations mainly characterise LTLE. Mental hallucinations and illusions are common in both. Olfactory and gustatory hallucinations are less common.

Subjective ictal symptoms of temporal lobe seizures, in order of prevalence, include:

- ascending epigastric aura
- experiential (mental or psychic) symptoms
- fear and panic
- déjà vu or jamais vu and their variations
- auditory hallucinations and illusions
- olfactory and gustatory hallucinations
- other symptoms.

Epigastric or visceral aura

Epigastric or visceral aura is by far the commonest symptom of mesial temporal lobe seizures.[40,44,45] It is defined by location, quality, duration, movement and associated symptoms in progression.

Location: It is usually felt in the upper half of the abdomen[44] with most patients pointing with the palm of one or both hands to a wide area between the end of the sternum and the umbilicus. Of hundreds of patients I have interrogated, I do not recall anyone pointing with a finger instead of the palm or lateralising to one side or the other. Less than 10% of 100 patients thoroughly studied by Van Buren (1963) pointed slightly lateral to the midline.[44]

Quality: Epigastric aura is often initially described as pain, but on further questioning is rarely pain. It is a strange 'difficult-to-describe' sensation in that area for which the most common description I get is as 'if the organs inside are squeezed and twisted'. Other descriptions are of emptiness, rolling, turning, whirling, tenderness, fluttering, butterflies, pressure, burning, nausea, emptiness and their variations.[44] Genuine pain, sometimes excruciating, is exceptional, but does occur.

Duration: This is usually short, a few seconds, but becomes longer with the appearance of other symptoms as the seizure progresses. I am not aware of any report of *'epigastric status epilepticus'*, but it may occur:

A patient with typical MRI and PET scan evidence of right-sided hippocampal sclerosis had frequent seizures starting with an ascending abdominal sensation of discomfort in the stomach "as though being in a lift that stops abruptly". This often progressed to a feeling of disorientation and "shivering", and sometimes déjà vu prior to losing consciousness witnessed as: "stares and fiddles or drums with his fingers on a table". He also had clusters of the same "intense abdominal discomfort and a feeling of shivering" lasting for 2–5 minutes, becoming repetitive at intervals of 1 hour for approximately half a day to 2 days. Within that period lengthy attacks of more than half an hour occurred.

Movement: An ascending epigastric sensation is probably the most characteristic feature of this type of epileptic seizure. Irrespective of quality, this sensation often moves upwards in a slow or fast fashion (within seconds) and, interestingly, it is when it reaches the level of the throat that the patient loses consciousness. Downward movement towards the feet is exceptional.

Fear

Fear is the commonest aura after epigastric sensations in mesial temporal lobe seizures. It is an affective mental symptom. There are two aspects to this. Firstly, fear may be a symptom of a seizure itself. Secondly, fear may be the realistic and natural reaction to an impending convulsion heralded by an aura. In some cases, the one cannot be disentangled from the other, although in most patients fear is an evidenced ictal event.

The intensity and quality of ictal fear varies considerably between patients, though it is stereotypical in each individual. Most patients use the terms 'fear' and 'panic' synonymously. It is not directed towards any particular circumstance, event or person. It is just fear or panic that may be the first, and sometimes the only, ictal symptom.

"I am scared, I have my panic" a 5-year-old boy said during a 2-min video-EEG recorded seizure without other subjective or objective symptoms (Figure 12.2).

More often, fear appears with other symptoms at the beginning or during the course of the seizure.

It starts with my panic and that stomach feeling, and then I pass out.

Fear is not specific to only mesial temporal lobe seizures. Although it is mainly associated with amygdaloid, periamygdaloid and hippocampal stimulation, neocortical areas can also be responsible. A typical example is the fear of frontal lobe seizures. However, there is a major difference between the fear of temporal versus frontal lobe epilepsy:

Fear in mesial temporal lobe seizures is predominantly subjective "I am scared, I am in a terrible panic", which is not apparent to the observer. Conversely, in frontal seizures, 'fear' is predominantly expressive, such as 'his face is fearful'.

I have reached this conclusion after comparing relevant video EEG recordings of a significant number of patients. In temporal lobe seizures, patients feel intense fear or panic while, at the same time, they look relatively calm or their 'fearful' expression is disproportional to the intensity of their panic. Conversely, patients with frontal lobe seizures look so very terrified, which is disproportional to the actual subjective experience of fear. This differentiation should be expected: the temporal lobe is dealing with emotions/memory, while the frontal lobe dictates expression/movement.

Briefly, 'fear' is mainly *felt emotionally* in mesial temporal lobe seizures and mainly *expressed facially* in frontal seizures.

Experiential symptoms (mental, intellectual or psychic symptoms, dreamy states)

Experiential symptoms (also described as mental, intellectual or psychic symptoms, or dreamy states) of temporal lobe seizures are hallucinations, illusions or both. They may involve any faculty of the human mind: thinking, emotion, memory and recollection, chronological order, speed, sensation, reality and unreality, and their interactions with past, present and imaginary experiences. Events and experiences may be reproduced intact or disturbed: the present may be misplaced to the past, and the past to the present; real may be seen as unreal and vice versa; time may be speeded up or slowed down; and shape and other morphology may be natural or unnatural, and deformed or undistorted. Mental ictal symptoms may be very simple and natural, such as the 'déjà vu' phenomenon, a sensation of 'fear and panic' or a mild sense of depersonalisation such as "who am I?", that may also be experienced by normal people who do not have seizures. On other occasions, these symptoms may be more complicated with a complete distortion of time, space, morphology, direction, experience and normality.

The mental ictal manifestations of temporal lobe seizures typically combine elements of perception, memory and affect that, as in real life, are often encompassed together in a unified subjective symptom.[28] Perceptual, mnemonic or affective aberrations usually cluster in various combinations and various degrees of disturbance. However, one aberration may be more involved than another; sometimes, one may be exclusively affected and may occur in isolation. Depending on the predominant mental aberration, they are subdivided under various names, such as: *ideational* (impairment of thoughts), *dysmnesic* (impairment of memory), *affective* (emotional impairment)[46] and *dyscognitive* (impairment of perception, cognition).

Déjà vu

Déjà vu is another common symptom that is experienced exclusively as an ictal phenomenon in temporal lobe seizures. Déjà vu is a natural event that has been experienced by most normal people and the term is used in everyday life. In temporal lobe epilepsy, déjà vu is signified by the presence and the sequence of other epileptic events that may precede, coincide or follow it.

'Déjà vu' (already seen) is commonly used in a much broader sense, to include 'déjà entendu' (already heard) and 'déjà veçu' (already lived, experienced), as a false feeling of having experienced, seen and heard something before that is actually

Nomenclature issues

'Dreamy states', 'psychic or mental symptoms', 'intellectual aura' and 'experiential phenomena' are the terms most widely used to denote symptoms of temporal lobe seizures that uniquely relate to the patient's personality regarding identity, experience, emotion, thought and memory. These terms are not necessarily synonymous, because they are used in the relevant literature to encompass either limited or much wider ictal manifestations.

Hughlings Jackson[14;15;47;48] introduced the term 'dreamy state' in favour of 'intellectual aura' or 'psychical state'. He also used the word 'psychical' not as synonymous to the 'dreamy state', but to differentiate it from physical symptoms.

Peculiar mental state' are the words used by Holmes.[16]

Of these terms, 'psychic symptoms'[1] became popular first and 'dreamy state' second. Other terms used are 'mental aura' or 'mental symptoms' that may be illusionary or hallucinatory. 'Psychic' has inappropriate connotations and implications. Furthermore, these symptoms are transient mental, not psychic, aberrations. Patients have a clear insight that these are pathological symptoms for which they themselves seek medical advice. 'Experiential phenomena', introduced by Penfield[49] and masterly detailed by Gloor (1993)[31] and Bancaud et al. (1994),[33] may be an appropriate term for only those manifestations that are based on previously experienced events. It is of limited value for ictal mental symptoms that are not related to previous experiences or in certain common circumstances that defy such experiential links.

Definition

Déjà vu is defined as any subjectively inappropriate impression of familiarity of a present experience with an undefined past. Different mental components, such as memory, attention and perception, are associated with this distinct experience.

happening now. In déjà vu, the physical recognition is correct, but it is inappropriately connected with mental, emotional, experiential and timing processes that are associated with other physical presentations. The feeling of familiarity supervenes. It is mainly, a feeling of immense and vivid familiarity with the present situation irrespective of whether the content is visual, auditory or of any other physical presentation. The patient may say "that it is as if I have seen, heard or lived this before", but more often the expression is "it was so familiar to me".[33,50]

> Extreme familiarity with people and surroundings, as if I knew them well, as if they were close friends or relatives, intimate relations, as if it was my everyday experience. It is more of a feeling of knowing them well than of visual or auditory recognition and experience.

> Seizures start with a strong feeling of extreme familiarity with what he sees, hears or happens at the moment. The feeling is so intense and vivid that on one occasion when this happened while playing cards with his wife, he thought that he knew exactly the next sequence of cards to be played.

The precise origin of déjà vu is still controversial (see for review ref [50]). On the basis of intracranial EEG monitoring and stimulation studies, three possible sites of dysfunction have been proposed: (a) the mesial temporal lobe especially in the non-dominant hemisphere; (b) the superior lateral temporal cortex; and (c) a neuronal network that engages both mesial and lateral aspects of the temporal lobe. However, it is uncertain whether the temporal lobe disturbance is sufficient and necessary for the generation of déjà vu, since it is difficult to evaluate wider cortical regions using intracranial recordings. Based on PET scan studies, Adachi et al. (1999)[50] proposed that extensive cortical areas beyond the temporal lobe, such as the parietal and possibly other association areas, may be involved in the network that integrates the déjà vu experience. Involvement of the left hemisphere, irrespective of the side of ictal onset, seems to be of particular importance for the generation of the déjà vu experience.

Jamais vu, jamais entendu and jamais veçu

Jamais vu (never seen), jamais entendu (never heard) and jamais veçu (never experienced before) are similar as the jamais vu expressions for illusions "during which the subject's surroundings even when familiar are no longer recognised, although they are clearly perceived by the subject". Jamais vu is commonly used in a much broader sense to include jamais entendu and jamais veçu. It is a false feeling of unfamiliarity (has not been experienced, seen or heard) with something that has been previously encountered.

Jamais vu is much rarer than déjà vu, but it is well described by some patients with temporal lobe epilepsy. Similar to 'déjà vu/familiarity', in 'jamais vu/unfamiliarity', the feeling of unfamiliarity is stronger than the visual, auditory or other sensorial component. Visual, auditory and any other physical recognition is correct, but the connections to the mental and emotional processes associated with them are missing.

> I know that she is my mother but I do not feel that she is. Her features do not change. She is still my mother but I do not have the same human attachment to her. She is a stranger with the looks, the voice and the manners of my mother. She is a stranger.

Auditory hallucinations and illusions

Auditory hallucinations are attributed to lateral temporal lobe seizures, which are much less common than mesial temporal lobe seizures. They may be elementary or complex auditory hallucinations.

Elementary auditory hallucinations are crude and described as buzzing, ringing, hissing, fizzing, whistling, humming, shrilling, sizzling or clicking auditory sensations. High pitch noises are more frequently reported. They mainly originate from the activation of Heschl's auditory cortex in the superior temporal gyrus. For many patients, this 'buzz' is the aura and the start of the seizure itself.

> Here it is again. That buzzing in both ears. It is just buzz. I cannot describe it. A buzz. There is nothing else. No voice, no identifiable noise that simulates anything else, just a buzz.

Complex auditory hallucinations consist of voices, music or other sounds that may be familiar or unfamiliar, friendly or aggressive and offensive, clear or indefinable, meaningful or incomprehensible. Complex auditory hallucinations are rarely the first ictal symptom and they usually combine with other visual or mental ictal symptoms of the 'dreamy state'. These are mainly elicited by activation of the associated auditory cortex. Auditory hallucinations of hearing a voice are almost always without semantic content, even though the voice may sound familiar and may be identifiable.[31] The affective tone of the voice is, however, often recognised.

> "It is a clear voice of a woman, she says something that I do not remember", "conversations of people talking next door", "a hoarse voice of a man saying that I have to go", "sounds of human voices and animals", "I hear the same voice saying the same thing. I know it at the time but I can not recall it afterwards", "a voice filtered as if spoken through a handkerchief", "it is my own voice talking to myself", "voices through an amplifier or a loud speaker."

Hearing music, often the same piece for every seizure, is uncommon though it is frequently cited in the literature and can be reproduced during electrical stimulation studies. [18,51-53] A song, usually a nursery rhyme, may be more common than music.

Auditory illusions are altered perceptions and interpretations of sounds, voices and conversations in the actual environment during the seizure. This may refer to simple changes of intensity, resonance, spatial orientation, tone, echo and clarity or be more complicated. Sounds and voices may appear louder/deafening/ear-splitting or dim/faded, nearer or further away, clearer or disturbed, higher or lower pitched, echoed and variations of all of these.

> "the voices fade away", "my hearing is heightened so I can hear everything loud and high pitched", "as if talking from a distance", "the voices become hoarse", "a woman's voice sounds like a man's voice or like that of an animal", "the sounds become so intense as if somebody has put the radio at maximum volume next to your ears", "I hear the echo of the voices", "as if you are in an empty church, you hear the sounds and their echoes."

Olfactory and gustatory hallucinations

Olfactory epileptic auras are rare, constituting about 0.9% of all auras, and are typically, but not necessarily, unpleasant.[54-56] The amygdala is the most likely symptomatogenic zone of olfactory auras. Tumours[54] and hippocampal sclerosis[56] are common causes.

> "a strong smell of gas or something like this", "a smell of rotten leaves", "a smell of perfume", "a peculiar odour that I can not describe".

Gustatory epileptic auras are hallucinations of taste that are usually unpleasant (rotten food) or a strange taste. They are usually generated in the insula or superior Sylvian bank.[55,57,58]

> "a strange taste of food in my mouth", "a taste of burnt food", "a taste of rotten food", "taste of funny food in my mouth."

Visual hallucinations and illusions

Visual hallucinations and visual illusions are detailed in the discussion of occipital lobe epilepsies.

Elementary visual hallucinations originate in the visual cortex. They do not feature in temporal lobe seizures except after secondary spread to the occipital lobes.

Complex visual hallucinations originate from the occipito-parietal-temporal junction and therefore may be part of any seizure that starts from or spreads to this area.

Complex visual hallucinations may take the form of persons, animals, objects, figures or scenes. They may be static or moving, real or unreal, normal or distorted in size, shape and dimension. They often progress to more complex visual hallucinatory experiences. They may be familiar or unfamiliar, friendly, frightening or grotesque. They may or may not be related with a past visual experience or connected with past events. In two patients reported by Penfield and associates,[59,60] habitual complex visual hallucinations could be elicited by stimulation of the right posterior temporal regions.

An influential report on this subject has been written by Lance (1976)[61] and the topic has been effectively reviewed by Kolmel (1993).[62]

Gordon Holmes (1927),[16] in differentiating visual hallucinations of occipital from temporal lobe epilepsy, clearly stated:

> "More complicated subjective visual phenomena associated with local lesions in the neighbourhood of the uncus of the temporal lobe are different in origin and nature to those of occipital epilepsy. These uncinate epileptic seizures frequently begin with subjective smells and tastes, which are almost invariably of an unpleasant, usually of an extremely disagreeable, character; often there is, too, an epigastric sensation which may account to actual nausea. Then comes that peculiar mental state which Jackson called the 'dreamy state' or 'intellectual aura' characterised by a feeling of unreality of the present or familiarity with the events of the moment as though they had been experienced before. Often visions, which the patient associates with the past come up. A patient whom I had under observation always saw, in this stage a woman with a red cloak approaching nearer and nearer until, as the spectre reached her, she lost consciousness. In other cases, the vision may be of a scene tinted with a tone of familiarity, a building or a similar object. In such cases the visual hallucinations, for to these the term hallucination can be applied, is only part of the intellectual aura of Jackson and is obviously the result of more complicated cerebral and psychological processes than the perception and projection of lights and colour."

Usually, auditory and visual hallucinations occur together. These are complex hallucinations of a scene, people, animals, objects, voices, music or the noise of a train. The content of these hallucinations usually appears familiar, but it may be entirely strange or unidentifiable.

Ictal urinary urge

Ictal urinary urge indicates seizure onset in the non-dominant temporal lobe.[63] Six patients with temporal lobe seizures characterised by an aura of ictal urinary urge were recently described.[63] In ictal single photon emission computed tomography (SPECT) of two patients, there was hyperperfusion of the insular cortex, indicating a critical role of the insula in the generation of the urinary urge.

OBJECTIVE ICTAL SYMPTOMS

Objective ictal symptoms of temporal lobe epilepsy usually occur when consciousness is impaired. The patient is seldom aware of them. They are described by witnesses or captured on video recordings.

Objective ictal symptoms in order of prevalence include:

- Automatisms
- Autonomic disturbances
- Speech disturbances
- Head and eye deviation as well as dystonic postures

- Motor arrest with staring
- Unilateral ictal paresis
- Unilateral eyelid blinking
- Ictal vomiting

In general, nearly all of these ictal symptoms are not specific to temporal lobe seizures. Recent reviews and reports of temporal lobe epilepsy have emphasised objective symptoms only because of their lateralising value.

Automatisms

Oro-alimentary automatisms, which are often followed by simple gestural automatisms, are characteristic of MTLE *only if* preceded by epigastric aura, fear and mental symptoms of the 'dreamy state' of Jackson, alone or in combination.[34,37,39,64-67] Oro-alimentary automatisms are more likely to begin in the first part of a complex focal seizure after the aura . They are attributed to seizures originating from the amygdala and periamygdaloid region, and not from the hippocampus. However, hippocampal after-discharges invariably spread to the amygdala, which explains the high prevalence of these automatisms in MTLE.

Simple automatisms, devoid of behavioural changes, are of no diagnostic significance in temporal lobe epilepsy. They are among the commonest symptoms in childhood and juvenile absence epilepsy. They are differentiated by clustering of other symptoms, duration and EEG manifestations.

Verbal automatisms of coherent speech are associated with seizure onset in the non-dominant hemisphere.[38,70] Ictal vocalisation probably has no lateralising value.[70] Both ictal vocalisation and verbal automatisms can occur in extratemporal epilepsies, such as frontal lobe seizures; they often occur in childhood and juvenile absence epilepsy.[71]

Definitions of automatisms

Automatisms are coordinated involuntary simple movements or more complex acts performed by a patient who is unaware of them, because consciousness is sufficiently impaired. The patient is totally amnesic of this behaviour.

Automatisms are defined by the ILAE as "A more or less coordinated, repetitive, motor activity usually occurring when cognition is impaired and for which the subject is usually amnesic afterwards. This often resembles a voluntary movement, and may consist of inappropriate continuation of ongoing preictal motor activity."[68]

According to Jackson "They have one common character – they are automatic; they are done unconsciously, and the agent is irresponsible. Hence, I use the term mental automatism."[47;69]

In the *Dictionary of Epilepsy*[46] automatisms are "more or less coordinated adapted (eupractic or dyspractic) involuntary motor activity occurring during the state of clouding of consciousness either in the course of, or after an epileptic seizure, and usually followed by amnesia for the event. The automatism may be simply a continuation of an activity that was going on when the seizure occurred, or, conversely, a new activity developed in association with the ictal impairment of consciousness. Usually, the activity is commonplace in nature, often provoked by the subject's environment, or by his sensations during the seizure: exceptionally, fragmentary, primitive, infantile, or antisocial behaviour may occur."

Automatisms may be simple or complex.

I. Simple automatisms, devoid of behavioural changes, manifest with simple involuntary movements and include:

Oro-alimentary automatisms: lip smacking, lip pursing, chewing, licking, tooth grinding or swallowing

Vocal: single or repetitive utterances consisting of sounds such as grunts or shrieks

Verbal: single or repetitive utterances consisting of words, phrases or brief sentences, such as uttering, shouting, talking or singing words, sentences or phrases

Gestural: often unilateral: (a) fumbling or exploratory movements with the hand directed towards self or environment; fiddling, fumbling, picking, tapping, patting or plucking, rubbing or scratching the face and other gestural movements; and (b) movements resembling those intended to lend further emotional tone to speech

Ambulatory automatisms: well coordinated acts, such as walking straight or in circles, continuing cycling or even driving

Manual or pedal: bilateral or unilateral fumbling, tapping, manipulating movements

Mimetic: facial expression suggesting an emotional state, often fear[68]

II. Complex (behavioural)automatisms: rich in behavioural changes with complex acts performed without apparent awareness. Semi-purposeful or well-organised exploratory or inappropriate behavioural manifestations, such as embarrassing actions, undressing in public, chewing objects that are not edible, wandering or running inappropriately, or aggressive behavioural acts.

Automatisms may also be spontaneous or interactive

Spontaneous: stereotyped, involve only self, and are virtually independent of environmental influences

Interactive: not stereotyped, involve more than self, and are environmentally influenced.

Complex automatisms rich in behavioural aberrations are also common in temporal lobe epilepsy, and also occur in extratemporal seizures; they are exceptional in typical absence seizures.

Spitting, either as an ictal or postictal event,[72] and bicycling movements[73] are also common in extratemporal seizures.

Automatisms involving masturbation or other sexually related behaviour are uncommon, though often mentioned even in brief textbook reviews; I have never encountered them. Ictal penile erection and ejaculation are autonomic disturbances.[74,75]

It is generally considered that unilateral automatisms are ipsilateral to the seizure onset.[38] However, this has been debated by Elger (2000)[76] and it is not applicable in patients with bilateral independent temporal spikes.[77]

Language and speech ictal disturbances

In addition to vocal and verbal automatisms, speech arrest and language disturbances are frequent manifestations of temporal lobe seizures. The commonest of all is the inability to speak.

> "I know what is going on and I understand what they are saying, but I can not speak" is much more common than "I know what it is but I can not find the word".

Ictal aphasia and ictal speech arrest have been attributed to seizure onset in the language-dominant temporal lobe.[78] Clear ictal speech and quick recovery mainly characterise seizures of the non-dominant temporal lobe,[38,65] while postictal aphasia and prolonged recovery are mainly features of seizures of the dominant temporal lobe.[38]

Motor arrest, staring and temporal lobe absence

Motor and speech arrest together with staring and loss of consciousness may be the first objective symptom of a temporal lobe seizure. As a rule, they follow other subjective symptoms, but in around 10% of patients, they may occur alone from the beginning of the seizure. These symptoms are clinically similar to those of generalised absence seizures when examined in isolation. For this reason, this type of focal seizure is also called 'temporal lobe absence', a term that should be discouraged to avoid confusion with 'generalised absence seizures', which are completely different if other symptoms and duration are considered in their entirety.

The duration of motor arrest, staring and loss of consciousness varies, but usually lasts for 1 min. Occasionally, this may be the only manifestation of the seizure. The patient usually recovers without other concurrent symptoms, such as automatisms.

Motor manifestations

Motor manifestations include eye and head deviation, as well as dystonic postures that occur in around one-fifth of patients. These symptoms, which are also detailed in other chapters, are not specific to temporal lobe seizures. Thus, eye and head deviation is a common symptom in frontal and occipital lobe seizures. Dystonic postures are more often related to the frontal than temporal lobe.

Motor manifestations, despite their insignificance for pure anatomical localisation, are of value with respect to possible lateralisation:

Early and casual deviation of the eyes and head, in the setting of other more typical mesial temporal lobe ictal symptoms, may be ipsilateral to the epileptogenic focus.[38,79-81] Conversely, it is almost always contralateral if it occurs during the progression of the seizure, when it is also more violent and often followed by secondarily GTCS.[37]

Unilateral tonic or dystonic posturing of arm, leg and face was described by Ajmone-Marsan and Ralston[19] who called it 'larval M2e' to differentiate it from that of frontal lobe seizures. It is often associated with ipsilateral automatisms. It is reliably contralateral to the epileptogenic focus.[38]

Unilateral eyelid blinking is ipsilateral to the epileptogenic focus.[82]

Unilateral ictal paresis is contralateral to the origin of the seizure.[83]

AUTONOMIC DISTURBANCES AND ICTUS EMETICUS

Autonomic disturbances of any type are among the most frequent ictal symptoms of temporal lobe epilepsy.[84-88]

Cardiovascular symptoms, mainly tachycardia and arrhythmias, less often bradycardia, asystole or hypertension, are very common and may be a common cause of sudden death in temporal lobe epilepsies (Figure 12.3).[75,84,88-93]

A brief respiratory arrest, a sigh or a gasp is common in the initial part of complex focal seizures. Hyperpnoea, hypopnoea or even apnoea may occur in the late seizure phase.[75]

Mydriasis, sometimes asymmetrical, is a frequent symptom associated with the arrest reaction.[38,75] Miosis and hippus pupillae are also common.[75]

A feeling of 'shivering cold' is sometimes associated with piloerection.[75] Salivation is common, but lacrimation and nasal secretion are rare.[75]

There are occasional reports of penile erection, and even ejaculation or other sexual ictal manifestations.[74]

Flushing or more often pallor are commonly encountered.[75]

Ictus emeticus (nausea, retching and vomiting), and particularly ictal vomiting, is exceptional in adult patients with temporal lobe seizures, but very common in children with Panayiotopoulos syndrome.

Important clinical note on ictus emeticus in adults and children

In adults, there are no more than 30 reported cases of ictal vomiting, which predominantly emanates from the non-dominant temporal lobe and usually occurs after seizure onset, concurrently with other symptoms, and the patient is amnesic of the events.[77,94-97] Conversely, ictus emeticus in children is very common, usually occurs at the onset of the seizures and the patient has a good recollection of the event (see ictus emeticus in Panayiotopoulos syndrome page 235).[98-100]

Cardiac asystole in temporal lobe seizures

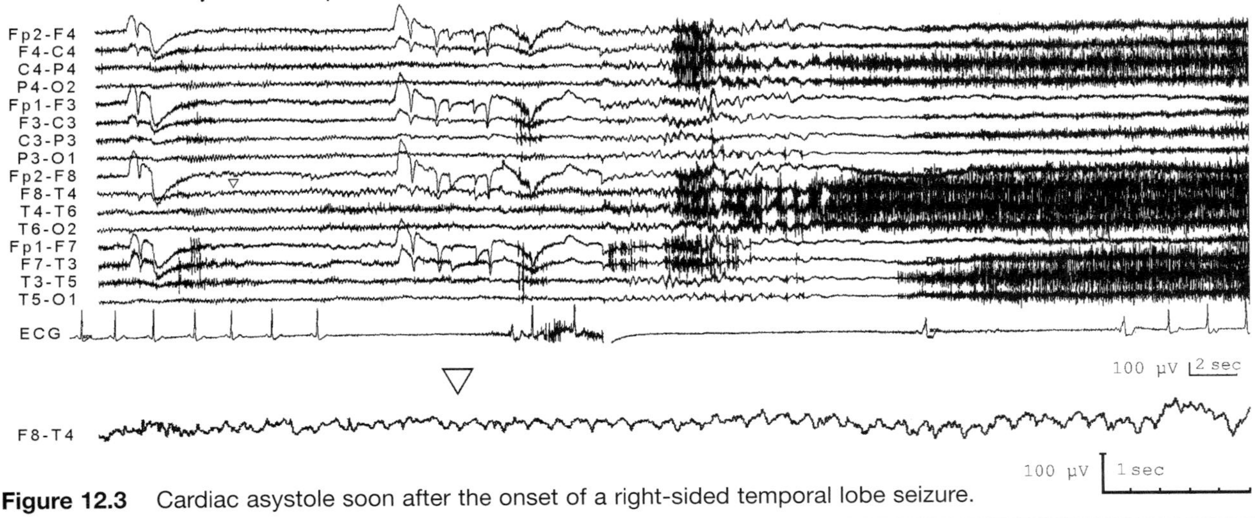

Figure 12.3 Cardiac asystole soon after the onset of a right-sided temporal lobe seizure.

The patient is a 60-year-old man with seizures of MTLE of recent onset. Seizures start with a vague feeling of ascending epigastric sensation. He never had GTCS. Brain MRI was normal.

Figure courtesy of Dr Michael Koutroumanidis, Department of Clinical Neurophysiology and Epilepsies, St. Thomas' Hospital, London, UK.

GELASTIC SEIZURES OF TEMPORAL LOBE EPILEPSY

Ictal laughter is rare, but has been well documented in over 34 cases of temporal lobe epilepsy.[101] It has been attributed mainly to right-[76] and less often to left-sided[102-104] extramesial seizures. Age at onset is variable with several cases starting in childhood. Gelastic seizures have been produced by stimulation of the temporobasal cortex in two candidates for surgery for non-gelastic seizures and explored with subdural electrodes.[105]

The clinical descriptions are variable; the laughter being natural or forced, unmotivated, associated or even reactional to a pleasant event or feeling.

The laughter commonly is devoid of any sensation and is accompanied by a break of contact. A few patients have described feelings of mirth associated with laughter[105-108] or an immediate environment felt to be amusing or distorted.[105,107] In one case, the seizures could be triggered by hyperextension of the back and, in another case, sexual sensation was reported prior to the development of laughter.[108]

In 50% of cases, other types of seizures occur concomitantly or precede the gelastic seizures.[101]

See also hypothalamic (gelastic) epilepsy.

AMNESIC SEIZURES

In pure amnesic seizures, the only clinical manifestation is an inability to retain in memory what occurs during the seizure. Other cognitive functions are preserved and patients interact normally with their physical and social environment.[109] Pure amnesic seizures of patients with temporal lobe epilepsy never represent the only type of seizure. This may suggest that they result from selective ictal inactivation of mesial temporal structures without neocortical involvement. Amnesic seizures occur most often in patients with neuropsychological and EEG evidence of bilateral dysfunction of mesial temporal lobe structures. More rarely, in unilateral dysfunction, amnesic seizures may be due to seizure discharge limited to the mesial temporal structures of both sides, probably as a result of contralateral spread from one to the other through the dorsal hippocampal commissure.[109]

CATAMENIAL TEMPORAL LOBE SEIZURES

Some women have exclusively catamenial seizures, which may demand different management.[110,111]

A 32-year-old businesswoman had had strictly catamenial simple focal seizures since 13 years of age. On the third premenstrual day, she would have 10–14 seizures, 5–6 the next day, then 1–3 the next day and none until the next month when the same pattern of events was repeated. The seizures are stereotyped and last for around 30 s. Suddenly, she has a feeling of extreme familiarity with people and her surroundings. She also has the feeling that people or animals look alike. All her senses (smell, hearing, skin) are heightened. There is no apparent impairment of consciousness. Postictally, she is tired and has severe bifrontal postictal headache, which may last for hours. These progressed to loss of consciousness and mild convulsions on only three occasions. Treatment with valproate and later with carbamazepine did not have any effect. She did not take any medication after the age of 18 years. From around 20 years of age, the seizures improved dramatically and there was no catamenial relation after starting hormonal contraception.

POSTICTAL SYMPTOMS

Postictal symptoms are common, often characteristic and may be of value in lateralising temporal lobe seizures. Such symptoms include mental and physical fatigue, drowsiness, headache, language aberrations, inability to concentrate and confusion to varying degrees that is often severe and associated with automatic behaviour of which the patient may be amnesic. Some patients may wander about in the streets, behaving normally or in a socially unacceptable manner, having no recollection of the events when they recover.

In an attempt to reorient to the current situation, an embarrassing smile, coughing, spitting or sighing are early postictal symptoms (Figure 12.2).[76,113]

Postictal symptoms may be disproportionately more severe than the ictal manifestations and may last for hours.

> "Soon, perhaps a minute, afterwards, his actions, or I should say the irrelevant-seeming actions, ceased; he replied correctly to simple questions, and told me that it was not necessary for me to go home with him. He, however, looked confused and seemed strange. When we got to his house a few yards away, I thought he was fully recovered, and, as I was thinking of making another room on the ground floor of my house, I took the opportunity of speaking to him about a third room there was on the ground floor of his house. Among other things he said he used to breakfast there. I was surprised when he afterwards, next day, told me that he remembered nothing from the time of being in my room consulting me (before the fit) to a little time after I left him at his own house".
>
> Jackson JH and Colman WS. 1898[15]

Marked postictal manifestations may follow seemingly mild attacks and vice versa.

> I am so drained and exhausted with irresistible drowsiness.
> I write the rest of my day off.

SIGNIFICANCE OF POSTICTAL SYMPTOMS IN LATERALISATION

Recent reports signified postictal aphasia and global disorientation as a lateralising symptom of the language dominant hemisphere.[38,65,66] Conversely, well-formed ictal speech and rapid return to baseline postictally occur in non-dominant temporal lobe seizures.[66] Contrary to these, Elger (2000)[76] found postictal aphasia in both right and left hippocampal epilepsy, "possibly due to the spread of seizure discharges from right to left".

Lateralised postictal motor deficits are contralateral to seizure origin.[38,83]

DIFFERENTIATING TEMPORAL LOBE SEIZURES FROM OTHER EXTRATEMPORAL SEIZURES ON THE BASIS OF POSTICTAL SYMPTOMS

Postictal symptoms are far more common after temporal lobe than extratemporal seizure onsets. Postictal confusional states and automatisms are exceptional in extratemporal seizures. In frontal lobe seizures, the patient immediately recovers after the fit with no postictal manifestations. In visual occipital seizures, the only postictal abnormality is a severe migraine-like headache that often follows[71].

DIAGNOSTIC PROCEDURES

Brain MRI is the most important diagnostic test required for all patients with temporal lobe epilepsy to detect symptomatic causes.[114-118] High resolution MRI may detect abnormalities in 90% of patients in neurosurgical series.

A brief reminder of catamenial epilepsy

"Catamenial epilepsy is often vaguely defined as the occurrence of seizures around the time of menses or an increase in seizures in relation to the menstrual cycle."[111] Catamenial seizures increase in approximately one-third of women with focal or generalised epilepsies, but only a small proportion of these patients suffer from pure catamenial epilepsy (i.e. seizures occurring only in relation to their menses). Catamenial epilepsy may be perimenstrual, periovulatory and luteal.[111]

The diagnosis is based on careful assessment of menstrual and seizure diaries, and characterisation of cycle type and duration.

Of a variety of mechanisms proposed, hormonal influences are the best established and exert significant effects on seizure threshold. Oestrogens have a proconvulsant effect, while progesterone has mainly anticonvulsant properties.[111]

However, in contrast to focal and secondarily GTCS, progesterone may exacerbate absence seizures and generalised spike and wave discharge (GSWD).[111;112]

The most common therapies proposed in small, uncontrolled or anecdotal reports include acetazolamide, cyclical use of benzodiazepines (mainly clobazam) or antiepileptic drugs (AEDs), and hormonal therapy.[111]

Magnetic resonance spectroscopy (MRS) offers valuable insights and is useful in the presurgical evaluation of patients. PET scanning and other functional brain imaging modalities are helpful for localisation.

The serum prolactin concentration may rise markedly 10 min after seizure onset in three-quarters of patients.[119]

ELECTROENCEPHALOGRAPHY

Interictal EEG of MTLE is identical to that detailed in hippocampal epilepsy (see page 378), irrespective of aetiology.[120-122] Briefly, in one-third of patients, the classical spike or sharp and slow wave is shown by the anterior temporal electrode (Figure 12.4), and the yield is increased with prolonged EEG recordings and sleep EEG.

In LTLE, spike and sharp wave complexes may be seen in the middle temporal electrode (Figure 12.5), but this is often indistinguishable from MTLE.

"Please, exclude temporal lobe epilepsy" is the commonest reason for requesting an EEG for any kind of transient behavioural aberration; it is often an impossible task.

About two-thirds of patients have a normal routine interictal EEG or show non-specific abnormalities with an excess of slow waves in one temporal lobe. Runs of monomorphic slow waves may be important for lateralisation and appear ipsilateral to seizure onset (Figure 12.4).[123-125] Furthermore, in patients with temporal lobe epilepsy whose MRI is either normal or suggestive of hippocampal sclerosis,

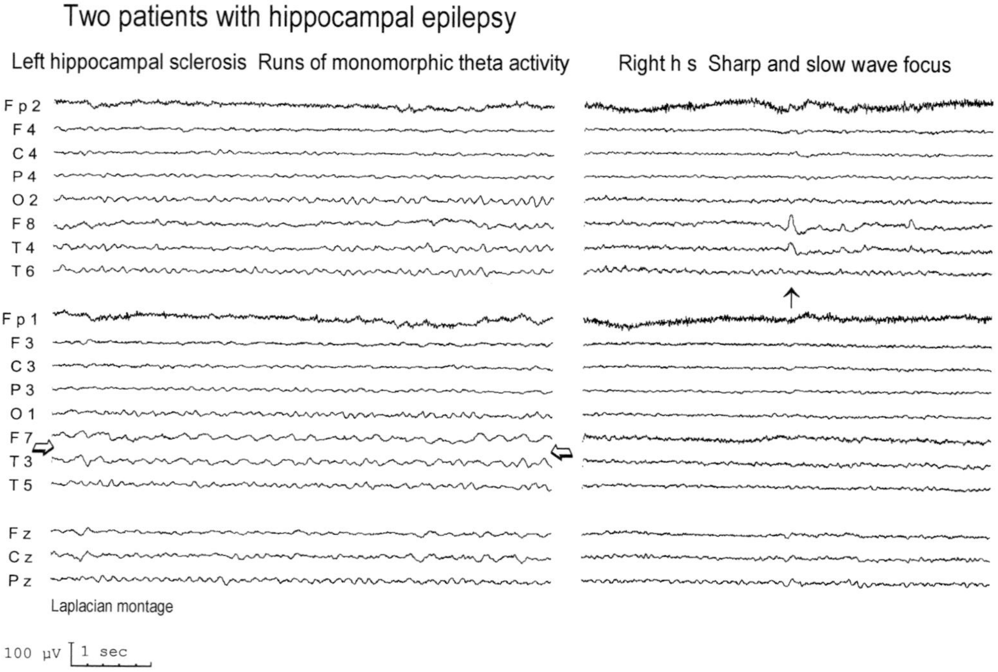

Figure 12.4 EEG samples from two patients with hippocampal epilepsy.

Left: Discrete runs of monomorphic theta activity are localised in the left anterior temporal regions in this patient with left hippocampal sclerosis. There were no spikes or other 'conventional' epileptogenic abnormalities.

Right: The conventional epileptogenic focus of sharp and slow wave complexes is localised in the right anterior temporal electrode. The patient had right hippocampal sclerosis.

interictal temporal delta activity has a lateralising value similar to that of temporal spiking.[125]

Ictal EEG as detailed in hippocampal epilepsy is not significantly different in either MTLE or LTLE.[126-128] It mainly consists of regional ipsilateral rhythmic 4–7-Hz activity (Figures 12.2 and 12.3). Less often, there is attenuation of the background rhythms and remission of the interictal spikes. In one study, the ictal EEG in LTLE revealed a lower mean frequency of lateralised rhythmic activity that frequently had a hemispheric distribution, whereas in MTLE seizures this was maximal over the ipsilateral temporal region.[113]

DIFFERENTIAL DIAGNOSIS

The typical temporal lobe seizures consisting of rising epigastric sensation, fear and progression to impairment of consciousness with oro-alimentary automatisms should be easy to diagnose.

DIFFERENTIATION FROM FRONTAL LOBE AND OTHER EXTRA-TEMPORAL SEIZURES

Although various ictal symptoms of temporal lobe epilepsy may also occur with a varying degree of frequency in extratemporal lobe seizures, the vast majority of temporal lobe epilepsy offers no difficulty in differential diagnosis if symptoms are properly analysed, synthetically and chronologically.

A single ictal symptom may predominate in one or another type of seizure from various locations, but makes no significant contribution to diagnosis. For example, head deviation can occur in seizures from any location, which are identified by other concurrent symptoms, such as elementary visual hallucinations in occipital seizures, epigastric and other auras in temporal lobe epilepsy, and stereotypical and rather violent jerks of the head in frontal lobe seizures.

Another example is dystonic motor manifestations that are common in both temporal and frontal lobe epilepsy. However, in frontal lobe seizures, these manifestations are usually the very first symptom; they are brief and often occur without severe impairment of consciousness, mainly during sleep and with no

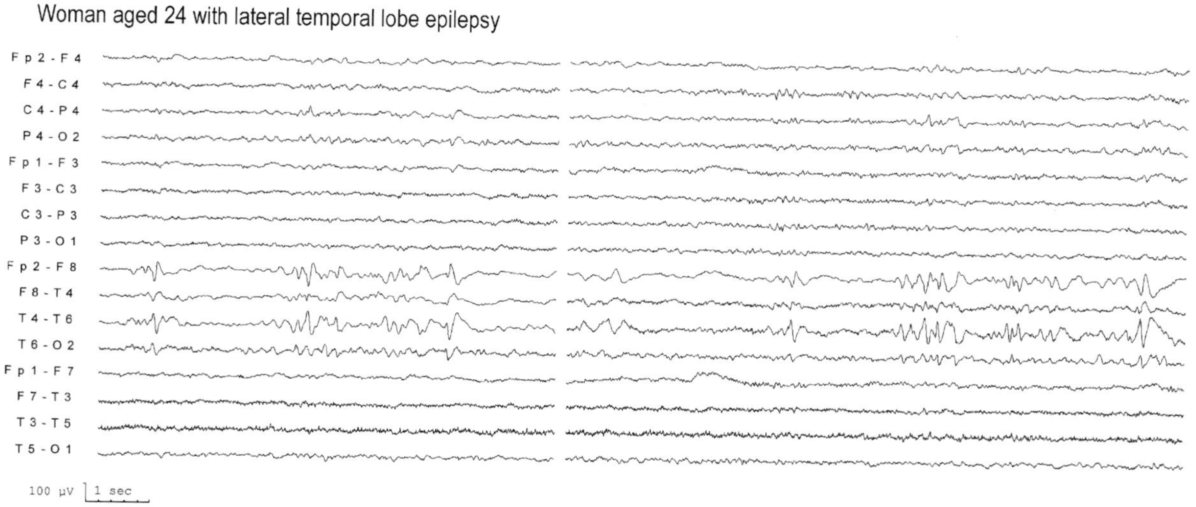

Figure 12.5 EEG of a woman aged 24 with LTLE. Note the marked focal abnormalities of slow waves and sharp–slow wave complexes around the right anterior-midtemporal regions.

postictal symptoms. There are no preceding symptoms of rising epigastric sensations, oro-alimentary automatisms, olfactory and gustatory hallucinations, or mental illusions and hallucinations.

The most frequent misdiagnosis is that of typical absence seizures in adults as temporal lobe seizures with which they have nothing else in common other than impairment of consciousness and automatisms.[129]

PROGNOSIS

The prognosis is largely, but not exclusively, cause related. Thus, of the established syndromes, familial temporal lobe epilepsy is usually mild (page 353), while hippocampal epilepsy may take a progressive course that can be successfully halted by appropriate neurosurgical procedures. However, even in cases with the same cause, such as hippocampal epilepsy, the prognosis can vary significantly from mild to severe (page 389). In community studies, it appears that 10–40% or more of patients with epileptic seizures of temporal lobe origin may go into remission.[130]

MANAGEMENT

Management comprises AEDs and/or neurosurgical excision of the epileptogenic region.

A recent practice parameter for temporal lobe epilepsy and localised neocortical resections[131,132] concludes:

"*The benefits of anteromesial temporal lobe resection for disabling complex partial seizures is greater than continued treatment with antiepileptic drugs, and the risks are at least comparable. For patients who are compromised by such seizures, referral to an epilepsy surgery center should be strongly considered. Further studies are needed to determine if neocortical seizures benefit from surgery, and whether early surgical intervention should be the treatment of choice for certain surgically remediable epileptic syndromes.*"[131,132]

MESIAL TEMPORAL LOBE EPILEPSY WITH HIPPOCAMPAL SCLEROSIS

HIPPOCAMPAL EPILEPSY

MTLE with hippocampal sclerosis (MTLE-HS) or hippocampal epilepsy is the commonest and one of the most distinct epileptic diseases/syndromes with defined underlying hippocampal pathology shown on MRI, clinical seizure types and post-resection seizure relief.[133,134] MTLE-HS has been the subject of a recent state-of-the art ILAE report.[134] Experts discussed the definition, natural history, pathological features, pathogenesis, electroclinical, neurophysiological, neuropsychological, and structural and functional imaging findings of MTLE-HS.

The clinical features and prognosis of MTLE-HS derive almost exclusively from neurosurgical series of cases that are medically intractable.[37,39,75,76,134-136] Therefore, they may not accurately represent the clinical spectrum of MTLE-HS, particularly with respect to severity and prognosis. The neurosurgical cases may represent the tip of the iceberg and the worst cases (about 20%). The vast majority of cases (80%) are not seen in these specialised neurosurgical centres, and some cases may be very mild and easily controlled with appropriate AEDs. I have seen an impressive number of professionals (physicians, nurses, solicitors, successful businessmen, teachers) and ordinary working class people that live a normal life, some with minor focal seizures, but others with an occasional secondary GTCS often controlled with AED monotherapy.

A 35-year-old man had an excellent work and health record as a fire-fighter and driver for 11 years despite numerous seizures from 31 years of age.

The onset of seizures was inconspicuous with brief episodes (lasting a few seconds) of "an empty feeling in the stomach" with no other symptoms. However, 2 years later, these occurred on a daily basis and were associated with a "daydream, you disappear in your own world for a moment, a second". He did not experience any overt loss of consciousness during these events, but he felt distant and he was told by his colleagues that he became aggressive. These episodes lasted a few seconds and rarely 1 min. He was investigated in a major teaching hospital for hypoglycaemia and cardiac dysrhythmia. EEG showed independent bitemporal abnormalities of slow and occasional sharp waves. MRI documented left-sided hippocampal atrophy. Nearly all the seizures were stopped with carbamazepine 400 mg daily. Following the diagnosis of temporal lobe epilepsy, he was made redundant from work.

A more complete clinical picture is expected to emerge now that MRI enables an in-vivo diagnosis of hippocampal sclerosis/atrophy (Figures 12.1 and 12.6).[137,138]

DEMOGRAPHIC DATA

Habitual hippocampal seizures typically begin in late childhood and early adolescence, mainly between 4 and 16 years of age.[37,87,134,139] Onset before 4 years of age is considered rare,[76] but certainly occurs[140] (see also Figure 12.2). Seizures of MTLE-HS start earlier than in other forms of temporal lobe epilepsy.[45] Both sexes are equally affected.[134]

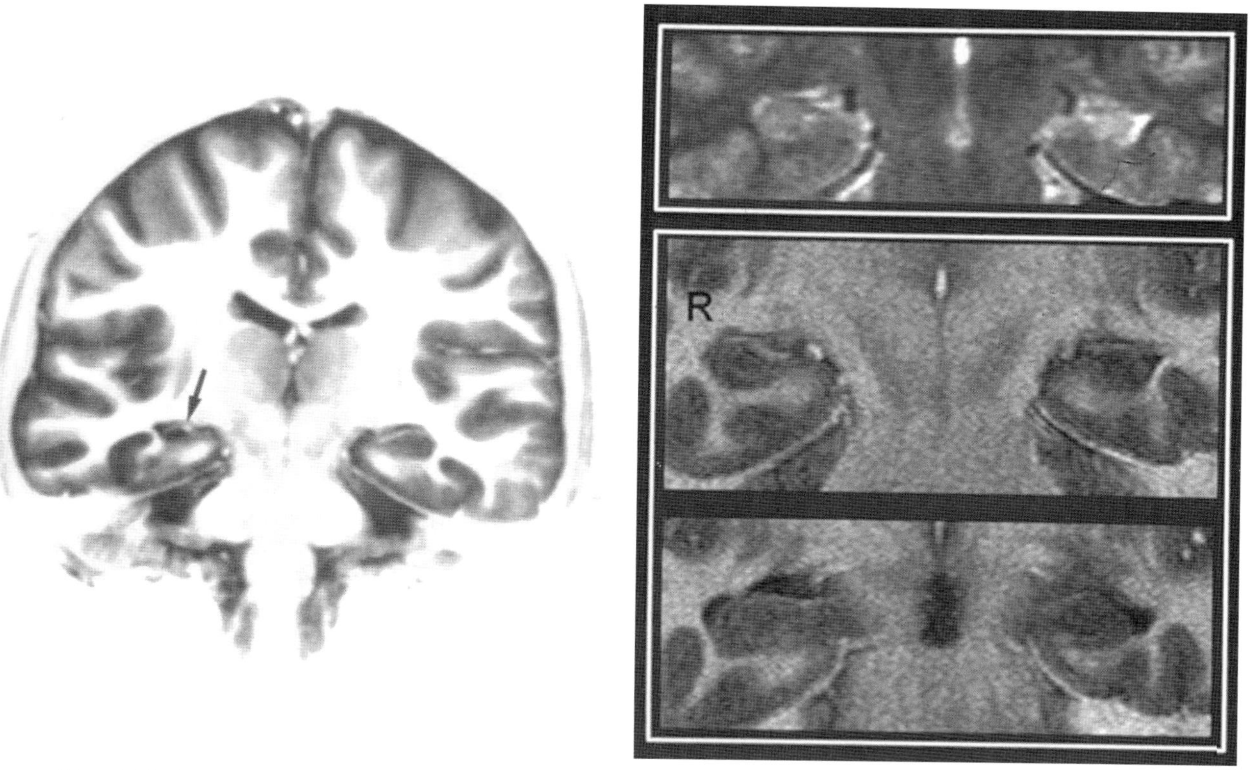

Figure 12.6 MRI findings in hippocampal sclerosis.

Left: Coronal T1-weighted MRI scan showing right hippocampal sclerosis (arrow).

Right: Coronal T2-weighted and magnified T1-weighted MRI scan showing left hippocampal sclerosis.

Figure courtesy of Professor John S Duncan and the National Society for Epilepsy MRI Unit, London, UK.

MTLE-HS is the more common epileptic disease/syndrome, but its exact incidence and prevalence is unknown.[4,5] It probably accounts for around 20% of patients with epilepsy and for 65% of patients with MTLE.[8] Of patients whose epileptogenic region is sufficiently well localised to one temporal lobe to warrant temporal lobectomy, 60–70% have hippocampal sclerosis.[141] The others have small alien tissue lesions, such as hamartomas or glial tumours, vascular and congenital malformations, and non-specific findings.

Similarly among children with temporal lobe epilepsy, 60% appear to have MTLE-HS.[142] However, in a recent study of 63 children with new-onset temporal lobe epilepsy, only 18 (29%) had MTLE-HS. The others had either cryptogenic/idiopathic (34 children with normal neuroimaging findings and no significant past history) or developmental (10 children with long-standing, non-progressive temporal lobe tumours and malformations) temporal lobe epilepsy.[143]

CLINICAL MANIFESTATIONS[37,39,75,76,135,136]

Patients with MTLE-HS usually have a previous history of initial precipitating incidents, including febrile seizures, trauma, hypoxia and intracranial infections, before 5 years of age and prior to the onset of their habitual non-febrile seizures.[40,134,142,144-149] Complex focal seizures or generalised convulsions are the initial non-febrile seizures that attract medical attention. As a rule, they are preceded by simple focal seizures that may have been considered, sometimes for years, as normal phenomena. Classically, the onset of habitual seizures occurs after a latent period from the initial precipitating incidents. However, some patients have no identifiable initial precipitating incidents, and some have habitual seizures that begin immediately after the initial precipitating incidents.[134]

Epigastric aura, fear and oro-alimentary automatisms are the most common ictal symptoms.

It starts with that strange stomach feeling and my panic, and then I pass out.

SIMPLE FOCAL SEIZURES

Simple focal seizures are the commonest and most frequent seizure type in MTLE-HS, and occur in more than 90% of patients.[35,37,38,40-43,45,65,70,76,78,133,136,150,151] The first symptom is always an aura. They mainly start with an ascending epigastric aura and less often with fear. Mental hallucinations and illusions of déjà vu and their variations occur, but not as commonly as in other extra-hippocampal epilepsies. Olfactory and gustatory hallucinations occur less often.

ILAE classification and definitions

The ILAE Commission (1989)[1] classifies MTLE-HS among other temporal lobe epilepsies under the name *'Amygdalo-hippocampal (mesiobasal limbic or rhinencephalic) seizures'* and describes them as follows:

"Hippocampal seizures are the most common form; the symptoms are those described in the previous paragraphs except that auditory symptoms may not occur. The interictal scalp EEG may be normal, may show interictal unilateral temporal sharp or slow waves, may show bilateral sharp or slow waves, synchronous or asynchronous. The intracranial interictal EEG may show mesial anterior temporal spikes or sharp waves. Seizures are characterized by rising epigastric discomfort, nausea, marked autonomic signs, and other symptoms, including borborygmi, belching, pallor, fullness of the face, flushing of the face, arrest of respiration, papillary dilatation, fear, panic, and olfactory-gustatory hallucinations."[1]

The new ILAE diagnostic scheme classifies MTLE with hippocampal sclerosis in limbic epilepsies (page 21).[2] The majority of expert contributors in the 2004 ILAE report consider MTLE-HS to represent a sufficient cluster of signs and symptoms to make up a syndromic diagnostic entity, but not a disease (despite common pathology).[134]

Clarifications on nomenclature

MTLE-HS is usually described under the heading 'MTLE', though only 65% of patients have mesial temporal lobe seizures due to hippocampal atrophy. The remainder is due to mesial temporal lobe pathology other than hippocampal sclerosis.

The term 'complex focal (partial) seizures' has been erroneously used as a synonym of 'temporal lobe epilepsy'.[2] Ictal impairment of consciousness in focal epilepsies is a symptom of either neocortical or limbic seizures.

Simple focal seizures may be the only seizure type, though they often progress to *complex focal seizures.*

Ascending epigastric or visceral aura is by far the more common aura (around 80% of cases), and the most characteristic of all other ictal symptoms of simple hippocampal seizures.

Ictal fear is in a distant second most common aura (around 20–30% of cases), but is not specific to hippocampal seizures alone.

Dreamy states,[47] *experiential phenomena,*[28] *intellectual aura, mental or psychic symptoms.* These events occur less often than epigastric aura and fear, and the patient may also have other subjective ictal symptoms, such as mental illusions and hallucinations of déjà vu, depersonalisation and their variations.

Unspecified somatic sensations or olfactory and gustatory hallucinations may occur. Elementary or complex visual and auditory hallucinations do not occur.[37]

Urgency to urinate is exceptional and is associated with right-sided foci.[63]

Language impairment during simple focal seizures has not been examined thoroughly. Most patients are able to understand conversations fully, but they are unable to speak or carry on conversations; they answer monosyllabically or with movements of the head or hands.

> I know well what they say, but I can not speak or I reply in the simplest possible way with 'yes' or 'no' until I am back to normal again in a minute or so.

Simple focal seizures may be the only seizure type, sometimes for years, and can vary in duration from "a few seconds to rarely 1–2 minutes". They may be entirely inconspicuous to the observer, though close relatives or friends are able to say when it happens.

> "He has it now", the relative points out. The patient and the EEG confirms it, but nothing significant can be detected on the video record of events.

Simple focal seizures frequently progress to complex focal seizures with mainly oro-alimentary automatisms.

COMPLEX FOCAL SEIZURES

In MTLE-HS, complex focal seizures usually emerge as a progression of simple focal seizures with gradual or abrupt impairment of consciousness that typically associates with oro-alimentary automatisms in about 70% of cases.[35,37–43,45,65,70,76,78,133,136,150–153]

The initial objective symptoms in this stage of impairment of consciousness are staring, motor restlessness or motor arrest, oro-alimentary automatisms and unforced head deviation. The patient has no recollection of this phase, but may still be responsive (70% of cases in one study).[76] Gestural automatisms, other forms of automatisms, vocalisations and dystonic posturing may occur soon after. Hypersalivation (left sided) is exceptional.

Complex focal seizures last for 2–3 min, occur on average once or twice a week and usually appear in clusters of two or three. They may also occur during sleep and, in some women, they are exclusively or predominantly catamenial.

Oro-alimentary automatisms consist of lip smacking, chewing, swallowing, licking and tooth-grinding movements. They are often followed by simple gestural automatisms. Oro-alimentary automatisms are characteristic of MTLE only if preceded by epigastric aura, fear and mental symptoms of the 'dreamy state' of Jackson, alone or in combination.

Gestural automatisms consist of fiddling, fumbling, picking, tapping, patting or plucking, rubbing or scratching the face and other gestural movements.

Autonomic manifestations of any type are among the most frequent ictal symptoms of MTLE-HS.[75,84–88,134] These manifestations include: pupillary dilatation and less commonly miosis;[38,75] cardiovascular symptoms, mainly tachycardia and arrhythmias and less often bradycardia, asystole or hypertension;[75,84,88-93] pallor and less commonly flushing;[75] and changes in respiratory rate and depth, mainly in the late seizure phase.[75]

There are occasional reports of penile erection, or even ejaculation, and other sexual ictal manifestations.[74,75]

LATERALISING SIGNS OF ICTAL SYMPTOMS

Dystonic posturing occurs in 20–30% of patients and is contralateral to the side of seizure onset.[38,136,154]

Head deviation early in the seizure is usually ipsilateral to the seizure focus, but head deviation late in the seizure is contralateral and often a prelude to generalisation.[38]

Ictal or postictal aphasia and prolonged recovery is mainly seen following seizures in the dominant temporal lobe,[38] while clear ictal speech and quick recovery mainly characterise seizures of the non-dominant temporal lobe.[38,65]

It is generally considered that unilateral automatisms are ipsilateral to the seizure onset.[38]

Although non-specific for right or left disease, impaired consciousness,[76] motion arrest,[76]escape automatisms[76] and fear[87,155] occur more often in patients with left rather than right mesial temporal sclerosis.

Hyperventilation during the seizure is rare and occurs in left mesial onset.[76]

Vocalisations,[76] motor restlessness,[76] staring,[76] oral automatisms,[38] pupillary dilatation,[38] impaired consciousness[38] or generalised rigidity[38] do not predict side of origin.

GENERALISED TONIC CLONIC SEIZURES

Secondarily GTCS are usually infrequent in patients receiving appropriate AEDs.[134] They are not uniform in their clinical presentation, but are more stereotyped in their final phases than the initial clinical signs of generalisation.[156] Some patients (probably around 10%) may never have GTCS.

PSYCHOMOTOR COMPLEX FOCAL STATUS EPILEPTICUS

Psychomotor complex focal status epilepticus features particularly in untreated patients with temporal lobe epilepsy. It is less common than the absence status epilepticus of idiopathic generalised epilepsy, but its prevalence may be underestimated.[157-159] It may be confused with transient global amnesia.[160,161]

POSTICTAL SYMPTOMS

Postictal symptoms of the mainly complex focal seizures in MTLE-HS are very frequent and often severe. They comprise mental and physical fatigue, drowsiness, headache, language aberrations, inability to concentrate and confusion of various degrees that may be severe and associated with automatic behaviour of which the patient may be amnesic.

I am more concerned by what follows than the fit itself.

Definitions

Psychomotor (complex focal) status epilepticus is characterised by continuous or rapidly recurring psychomotor (complex focal) seizures that may involve temporal or extratemporal regions. Cyclic disturbance of consciousness is characteristic of psychomotor status epilepticus of temporal lobe origin. The differential diagnosis from complex focal status epilepticus of frontal lobe origin remains a challenge (Figure 12.11).[162] In one-third of cases, a frontal lesion is revealed.[163]

NEUROLOGICAL, MENTAL STATE AND BEHAVIOUR

Neurological examination is usually normal; facial asymmetry contralateral to the epileptogenic zone may be apparent in some patients. Specific baseline and follow-up memory testing are necessary. The only clearly defined behavioural disturbance in MTLE-HS is a material-specific memory deficit, but this may also be seen in MTLE due to other mesial temporal lesions.[134] Many other psychiatric and psychological problems, especially depression, have been reported to be more prevalent in MTLE-HS, but inadequate information exists to determine the extent to which these disturbances are a direct biological result of either the hippocampal sclerosis or the mesial temporal seizures, a non-specific biological result of brain injury, or a consequence of external psychological and social factors.[134]

FEBRILE CONVULSIONS AND OTHER INITIAL PRECIPITATING EVENTS

One-third of patients with MTLE-HS have a previous history of prolonged febrile convulsions and many others have a history of cerebral insults in early life.[40,134,142,144-149]

Mathern et al. (1995)[147] found that 90% of patients have a history of complicated febrile convulsions or other initial precipitating events. The type of initial precipitating events and the patient's age at which it occurred are related to the clinicopathological features. Thus, patients with a prolonged febrile seizure before 5 years of age are likely to have unilateral hippocampal atrophy and a good neurosurgical response.[147,149]

AETIOLOGY

By definition all patients with MTLE-HS have hippocampal sclerosis. Conversely, hippocampal sclerosis is found in only two-thirds (65%) of patients with MTLE.[8-11] Hippocampal sclerosis is predominantly unilateral in about 80% of neurosurgical series, contralateral hippocampal EEG discharges are common and one-third of patients have functional and structural extrahippocampal abnormalities.[164,165] Other mesial temporal lobe structures may also be affected.[75,165]

'Dual pathology' is common[166,167] and includes microdysgenesis, temporal lobe malformations of cortical development and indolent tumours, such as DNET.[168] Patients with 'dual pathology' are more likely to have bilateral hippocampal atrophy.[166,167]

A genetic predisposition may be found in MTLE-HS, but this is not a uniform process:[134]

- There is an increased incidence of a family history of febrile convulsions and epilepsy (mainly generalised epilepsies).[145,169-171] The genetic predisposition for febrile seizures could be associated with especially severe seizures in some patients to produce hippocampal sclerosis and MTLE. Generalised epilepsy with febrile seizures plus (GEFS+) that leads to focal seizures could be an example of this.[134]
- Usually, there is no increased family history of similar hippocampal seizures and hippocampal sclerosis does not occur in clinically unaffected twins.[172] However, 18 of 52 asymptomatic individuals from 11 families with familial MTLE[173] had left-sided (11 subjects) or bilateral (7 subjects) hippocampal atrophy; 14 of these individuals had classical MRI signs of hippocampal sclerosis.[174] In these cases, the assumption is that the genetic defect may cause MTLE, which then leads to HS with or without febrile seizures.[134] The role of genes has been recently reviewed.[167,172]

- Sodium-channel defects in mice can cause hippocampal sclerosis, and it is possible that similar defects could have the same effect in humans leading to MTLE, with or without febrile seizures.[134]

HIPPOCAMPAL SCLEROSIS

A hypocellular and gliotic (thus the word 'sclerotic') hippocampus is the pathological substrate of MTLE-HS. Hippocampal sclerosis presents with a unique pattern of cellular loss that is not found in other brain diseases.[8]

- Selective regional hippocampal, mainly CA1, pyramidal cell loss occurs (> 30–50% of cases), predominantly involving the hilar region and dentate granule cells. Somatostatin and neuropeptide Y-containing hilar neurons are particularly susceptible. Preservation of the subiculum is pathognomonic.
- Gamma-aminobutyric acid (GABA) neurons and terminals are relatively well preserved. CA2 are relatively spared.
- Dispersion of dentate gyrus granule cells and sprouting of their axons (mossy fibres) that form aberrant monosynaptic excitatory feedback synapses on to the dendrites of granule cells.[8,175,176].[8,175,176]
- Changes in neuropeptide Y and somatostatin expression and reorganisation occur.[177]

HIPPOCAMPAL SCLEROSIS AND TEMPORAL LOBE EPILEPSY: CAUSE OR CONSEQUENCE?[178]

The cause of hippocampal sclerosis is unknown. There are two opposite views:

1. The traditional concept is that prolonged febrile convulsions and other cerebral insults in early life cause hippocampal sclerosis and hippocampal epilepsy. This is because:
   - one-third of patients with MTLE-HS have a previous history of prolonged febrile convulsions and many others have a history of cerebral insults in early life[40,142,144-148]
   - MRI studies demonstrate that prolonged and focal febrile convulsions produce acute hippocampal injury evolving to hippocampal atrophy.[179,180]
2. A current trend is that pre-existing hippocampal abnormalities predispose to febrile convulsions. If these are prolonged, they may cause further hippocampal damage evolving to mesial temporal sclerosis that may manifest with temporal lobe epilepsy.[179-181] This view is supported because:
   - the estimated risk for developing temporal lobe epilepsy subsequent to prolonged febrile seizures is negligible, probably 1/75,000 children per year[180,182]
   - MRI studies suggest that there is a subtle, pre-existing hippocampal malformation that may facilitate febrile convulsions and contribute to the development of subsequent hippocampal sclerosis.[179-181]

Opinions and results are divided with probably half in favour of the first and the other half in favour of the second assumption.

PATHOPHYSIOLOGY

How does this 'atrophic' and 'sclerotic' organ become one of the most powerful and common epileptogenic agents in human epilepsy?

The role of the hippocampus in epilepsy is due to synaptic remodelling and reorganisation of the hippocampal region. Enhanced sensitivity to glutamate may be important.[183] These changes predispose surviving hippocampal neurons to abnormal hypersynchronous discharges that then propagate to other limbic and non-limbic structures, producing the manifestations of complex focal seizures.

Babb (1999),[8] in an excellent review, on the subject concludes:

"The epileptic hippocampus has synaptic reorganisations, with GABA increasing the synchrony of firing thresholds and mossy fibres providing convergent excitation that then makes an otherwise cell-poor region fire a greater number of neurones for seizure initiation and propagation."[8]

Engel et al.,[184] in a recent review, summarised the current state of our knowledge as follows:

"Most current parallel human/animal invasive research indicates that epileptogenesis in MTLE-HS is initiated by specific types of cell loss and neuronal reorganisation, which results not only in enhanced excitation, but also in enhanced inhibition, predisposing to hypersynchronisation. Also, evidence is found for more than one type of ictal onset, and individual seizures can demonstrate a transition from one ictal mechanism to another. In vivo and in vitro parallel, reiterative investigations in patients with MTLE-HS, and in rats with intrahippocampal kainate-induced hippocampal seizures, have revealed the presence of interictal epileptiform events, termed ***'fast ripples'****, which appear to be unique in tissue capable of generating spontaneous seizures."*[184]

See also other recent reports.[175,184-191]

DIAGNOSTIC PROCEDURES

A clinical diagnosis of MTLE-HS demands confirmation with high-resolution MRI and EEG. CT brain scanning is unrewarding. Functional brain imaging provides insights in neurosurgical cases for which further information is required regarding lateralisation. Invasive intracranial recordings are necessary in exceptional cases.

BRAIN IMAGING

MRI is the most important investigational tool.[117,134]

With improvements in MRI techniques, modern MRI scanners are of sufficiently high resolution to allow in-vivo visualisation of hippocampal sclerosis in all patients.[137,138,192-195] Two-thirds of patients with MTLE have unilateral or bilateral hippocampal atrophy. In some patients, there is also evidence of other 'dual pathology', such as cortical malformations. In the other third, which by definition do not have MTLE-HS, MRI may be normal, but more usually reveals the structural cause responsible, such as a tumour (astrocytoma, ganglioglioma, dysembryoplastic neuroepithelial malformation), vascular abnormality (cavernous and venous angiomas, arteriovenous malformations), developmental abnormality (cortical malformations), atrophy or trauma. The sensitivity of MRI in the diagnosis of tumours and other lesions of the temporal lobe is estimated to be around 90%,[137] but this will soon be exceeded.[138]

In straightforward cases of incontrovertible unilateral MTLE-HS confirmed by MRI, other tests may be unnecessary. However, it should be remembered that:

MRI evidence of hippocampal sclerosis is not necessarily related to seizure severity and may occur in individuals who never had seizures.[174]

18F-deoxyglucose positron emission tomography (FDG-PET) usually demonstrates ipsilateral hypometabolism if interictal or hypermetabolism if ictal (Figure 3.10). The abnormality of the affected temporal lobe appears much wider on FDG-PET than MRI.[196,197] Interictal bitemporal PET hypometabolism of proven unilateral MRI hippocampal sclerosis is important and may reflect an advanced stage of the disease process. Half of these patients (53%) have bilateral independent seizure onset, longer disease duration and a poorer memory performance in the Wada test.[198]

[11 C] flumazenil PET is more sensitive than FDG-PET and a useful tool for investigating the hippocampal damage in vivo, even in patients with no remarkable hippocampal abnormalities on quantitative MRI.[199] Results show a good correlation with the severity of reduced hippocampal volume, T2 prolongation, and histologically assessed neuronal loss and astrogliosis.[199] 11C-flumazenil PET with correction for focal-volume effect[200] reliably detects in-vivo reductions in central benzodiazepine receptor binding on the remaining neurons in the sclerotic hippocampi of patients with MTLE-HS.

SPECT is not as good for interictal studies, though ictal and postictal SPECT patterns are useful and reasonably reliable (Figure 3.8).[201]

New methodologies are nearly impossible to follow, and any reference to them made today would become obsolete within a few months._

Proton magnetic resonance spectroscopic imaging (1H-MRSI) of N-acetyl-aspartate, creatine and choline can accurately lateralise MTLE. It is less accurate in extratemporal epilepsy.[118,202-207] 1H-MRSI demonstrates a decreased relative resonance:intensity ratio of the neuronal marker N-acetylaspartate:creatine and phosphocreatine (NAA/Cr) in the affected hippocampus. 1H-MRSI may be valuable in neurosurgical cases with bilateral hippocampal atrophy. In one study, discriminant features associated with favourable surgical outcome were: (a) concordant 1H-MRSI lateralisation; (b) a greater side-to-side asymmetry of NAA/Cr; and (c) an absence of contralateral posterior NAA/Cr reduction.[208] Recently, ^{31}P nuclear magnetic resonance spectroscopic imaging, using very high strength magnets, has been shown to be useful.[209]

Important points on diagnostic procedures

- High resolution MRI provides in-vivo visualisation of hippocampal sclerosis in nearly all patients.
- A single routine interictal EEG is more likely to be normal (two-thirds of patients) than show the classical spike–wave focus in the anterior temporal lobe electrode (one-third of patients).

INTERICTAL ELECTROENCEPHALOGRAPHY

Routine interictal EEG shows the classical sharp or spike and slow-wave focus in nearly one-third of patients (Figure 12.4). Thus, in two-thirds of patients with MTLE-HS, a single, routine, 30-min EEG recording may be normal or show mild and non-specific abnormalities. The yield is doubled in repeat EEG, particularly when a longer sleep recording is made. Epileptiform abnormalities nearly always occur during prolonged monitoring.[210]

The characteristic interictal EEG abnormality consists of high-amplitude spike or sharp and slow wave complexes, either single or in clusters, localised in the anterior temporal electrode (Figure 12.4). These traditional 'epileptogenic complexes', when present, are unilateral in two-thirds of patients and occur independently, on the right or left, in the other third.[75,210] They focus maximum in the basal derivations and they are best seen with sphenoidal, earlobe or true temporal derivations.[211]

Regional temporal lobe interictal runs of slow waves, which are of lateralising value, are recorded in about 50% of patients (Figure 12.4).[123-125] Though not traditionally considered 'epileptogenic', runs of monomorphic slow waves occur more often than the spike itself.[123-125]

Bilateral GSWD do not occur, though occasionally bilateral fronto-polar spikes may be seen.

ICTAL ELECTROENCEPHALOGRAPHY

The ictal scalp EEG may be 'normal' or inconclusive in around 60% of cases at seizure onset in MTLE-HS.

A typical ictal EEG pattern consists of rhythmic, crescendo-like theta activity with decreasing frequency and increasing amplitude (Figure 12.2). It first appears over the affected temporal lobe, usually starts around 30 s prior to subjective or objective clinical seizure manifestations, and commonly spreads to the neighbouring and other regions (Figures 12.2 and 12.3).[75] Rhythmic waxing-waning theta activity is also often encountered in scalp EEG, either lateralised with a maximum over temporal areas or not lateralised.[134]

Onset with regional attenuation of background rhythms and disappearance of the interictal spikes is less common.[75] Such EEG flattening can occur either as a diffuse pattern or with predominance over one temporal region.

Unlike seizures from other locations, there are no fast spikes or fast rhythmic discharges in the ictal EEG of hippocampal seizures and spikes are relatively absent.

Simultaneous EEG and clinical onsets are uncommon.[103] In the study of Williamson et al.,[210] ictal scalp EEG changes were rarely detected at the time of clinical seizure onset, but lateralised build-up of rhythmic seizure activity during the seizure occurred in 80% of patients. However, in 13% of patients, the scalp EEG seizure build-up was contralateral to the side of seizure origin, as subsequently determined by depth EEG and curative surgery.

INVASIVE ELECTROENCEPHALOGRAPHY

Concordant outpatient EEG and unilateral MRI hippocampal atrophy would obviate the need for in-patient EEG monitoring.[193]

Invasive EEG with depth implanted electrodes, subdural strips or grids and foramen ovale electrodes, alone or in combination, are now rarely needed, because precise localisation is usually possible following the improvements in non-invasive methodology, particularly MRI and functional brain imaging.[134,192-195,212] However, they are still used when it is uncertain on which side mesial temporal ictal onset occurs or neocortical ictal onset has not been excluded. Direct recording from the hippocampus shows a 'hypersynchronous hippocampal discharge pattern' followed by low amplitude, high frequency, recruiting rhythm of more than 20 Hz.[75,196] A low voltage, fast discharge is the second most common pattern.

OTHER ENCEPHALOGRAPHIC METHODOLOGIES

Non-linear analysis of intracranial EEG activities can detect a 'pre-ictal phase preceding the epileptic seizure.[213]

Whole-head magnetoencephalography may be a valuable non-invasive method; it distinguishes between mesial and lateral temporal seizure onset zones and identifies the spatial relationship of the structural lesion to the irritative zone.[214]

DIFFERENTIAL DIAGNOSIS

MTLE-HS needs to be differentiated from non-epileptic conditions and from seizures arising from other brain locations (Table 12.1).

- *Non-epileptic conditions.* The diagnosis of hippocampal seizures should be suspected from their very brief duration, the ascending character of the epigastric sensations, the occasional nocturnal appearance and often an associated feeling of depersonalisation. However, simple focal seizures of epigastric aura and 'panic attacks' are unlikely to raise suspicion of epilepsy in either the patient or the general physician (Figure 12.2). These patients are often investigated for gastroenterological and psychological disorders[215] or hypoglycaemia until more salient seizure features appear with the development of complex focal seizures and secondarily GTCS. Patients are often reassured by normal relevant tests or told that their symptoms are the result of anxiety. It is rare, at this stage, that a general physician would request an EEG, but again, if this normal (as is the case in two-thirds of patients), a diagnosis of stress-related events would be reinforced.

Pseudo-seizures may be difficult to differentiate. An increase in serum prolactin level postictally may be helpful in differentiating between epileptic seizures and 'pseudo-seizures'.[216]

- *Mesial temporal epilepsy with aetiologies other than hippocampal sclerosis:* The differential diagnosis of hippocampal from other MTLE is practically impossible without MRI, with the possible exception of olfactory-gustatory hallucinations, which may be more often associated with tumoural MTLE.[134]
- *Hippocampal versus other temporal lobe seizures:* The epigastric aura and early oro-alimentary automatisms predominate in MTLE compared with other neocortical temporal lesions. Conversely, MTLE-HS is unlikely when seizures manifest with early focal motor, somatosensory, visual or auditory ictal symptoms, frequent secondarily GTCS or occur in patients with neurological or cognitive deficits other than memory impairment.
- *Hippocampal versus mesial familial temporal lobe epilepsy (MFTLE):* The main differentiating features in favour of mesial familial temporal lobe epilepsy are:
  - onset in teenage or early adult life and familial occurrence
  - no febrile convulsions or other initial precipitating events
  - no ictal symptoms of rising epigastric aura
  - mild and infrequent seizures that may remit
  - usually normal MRI.
- *Typical absence seizures* are more likely to be misdiagnosed as complex focal seizures than vice versa.

PROGNOSIS

Despite the high prevalence and known pathology, the prognosis and many other important aspects of MTLE-HS are largely unknown.

Table 12.1 Mesial versus lateral temporal lobe epilepsy

	Mesial TLE	**Lateral TLE**
Epigatric auras, fear and early oroalimentary automatisms	Predominate	Rare
Non-specific auras, early focal motor, somatosensory, visual or auditory symptoms	Rare	Predominate
Contralateral hand dystonia	Common	Rarer
Early clonic activity following automatisms	Rare	Common
GTCS	Infrequent	Frequent
History of febrile seizures	Predominates	Rare
Interictal EEG	Ipsilateral anterior temporal spikes	Middle and posterior temporal spikes
MRI	Hippocampal sclerosis	Neocortical lesions such as malformations of cortical development

NEUROSURGICAL SERIES

The neurosurgical cases show a specific clinical pattern.[37,39,75,76,135,136] Seizures are initially relatively well controlled with AED for several years (silent period).[134] Seizures relapse in adolescence or early adulthood, occurring several times per week or usually several times per month, and become refractory to medication. Memory and behavioural disturbances may occur. Neurosurgery is probably mandatory at this stage, because spontaneous remission is unlikely, drugs do not work and polypharmacy makes it worse.

COMMUNITY STUDIES

Community-based studies have shown that 10–40% or more of patients with epileptic seizures of temporal lobe origin may go into remission.[130] I have tried to understand and give a gross estimate of the prognosis in MTLE-HS by reviewing the literature, my database and asking other epileptologists. I reached the following conclusions, which may roughly indicate the spectrum of MTLE-HS.

- About 50% are intractable cases that require neurosurgical evaluation and management, though only 10% or less of these patients benefit.
- Around 30% of patients are relatively well controlled with appropriate AEDs. These patients may have simple or complex focal seizures, and occasional GTCS that interfere with their daily life, but not to a degree that makes it intolerable. They are handicapped, but they may still function adequately within their families and their jobs. How many of these patients need or would accept neurosurgical intervention is uncertain.
- The other 20% of patients are otherwise normal, with occasional simple or complex focal seizures for which they may be treated or untreated. These patients may come to our attention because of an occasional GTCS, a lengthy or severe complex focal seizure or an EEG performed for reasons other than epilepsy.

IS HIPPOCAMPAL EPILEPSY A PROGRESSIVE DISEASE?

Whether hippocampal epilepsy is a progressive disease is a highly debatable and controversial matter.[134] In most patients, MTLE-HS may not have a progressive course as indicated by community studies and clinical experience. Further, hippocampal atrophy remains stable over the duration of temporal lobe onset seizure disorders.[217] Miller et al. (2000)[218] used proton MRSI to measure NAA/Cr ratios in the temporal lobes of five consecutive children with newly diagnosed temporal lobe epilepsy compared with another five children of similar age that suffered from intractable temporal lobe epilepsy. They found that the severity of the neuronal dysfunction in children with newly diagnosed temporal lobe epilepsy was at least as severe as in those with intractable temporal lobe epilepsy, implying that the neuronal abnormalities occurred before the clinical manifestations.

The neurosurgical patients may be derailed cases of MTLE-HS. This may be a common, but not a defining situation. Engel et al. (1997)[37] favour a progressive course for the neurosurgical cases for the following reasons:

- Cell death and neuronal reorganisation probably continue with recurrent seizures.[8,147]
- There is a long silent period between the time risk factors (febrile convulsions) appear and the onset of habitual seizures. Similarly, medical intractability may develop long after relevant control of seizures with medication.[40]
- Persistence of simple focal seizures (auras) after extensive mesial temporal lobe resection is correlated with the duration of epilepsy before surgery, and may indicate that wider brain areas than the sclerotic hippocampus are epileptogenic.[37]

MANAGEMENT

Medical treatment of MTLE-HS with AEDs may be relatively effective in 80% of patients; for the other 20% and probably many more with intractable seizures, neurosurgical resection of the offending epileptogenic region is usually successful.

ANTIEPILEPTIC DRUG TREATMENT

Drug treatment is similar to that for any other type of focal seizure.

Of the older drugs, carbamazepine or phenytoin monotherapy is the most appropriate. *Carbamazepine* is superior for controlling focal seizures in more than 70% of patients (10% of the patients develop idiosyncratic reactions).

Phenytoin is as effective as carbamazepine, but its use is falling dramatically in developed countries, mainly because of chronic toxicity.

Phenobarbitone and primidone are less efficacious and have been practically eliminated from use, mainly because of their adverse effects on cognition.

Clobazam, though often highly beneficial in selective cases, is rarely used as continuous AED treatment. Clobazam is, however, worth trying in patients who do not respond or those who develop side effects, such allergic reactions to other drugs.

Valproate, though a superior drug for generalised epilepsies, is inferior in focal epilepsies with significant concerns in the treatment of women.

The new AEDs, in order of my preference, are as follows:

1. Oxcarbazepine, possibly of equal efficacy with carbamazepine but with fewer idiosyncratic reactions, is probably the AED of first choice in monotherapy. Its use in polytherapy is less advantageous.
2. Levetiracetam is becoming increasingly popular. It is the first choice AED in adjunctive treatment, because of its combination of high efficacy, comparative poverty of adverse reactions, lack of drug–drug interactions, novel mechanism of action and rapid titration.
3. Lamotrigine may work extremely well in some patients. It is one of the best drugs in terms of lack of cognitive adverse effects, but its efficacy is low and idiosyncratic reactions, which may be fatal in exceptional cases, are a realistic threat.
4. Topiramate is the most efficacious of the new drugs, but significant concerns about serious and multiple adverse reactions hinder its use.
5. Zonisamide is used extensively in Japan and may become more popular in other countries.
6. Tiagabine is being used cautiously, because of moderate efficacy and adverse reactions.
7. Gabapentin is largely ineffective, even in high doses.

If treatment with one or two of the main AEDs fails, the chances of achieving medical control in MTLE-HS are negligible. Polypharmacy with more than two or three AEDs, even when rational, will add more misery, memory problems and drowsiness rather than any benefit.[219,220] These patients, even in childhood,[221] need urgent evaluation for neurosurgical treatment for which they are the best candidates of all symptomatic focal epilepsies, and the most likely to have excellent and sustained benefit.

NEUROSURGICAL TREATMENT

With early surgical intervention, patients with MTLE-HS have an excellent chance of cure and a subsequent normal life.[134]

MTLE-HS responds well to temporal lobe surgery, regardless of whether resection of the anterior two-thirds of the temporal lobe or a selective amygdalohippocampectomy is performed.[37,75,134,167,222-225] Cognitive outcome is better after amygdalohippocampectomy, which is the procedure of first choice when pathology is confined to mesial structures.[76]

After anterior temporal lobe resection with hippocampectomy, around 60% of patients will be seizure free even after all AEDs have been withdrawn, 20% will need to continue with AEDs and may have reduced numbers of seizures, 10% will have no benefit, and 10% may have neurosurgical complications and get worse. Significant neurosurgical complications rarely occur.[226]

There is no consensus as to how much of the hippocampus should be removed.[134] It has not yet been determined whether all patients require a maximal hippocampal resection. The amount of hippocampal resection is often determined intraoperatively by the extent of electrocorticographic interictal epileptiform abnormalities, allowing for sparing of possibly functionally important hippocampus.[227]

In general, "the benefits of anteromesial temporal lobe resection for disabling complex partial seizures of temporal lobe epilepsy is greater than continued treatment with antiepileptic drugs, and the risks are at least comparable".[131,132]

The quality of life following surgical treatment depends on psychosocial factors, and pre-existing vocational and interpersonal skills.[228] Attention to psychosocial and possibly memory deficits is of paramount importance. Appropriate rehabilitation following successful surgery is needed; some patients find it difficult to adjust to a new life 'without epilepsy'.

Interesting historical note

It is amazing that MTLE-HS, the most frequent and provocative focal epilepsy escaped recognition until around 1953.[229] Until then, focal seizures were attributed to damage of neocortical brain regions for which excisional neurosurgery was utilised. The atrophic hippocampus was ignored.

MESIAL TEMPORAL LOBE EPILEPSY DEFINED BY SPECIFIC AETIOLOGIES OTHER THAN HIPPOCAMPAL SCLEROSIS

In MTLE with aetiologies other than hippocampal sclerosis,[37,39,75,76,135,136] seizure symptomatology is the same irrespective of cause and location within the mesial temporal lobe structures. MRI commonly identifies structural causes.

CLINICAL MANIFESTATIONS

The overall view is that seizure symptomatology is the same irrespective of cause and location within the mesial temporal lobe structures. Thus, seizures of hippocampal sclerosis are considered indistinguishable from those caused by other lesions in the mesial temporal lobe. Their differentiation is also practically impossible with surface EEG. High resolution MRI provides anatomical evidence of localisation in nearly all symptomatic cases. The sensitivity of MRI in the diagnosis of tumours and other lesions of the temporal lobe is estimated to be around 90%,[137] but this will soon be exceeded.

AETIOLOGY

Structural causes comprise malignant and benign tumours (astrocytomas, gangliogliomas, dysembryoplastic neuroepithelial malformations), vascular abnormalities (cavernous and venous angiomas, arteriovenous malformations), malformations of cortical development, trauma and other injuries, viral and other infective agents, and cerebrovascular disease.[7,143]

MANAGEMENT

Drug treatment is similar to that for any other type of focal seizure.

Neurosurgical intervention often provides an excellent chance of cure and a subsequent normal life in certain pathological conditions of LTLE.

LATERAL TEMPORAL LOBE EPILEPSY

Lateral temporal lobe epilepsy [1,76,113,136] is neocortical as opposed to MTLE, which is limbic.

CLINICAL MANIFESTATIONS

Simple seizures of LTLE are characterised by auditory hallucinations (ringing, humming, clicking, unspecified noises) or illusions, vestibular phenomena, mental illusions and hallucinations of the dreamy states and visual misperceptions. Language disturbances occur in dominant hemisphere focus.

Motor ictal symptoms include clonic movements of facial muscles, grimacing, finger and hand automatisms, dystonic posturing of an upper extremity, leg automatisms, restlessness and unformed vocalisations. Rotation of the whole body is common and of value in differentiating LTLE from MTLE.

Symptoms may progress to complex focal seizures by spreading to mesial temporal or extratemporal structures. Impairment of consciousness is not as pronounced as in MTLE.[76]

See also lateral (autosomal dominant) familial temporal lobe epilepsy (see page 355).

AETIOLOGY

The structural causes of LTLE are similar to those of MTLE apart from hippocampal sclerosis.

DIAGNOSTIC PROCEDURES

MRI often determines structural causes of LTLE (Figure 12.7).

Scalp interictal EEG shows unilateral or bilateral midtemporal or posterior temporal spikes (Figure 12.5).[1,76]

DIFFERENTIAL DIAGNOSIS

Lateral temporal lobe seizures usually lack the features commonly exhibited in MTLE, as detailed in Table 12.1.

Gil-Nagel and Risinger (1997)[136] compared the ictal features of 16 patients with hippocampal epilepsy with those of 19 patients with extra-hippocampal temporal lobe seizures associated with a small tumour in the lateral or inferior temporal cortex. The association of a prior history of febrile convulsions, epigastric aura and early oral automatisms with hippocampal epilepsy was statistically significant. Conversely, an aura with experiential content and early motor involvement of the contralateral upper extremity without oral automatisms was significantly associated with extra-hippocampal temporal lobe epilepsy. Arrest reaction, vocalisation, speech, facial grimace, postictal cough, late oral automatisms and late motor involvement of the contralateral arm and hand occurred with similar frequency in both groups.

Foldvary et al. (1997)[113] compared eight patients with LTLE and 20 patients with MTLE. MTLE patients were younger at the onset of habitual seizures and more likely to have a prior history of febrile seizures, CNS infection,

---

The ILAE (1989) definition for lateral temporal lobe seizures is:[1]

'Simple seizures characterized by auditory hallucinations or illusions or dreamy states, visual misperceptions, or language disorders in case of language dominant hemisphere focus. These may progress to complex focal seizures if propagation to mesial temporal or extratemporal structures occurs. The scalp EEG shows unilateral or bilateral midtemporal or posterior temporal spikes which are most prominent in the lateral derivations."[1]

perinatal complications or head injury. LTLE seizures lacked the features commonly exhibited in MTLE, including automatisms, contralateral dystonia, searching head movements, body shifting, hyperventilation and postictal cough or sigh.

Elger (2000)[76] reported that, in LTLE, auras are rare and variable (15%). Motor ictal symptoms include clonic movements of the facial muscles, grimacing, finger and hand automatisms, dystonic posturing of an upper extremity, oro-alimentary automatisms, leg automatisms, restlessness and unformed vocalisations. He emphasised that rotation of the whole body is frequent and of value in differentiating LTLE from MTLE. Eye blinking, aggressive behaviour, dystonic posturing, early or late oro-alimentary automatisms and hypersalivation, which are common in MTLE, did not occur in epilepsy of non-mesial onset. Further, impairment of consciousness was not as pronounced as in MTLE.

MANAGEMENT

Drug treatment is similar to that for any other type of focal seizure.

Neurosurgical treatment provides an excellent chance of cure and a subsequent normal life in certain pathological conditions of LTLE.

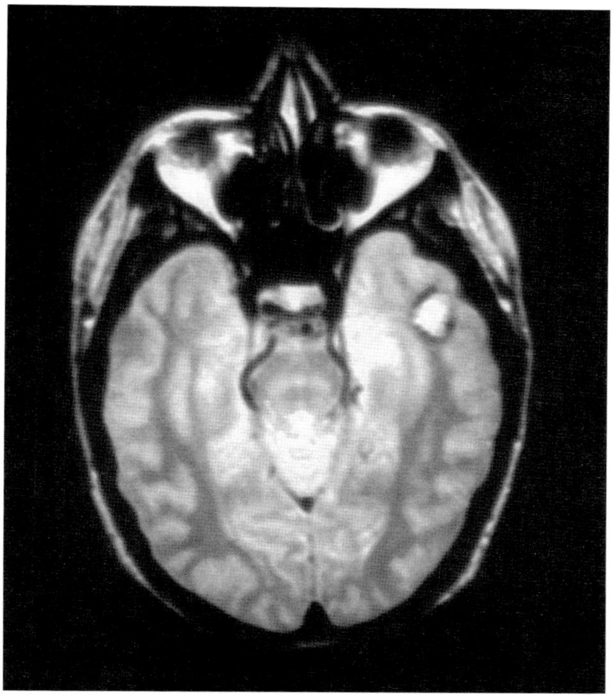

Figure 12.7 Axial proton density-weighted MRI showing left temporal lobe cavernoma in a patient with LTLE.

Figure courtesy of Professor John S Duncan and the National Society for Epilepsy MRI Unit.

FRONTAL LOBE EPILEPSIES

Frontal lobe epilepsies manifest with seizures originating from a primary epileptic focus anywhere within the frontal lobe. The clinical and EEG manifestations vary greatly and depend on the origin and spread of the epileptogenic focus.[230-240] The frontal lobe occupies 40% of the cerebral cortex and is the largest of the brain lobes. On the basis of cyto-architectural and functional studies, the frontal lobe can be subdivided into the primary motor cortex, premotor cortex, prefrontal cortex, and the limbic and paralimbic cortices,[236] with distinct cortico-subcortical organisations and immense connections with the temporal and parietal cortices.[233,241] Complex and varied patterns in the spread of seizure discharges explain the variability in the clinical and EEG manifestations of frontal lobe seizures.[232,242] Also, exact localisation is often hindered because of the rapid propagation of seizures within the frontal lobe from and to extrafrontal areas. It is difficult to assign the origin of seizures with pre- and post-central symptomatology to the frontal or parietal lobe. Such overlap to adjacent anatomical regions also occurs in opercular epilepsy.[1]

Seizures arising from the primary motor cortex and the supplementary motor area (SMA; Figures 12.8 and 12.9) have been relatively well defined, but seizures generated in other regions of the frontal lobe are less well specified.

DEMOGRAPHIC DATA

Frontal lobe epilepsies may start at any age and both sexes are equally affected. They are probably rare, accounting for about 1–2% of all epilepsies, though they are second in prevalence, after temporal lobe epilepsies, in neurosurgical series. In a prospective community-based study,[243] the prevalence of frontal seizures (22.5%) among focal epilepsies was comparable to that of temporal lobe (27%) and central sensorimotor (32.5%) localisation. Seizure onset from the frontotemporal (5.6%), parietal (6.3%) or posterior cortex (6.3%) was less common.[243]

CLINICAL MANIFESTATIONS

According to their origin within the frontal lobe, various seizure patterns have been recognised though multiple frontal areas may be involved. Rapid and specific seizure types may not be discernible.[1] Motor manifestations are more common and the most characteristic ictal symptom occurring in 90% of seizures.

The following are the most common frontal lobe seizures.

SEIZURES FROM THE MOTOR CORTEX

Seizures from the motor cortex are mainly simple focal motor seizures. Symptoms depend on the side and topography of the area involved. Focal motor seizures (with or without march) originate from the contralateral precentral gyrus. In the lower pre-Rolandic area, there may be speech arrest, vocalisation or dysphasia, tonic-clonic movements of the face on the contralateral side, or swallowing. In the paracentral lobule, tonic movements of the foot may occur, which may be ipsilateral or contralateral. Seizures often progress to secondarily generalisation. Postictal Todd's paralysis is frequent.

Simple focal motor clonic or tonic-clonic seizures with or without Jacksonian march.

These seizures manifest with localised, rhythmic or arrhythmic, clonic movements that may affect the thumb only, the thumb and ipsilateral side of the lips, the hand, the whole arm or any other body part contralateral to the focus. Distal segments are more frequently affected than proximal segments. The hand (mainly the thumb) and face (mainly the lips) are preferentially affected because of their larger cortical representation (homunculus of Penfield). These ictal motor manifestations may remain highly localised for the whole of the seizure or march in an ordinary anatomical fashion to neighbouring motor regions, which constitute the classical Jacksonian (or Bravais-Jackson) seizure.

> Usually there are a few jerks of the right corner of my mouth and the right thumb. That is all. However, the jerks may become more intense and spread gradually to my eye and my fingers on the same side. Then my elbow and shoulder also start jerking violently and this may also go to my leg. The whole right side of my body is jerking and jerking, and there is nothing I can do before this stops suddenly or I lose consciousness and I have whole body convulsions.

Myoclonic seizures that may be unilateral or bilateral are predominantly facial or distal in the limbs. Epilepsia partialis continua of Kozhevnikov is one type of myoclonic seizure.

Tonic postural motor seizures associated with clonic movements are asymmetric, unilateral or bilateral.

ILAE classification and definitions

The seizures and some syndromes of frontal lobe epilepsy have been well described in the 1989 ILAE classification among the *localisation-related (focal, local, partial) epilepsies and epileptic syndromes, and defined as follows:*[1]

"Frontal lobe epilepsies are characterized by simple partial, complex partial, secondarily generalized seizures or combinations of these. Seizures often occur several times a day and frequently occur during sleep. Frontal lobe partial seizures are sometimes mistaken for psychogenic seizures. Status epilepticus is a frequent complication.

General characteristics

Features strongly suggestive of the diagnosis include:

1. Generally short seizures.
2. Complex partial seizures arising from the frontal lobe, often with minimal or no postictal confusion.
3. Rapid secondary generalization (more common in seizures of frontal than of temporal lobe epilepsy).
4. Prominent motor manifestations which are tonic or postural.
5. Complex gestural automatisms frequent at onset.
6. Frequent falling when the discharge is bilateral.

A number of seizure types are described below; however, multiple frontal areas may be involved rapidly and specific seizure types may not be discernible.

Supplementary motor seizures. In supplementary motor seizures, the seizure patterns are postural, focal tonic, with vocalization, speech arrest, and fencing postures.

Cingulate. Cingulate seizure patterns are complex partial with complex motor gestural automatisms at onset. Autonomic signs are common, as are changes in mood and affect.

Anterior frontopolar region. Anterior frontopolar seizure patterns include forced thinking or initial loss of contact and adversive movements of head and eyes, with possible evolution including contraversive movements and axial clonic jerks and falls and autonomic signs.

Orbitofrontal. The orbitofrontal seizure pattern is one of complex partial seizures with initial motor and gestural automatisms, olfactory hallucinations and illusions, and autonomic signs.

Dorsolateral. Dorsolateral seizure patterns may be tonic or, less commonly, clonic with versive eye and head movements and speech arrest.

Opercular. Opercular seizure characteristics include mastication, salivation, swallowing, laryngeal symptoms, speech arrest, epigastric aura, fear, and autonomic phenomena. Simple partial seizures, particularly partial clonic facial seizures, are common and may be ipsilateral. If secondary sensory changes occur, numbness may be a symptom, particularly in the hands. Gustatory hallucinations are particularly common in this area.

Motor cortex. Motor cortex epilepsies are mainly characterized by simple partial seizures, and their localization depends on the side and topography of the area involved. In cases of the lower prerolandic area there may be speech arrest, vocalization or dysphasia, tonic-clonic movements of the face on the contralateral side, or swallowing. Generalization of the seizure frequently occurs. In the rolandic area, partial motor seizures without march or jacksonian seizures occur, particularly beginning in the contralateral upper extremities. In the case of seizures involving the paracentral lobule, tonic movements of the ipsilateral foot may occur as well as the expected contralateral leg movements. Postictal or Todd's paralysis is frequent."[1]

"In frontal lobe epilepsies, the interictal scalp recordings may show (a) no abnormality; (b) sometimes background asymmetry, frontal spikes or sharp waves; or (c) sharp waves or slow waves (either unilateral or frequently bilateral or unilateral multiobar. Intracranial recordings can sometimes distinguish unilateral from bilateral involvement.

In frontal lobe seizures, various EEG patterns can accompany the initial clinical symptomatology. Uncommonly, the EEG abnormality precedes the seizure onset and then provides important localizing information, such as: (a) frontal or multilobar, often bilateral, low-amplitude fast activity, mixed spikes, rhythmic spikes, rhythmic spike waves, or rhythmic slow waves; or (b) bilateral high amplitude single sharp waves followed by diffuse flattening. Depending on the methodology, intracranial recordings may provide additional information regarding the chronologic and spatial evolution of the discharges; localization may be difficult." [1]

Frontal lobe epilepsies other than epilepsia partialis continua and Kozhevnikov-Rasmussen syndrome have not been detailed in the new ILAE diagnostic scheme. [10]

SEIZURES FROM THE SUPPLEMENTARY SENSORIMOTOR AREA

Seizures from the SMA have distinct and characteristic clustering of symptoms, and are usually stereotyped (Figure 12.9).[244–249]

Hypermotor seizures[250] of bizarre bilateral, asymmetric tonic posturing and movements

The characteristic hypermotor seizure of SMA consists of sudden and explosive, bilateral and asymmetric tonic posturing of limb girdles at shoulder and pelvis often with contraversion of the eyes and head, vocalisation or speech arrest.

'Fencing posturing'[251] is the best known descriptive term for these SMA seizures, though it may not be common.[249] In fencing posturing, one arm is raised and semi-extended above the head, while the other remains by the body semi-flexed at the elbow. Bilateral asymmetrical posturing is the most common.

M^2E posture is another term used to describe flexion of the elbow of one arm, abduction of the shoulder to 90^0, with associated external rotation.[19] The head looks at the postured hand, and the opposite arm shows slight flexion. The leg ipsilateral to the involved arm extends, while the opposite leg flexes at the hip and knee.

Posturing is extremely variable among patients with SMA seizures, but it is stereotypical for each individual patient.

This variability of hypermotor seizures is reflected well by other descriptive terms of SMA seizures, such as:

- complex gestural automatisms,
- extreme motor restlessness,
- complex motor automatisms and agitation,
- frenetic complex motor automatisms of both arms and legs,
- intensely affective vocal and facial expression associated with powerful bimanual-bipedal and axial activity,
- repetitive rhythmical and postural movements accompanied by bizarre vocalisation,
- complex motor automatisms with kicking and thrashing, complex and global gesticulations.

Somatosensory or other ill-defined auras (not epigastric), vocalisations and speech arrest are common ictal manifestations of SMA seizures.

Somatosensory auras are described by more than half and probably about 80%[253] of patients, mainly at onset. Unilateral somatosensory sensations usually accurately predict contralateral lateralisation.[254] Cephalic sensations are probably more common.[253] Auras are described as:

> pressure on the chest, difficult to breathe, floating away, paraesthesia of a hand, dizziness and light headedness, cephalalgia or electrical sensation in the head, discharge in the whole body, sensation of body heat, feeling of coldness or heat in the back and the head, vertebral column shivering, moving outside oneself, crawling sensation in both, one leg or somewhere in the body.[250,253,255,256]

Epigastric auras do not occur.

Vocalisations: One-third of patients manifest with vocalisations that may vary from a brief deep breath or air expiration and palilalic vocalisations to the most bizarre, loud and scaring noises.

Speech arrest is a well-documented and frequent ictal manifestation. Pure paroxysmal speech arrest without other motor activity is exceptional.

Definition of hypermotor seizures

Hypermotor seizures consist of "complex, organised movements which affect mainly the proximal portions of the limbs and lead to a marked increase in motor activity. Consciousness may be preserved. They are most frequently associated with frontal lobe epilepsy".[250,252]

Consciousness is usually well preserved; as a rule, these are simple focal seizures. Other characteristics of seizures from the SMA are:

- abrupt onset and abrupt termination
- nocturnal circadian distribution; rarely occur in awake states
- high frequency, sometimes many per night
- lack of postictal confusion.

SEIZURES FROM OTHER FRONTAL LOBE REGIONS

Seizures from other frontal lobe regions are less common and are, topographically: cingulate, anterior frontopolar, orbitofrontal, dorsolateral and opercular seizures.[1]

OTHER FRONTAL LOBE SEIZURES OF PARTICULAR CLINICAL INTEREST

The following frontal seizures are of particular clinical interest:

a. *'Frontal absences'* are similar and often indistinguishable from generalised absence seizures in their clinical and EEG manifestations (Figure 12.10).[257,258]

b. *Seizures characterised by unusual symptoms of 'forced thinking' and 'forced acts'.* The patient is forced into an obsessive thought *(forced thinking)* associated with a fairly well-adapted attempt to act on this thought (*forced acts*),[49,49,51,51] with *'eye-directed automatisms'* and *'pseudo-compulsive behaviour'.* These seizures emanate from the dorsolateral intermediate frontal lobe. French investigators vividly described the seizures as follows:[232,238,259-261]

"Gaze and gestures of the upper limbs appear to be attracted by some object in the immediate environment, which orients a pseudo-intentional sequence of catching, touching, putting in order, or playing with the hands. Aggressive facial expression

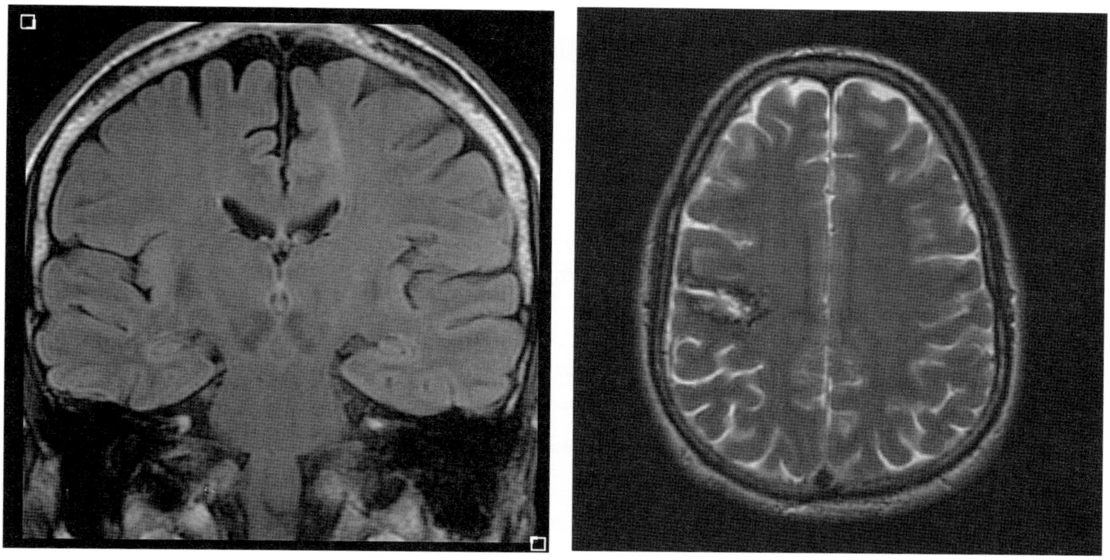

Figure 12.8 MRI in two patients with symptomatic frontal lobe epilepsy.

Left: Coronal FLAIR MRI showing focal cortical dysplasia in the supplementary motor area of the left frontal lobe. Note the tail extending down towards the frontal horn of the lateral ventricle. This patient was 60 years old and had had left SMA seizures for 7 years. All previous MRI studies were negative.

Figure courtesy of Professor John S Duncan and the National Society for Epilepsy MRI Unit, London, UK.

Right: Axial T2-weighted MRI showing an heterogeneous lesion in the left precentral area. The signal changes are consistent with haemosiderosis suggestive of a cavernous angioma.

Figure courtesy of Dr Ruben Kuzniecky, NYU Epilepsy Center, New York, USA.

and complex vocalisation (menaces, insults, obscenities) precede a sequential gestural pattern such as standing up, then running around the table, spitting, tapping on the table, seemingly speaking to somebody; or jumping or pedalling movements with rhythmic joyful vocalisation. Their onset is often marked by alternating head deviations as if oriented towards an external stimulus... In other cases, they consist of much more complex and bizarre gesticulations, seemingly aimless, or apparently running away from some frightening situation, possibly as a reaction to 'unconscious' hallucinations. Often occurring during sleep, they are characterised by a facial expression of fear or terror, a powerful vocalisation (screaming), agitation of the upper limbs as if struggling or tearing out something, manipulation of the genitals accompanying pelvic movements, pedalling movements, or kicking."[232,238,259-261]

Tonic deviation of the eyes preceding head deviation (frontal eye field involvement) may occur independently or in association with these strange symptoms.[232,238,261]

The patient is compulsively 'forced to fix on something with the eyes', 'the brain commands him to do something that he should not do', 'a sensation of being forced to open the eyes'. This is often associated with forced bizarre actions of hypermotor seizures.

A 30-year-old man, holder of a karate black belt, had a cluster of 30–50 such seizures while dozing in the waiting room of my clinic. Each seizure, which lasted for 10–15 s, was of sudden onset and termination. His facial expression was very aggressive and he would perform various karate acts, often kicking or punching objects in the office (without damaging them), with simultaneous and irregular roaring and other vocalisations. Immediately, after each attack, he would go back and sit in his chair, and fully aware of what was happening he would then apologise, "I can not resist doing this. It will be OK after a while", before jumping off again to perform a similar enforced act. The staff and the other patients were terrified and maintained a safe distance from him, while I had to put on a brave face to approach him until he recovered.

c. *Gelastic seizures of frontal lobe origin.*[101,262] There are around 15 well-documented cases of gelastic seizures originating from the frontal lobe. Onset is usually before the age of 6 years, but may start in adulthood in one-third of

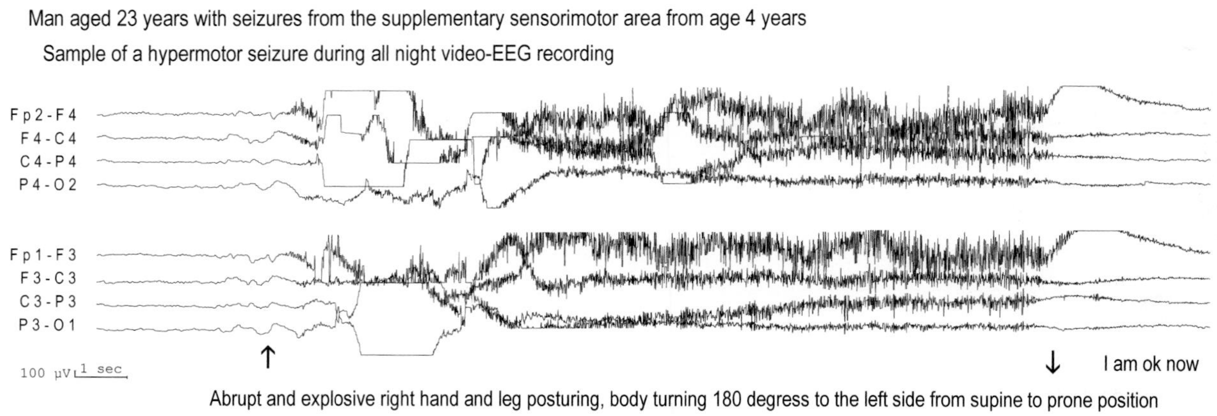
Man aged 23 years with seizures from the supplementary sensorimotor area from age 4 years
Sample of a hypermotor seizure during all night video-EEG recording
Fp2-F4
F4-C4
C4-P4
P4-O2
Fp1-F3
F3-C3
C3-P3
P3-O1
100 µV 1 sec
I am ok now
Abrupt and explosive right hand and leg posturing, body turning 180 degress to the left side from supine to prone position

Figure 12.9 Hypermotor seizure of the sensorimotor supplementary area.

Sample from one of 10 stereotypical hypermotor seizures recorded during an all-night video EEG. Note the abrupt and explosive character of the seizure, which lasted for only 14 s. There are no discernible ictal EEG abnormalities, though occasionally some bilateral slow waves precede the onset of the seizures. Frequent EEGs, ictal and interictal, over a 20-year-period, failed to reveal any conventional epileptogenic abnormalities.

The patient is an intelligent man who has experienced numerous nocturnal hypermotor seizures from the age 4 years. He is fully aware of the attacks, but he can not speak during them, though he hears and understands. He has a somatosensory aura of "a tight sensation in my chest and a feeling that I can not breathe as all the holes of my body are closed". All possible drug treatments had failed. High resolution brain MRI and PET scans were normal.

patients. Most lesions commonly involve the cingulate gyrus. Laughter is described as unnatural and mirthless. The duration of the seizure is brief, lasting from less than 30 s to less than 2 min. Other types of seizures may predate or follow the gelastic attacks.

See also hypothalamic (gelastic) epilepsy on page 193.

d. *Negative motor seizures* manifest with ictal loss of localised muscle power or inability to produce a voluntary movement.

Focal status epilepticus of frontal lobe origin

Focal (non-convulsive) status epilepticus of frontal lobe origin is of undetermined prevalence.[162,163] It manifests with prolonged impairment of consciousness and inappropriate behaviours (Figure 12.11). Symptoms fluctuate in intensity and severity over time. Concurrent turning of the head and focal jerking may occur. It commonly ends with GTCS. Ictal EEG shows repetitive frontopolar, frontocentral and frontotemporal epileptiform discharges with unilateral emphasis. It is difficult to differentiate from frontal or idiopathic absence status epilepticus without EEG (Figure 12.11).

Thomas et al. (1999)[163] described two types of frontal lobe status epilepticus. The first and more common type manifests with mood disturbances with affective disinhibition or affective indifference, which are associated with subtle impairment of cognitive functions without overt confusion. The EEG shows a unilateral frontal ictal pattern and normal background activity. In the second type, impaired consciousness is associated with bilateral, asymmetric frontal EEG discharges on an abnormal background. The response to intravenous benzodiazepines is poor, while intravenous phenytoin successfully controls seizures in most patients.[163]

AETIOLOGY

Frontal lobe epilepsies may be symptomatic, probably symptomatic or idiopathic. Two-thirds of patients in neurosurgical series are symptomatic[261] as a result of malformation of cortical development (57.4%), tumours (16.4%), and trauma and other lesions (26.2%).[263]

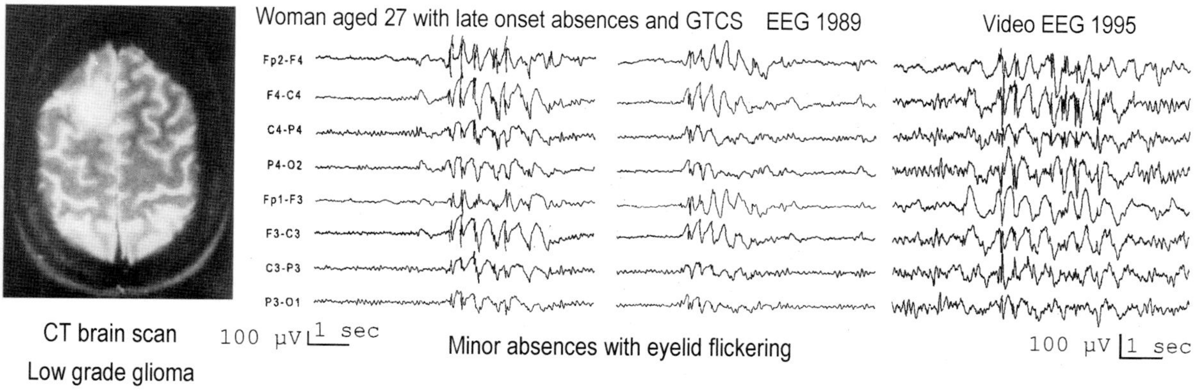

Figure 12.10 Typical absence seizures of late onset due to frontal lobe glioma.

Left: Brain imaging showing a right-sided frontal glioma in a woman who started having absences at 28 years of age (1989).

Middle right and left: Initially, the EEG GSWD were entirely symmetrical; there was nothing to suggest that these were symptomatic absences. Clinically, during the GSWD, the woman made minor and occasional errors on breath counting, with consistent eyelid flickering. In her daily life, these were manifested as "losing control of thoughts, repeating simple phrases and occasional mild jerking of the head to the right". This could last for a few seconds to a minute and once she had non-convulsive status epilepticus with mild confusion and expressive dysphasia.

Right: Video EEG 6 years later showed that she continued to have similar GSWD with right-sided asymmetry

Of the idiopathic forms, autosomal dominant, nocturnal, frontal lobe epilepsy is detailed in Chapter 11.

DIAGNOSTIC PROCEDURES

High resolution brain MRI is mandatory. This reveals abnormalities in around two-thirds of patients.

Functional neuroimaging and magnetoencephalograpy are important for localisation.[264]

Ictal and interictal surface EEG has a notoriously low yield. Normal EEG is often misinterpreted as evidence of non-epileptic attacks.

Serum prolactin concentration (> 700 μU/ml) may be raised after frontal lobe seizures, with or without secondarily GTCS. However, failure of prolactin levels to rise does not help in the clinical differentiation of frontal lobe complex focal seizures from psychogenic attacks.

MRI

High resolution MRI detects abnormalities in 67% of patients with frontal lobe epilepsy as opposed to 79% in temporal lobe epilepsy. The overall sensitivity and accuracy of MRI is around 50% in neurosurgical series, but will become higher with new MRI technologies (Figure 12.8). This figure is similar to qualitative linear (routine) analysis of FDG-PET. Quantitative normalised analysis of FDG-PET scans have 96% sensitivity and 74–78% accuracy, and also detects 81% of abnormalities in non-lesional cases.[265]

MRS may be useful in the presurgical evaluation of patients with frontal lobe epilepsy.[266]

ELECTROENCEPHALOGRAPHY

Interictal and ictal surface EEG is often unhelpful in the diagnosis of frontal lobe epilepsies. They are often normal (50–60% of cases), particularly when seizures originate from the medial frontal regions. The EEG of patients with lateral

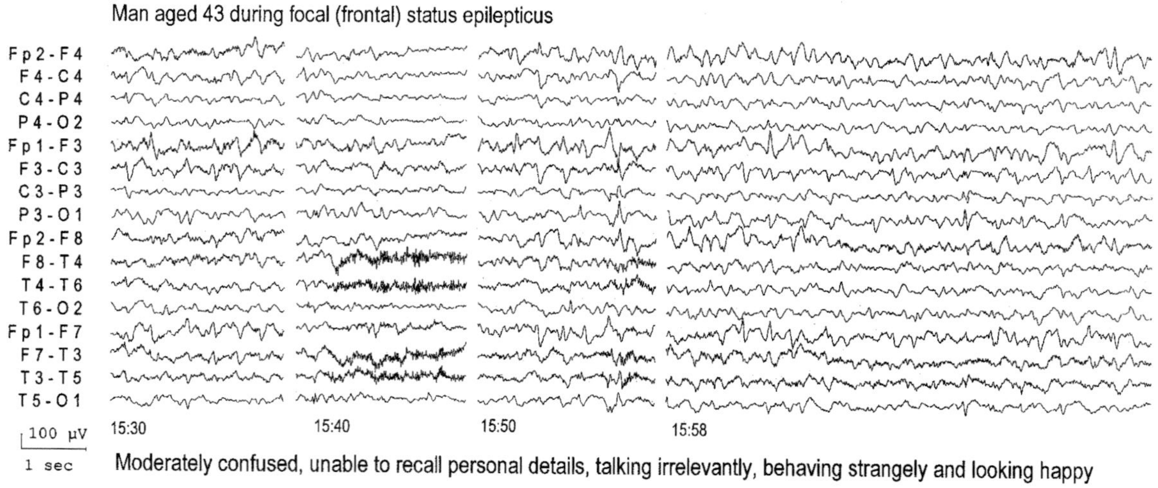

Figure 12.11

Video EEG of a 43-year-old man during complex focal status epilepticus of frontal lobe origin. He was confused, disorientated in time and place, with bizarre behaviour, laughing and making inappropriate jokes.
Note: (a) the frequent, but irregular, appearance of sharp–slow wave complexes, which are mainly localised in the bifrontal electrodes with left-sided preponderance; (b) the relative preservation of alpha activity; and (c) brief discontinuation of the ictal discharge.
The numbers show the actual time of the recording.

seizures is far more revealing than that of mesial frontal seizures (Figure 12.11). Prolonged video EEG recording increases the EEG yield.[267]

The video EEG of one of my patients with tens of clinical SMA seizures was entirely normal over two nights, except for a single, left frontal, giant sharp and slow wave that occurred only once.

The EEG, both interictal and ictal, is usually normal in seizures originating from the mesial frontal regions, a factor that contributes to misdiagnosis.[1,239,263,268]

If abnormal, interictal EEGs may show background asymmetry, frontal spikes or sharp waves (either unilateral or frequently bilateral or unilateral multilobar).[1] Generalised discharges of 3-Hz spike–waves may occur with or without evidence of secondary bilateral synchrony.

Abnormal ictal EEG patterns consist of:

- frontal or multilobar, often bilateral, low amplitude, fast activity, mixed spikes, rhythmic spikes, rhythmic spike waves, or rhythmic slow waves (Figure 12.12). Ictal, fast, rhythmic paroxysms may be of very high frequency (> 50 Hz) and low amplitude requiring specialised recording systems with fast sampling rates and high sensitivity.[269]
- bilateral high amplitude single sharp waves followed by diffuse flattening. Uncommonly, this EEG abnormality precedes the seizure onset providing important localising information.[1,270]

Even when EEG is abnormal, its localisation value is often unreliable without focal ictal paroxysmal patterns at seizure onset. This is probably because of

- early seizure spread within and outside the frontal lobe
- widespread distribution of the epileptogenic brain tissue
- secondary bilateral synchrony and secondary epileptogenesis.

Though seizures predominate in sleep, sleep organisation is normal.

DIFFERENTIAL DIAGNOSIS

The typical motor seizure with or without Jacksonian march is unlikely to impose any diagnostic difficulties. However, hypermotor seizures with the bizarre movements, posturing and vocalisations are frequently misdiagnosed as pseudoseizures[271] or other episodic movement disorders.[240,249] Usually, normal interictal and often ictal EEG reinforces this error. Nowadays, this should be an unlikely misdiagnosis, because the constellation of hypermotor seizures is probably unique with their sudden onset and termination, stereotypical appearance in each patient and nocturnal occurrence in clusters.

Differentiation from non-epileptic paroxysmal movement disorders

Frontal lobe hypermotor seizures should be differentiated from non-epileptic paroxysmal movement disorders,[272-274]such as:

- Psychogenic movement disorders[275]
- Familial paroxysmal dystonic choreoathetosis[276]
- Paroxysmal kinesigenic choreoathetosis[277-279]
- Episodic ataxia type 1.[273,280-283]

Familial paroxysmal dystonic choreoathetosis[276] is a non-epileptic hyperkinetic movement disorder characterised by attacks of involuntary chorea, dystonia and ballism with onset in childhood. Attacks typically last from half an hour to several hours (with no signs of abnormality between attacks) and may occur several times each week. There is no impairment of consciousness and the EEG is normal during the episodes. Attacks are precipitated by a variety of factors, including caffeine, alcohol and emotion. Contrary to frontal lobe seizures, attacks in familial paroxysmal dystonic choreoathetosis can be relieved by short periods of sleep in most subjects.

Non-epileptic paroxysmal kinesigenic choreoathetosis is characterised by recurrent, brief attacks of involuntary movements induced by sudden voluntary movements.[277,278,284,285] The involuntary movements combine tonic, dystonic and choreoathetoid features on one or both sides. They are often associated with dysarthria, upward gaze and sensory aura. Consciousness is entirely intact. Their duration is usually 10–30 s and no more than 3 min. The EEG during the attacks is normal. There may be tens of attacks per day in more than 5% of patients. Onset is in the mid-teens with a range of 5–16 years. Most patients respond well to AEDs, such as carbamazepine, phenytoin or phenobarbitone.[286] In nearly all patients, spontaneous remissions occur between 20 and 30 years of age.

Paroxysmal kinesigenic choreoathetosis is distinct from reflex epilepsy. However, patients may have a history of benign infantile seizures between the ages of 3 and 8 months.[287] There are no differences in the clinical presentation of cases with and without infantile seizures.[287] In addition, there may be a family history of epileptic seizures in 8% of cases.

Episodic ataxia type 1: Of the various types of episodic ataxias,[280-283] only type 1 may impose problems in differential diagnosis. In episodic ataxia type 1, patients

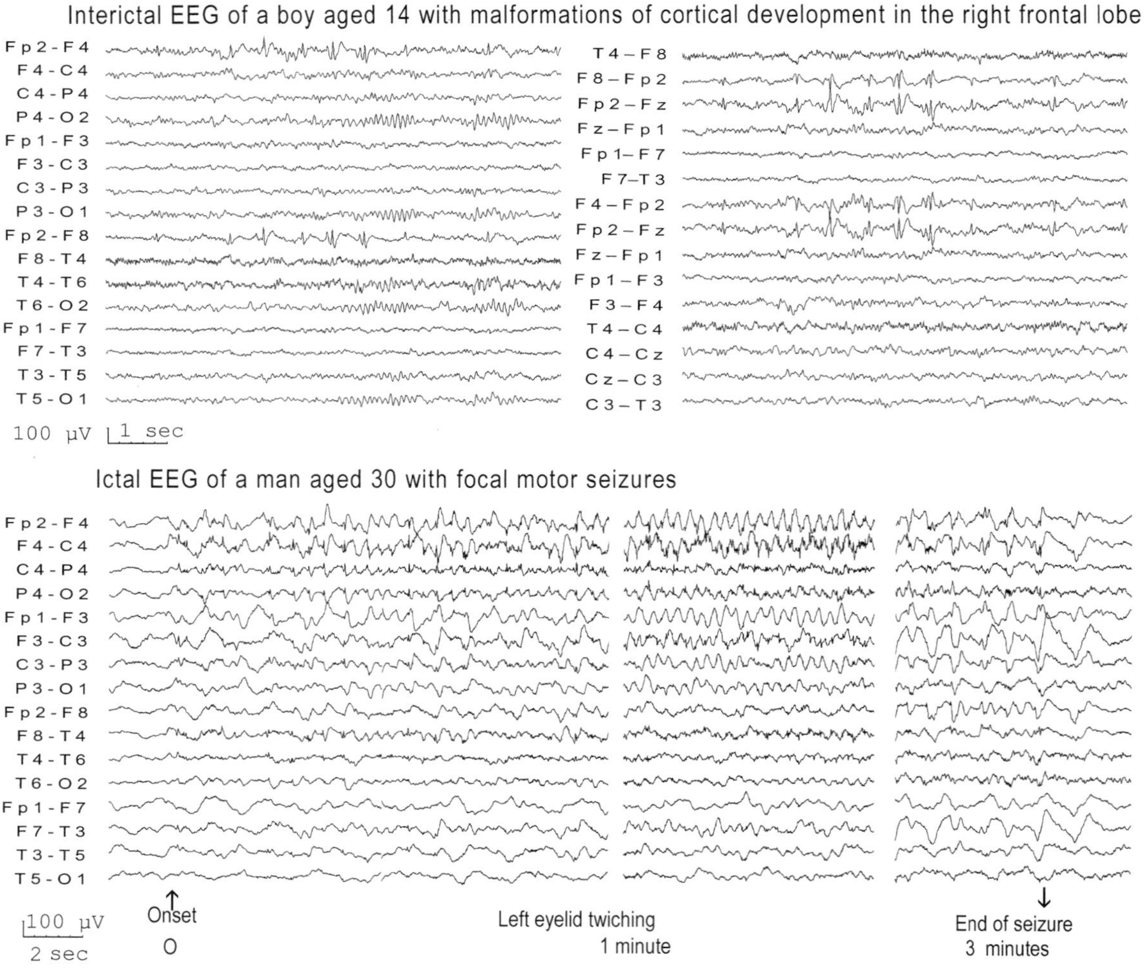

Figure 12.12

Top: Interictal EEG of a 14-year-old child with malformations of cortical development in the dorsolateral aspect of the right frontal lobe. The same EEG sample is presented in different montages. Note frequent clusters of high amplitude spikes intermixed with slow waves in the right frontopolar electrode (Fp2).

Bottom: Ictal EEG of a 30-year-old patient with left-sided focal motor seizures.

suffer from brief attacks of ataxia and dysarthria, lasting seconds to minutes, often associated with continuous inter-attack myokymia. Attacks are diurnal and may occur several times per day. The EEG is frequently abnormal and patients may also have seizures. Episodic ataxia type 1 is a rare, autosomal dominant, potassium channelopathy caused by at least 10 different point mutations in the *KCNA1* gene on chromosome 12p13.

Differentiation from sleep disorders

Hypermotor seizures may be mistaken for pavor nocturnus in children or rapid-eye-movement behaviour disorder. However, the lack of dream recall, the stereotyped movements and occasional secondarily GTCS are useful distinguishing features.

So-called 'paroxysmal nocturnal dystonia or hypnogenic paroxysmal dystonia' is frontal lobe epilepsy.

Differentiation from other seizures

Temporal lobe seizures: Oro-alimentary automatisms, fear, olfactory and gustatory hallucinations, 'absence' with no focal symptoms, experiential phenomena and visual illusions favour temporal lobe seizures.[64]

Symptomatic frontal lobe absences may have similar clinical and EEG features to typical absence seizures (Figure 12.10).[288-290]

MANAGEMENT

The focal seizures of frontal lobe epilepsies are usually resistant to AEDs, but they usually protect patients against secondarily GTCS. Drug treatment is similar to that for any other type of focal seizure.

Neurosurgery has limited success.[247,291] Presurgical MRI is a an important predictor of surgical outcome. Focal frontal lobe MRI lesions and pathological abnormalities correlate strongly with good outcome. In contrast, less favourable results are reported in patients with normal MRI and gliosis or no pathological abnormality on pathological examination. Multilobar MRI abnormalities have the poorest outcome.

Surface EEG and location has no predictive value in neurosurgical cases. However, generalised epileptiform discharges and generalised interictal slow activity indicates a poor neurosurgical outcome.[263] The absence of generalised EEG signs is the most predictive variable for a seizure-free outcome in neurosurgery for frontal lobe epilepsy.[263]

EPILEPSIA PARTIALIS CONTINUA OF KOZHEVNIKOV

Epilepsia partialis continua of Kozhevnikov is rightly considered as a type of seizure/status epilepticus caused by various heterogeneous conditions in children and adults.[292-299]

DEMOGRAPHIC DATA

Onset occurs at any age from the very young to the very old, but probably before 16 years of age in one-third of cases. Both sexes are equally affected. Prevalence is extremely small, probably less than one per million population.[295]

CLINICAL MANIFESTATIONS

The cardinal and defining symptom of epilepsia partialis continua is "spontaneous regular or irregular clonic muscle twitching of cerebral cortical origin, sometimes aggravated by action or sensory stimuli, confined to one part of the body, and continuing for a period of hours, days, or weeks".[292] Epilepsia partialis continua is a prolonged segmental myoclonic seizure lasting a few milliseconds repeated nearly every second for hours, days or months. The twitching is limited to a muscle or a small group of contiguous or unrelated muscles on one side of the body. Agonist and antagonist muscles are simultaneously contracted. Facial and hand muscles are preferentially affected.

The chronic focal epileptic muscle twitching of epilepsia partialis continua is characterised by location, frequency, intensity, duration and coexistence with other types of more conventional seizures.[255,295,296,299-301] Activation, reflex, by movement or other means, is characteristic in some patients.[292,294,295]

Location: Epilepsia partialis continua may involve one muscle or a small muscle group of agonists and antagonists. These may be in the same region (corner of the mouth, thumb and other fingers) or occur simultaneously in other locations on the same side without direct anatomical continuity. Thus, a patient may stereotypically experience twitching of the eyelid and the shoulder or abdominal muscles simultaneously, leaving other facial or limb muscles unaffected. Facial and distal muscles of the upper limbs are more commonly affected than proximal or leg musculature. Truncal muscles on one side, such as the rectus abdominus,[302] teres major[295] or other muscles, may be involved.

Epilepsia partialis continua that involves both sides of the body alternately is exceptional.[303]

Frequency: Typically every jerk occurs about once every second or so. In one quantitative study, 33% of patients experienced 10 jerks/min, 19% 10–20 jerks/min and 14% less than 20 jerks/min.[295] Epilepsia partialis continua usually persists during slow wave sleep, though is often of diminished frequency and intensity. It may be reduced or exaggerated during REM.[304-307]

Intensity: Commonly the jerks in epilepsia partialis continua are not violent and the patient, though distressed, can tolerate them well. Intensity varies from nearly inconspicuous to clearly visible repetitive rapid movements of the affected parts.

Duration is, by definition, for hours, days, weeks or months, though each jerk lasts for only a few milliseconds.[292]

Activation: That epilepsia partialis continua is sometimes 'aggravated by action or sensory stimuli' is a defining characteristic, though not in all patients.[292] Movement or other means of activation of the affected muscles may be a characteristic feature in some patients.[294]

Other type of seizures: About 60% of patients exhibit, in addition to epilepsia partialis continua, other types of seizures, such as motor focal seizures or secondarily GTCS and, more rarely, complex focal seizures.[255,295,296,299,300] These may occur independently, precede or follow the appearance of epilepsia partialis continua. More often motor focal seizures are interspersed with epilepsia partialis continua.

ILAE classification and definition

The ILAE Commission considers epilepsia partialis continua as *"Kozhevnikov syndrome type 1"*[1] and defines it as follows: "This type represents a particular form of rolandic partial epilepsy in both adults and children and is related to a variable lesion of the motor cortex. Its principal features are:

(a) motor partial seizures, always well localised;

(b) often late appearance of myoclonus in the same site where somatomotor seizures occur;

(c) an EEG with normal background activity and a focal paroxysmal abnormality (spikes and slow waves);

(d) occurrence at any age in childhood and adulthood;

(e) frequently demonstrable aetiology (tumor, vascular); and

(f) no progressive evolution of the syndrome (clinical, electroencephalographic or psychological, except in relation to the evolution of the causal lesion). This condition may result from mitochondrial encephalopathy (MELAS)."[1]

Certain aspects of the differences between the ILAE Commission of 1985/1989[1] and the ILAE Task Force[2] have been detailed on page 8. Rightly, the new diagnostic scheme recognised *Epilepsia partialis continua of Kozhevnikov* as a seizure type and not as as syndrome.[2]

Neurological signs and symptoms: Varying degrees of muscle weakness and neurological signs occur during epilepsia partialis continua.[255,296,299] Permanent neurological and mental deficits may be static or progressive, and precede or follow the appearance of epilepsia partialis continua.

Patients with localised neoplastic, vascular or infectious brain lesions may have neurological deficits and isolated seizures prior to the onset of the focal status.[255] In non-ketotic hyperglycaemia or drug-induced epilepsia partialis continua, the onset is sudden.[294]

AETIOLOGY

There are multiple and diverse causes of epilepsia partialis continua, such as focal or multifocal brain lesions, systemic diseases affecting the brain and metabolic or other derangements (Table 12.2). Kozhevnikov-Rasmussen syndrome and malformations of cortical development are the main causes in children. Cerebrovascular disease and brain space-occupying lesions are the main causes in adults. Non-ketotic hyperglycaemia is the most common reversible cause. Other metabolic, mitochondrial or hereditary disorders are well described. Dereux (1955),[308] in a thesis comprising 102 cases, found that more than 50% were caused by an 'encephalitic process'. Rasmussen et al. (1958) described three children with epilepsia partialis continua, progressive hemiparesis, cognitive impairment and pathological changes of chronic encephalitis.

Russian spring-summer tick-borne encephalitis is a rare cause that occurs in

Table 12.2 Causes of epilepsia partialis continua

Chronic or acute encephalitis	Kozhevnikov-Rasmussen syndrome Acute encephalitis including tick-borne encephalitis Human immunodeficiency virus infection Renal and hepatic encephalopathy Anti-Hu-associated paraneoplastic encephalomyelitis
Mitochondrial disorders	
Creutzfeldt-Jakob disease	
Metabolic disturbances	Non-ketotic hyperglycaemic diabetes mellitus, particularly when associated with hyponatraemia Alpers syndrome Kufs' disease NADH-coenzyme Q reductase deficiency
Lesional diseases of the brain	Cerebrovascular disease, brain tumour, abscess, trauma, metastasis, granuloma, cysticercosis, haemorrhage, infarct, arteriovenous malformation and cortical vein thrombosis Malformations of cortical development Multiple sclerosis
Drugs	Penicillin and azlocillin-cefotaxime (and the old contrast media metrizamide) may induce epilepsia partialis continua
Unknown (20%)	

endemic areas. This condition is overemphasised based on the erroneous assumption[309] that it caused the cases of epilepsia partialis continua described by Kozhevnikov (see review in ref [310]).

PATHOPHYSIOLOGY

The current consensus is that epilepsia partialis continua is of cortical origin and emanates mainly in the primary motor cortex. However, in all series, also utilising sophisticated neurophysiological techniques, there is a minority of patients in whom the cortical origin of epilepsia partialis continua can not be documented. For example, in the study of Cockerell et al. (1996),[295] of 16 patients who underwent detailed clinical and neurophysiological assessments, only six had direct EEG and EMG evidence of a cortical origin of their jerks; five patients had indirect evidence of a cortical origin, two did not have myoclonus of cortical origin but of some other source (brainstem and basal ganglia) and the origin in the remaining three patients was uncertain.[295]

DIAGNOSTIC PROCEDURES

The yield of investigative procedures is cause dependent. Around two-thirds of patients have abnormal brain MRI scans and EEG, which get worse in progressive disorders such as Kozhevnikov-Rasmussen syndrome. Ictal EEG may or may not show epileptiform abnormalities concomitant with the jerks (Figures 12.13 and 12.14). Typically, jerk-locked back-averaged cortical potentials appear in the contralateral primary motor area preceding the jerks by a few milliseconds, sensory evoked potentials are of high amplitude (Figure 12.15) and there is a rostro-caudal pattern of muscle recruitment with co-contraction of agonist and antagonist muscles. PET and SPECT scans often localise the abnormal region, but they are not specific. Screening for metabolic and mitochondrial disorders may be necessary and a few cases are of unknown origin.

DIFFERENTIAL DIAGNOSIS

Epilepsia partialis continua should not be difficult to diagnose on clinical grounds. There are not many other conditions that exhibit the characteristic segmental, continuous muscle twitching of this type. EEG may or may not be useful. A normal ictal EEG is not against this diagnosis. Brain imaging may or may not be abnormal. The main difficulty is to differentiate the genuine cortical from the non-cortical cases, and this is often a formidable task without appropriate neurophysiological examinations (jerk-locked back averaging, somatosensory evoked responses and sequential EMG). In clinical terms, the coexistence of other types of focal epileptic seizures practically identifies cortical epilepsia partialis continua.

Tremors, ticks and extrapyramidal disorders emphasised in relevant reviews or reports rarely, if ever, have this constant, unilateral and highly localised appearance of epilepsia partialis continua. However, difficulties may be imposed by 'hemifacial spasm', which is probably due to ipsilateral facial nerve root compression and segmental demyelination. Hemifacial spasm, like epilepsia partialis continua, manifests with unilateral painless irregular and continuous clonic twitching of the facial muscles. It affects mainly women, aged 50–60 years, without known antecedent causes other than Bell's palsy in a few cases. The spasms usually begin in the orbicularis oculi and gradually spread to other facial muscles and the platysma of the face. Like epilepsia partialis continua, facial spasms may be induced or aggravated by voluntary and reflex movements of the face.[311]

A 50-year-old woman had nearly continuous twitching in the left side of the face for 2 months. The diagnosis of hemifacial spasms was made by eminent neurologists. However, MRI and subsequent surgery revealed a large glioblastoma in the right side of the brain.

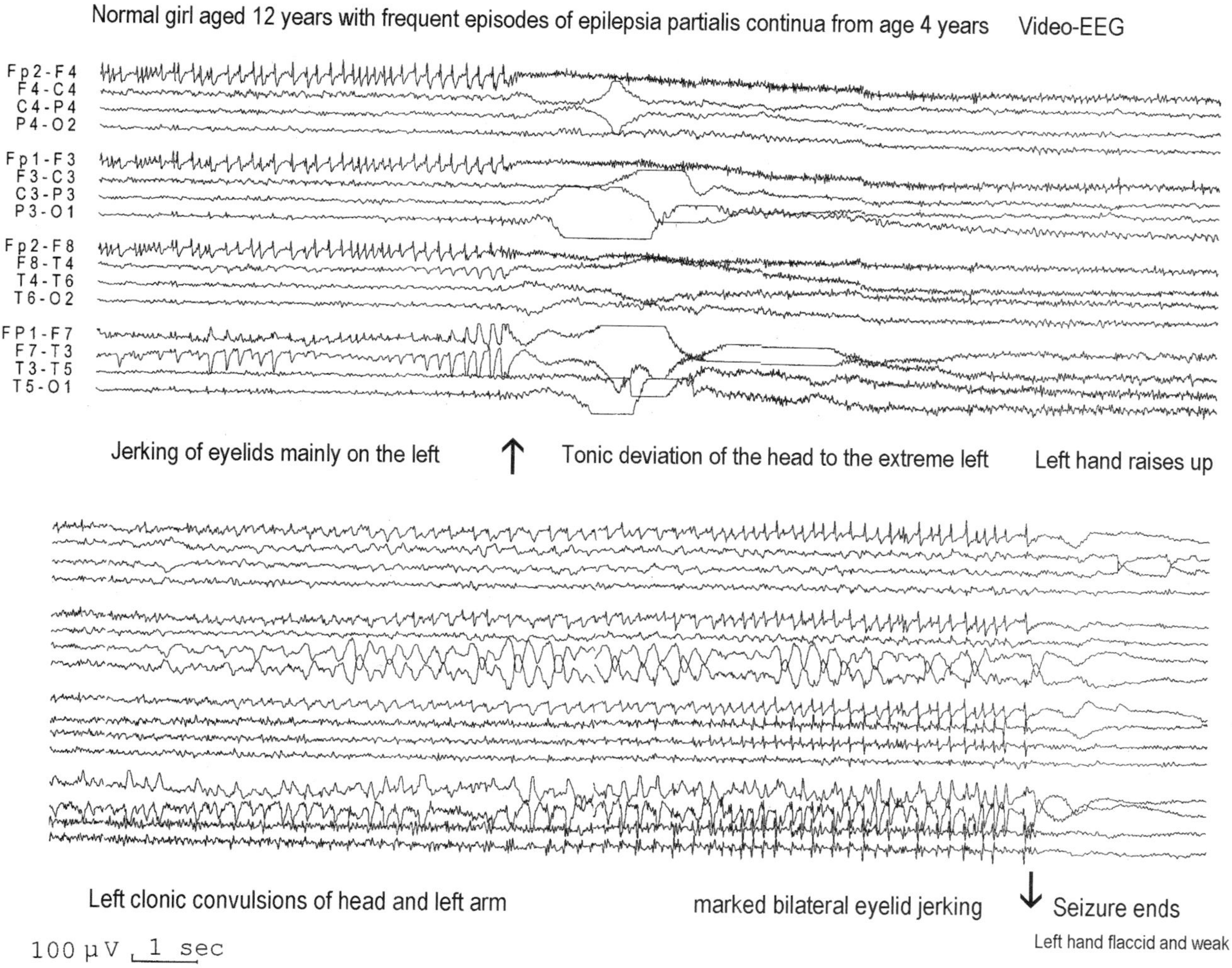

Figure 12.13 Epilepsia partialis continua of 3 days' duration, ending with hemiconvulsions.

Sample from a video EEG of a girl aged 12 years. She has epilepsia partialis continua, which started at the age of 4 years and continues to date with increasing frequency and duration. Fast (3–10 Hz) twitching of the left eyelids occurs simultaneously with the left rectus abdominis (she points close to the midline by the umbilicus) and a muscle in the armpit (probably the latissimus dorsi). This lasts from hours to 2–3 days and is continuous day and night. This is interspersed with left-sided, focal tonic-clonic motor seizures mainly affecting the face and upper limb. Additionally, there is postictal, and probably ictal, left hemiparesis mainly of the upper limb. She does not lose consciousness during these attacks and communicates well. She is also able to understand, but can not speak, during the focal motor seizures. She has never had a full-blown GTCS.
Initially, the seizures occurred once or twice per year, but now occur every 2 weeks. Neurological and mental status is normal. High resolution brain MRI was normal. All appropriate tests for metabolic or other diseases associated with epilepsia partialis continua were normal. Drug treatments have failed; only rectal diazepam provides temporary relief during the attacks.
Differential diagnosis: Epilepsia partialis continua is a non-specific seizure type that may occur in a number of diverse conditions and have a number of different causes. In a child, the first syndrome that comes to mind is Kozhevnikov-Rasmussen chronic encephalitis. However, her good clinical status over the years, as well as the normal MRI and the lack of background EEG abnormalities, is rather against this diagnosis though some unusual cases in which deterioration occurs 10 years after onset of epilepsia partialis continua have been recorded.

Once the diagnosis of epilepsia partialis continua is made, the underlying cause should be thoroughly sought with clinical and investigative means mandated by the causative factors listed in Table 12.2.

PROGNOSIS

Epilepsia partialis continua is a symptom of a group of heterogeneous disorders that may be progressive, static or reversible (Table 12.2). Therefore, the long-term prognosis is cause-dependent and is usually poor. Most patients will continue with intractable epilepsia partialis continua and also develop neurological and mental defects.

Only a few patients may have a remission. Drug-induced epilepsia partialis continua disappears following the removal of the offending agent. Similarly, epilepsia partialis continua occurring in the setting of non-ketotic hyperglycaemia is reversible once the metabolic defect is corrected.

MANAGEMENT

Epilepsia partialis continua is resistant to treatment with AEDs. Clonazepam, valproate, carbamazepine and new broad-spectrum AEDs, such as levetiracetam and topiramate, are probably the most effective.

Successful treatment with multiple subpial transections has been reported in only a minority of operated patients.[295,298]

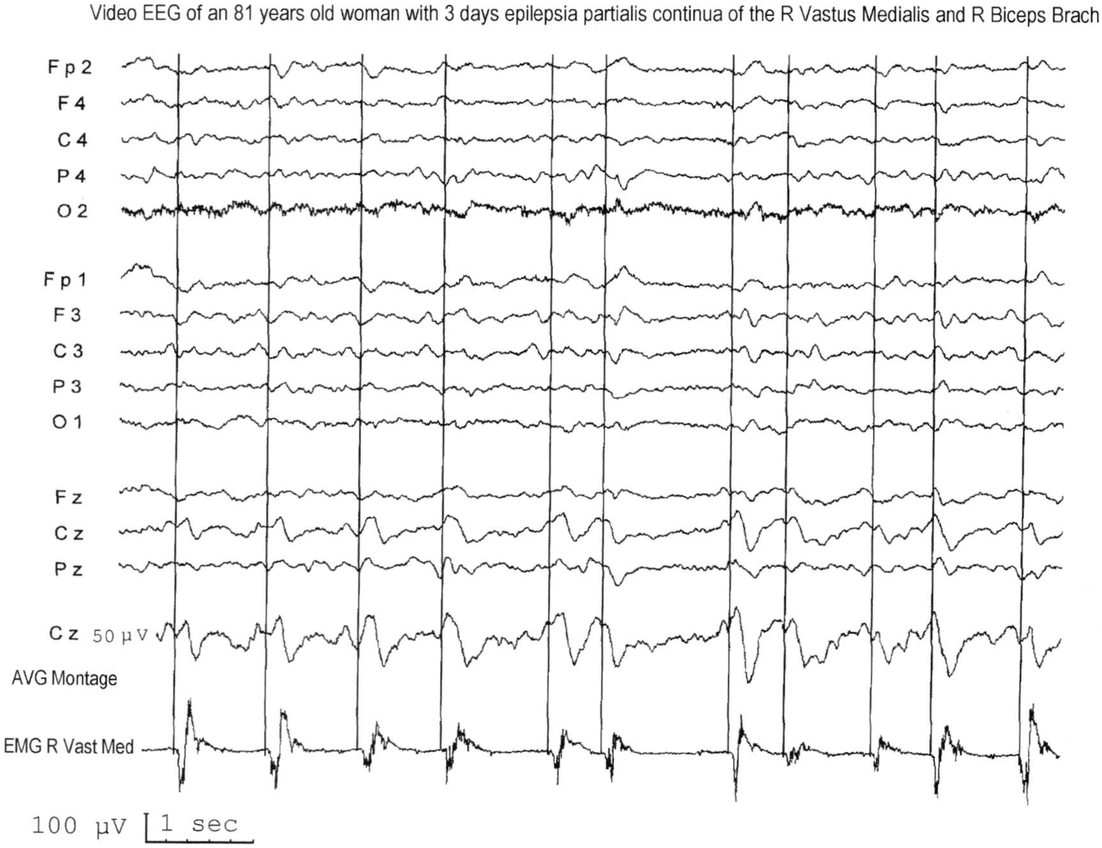

Figure 12.14 Epilepsia partialis continua of 3 days' duration in an elderly woman in a coma. The right vastus medialis and right biceps brachius muscles were involved. Note that the only concurrent EEG abnormality during the jerking of the right vastus medialis muscle was apparent only in the central midline electrode.

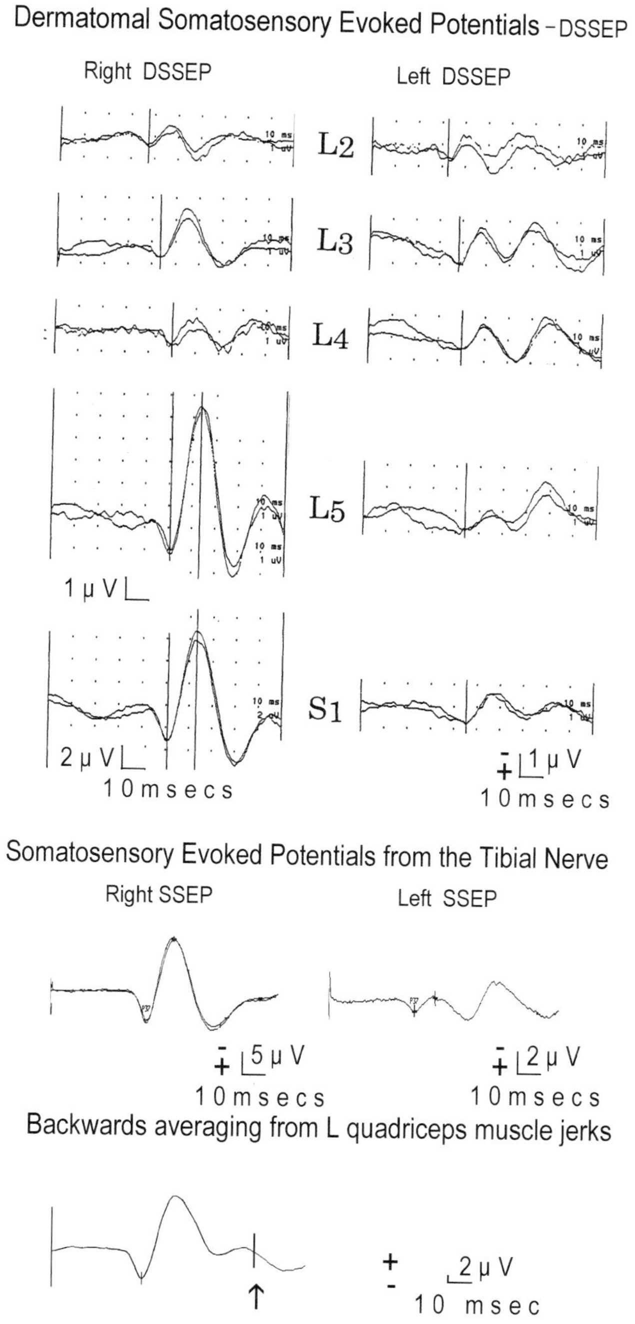

Figure 12.15

Neurophysiological investigations in a man aged 26 years with onset of epilepsia partialis continua at the age of 25. This consisted of continuous and arrhythmic twitching of various muscles of the left leg and particularly the toes. There was great variation in intensity, spread and severity. It was exaggerated on dorsiflexion of the foot and improved when resting. On five occasions, this progressed in a Jacksonian manner to GTCS. The clonic movements of the toes spread to the foot and then to the knee for 5 min prior to GTCS. On neurological examination, there were mild pyramidal signs of the left leg. All possible tests to discover the cause of this were negative, including high resolution MRI and PET scanning, and CSF with appropriate metabolic screening. Mitochondrial disease was also excluded. After a short course of steroids and drug treatment with mainly clonazepam, the situations improved dramatically. Ten years later, he is well though has some infrequent clusters of irregular twitching of the toes of the left leg and is still on clonazepam.

Top and middle: Dermatomal and somatosensory potentials are gigantic on the right side (from stimulation of the left). Note that the maximum amplitude of the dermatomal potentials is obtained when the S1 dermatome is stimulated.

Bottom: Jerk-locked back-averaged cortical potentials appear in the contralateral primary motor area preceding the jerks by 25 ms (positive peak).

PARIETAL LOBE EPILEPSIES

Parietal lobe epilepsies manifest with seizures originating from a primary epileptic focus anywhere within the parietal lobe.[1,312-324]

The clinical seizure characteristics, EEG findings and results of neuroimaging studies have been established mainly in neurosurgical series of patients with a carefully documented seizure of parietal lobe origin.[312-314,318,319,321-324] The report by Kim et al. (2004)[324] is an excellent description of the modern approach to parietal lobe epilepsies.

DEMOGRAPHIC DATA

Parietal lobe epilepsies may start at any age. Both sexes are equally affected. Age at onset is much later in patients with tumours[319] than in those without tumours.[318] Parietal lobe epilepsy is relatively rare and probably accounts for 6% of all focal epilepsies in neurosurgical series.[325] In one report, they were twice as common as occipital lobe seizures.[315]

CLINICAL MANIFESTATIONS

Seizures emanating from the parietal lobes are mainly *simple focal* without impairment of consciousness. They manifest with subjective symptoms (auras), which are, in order of prevalence:

- somatosensory
- somatic illusions (subjective disturbances of body image)
- vertiginous
- visual illusions or complex formed visual hallucinations
- receptive or conductive linguistic disturbances.

Clinical seizure manifestations are usually related to the epileptogenic location, anterior or posterior, of the dominant or non-dominant parietal lobe. Onset with sensorimotor symptoms is usually associated with anterior parietal lobe foci, whereas more complex symptomatology emanates from posterior parietal lobe regions. Approximately 50% of patients experience more than one type of seizure.[324]

ILAE classification and definitions

Parietal lobe epilepsies have not yet been detailed in the new ILAE diagnostic scheme.[10] The 1989 ILAE Commission classifies parietal lobe epilepsies among the *localisation-related (focal, local, partial) epilepsies and epileptic syndromes*, but describes parietal seizures rather than parietal lobe syndromes:[1]

"Parietal lobe epilepsy syndromes are usually characterized by simple partial and secondarily generalized seizures. Most seizures arising in the parietal lobe remain as simple partial seizures, but complex partial seizures may arise out of simple partial seizures and occur with spread beyond the parietal lobe. Seizures arising from the parietal lobe have the following features: Seizures are predominantly sensory with many characteristics. Positive phenomena consist of tingling and a feeling of electricity, which may be confined or may spread in a Jacksonian manner. There may be a desire to move a body part or a sensation as if a part were being moved. Muscle tone may be lost. The parts most frequently involved are those with the largest cortical representation (e.g., the hand, arm, and face). There may be tongue sensations of crawling, stiffness, or coldness, and facial sensory phenomena may occur bilaterally. Occasionally, an intraabdominal sensation of sinking, choking, or nausea may occur, particularly in cases of inferior and lateral parietal lobe involvement. Rarely, there may be pain, which may take the form of a superficial burning dysaesthesia, or a vague, very severe, painful sensation. Parietal lobe visual phenomena may occur as hallucinations of a formed variety. Metamorphopsia with distortions, shortenings, and elongations may occur, and are more frequently observed in cases of nondominant hemisphere discharges. Negative phenomena include numbness, a feeling that a body part is absent, and a loss of awareness of a part or a half of the body, known as somatoagnosia. This is particularly the case with nondominant hemisphere involvement. Severe vertigo or disorientation in space may be indicative of inferior parietal lobe seizures. Seizures in the dominant parietal lobe result in a variety of receptive or conductive language disturbances. Some well lateralised genital sensations may occur with paracentral involvement. Some rotatory or postural motor phenomena may occur. Seizures of the paracentral lobule have a tendency to become secondarily generalized."

SOMATOSENSORY SEIZURES

Somatosensory seizures are by far the most common type (around two-thirds of cases).[319]

Quality: Various types of paraesthetic, dysaesthetic and painful sensations are described, such as tingling, numbness, thermal, burning, tickling, pricking, creeping, tight, crawling, electric and their variations. Tingling may be the most characteristic symptom (76% in one study).[326] There may be tongue sensations of crawling, stiffness or coldness. The same patient may experience different types of sensation in different seizures.

> They all start with a tingling sensation around the left side of my lip. This lasts for 10–20 s before spreading to my left arm. Then I lose coordination and power in my left arm, which may start convulsing with little if any manifestations from my leg. The whole seizure lasts for approximately 1½ min. During this time, I am able to talk and understand.

Pain, sometimes excruciating, is experienced by 25% of patients with somatosensory seizures.[315,318,319,322,327,328] Pain is usually unilateral, but may be cephalic or abdominal.[327] When lateralised, the painful symptoms are contralateral to the side of seizure origin.[327]

Symptom location: The face (mainly lips and tongue), hand (mainly thumb) and arm that have the largest cortical representation (homunculus of Penfield) are more likely to be involved. Facial sensory phenomena may occur bilaterally.[329] Symptoms may be static and remain confined to their region of origin during the whole seizure (40% of cases). Somatosensory symptoms often march in a manner similar to the Jacksonian motor seizure. A bilateral or discontiguous manner of spread is rarer. Unilateral somatosensory seizures are usually contralateral to the epileptogenic zone. Seizures ipsilateral to the side of seizure origin are exceptional.[313]

> It is numbness or a hot feeling restricted to the corner of my left lip of the size of no more than a 2-pence piece. This lasts for 1–3 s and comes approximately once every week. On rare occasions, this numbness spreads to my left hand for a second and at the same time I am unable to articulate words. This also may be followed by 'shaking of the lips'. On eight occasions in 14 years, this was followed by convulsions.

Ictal sensations in the genital areas and the rectum, and orgasmic seizures are infrequent, but patients may be embarrassed to report them.[1,315,319,330,331] Postictal or peri-ictal true masturbation may happen.[330] Sexual dyspraxic automatisms (i.e. fondling the genitals) occur only in the postictal phase of seizures.

Objective ictal somatosensory deficits: Objectively demonstrable transient somatosensory deficits may be common if tested during the seizure. For example, a patient of Penfield, while undergoing electrocorticography under local anaesthesia, had an electrically induced seizure restricted to the parietal lobe.[51] The patient was unaware of any specific symptoms, but two-point discrimination was impaired in the contralateral hand and returned to normal at seizure termination.

DISTURBANCES OF BODY IMAGE AND SOMATIC ILLUSIONS

Disturbances of body image and somatic illusions are the second most common ictal symptoms of parietal lobe seizures. They include illusions of distorted posture, limb position or movement, a feeling that an extremity or a body part is alien or absent, dissociations and misperceptions of location and body part identity. Patients describe sensations of twisting, swelling, shrinking, turning or movement in one extremity or in the body, a feeling that one leg is absent and displacement of a limb or the body:

> Having my body bend toward the left, I just sort of swayed.[318,319]

Most patients have paraesthesia associated with these illusions. Ictal somatosensory hallucinations are rare.[25,51]

Ictal somatic illusions probably reflect seizure discharges in the inferior parietal lobule and superior part of the postcentral gyrus of the non-dominant hemisphere.[315]

Somatoagnosia (from the Greek words *soma* [body] and *agnosia* [ignorance]) is the inability to recognise the affected body part as one's own. Somatoagnosia and most of the somatic sensations occur more frequently with dysfunction of the non-dominant cerebral hemisphere.[332-334] Ictal *limb agnosia* (sudden loss of sensation in a limb) and phantom limb sensations (the sense that the limb is in a position that is not the true position) probably originate in the posterior parietal region.[335,336] Neglect is more commonly associated with the right rather than the left inferior parietal lobe. These auras may reflect ictal impairment *'in the body image mechanism of the posterior parietal lobe'*.[335]

Illusions of movement are often typical of parietal lobe seizures,[337,338] while the sensation of a desire to move emanates from the precentral gyrus.[339]

Other ictal subjective symptoms

Vertigo and other vertiginous sensations of an illusion of rotatory body movement are well reported and probably about 10% as ictal manifestations of parietal lobe seizures.[315,318,319,340] They are elicited predominantly from the temporo-parietal border.[17,341]

Visual illusions and complex formed visual hallucinations occur in about 12% of patients with parietal lobe epilepsy. Images may be larger or smaller, close or far away, or moving though static. Ictal visual illusions, such as *micropsia, metamorphopsia, autoscopia* and *palinopsia*, most likely emanate from the non-dominant parietal regions.

Linguistic disturbances: Dominant temporal-parietal lobe seizures are associated with a variety of linguistic disturbances, alexia with agraphia and significant calculation defects. Non-dominant parietal-occipital-temporal seizure activity usually results in significant spatial disturbances.

Inhibitory motor seizures, ictal hemiplegia[322] or *negative motor manifestations*, including drop attacks,[318] are exceptional. An inability to move one extremity or a feeling of weakness in the hand contralateral to the epileptogenic zone may be more common than reported.[319]

> On most occasions my left hand becomes numb, but in a few other instances, it becomes heavy and I am unable to move it for a minute or so.

Seizure spreading to extraparietal regions

Simple focal seizures often spread to extraparietal regions producing unilateral focal clonic convulsions (57% of patients), head and eye deviation (41% of patients), tonic posturing of usually one extremity (28% of patients) and automatisms (21% of patients).

Most patients also suffer from secondarily GTCS, but these are usually infrequent.[324]

Duration of seizures

The duration of seizures varies from a few seconds to 1–2 min.[316] Prolonged isolated sensory auras comparable to *epilepsia partialis continua*, but without any motor manifestations, have been reported[51,318,319] and this condition may be misdiagnosed as non-epileptic psychogenic seizures.[342]

Postictal manifestations

Postictal manifestations are usually short,[316] though Todd's paralysis (22%) and dysphasia (7%) may be common.[318]

Epileptogenic localisation

Seizures of the primary sensory cortex typically produce contralateral positive or negative symptoms. However, focal sensorimotor phenomena at the onset also occur with seizures emanating from posterior parietal regions.[325] This means that the primary epileptogenic focus is clinically silent and that symptoms are produced by spreading of the ictal discharge to the eloquent ictal symptomatogenic zone of the postcentral gyrus.[51,324] Bilateral sensory symptoms usually derive from the secondary sensory area.[51,342]

Ictal sensations in the genital areas usually emanate from the parietal paracentral lobule.[1,315,318] Ictal pain is usually reproduced by stimulating area 5a, behind the postcentral gyrus.[318,319,343,344]

Precipitating factors

Seizures may be provoked by movements of the affected part of the body, tapping or other somatosensory stimuli.[345,346] These are exceptional in neurosurgical series.[318]

In one patient, seizures frequently occurred when she was trying to open a container or package.[313,322,327]

Accidental finger amputation resulted in seizure control in a boy whose seizures included ictal sensory loss in one arm provoked by using cutlery while eating.[347]

Sensorimotor seizures may also be triggered by music[348] or toothbrushing.[349]

Giant EEG spikes evoked by somatosensory stimuli in benign childhood seizure susceptibility syndrome are detailed on page 255.

AETIOLOGY

The aetiology is diverse and includes symptomatic (Figure 12.16), probably symptomatic and idiopathic causes.

Of 82 non-tumoural patients with parietal lobe epilepsy, 43% had a history of head trauma, 16% a history of birth trauma and the cause was unknown in 20%.[318] The remaining 21% had a history of encephalitis, febrile convulsions, gunshot wounds to the head, forme fruste of tuberous sclerosis, hamartoma, vascular malformations, tuberculoma, arachnoid or porencephalic cysts, microgyria and post-traumatic thrombosis of the middle cerebral artery.[318] Of the tumours, astrocytomas (62%) were more common than meningiomas (14%), hemangiomas (9%), oligodendrogliomas (9%) and ependymoblastomas (3%).[319] However, patients with more aggressive tumours, such as glioblastomas, are unlikely to feature in these series.

In reports with MRI, lesions were small, indolent or non-progressive and could have been found only on pathological examination.[313,314] Malformations of cortical development, mild or severe, are probably the most common cause.[324,326]

DIAGNOSTIC PROCEDURES

Neurological examination is usually normal in patients with non-tumoural parietal lobe epilepsy or the abnormalities are mild. Sensory deficits, such as impaired two-point discrimination or stereoagnosia (of which patients may be unaware), mild limb atrophy and inferior quadrantic visual field defects, should be sought. Patients should also be examined for disturbances of written language, aphasia, spatial orientation and right-left disorientation.[325,326] Patients with tumoural parietal lobe epilepsy have similar neurological deficits, but mild contralateral weakness is common (38%), while unilateral limb atrophy is exceptional.[319]

Brain imaging, preferably with high resolution MRI, is mandatory for any patient with parietal lobe epilepsy and may be abnormal in around 60% of patients (Figure 12.16).[319] Other brain imaging modalities, such as FDG-PET and ictal SPECT, are useful in neurosurgical evaluations.[324]

ELECTROENCEPHALOGRAPHY

Interictal EEG

Surface interictal EEG may be normal, non-specific, or even misleading.[313,324] In symptomatic patients, localised slow waves may be the only interictal abnormality

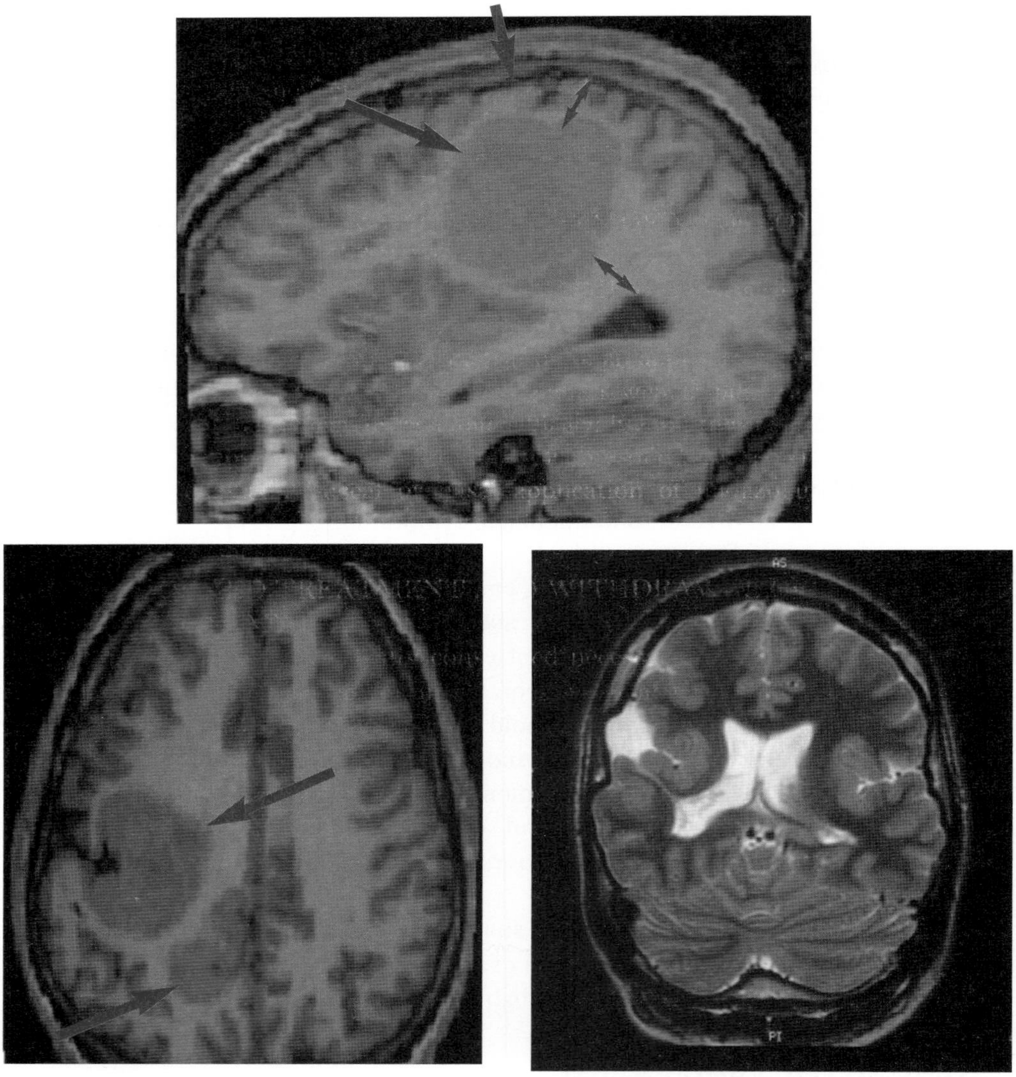

Figure 12.16

Top: Coronal and axial T1-weighted MRI demonstrating parietal subcortical heterotopia (arrows).
Bottom left: Coronal T2-weighted MRI demonstrating bilateral perisylvian polymicrogyria.

Figure courtesy of Professor John S Duncan and the National Society for Epilepsy MRI Unit, London, UK.

Bottom right: Coronal inverted T2-weighted MRI demonstrating abnormal signal changes (post-traumatic in nature) in the left parietal lobe involving the white matter.

Figure courtesy of Dr Ruben Kuzniecky, NYU Epilepsy Center, New York, USA.

(Figure 12.17).[318,319] Epileptiform abnormalities, if they occur, may appear in areas other than the parietal regions, involving frontal, temporal or occipital electrodes.[313-315,318,319,324] Of patients with intractable parietal lobe epilepsy, 16% do not have epileptiform discharges.[318] In these patients, secondary bilateral synchrony may be common (32%).[318] Interictal spikes, if present, should be interpreted cautiously regarding localisation.[346]

In one report,[313] scalp EEGs correctly localised the side and region of seizure onset in only 1 of 11 patients in whom lesions had been detected with MRI. Three additional patients with congruent parietal localisation on scalp EEG had additional misleading EEG findings.

ICTAL EEG

The ictal EEG may be normal in 80% of simple focal sensory seizures.[326] The prevalence of scalp EEG changes in simple focal seizures with predominant sensory symptoms is only 15%, as opposed to 33% when motor symptoms are present.[350]

Localised parietal seizure onset is rare (11%).[313,318] Ictal onset may be distant from the area of the predominant interictal spiking,[329] and ictal EEG patterns are occasionally difficult to interpret,[346] particularly when seizures rapidly become generalised.

POSTICTAL EEG

Postictal EEG may have some localising value when focal slow wave attenuation of background activity or spike activation occur.[351]

DIFFERENTIAL DIAGNOSIS

Simple somatosensory seizures, alone whether brief or prolonged, are a challenging proposition. Even if reported, they are likely to be misdiagnosed as non-epileptic psychogenic fits, transient ischaemic attacks or migraine with aura, in that order. Commonly, it is only when they progress to motor symptoms or impairment of consciousness that genuine seizures are suspected and appropriate investigations are initiated.

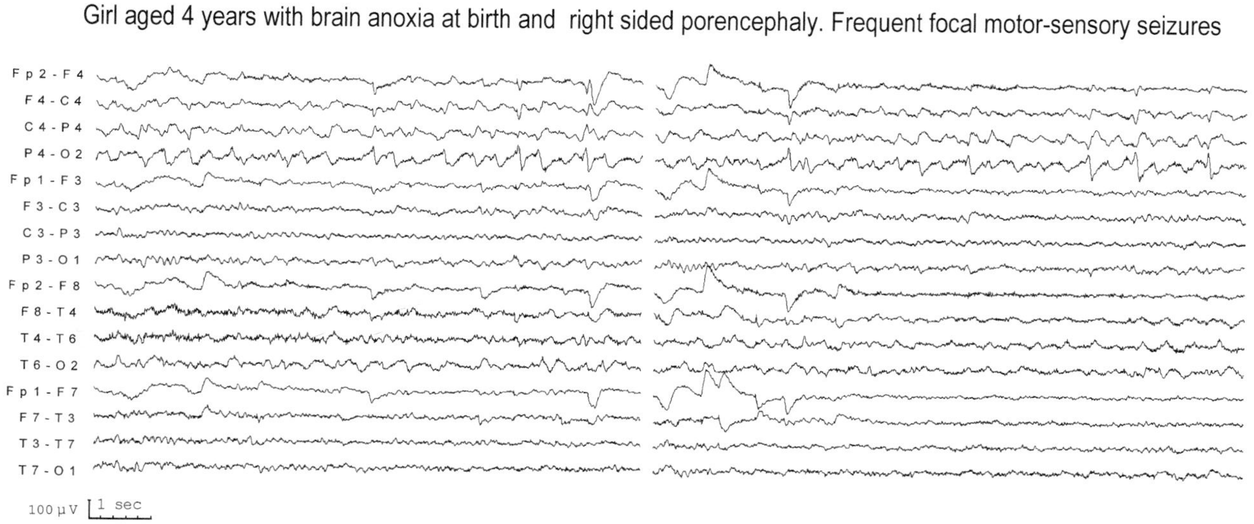

Figure 12.17 Interictal EEG of a 5-year-old girl with extensive right-sided porencephaly due to brain anoxia at birth. Severe right sided abnormalities of spikes, sharp and slow waves are mainly focused around the parietal regions. Clinically she had frequent and intractable focal sensory-motor seizures.

Differentiating pure somatosensory seizures from non-epileptic psychogenic seizures or psychiatric disturbances may be extremely difficult;[342] even ictal EEG changes are not seen in 80% of patients.[326] Ictal pain, sensory epilepsia partialis continua, and genital and orgasmic manifestations are unlikely to be diagnosed as epileptic seizures. Sensory Jacksonian seizures may imitate migraine with sensory aura.[352] In older patients, transient ischaemic attacks are the most likely diagnostic error.

MANAGEMENT

Drug treatment is similar to that for any other type of focal seizures and is usually effective.

In intractable cases, neurosurgery after appropriate modern presurgical evaluation is associated with a high proportion of patients achieving a seizure-free state or remarkable improvement (> 65%).[318,324] MRI abnormality, concordance of different diagnostic modalities and completeness of resection of the epileptogenic zone correlates with better outcome.[313,314,323,324]

However, because the parietal lobe contains highly eloquent areas, resection may lead to deficits in vision, language, praxis, attention and higher cortical function, which make surgical resection problematic.[324]

OCCIPITAL LOBE EPILEPSIES*

Occipital seizures originate from an epileptic occipital focus that is triggered spontaneously or by external visual stimuli.[315,317,328,353-358] These epilepsies may be idiopathic, symptomatic or probably symptomatic.

DEMOGRAPHIC DATA

Symptomatic occipital seizures may start at any age and at any stage after or during the course of the underlying causative disorder. Idiopathic occipital epilepsy usually starts in late childhood (see page 249). Occipital epilepsies account

*This section is primarily based on an extensive review from ancient to current times, studies and numerous illustrative cases in a previous monograph of mine, which I have updated appropriately.[328,359-361]

ILAE classification and definitions

The 1989 ILAE Commission classifies occipital lobe epilepsies among the *localisation-related (focal, local, partial) epilepsies and epileptic syndromes*, but describes occipital seizures rather than occipital lobe syndromes:[1] "Occipital lobe epilepsy syndromes are usually characterized by simple partial and secondarily generalised seizures. Complex partial seizures may occur with spread beyond the occipital lobe. The frequent association of occipital lobe seizures and migraine is complicated and controversial. The clinical seizure manifestations usually, but not always, include visual manifestations. Elementary visual seizures are characterized by fleeting visual manifestations which may be either negative (scotoma, hemianopsia, amaurosis) or, more commonly, positive (sparks or flashes, phosphenes). Such sensations appear in the visual field contralateral to the discharge in the specific visual cortex, but can spread to the entire visual field. Perceptive illusions, in which the objects appear to be distorted, may occur. The following varieties can be distinguished: a change in size (macropsia or micropsia), or a change in distance, an inclination of objects in a given plane of space and distortion of objects or a sudden change of shape (metamorphopsia). Visual hallucinatory seizures are occasionally characterized by complex visual perceptions (e.g. colourful scenes of varying complexity). In some cases, the scene is distorted or made smaller, and in rarer instances, the subject sees his own image (heautoscopy). Such illusional and hallucinatory visual seizures involve epileptic discharge in the temporo-parieto-occipital junction. The initial signs may also include tonic and/or clonic contraversion of eyes and head or eyes only (oculoclonic oroculogyric deviation), palpebral jerks, and forced closure of eyelids. Sensation of ocular oscillation or of the whole body may occur. The discharge may spread to the temporal lobe, producing seizure manifestations of either lateral posterior temporal or hippocampoamygdala seizures. When the primary focus is located in the supracalcarine area, the discharge can spread forward to the suprasylvian convexity or the mesial surface, mimicking those of parietal or frontal lobe seizures. Spread to contralateral occipital lobe may be rapid. Occasionally the seizure tends to become secondarily generalized."[1] Occipital lobe epilepsies have not yet been detailed in the new ILAE diagnostic scheme.

for around 5–10% of all epilepsies.[328] In neurosurgical series, the prevalence is about 5%,[355] which is comparable to the 6% seen in demographic studies.[362]

CLINICAL MANIFESTATIONS

Ictal clinical symptoms of occipital lobe epilepsies are subjective, objective or both. The cardinal symptoms are mainly visual and oculomotor.

Visual subjective symptoms include:

- elementary and less often complex visual hallucinations
- blindness
- visual illusions
- pallinopsia
- sensory hallucinations of ocular movements.

Ocular subjective symptoms comprise:

- ocular pain.

Ictal objective oculomotor symptoms are:

- tonic deviation of the eyes (pursuit-like rather than oculotonic)
- oculoclonic movements or nystagmus
- repetitive eyelid closures or eyelid fluttering.

Some of these ictal manifestations, such as elementary visual hallucinations, are generated in the primary visual cortex; others, such as visual illusions, emanate from the neighbourhood of the occipital-parietal and occipito-temporal regions. Seizures may spread from the occipital to other more anterior regions of the brain generating symptoms from the temporal, parietal and frontal lobes and secondarily hemi- or generalised convulsions. Ictal or postictal headache is frequently associated with occipital seizures.

Elementary visual hallucinations

Elementary visual hallucinations are the most common, characteristic and well-defined ictal symptoms of occipital lobe seizures (Figure 12.18). They are usually the first, and often the only, ictal symptom during a seizure and may progress to other occipital and extra-occipital manifestations and convulsions.

Elementary visual hallucinations of visual seizures are mainly coloured and circular, develop rapidly within seconds and are brief in duration (Figure 12.18). They often appear in the periphery of a temporal visual hemifield, becoming larger and multiplying in the course of the seizure, and frequently moving horizontally towards the other side. They are fundamentally different to the visual aura of migraine for which they are often mistaken.[357,363,364]

Panayiotopoulos has studied the elementary visual hallucinations of idiopathic and symptomatic occipital seizures in a qualitative and quantitative chronological manner,[357,364] differentiated them from the visual aura of migraine[365,366] and reviewed them exhaustively from ancient times.[359] The main conclusions of these studies are briefly described here.

Ictal elementary visual hallucinations (Figure 12.18) are defined by colour, shape, size, location, movement, speed of appearance and duration, frequency and associated symptoms of progression.

Colour, shape and size: The predominant patterns are coloured, usually multicoloured, and circular. Bright red, yellow, blue and green prevail. Shapes are mainly circular, spots, circles and balls. Individual elements are multiple and rarely single. Their size varies from *'spots'* to rarely the size of a *'small ball'*.

Coloured, square, triangular and rectangular or star-like shapes, alone or in combination with circular patterns are less frequent. Flashing or flickering achromatic lights, shades or non-circular patterns are rare. The components of visual hallucinations increase in number, size or both with progression of the seizure, particularly prior to other non-visual symptoms.

Multicoloured blue, yellow and red, circular flickering patterns closely packed together and multiplying in the left lateral hemifield. Then it seems that the environment moves slowly and stepwise from left to right.

A 'rainbow' of all colours with dust blocks of shadow-like bricks in the periphery of the right eye.

Location: Their location at onset is usually unilateral, mainly in the temporal visual hemifield (Figure 12.18). They may appear in a normal, blind or damaged hemifield.[367] Central or undefined localisation occurs in 10–30% of patients.

Movement: The components of elementary visual hallucinations usually multiply and become larger without any particular movement other than changing positions and luminance within their visual territory (Figure 12.18). Flickering or flashing is common. Movement towards the centre of vision or the other side is less common. Rarely, the movement is spinning, circling, rotatory, random, approaching or moving away from the patient.[51,367,368]

"Visual movement was more frequently present than absent. The image might remain still, but more often it moved slowly in a certain direction or it danced, flickered, or whirled."[369]

"There are 3–4 concentric spherical rings of red and yellow moving from the left to the right of my vision, and repeating the same course again and again after their disappearance on the right". [328]

Lateralisation: The side of unilateral elementary visual hallucinations is *contralateral* to the epileptogenic focus (Figure 12.18). Conversely, this is *ipsilateral* to the epileptogenic focus for unilateral visual hallucinations moving horizontally towards the other side.[368,370]

Vision: Ictally, vision may be obscured only in the area occupied by the visual hallucinations. However, some patients may be even able to read through them. Blurring of vision at onset, with or without visual hallucinations, may be a common mild form of visual seizure if investigated.

The additional notable symptom that I suffer is clusters of momentary left visual field disturbances "like a momentary flickering or blurring of vision (always in the left temporal field only)". Several of these moments can occur within, for example, a 10 min period and then several again over a similar period 1 or more hours later.

My sight deteriorates very slightly before the visual aura, but flashing does not start. It is a reduction of visual awareness of around 10%.

Duration: Visual seizures develop rapidly within seconds and they are usually brief, lasting from a few seconds to 1–3 min, rarely longer.[357,364,365] Exceptionally, they last for 20–150 minutes, sometimes constituting *focal visual status epilepticus* without other ictal symptoms.[16,359,371,372]

As a rule, elementary visual hallucinations are longer prior to secondarily generalisation.

Frequency and circadian distribution: Visual seizures occur, often in multiple clusters, daily or weekly. Commonly, several may occur per day. They are usually diurnal, but some patients often wake up with elementary visual hallucinations.

I would wake up from sleep either with elementary visual hallucinations or with white blindness (all white), before a generalised convulsion.

Stereotypic appearance: Ictal symptoms of elementary visual hallucinations are stereotyped, particularly at onset, in all aspects other than duration. Exceptionally, the same patient may experience different types of seizures.

Progression to other occipital or non-occipital seizure manifestations: Elementary visual hallucinations may be the only seizure manifestation, but they often progress to other ictal symptoms, such as complex visual hallucinations, oculoclonic seizures, tonic deviation of the eyes, eyelid fluttering or repetitive eye closures, impairment of consciousness, experiential phenomena, hemi-anaesthesia, and unilateral or generalised convulsions. On other occasions, they progress to extra-occipital seizure manifestations by spread to the temporal, frontal or parietal regions.

> Bright, multicoloured, blue, red, yellow and green spots of light in the periphery of the right eye multiply rapidly and occupy the whole right visual field, though I can see through them. They cause me a pleasant feeling 'because of the colours'. These are sometimes followed by distortion of the surrounding objects and persons as if 'through the mirrors of a theme park'.

> A spinning ball filled with mainly red and yellow colours on the right. This could be followed by visions of distorted bodies.

Complex visual hallucinations, visual illusions and other symptoms from more anterior ictal spreading

Complex visual hallucinations, visual illusions and other symptoms from more anterior ictal spreading mainly occur in progression of the seizure that may terminate with hemiconvulsions or generalised convulsions. They may be the first ictal symptom, but more often follow elementary visual hallucinations.

Complex visual hallucinations may take the form of persons, animals, objects, figures or scenes. They may be familiar or unfamiliar, friendly or frightening, and simple or grotesque. They may appear in a small or large area of a hemifield, or in the centre and the whole of the visual field. They may be static, move horizontally, expand or shrink, approach or move away. In patients with visual field defects due to structural brain lesions, complex visual hallucinations appear in the defective visual field. Complex visual hallucinations of occipital seizures do not have the emotional and complicated character of temporal lobe seizures.[357,364,381]

> Sudden awareness of rapidly oscillating, vague, dark, disproportionate, face-like, frightening figures moving forwards and backwards in the temporal field of my left eye.

An interesting, but extremely rare ictal complex visual hallucination is *autoscopia (or heautoscopy)*, which means viewing his own image/viewing himself.[382,383] This mirror self image looks 'real' and is usually undistorted, silent, brief or recurrent, from the present time or from the past, framed or performing complex tasks.

Complex visual hallucinations including ictal autoscopia probably originate

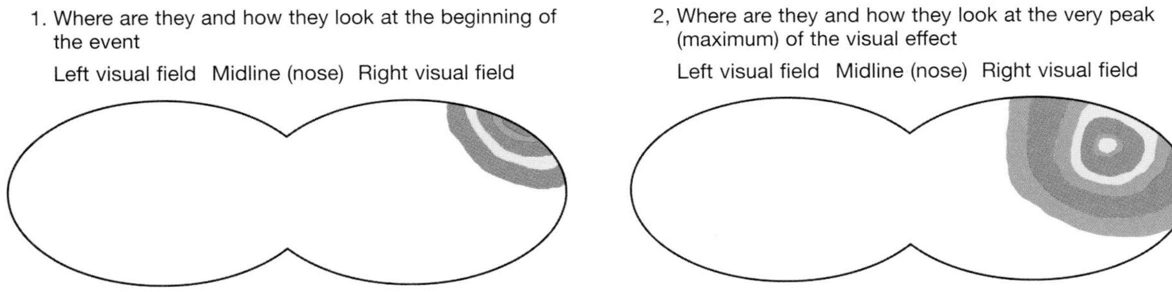
1. Where are they and how they look at the beginning of the event
Left visual field Midline (nose) Right visual field
2, Where are they and how they look at the very peak (maximum) of the visual effect
Left visual field Midline (nose) Right visual field

Figure 12.18 Visual seizures as perceived and drawn by a patient with an interesting form of symptomatic occipital epilepsy (case detailed in ref [373]).

From Panayiotopoulos (1999)[357] with the permission of the Editor of *Epileptic Disorders*.

from occipito-parietal and occipito-temporal junction areas.

Visual illusions are misinterpretations, false percepts, of real external images. These distorted images (*metamorphopsia*) involve changes in size, dimension, shape, proportions, position, colour, illumination and movement, alone or in combination. Changes in perception of object size are common, the percepts being smaller *(micropsia)* or larger *(macropsia)* than the real image. Objects may be distorted in shape, pulled, compressed or rotated in lateral or vertical directions. They may appear in black and white *(achromatopsia),* in one colour *(monochromopsia),* hazy and dark or highly illuminated and bright. Motion and speed may be affected with or without distortion of direction (horizontal, vertical or rotated, approaching or moving away). Movement is faster or slower. Moving objects may appear stationary and vice versa.

Visual illusions also entail changes in spatial interpretation affecting stereoscopic vision.

> "Far objects appear near, near ones far, and convex ones concave, or vice versa."[384]

Ictal visual illusions may occupy part or the whole visual field, and are probably more likely to be associated with symptomatic than with idiopathic occipital seizures.

Palinopsia

Palinopsia, that is persistence or recurrence of visual images after the exciting stimulus has been removed, is an interesting form of visual illusion associated with right posterior parieto-temporal lesions.

> He looked at a small video display unit and, after he looked away, the image of the screen persisted in the right upper corner of his vision and nearly simultaneously, started flashing at a rate of 3–5 Hz for 2 s. This was followed by visual illusions of the walls and the passengers closing in on him, ending within 5 s with GTCS.

Sensory hallucinations of ocular movements

Sensory hallucinations of ocular movements, that is a sensation of ocular movement in the absence of detectable motion, is rare.

> "This involuntary movement of the eyes to the left and at a slight tilt upwards causes the pain described above. The motion to the left seems out of your control. It can be resisted but this adds to nausea and general pain." Neither he nor the witnesses could confirm any such movement of the eyes.

Ictal blindness (ictal amaurosis)

Terminology

Autoscopia (or heautoscopy) means viewing his/her own image, viewing himself.[374,375]

Fortification spectra in migraine are visual hallucinations with similarities to the bastioned, star-patterned, pentagonal fortifications and not of the castellated appearances of battlements.[376,377] A bastion is a projecting part of a fortification, consisting of an earthwork in the form of an irregular pentagon, having its base in the main line or at an angle of the fortification. Spectrum is used by Gowers[378] "to mean apparition and not a coloured band of light."

Pallinopsia (visual persevereness) is the persistence or recurrence of visual images after the exciting stimulus has been removed.

Percept is the mental image or product of perception of any object in space.

Phosphenes are subjective sensations of light due to non-luminous stimulation of the retina. Phosphenes are also used to denote visual percepts from stimulation of the visual cortex with an electrical stimulus, in which case they are usually coloured spots or circles.[379]

Photopsias (*phos* = light, *opsis* = appearance) are unformed flashes of light and sparks.

Scintillating (*scintilla* = spark) *scotoma* (*skotos* = darkness) is also used because of the sparking appearance of the visual hallucinations of migraine (brilliant flashes of light in the periphery of dark areas in the visual fields).

Teichopsia (*teichos* = town wall, *opsis* = appearance) was coined by Airy[380] "to represent the bastioned form of transient hemiopsia which I have been describing, not without a reminiscence of some words of Tennyson's:

as yonder walls
Rose slowly to a music slowly breathed,
A cloud that gathered shape."

Visual hallucinations are subjectively experienced images in the absence of an actual external stimulus:

<u>Elementary</u> *visual hallucinations* consist of simple, usually geometric forms, spots or lines.

<u>Complex</u> *visual hallucinations* consist of objects, faces or scenes.

Visual illusions are misinterpreted false percepts of real images.

Ictal blindness (ictal amaurosis) may follow the visual hallucinations and progress to other epileptic symptoms, but often occurs as a starting or the only ictal seizure manifestation with abrupt onset.[357,359,364,366,385]

> I usually have millions of small, very bright, mainly blue and green coloured, circular spots of light, which appear on the left side and sometimes move to the right, but on one occasion suddenly everything went black, I could not see and I had to ask other swimmers to show me the direction to the beach.[328,386]

The duration of ictal blindness is usually longer (3–5 minutes) than ictal visual hallucinations; occasionally, blindness may last for hours or days *(status epilepticus amauroticus)*.[387-389] Ictal blindness and less frequently ictal hemianopia occur in one-third of patients with symptomatic and two-thirds of patients with idiopathic occipital epilepsy.

An interesting rare variation of ictal blindness is *'white ictal blindness'*.[357,359] The patient can not see because everything is white.

> I can not see, like a white sheet in front of my eyes.
>
> It is all white.

Blurring of vision as an initial seizure manifestation prior to visual hallucinations may be common if investigated.[357,364,381]

> It starts with a momentary flickering or blurring of vision (always in the left temporal field only) (case 7.2 in ref [328]).
>
> My sight deteriorates very slightly as it does before the aura, but flashing does not start. It is a reduction of visual awareness of around 10% (case 30 in ref [328]).

Tonic deviation of the eyes, oculoclonic seizures and epileptic nystagmus

Tonic deviation of the eyes often, but not necessarily, followed by ipsilateral turning of the head is the most common (40–50% of cases) non-visual symptom of occipital seizures. This is similar to a voluntary, pursuit-like turning of the eyes to one side. This usually follows visual symptoms and mainly elementary visual hallucinations, but it may also occur from seizure onset. Consciousness is often, but not invariably, impaired when eye deviation occurs.

The epileptogenic focus is more likely to be contralateral to the movement of the head and the eyes if consciousness is not impaired.

Ictal nystagmus (epileptic nystagmus) is mainly horizontal and rarely vertical. The quick phase of the nystagmus is opposite to the epileptic focus, in the same direction of eye and head deviation, which may coexist, precede or follow.

Repetitive eyelid closures, eyelid fluttering and eyelid blinking

Repetitive eyelid closures, eyelid fluttering and eyelid blinking is an interesting ictal clinical symptom of symptomatic and idiopathic occipital epilepsy. It usually occurs after the phase of visual hallucinations, at a stage when consciousness is impaired and heralds the impending secondarily generalised convulsions. However, it may also occur alone, be inconspicuous in appearance and not be suspected as a seizure event, documented only by video EEG recordings in occipital photosensitive patients.

Eyelid opening, or 'eyes widely opened', is another well-described symptom in occipital epilepsy, but may also be a symptom associated with other cerebral locations. Widened palpebral fissures with fixed staring and dilated pupils are among the typical symptoms of mesial temporal lobe seizures.[390]

Consciousness

Consciousness is not impaired during the elementary and complex visual hallucinations, blindness and other subjective occipital seizure symptoms, but may be disturbed or lost in the course of the seizure, usually at the time of eye deviation or eye closure, and generally prior to convulsions.

Ictal or postictal headache

Ictal or postictal headache is frequently associated with occipital seizures.[357,359,364,366] Ictal pain is mainly orbital. It is described as a sharp, stabbing, retro-orbital pain, a sensation of bifrontal pressure, a vague ache in the head or a sensation of electricity.

> The visual hallucinations consist of vivid, flashing multicoloured lights and circular patterns that occupy and obscure my vision. Severe unilateral throbbing headache follows 1–2 min later, lasts for hours and it is often associated with vomiting (case 7.1 in ref [328]).

Postictal headache, often indistinguishable from migraine, is far more common in occipital (occurring in more than 50% of cases) than in any other focal epilepsy,[391,392] and may occur even after brief visual seizures.[357,364] Also, postictal headache often occurs 3–15 min from the end of the visual seizure, a situation known in migraine as the *'asymptomatic interval'* between the end of migraine aura and the onset of headache.[393]

Postictal hemianopia may occur.

> When the visual hallucinations ceased completely, I had almost no vision in the left eye, only blackness (case 7.2 in ref [328]).

Seizure spreading

Seizures may spread from the occipital to other more anterior regions of the brain, generating symptoms from the temporal, parietal and frontal lobes and secondarily hemi- or generalised convulsions. Infra-calcarine occipital foci will propagate to the temporal lobe causing complex focal seizures, while supra-calcarine foci tend to propagate to the parietal and frontal areas giving rise to predominantly motor seizures.

Progression to temporal lobe seizure symptomatology is rather exceptional in idiopathic cases.

AETIOLOGY

Aetiology may be idiopathic, structural or metabolic.[357,359,364,366]

In symptomatic occipital epilepsy, lesions may be congenital, residual or progressive resulting from vascular, neoplastic, metabolic, hereditary, congenital, inflammatory, parasitic, systemic diseases and infections. Malformations of cortical development are a common cause, which is being increasingly recognised with MRI, as it is the case today in all focal symptomatic or probably symptomatic epilepsies (Figure 12.8).[355]

Metabolic or other derangements, such as eclampsia, may have a particular predilection for the occipital lobes and cause either occipital *'seizures that do not require a diagnosis of epilepsy'* or permanent occipital lesions leading to symptomatic occipital epilepsy.[394] There is an interesting association between coeliac disease (CD) and occipital lobe epilepsy.[395] Occipital seizures may be the first manifestation of a devastating course, as in Lafora disease for example,[396-398] or mitochondrial disorders.[399]

COELIAC DISEASE AND OCCIPITAL EPILEPSY

The association between occipital seizures and CD, with or without bilateral occipital calcifications, has been well documented, mainly by Italian authors. The book *'Epilepsy and other neurological disorders in celiac disease'*[400] is highly recommended.

Diverse epileptic conditions with onset in childhood and early adolescence have been reported in patients with symptomatic or asymptomatic CD. These conditions include severe epilepsies, such as Lennox-Gastaut syndrome, and myoclonic epilepsies with ataxia, but more commonly symptomatic occipital epilepsy.

Age at onset of epilepsy is 1–28 years, and most commonly between 4 and 13 years. Occipital seizures are by far the commonest, though other focal fits, GTCS and absences may occur from the onset of epilepsy. In most patients, seizures start before the detection of CD and the institution of a gluten-free diet (GFD). GFD seems to control the seizures if started soon after the onset of epilepsy and early in childhood. However, seizures may also start after GFD, in which case they are more likely to be symptomatic, drug-resistant occipital epilepsy manifesting mainly with elementary visual hallucinations. A few cases may have a benign course, but the majority progress to other seizure types and an epileptic encephalopathy with delayed mental development, despite an initial relatively good response to treatment. The severity of the epileptic seizures is not proportional to the severity of the cerebral calcifications.

EEG abnormalities initially consist mainly of occipital paroxysms, occipital spikes or generalised discharges. Activation of occipital spikes by intermittent photic stimulation (IPS) is not uncommon. Multispike discharges in the sleep EEG often betray their symptomatic character.

A history of gastrointestinal symptoms, nutritional problems, a positive family history of CD and an atypical Sturge-Weber syndrome without a cutaneous naevus should raise the possibility of this syndrome. Occipital seizures in Sturge-Weber syndrome are rare.

ECLAMPSIA AND OCCIPITAL SEIZURES

There is a selective vulnerability of the occipital lobes to eclamptic hypertensive encephalopathy. Neurological symptoms of eclampsia include seizures, headache, blindness and impairment of consciousness. Seizures may be GTCS or focal visual seizures with secondarily GTCS. Seizures persisting after recovery from eclampsia are rare.[394] Recent reports indicate that eclampsia may also be a risk factor for MTLE-HS.[401]

LAFORA DISEASE AND OCCIPITAL SEIZURES

Lafora disease is an autosomal recessive disorder among the progressive myoclonic epilepsies, characterised by the presence of Lafora bodies (periodic acid–Schiff-positive diastase-resistant polyglucosan inclusions) found in the brain, skin, liver and other body tissues.[402] The disease is caused by mutations in the *EPM2A* gene on chromosome 6q24. Onset of the disease is around the age of 14 years (common range 8–18 years), mainly with occipital seizures, myoclonic jerks and GTCS. Occipital seizures occur in 30–50% of patients, may be spontaneous or photically induced, and consist of complex and elementary visual hallucinations. In the initial stages, Lafora disease may imitate idiopathic generalised epilepsies, with myoclonic jerks, GTCS and generalised discharges of polyspikes and slow waves that are spontaneous or photically induced, and a relatively normal EEG background. Occipital involvement is indicated by occipital polyspikes and visual seizures, but these rarely occur without coexisting myoclonic seizures, GTCS and EEG generalised discharges that are also often induced by IPS. Background EEG may be abnormal before onset of seizures, but may also be normal in the initial stages of the disease. Cognitive decline is relentless either before or soon, within months, after the onset of seizures, and death is unavoidable within 1–10 years.

Lafora disease should be suspected when the onset of occipital seizures is combined or followed by myoclonus and progressive mental decline.

PATHOPHYSIOLOGY

Elementary visual hallucinations are generated from the primary visual cortex, complex visual hallucinations from the occipito-parietal-temporal junction areas, and visual illusions from the non-dominant parietal regions.[328]

Ictal blindness is probably due to contralateral seizure spread to involve both occipital lobes or to inhibition of the visual cortex by the seizure discharge.[403]

Because of the frequent occurrence of postictal headache in occipital epilepsy, it is reasonable to suggest that occipital seizures often generate migraine-like attacks and that the occipital lobes are preferentially associated with the trigeminovascular or brainstem mechanisms responsible for migraine headache.[404] Postictal headache of occipital seizures may be related to serotonergic mechanisms and respond to oral sumatriptan.[405] Another similarity with migraine is that postictal headache often occurs 3–15 minutes from the end of the visual seizure, a situation described in migraine as the *'asymptomatic interval'* between the end of migraine aura and the onset of headache.[393]

Thus, the *'occipital seizure-migraine'* sequence[357,364,366,406] appears to be much more common than the previously prevailing view of *'migraine visual aura triggering epileptic seizures'* or *'migraine-epilepsy syndromes'*.[407-409]

DIAGNOSTIC PROCEDURES

The discovery of the underlying cause in symptomatic occipital epilepsies may require haematology and biochemistry screening for metabolic disorders, molecular DNA analysis, or even skin or other tissue biopsy.[328] High resolution MRI is necessary in all patients with occipital lobe epilepsy (Figure 12.19).[328] Unsuspected residual or progressive lesions, tumours, vascular malformations and malformations of cortical development are all detected by MRI. CT scanning is far inferior to MRI and insensitive to focal cortical dysplasia. Conversely, the calcifications of CD may be missed with MRI, but this is rare. Functional brain imaging for localisation is of practical value in neurosurgical cases.[410]

ELECTROENCEPHALOGRAPHY

EEG is essential, but certain limitations should be recognised.

Interictal EEG

In symptomatic cases, the background EEG is usually abnormal with posterior lateralised slow waves. Unilateral occipital spikes or fast multiple spikes and, occasionally, occipital paroxysms occur. There may be occipital photosensitivity.[328] Worsening of the background EEG is significant in the diagnosis of progressive causes.

In idiopathic cases, such as Gastaut-type idiopathic childhood occipital epilepsy and photosensitive occipital epilepsy, the background interictal EEG is normal.[328] Occipital spikes and occipital paroxysms, spontaneous, evoked or both, are often abundant. They disappear with age frequently long after cessation of the occipital seizures.

Ictal EEG

Surface ictal EEG in occipital seizures, irrespective of cause, usually manifests with paroxysmal fast activity, fast spiking or both, localised in the occipital regions with occasional gradual anterior spreading and generalisation with irregular spike wave discharges or monomorphic spike and wave activity. Brief occipital flattening may be seen before the fast rhythmic pattern. Often, in patients with symptomatic occipital lobe epilepsy, the ictal discharge is more widespread (regional) rather than of a precise occipital localisation. Usually, there is no postictal localised slow activity unless the seizure is prolonged or progresses to secondarily GTCS.

In one-third of patients (30%), the ictal surface EEG does not show any appreciable changes in occipital seizures.[328]

DIFFERENTIAL DIAGNOSIS

Occipital seizures should not be difficult to diagnose, but should be first differentiated from migraine, normal phenomena and psychogenic or other causes unrelated to seizures.[328]

Differentiating visual seizures from migraine

Visual aura of migraine:

> "I was startled by a single, shadowy appearance at the outside corner of the field of vision of the left eye. It gradually advanced into the field of view and then appeared to be a pattern of straight-lined angular forms, very much in general aspects like the drawing of a fortification, with salient and re-entering angles, bastions and ravelins with some suspicion of faint lines of colour between the dark lines."
>
> Sir JFW Herschel (1866)[376]

Visual seizure:

> "They commenced with the appearance of several small spheres, white in the centre with an intermediate zone of blue and outside this a ring of red, immediately to the left of the point at which the patient gazed; from here they moved either at a uniform rate or in jerks to the left and downwards...In all attacks the eyes deviated towards the left and the head turned in the same direction as soon as the visual spectra appeared."
>
> G Holmes (1927)[16]

Misdiagnosis of visual seizures as migraine appears to be high though their differentiation should not be difficult.[328,357,364] Occipital seizures manifesting with elementary visual hallucinations, blindness and headache, alone or in combination, may imitate migraine, which is the reason that they are often mistaken as migraine with aura, acephalgic or basilar migraine (Table 12.3).[328,357,364] Even lesional occipital epilepsy is often misdiagnosed as migraine and, on many occasions, visual

A

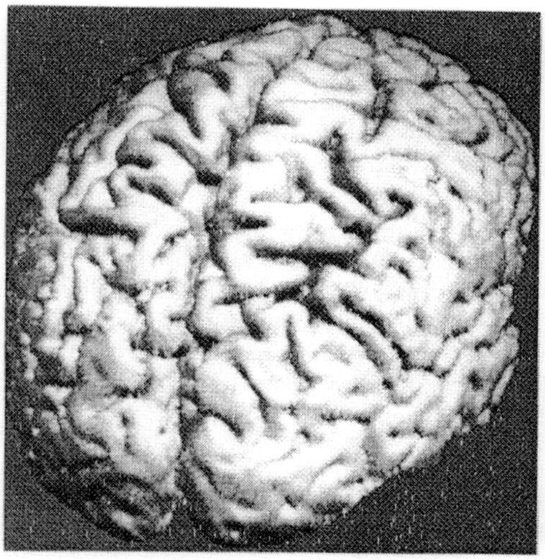

B

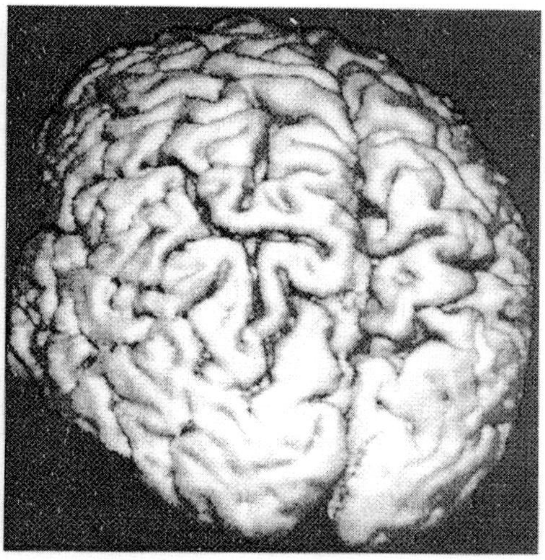

Figure 12.19 Patient with visual seizures and focal status epilepticus of occipital lobe epilepsy.[369] Three dimensional reconstruction of the brain demonstrating abnormal gyral patterns on the right.

A. Surface rendering of cortex viewed from right posterosuperior occipital aspect, demonstrating abnormally enlarged gyral pattern.

B: Surface rendering of cortex viewed from left posterosuperior occipital aspect, with normal gyral pattern shown for comparison.

From Walker et al. (1995)[369] with the permission of the authors and the Editor of *Epilepsia*.

seizures are considered as visual aura of migraine, thus limiting their prognostic significance regarding continuation of treatment.[357] The following are quotes from medical referrals of patients with visual seizures:

"This patient has visual migraine-like disturbances, such as teichopsias."

"Scintillating scotoma or sparkling scotoma of migraine."

"Migrainous aura before the fit."

There are two main reasons that visual seizures are misdiagnosed as migraine.[357,359,364,366] *Firstly,* visual seizures are not examined in a comprehensive manner; instead they are abbreviated to terms such as *'scintillating scotoma'* or *'teichopsia'*, which often do not represent the actual description of the patients. *Secondly,* their differential diagnostic criteria have only recently been adequately studied and addressed by Panayiotopoulos.[357,363,364] The diagnosis of visual seizures may comfortably rely on clinical criteria only; other investigative procedures are essential, but even ictal EEG may not identify one-third or more of cases.

Factors contributing to error in the diagnosis of visual seizures

The major contributory factor to error is that the description of visual hallucinations is often abbreviated in terms such as fortification spectrum, teichopsia, scintillating scotoma, phosphenes and their variations.[363] Their meaning does not always represent the actual descriptions, which should be meticulously requested. Erroneously, they are frequently unquestionably equated with migraine.

The quality and the chronological sequence of ictal elementary visual hallucinations are markedly different from the visual aura of migraine. Visual seizures and the visual aura of migraine may imitate each other, but their true identity can not easily escape clinical scrutiny.

Though brief duration is significant, there are many more clinical manifestations to differentiate visual seizures from the visual aura of migraine (Table 12.3).

Diagnostic clues

As a rule, brief (< 1 min), elementary visual hallucinations that develop rapidly within seconds, with coloured and circular patterns and daily frequency are probably pathognomonic of visual seizures, despite severe headache and vomiting that may follow. EEG may be normal, show non-specific abnormalities or reveal slow focal or occipital spikes. A high resolution MRI is mandatory as it may detect a structural lesion requiring early attention and management.

The visual aura of migraine with aura and acephalgic migraine are adequately studied and illustrated in all relevant textbooks and publications. In one of the most detailed, a nosographic analysis[411] describes migraine visual aura as:

"started as a flickering, uncoloured, zigzag line in the centre of the visual field and affected the central vision. It gradually progressed over > 4 min, usually lasting < 30

Clarifications on migraine and epilepsy

Migraine and epilepsy are the commonest neurological disorders. The prevalence of migraine is probably around 6% in men and three times more common in women. The prevalence of epilepsy is around 0.5%, and men and women are equally affected. If there was a relation between them, this would be obvious in our everyday neurological practice. It would not be revealed only through obscure and complicated cases with bizarre symptomatology. It would be simple and common. It is not. The problem is that occipital seizures are not appropriately differentiated from migraine and, therefore, they are often erroneously diagnosed as migraine.

Seizures may be triggered from a migrainous event or caused by a migraine-stroke, but this is rare. There should be no doubt that a cerebral infarct due to severe migraine can be responsible for symptomatic seizures. Also, there should be no reason that epileptic seizures, so vulnerable to extrinsic and intrinsic precipitating factors, could not also be susceptible to cortical changes introduced by migraine. Thus a migrainous attack may also be able to trigger epileptic seizures in susceptible individuals. However, both these cases are rare. In my opinion, the commonest reason for their association is the coincidence of two of the more common neurological disorders, and an erroneous interpretation of epileptic seizures as migraine, and less often vice versa. The emerging and more realistic concept of occipital seizures triggering migrainous headache needs consideration and exploration. More importantly, patients with daily visual seizures that may progress to convulsions merit a precise diagnosis and appropriate treatment, probably with carbamazepine. Most of these patients with visual seizures are misdiagnosed as migraine with aura, basilar migraine, acephalgic migraine or migralepsy, simply because physicians are not properly informed about the differential diagnostic criteria. As a result, diagnosis, appropriate investigations and treatment may be delayed for years. There are numerous published reports of such misdiagnosis.

> min, towards the periphery of one hemifield and often left a scotoma. The total duration of visual auras was 60 min. Only four patients had exclusively acute onset visual aura." [411]

Furthermore, migraine visual aura:

- rarely has daily frequency
- non-visual ictal occipital symptoms, such as eye and head deviation, and repetitive eyelid repetitive do not occur
- it is debatable and probably exceptional to progress to non-visual epileptic seizures.

Less typical features of migraine visual aura, such as spots, circles and beads, with or without colours, may be experienced during the migraine visual aura, but usually they are not dominant. More importantly, clustering of other symptoms, as above, betrays their migraine nature.

Based on the results of my studies, my thesis is that the visual aura of migraine is entirely different from that of visual seizures when all their components are synthesised together (Table 12.3).

Basilar migraine of Bickerstaff[412,413] is characterised by transient and fully reversible symptoms of aura, indicating focal dysfunction of the brainstem, the

Table 12.3 Differential diagnosis of occipital seizures from basilar migraine or migraine with aura.

	Occipital epilepsy	Migraine with aura	Basilar migraine
Visual hallucinations			
Duration for seconds to a minute	Exclusive	None	None
Duration for 1–3 minutes	Frequent	Rare	Rare
Duration for 4–30 minutes	Rare	As a rule	As a rule
Daily in frequency	As a rule	Rare	None
Mainly coloured circular patterns	As a rule	Rare	Exceptional
Mainly achromatic or black and white linear patterns	Exceptional	As a rule	Rare
Moving to the opposite side of the visual field	Exclusive	None	None
Expanding from the centre to the periphery of a visual hemifield	Rare	As a rule	Frequent
Evolving to blindness	Rare	Rare	As a rule
Evolving to tonic deviation of eyes	Exclusive	None	None
Evolving to impairment of consciousness without convulsions	Frequent	Rare	Frequent
Evolving to impairment of consciousness with convulsions	Frequent	Exceptional	Rare
Associated with post-ictal/post-critical headache	Frequent	As a rule	Frequent
Blindness and hemianopia			
Without other preceding or following symptoms	Frequent	None	Frequent
Other neurological symptoms			
Brain stem symptoms	None	None	Exclusive
Post-ictal/post-critical vomiting	Rare	Frequent	Frequent
Post-ictal/post-critical headache			
Post-ictal or post-critical severe headache	Frequent	As a rule	Frequent

Modified from Panayiotopoulos (1999)[357] with the permission of the editor of *Epileptic Disorders*.

occipital lobes or both, followed by headache.[361] Common neurological symptoms of aura include visual manifestations, dizziness, vertigo and tinnitus, ataxia, bilateral weakness and dysaesthesia, diplopia, dysarthria and decreased hearing. Visual symptoms mainly consist of dimming of vision, blindness, tunnel vision, hemianopia and scotomata. Elementary visual hallucinations are usually bilateral, described as *'teichopsia', 'flashes or blobs of light', 'coloured figures'* or *'dysmorphopsia'*. Aura symptoms develop gradually over 4 min and last for less than 30 min to 1 hour. Impairment or loss of consciousness without convulsions may occur in one-quarter of patients between the aura and the headache phase.

> "The loss of consciousness is described as curiously slow in onset – never abrupt, and never causing the patient to fall or to be injured. A dreamlike state sometimes precedes impairment of consciousness. The degree of impairment of consciousness was never profound but the patients were never unrousable; on vigorous stimulation they could be aroused to cooperate but they returned to unconsciousness when the stimulation ceased."[413]

Attacks of basilar migraine are usually infrequent and, over the years, they may cease or be replaced by common migraine with or without aura.[361]

Migralepsy versus epilepsy-migraine: Migralepsy, migra(ine) and (epi)lepsy, is a term used to denote "a seizure that may be a composite of symptoms encountered in epilepsy and migraine".[18,414] The term intercalated seizures is used to denote epileptic seizures occurring between the migrainous aura and the headache phase of migraine.[415] There should be no reason that epileptic seizures, which are so vulnerable to precipitating factors, could not be susceptible to cortical changes induced by migraine. However, this is exceptional considering that migraine and epilepsy are the most common brain diseases. According to a recent review, most of the reported cases are likely to be genuine occipital seizures imitating migraine aura.[357,364] Of the most influential cases that I have detailed,[357,364] two of three *'migralepsy'* patients,[18] one case of *'basilar migraine and epilepsy'*[416] and one boy with *'juvenile migraine with epilepsy'*,[417] all had symptoms of visual seizures as defined in this book, which were interpreted as migraine aura. The patient of Barlow[417] with symptomatic occipital epilepsy may be indicative.

> This boy at age 13 years, "While ski-ing he saw blue to the right associated with blurred vision that lasted for a few seconds", after which he vomited, became confused for 30 minutes, followed by severe throbbing headache. Subsequently he had occasional "episodes of similar visual disturbance" diagnosed as juvenile migraine and successfully treated with phenytoin. An arteriovenous malformation was found in the left occipital lobe. "Visual scotomata accompanied by flashing lights that only occasionally were followed by headache" continued postoperatively.

None of 1550 patients I have studied had any evidence of seizures developing from migraine aura, though this was often the initial erroneous diagnosis on referral.[357] Conversely, postictal headache and other migraine-like symptoms frequently occurred after occipital seizures. However, an incontrovertible diagnosis may be difficult in some equivocal cases.

> A 38-year-old man who, while working with the computer, saw flashing lights in between his eyes. They were moving for a few centimetres upwards and to the right repetitively. Gradually the intensity of the light and the area increased over the next 30 min obscuring his vision. This ended with a GTCS as he was entering the examination room of his general practitioner, which he had walked to for help. He had never had similar symptoms, seizures or migraine in the past. MRI was normal. EEG showed minor non-specific abnormalities.

The concept of migralepsy and its synonymous intercalated seizures or of an epilepsy–migraine sequence needs re-evaluation based on accurate diagnosis. In most instances, it is seizures imitating migraine.

Misconceptions

There is a misconception that there is a syndrome of *'basilar migraine with EEG occipital paroxysms'*, which is perpetuated in every relevant publication and textbook to date. Retrospective analysis of cases described as *"basilar migraine with occipital paroxysms"*[386,418,419] showed that these patients genuinely suffer from idiopathic occipital epilepsy.[328,420]

Differentiating ictal deviation of the eyes of occipital versus extra-occipital origin

I am not aware of any study that has compared ictal deviation of the eyes, head or both of occipital origin with that of extra-occipital origin. The following conclusions are derived from my personal experience, supplemented by relevant reports in the literature.

In occipital epilepsy, the deviation of the eyes is usually pursuit-like or tonic, rarely clonic and different to the oculoclonic ictal symptoms that are often seen in focal motor seizures of extra-occipital, mainly frontal origin. Occipital oculotonic seizures are similar to a voluntary, pursuit-like turning of the eyes to one side that, by itself, could not be considered as an abnormal movement by witnesses. They usually follow visual symptoms and mainly elementary visual hallucinations, but may also occur ab initio. At this stage, consciousness is often but not invariably impaired. This phase may progress to unilateral clonic seizures of the face and the extremities, with or without progressing to GTCS.

Conversely, ictal eye movements of extra-occipital origin are more violent and look unnatural. Ipsilateral eyelid tonic or clonic convulsions are commonly associated with upward deviation of the eyeballs. It is simultaneous, and precedes or follows tonic or clonic convulsions of other facial, neck and shoulder muscles of the same side (e.g. as in hemifacial Rolandic seizures).

Differentiating idiopathic from symptomatic occipital epilepsy

Differentiation between symptomatic and idiopathic occipital epilepsy is essential with regard to prognosis and management.

The visual seizures of symptomatic versus idiopathic occipital epilepsy are indistinguishable.[357] The only difference is that symptomatic visual seizures more frequently progress to other extra-occipital seizure manifestations and mainly temporal lobe seizures. Though progression to ictal motor manifestations may be common in both, temporal lobe symptoms are nearly exclusively seen in symptomatic occipital epilepsy. A normal neurological state (including visual fields) and brain imaging may be misleading, and suggest an idiopathic cause without high resolution MRI using the new generation scanners.[328,355]

PROGNOSIS

Frequency, severity and response to treatment vary considerably from good to intractable or progressive, mainly depending on the underlying cause and extent of the lesions.[328]

MANAGEMENT

AED treatment is similar to that for any other type for focal seizures, is usually effective and should be initiated as soon as possible.[328] Carbamazepine is the drug of choice.

The postictal headache of occipital seizures may be related to serotonergic mechanisms and responds to oral sumatriptan. [405]

Neurosurgery is performed for selective symptomatic cases and may be effective in around 70% of patients with 30% becoming seizure free.[312,321,403,421]

THE DRUG TREATMENT OF FOCAL EPILEPSIES

The treatment of focal epilepsies of any cause begins first with AEDs. If this fails, neurosurgical options are now becoming more widely available and are often life saving for symptomatic and probably symptomatic epilepsies (see individual syndromes).

Existing evidence indicates that 15[422]–30%[423] of those with newly diagnosed focal epilepsy (of any cause) fail to achieve reasonably sustained remission with optimal antiepileptic medication. The figure is significantly higher (35%) for those with symptomatic focal epilepsy.[422] Of those failing to respond, 25–50% develop intractable disease, that is continuation of seizures beyond 2–3 years, despite optimal AED treatment. In one large study, complex focal seizures were controlled in only 16–43% of patients, compared with 48–53% in those with only secondarily GTCS at 1 year.[424]

AED treatment in focal epilepsies has been detailed in recent books[425-430] and reviews,[431-445] although the conclusions of experts sometimes differ significantly. My recommendations, based on the procedures explained in Chapter 4 (page 59), are fairly pragmatic, combining evidence-based medicine with clinical experience. Details for each AED can be found in Chapter 14 in the pharmacopoeia (page 497).

ANTIEPILEPTIC DRUGS EFFECTIVE FOR FOCAL SEIZURES

Carbamazepine and phenytoin are the superior old AEDs in the treatment of focal seizures. According to evidence-based medicine, all new AEDs entered into randomised controlled trials (RCT) have approximately equal efficacy to carbamazepine, phenytoin and valproate in controlling focal seizures, but are better tolerated.[431,432,446] The reality in clinical practice often contradicts these conclusions for many reasons.[431,447,448] It is extremely difficult to find a balance. There is a significant and rapidly changing swing with the increasing experience obtained from the clinical application of licensed new drugs and the introduction of new antiepileptic agents. The following may be applicable at the *present time*.

EVIDENCE-BASED MEDICINE

Overall, RCTs in patients with focal seizures with or without secondarily GTCS have shown the following.

- In head-to-head comparisons of old AEDs (phenobarbitone, primidone, phenytoin and carbamazepine), overall treatment success was highest with carbamazepine or phenytoin, intermediate with phenobarbitone and lowest with primidone.[424] Carbamazepine provided complete control of focal seizures more often than primidone or phenobarbitone. The control of GTCS and the proportion of patients rendered seizure free (48–63%) did not differ significantly with the various AEDs. The differences in the failure rates were explained primarily by their adverse reactions.[424]
- In head-to-head comparisons of carbamazepine with valproate, carbamazepine provided better control of complex focal seizures and had fewer long-term adverse effects than valproate.[449] Both drugs were comparably effective for the control of secondarily GTCS.[449] These conclusions have been confirmed in a recent meta-analysis report.[450]

- "The new AEDs gabapentin, lamotrigine, levetiracetam, oxcarbazepine, tiagabine, topiramate, vigabatrin and zonisamide are of nearly equal efficacy to carbamazepine, phenytoin and valproate (phenobarbitone and clobazam have not been used in recent RCT)."[431,432,446] Comparatively, topiramate and levetiracetam have the highest efficacy, while lamotrigine and gabapentin are the least efficacious (Table 12.4 andFigure 12.20).

New AEDs are "better tolerated, with few adverse effects, minimal drug interactions, and a broad spectrum of activity".[431,432,446,458] However, this generalisation needs clarification (Table 12.4). Only a few of the new AEDs, such as levetiracetam, fulfil these conclusions. Conversely, certain other new AEDs, such as topiramate have adverse reactions that are worse than those of carbamazepine. Lamotrigine, oxcarbamazepine and topiramate have clinically significant drug–drug interactions. Gabapentin and tiagabine have a narrow spectrum of antiepileptic activity and they are contraindicated in generalised epilepsies (Table 12.4).

There are no direct head-to-head comparisons between new AEDs. Therefore, the comparative efficacy and tolerability of new AEDs is deduced from meta-analyses of RCTs (Figure 12.21).[430,459-461] A reliable way of comparing new AEDs is to display the odds ratios for efficacy and tolerability in the same graph (Figure 12.20). Efficacy is assessed by the odds ratio for a 50% seizure reduction, which is defined as the probability of a patient being a ≥ 50% responder with the test AED divided by the probability of being a ≥ 50% responder with placebo. The more effective the AED tested, the bigger is the numerical value of the odds ratio and the higher the position of the AED in the histogram in Figure 12.20. A numerical value of unity indicates that there is an equal probability of a patient being a ≥ 50%

Table 12.4 Order of priority of new AEDs in intractable focal epilepsies.

AED name	Efficacy[451]	Tolerability[451]	Serious adverse events[452]	Drug–drug interactions[453] including hormonal contraception	Pharmacokinetics [453]	Titration	Need for laboratory testing	Mechanism of action
Levetiracetam	High	Excellent	No	No	Ideal[454]	Fast	Minimal	Novel SV2A-ligand [455]
Lamotrigine	Low	Excellent	Yes	Yes*	Poor	Very slow	Maximal	↓Na^+
Topiramate	High	Poor	Yes	Yes	Satisfactory	Very slow	Maximal	Multiple
Oxcarbazepine	Medium	Poor	Yes	Yes	Poor	Slow	Maximal	↓Na^+
Zonisamide	Medium	Good	Yes	No	Satisfactory	Slow	Maximal	Multiple
Tiagabine	Medium	Good	Yes	Yes*	Poor	Slow	Minimal	↑GABA
Gabapentin	Low	Excellent	No	No	Ideal	Fast	Minimal	Multiple

* Their plasma levels are increased or decreased depending on the concurrent AED. Notable is the effect of hormonal contraception[456] and pregnancy[457] on lamotrigine, which significantly lower (more than half) lamotrigine levels.[457] Frequent lamotrigine level monitoring and appropriate dose adjustments are advised in the period before and during pregnancy and after delivery, especially in women on lamotrigine monotherapy to avoid breakthrough seizures mainly during the first trimester of pregnancy (if lamotrigine levels are not corrected) or toxic effects postpartum (if lamotrigine levels had been adjusted during pregnancy but not after delivery).[457]

responder, either with the tested AED or placebo. The tolerability and safety of AEDs is usually assessed by the odds ratio of premature withdrawal from the RCT. AEDs with small odds ratios are better tolerated and further on the right in the histogram. An odds ratio of unity indicates that the probability for withdrawal is equal for the tested AED and the placebo.

CLINICAL PRACTICE IN DEVELOPED COUNTRIES

Old antiepileptic drugs in developed countries

Carbamazepine is the superior drug for controlling focal seizures in more than 70% of patients (10% of patients develop idiosyncratic reactions). Valproate, a superior drug in generalised epilepsies, is inferior in focal epilepsies, with significant concerns in the treatment of women. Use of phenytoin, which is as effective as carbamazepine, is falling dramatically, mainly because of chronic toxicity. Phenobarbitone and primidone, which are less efficacious, have been practically eliminated, mainly because of their adverse effects on cognition. Clobazam, though often highly beneficial in selective cases, is rarely used as continuous AED treatment and it is not licensed in the USA.

New antiepileptic drugs in developed countries

Oxcarbazepine, which is probably of equal efficacy to carbamazepine and possibly with less idiosyncratic reactions, is gaining some ground.[474] Levetiracetam has become increasingly more popular, because of a combined high efficacy, comparative poverty of adverse reactions, lack of drug–drug interactions and rapid titration. Topiramate is very efficacious, but with serious and numerous adverse reactions that reduce its value. Lamotrigine is relatively widely used despite relatively low efficacy in RCTs, often severe idiosyncratic reactions and drug–drug interactions. Gabapentin has very weak antiepileptic efficacy and rarely achieves satisfactory control of seizures,[430] but it is has become popular in the USA, where it has been promoted for many off-label uses, mainly neurogenic pain. Zonisamide has been used widely in Japan in intractable focal epilepsies. Tiagabine is used cautiously, because of fears of adverse reactions, such as non-convulsive status epilepticus. Vigabatrin has been practically discarded in the treatment of

Note on the use of valproate and clobazam in focal epilepsies

Valproate is the superior AED for generalised epilepsies, but its use as monotherapy in focal epilepsies is debated. The assessment of RCTs[450] that valproate is of nearly equal efficacy to carbamazepine in focal epilepsies contradicts the experience in clinical practice that valproate is not the appropriate AED for focal seizures. There are many reasons for this contradiction. Firstly, in RCTs, "Misclassification of patients may have confounded the results … The age distribution of adults classified as having generalised seizures indicated that significant numbers of patients may have had their seizures misclassified."[450] Secondly, "systematic reviews cannot upgrade poor primary research. Also, a major hurdle is that of publication bias, as trials with a positive result are more likely to be published than those with a negative result.[462] It is not surprising that a review of trials with positive results will come up with a positive answer."[460]

Personally, after consistent failures to introduce valproate as monotherapy in focal seizures, I rarely use it and only adjunctively in patients with focal and secondarily GTCS because of the following: effective required doses of valproate are much higher for focal than generalised epilepsies; side effects, particularly in some women, make its use extremely problematic;.currently, there are other more effective and safer drugs for focal seizures.

Clobazam in the treatment of focal epilepsies

Based on recent evidence, clobazam is a very useful AED both as monotherapy and polytherapy, though it is not licensed in the USA.[463-473] It is neglected in current clinical practice mainly because it is erroneously considered of high dependence for all patients, of similar effectiveness regarding seizure type to that of clonazepam and because it is a benzodiazepine. Clobazam is a very useful drug that should be tried in all intractable patients with focal seizures that fail to respond to other AEDs. Tolerance to clobazam has been overemphasised. The truth is in between and many patients may remain seizure free despite continuing use.[464,473]

A 23-year-old man with intractable temporal lobe epilepsy failed to respond to any appropriate medication. While waiting for neurosurgical evaluation, 20 mg of clobazam nocte was added with a miraculous effect. He has remained seizure free for 7 years.

epilepsies, because of common and often irreversible visual field defects. Currently, the use of vigabatrin is limited to infantile spasms.

CLINICAL PRACTICE IN DEVELOPING COUNTRIES
Phenytoin, carbamazepine and phenobarbitone are by far the most common main antiepileptic agents for treating focal epilepsies, either as monotherapy or polytherapy).

MONOTHERAPY OF FOCAL EPILEPSIES

Monotherapy is the primary aim in all, and therefore also focal, epilepsies.

Carbamazepine remains the first choice AED in focal seizures, but over 10% of patients develop acute idiosyncratic reactions (mainly rash). In numerous comparative studies, no other drug showed better efficacy than carbamazepine in focal seizures, although some new AEDs were better tolerated.

If treatment with carbamazepine in maximal tolerated doses fails, other pragmatic options include, of the old AEDs, phenytoin and, of the new AEDs, oxcarbazepine, levetiracetam, lamotrigine, topiramate and zonisamide (in order of preference). Personally, I also use clobazam in selected cases and I do not recommend valproate.

Phenytoin, despite its high efficacy, may not be tolerated by 10–20% of patients, because of idiosyncratic reactions, which may be fatal in exceptional cases. Long-term use is associated with unacceptable adverse reactions, including dysmorphic features.

Phenobarbitone and primidone are still very useful AEDs, particularly when cost is of concern. Their use is often barred by cognitive adverse reactions.

All new AEDs have shown a variable degree of efficacy (Figure 12.20), tolerability (Figure 12.20), safety profile, pharmacokinetics and drug–drug interactions, which should be taken into account when choosing one drug over another and which may be in the following order of priority: oxcarbazepine, levetiracetam, lamotrigine, topiramate, gabapentin and zonisamide.

Oxcarbazepine should probably be the drug of first choice by virtue of similar efficacy to carbamazepine, evidence-based documentation and length of experience; it is the first of the new AEDs to achieve FDA approval as monotherapy in focal seizures.

Of all other new AEDs only levetiracetam, lamotrigine and topiramate have the potential to be monotherapy in focal seizures.

RATIONAL POLYTHERAPY

Rational polytherapy* is often needed for the treatment of intractable focal epilepsies. The decision for polytherapy should first examine the possible/probable reasons why the monotherapy failed. These should thoroughly examine the following possibilities, which often require re-evaluation of the diagnosis (genuine epileptic seizures? and what type of seizures?).

- The patient does not suffer from epileptic seizures.
- The patient has both genuine epileptic and non-epileptic seizures.
- The patient has generalised seizures and not focal seizures.
- The AED used as monotherapy was not suitable for the particular type of seizures or had weak efficacy.

Non-compliance, which varies from unwillingness to take medication to occasionally forgetting or missing the AED dose. The latter is often improved with the use of AED-monitored dosage systems, which are widely available through pharmacies. These are useful even for patients who comply well, but who often may be uncertain whether or not they have taken their medication.

*The word *"rational"* has been used in conjunction with "polytherapy" in order to emphasise that this can also be *irrational* and *hazardous* if a diagnosis is incorrect and anti-epileptic drug indications/contraindications are violated.[475] Conversion from polytherapy to monotherapy should also be *rational*.[476]

In polytherapy, initially, a second drug is added to the first line agent, which had demonstrated acceptable but insufficient efficacy, tolerability or both in monotherapy. Adding a new AED with another one to three AEDs that have already partially or totally failed or have made the situation worse is a formidable physician's task for a disappointed and frustrated patient. The choice of a second or sometimes a third AED depends on many factors such as efficacy, adverse effects, interactions with other drugs and mode of action (Table 12.4). Polytherapy with more than three drugs is discouraged because adverse reactions become more prominent with little if any seizure improvement.

Of the old AEDs, carbamazepine, phenytoin, valproate and phenobarbital (in that order of importance and priority) are the most valuable either as monotherapy or polytherapy and particularly when cost is of concern.

Carbamazepine is currently the gold standard for controlling focal seizures in more than 70% of patients (10% of the patients develop idiosyncratic reactions). Valproate, the gold standard in generalised epilepsies, is inferior in focal epilepsies, with significant concerns in the treatment of women. The usage of phenytoin, which is as effective as carbamazepine, is dramatically decreasing because of mainly chronic toxicity. Phenobarbitone and primidone, which are less efficacious, have been practically eliminated in developed countries, mainly because of their adverse effects on cognition.

Of the new AEDs, the consensus, including the recent American QS&TTA assessment,[477] is that all of them are appropriate for adjunctive treatment in refractory focal epilepsies with or without secondarily GTCS.

It is appropriate to use gabapentin, lamotrigine, tiagabine, topiramate, oxcarbazepine, levetiracetam and zonisamide as add-on therapy in patients with refractory focal epilepsy.[477]

Guidance that gives the physician a list of options is unsatisfactory in practice. The clinician's important question is:

'In what order of priority the new AEDs should be used?'

The ideal profile of an antiepileptic drug for polytherapy purposes[478] is that it:

1. is effective

2. has a low incidence of adverse effects

3. causes no pharmacokinetic interactions

4. favourably combines with drugs with different mechanisms of action

5. needs minimal laboratory monitoring

6. needs as little as possible titration.

Thus, the order of priority of the new add-on AED is determined by the following factors.

- **Strength of efficacy.** The more efficacious a drug the more likely it is to control seizures and, if successful, withdrawal of other concomitant AEDs may be possible without losing seizure control and, in some cases, with improved seizure control (Figure 12.20).[476] Seizure-free status is the ultimate, often achievable, goal of treatment and this should be precisely evaluated in any RCT and relevant formal practice parameter recommendations.[479]

- **Safety and tolerability.** This includes adverse reactions and particularly those that may be serious and may outweigh any beneficial effect achieved by a reduction in seizures (Table 12.4 and Figure 12.20). Topiramate is probably the worst of all new broad spectrum AEDs because of multiple and severe adverse reactions.

- **Interactions with other antiepileptic drugs, whether pharmacokinetic, pharmacodynamic or both, are particularly unwanted in polytherapy** (Table 12.4).[478] Raising the levels of concomitant AEDs and pharmacodynamic interactions may lead to toxic effects. Conversely, decreasing their levels may increase and worsen seizures causing a vicious circle in clinical management. With the exception of levetiracetam and[454] gabapentin, all other new AEDs exhibit sometimes complex undesirable drug–drug interactions.[453] Lamotrigine is amongst the worst of all new AEDs from that point. It requires different dosage and titration schemes when combined with hepatic enzyme-inducers and when combined with valproate. Concomitant administration of carbamazepine with lamotrigine enhances each drug's side-effect profile as the result of pharmacodynamic interactions.

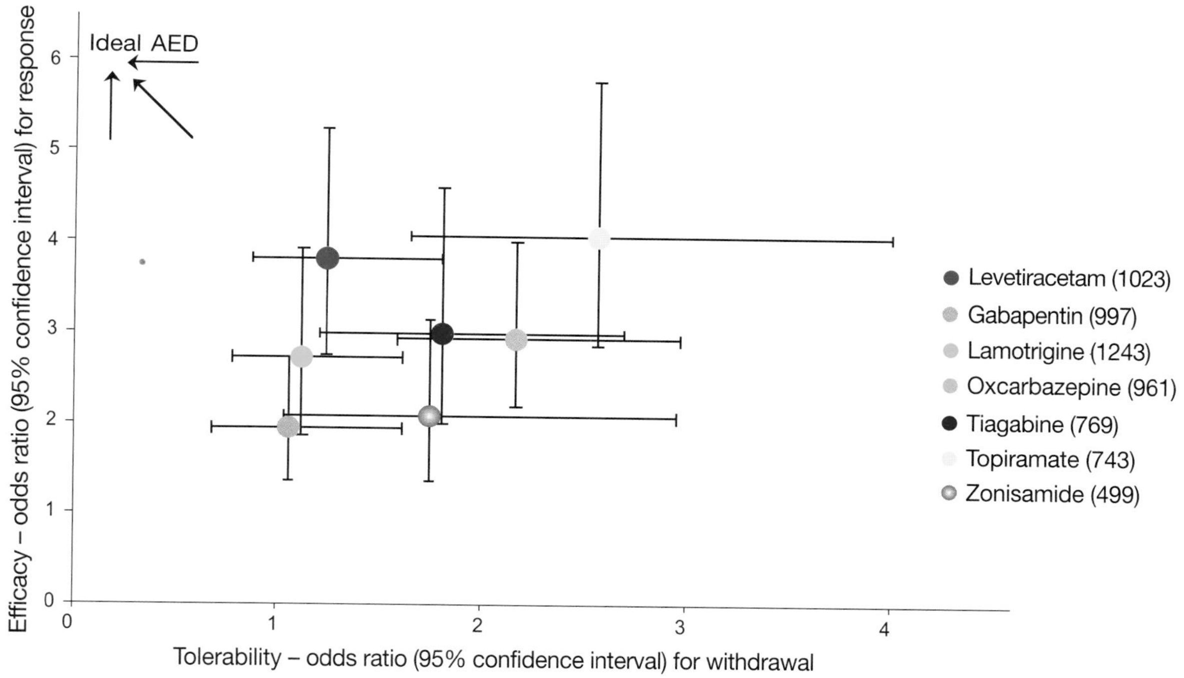

Figure 12.20 Comparison of odds ratios, with 95% confidence intervals, for the efficacy (responder rates) and tolerability (withdrawal rates) of new AEDs in a meta-analysis of published RCTs.[461]

The numbers of patients included in the studies are in parentheses. AEDs in the left upper corner (levetiracetam) are of comparatively higher efficacy and excellent tolerability. AEDs towards the bottom of the histogram (lamotrigine and gabapentin) are of low efficacy. AEDs towards the right of the histogram are poorly tolerated (topiramate and oxcarbazepine).

- **Different mechanisms of action in relation to other concurrent AEDs** (Table 4.5, page 70).[478,480] Antiepileptic drug–drug interactions may be purely additive, antagonistic or synergistic. AEDs with the same mechanism of action would be expected to be additive, while combining AEDs with different mechanisms of action may have synergistic efficacy.[478,480] A review of clinical studies suggested that a combination of a sodium channel blocker with a drug that increases the GABAergic neurotransmission or that has multiple mechanisms is generally more effective than a combination of two sodium channel blockers.[480] An AED is unlikely to have better success and more likely to have additive adverse reactions if added to another AED with the same mechanism of action.[480] Levetiracetam appears to have a unique mode of action (Figure 12.21).
- **Need for less laboratory monitoring** (Table 12.4). This refers firstly to monitoring of the serum AED levels of the added AED or the co-medications that may be affected, such as with lamotrigine or topiramate added to carbamazepine and, secondly, blood or other tests needed for detecting possible adverse drug reactions such as hypernatraemia with oxcarbazepine, metabolic acidosis for topiramate and zonisamide. More laboratory testing may mean less compliance, more expenses and more uncomfortable situations for patients.
- **The need for as little as possible titration** (Table 12.4). Very slow titration may mean more seizures that may also be traumatic. Levetiracetam and gabapentin are nearly ideal from that point of view with their starting dose often equalling the effective maintenance dose. Conversely, lamotrigine and topiramate are inferior requiring 6-8 weeks of low dose and slow titration in order to reach reasonable therapeutic levels.

Taking all these parameters together levetiracetam is much superior to all other new AEDs (Tables 4.3, 4.4, 4.5, 4.6, 4.7 and 12.4 and Figure 12.20).

Levetiracetam

- It is highly efficacious and has the most favourable 'responder-withdrawal ratio' of any other new AED (Figure 12.20 and Table 12.4).[433,481] It reduces the

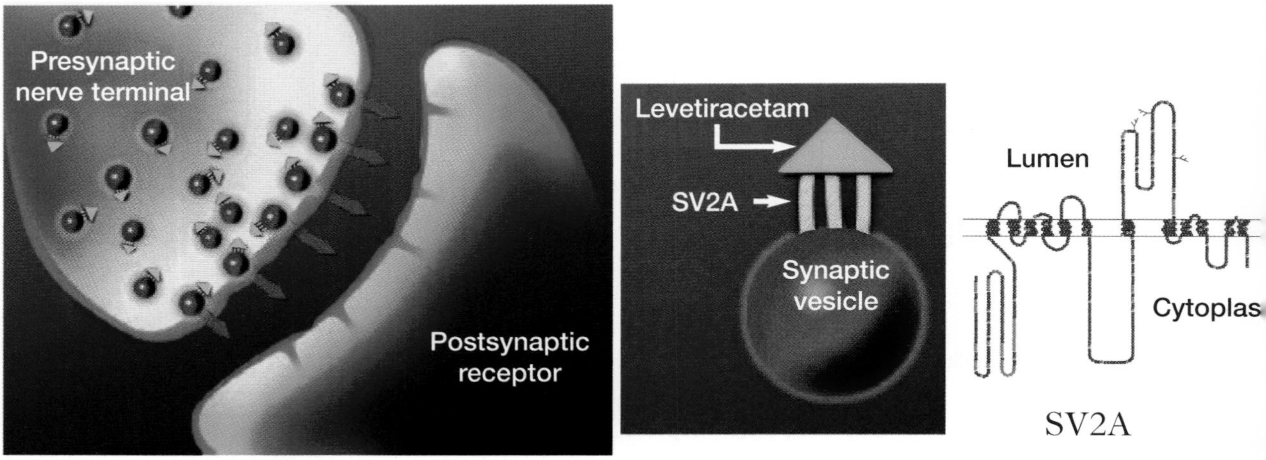

Figure 12.21 Synaptic vesicle protein 2A, the binding site of levetiracetam.

Levetiracetam is the first and only AED found to bind to synaptic vesicle protein 2A (SV2A).[455] SV2A binding inhibits abnormal bursting in epileptic circuits, which may inhibit the occurrence of seizures.

Figure courtesy of UCB Pharma

frequency of simple and complex focal seizures and demonstrates a specific, independent reduction of secondarily GTCS.[482] Furthermore, in RCTs of intractable focal epilepsies *the highest percentage of seizure free status was achieved with* levetiracetam (9%) than any other of the new AEDs (0-5%). In the largest single-tertiary centre cohort of 811 patients with 'chronic epilepsy' taking levetiracetam, almost half of patients achieved a period of reduction in seizure frequency of ≥ 50%, with nearly one in five achieving a period of seizure freedom.[483] Two-thirds of patients were continuing levetiracetam therapy at last follow-up. Impressively, seizure freedom was attained in 120/654 (18%) patients with cryptogenic or symptomatic focal epilepsy and 15/68 (22%) patients with IGE. Forty-six patients achieved levetiracetam monotherapy, and 26 of these had periods of seizure freedom ranging from 2-35 months (mean 13 months, median 11 months).[483]

- It is considered as one of the most adverse reaction-free AED.[484]
- The regulatory approved starting dose of 1000 mg/day is often therapeutic.
- It does not have drug–drug interactions with concomitant medications.[453,485] It does not influence other AEDs in a clinically meaningful way and, conversely, other drugs do not interfere with the pharmacokinetics of levetiracetam.
- It has a novel mechanism of action, which is different to all other old and new AEDs (Figure 12.21).
- The need for laboratory tests is minimal if any.

A 25-year-old woman had surgery for drug-resistant focal epilepsy due to left temporal lobe cavernoma at age 21 years. There was no improvement: she continued having four complex focal seizures per week and one GTCS per month despite appropriate combinations of all available AEDs being tried. A breakthrough in her life came when levetiracetam was added. She is now seizure free and obtained her driving licence on 1500 mg of levetiracetam daily and carbamazepine at reducing doses of 200 mg twice daily (case of Professor J. W. A. S. Sander).

Next to levetiracetam, the other new AEDs are in the following order of priority.

1. *Lamotrigine* is one of the best AEDs regarding cognitive adverse effects, but is of low efficacy in RCTs of refractory patients with focal seizures. Frequent idiosyncratic reactions, which rarely may be fatal, are a realistic threat.[486] Other significant disadvantages are drug-drug interactions including with hormonal contraception and the effect of pregnancy on lamotrigine plasma concentration[487] and slow titration.
2. *Topiramate*, despite its significant efficacy, is characterised by frequent and sometimes serious adverse reactions such as nephrolithiasis, open angle glaucoma, hypohidrosis, metabolic acidosis, weight loss and language dysfunction.[452] Metabolic acidosis in children may have a predictable detrimental growth and bone-related sequelae in long-term use. It is the worst tolerated AED in comparative RCTs (Figure 12.20). Drug-drug interactions including hormonal contraception are an additional disadvantage.
3. *Oxcarbazepine* is amongst the first choice AEDs as monotherapy and it is the first of the new AEDs to achieve FDA approval for this indication in children. However, oxcarbazepine does not have high priority in co-medication with carbamazepine and phenytoin because of drug–drug interactions and added adverse reactions.
4. *Gabapentin* is of very low efficacy in RCTs (Figure 12.20) and the clinical experience of most epileptologists with gabapentin,[451] which I share, is disappointing.

The therapeutic efficacy of gabapentin is weak in relation to other AEDs, the number of responders is disappointingly low even when higher doses are used and it is unusual for patients with severe focal epilepsies to derive much benefit. [451]

5. *Zonisamide:* one of the most popular drugs in Japan but with significant drug-drug interactions and side effects some of which may be severe such hypohidrosis and hyperthermia or Stevens-Johnson syndrome. Nephrolitiasis occurred in 4% of patients in a USA study.[488]
6. *Tiagabine:* treatment emergent non-convulsive status epilepticus has been reported in a significant number of patients. Its role is probably in the treatment of severe forms of focal epilepsies that failed to respond to other AEDs combinations. It is contraindicated in IGEs.
7. *Vigabatrin:* Its use in epilepsies, other than West syndrome, is very restricted due to the high risk of irreversible visual field defects. It is contraindicated in IGEs. Tiagabine and vigabatrin are two GABAergic drugs that are contraindicated in IGEs. They induce (not treat) absences and absence status epilepticus.[479,489]
8. *Pregabalin:* It is probably too early to make any predictions for the role of pregabalin in the treatment of focal epilepsies. However, the high incidence of weight gain[490] (consider the decline in the use of valproate because of this side effect and its causative relation with polycystic ovaries in women), treatment emergent myoclonic jerks [490,491] and similarities with gabapentin[492] are not promising signs.

   Weight gain appears to be significant even in RCTs of short duration involving active treatment with pregabalin. In one such RCT mean weight gain from baseline to termination (12 weeks) appeared to be dose related and ranged from 0.50 kg in the 50 mg/day treatment group to 2.28 kg in the 600 mg/day treatment group (12.4% of patients).[493] Future RCTs are expected to determine whether weight gain with pregabalin is progressive with continuing use of this agent.

   The pro-myoclonic action of pregabalin is even more disquieting. Four of 19 patients (21%) with intractable focal seizures developed myoclonic jerks in a RCT when pregabalin was added to other AEDs.[491] Though the prevalence of pregabalin-induced myoclonus was found to be much lower (2% of patients) in another recent RCT (2% of patients with focal seizures)[490] this is a warning sign against its use in generalised epilepsies (in which myoclonus is often a prominent symptom to treat) or at its best it indicates a narrow antiepileptic spectrum of pregabalin similar to that of gabapentin.

REFERENCES

1. Commission on Classification and Terminology of the International League Against Epilepsy. Proposal for revised classification of epilepsies and epileptic syndromes. *Epilepsia* 1989;**30**:389-99.
2. Engel J, Jr. A proposed diagnostic scheme for people with epileptic seizures and with epilepsy: Report of the ILAE Task Force on Classification and Terminology. *Epilepsia* 2001;**42**:796-803.
3. Hauser WA. Incidence and prevalence of epilepsy. In Engel JJ, Pedley TA, eds. *Epilepsy: A comprehensive Textbook*, pp 47-57. Philadelphia: Lippincott-Raven Publishers, 1997.
4. Crawford PM. Epidemiology of intractable focal epilepsy. In Oxbury JM, Polkey CE, Duchowny M, eds. *Intractable focal epilepsy*, pp 25-40. London: W.B.Saunders, 2000.
5. Wiebe S. Epidemiology of temporal lobe epilepsy. *Can J Neurol Sci.* 2000;**27 Suppl 1**:S6-10.
6. Sisodiya SM. Malformations of cortical development: burdens and insights from important causes of human epilepsy. *Lancet Neurol.* 2004;**3**:29-38.
7. Mathern GW, Babb TL, Pretorius JK, Melendez M, Levesque MF. The pathophysiologic relationships between lesion pathology, intracranial ictal EEG onsets, and hippocampal neuron losses in temporal lobe epilepsy. *Epilepsy Res* 1995;**21**:133-47.
8. Babb TL. Synaptic reorganizations in human and rat hippocampal epilepsy. *Adv Neurol* 1999;**79**:763-79.
9. Wolf HK, Campos MG, Zentner J, Hufnagel A, Schramm J, Elger CE *et al.* Surgical pathology of temporal lobe epilepsy. Experience with 216 cases. *J Neuropathol Exp Neurol* 1993;**52**:499-506.
10. Wolf HK, Zentner J, Hufnagel A, Campos MG, Schramm J, Elger CE *et al.* Morphological findings in temporal lobe epilepsy: experience with 216 consecutive surgical specimens. *Verh Dtsch Ges Pathol.* 1994;**78**:438-42.
11. Wolf HK, Aliashkevich AF, Blumcke I, Wiestler OD, Zentner J. Neuronal loss and gliosis of the amygdaloid nucleus in temporal lobe epilepsy. A quantitative analysis of 70 surgical specimens. *Acta Neuropathol.(Berl)* 1997;**93**:606-10.
12. Bouchet C, Cazauvieilh JB. De l'épilepsie considéré dans ses rapports avec l'aliénation mentale. *Arch Gen Med* 1825;**9**:510-42.
13. Gowers WR. Epilepsies and other chronic convulsive diseases. Their causes, symptoms and treatment. London: Churchill JA, 1881.
14. Jackson JH. On a particular variety of epilepsy ("intellectual aura"), one case with symptoms of organic brain disease. *Brain* 1888;**11**:179-207 (In: Taylor J, ed. *Selected writings of John Hughlings Jackson.* London: Hodder and Stoughton 1958:385-405).
15. Jackson JH,.Colman WS. Case of epilepsy with tasting movements and "dreaming state"-very small patch of softening in the left uncinate gyrus. *Brain* 1898;**21**:580-90 (In: Taylor J, ed. *Selected writings of John Hughlings Jackson.* London: Hodder and Stoughton 1958:458-463).
16. Holmes G. Sabill memorial oration on focal epilepsy. *Lancet* 1927;**i**:957-62.
17. Penfield W, Kristiansen K. Epileptic seizure patterns. Springfield,IL: Charles C Thomas, 1951.
18. Lennox WG, Lennox MA. Epilepsy and related disorders. Boston: Little,Brown & Co., 1960.
19. Ajmone-Marsan C, Ralston BL. The epileptic seizure:its functional morphology and diagnostic significance. A clinical-electrographic analysis of metrazol-induced attacks. Springfield,Illinois: Charles C. Thomas, 1957.
20. Baldwin M, Bailey P. Temporal lobe epilepsy. Springfield,Ill: Charles C. Thomas, 1958.
21. Ajmone-Marsan C,.Abraham K. A seizure atlas. *Electroencephalogr Clin Neurophysiol* 1960;**(Suppl 15)**:1-215.
22. Aird RB, Venturini AM, Spielman PM. Antecedents of temporal lobe epilepsy. *Arch Neurol* 1967;**16**:67-73.
23. Aird RB, Crowther DL. Temporal lobe epilepsy in childhood. Clinical expressions observed in 125 affected children. *Clin Pediatr* 1970;**9**:409-15.
24. Currie S, Heathfield KW, Henson RA, Scott DF. Clinical course and prognosis of temporal lobe epilepsy. A survey of 666 patients. *Brain* 1971;**94**:173-90.
25. Daly DD. Ictal clinical manifestations of complex partial seizures. *Adv Neurol* 1975;**11**:57-83.
26. Penry JK. Perspectives in complex partial seizures. *Adv Neurol* 1975;**11**:1-14.
27. Penfield W. The mystery of the mind. Princeton,New Jersey: Princeton University Press, 1975.
28. Gloor P, Olivier A, Quesney LF, Andermann F, Horowitz S. The role of the limbic system in experiential phenomena of temporal lobe epilepsy. *Ann Neurol* 1982;**12**:129-44.
29. Ounsted C, Lindsay J, Richards P. Temporal lobe epilepsy.A biographical study 1948-1986. London: MacKeith Press, 1988.
30. Bruton CJ. The neuropathology of temporal lobe epilepsy. Oxford: Oxford Press, 1988.
31. Gloor P. Experiential phenomena of temporal lobe epilepsy. Facts and hypotheses. *Brain* 1990;**113**:1673-94.
32. Wieser HG. Ictal manifestations of temporal lobe seizures. *Adv Neurol* 1991;**55**:301-15.
33. Bancaud J, Brunet-Bourgin F, Chauvel P, Halgren E. Anatomical origin of deja vu and vivid 'memories' in human temporal lobe epilepsy. *Brain* 1994;**117**:71-90.
34. Kotagal P, Luders HO, Williams G, Nichols TR, McPherson J. Psychomotor seizures of temporal lobe onset: analysis of symptom clusters and sequences. *Epilepsy Research* 1995;**20**:49-67.
35. Wieser HG. Electroclinical features of the psychomotor seizure:A stereoelectroencephalographic study of ictal symptoms and chronotopographical seizure patterns including clinical effects of intracerebral stimulation. Stuttgard: Gustav Fischer, 1983.
36. Luders H, Lesser RP. Epilepsy. Electroclinical syndromes. Berlin Heidelberg: Springer-Verlag, 1987.
37. Engel J, Jr., Williamson PD, Wieser HG. Mesial temporal lobe epilepsy. In Engel JJ, Pedley TA, eds. *Epilepsy: A comprehensive Textbook*, pp 2417-26. Philadelphia: Lippincott-Raven Publishers, 1997.
38. Williamson PD, Thadani VM, French JA, Darcey TM, Mattson RH, Spencer SS *et al.* Medial temporal lobe epilepsy: videotape analysis of objective clinical seizure characteristics. *Epilepsia* 1998;**39**:1182-8.
39. Williamson PD. Mesial temporal lobe epilepsy. In Gilman S, ed. *Medlink*, San Diego CA: Arbor Publishing, 2004.
40. French JA, Williamson PD, Thadani VM, Darcey TM, Mattson RH, Spencer SS *et al.* Characteristics of medial temporal lobe epilepsy: I. Results of history and physical examination. *Ann Neurol* 1993;**34**:774-80.
41. Gonzalez-Pal S, Faure A, Quintana J, Fabelo R, Dominguez ME, Gomez-Plasencia R *et al.* Frontal lobe dysfunction in patients with epilepsy and chronic psychosis. *Rev Neurol* 1999;**28**:219-23.
42. Sperling MR, Lieb JP, Engel J, Jr., Crandall PH. Prognostic significance of independent auras in temporal lobe seizures. *Epilepsia* 1989;**30**:322-31.
43. Sperling MR,.O'Connor MJ. Auras and subclinical seizures: characteristics and prognostic significance. *Ann Neurol* 1990;**28**:320-8.
44. van Buren JM. The abdominal aura: a study of abdominal sensations occurring in epilepsy and produced by depth stimulation. *Electroencephalogr Clin Neurophysiol* 1963;**15**:1-19.
45. Duncan JS, Sagar HJ. Seizure characteristics, pathology, and outcome after temporal lobectomy. *Neurology* 1987;**37**:405-9.
46. Gastaut H. Dictionary of epilepsies. Part I:Definitions. Geneva: World Health Organisation, 1973.
47. Jackson JH. On the anatomical, physiological and pathological investigation of the epilepsies. *West Riding Lunatic Asylum Medical Reports* 1873;**3**:315-39 (In: Taylor J, ed. *Selected writings of John Hughlings Jackson.* London: Hodder and Stoughton 1958 :90-111).
48. Jackson JH. On right or left-sided spasm at the onset of epileptic paroxysms, and on crude sensation warnings, and elaborate mental states. *Brain* 1880;**iii**:192- (In: Taylor J, ed. *Selected writings of John Hughlings Jackson.* London: Hodder and Stoughton 1958:308-317).
49. Penfield W,.Perot P. The brain's record of auditory and visual experience. *Brain* 1963;**86**:595-696.
50. Adachi N, Koutroumanidis M, Elwes RD, Polkey CE, Binnie CD, Reynolds EH *et al.* Interictal 18FDG PET findings in temporal lobe epilepsy with deja vu. *J Neuropsychiatry Clin Neurosci.* 1999;**11**:380-6.
51. Penfield W, Jasper HH. Epilepsy and the functional anatomy of the human brain. Boston: Little, Brown & Co., 1954.

52. Wieser HG,.Mazzola G. Musical consonances and dissonances: are they distinguished independently by the right and left hippocampi? *Neuropsychologia* 1986;**24**:805-12.
53. Wieser HG,.Walter R. Untroubled musical judgement of a performing organist during early epileptic seizure of the right temporal lobe. *Neuropsychologia* 1997;**35**:45-51.
54. Acharya V, Acharya J, Luders H. Olfactory epileptic auras. *Neurology* 1998;**51**:56-61.
55. Ebner A, Kerdar MS. Olfactory and gustatory auras. In Luders HO, Noachtar S, eds. *Epileptic seizures. Pathophysiology and clinical semiology*, pp 313-9. New York: Churchill Livingstone, 2000.
56. Chen C, Shih YH, Yen DJ, Lirng JF, Guo YC, Yu HY *et al.* Olfactory auras in patients with temporal lobe epilepsy. *Epilepsia* 2003;**44**:257-60.
57. Badalian LO, Temin PA, Mukhin KI, Askochenskaia TI, Shnaidman RV, Korshunov SV. Temporal-lobe epilepsy with psychosensory and gustatory attacks. *Zh Nevropatol Psikhiatr Im S S Korsakova* 1993;**93**:17-9.
58. Hausser-Hauw C,.Bancaud J. Gustatory hallucinations in epileptic seizures. Electrophysiological, clinical and anatomical correlates. *Brain* 1987;**110**:339-59.
59. Nagy Z,.Esiri MM. Neuronal cyclin expression in the hippocampus in temporal lobe epilepsy. *Exp Neurol* 1998;**150**:240-7.
60. Yanez A, Morales E, Galdames D, Aguilera L, Faure E, Ortiz V *et al.* Temporal lobectomy in refractory partial epilepsy. Report of 4 cases. *Rev Med Chil.* 1994;**122**:186-92.
61. Lance JW. Simple formed hallucinations confined to the area of a specific visual field defect. *Brain* 1976;**99**:719-34.
62. Kolmel HW. Visual illusions and hallucinations. *Baillieres Clinical Neurology* 1993;**2**:243-64.
63. Baumgartner C, Groppel G, Leutmezer F, Aull-Watschinger S, Pataraia E, Feucht M *et al.* Ictal urinary urge indicates seizure onset in the nondominant temporal lobe. *Neurology* 2000;**55**:432-4.
64. Manford M, Fish DR, Shorvon SD. An analysis of clinical seizure patterns and their localizing value in frontal and temporal lobe epilepsies. *Brain* 1996;**119**:17-40.
65. Dantas FG, Yacubian EM, Jorge CL, Pedreira CC, Bueno JF, Valerio RM. Clinical and EEG analysis of mesial and lateral temporal lobe seizures. *Arq Neuropsiquiatr.* 1998;**56**:341-9.
66. Fakhoury T, Abou-Khalil B, Peguero E. Differentiating clinical features of right and left temporal lobe seizures. *Epilepsia* 1994;**35**:1038-44.
67. Duchowny M, Jayakar P, Resnick T, Levin B, Alvarez L. Posterior temporal epilepsy: electroclinical features. *Ann Neurol* 1994;**35**:427-31.
68. Blume WT, Luders HO, Mizrahi E, Tassinari C, van Emde BW, Engel J, Jr. Glossary of descriptive terminology for ictal semiology: report of the ILAE task force on classification and terminology. *Epilepsia* 2001;**42**:1212-8.
69. Jackson HJ. On temporary mental disorders after epilepsy paroxysms. *West Riding Lunatic Asylum Medical Reports* 1875;**v**:-(In: Taylor J, ed. *Selected writings of John Hughlings Jackson.* London: Hodder and Stoughton 1958: 119-134).
70. Yen DJ, Su MS, Yiu CH, Shih, Kwan SY, Tsai CP *et al.* Ictal speech manifestations in temporal lobe epilepsy: a video- EEG study. *Epilepsia* 1996;**37**:45-9.
71. Panayiotopoulos CP. A clinical guide to epileptic syndromes and their treatment. Oxford: Bladon Medical Publishing, 2002.
72. Hecker A, Andermann F, Rodin EA. Spitting automatism in temporal lobe seizures with a brief review of ethological and phylogenetic aspects of spitting. *Epilepsia* 1972;**13**:767-72.
73. Sussman NM, Jackel RA, Kaplan LR, Harner RN. Bicycling movements as a manifestation of complex partial seizures of temporal lobe origin. *Epilepsia* 1989;**30**:527-31.
74. Remillard GM, Andermann F, Testa GF, Gloor P, Aube M, Martin JB *et al.* Sexual ictal manifestations predominate in women with temporal lobe epilepsy: a finding suggesting sexual dimorphism in the human brain. *Neurology* 1983;**33**:323-30.
75. Wieser HG, Hajek M, Gooss A, Aguzzi A. Mesial temporal lobe epilepsy syndrome with hippocampal and amygdala sclerosis. In Oxbury JM, Polkey CE, Duchowny M, eds. *Intractable focal epilepsy*, pp 131-58. London: W.B.Saunders, 2000.
76. Elger CE. Semeiology of temporal lobe seizures. In Oxbury JM, Polkey CE, Duchowny M, eds. *Intractable focal epilepsy*, pp 63-8. London: W.B.Saunders, 2000.
77. Serles W, Pataraia E, Bacher J, Olbrich A, Aull S, Lehrner J *et al.* Clinical seizure lateralization in mesial temporal lobe epilepsy: differences between patients with unitemporal and bitemporal interictal spikes. *Neurology* 1998;**50**:742-7.
78. Abou-Khalil B, Welch L, Blumenkopf B, Newman K, Whetsell WO, Jr. Global aphasia with seizure onset in the dominant basal temporal region. *Epilepsia* 1994;**35**:1079-84.
79. Esclapez M,.Houser CR. Up-regulation of GAD65 and GAD67 in remaining hippocampal GABA neurons in a model of temporal lobe epilepsy. *J Comp Neurol* 1999;**412**:488-505.
80. Fernandez Torre JL, Alarcon G, Binnie CD, Polkey CE. Comparison of sphenoidal, foramen ovale and anterior temporal placements for detecting interictal epileptiform discharges in presurgical assessment for temporal lobe epilepsy. *Clin Neurophysiol.* 1999;**110**:895-904.
81. Kotagal P, Luders H, Morris HH, Dinner DS, Wyllie E, Godoy J *et al.* Dystonic posturing in complex partial seizures of temporal lobe onset: a new lateralizing sign. *Neurology* 1989;**39**:196-201.
82. Benbadis SR, Kotagal P, Klem GH. Unilateral blinking: a lateralizing sign in partial seizures. *Neurology* 1996;**46**:45-8.
83. Oestreich LJ, Berg MJ, Bachmann DL, Burchfiel J, Erba G. Ictal contralateral paresis in complex partial seizures. *Epilepsia* 1995;**36**:671-5.
84. Ansakorpi H, Korpelainen JT, Suominen K, Tolonen U, Myllyla VV, Isojarvi JI. Interictal cardiovascular autonomic responses in patients with temporal lobe epilepsy. *Epilepsia* 2000;**41**:42-7.
85. O'Donovan C.A., Burgess RC, Lueders H. Autonomic auras. In Luders HO, Noachtar S, eds. *Epileptic seizures. Pathophysiology and clinical semiology*, pp 320-35. New York: Churchill Livingstone, 2000.
86. Toichi M, Murai T, Sengoku A, Miyoshi K. Interictal change in cardiac autonomic function associated with EEG abnormalities and clinical symptoms: a longitudinal study following acute deterioration in two patients with temporal lobe epilepsy. *Psychiatry Clin Neurosci.* 1998;**52**:499-505.
87. Gleizer MA, Karlov VA. Autonomic dysfunction in patients with temporal lobe epilepsy. *Zh Nevropatol Psikhiatr Im S S Korsakova* 1988;**88**:11-5.
88. Saleh Y, Kirchner A, Pauli E, Hilz MJ, Neundorfer B, Stefan H. Temporal lobe epilepsy: effect of focus side on the autonomic regulation of heart rate?. *Nervenarzt* 2000;**71**:477-80.
89. Schernthaner C, Lindinger G, Potzelberger K, Zeiler K, Baumgartner C. Autonomic epilepsy—the influence of epileptic discharges on heart rate and rhythm. *Wien Klin.Wochenschr.* 1999;**111**:392-401.
90. Blumhardt LD, Smith PE, Owen L. Electrocardiographic accompaniments of temporal lobe epileptic seizures. *Lancet* 1986;**1**:1051-6.
91. Delamont RS, Julu PO, Jamal GA. Changes in a measure of cardiac vagal activity before and after epileptic seizures. *Epilepsy Res* 1999;**35**:87-94.
92. Massetani R, Strata G, Galli R, Gori S, Gneri C, Limbruno U *et al.* Alteration of cardiac function in patients with temporal lobe epilepsy: different roles of EEG-ECG monitoring and spectral analysis of RR variability. *Epilepsia* 1997;**38**:363-9.
93. Scott CA, Fish DR. Cardiac asystole in partial seizures. *Epilep Disord.* 2000;**2**:89-92.
94. Baumgartner C, Olbrich A, Lindinger G, Pataraia E, Groppel G, Bacher J *et al.* Regional cerebral blood flow during temporal lobe seizures associated with ictal vomiting: an ictal SPECT study in two patients. *Epilepsia* 1999;**40**:1085-91.
95. Chen C, Yen DJ, Yiu CH, Shih YH, Yu HY, Su MS. Ictal vomiting in partial seizures of temporal lobe origin. *Eur.Neurol* 1999;**42**:235-9.
96. Schauble B, Britton JW, Mullan BP, Watson J, Sharbrough FW, Marsh WR. Ictal vomiting in association with left temporal lobe seizures in a left hemisphere language-dominant patient. *Epilepsia* 2002;**43**:1432-5.
97. Koutroumanidis M. Ictal vomiting in association with left temporal lobe seizures in a left hemisphere language-dominant patient. *Epilepsia* 2003;**44**:1259.
98. Panayiotopoulos CP. Vomiting as an ictal manifestation of epileptic seizures and syndromes. *J Neurol Neurosurg Psychiatr* 1988;**51**:1448-51.
99. Panayiotopoulos CP. Panayiotopoulos syndrome. *Lancet* 2001;**358**:68-9.
100. Panayiotopoulos CP. Autonomic seizures and autonomic status epilepticus peculiar to childhood: diagnosis and management. *Epilepsy Behav.* 2004;**5**:286-95.

101. Tassinari CA, Riguzzi P, Rizzi R, Passarelli D, Volpi L. Gelastic seizures. In Tuxhorn I, Holthausen H, Boenigk H, eds. *Paediatric epilepsy syndromes and their surgical treatment*, pp 429-46. London: John Libbey & Comapny Ltd, 1997.
102. Mitchell A,.Penman MF. Temporal lobectomy: an increasingly viable option for seizure patients. *Axone.* 1989;**10**:69-71.
103. Risinger MW, Engel J, Jr., Van Ness PC, Henry TR, Crandall PH. Ictal localization of temporal lobe seizures with scalp/sphenoidal recordings. *Neurology* 1989;**39**:1288-93.
104. Brorson JR, Brewer K. St Paul and temporal lobe epilepsy. *J Neurol Neurosurg Psychiatry* 1988;**51**:886-7.
105. Arroyo S, Lesser RP, Gordon B, Uematsu S, Hart J, Schwerdt P *et al.* Mirth, laughter and gelastic seizures. *Brain* 1993;**116**:757-80.
106. Gascon GG,.Lombroso CT. Epileptic (gelastic) laughter. *Epilepsia* 1971;**12**:63-76.
107. Lehtinen LO, Kivalo A. Laughter epilepsy. *Acta Neurol Scand* 1965;**41**:255-8.
108. Jacome DE, McLain LW, Jr., FitzGerald R. Postural reflex gelastic seizures. *Arch Neurol* 1980;**37**:249-51.
109. Palmini AL, Gloor P, Jones-Gotman M. Pure amnestic seizures in temporal lobe epilepsy. Definition, clinical symptomatology and functional anatomical considerations. *Brain* 1992;**115**:749-69.
110. Bauer J, Ghane Y, Flugel D, Wildt L, Stefan H. Etiology, follow-up and therapy of seizure clusters in temporal lobe epilepsy and catamenial epileptic seizures. *Schweiz Arch Neurol Psychiatr.* 1992;**143**:117-34.
111. Foldvary-Schaefer N,.Falcone T. Catamenial epilepsy: pathophysiology, diagnosis, and management. *Neurology* 2003;**61**:S2-15.
112. Grunewald RA, Aliberti V, Panayiotopoulos CP. Exacerbation of typical absence seizures by progesterone. *Seizure* 1992;**1**:137-8.
113. Foldvary N, Lee N, Thwaites G, Mascha E, Hammel J, Kim H *et al.* Clinical and electrographic manifestations of lesional neocortical temporal lobe epilepsy. *Neurology* 1997;**49**:757-63.
114. Antel SB, Li LM, Cendes F, Collins DL, Kearney RE, Shinghal R *et al.* Predicting surgical outcome in temporal lobe epilepsy patients using MRI and MRSI. *Neurology* 2002;**58**:1505-12.
115. Briellmann RS, Berkovic SF, Syngeniotis A, King MA, Jackson GD. Seizure-associated hippocampal volume loss: a longitudinal magnetic resonance study of temporal lobe epilepsy. *Ann Neurol.* 2002;**51**:641-4.
116. Duncan JS. Neuroimaging. In Duncan JS, Sisodiya S, Smalls JE, eds. *Epilepsy 2001. From science to patient*, pp 173-216. Oxford: Meritus Communications, 2001.
117. Cendes F. Radiological evaluation of hippocampal sclerosis. In Oxbury JM, Polkey CE, Duchowny M, eds. *Intractable focal epilepsy*, pp 571-94. London: W.B.Saunders, 2000.
118. Li LM, Caramanos Z, Cendes F, Andermann F, Antel SB, Dubeau F *et al.* Lateralization of temporal lobe epilepsy (TLE) and discrimination of TLE from extra-TLE using pattern analysis of magnetic resonance spectroscopic and volumetric data. *Epilepsia* 2000;**41**:832-42.
119. Meierkord H, Shorvon S, Lightman S, Trimble M. Comparison of the effects of frontal and temporal lobe partial seizures on prolactin levels. *Arch Neurol* 1992;**49**:225-30.
120. Malow BA, Selwa LM, Ross D, Aldrich MS. Lateralizing value of interictal spikes on overnight sleep-EEG studies in temporal lobe epilepsy. *Epilepsia* 1999;**40**:1587-92.
121. Pataraia E, Lurger S, Serles W, Lindinger G, Aull S, Leutmezer F *et al.* Ictal scalp EEG in unilateral mesial temporal lobe epilepsy. *Epilepsia* 1998;**39**:608-14.
122. Cascino GD, Trenerry MR, So EL, Sharbrough FW, Shin C, Lagerlund TD *et al.* Routine EEG and temporal lobe epilepsy: relation to long-term EEG monitoring, quantitative MRI, and operative outcome. *Epilepsia* 1996;**37**:651-6.
123. Koutroumanidis M, Binnie CD, Panayiotopoulos CP. Positron emission tomography in partial epilepsies: the clinical point of view. *Nucl Med Commun.* 1998;**19**:1123-6.
124. Koutroumanidis M, Binnie CD, Elwes RD, Polkey CE, Seed P, Alarcon G *et al.* Interictal regional slow activity in temporal lobe epilepsy correlates with lateral temporal hypometabolism as imaged with 18FDG PET: neurophysiological and metabolic implications. *J Neurol Neurosurg Psychiatry* 1998;**65**:170-6.
125. Koutroumanidis M, Martin-Miguel C, Hennessy MJ, Akanuma N, Valentin A, Alarcon G *et al.* Interictal temporal delta activity in temporal lobe epilepsy: correlations with pathology and outcome. *Epilepsia* 2004;**45**:1351-67.
126. Sakai Y, Nagano H, Sakata A, Kinoshita S, Hamasaki N, Shima F *et al.* Localization of epileptogenic zone in temporal lobe epilepsy by ictal scalp EEG. *Seizure.* 2002;**11**:163-8.
127. Sadler M,.Desbiens R. Scalp EEG in temporal lobe epilepsy surgery. *Can J Neurol Sci.* 2000;**27 Suppl 1**:S22-S28.
128. Schulz R, Luders HO, Hoppe M, Tuxhorn I, May T, Ebner A. Interictal EEG and ictal scalp EEG propagation are highly predictive of surgical outcome in mesial temporal lobe epilepsy. *Epilepsia* 2000;**41**:564-70.
129. Panayiotopoulos CP, Chroni E, Daskalopoulos C, Baker A, Rowlinson S, Walsh P. Typical absence seizures in adults: clinical, EEG, video-EEG findings and diagnostic/syndromic considerations. *J Neurol Neurosurg Psychiatr* 1992;**55**:1002-8.
130. Hauser WA. The natural history of temporal lobe epilepsy. In Luders HO, ed. *Epilepsy surgery*, pp 133-41. New York: Raven Press, 1992.
131. Engel J, Jr., Wiebe S, French J, Sperling M, Williamson P, Spencer D *et al.* Practice parameter: temporal lobe and localized neocortical resections for epilepsy: report of the Quality Standards Subcommittee of the American Academy of Neurology, in association with the American Epilepsy Society and the American Association of Neurological Surgeons. *Neurology* 2003;**60**:538-47.
132. Engel J, Jr., Wiebe S, French J, Sperling M, Williamson P, Spencer D *et al.* Practice parameter: temporal lobe and localized neocortical resections for epilepsy. *Epilepsia* 2003;**44**:741-51.
133. Engel J, Jr. Recent advances in surgical treatment of temporal lobe epilepsy. *Acta Neurol Scand.Suppl* 1992;**140**:71-80.
134. Wieser HG. ILAE Commission Report. Mesial temporal lobe epilepsy with hippocampal sclerosis. *Epilepsia* 2004;**45**:695-714.
135. Engel J, Jr., (ed). Surgical treatment of the epilepsies. New York: Raven, 1993.
136. Gil-Nagel A, Risinger MW. Ictal semiology in hippocampal versus extrahippocampal temporal lobe epilepsy. *Brain* 1997;**120**:183-92.
137. Mohamed A,.Luders HO. Magnetic resonance imaging in temporal lobe epilepsy: usefulness for the etiological diagnosis of temporal lobe epilepsy. *Neurol Med Chir (Tokyo)* 2000;**40**:1-15.
138. Hogan RE, Wang L, Bertrand ME, Willmore LJ, Bucholz RD, Nassif AS *et al.* MRI-based high-dimensional hippocampal mapping in mesial temporal lobe epilepsy. *Brain* 2004.
139. Frost JJ, Mayberg HS, Fisher RS, Douglass KH, Dannals RF, Links JM *et al.* Mu-opiate receptors measured by positron emission tomography are increased in temporal lobe epilepsy. *Ann Neurol* 1988;**23**:231-7.
140. Kanos CC, Davies KG, O'Brien T, DohanJr FC, Jr. Hippocampal Sclerosis in a Two-Year-Old with Temporal Lobe Epilepsy: Case Report with Pathological Confirmation. *Pediatr Neurosurg.* 2000;**32**:316-20.
141. Babb TL, Brown WJ. Pathological findings in epilepsy. In Engel J, Jr., ed. *Surgical treatment of the epilepsies*, pp 511-40. New York: Raven, 1987.
142. Harvey AS, Grattan-Smith JD, Desmond PM, Chow CW, Berkovic SF. Febrile seizures and hippocampal sclerosis: frequent and related findings in intractable temporal lobe epilepsy of childhood. *Pediatr Neurol* 1995;**12**:201-6.
143. Harvey AS, Berkovic SF, Wrennall JA, Hopkins IJ. Temporal lobe epilepsy in childhood: clinical, EEG, and neuroimaging findings and syndrome classification in a cohort with new-onset seizures. *Neurology* 1997;**49**:960-8.
144. Cendes F, Cook MJ, Watson C, Andermann F, Fish DR, Shorvon SD *et al.* Frequency and characteristics of dual pathology in patients with lesional epilepsy. *Neurology* 1995;**45**:2058-64.
145. Falconer MA. Genetic and related aetiological factors in temporal lobe epilepsy. A review. *Epilepsia* 1971;**12**:13-31.
146. Maher J,.McLachlan RS. Febrile convulsions. Is seizure duration the most important predictor of temporal lobe epilepsy? *Brain* 1995;**118**:1521-8.
147. Mathern GW, Babb TL, Vickrey BG, Melendez M, Pretorius JK. The clinical-pathogenic mechanisms of hippocampal neuron loss and surgical outcomes in temporal lobe epilepsy. *Brain* 1995;**118**:105-18.
148. O'Connor WM, Masukawa L, Freese A, Sperling MR, French JA, O'Connor MJ. Hippocampal cell distributions in temporal lobe epilepsy: a comparison between patients with and without an early risk factor. *Epilepsia* 1996;**37**:440-9.
149. Ohtsu M, Oguni H, Awaya Y, Osawa M. Clinical and EEG analysis of initial status epilepticus during infancy in patients with mesial temporal lobe epilepsy. *Brain Dev.* 2002;**24**:231-8.

150. Delgado-Escueta AV,.Walsh GO. Type I complex partial seizures of hippocampal origin: excellent results of anterior temporal lobectomy. *Neurology* 1985;**35**:143-54.

151. Dill R,.Gullotta F. Pathomorphologic findings in temporal lobe epilepsy. A contribution to the question of ganglioblastomas. *Schweiz Arch Neurol Neurochir Psychiatr.* 1970;**106**:241-55.

152. O'Brien TJ, Kilpatrick C, Murrie V, Vogrin S, Morris K, Cook MJ. Temporal lobe epilepsy caused by mesial temporal sclerosis and temporal neocortical lesions. A clinical and electroencephalographic study of 46 pathologically proven cases. *Brain* 1996;**119**:2133-41.

153. Mayanagi Y, Watanabe E, Kaneko Y. Mesial temporal lobe epilepsy: clinical features and seizure mechanism. *Epilepsia* 1996;**37 Suppl 3**:57-60.

154. Szkiladz E, Bacia T, Bidzinski J, Checinski S, Rakowicz M. Somatosensory potentials evoked by stimulation of the median nerves recorded during the operation from the surface of the cerebral cortex in patients with temporal lobe epilepsy. *Neurol Neurochir Pol.* 1989;**23**:355-62.

155. Dennis M, Farrell K, Hoffman HJ, Hendrick EB, Becker LE, Murphy EG. Recognition memory of item, associative and serial-order information after temporal lobectomy for seizure disorder. *Neuropsychologia* 1988;**26**:53-65.

156. Jobst BC, Williamson PD, Neuschwander TB, Darcey TM, Thadani VM, Roberts DW. Secondarily generalized seizures in mesial temporal epilepsy: clinical characteristics, lateralizing signs, and association with sleep-wake cycle. *Epilepsia* 2001;**42**:1279-87.

157. Lugaresi E, Pazzaglia P, Tassinari CA. Differentiation of "Absence Status" and "Temporal Lobe Status". *Epilepsia* 1971;**12**:77-87.

158. Shorvon SD. Status epilepticus:its clinical features and treatment in children and adults. Cambridge: Cambridge University Press, 1994.

159. Burneo JG, Knowlton RC, Gomez C, Martin R, Kuzniecky RI. Confirmation of nonconvulsive limbic status epilepticus with the sodium amytal test. *Epilepsia* 2003;**44**:1122-6.

160. Duncan MB, Maccario M. Transient global amnesia, epilepsy, and migraine: diagnostic comparisons and distinctions. *Military Medicine* 1989;**154**:424-7.

161. Kopelman MD, Panayiotopoulos CP, Lewis P. Transient epileptic amnesia differentiated from psychogenic "fugue": neuropsychological, EEG, and PET findings. *J Neurol Neurosurg Psychiatr* 1994;**57**:1002-4.

162. Licht EA,.Fujikawa DG. Nonconvulsive status epilepticus with frontal features: quantitating severity of subclinical epileptiform discharges provides a marker for treatment efficacy, recurrence and outcome. *Epilepsy Res.* 2002;**51**:13-21.

163. Thomas P, Zifkin B, Migneco O, Lebrun C, Darcourt J, Andermann F. Nonconvulsive status epilepticus of frontal origin. *Neurology* 1999;**52**:1174-83.

164. Koepp MJ, Richardson MP, Labbe C, Brooks DJ, Cunningham VJ, Ashburner J *et al.* 11C-flumazenil PET, volumetric MRI, and quantitative pathology in mesial temporal lobe epilepsy. *Neurology* 1997;**49**:764-73.

165. Kuzniecky R, Bilir E, Gilliam F, Faught E, Martin R, Hugg J. Quantitative MRI in temporal lobe epilepsy: evidence for fornix atrophy. *Neurology* 1999;**53**:496-501.

166. Kuzniecky R, Ho SS, Martin R, Faught E, Morawetz R, Palmer C *et al.* Temporal lobe developmental malformations and hippocampal sclerosis: epilepsy surgical outcome. *Neurology* 1999;**52**:479-84.

167. Engel J, Jr., Cascino GD, Shields WD. Surgically remediable syndromes. In Engel JJ, Pedley TA, eds. *Epilepsy: A comprehensive Textbook*, pp 1687-96. Philadelphia: Lippincott-Raven Publishers, 1997.

168. Raymond AA, Fish DR, Boyd SG, Smith SJ, Pitt MC, Kendall B. Cortical dysgenesis: serial EEG findings in children and adults. *Electroencephalogr Clin Neurophysiol* 1995;**94**:389-97.

169. Falconer MA. Discussion on the surgery of temporal lobe epilepsy:syrgical and pathologica aspects. *Proc Royal Soc Medicine* 1953;**44**:971-5.

170. Falconer MA. Mesial temporal (Ammon's horn) sclerosis as a common cause of epilepsy. Aetiology, treatment, and prevention. *Lancet* 1974;**2**:767-70.

171. Loiseau P,.Beaussart M. Hereditary factors in partial epilepsy. *Epilepsia* 1969;**10**:23-31.

172. Berkovic SF,.Jackson GD. The hippocampal sclerosis whodunit: enter the genes [editorial]. *Ann Neurol* 2000;**47**:557-8.

173. Kobayashi E, Lopes-Cendes I, Guerreiro CA, Sousa SC, Guerreiro MM, Cendes F. Seizure outcome and hippocampal atrophy in familial mesial temporal lobe epilepsy. *Neurology* 2001;**56**:166-72.

174. Kobayashi E, Li LM, Lopes-Cendes I, Cendes F. Magnetic resonance imaging evidence of hippocampal sclerosis in asymptomatic, first-degree relatives of patients with familial mesial temporal lobe epilepsy. *Arch Neurol.* 2002;**59**:1891-4.

175. Proper EA, Oestreicher AB, Jansen GH, Veelen CW, van Rijen PC, Gispen WH *et al.* Immunohistochemical characterization of mossy fibre sprouting in the hippocampus of patients with pharmaco-resistant temporal lobe epilepsy. *Brain* 2000;**123**:19-30

176. Sutula T, Cascino G, Cavazos J, Parada I, Ramirez L. Mossy fiber synaptic reorganization in the epileptic human temporal lobe. *Ann Neurol* 1989;**26**:321-30.

177. de Lanerolle NC, Kim JH, Robbins RJ, Spencer DD. Hippocampal interneuron loss and plasticity in human temporal lobe epilepsy. *Brain Res* 1989;**495**:387-95.

178. Jefferys JG. Hippocampal sclerosis and temporal lobe epilepsy: cause or consequence? [editorial]. *Brain* 1999;**122**:1007-8.

179. Scott RC. Childhood status epilepticus:structural consequences and assessment of a novel treatment. PhD Thesis. Institute of child health.University College London Medical School, 1999.

180. VanLandingham KE, Heinz ER, Cavazos JE, Lewis DV. Magnetic resonance imaging evidence of hippocampal injury after prolonged focal febrile convulsions. *Ann Neurol* 1998;**43**:413-26.

181. Fernandez G, Effenberger O, Vinz B, Steinlein O, Elger CE, Dohring W *et al.* Hippocampal malformation as a cause of familial febrile convulsions and subsequent hippocampal sclerosis. *Neurology* 1998;**50**:909-17.

182. Berg AT, Shinnar S, Levy SR, Testa FM. Childhood-onset epilepsy with and without preceding febrile seizures. *Neurology* 1999;**53**:1742-8.

183. Brines ML, Sundaresan S, Spencer DD, de Lanerolle NC. Quantitative autoradiographic analysis of ionotropic glutamate receptor subtypes in human temporal lobe epilepsy: up-regulation in reorganized epileptogenic hippocampus. *Eur J Neurosci.* 1997;**9**:2035-44.

184. Engel J, Jr., Wilson C, Bragin A. Advances in understanding the process of epileptogenesis based on patient material: what can the patient tell us? *Epilepsia* 2003;**44 Suppl 12**:60-71.

185. Bragin A, Engel J, Jr., Wilson CL, Fried I, Mathern GW. Hippocampal and entorhinal cortex high-frequency oscillations (100—500 Hz) in human epileptic brain and in kainic acid—treated rats with chronic seizures. *Epilepsia* 1999;**40**:127-37.

186. Stoffel-Wagner B, Beyenburg S, Watzka M, Blumcke I, Bauer J, Schramm J *et al.* Expression of 5alpha-reductase and 3alpha-hydroxisteroid oxidoreductase in the hippocampus of patients with chronic temporal lobe epilepsy. *Epilepsia* 2000;**41**:140-7.

187. Suckling J, Roberts H, Walker M, Highley JR, Fenwick P, Oxbury J *et al.* Temporal lobe epilepsy with and without psychosis: exploration of hippocampal pathology including that in subpopulations of neurons defined by their content of immunoreactive calcium-binding proteins. *Acta Neuropathol.(Berl)* 2000;**99**:547-54.

188. Hinterkeuser S, Schroder W, Hager G, Seifert G, Blumcke I, Elger CE *et al.* Astrocytes in the hippocampus of patients with temporal lobe epilepsy display changes in potassium conductances. *Eur J Neurosci.* 2000;**12**:2087-96.

189. Kashihara K, Akiyama K, Kodama M, Kohira I, Abe K. Temporal changes in expression of neuronal nitric oxide synthase mRNA in the rat hippocampus associated with kainate-induced seizures. *Neurol Res* 2000;**22**:409-12.

190. Nagerl UV, Mody I, Jeub M, Lie AA, Elger CE, Beck H. Surviving granule cells of the sclerotic human hippocampus have reduced Ca(2+) influx because of a loss of calbindin-D(28k) in temporal lobe epilepsy. *J Neurosci.* 2000;**20**:1831-6.

191. Cavazos JE, Jones SM, Cross DJ. Sprouting and synaptic reorganization in the subiculum and CA1 region of the hippocampus in acute and chronic models of partial-onset epilepsy. *Neuroscience* 2004;**126**:677-88.

192. Moser DJ, Bauer RM, Gilmore RL, Dede DE, Fennell EB, Algina JJ *et al.* Electroencephalographic, volumetric, and neuropsychological indicators of seizure focus lateralization in temporal lobe epilepsy. *Arch Neurol* 2000;**57**:707-12.

193. Cendes F, Li LM, Watson C, Andermann F, Dubeau F, Arnold DL. Is ictal recording mandatory in temporal lobe epilepsy? Not when the interictal electroencephalogram and hippocampal atrophy coincide. *Arch Neurol* 2000;**57**:497-500.

194. Kuzniecky RI, Jackson GD. Magnetic resonance in epilepsy. New York: Raven Press, 1995.
195. Ho SS, Kuzniecky RI, Gilliam F, Faught E, Bebin M, Morawetz R. Congenital porencephaly and hippocampal sclerosis. Clinical features and epileptic spectrum. *Neurology* 1997;**49**:1382-8.
196. Henry TR, Mazziotta JC, Engel J, Jr., Christenson PD, Zhang JX, Phelps ME *et al.* Quantifying interictal metabolic activity in human temporal lobe epilepsy. *J Cereb Blood Flow Metab* 1990;**10**:748-57.
197. Hajek M, Antonini A, Leenders KL, Wieser HG. Mesiobasal versus lateral temporal lobe epilepsy: metabolic differences in the temporal lobe shown by interictal 18F-FDG positron emission tomography. *Neurology* 1993;**43**:79-86.
198. Koutroumanidis M, Hennessy MJ, Seed PT, Elwes RD, Jarosz J, Morris RG *et al.* Significance of interictal bilateral temporal hypometabolism in temporal lobe epilepsy. *Neurology* 2000;**54**:1811-21.
199. Lamusuo S, Pitkanen A, Jutila L, Ylinen A, Partanen K, Kalviainen R *et al.* [11 C]Flumazenil binding in the medial temporal lobe in patients with temporal lobe epilepsy: correlation with hippocampal MR volumetry, T2 relaxometry, and neuropathology. *Neurology* 2000;**54**:2252-60.
200. Koepp MJ, Hammers A, Labbe C, Woermann FG, Brooks DJ, Duncan JS. 11C-flumazenil PET in patients with refractory temporal lobe epilepsy and normal MRI. *Neurology* 2000;**54**:332-9.
201. Ho SS, Berkovic SF, McKay WJ, Kalnins RM, Bladin PF. Temporal lobe epilepsy subtypes: differential patterns of cerebral perfusion on ictal SPECT. *Epilepsia* 1996;**37**:788-95.
202. Meiners LC, van der GJ, van Rijen PC, Springorum R, de Kort GA, Jansen GH. Proton magnetic resonance spectroscopy of temporal lobe white matter in patients with histologically proven hippocampal sclerosis. *J Magn Reson Imaging* 2000;**11**:25-31.
203. Chu WJ, Kuzniecky RI, Hugg JW, Abou-Khalil B, Gilliam F, Faught E *et al.* Statistically driven identification of focal metabolic abnormalities in temporal lobe epilepsy with corrections for tissue heterogeneity using 1H spectroscopic imaging. *Magn Reson Med* 2000;**43**:359-67.
204. Hetherington H, Kuzniecky R, Pan J, Mason G, Morawetz R, Harris C *et al.* Proton nuclear magnetic resonance spectroscopic imaging of human temporal lobe epilepsy at 4.1 T. *Ann Neurol* 1995;**38**:396-404.
205. Kuzniecky R, Hugg JW, Hetherington H, Butterworth E, Bilir E, Faught E *et al.* Relative utility of 1H spectroscopic imaging and hippocampal volumetry in the lateralization of mesial temporal lobe epilepsy. *Neurology* 1998;**51**:66-71.
206. Namer IJ, Bolo NR, Sellal F, Nguyen VH, Nedelec JF, Hirsch E *et al.* Combined measurements of hippocampal N-acetyl-aspartate and T2 relaxation time in the evaluation of mesial temporal lobe epilepsy: correlation with clinical severity and memory performances. *Epilepsia* 1999;**40**:1424-32.
207. Capizzano AA, Vermathen P, Laxer KD, Matson GB, Maudsley AA, Soher BJ *et al.* Multisection proton MR spectroscopy for mesial temporal lobe epilepsy. *Am J Neuroradiol.* 2002;**23**:1359-68.
208. Li LM, Cendes F, Antel SB, Andermann F, Serles W, Dubeau F *et al.* Prognostic value of proton magnetic resonance spectroscopic imaging for surgical outcome in patients with intractable temporal lobe epilepsy and bilateral hippocampal atrophy. *Ann Neurol* 2000;**47**:195-200.
209. Chu WJ, Hetherington HP, Kuzniecky RI, Simor T, Mason GF, Elgavish GA. Lateralization of human temporal lobe epilepsy by 31P NMR spectroscopic imaging at 4.1 T. *Neurology* 1998;**51**:472-9.
210. Williamson PD, French JA, Thadani VM, Kim JH, Novelly RA, Spencer SS *et al.* Characteristics of medial temporal lobe epilepsy: II. Interictal and ictal scalp electroencephalography, neuropsychological testing, neuroimaging, surgical results, and pathology. *Ann Neurol* 1993;**34**:781-7.
211. Sadler RM, Blume WT. Significance of bisynchronous spike-waves in patients with temporal lobe spikes. *Epilepsia* 1989;**30**:143-6.
212. Spencer SS, McCarthy G, Spencer DD. Diagnosis of medial temporal lobe seizure onset: relative specificity and sensitivity of quantitative MRI. *Neurology* 1993;**43**:2117-24.
213. Le Van QM, Adam C, Martinerie J, Baulac M, Clemenceau S, Varela F. Spatio-temporal characterizations of non-linear changes in intracranial activities prior to human temporal lobe seizures. *Eur J Neurosci.* 2000;**12**:2124-34.
214. Baumgartner C, Pataraia E, Lindinger G, Deecke L. Neuromagnetic recordings in temporal lobe epilepsy. *J Clin Neurophysiol.* 2000;**17**:177-89.
215. Meyer MA, Zimmerman AW, Miller CA. Temporal lobe epilepsy presenting as panic attacks: detection of interictal hypometabolism with positron emission tomography. *J Neuroimaging* 2000;**10**:120-2.
216. Lin YY, Su MS, Yiu CH, Shih YH, Yen DJ, Kwan SY *et al.* Relationship between mesial temporal seizure focus and elevated serum prolactin in temporal lobe epilepsy. *Neurology* 1997;**49**:528-32.
217. Trenerry MR, Jack CR, Jr., Sharbrough FW, Cascino GD, Hirschorn KA, Marsh WR *et al.* Quantitative MRI hippocampal volumes: association with onset and duration of epilepsy, and febrile convulsions in temporal lobectomy patients. *Epilepsy Res* 1993;**15**:247-52.
218. Miller SP, Li LM, Cendes F, Caramanos Z, Rosenblatt B, Shevell MI *et al.* Neuronal dysfunction in children with newly diagnosed temporal lobe epilepsy. *Pediatr Neurol* 2000;**22**:281-6.
219. Engel J, Jr. Introduction to temporal lobe epilepsy. *Epilepsy Res* 1996;**26**:141-50.
220. Engel J, Jr. Clinical evidence for the progressive nature of epilepsy. *Epilepsy Res Suppl* 1996;**12**:9-20.
221. Blume WT,.Hwang PA. Pediatric candidates for temporal lobe epilepsy surgery. *Can J Neurol Sci.* 2000;**27 Suppl 1**:S14-S19.
222. Polkey CE. Temporal lobe resections. In Oxbury JM, Polkey CE, Duchowny M, eds. *Intractable focal epilepsy*, pp 667-95. London: W.B.Saunders, 2000.
223. Engel J, Jr. The timing of surgical intervention for mesial temporal lobe epilepsy: a plan for a randomized clinical trial. *Arch Neurol* 1999;**56**:1338-41.
224. Polkey CE. Surgical treatment of epilepsy. *Lancet* 1990;**336**: 553-5.
225. Hennessy MJ, Elwes RD, Rabe-Hesketh S, Binnie CD, Polkey CE. Prognostic factors in the surgical treatment of medically intractable epilepsy associated with mesial temporal sclerosis. *Acta Neurol Scand.* 2001;**103**:344-50.
226. Hennessy MJ, Langan Y, Elwes RD, Binnie CD, Polkey CE, Nashef L. A study of mortality after temporal lobe epilepsy surgery. *Neurology* 1999;**53**:1276-83.
227. McKhann GM, Schoenfeld-McNeill J, Born DE, Haglund MM, Ojemann GA. Intraoperative hippocampal electrocorticography to predict the extent of hippocampal resection in temporal lobe epilepsy surgery. *J Neurosurg.* 2000;**93**:44-52.
228. Mizrahi EM, Kellaway P, Grossman RG, Rutecki PA, Armstrong D, Rettig G *et al.* Anterior temporal lobectomy and medically refractory temporal lobe epilepsy of childhood. *Epilepsia* 1990;**31**:302-12.
229. Falconer MA. Discussion on the surgery of temporal lobe epilepsy:surgical and pathological aspects. *Proc Royal Soc Medicine* 1953;**44**:971-5.
230. Salanova V, Morris HH, Van Ness P, Kotagal P, Wyllie E, Luders H. Frontal lobe seizures: electroclinical syndromes. *Epilepsia* 1995;**36**:16-24.
231. Chauvel P, Delgado-Escueta AV, Halgren E, Bancaud J. Frontal lobe seizures and epilepsies. *Adv Neurol* 1992;1-750.
232. Bancaud J,.Talairach J. Clinical semiology of frontal lobe seizures. *Adv Neurol* 1992;**57**:3-58.
233. Jasper H, Riggio S, Goldman-Rakie P. Epilepsy and the functional anatomy of the frontal lobe. New York:Raven Press,1995.
234. Chauvel P, Kliemann F, Vignal JP, Chodkiewicz JP, Talairach J, Bancaud J. The clinical signs and symptoms of frontal lobe seizures. Phenomenology and classification. *Adv Neurol* 1995;**66**:115-25.
235. Williamson PD. Frontal lobe epilepsy. Some clinical characteristics. *Adv Neurol* 1995;**66**:127-50.
236. Kotagal P,.Arunkumar GS. Lateral frontal lobe seizures. *Epilepsia* 1998;**39 Suppl 4**:S62-S68.
237. Niedermeyer E. Frontal lobe epilepsy: the next frontier. *Clin Electroencephalogr.* 1998;**29**:163-9.
238. Bartolomei F, Chauvel P. Seizure symptoms and cerebral localization:frontal lobe and rolandic seizures. In Oxbury JM, Polkey CE, Duchowny M, eds. *Intractable focal epilepsy*, pp 55-62. London: W.B.Saunders, 2000.
239. Blume WT, Ociepa D, Kander V. Frontal lobe seizure propagation: scalp and subdural EEG studies. *Epilepsia* 2001;**42**:491-503.
240. Sinclair DB, Wheatley M, Snyder T. Frontal lobe epilepsy in childhood. *Pediatr Neurol.* 2004;**30**:169-76.

241. Goldman-Rakie, P. Anatomical and functional circuits in prefrontal cortex of non-human primates. Relevance to epilepsy. *Adv Neurol* 1995;**66:** 51-65.

242. Rasmussen T. Characteristics of a pure culture of frontal lobe epilepsy. *Epilepsia* 1983;**24**:482-93.

243. Manford M, Hart YM, Sander JW, Shorvon SD. National General Practice Study of Epilepsy (NGPSE): partial seizure patterns in a general population. *Neurology* 1992;**42**:1911-7.

244. Laich E, Kuzniecky R, Mountz J, Liu HG, Gilliam F, Bebin M *et al.* Supplementary sensorimotor area epilepsy. Seizure localization, cortical propagation and subcortical activation pathways using ictal SPECT. *Brain* 1997;**120**:855-64.

245. Baumgartner C, Flint R, Tuxhorn I, Van Ness PC, Kosalko J, Olbrich A *et al.* Supplementary motor area seizures: propagation pathways as studied with invasive recordings. *Neurology* 1996;**46**:508-14.

246. King DW,.Smith JR. Supplementary sensorimotor area epilepsy in adults. *Adv Neurol* 1996;**70**:285-91.

247. Spencer DD, Schumacher J. Surgical management of patients with intractable supplementary motor area seizures. The Yale experience. *Adv Neurol* 1996;**70**:445-50.

248. Connolly MB, Langill L, Wong PK, Farrell K. Seizures involving the supplementary sensorimotor area in children: a video-EEG analysis. *Epilepsia* 1995;**36**:1025-32.

249. So NK. Supplementary motor area epilepsy:the clinical syndrome. In Wolf P, ed. *Epileptic seizures and syndromes*, pp 299-317. London: John Libbey & Company Ltd, 1994.

250. Holthausen H, Hoppe M. Hypermotor seizures. In Luders HO, Noachtar S, eds. *Epileptic seizures. Pathophysiology and clinical semiology*, pp 439-48. New York: Churchill Livingstone, 2000.

251. Penfield W. The supplementary motor area in the cerebral cortex of man. *Arch Psychiatr.*1950;**185**: 670-4.

252. Luders HO, Noachtar S, Burgess RC. Semiologic classification of epileptic seizures. In Luders HO, Noachtar S, eds. *Epileptic seizures. Pathophysiology and clinical semiology*, pp 263-85. New York: Churchill Livingstone, 2000.

253. Marchesi GF, Macchi G, Cianchetti C, Chinzari P. Supplementary motor areas in the cat: electrophysiological studies of the suprasylvian and ectosylvian regions. *Boll Soc Ital Biol Sper.* 1972;**48**:70-4.

254. Van Ness PC, Bleasel A, Tuxhorn I. Supplementary motor seizures: localization of the epileptogenic zone. In Wolf P, ed. *Epileptic seizures and syndromes*, pp 319-30. London: John Libbey & Company Ltd, 1994.

255. Bancaud J. Kojewnikow's syndrome (epilepsia partialis continua) in children. In Roger J, Bureau M, Dravet C, Dreifuss FE, Perret A, Wolf P, eds. *Epileptic syndromes in infancy, childhood and adolescence*, pp 363-74. London: John Libbey, 1992.

256. Foerster O, Penfield W. The structural basis of traumatic epilepsy and results of radical operation. *Assoc Res Nev Ment Dis* 1929; **7**: 569-91.

257. Gastaut H, Jasper H, Bancaud J, Waltregny A, eds. The physiopathogenesis of the epilepsies. Springfield,Illinois: Charles C Thomas, 1969.

258. Bancaud J. Physiopathogenesis of generalised epilepsies of organic nature (stereo-electroencephalographic study). In Gastaut H, Jasper H, Bancaud J, Waltregny A, eds. *The physiopathogenesis of the epilepsies*, pp 158-85. Springfield: Charles C Thomas, 1969.

259. Quesney LF, Constain M, Rasmussen T. Seizures from the dorsolateral frontal lobe. *Adv Neurol* 1992;**57**:233-43.

260. Geier S, Bancaud J, Talairach J, Bonis A, Szikla G, Enjelvin M. The seizures of frontal lobe epilepsy. A study of clinical manifestations. *Neurology* 1977;**27**:951-8.

261. Chauvel P, Bancaud J. The spectrum of frontal lobe seizures:with a note of frontal lobe syndromatology. In Wolf P, ed. *Epileptic seizures and syndromes*, pp 331-4. London: John Libbey & Company Ltd, 1994.

262. Sartori E, Biraben A, Taussig D, Bernard AM, Scarabin JM. Gelastic seizures: video-EEG and scintigraphic analysis of a case with a frontal focus; review of the literature and pathophysiological hypotheses. *Epilep Disord.* 1999;**1**:221-8.

263. Janszky J, Jokeit H, Schulz R, Hoppe M, Ebner A. EEG predicts surgical outcome in lesional frontal lobe epilepsy. *Neurology* 2000;**54**:1470-6.

264. Genow A, Hummel C, Scheler G, Hopfengartner R, Kaltenhauser M, Buchfelder M *et al.* Epilepsy surgery, resection volume and MSI localization in lesional frontal lobe epilepsy. *Neuroimage.* 2004;**21**:444-9.

265. Engel J, Jr., Henry TR, Swartz BE. Positron emission tomography in frontal lobe epilepsy. *Adv.Neurol* 1995;**66**:223-38.

266. Czapinski P,Terczynski A. Intravenous valproic acid administration in status epilepticus. *Neurol Neurochir Pol.* 1998;**32**:11-22.

267. Hopkins H. The time of appearance of epileptic seizures in relation to age, duration and type of the syndrome. *J Nerv Ment Dis* 1933;**77**:153-62.

268. Ferri R, Stam CJ, Lanuzza B, Cosentino FI, Elia M, Musumeci SA *et al.* Different EEG frequency band synchronization during nocturnal frontal lobe seizures. *Clin Neurophysiol.* 2004;**115**:1202-11.

269. Allen PJ, Fish DR, Smith SJ. Very high-frequency rhythmic activity during SEEG suppression in frontal lobe epilepsy. *Electroencephalogr Clin Neurophysiol.* 1992;**82**:155-9.

270. Bautista RE, Spencer DD, Spencer SS. EEG findings in frontal lobe epilepsies. *Neurology* 1998;**50**:1765-71.

271. Williamson A, Spencer SS, Spencer DD. Depth electrode studies and intracellular dentate granule cell recordings in temporal lobe epilepsy. *Ann Neurol* 1995;**38**:778-87.

272. Fahn S. The early history of paroxysmal dyskinesias. *Adv Neurol.* 2002;**89**:377-85.

273. Jankovic J, Demirkiran M. Classification of paroxysmal dyskinesias and ataxias. *Adv Neurol.* 2002;**89**:387-400.

274. Guerrini R. Idiopathic epilepsy and paroxysmal dyskinesia. *Epilepsia* 2001;**42 Suppl 3**:36-41.

275. LeWitt PA. Psychogenic movement disorders. In Gilman S, ed. *Neurobase*, San Diego SA: Arbor Publishing Corp, 2000.

276. Matsuo H, Kamakura K, Matsushita S, Ohmori T, Okano M, Tadano Y *et al.* Mutational analysis of the anion exchanger 3 gene in familial paroxysmal dystonic choreoathetosis linked to chromosome 2q. *Am J Med Genet.* 1999;**88**:733-7.

277. Houser MK, Soland VL, Bhatia KP, Quinn NP, Marsden CD. Paroxysmal kinesigenic choreoathetosis: a report of 26 patients. *J Neurol* 1999;**246**:120-6.

278. Sadamatsu M, Masui A, Sakai T, Kunugi H, Nanko S, Kato N. Familial paroxysmal kinesigenic choreoathetosis: an electrophysiologic and genotypic analysis. *Epilepsia* 1999;**40**: 942-9.

279. Tomita H, Nagamitsu S, Wakui K, Fukushima Y, Yamada K, Sadamatsu M *et al.* Paroxysmal kinesigenic choreoathetosis locus maps to chromosome 16p11.2- q12.1. *Am J Hum Genet.* 1999;**65**:1688-97.

280. Escayg A, De Waard M, Lee DD, Bichet D, Wolf P, Mayer T *et al.* Coding and noncoding variation of the human calcium-channel beta4- subunit gene CACNB4 in patients with idiopathic generalized epilepsy and episodic ataxia. *Am.J Hum Genet.* 2000;**66**:1531-9.

281. Boland LM, Price DL, Jackson KA. Episodic ataxia/myokymia mutations functionally expressed in the Shaker potassium channel. *Neuroscience* 1999;**91**:1557-64.

282. Denier C, Ducros A, Vahedi K, Joutel A, Thierry P, Ritz A *et al.* High prevalence of CACNA1A truncations and broader clinical spectrum in episodic ataxia type 2. *Neurology* 1999;**52**:1816-21.

283. Zuberi SM, Eunson LH, Spauschus A, De Silva R, Tolmie J, Wood NW *et al.* A novel mutation in the human voltage-gated potassium channel gene (Kv1.1) associates with episodic ataxia type 1 and sometimes with partial epilepsy. *Brain* 1999;**122**: 817-25.

284. Lance JW. Familial paroxysmal dystonic choreoathetosis and its differentiation from related syndromes. *Ann Neurol* 1977;**2**:285-93.

285. Hayashi R, Hanyu N, Yahikozawa H, Yanagisawa N. Ictal muscle discharge pattern and SPECT in paroxysmal kinesigenic choreoathetosis. *Electromyogr Clin Neurophysiol.* 1997;**37**:89-94.

286. Wein T, Andermann F, Silver K, Dubeau F, Andermann E, Rourke-Frew F *et al.* Exquisite sensitivity of paroxysmal kinesigenic choreoathetosis to carbamazepine. *Neurology* 1996;**47**:1104-6.

287. Hamada Y, Hattori H, Okuno T. Eleven cases of paroxysmal kinesigenic choreoathetosis; correlation with benign infantile convulsions. *No To Hattatsu* 1998;**30**:483-8.

288. Ferrie CD, Giannakodimos S, Robinson RO, Panayiotopoulos CP. Symptomatic typical absence seizures. In Duncan JS, Panayiotopoulos CP, eds. *Typical absences and related epileptic syndromes*, pp 241-52. London: Churchill Communications Europe, 1995.

289. Kudo T, Sato K, Yagi K, Seino M. Can absence status epilepticus be of frontal lobe origin? *Act Neurol Scand* 1995;**92**:472-7.

290. Pavone A,.Niedermeyer E. Absence seizures and the frontal lobe. *Clin Electroencephalogr.* 2000;**31**:153-6.
291. Olivier A. Surgery of frontal lobe epilepsy. *Adv Neurol* 1995;**66**:321-48.
292. Obeso JA, Rothwell JC, Marsden CD. The spectrum of cortical myoclonus. From focal reflex jerks to spontaneous motor epilepsy. *Brain* 1985;**108**:193-24.
293. Bancauc J. Kojewnikow's syndrome (epilepsia partialis continua) in children :Up-date. In Roger J, Bureau M, Dravet C, Dreifuss FE, Perret A, Wolf P, eds. *Epileptic syndromes in infancy, childhood and adolescence*, pp 374-9. London: John Libbey, 1992.
294. Schomer DL. Focal status epilepticus and epilepsia partialis continua in adults and children. *Epilepsia* 1993;**34 Suppl 1**: S29-36.
295. Cockerell OC, Rothwell J, Thompson PD, Marsden CD, Shorvon SD. Clinical and physiological features of epilepsia partialis continua. Cases ascertained in the UK. *Brain* 1996;**119**:393-407.
296. Biraben A, Chauvel P. Epilepsia Partialis Continua. In Engel JJ, Pedley TA, eds. *Epilepsy: A comprehensive Textbook*, pp 2447-53. Philadelphia: Lippincott-Raven Publishers, 1997.
297. Shigeto H, Tobimatsu S, Morioka T, Yamamoto T, Kobayashi T, Kato M. Jerk-locked back averaging and dipole source localization of magnetoencephalographic transients in a patient with epilepsia partialis continua. *Electroencephalogr Clin Neurophysiol.* 1997;**103**:440-4.
298. Molyneux PD, Barker RA, Thom M, van Paesschen W, Harkness WF, Duncan JS. Successful treatment of intractable epilepsia partialis continua with multiple subpial transections. *J Neurol Neurosurg Psychiatry* 1998;**65**:137-8.
299. Wieser HG. Epilepsia partialis continua. In Gilman S, ed. *Medlink*, San Diego SA: Arbor Publishing Corp, 2004.
300. Caraballo R, Tenembaum S, Cersosimo R, Pomata H, Medina C, Soprano AM *et al.* Rasmussen syndrome. *Rev Neurol* 1998;**26**:978-83.
301. Thomas JE, Reagan TJ, Klass DW. Epilepsia partialis continua. A review of 32 cases. *Arch Neurol* 1977;**34**:266-75.
302. Rosenbaum DH,.Rowan AJ. Unilateral truncal seizures: frontal origin. *Epilepsia* 1990;**31**:37-40.
303. Silver K, Andermann F, Meagher-Villemure K. Familial alternating epilepsia partialis continua with chronic encephalitis: another variant of Rasmussen syndrome? *Arch Neurol.* 1998;**55**:733-6.
304. Wieser HG, Graf HP, Bernoulli C, Siegfried J. Quantitative analysis of intracerebral recordings in epilepsia partialis continua. *Electroencephalogr Clin Neurophysiol.* 1978;**44**:14-22.
305. Perniola T, Sforza E, Rodriguez M, Margari L. Neurophysiological follow-up in a case of chronic progressive epilepsia partialis continua of childhood. *Ital J Neurol Sci.* 1989;**10**:369-76.
306. Velasco M, Velasco F, Alcala H, Diaz de Leon AE. Wakefulness-sleep modulation of EEG-EMG epileptiform activities: a quantitative study on a child with intractable epilepsia partialis continua. *Int J Neurosci.* 1990;**54**:325-37.
307. Ambrosetto C, Lugaresi E, Tassinari CA. The evolution of physiological sleep in states of epilepsia partialis continuans. *Electroencephalogr Clin Neurophysiol.* 1967;**23**:186-7.
308. Dereux J. Le syndrome de Kojewnikow (epilepsie partialis continue). Paris: Thesis, 1955.
309. Andermann F, Hart Y. Rasmussen's syndrome. In Gilman S, ed. *Medlink Neurology*, San Diego SA: 2004.
310. Panayiotopoulos CP, Andermann F. Kozhevnikov-Rasmussen syndrome and the new proposal on classification. *Epilepsia* 2002;**43**:948-50.
311. Adams RD, Victor M, Ropper AH. Principles of Neurology. New York: McGraw-Hill, 1997.
312. Rasmussen T. Surgery for central, parietal and occipital epilepsy. *Can J Neurol Sci.* 1991;**18**:611-6.
313. Williamson PD, Boon PA, Thadani VM, Darcey TM, Spencer DD, Spencer SS *et al.* Parietal lobe epilepsy: diagnostic considerations and results of surgery. *Ann Neurol* 1992;**31**: 193-201.
314. Cascino GD, Hulihan JF, Sharbrough FW, Kelly PJ. Parietal lobe lesional epilepsy: electroclinical correlation and operative outcome. *Epilepsia* 1993;**34**:522-7.
315. Sveinbjornsdottir S, Duncan JS. Parietal and occipital lobe epilepsy: a review. *Epilepsia* 1993;**34**:493-521.
316. Ho SS, Berkovic SF, Newton MR, Austin MC, McKay WJ, Bladin PF. Parietal lobe epilepsy: clinical features and seizure localization by ictal SPECT. *Neurology* 1994;**44**:2277-84.
317. Williamson PD. Seizures with origin in the occipital or parietal lobes. In Wolf P, ed. *Epileptic seizures and syndromes*, pp 383-90. London: John Libbey & Company Ltd, 1994.
318. Salanova V, Andermann F, Rasmussen T, Olivier A, Quesney LF. Parietal lobe epilepsy. Clinical manifestations and outcome in 82 patients treated surgically between 1929 and 1988. *Brain* 1995;**118**:607-27.
319. Salanova V, Andermann F, Rasmussen T, Olivier A, Quesney LF. Tumoural parietal lobe epilepsy. Clinical manifestations and outcome in 34 patients treated between 1934 and 1988. *Brain* 1995;**118**:1289-304.
320. Abou-Khalil B, Fakhoury T, Jennings M, Moots P, Warner J, Kessler RM. Inhibitory motor seizures: correlation with centroparietal structural and functional abnormalities. *Act Neurol Scand* 1995;**91**:103-8.
321. Olivier A, Boling W, Jr. Surgery of parietal and occipital lobe epilepsy. *Adv.Neurol* 2000;**84**:533-75.
322. Siegel AM, Williamson PD. Parietal lobe epilepsy. *Adv Neurol* 2000;**84**:189-99.
323. Kasowski HJ, Stoffman MR, Spencer SS, Spencer DD. Surgical management of parietal lobe epilepsy. *Adv Neurol.* 2003;**93**: 347-56.
324. Kim DW, Lee SK, Yun CH, Kim KK, Lee DS, Chung CK *et al.* Parietal lobe epilepsy: the semiology, yield of diagnostic workup, and surgical outcome. *Epilepsia* 2004;**45**:641-9.
325. Rasmussen T. Surgery for epilepsy arising in regions other than the temporal and frontal lobes. *Adv Neurol* 1975;**8**:207-26.
326. Tuxhorn I, Kerdar MS. Somatosensory auras. In Luders HO, Noachtar S, eds. *Epileptic seizures. Pathophysiology and clinical semiology*, pp 286-97. New York: Churchill Livingstone, 2000.
327. Siegel AM, Williamson PD, Roberts DW, Thadani VM, Darcey TM. Localized pain associated with seizures originating in the parietal lobe. *Epilepsia* 1999;**40**:845-55.
328. Panayiotopoulos CP. Benign childhood partial seizures and related epileptic syndromes. London: John Libbey & Company Ltd, 1999.
329. Blume WT, Jones DC, Young GB, Girvin JP, McLachlan RS. Seizures involving secondary sensory and related areas. *Brain* 1992;**115**:1509-20.
330. Stoffels C, Munari C, Bonis A, Bancaud J, Talairach J. Genital and sexual manifestations occurring in the course of partial seizures in man. *Rev Electroencephalogr Neurophysiol Clin* 1980;**10**:386-92.
331. Calleja J, Carpizo R, Berciano J. Orgasmic epilepsy. *Epilepsia* 1988;**29**:635-9.
332. Grand'Maison F, Reiher J, Lebel ML, Rivest J. Transient anosognosia for episodic hemiparesis: a singular manifestation of TIAs and epileptic seizures. *Can J Neurol Sci.* 1989;**16**:203-5.
333. Heilman KM, Howell GJ. Seizure-induced neglect. *J Neurol Neurosurg Psychiatry* 1980;**43**:1035-40.
334. Schwartz TH, Resor SR, Jr., De La PR, Goodman RR. Functional magnetic resonance imaging localization of ictal onset to a dysplastic cleft with simultaneous sensorimotor mapping: intraoperative electrophysiological confirmation and postoperative follow-up: technical note. *Neurosurgery* 1998;**43**:639-44.
335. Russell WR, Whitty CWM. Studies in traumatic epilepsy. 2. Focal motor and somatic sensory fits: A study of 85 cases. *J Neurol Neurosurg Psychiatr* 1953;**16**:73-97.
336. Mauguiere F, Courjon J. Somatosensory epilepsy. A review of 127 cases. *Brain* 1978;**101**:307-32.
337. Fish DR, Gloor P, Quesney FL, Olivier A. Clinical responses to electrical brain stimulation of the temporal and frontal lobes in patients with epilepsy. Pathophysiological implications. *Brain* 1993;**116**:397-414.
338. Palmini A,.Gloor P. The localizing value of auras in partial seizures: a prospective and retrospective study. *Neurology* 1992;**42**:801-8.
339. Penfield W,.Boldrey E. Somatic motor and sensory representation in the cerebral cortex of man as studied by electrical stimulation. *Brain* 1937;**60**:389-443.
340. Fujino O, Hashimoto K, Enokido H, Komatsuzaki H, Fujita T, Takaishi Y *et al.* Epileptic vertiginous seizure in a Japanese boy: a case report. *No To Hattatsu* 1996;**28**:515-9.
341. Kogeorgos J, Scott DF, Swash M. Epileptic dizziness. *B Med J* 1981;**282**:687-9.
342. Lesser RP, Lueders H, Conomy JP, Furlan AJ, Dinner DS. Sensory seizure mimicking a psychogenic seizure. *Neurology* 1983;**33**:800-2.

343. Foerster O. The cerebral cortex in man. *Lancet* 1931;**2**: 309-12.
344. Penfield W, Gage L. Cerebral localization of epileptic manifestations. *Arch Neurol Psychiatry* 1933;**30**:709-27.
345. Vignal JP, Biraben A, Chauvel PY, Reutens DC. Reflex partial seizures of sensorimotor cortex (including cortical reflex myoclonus and startle epilepsy). *Adv Neurol* 1998;**75**:207-26.
346. Van Ness PC, Lesser RP, Duchowny MS. Simple sensory seizures. In Engel JJ, Pedley TA, eds. *Epilepsy: A comprehensive textbook*, pp 533-42. 1997.
347. Reder AT,Wright FS. Epilepsy evoked by eating: the role of peripheral input. *Neurology* 1982;**32**:1065-9.
348. Sutherling WW, Hershman LM, Miller JQ, Lee SI. Seizures induced by playing music. *Neurology* 1980;**30**:1001-4.
349. Koutroumanidis M, Pearce R, Sadoh DR, Panayiotopoulos CP. Tooth brushing-induced seizures: a case report. *Epilepsia* 2001;**42**:686-8.
350. Devinsky O, Kelley K, Porter RJ, Theodore WH. Clinical and electroencephalographic features of simple partial seizures. *Neurology* 1988;**38**:1347-52.
351. Kaibara M,.Blume WT. The postictal electroencephalogram. *Electroencephalogr Clin Neurophysiol* 1988;**70**:99-104.
352. Poeck K. Differential diagnosis of "migraine accompagnee" and sensory Jacksonian seizures. *Dtsch Med Wochenschr.* 1972;**97**:637-41.
353. Andermann F, Beaumanoir A, Mira E, Roger J, Tassinari CA, eds. Occipital seizures and epilepsies in children. London: John Libbey & Company Ltd, 1993.
354. Salanova V, Andermann F, Rasmussen TB. Occipital lobe epilesy. In Wyllie E, ed. *The treatment of epilepsy*, pp 533-40. Philadelphia: Lee & Febiger, 1993.
355. Kuzniecky R, Gilliam F, Morawetz R, Faught E, Palmer C, Black L. Occipital lobe developmental malformations and epilepsy: clinical spectrum, treatment, and outcome. *Epilepsia* 1997;**38**:175-81.
356. Kuzniecky R. Symptomatic occipital lobe epilepsy. *Epilepsia* 1998;**39 Suppl 4**:S24-31.
357. Panayiotopoulos CP. Visual phenomena and headache in occipital epilepsy: a review, a systematic study and differentiation from migraine. *Epilep Disord.* 1999;**1**:205-16.
358. Taylor I, Scheffer IE, Berkovic SF. Occipital epilepsies: identification of specific and newly recognized syndromes. *Brain* 2003;**126**:753-69.
359. Panayiotopoulos CP. Occipital seizures and related epileptic syndromes. In Panayiotopoulos CP, ed. *Benign childhood partial seizures and related epileptic syndromes*, pp 101-228. London: John Libbey & Company Ltd, 1999.
360. Panayiotopoulos CP. Idiopathic photosensitive occipital spikes seizures. In Panayiotopoulos CP, ed. *Benign childhood partial seizures and related epileptic syndromes*, pp 241-55. London: John Libbey & Company Ltd, 1999.
361. Panayiotopoulos CP. Basilar migraine: a review. In Panayiotopoulos CP, ed. *Benign childhood partial seizures and related epileptic syndromes*, pp 303-8. London: John Libbey & Company Ltd, 1999.
362. Manford M, Hart YM, Sander JW, Shorvon SD. The National General Practice Study of Epilepsy. The syndromic classification of the International League Against Epilepsy applied to epilepsy in a general population. *Arch Neurol.* 1992;**49**:801-8.
363. Panayiotopoulos CP. Elementary visual hallucinations in migraine and epilepsy. *J Neurol Neurosurg.Psychiatry* 1994;**57**:1371-4.
364. Panayiotopoulos CP. Elementary visual hallucinations, blindness, and headache in idiopathic occipital epilepsy: differentiation from migraine. *J Neurol Neurosurg Psychiatry* 1999;**66**:536-40.
365. Panayiotopoulos CP. Idiopathic childhood occipital epilepsies. In Roger J, Bureau M, Dravet C, Genton P, Tassinari CA, Wolf P, eds. *Epileptic syndromes in infancy, childhood and adolescence (3rd edn)*, pp 203-27. London: John Libbey & Co Ltd, 2002.
366. Panayiotopoulos CP. Differentiating occipital epilepsies from migraine with aura, acephalgic migraine and basilar migraine. In Panayiotopoulos CP, ed. *Benign childhood partial seizures and related epileptic syndromes*, pp 281-302. London: John Libbey & Company Ltd, 1999.
367. Russell WR,Whitty CWM. Studies in traumatic epilepsy 3. Visual fits. *J Neurol Neurosurg Psychiatr* 1955;**18**:79-96.
368. Ludwig BI, Marsan CA. Clinical ictal patterns in epileptic patients with occipital electroencephalographic foci. *Neurology* 1975;**25**:463-71.
369. Penfield W, Rasmussen T. The cerebral cortex of man:A clinical study of localisation of function. New York: The Macmillan Company, 1957.
370. Babb TL, Halgren E, Wilson C, Engel J, Crandall P. Neuronal firing patterns during the spread of an occipital lobe seizure to the temporal lobes in man. *Electroencephalogr Clin Neurophysiol* 1981;**51**:104-7.
371. Guerrini R, Dravet C, Genton P, Bureau M, Bonanni P, Ferrari AR *et al.* Idiopathic photosensitive occipital lobe epilepsy. *Epilepsia* 1995;**36**:883-91.
372. Walker MC, Smith SJ, Sisodiya SM, Shorvon SD. Case of simple partial status epilepticus in occipital lobe epilepsy misdiagnosed as migraine: clinical, electrophysiological, and magnetic resonance imaging characteristics. *Epilepsia* 1995;**36**:1233-6.
373. Thom M, Moran NF, Plant GT, Stevens JM, Scaravilli F. Cortical dysplasia with angiodysgenesis and chronic inflammation in multifocal partial epilepsy. *Neurology* 1999;**52**:654-7.
374. Maillard L, Vignal JP, Anxionnat R, TaillandierVespignani L. Semiologic value of ictal autoscopy. *Epilepsia* 2004;**45**:391-4.
375. Blanke O, Landis T, Spinelli L, Seeck M. Out-of-body experience and autoscopy of neurological origin. *Brain* 2004;**127**:243-58.
376. Herschel JFW. Familiar lectures on scientific aspects. pp 406L ondon: Alexander Straham, 1866.
377. Plant GT. The fortification spectra of migraine. *B MJ* 1986; **293**:1613-7.
378. Gowers W R. Subjective sensations of sight and sound; Abiotrophy and other lectures. Philadelphia; P.Blackinston's Son & Co, 1904.
379. Schmidt EM, Bak MJ, Hambrecht FT, Kufta CV, O'Rourke DK, Vallabhanath *et al.* Feasibility of a visual prosthesis for the blind based on intracortical microstimulation of the visual cortex. *Brain* 1996;**119**:507-22.
380. Airy H. On a distinct form of transient hemiopsia. *Philos Trans R Soc Lond* 1870;**160**:247-70.
381. Bien CG, Benninger FO, Urbach H, Schramm J, Kurthen M, Elger CE. Localizing value of epileptic visual auras. *Brain* 2000;**123**:244-53.
382. Maillard L, Vignal JP, Anxionnat R, TaillandierVespignani L. Semiologic value of ictal autoscopy. *Epilepsia* 2004;**45**:391-4.
383. Blanke O, Landis T, Spinelli L, Seeck M. Out-of-body experience and autoscopy of neurological origin. *Brain* 2004;**127**:243-58.
384. Critchley M. Butterworths Medical Dictionary. London:Butterworth & Co (Publishers) Ltd, 1986.
385. Shahar E, Barak S. Favorable outcome of epileptic blindness in children. *J Child Neurol.* 2003;**18**:12-6.
386. Panayiotopoulos CP. Basilar migraine? Seizures, and severe epileptic EEG abnormalities. *Neurology* 1980;**30**:1122-5.
387. Ayala G. Status epilepticus amauroticus. *Boll Accad Med Roma* 1929;**55**:288-90.
388. Barry E, Sussman NM, Bosley TM, Harner RN. Ictal blindness and status epilepticus amauroticus. *Epilepsia* 1985;**26**:577-84.
389. Sawchuk KS, Churchill S, Feldman E, Drury I. Status epilepticus amauroticus. *Neurology* 1997;**49**:1467-9.
390. Williamson PD, Engel JJr. Complex partial seizures. In Engel JJr, Pedley TA, eds. *Epilepsy: A comprehensive textbook*, pp 557-66. Philadelphia: Lippincott-Raven Publishers, 1997.
391. Ito M, Adachi N, Nakamura F, Koyama T, Okamura T, Kato M *et al.* Multi-center study on post-ictal headache in patients with localization-related epilepsy. *Psychiatry Clin Neurosci.* 2003;**57**:385-9.
392. Ito M, Adachi N, Nakamura F, Koyama T, Okamura T, Kato M *et al.* Characteristics of postictal headache in patients with partial epilepsy. *Cephalalgia* 2004;**24**:23-8.
393. Blau JN. Classical migraine: symptoms between visual aura and headache onset. *Lancet* 1992;**340**: 355-6.
394. Plazzi G, Tinuper P, Cerullo A, Provini F, Lugaresi E. Occipital lobe epilepsy: a chronic condition related to transient occipital lobe involvement in eclampsia. *Epilepsia* 1994;**35**:644-7.
395. Gobbi G, Bertani G, Italian Working Group on Coeliac Disease and Epilepsy. Coeliac disease and epilepsy. In Gobbi G, Andermann F, Naccarato S, Banchini G, eds. *Epilepsy and other neurological disorders in coeliac disease*, pp 65-79. London: John Libbey & Company Ltd, 1997.
396. Berkovic SF. Progressive myoclonuc epilepsies. In Engel JJr, Pedley TA, eds. *Epilepsy: A comprehensive textbook*, pp 2455-68. Philadelphia: Lippincott-Raven Publishers, 1997.

397. Roger J, Genton P, Bureau M, Dravet C. Progressive myoclonus epilepsies in childhood and adolescence. In Roger J, Bureau M, Dravet C, Dreifuss FE, Perret A, Wolf P, eds. *Epileptic syndromes in childhood and adolescence*, pp 381-400. London: John Libbey & Company Ltd, 1992.
398. Minassian BA. Lafora's disease: towards a clinical, pathologic, and molecular synthesis. *Pediatr Neurol.* 2001;**25**:21-9.
399. Hirano M, DiMauro S. Primary Mitochondrial Diseases. In Engel JJr, Pedley TA, eds. *Epilepsy. A comprehensive textbook*, pp 2563-70. Philadelphia: Lippincott-Raven, 1997.
400. Gobbi, G, Andermann, F, Naccarato, S, and Banchini, G. eds. Epilepsy and other neurological disorders in coeliac disease. London;John Libbey & Company Ltd, 1997.
401. Lawn N, Laich E, Ho S, Martin R, Faught E, Knowlton R *et al.* Eclampsia, hippocampal sclerosis, and temporal lobe epilepsy: accident or association? *Neurology* 2004;**62**:1352-6.
402. Minassian BA. Progressive myoclonus epilepsy with polyglucosan bodies: Lafora disease. *Adv Neurol* 2002;**89**:199-210.
403. Salanova V, Andermann F, Olivier A, Rasmussen T, Quesney LF. Occipital lobe epilepsy: electroclinical manifestations, electrocorticography, cortical stimulation and outcome in 42 patients treated between 1930 and 1991. Surgery of occipital lobe epilepsy. *Brain* 1992;**115**:1655-80.
404. Welch KM. Pathogenesis of migraine. *Semin Neurol* 1997;**17**:335-41.
405. Ogunyemi A, Adams D. Migraine-like symptoms triggered by occipital lobe seizures: response to sumatriptan. *Can J Neurol Sci.* 1998;**25**:151-3.
406. Panayiotopoulos CP. Difficulties in differentiating migraine and epilepsy based on clinical and EEG findings. In Andermann F, Lugaresi E, eds. *Migraine and epilepsy*, pp 31-46. Boston: Butterworths, 1987.
407. Andermann F, Zifkin B. The benign occipital epilepsies of childhood: an overview of the idiopathic syndromes and of the relationship to migraine. *Epilepsia* 1998;**39 Suppl 4**:S9-23.
408. Hart YM, Andermann F. Migraine aura, seizures, and temporal lobe epilepsy. *Adv Neurol* 1999;**81**:145-52.
409. Andermann F. Migraine and the benign partial epilepsies of childhood:evidence for an association. *Epilep Disord.* 2000;**2 (Suppl 1)**:S37-S39.
410. Kim SK, Lee DS, Lee SK, Kim YK, Kang KW, Chung CK *et al.* Diagnostic performance of [18F]FDG-PET and ictal [99mTc]-HMPAO SPECT in occipital lobe epilepsy. *Epilepsia* 2001;**42**:1531-40.
411. Russell MB, Olesen J. A nosographic analysis of the migraine aura in a general population. *Brain* 1996;**119**:355-61.
412. Bickerstaff ER. Basilar artery migraine. *Lancet* 1961;**i**:15-7.
413. Bickerstaff ER. Impairment of consciousness in migraine. *Lancet* 1961;**ii**:1057-9.
414. Marks DA, Ehrenberg BL. Migraine-related seizures in adults with epiiepsy, with EEG correlation. *Neurology* 1993;**43**:2476-83.
415. Terzano MG, Parrino L, Pietrini V, Galli L. Migraine-epilepsy syndrome:intercalated seizures in benign occipital epilepsy. In Andermann F, Beaumanoir A, Mira L, Roger J, Tassinari CA, eds. *Occipital seizures and epilepsies in children*, pp 93-9. London: John Libbey & Company Ltd, 1993.
416. Slatter KH. Some clinical and EEG findings in patients with migraine. *Brain* 1968;**91**:85-98.
417. Barlow CF. Headaches and migraine in childhood. Oxford; Blackwell Scientific Publications Ltd, 1984.
418. Camfield PR, Metrakos K, Andermann F. Basilar migraine, seizures, and severe epileptiform EEG abnormalities. *Neurology* 1978;**28**:584-8.
419. De Romanis F, Buzzi MG, Assenza S, Brusa L, Cerbo R. Basilar migraine with electroencephalographic findings of occipital spike-wave complexes: a long-term study in seven children. *Cephalalgia* 1993;**13**:192-6.
420. Panayiotopoulos CP. Basilar migraine. *Neurology* 1991;**41**:1707.
421. Williamson PD, Thadani VM, Darcey TM, Spencer DD, Spencer SS, Mattson *et al.* Occipital lobe epilepsy: clinical characteristics, seizure spread patterns, and results of surgery. *Ann Neurol* 1992;**31**:3-13.
422. Kramer G. The limitations of antiepileptic drug monotherapy. *Epilepsia* 1997;**38 Suppl 5**:S9-S13.
423. Cockerell OC, Johnson AL, Sander JW, Shorvon SD. Prognosis of epilepsy: a review and further analysis of the first nine years of the British National General Practice Study of Epilepsy, a prospective population-based study. *Epilepsia* 1997;**38**:31-46.
424. Mattson RH, Cramer JA, Collins JF, Smith DB, Delgado-Escueta AV, Browne TR *et al.* Comparison of carbamazepine, phenobarbital, phenytoin, and primidone in partial and secondarily generalized tonic-clonic seizures. *N Engl J Med* 1985;**313**:145-51.
425. Wyllie E, ed. The treatment of epilepsy. Principles and Practice. 1993.
426. Shorvon S, Dreifuss FE, Fish D, Thomas D, eds. The treatment of epilepsy. Oxford: Blackwell Science Ltd, 1996.
427. Oxbury JM, Polkey CE, Duchowny M, (eds. Intractable focal epilepsy. London: W.B.Saunders, 2000.
428. Shorvon, S. Handbook of epilepsy treatment. Oxford, Blackwell Science, 2000.
429. Pellock JM, Dodson WE, Bourgeois BFDe. Pediatric epilepsy. New York: Demos, 2001.
430. Shorvon S, Perucca E, Fish D, Dodson E. The treatment of epilepsy (2nd edition). In Shorvon S, Perucca E, Fish D, Dodson E, eds. *The treatment of epilepsy (2nd edition)*, pp 1-913. Oxford: Blackwell Publishing, 2004.
431. Leach JP, Marson T, Chadwick D. New antiepileptic drugs: revolution or marketing spin? *Practical Neurology* 2001;**1**:70-81.
432. Marson AG, Chadwick DW. New drug treatments for epilepsy. *J Neurol Neurosurg Psychiatry* 2001;**70**:143-7.
433. Marson AG, Hutton JL, Leach JP, Castillo S, Schmidt D, White S *et al.* Levetiracetam, oxcarbazepine, remacemide and zonisamide for drug resistant localization-related epilepsy: a systematic review. *Epilepsy Res.* 2001;**46**:259-70.
434. Baulac M. New antiepileptic drugs: new therapeutic options. *Rev Neurol (Paris)* 2002;**158**:46-54.
435. Bialer M, Walker MC, Sander JW. Pros and cons for the development of new antiepileptic drugs. *CNS.Drugs* 2002;**16**:285-9.
436. Bialer M. New antiepileptic drugs currently in clinical trials: is there a strategy in their development? *Ther Drug Monit.* 2002;**24**:85-90.
437. Brunbech L, Sabers A. Effect of antiepileptic drugs on cognitive function in individuals with epilepsy: a comparative review of newer versus older agents. *Drugs* 2002;**62**:593-604.
438. Duncan JS. The promise of new antiepileptic drugs. *Br J Clin Pharmacol.* 2002;**53**:123-31.
439. Hachad H, Ragueneau-Majlessi I, Levy RH. New antiepileptic drugs: review on drug interactions. *Ther Drug Monit.* 2002;**24**:91-103.
440. Leppik IE. Three new drugs for epilepsy: levetiracetam, oxcarbazepine, and zonisamide. *J Child Neurol.* 2002;**17 Suppl 1**:S53-S57.
441. Perucca E. Marketed new antiepileptic drugs: are they better than old-generation agents? *Ther Drug Monit.* 2002;**24**:74-80.
442. Schwabe SK. Challenges in the clinical development of new antiepileptic drugs. *Ther Drug Monit.* 2002;**24**:81-4.
443. Temple RJ,.Himmel MH. Safety of newly approved drugs: implications for prescribing. *JAMA* 2002;**287**:2273-5.
444. Weinstein SL, Conry J. New antiepileptic drugs: comparative studies of efficacy and cognition. *Curr Neurol Neurosci Rep.* 2002;**2**:134-41.
445. Bialer M, Johannessen SI, Kupferberg HJ, Levy RH, Loiseau P, Perucca E. Progress report on new antiepileptic drugs: a summary of the Fifth Eilat Conference (EILAT V). *Epilepsy Res.* 2001;**43**:11-58.
446. Smith D, Chadwick D. The management of epilepsy. *J Neurol Neurosurg Psychiatry* 2001;**70 Suppl 2**:II15-II21.
447. Walker MC, Sander JW. The impact of new antiepileptic drugs on the prognosis of epilepsy: seizure freedom should be the ultimate goal. *Neurology* 1996;**46**:912-4.
448. Walker MC, Sander JW. Difficulties in extrapolating from clinical trial data to clinical practice: the case of antiepileptic drugs. *Neurology* 1997;**49**:333-7.
449. Mattson RH, Cramer JA, Collins JF. A comparison of valproate with carbamazepine for the treatment of complex partial seizures and secondarily generalized tonic- clonic seizures in adults. The Department of Veterans Affairs Epilepsy Cooperative Study No. 264 Group. *NEJM* 1992;**327**:765-71.
450. Marson AG, Williamson PR, Clough H, Hutton JL, Chadwick DW. Carbamazepine versus Valproate Monotherapy for Epilepsy: A Meta-analysis. *Epilepsia* 2002;**43**:505-13.
451. Shorvon SD. The choice of drugs and approach to drug treatments in partial epilepsy. In Shorvon S, Perucca E, Fish D, Dodson E, eds. *The treatment of epilepsy (2nd edition)*, pp 317-33. Oxford: Blackwell Publishing, 2004.

452. French JA, Kanner AM, Bautista J, Abou-Khalil B, Browne T, Harden CL *et al.* Efficacy and tolerability of the new antiepileptic drugs I: treatment of new onset epilepsy: report of the Therapeutics and Technology Assessment Subcommittee and Quality Standards Subcommittee of the American Academy of Neurology and the American Epilepsy Society. *Neurology* 2004;**62**:1252-60.

453. Patsalos PN, Perucca E. Clinically important drug interactions in epilepsy: interactions between antiepileptic drugs and other drugs. *Lancet Neurol.* 2003;**2**:473-81.

454. Patsalos PN. Clinical pharmacokinetics of levetiracetam. *Clin Pharmacokinet.* 2004;**43**:707-24.

455. Lynch BA, Lambeng N, Nocka K, Kensel-Hammes P, Bajjalieh SM, Matagne A *et al.* The synaptic vesicle protein SV2A is the binding site for the antiepileptic drug levetiracetam. *Proc Natl Acad Sci.U.S.A* 2004;**101**:9861-6.

456. Tran TA, Leppik IE, Blesi K, Sathanandan ST, Remmel R. Lamotrigine clearance during pregnancy. *Neurology* 2002;**59**:251-5.

457. de Haan GJ, Edelbroek P, Segers J, Engelsman M, Lindhout D, Devile-Notschaele M *et al.* Gestation-induced changes in lamotrigine pharmacokinetics: a monotherapy study. *Neurology* 2004;**63**:571-3.

458. LaRoche SM, Helmers SL. The new antiepileptic drugs: scientific review. *JAMA* 2004;**291**:605-14.

459. Marson AG, Kadir ZA, Chadwick DW. New antiepileptic drugs: a systematic review of their efficacy and tolerability. *BMJ* 1996;**313**:1169-74.

460. Marson AG. Meta-analysis of antiepileptic drug trials. In Duncan JS, Sisodiya S, Smalls JE, eds. *Epilepsy 2001. From science to patient*, pp 317-28. Oxford: Meritus Communications, 2001.

461. Hovinga CA. Levetiracetam: a novel antiepileptic drug. *Pharmacotherapy* 2001;**21**:1375-88.

462. Cochrane AL. Effectiveness and efficiency:Random reflections on health services. Cambridge: Cambridge University Press, 1989.

463. Montenegro MA, Cendes F, Noronha AL, Mory SB, Carvalho MI, Marques LH *et al.* Efficacy of clobazam as add-on therapy in patients with refractory partial epilepsy. *Epilepsia* 2001;**42**:539-42.

464. Barcs G, Halasz P. Effectiveness and tolerance of clobazam in temporal lobe epilepsy. *Acta Neurol Scand.* 1996;**93**:88-93.

465. Sheth RD, Ronen GM, Goulden KJ, Penney S, Bodensteiner JB. Clobazam for intractable pediatric epilepsy. *J Child Neurol* 1995;**10**:205-8.

466. Singh A, Guberman AH, Boisvert D. Clobazam in long-term epilepsy treatment: sustained responders versus those developing tolerance. *Epilepsia* 1995;**36**:798-803.

467. Remy C. Clobazam in the treatment of epilepsy: a review of the literature. *Epilepsia* 1994;**35 Suppl 5**:S88-S91.

468. Schmidt D. Clobazam for treatment of intractable epilepsy: a critical assessment. *Epilepsia* 1994;**35 Suppl 5**:S92-S95.

469. Buchanan N. Clobazam in the treatment of epilepsy: prospective follow-up to 8 years. *J R Soc Med* 1993;**86**:378-80.

470. Munn R, Farrell K. Open study of clobazam in refractory epilepsy. *Pediatr Neurol* 1993;**9**:465-9.

471. Canadian Clobazam Cooperative Group. Clobazam in treatment of refractory epilepsy: the Canadian experience. A retrospective study. *Epilepsia* 1991;**32**:407-16.

472. Canadian Study Group for Childhood Epilepsy.Clobazam has equivalent efficacy to carbamazepine and phenytoin as monotherapy for childhood epilepsy. *Epilepsia* 1998;**39**:952-9.

473. Bawden HN, Camfield CS, Camfield PR, Cunningham C, Darwish H, Dooley JM *et al.* The cognitive and behavioural effects of clobazam and standard monotherapy are comparable. Canadian Study Group for Childhood Epilepsy. *Epilepsy Res* 1999;**33**:133-43.

474. Glauser TA. Oxcarbazepine in the treatment of epilepsy. *Pharmacotherapy* 2001;**21**:904-19.

475. Schmidt D. Modern management of epilepsy: Rational polytherapy. *Baillieres Clin Neurol* 1996;**5**:757-63.

476. Baulac M. Rational conversion from antiepileptic polytherapy to monotherapy. *Epileptic Disord.* 2003;**5**:125-32.

477. French JA, Kanner AM, Bautista J, Abou-Khalil B, Browne T, Harden CL *et al.* Efficacy and tolerability of the new antiepileptic drugs II: treatment of refractory epilepsy: report of the Therapeutics and Technology Assessment Subcommittee and Quality Standards Subcommittee of the American Academy of Neurology and the American Epilepsy Society. *Neurology* 2004;**62**:1261-73.

478. Schmidt D, Elger C, Holmes GL. Pharmacological overtreatment in epilepsy: mechanisms and management. *Epilepsy Res.* 2002;**52**:3-14.

479. Panayiotopoulos CP, Benbadis SR, Covanis A, Dulac O, Duncan JS, Eeg-Olofsson O *et al.* Efficacy and tolerability of the new antiepileptic drugs; commentary on the recently published practice parameters. *Epilepsia* 2004;**45**:1646-9.

480. Deckers CL, Knoester PD, de Haan GJ, Keyser A, Renier WO, Hekster YA. Selection criteria for the clinical use of the newer antiepileptic drugs. *CNS.Drugs* 2003;**17**:405-21.

481. Briggs DE, French JA. Levetiracetam safety profiles and tolerability in epilepsy patients. *Expert Opin Drug Saf* 2004;**3**:415-24.

482. Leppik IE, Biton V, Sander JW, Wieser HG. Levetiracetam and Partial Seizure Subtypes: Pooled Data from Three Randomized, Placebo-controlled Trials. *Epilepsia* 2003;**44**:1585-7.

483. Depondt C, Yuen ACW, Mula M, Liu RSN, Mitchell TN, Bell GS *et al.* Long-term retention and efficacy of levetiracetam in a large cohort of patients with chronic epilepsy. *Epilepsia* 2004;**45 (Suppl 7)**:1.315.

484. Cramer JA, Arrigo C, Van Hammee G, Gauer LJ, Cereghino JJ. Effect of levetiracetam on epilepsy-related quality of life. N132 Study Group. *Epilepsia* 2000;**41**:868-74.

485. Patsalos PN. Levetiracetam. *Reviews in Contemporay Pharmacology* 2004;**13**:1-168.

486. Guberman AH, Besag FM, Brodie MJ, Dooley JM, Duchowny MS, Pellock JM *et al.* Lamotrigine-associated rash: risk/benefit considerations in adults and children. *Epilepsia* 1999;**40**:985-91.

487. Sabers A, Ohman I, Christensen J, Tomson T. Oral contraceptives reduce lamotrigine plasma levels. *Neurology* 2003;**61**:570-1.

488. Leppik IE. Zonisamide. *Epilepsia* 1999;**40 Suppl 5**:S23-S29.

489. Panayiotopoulos CP. Idiopathic generalised epilepsies. In Panayiotopoulos CP, ed. *A guide to epileptic syndromes and their treatment*, pp 114-60. Oxford: Bladon Medical Publishing, 2002.

490. Arroyo S, Anhut H, Kugler AR, Lee CM, Knapp LE, Garofalo EA *et al.* Pregabalin Add-on Treatment: A Randomized, Double-blind, Placebo-controlled, Dose-Response Study in Adults with Partial Seizures. *Epilepsia* 2004;**45**:20-7.

491. Huppertz HJ, Feuerstein TJ, Schulze-Bonhage A. Myoclonus in epilepsy patients with anticonvulsive add-on therapy with pregabalin. *Epilepsia* 2001;**42**:790-2.

492. Fink K, Dooley DJ, Meder WP, Suman-Chauhan N, Duffy S, Clusmann H *et al.* Inhibition of neuronal Ca(2+) influx by gabapentin and pregabalin in the human neocortex. *Neuropharmacology* 2002;**42**:229-36.

493. French JA, Kugler AR, Robbins JL, Knapp LE, Garofalo EA. Dose-response trial of pregabalin adjunctive therapy in patients with partial seizures. *Neurology* 2003;**60**:1631-7.

13 REFLEX SEIZURES AND REFLEX EPILEPSIES

Epileptic seizures can arise in a 'spontaneous' unpredictable fashion without detectable precipitating factors, or they can be provoked by certain recognisable stimuli.

Factors and stimuli that contribute towards the initiation of a seizure are provided by the internal and external environment of the subject.[1] Hormones, electrolytes, state of consciousness and body temperature are examples of internal factors that alter the epileptogenic threshold. External stimuli may be sensory, electrical or biochemical. A complex interaction between external and internal factors may explain why the effectiveness of a well-defined seizure-precipitating stimulus may vary and why a patient may experience both 'spontaneous' and 'reflex' seizures.

Reflex or stimulus-sensitive or triggered or sensory-evoked epileptic seizures are synonyms denoting epileptic seizures, which are consistently elicited by a specific stimulus. *'Epilepsies characterised by seizures with specific modes of precipitation'* is the term used in the 1989 ILAE classification.[2] *'Reflex'* is the preferred name in the new ILAE diagnostic scheme.[3]

Reflex seizures have a prevalence of 4–7% among patients with epilepsies.[4-6] Aetiologically, reflex seizures are idiopathic, symptomatic or probably symptomatic.

Reflex epilepsies are determined by the *specific precipitating stimulus* and the *clinical/EEG response.*[4-6]

ILAE definition of reflex seizures

The 1989 ILAE classification[2] defines precipitating seizures and precipitating factors as follows:

"Precipitated seizures are those in which environmental or internal factors consistently precede the attacks and are differentiated from spontaneous epileptic attacks in which precipitating factors cannot be identified. Certain nonspecific factors (e.g., sleeplessness, alcohol or drug withdrawal, or hyperventilation) are common precipitators and are *not specific* modes of seizure precipitation. In certain epileptic syndromes, the seizures clearly may be somewhat more susceptible to nonspecific factors, but this is only occasionally useful in classifying epileptic syndromes. An epilepsy characterized by specific modes of seizure precipitation, however, is one in which a consistent relationship can be recognized between the occurrence of one or more definable nonictal events and subsequent occurrence of a specific stereotyped seizure. Some epilepsies have seizures precipitated by specific sensation or perception (the reflex epilepsies) in which seizures occur in response to discrete or specific stimuli. These stimuli are usually limited in individual patients to a single specific stimulus or a limited number of closely related stimuli. Although the epilepsies which result are usually generalised and of idiopathic nature, certain partial seizures may also occur following acquired lesions, usually involving tactile or proprioceptive stimuli."[2]

Reflex seizures are "Objectively and consistently demonstrated to be evoked by a specific afferent stimulus or by activity of the patient. Afferent stimuli can be: elementary, i.e. unstructured (light flashes, startle, a monotone) or elaborate i.e. structured. Activity may be elementary, e.g. motor (a movement); or elaborate, e.g. cognitive function (reading, chess playing), or both (reading aloud)."[7]

Reflex epilepsy syndrome is "A syndrome in which all epileptic seizures are precipitated by sensory stimuli. Reflex seizures that occur in focal and generalized epilepsy syndromes that are also associated with spontaneous seizures are listed as seizure types. Isolated reflex seizures can also occur in situations that do not necessarily require a diagnosis of epilepsy. Seizures precipitated by other special circumstances, such as fever or alcohol withdrawal, are not reflex seizures."[3]

Note from the author:

(a). In the definition of reflex epilepsy syndromes 'all seizures are precipitated by sensory stimuli' may be too restrictive. Most patients also suffer from spontaneous seizures. Should *'all'* be replaced by *'all or nearly all'*?

(b). The term *'precipitating stimulus'* should be differentiated from *'facilitating stimulus'*. In certain patients with idiopathic generalised epilepsy (IGE), for example, EEG discharges or seizures may increase during intermittent photic stimulation (IPS) *(facilitating stimulus)*, but these are not consistently evoked by IPS (as would be expected with *precipitating stimuli*).

THE PRECIPITATING STIMULUS

The stimulus evoking an epileptic seizure is specific for a given patient and may be extrinsic, intrinsic or both.

I. Extrinsic stimuli are:

- simple, such as flashes of light, elimination of visual fixation and tactile stimuli
- complex, such as reading or eating.

The latency from the stimulus onset to the clinical or EEG response is typically short (1–3 s) with simple stimuli and long (usually many minutes) with complex stimuli.

II. Intrinsic stimuli are:

- elementary, such as movements
- elaborate, such as those involving higher brain function, emotions and cognition (thinking, calculating, music, or decision-making).

THE RESPONSE TO THE STIMULUS

The response to the stimulus consists of clinical and EEG manifestations, alone or in combination. EEG activation may be subclinical only, that is without overt clinical manifestations. Conversely, ictal clinical manifestations may be triggered without conspicuous surface EEG changes.

Reflex seizures may be:

- generalised, such as absences, myoclonic jerks or generalised tonic clonic seizures (GTCS)
- focal, such as visual, motor or sensory.

Reflex generalised seizures occur either independently or within the broad framework of certain epileptic syndromes. The same patient in response to the same specific stimulus may have absences, myoclonic jerks and GTCS alone, or in various combinations. Usually, absences and myoclonic jerks precede the occurrence of GTCS. Patients may have reflex and spontaneous seizures.

Myoclonic jerks are by far the most common, and manifest in the limbs and trunk or regionally, such as in the jaw muscles (reading epilepsy) or the eyelids (eyelid myoclonia with absences).

GTCS may occur ab initio constituting the first clinical response or more commonly they follow a cluster of absences or myoclonic jerks. Secondarily GTCS to focal, simple or complex, seizures are much less common than primarily GTCS. Reflex absence seizures are common constituting the response to a variety of specific stimuli, such as photic, pattern, fixation-off, proprioceptive, cognitive, emotional or linguistic.[8] It is recognised that absences are also common in self-induction.

Focal seizures are exclusively seen in certain types of reflex focal or lobular epilepsy, such as visual seizures of photosensitive lobe occipital epilepsy or complex focal temporal lobe seizures of musicogenic epilepsy.

The electroclinical events may be strictly limited to the stimulus-related receptive brain region only (such as photically-induced EEG occipital spikes), spread to other cortical areas (such as in photosensitive focal seizures that propagate in extra-occipital areas) or become generalised (e.g. in photoparoxysmal responses of IGE). Further, the electroclinical response to a specific stimulus may correspond to activation of regions other than those of the relevant receptive area, such as in primary reading epilepsy, which manifests with jaw myoclonic jerks. Conversely, reading may elicit electroclinical events strictly confined to the brain regions subserving reading, such as alexia associated with focal ictal EEG paroxysms. There is great variability in the interindividual responses to the same stimulus.

The role of the EEG is fundamental in establishing the precipitating stimulus in reflex epilepsies, because it allows subclinical EEG, or minor clinical ictal events to be reproduced on demand by application of the appropriate stimulus. However, there are cases in which the stimulus–seizure relationship is difficult to document as in video game-induced seizures (VGS; page 455). Only 70% of these patients have EEG confirmation of photosensitivity with photoparoxysmal responses (PPR) on IPS and, in the other 30%, seizures may be due to a single or a variety of other precipitating or facilitating stimuli. Sleep deprivation, mental concentration, fatigue, excitement, borderline threshold to photosensitivity, fixation-off sensitivity (FOS), proprioceptive stimuli (praxis), or more complex visual or auditory stimuli, alone or in combination, are all possibilities that are difficult to document objectively with EEG.[9-11] There are also epileptic syndromes in which EEG 'epileptogenic activity' is consistently elicited by a specific stimulus with no apparent clinical relevance. This is exemplified by certain cases of benign focal childhood seizures in which somatosensory (tapping) or visual (elimination of fixation and central vision) stimuli consistently elicit spike activity, though these children appear to have *'unprovoked'* seizures, which mainly occur during sleep.[11]

Table 13.1 lists the types of precipitating stimuli, reflex seizures and epileptic syndromes according to the new ILAE diagnostic scheme.[3]

Table 13.2 is an analytical list of reflex seizures, related reflex epileptic syndromes and their precipitating stimuli. Some of these, such as photosensitivity, are well known and common, but others are extremely rare in humans, though they may be common in animals, such as audiogenic seizures.

In this chapter, common and principal forms of simple and complex reflex seizures and epilepsies are reviewed with particular emphasis on the syndromes listed in the new ILAE diagnostic scheme.[3] Classical references or reviews are cited for the remainder.

Visually induced seizures and epilepsies are the commonest of the reflex epilepsies.[4-6;12-15] Visual seizures are triggered by the physical characteristics of the visual stimuli and not by their cognitive effects. Photosensitivity and pattern sensitivity are the two main categories (with frequent overlap) of simple reflex epilepsies in which there is a short time interval (typically within seconds) between stimulus and response. These are detailed below.

Table 13.1 Precipitating stimuli and reflex seizures/syndromes listed in the new ILAE classification scheme[3]

Precipitating stimuli for reflex seizures	Reflex seizures
Visual stimuli	Reflex seizures in generalised epilepsy syndromes
Flickering light	Reflex seizures in focal epilepsy syndromes
– colour to be specified when possible	
Patterns	**Reflex epilepsies**
Other visual stimuli	Idiopathic photosensitive occipital lobe epilepsy
Thinking	Other visual sensitive epilepsies
Music	Primary reading epilepsy
Eating	Startle epilepsy
Praxis	
Somatosensory	**Conditions with epileptic seizures that do not require a diagnosis of epilepsy**
Proprioceptive	Reflex seizures
Reading	
Hot water	
Startle	

Modified from Engel (2001)[3] with the permission of the author and the Editor of *Epilepsia*

PHOTOSENSITIVE SEIZURES AND EPILEPTIC SYNDROMES

Photosensitivity, the propensity to seizures induced by light, is a genetically determined trait that may be asymptomatic throughout life or manifest with epileptic seizures.[12;15;60-62]

'Photosensitive epilepsy' is a broad term comprising all forms of heterogeneous epilepsies in which seizures are triggered by photic stimulation. It is not an epilepsy syndrome. EEG photosensitivity, that is provocation of PPR by IPS (Figure 13.1), may or may not be associated with clinical photosensitivity. Some recognised syndromes of IGE, such as juvenile myoclonic epilepsy, show a high incidence of clinical or EEG photosensitivity. A high prevalence of photosensitivity is also found in certain forms of severe epilepsy, such as Dravet syndrome (70%),[63] Unverricht-Lundborg (90%)[64] and other progressive myoclonic epilepsies.[64]

DEMOGRAPHIC DATA

Photosensitive seizures and epilepsies affect 1 in 4,000 of the population (5% of patients with epileptic seizures); two-thirds are women and the peak age at onset is 12–13 years.[12;65] The overall annual incidence of cases with a newly presenting seizure and unequivocal photosensitivity in the UK was 1.1 per 100,000 and 5.7 per 100,000 in the 7–19-year age group.[66;67] Clinical photosensitivity was found in 2% of patients of all ages presenting with seizures and 10% of patients presenting with seizures in the 7–19-year age range.[66;67]

In healthy males aged 17–25 years, EEG photosensitivity is very low (0.35%).[68]

Table 13.2 Reflex seizures, related reflex epilepsies and the precipitating stimuli (for details see refs [4;5])

I. Somatosensory stimuli

1. *Exteroceptive somatosensory stimuli*
a. Tapping epilepsy and benign childhood epilepsy with somatosensory evoked spikes[16-19]
b. Sensory (tactile) evoked idiopathic myoclonic seizures in infancy[20]
c. Toothbrushing epilepsy[21;22]

2. *Complex exteroceptive somatosensory stimuli*
a. Hot water epilepsy[23-26]

3. *Proprioceptive somatosensory stimuli*
a. Seizures induced by movements[27]
b. Seizures induced by eye closure and/or eye movements[28]
c. Paroxysmal kinesiogenic choreoathetosis[29]
d. Seizures induced by micturition[30;31]

4. Complex proprioceptive stimuli
a. Eating epilepsy[32;33]

II. Visual stimuli

1. *Simple visual stimuli*
a. Photosensitive epilepsies[12] (including self-induced photosensitive epilepsy)[12;15;34;35]
b. Pattern-sensitive epilepsies[12;36;37] (including self-induced pattern-sensitive epilepsy)[15;34;38]
c. Fixation-off sensitive epilepsies[39]
d. Scotogenic epilepsy[39]

2. Complex visual stimuli and language processing (language-induced seizures)
a. Reading epilepsy[40-44]
b. Graphogenic epilepsy[45;46]

III. Auditory, vestibular, olfactory and gustatory stimuli[1;27]
a. Seizures induced by pure sounds or words[27]
b. Audiogenic seizures [47]
c. Musicogenic epilepsy (and singing epilepsy)[48;49]
d. Telephone-induced seizures[50]
e. Olfacto-rhinoencephalic epilepsy[4]
f. Eating epilepsy triggered by tastes[33]
g. Seizures triggered by vestibular and auditory stimuli[27]

IV. High-level process induced seizures (cognitive, emotional, decision-making tasks and other complex stimuli)[1]
a. Thinking (noogenic) epilepsy[51;52]
b. Reflex decision-making epilepsy[53;54]
c. Epilepsia arithmetica (mathematica)[55]
d. Emotional epilepsies[56;57]
e. Startle epilepsy[58;59]

Modified from Panayiotopoulos (1996)[6] with the permission of the Editor S. Wallace and the Publishers Chapman & Hall

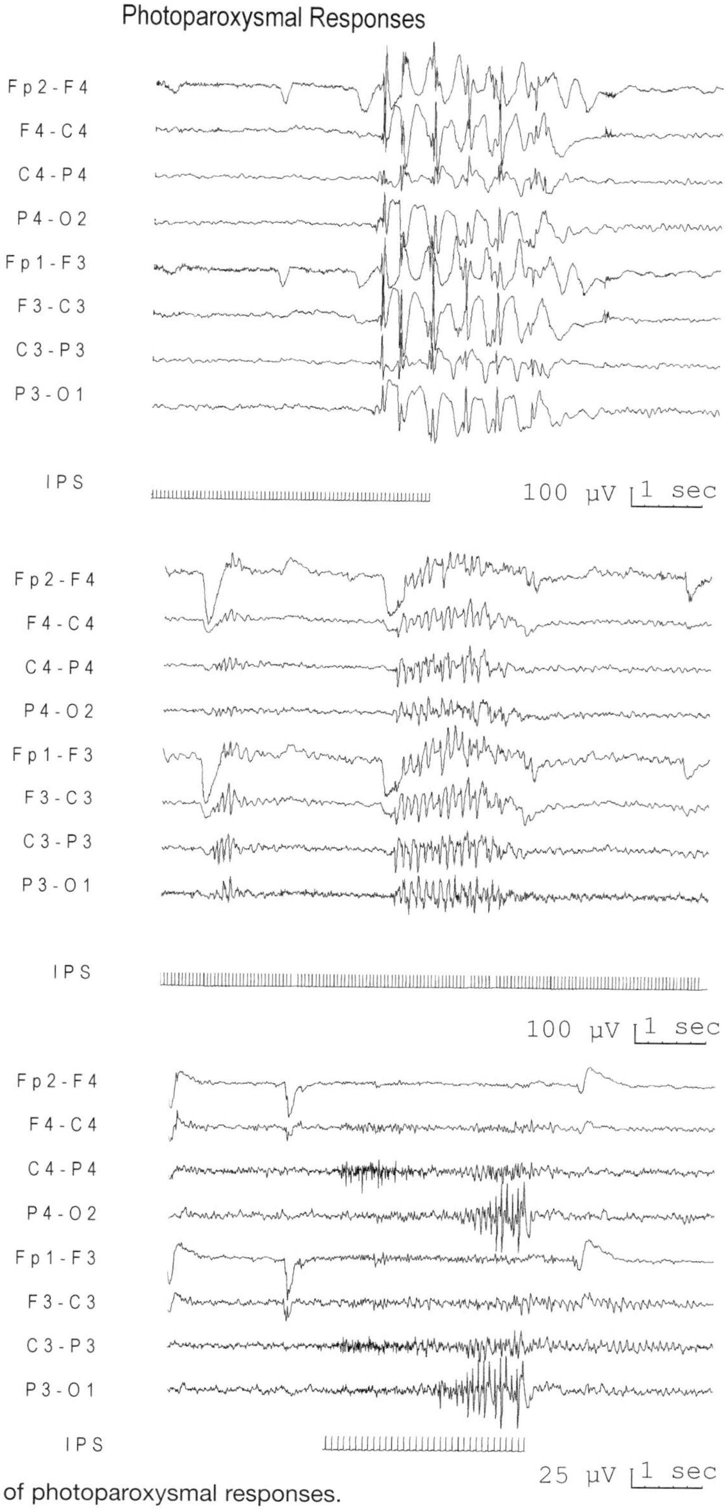

Figure 13.1 Examples of photoparoxysmal responses.

Top: Generalised 3–4 Hz spike/polyspike–waves associated with an absence. The discharge outlasts the duration of the stimulus.
Middle: Generalised polyspike discharge in a patient with symptomatic spontaneous and photically induced mainly GTCS, which are resistant to appropriate anti-epileptic medication. This type of discharge is usually associated with myoclonic jerks, which did not feature in this case. Note that the discharge occurs only after eye-blinks or eye-closure, and does not outlast the stimulus train.
Bottom: Typical occipital spikes time-locked to each flash of IPS. The patient is a woman with idiopathic occipital epilepsy (probably a variant of Gastaut-type childhood occipital epilepsy), who never had attacks precipitated by lights (case report in ref [69]).

CLINICAL MANIFESTATIONS

Clinical manifestations vary considerably depending on the underlying syndrome and severity of photosensitivity. Of patients with clinical seizures and EEG PPR, 42% have only photically induced seizures without spontaneous seizures (pure photosensitive epilepsy), 40% have spontaneous and photosensitive seizures, and the remaining 18% have spontaneous seizures only.[11;12;70-72]

In photosensitive epilepsy, generalised seizures are far more common than occipital seizures; any other focal seizures from other than occipital brain regions are exceptional ab initio.

GENERALISED SEIZURES

Myoclonic jerks, GTCS and absences, in their order of prevalence, can occur in photosensitive patients. Some subjects may have only one type, but most suffer from any combination, particularly myoclonic jerks and GTCS.

The fact that myoclonic jerks are by far the most common may appear to contradict the common view that GTCS prevail.[12] Thus, GTCS are reported far more frequently (55–84%) than absences (6–20%), focal seizures (2.5%) and myoclonic jerks (2–8%).[12] This prevalence is based on clinical historical evidence, which is likely to overexaggerate GTCS in relation to minor seizures, though these predominate. During PPR, 75% of patients experience impairment of consciousness or show motor symptoms, such as involuntary opening of the eyes or jerking, but only two-thirds of these are documented in the clinical history.[71;73] In my personal experience with video EEG of over 300 patients, PPR commonly induced eyelid manifestations (a blink, eyelid fluttering, flickering or myoclonia) and less often myoclonic jerks of the head, eyes, body or limbs. Absence seizures followed in prevalence. Only one patient had an accidental GTCS. Patients are often unaware of the minor seizures, though some of these may also be violent. These facts have been illustrated on many occasions in this book (e.g. see pages 280–4).

OCCIPITAL FOCAL SEIZURES

Photically induced occipital focal seizures are far less common than generalised seizures, but much more frequent than originally appreciated after the use of IPS in EEG testing. These may occur alone or progress to symptoms from other brain locations and GTCS.

Extra-occipital focal seizures from onset are exceptional.[74]

SUBJECTIVE SYMPTOMS DURING PHOTOPAROXYSMAL RESPONSES

A significant number of patients complain of subjective symptoms during PPR, such as dizziness, orbital pain, nausea, fear and unpleasant sensations, which are not usually ictal phenomena.[13;75] Many patients can not tolerate light at all. The monograph of Wilkins on visual stress caused by lights and patterns is highly recommended.[13]

An historical clarification

There are many reported versions of the first recorded provocation of fits with light stimulation. This refers to Apuleius in his book "Apologia" (around 125 AD) on a speech defending himself against an accusation that he was practising magic on a young slave Thallus who had a collapse in front of Apuleius. Apuleius pointed out that Thallus suffered from epilepsy: "Again the spinning of a potter's wheel will easily infect a man suffering from this disease with its own giddiness The sight of its rotations weakens his already feeble mind, and the potter is far more effective than the magician for casting epileptics into convulsions".

The potters' wheels at the times of Apuleius (who was Roman and not Greek) were solid (not spoked) and therefore could not produce intermittent light stimulation.[109]

PRECIPITATING FACTORS

By definition, all patients are sensitive to flickering lights. Many artificial or natural light sources can provoke epileptic seizures.[76] In order of prevalence, video games, television, computer visual display units, discotheques and natural flickering light are common triggers.

VIDEO GAME-INDUCED SEIZURES

Video games are a relatively new means of inducing epileptic seizures. Since the first description of *'space invader epilepsy'* in 1981,[77] they have now reached epidemic proportions.[78] The risk has been highlighted in media reports and manufacturers now warn of the risks.

There is clearly heterogeneity in seizure types, seizure syndromes, precipitating and facilitating factors, and underlying mechanisms.

Video game-induced seizures (VGS) can occur not only with games using an interlaced video monitor (television), but also with small hand-held liquid crystal displays and non-interlaced 70-Hz arcade games.[9;15;66;78-82] Most patients (87%) are 7–19 years of age and there is a preponderance of boys, probably because more boys than girls play video games.

Two-thirds of patients suffer from generalised seizures and the majority of them suffer from various syndromes of IGE. The other third have occipital seizures with or without photosensitivity. Other types of focal seizures are exceptional.

There are many mechanisms by which video games may induce seizures. These are:

- photosensitivity
- pattern sensitivity
- emotional and cognitive excitation (excitement or frustration)
- proprioceptive stimulation (movement/praxis).

Fatigue, sleep deprivation and prolonged playing are facilitating factors.

Photosensitive patients with VGS

Photosensitivity, which often combines with pattern sensitivity, is the main provocative factor in VGS. However, only 70% of patients with well-documented VGS that was not an incidental association are photosensitive on IPS.

Non-photosensitive patients with VGS

One-third of patients is not photosensitive in the sense that appropriate IPS does not evoke PPR. Four particular groups of non-photosensitive patients with VGS have been identified.

Idiopathic generalised epilepsy without photosensitivity: This group consists of patients with various forms of IGE with spontaneous seizures who also have VGS, though they are not photosensitive on IPS testing. One-third of VGS in non-photosensitive patients probably occur in these patients. Cognitive and emotional factors seem crucial provocative agents.

> This 45-year-old man with well-controlled juvenile absence epilepsy is a typical patient. On five occasions, he had a GTCS at the same point in a car-racing video game. The seizures all happened just when he was about to crash the car.

Idiopathic occipital lobe epilepsy: This group consists of patients with focal occipital seizures manifesting with ictal visual hallucinations, visual deficits or both. These patients are generally not photosensitive in the laboratory, but have

---

Terminology

The term *'video-game epilepsy'*, with the connotation of a single epilepsy syndrome, might not be the most appropriate. Since many patients have only single seizures, *'video game-induced seizures* is a more accurate term.

spontaneous occipital spikes in their resting EEG. This group probably accounts for two-thirds of VGS in non-photosensitive patients.[9] The seizure-provoking mechanism is unknown, but may be related to an association with playing games in arcades.

Low-threshold to seizures: This is a newly identified group of patients who have a single seizure, or at most two or three seizures, while playing video games.[9;10] They are young adults rather than teenagers. Their EEG is normal in all respects. VGS occur when a number of factors precipitating and facilitating seizures cluster together at the same time. These factors are sleep deprivation, thirst, hunger, mental and emotional heightening, and prolonged playing of exciting and provocative video games. In such patients, it is unlikely that one of these provocative factors on its own is sufficient to initiate seizures, but that a number of them together is.

> A 23-year-old professional man, who had two GTCS, one preceded by an absence seizure, while playing different video games is a typical patient. Three EEG examinations, including IPS and pattern stimuli, have been normal. Fatigue, prolonged playing, hunger and thirst were identified as possible factors.

Pure pattern epilepsy without photosensitivity: This type of VGS may be extremely rare.[83]

VGS should not be equated with photosensitivity alone. One-third of patients with VGS is not photosensitive.

The practical implication of this is that not all patients who have seizures while playing video games will be helped by the advice recommended for photosensitive patients. A thorough clinical and EEG evaluation is needed to identify likely precipitating factors and enable individual guidelines to be offered.

The risk of VGS in non-photosensitive patients with spontaneous seizures is practically nil. By and large, VGS in these patients represents a chance occurrence, although each individual should be carefully assessed.[84]

TELEVISION EPILEPSY

Television epilepsy is not a particular epileptic syndrome. It refers to seizures induced by television viewing in photosensitive patients. Television-induced seizures mainly affect children aged 10–12 years. There is a two-fold preponderance of girls. Seizures are more likely to occur when the patient is watching a faulty (i.e. flickering) television set or at a close distance to the screen. Programmes with flickering lights are particularly dangerous and occasionally their effect on eliciting seizures may reach epidemic proportions;[15;85] appropriate broadcasting guidelines have been successful in reducing the risks.[86] Whether the television is monochrome or colour does not appear to influence the provocative effect.[87;88]

Many patients have television-induced myoclonic jerks long before a television-induced GTCS occur. Myoclonic jerks often precede GTCS.

> First she jerked a few times, head and hands, and then she had the convulsions. I thought she was electrocuted by an electric fault in the television.

A substantial number of these patients also have spontaneous attacks. In *pure television epilepsy*, one or a few overt television-induced seizures occur without evidence of any other type of spontaneous seizure or seizures induced by other precipitating factors.

In 10% of cases, patients feel they are *"being drawn like a magnet"* and, when they get sufficiently close to the television screen, they have GTCS. This is called *"compulsive attraction"*.

> He was watching television and then suddenly, off he goes towards the set, eyes fixed on the picture, and he had the fit a few inches away from the screen.

I do not know what happens. My eyes were suddenly fixed on the picture, I could not move them away...

Technical aspects and explanations of television-induced seizures

The difference in the frequency of the alternating current (AC) in the mains electricity supply explains why proportionally more people have television-induced seizures in Europe and Japan than in the USA. IPS at 25 Hz is more epileptogenic than at 30 Hz.

A television picture consists of two frames of horizontal lines that intercalate and alternate at the half the frequency of the mains AC supply. They are produced by changes in the intensity of the spot of light that draws the lines across the television, and these lines are drawn alternately (i.e. the first, third, fifth, etc., then the second, fourth, sixth, etc.). Where the mains AC frequency is 50 Hz (e.g. Europe and Japan), each alternate set of lines takes 0.02 s to complete, and the two lines produce an alternating flicker at 25 Hz. Where the mains AC frequency is 60 Hz, as in the USA, this flicker has a frequency of 30 Hz.

Television-induced seizures are more likely to occur when the set is being watched from a close distance, less than 1 metre away from the screen.
The main reasons for this are that, at this distance:[87;88]

- the intensity of the stimulus is increased
- the two halves of the television scans can be resolved and therefore produce a 25-Hz flicker to which the majority of patients are usually sensitive; patients with PPR at 50 Hz are much less likely to have seizures while watching at a normal distance than those with PPR at 25 Hz[87-89]
- the retina, and therefore the number of neurons, stimulated receives the maximal stimulation.

SELF-INDUCED SEIZURES

Self-induction is a mode of seizure precipitation employed by entirely normal or mentally handicapped patients to produce seizures for themselves.[90] Manoeuvres for self-induction aim to provoke a seizure by producing optimal conditions of stimulation by flickering light (self-induced photosensitive epilepsy),[35;91-93] patterns (self-induced pattern-sensitive epilepsy)[38;94], proprioceptive stimuli[95] or higher brain functions (self-induced noogenic epilepsy).[52;96]

PREVALENCE OF SELF-INDUCED SEIZURES

Deliberately self-induced seizures are rare. They are far more common in photosensitive individuals.[34;35;93;97] The exact prevalence of self-induced photosensitive seizures is difficult to determine and probably significantly over-estimated.[35]

In my experience of 442 patients with onset of afebrile seizures between birth and 15 years of age, only five (1.3%) had self-induced seizures.[98] All were photosensitive, but one was using patterns, not light for self-induction.[38] Of the other four self-induced photosensitive patients, three were 'hand wavers' and one was rolling the television picture for self-induction. Three were of normal intelligence and development. Two of the normal 'hand wavers', followed up to the age of 23 years, had discontinued self-induction, but lights may have been a fascinating aspect in their life; one became a disc jockey. It is from them that I learned how 'self-induction' is discovered and the pleasant experience they got from it.

A higher prevalence is probably due to reports of self-induced photosensitive epilepsy in cases with:

a. 'self-induced' behaviours without evidence that these were wilful or consciously generated

b. early forced eyelid blinking and flutter, eyelid jerks and oculoclonic activity though these may be either ictal manifestations of occipital lobe seizures or over-exaggerated normal responses of 'attraction movements' when light is presented, and other manifestations of the optic fixation reflexes when volitional movements of the eyes are unattainable or weak[35;99]. "Blinking also functions as a complex indicator of phasic responses to stress such as that produced by listening to emotionally laden words".[100]

The following descriptions may be arbitrarily taken as indirect evidence of self-induction despite the fact that this is strongly denied by the patients.

> "The sun seems to do something to make me to look at it... I do not know...It does not give me any pleasure...I can not help it in one way, but when I think to stop it, I stop... do not go out and sit in the sun..."[101]

> "The mother of a medical practitioner, whenever she went into the sunlight her head went back and she blinked. A fleeting blankness of expression was recognisable. In addition, she had suffered from three major convulsions 20, 17 and 2 years ago. These occurred after periods of overwork and stress."[101]

> "I will be looking over there and the sunshine will be coming through on that side. And my head, without me even knowing, automatically turns, I can not stop it. It goes like this and my head has an automatic reaction to go back to the sunlight and my eyes start flickering and I try to pull myself away..."[35]

Also, whether compulsive attraction to television or bright sun is mainly an attempt at self-induction, part of the seizure or an enhanced normal optic fixation reflex is disputed.[35]

See self-induced photosensitivity in Jeavons syndrome (see page 478).

CLINICAL MANIFESTATIONS

Absences and myoclonic jerks are the commonest seizures in self-induction. A GTCS, when it occurs, is usually an accidental event, which was not desired. This is followed by deliberately self-induced absences or jerks.

The objective of self-induced seizures is relief of tension and anxiety, and escape from a disturbing situation.

> "I like it, it relieves tension..."

> "I do not actually deliberately go out to find some bright light, but if I find it I am happy.... In a way, it is a play between me and the sun... It is a mixture of feelings. On the one hand I do not want to do it, but on the other hand it is releasing something...No, it is not sexual. . I know it is strange..."[102]

It is less often highly pleasurable.

> It is like Christmas presents.

Sexual and masturbatory connotations are exceptional.[103]

MANOEUVRES FOR SELF-INDUCTION IN PHOTOSENSITIVE EPILEPSY

The best known manoeuvre for self-induction is looking at a bright light source, usually the sun, and voluntarily waving the abducted fingers in front of the eyes (sunflower syndrome)[97] in order to produce optimal IPS. It has also been well documented that some photosensitive patients may self-induce seizures by repetitive opening and closing of the eyes in front of a bright light source. Some patients combine both waving of the fingers and repetitive eyelid blinking which is the most effective stimulation. Other patients achieve IPS and self-induced seizures with lateral or vertical rhythmic movements of the head, making the television picture roll, quickly changing television channels while watching from a close distance or, more recently, playing video games.[9]

The discovery of the self-induced technique by patients is usually accidental:[91]

> I was playing football on a sunny day. I got the pleasant feeling when I tried to get my hair away from falling in front of my eyes.

AETIOLOGY OF PHOTOSENSITIVE EPILEPSY

Photosensitivity is genetically determined.[60;61;104] In particular the genetic basis for PPR is well documented. Monozygotic twin studies have shown an almost 100% concordance. Family studies indicate a sibling risk between 20 and 50%, the latter when siblings are studied between 5-15 years of age with one of the parents also being affected. These indicate autosomal dominant inheritance with age-related reduced penetrance in PPR-positive patients with seizures and non-seizure subjects. However, PPR also occur in a number of autosomal recessive diseases.[104]

In a large and lengthy study, 32 clinically photosensitive mothers had 67 children during the follow-up period.[105] In the last update, 13 children (20%) had PPR and 4 also had photosensitive seizures induced in the outside environment. Nine of the children have been found not to be photosensitive nor have they had seizures.

In a recent study of 16 multiplex families with PPR, empirical genome-wide significance for linkage was found for two chromosomes 7q32 and 16p13.[106] According to the authors these two susceptibility loci for PPR, may be related to the underlying myoclonic epilepsy phenotype present in the families studied.

A European consortium on the genetic analysis of photosensitivity and visual sensitive epilepsies is underway.

PATHOPHYSIOLOGY OF PHOTOSENSITIVE EPILEPSY

Photosensitivity results from functional abnormalities in the cortical mechanisms that control the response to strong visual stimulation.[107] It is now well documented that the visual cortex is the primary site of epileptogenesis in occipital photosensitivity and pattern seizure sensitivity.[6;13;62;72;107-110] This is also true for the onset of epileptogenicity in syndromes of IGE and photically-induced generalised seizures, though this has not been elucidated. It is possible that, in other forms of photosensitivity (eyelid myoclonia with absences may be an example), the onset is in the frontal regions, as is the case in the photosensitive baboon *Papio papio*.[111]

The pathophysiology of human photosensitivity has gone through several stages. Initially, the predominant view was that it is *'centrencephalic' (generalised epilepsy)* with the non-specific thalamocortical reticular system activated from the lateral geniculate body.[112;113] This view, which dominated the literature at that time, was mainly based on the findings that PPR are usually synchronous and generalised (Figures 13.1, and 13.2).[113] The first clear evidence of the occipital origin of PPR came from our studies of photically-induced occipital spikes often preceding generalised PPR (Figure 13.3).[109;110;114] This has now been confirmed with elaborate documentation of the primary role of the visual cortex in photic and pattern stimulation.

Evidence that occipital spikes are preferentially elicited in photosensitive patients documents the primary or exclusive role of the occipital cortex in the initiation of photically induced seizures.[109;110;114] This may be the only cortical region involved as in occipital photosensitive seizures or the initial trigger zone of generalised photosensitive epilepsy.

The visual stimuli eliciting occipital spikes depend on the number of flashes of light per second (or the number of pattern image changes per second), spatial frequency, orientation, contrast and the line width ratio.[12] All these factors indicate that the visual cortex is involved and this is the earliest site at which integration occurs.[12]

FAILURE OF INHIBITORY OR EXCITATORY MECHANISMS OR BOTH?
The IPS flash time-locked occipital spikes appear on the descending arm of the P_{100} component of the VER.[109;110;114] This, we postulated, was a failure of postsynaptic inhibition.[109;110;114] However, the findings that "the P_{100} VER component is enhanced in photosensitive patients and that valproate slightly reduces its amplitude, while occipital spikes are unaffected" were interpreted as evidence of "at least normal, if not supranormal post-inhibitory potentials", which suggests that the occipital spikes represent an excitatory phenomenon, rather than a failure of inhibition.[12] This latter view was challenged in a more recent study. [115].

Neurotransmitters

A selective dopaminergic mechanism in human epileptic photosensitivity has been postulated. [116;117] Apomorphine, a dopamine receptor agonist, blocked PPR in patients with IGE and this effect was not modified by naloxone, a specific opiate antagonist, thus suggesting that apomorphine acts on cerebral dopaminergic receptors.[116;117] Conversely, apomorphine did not block spontaneous GSWD in patients with non-photosensitive IGE.[116]

Pathophysiology of photosensitive epilepsy in animals

Photosensitive *Papio papio* baboons have long been used as an animal model of photosensitive epilepsy.[118-120] They suffer from IPS-induced myoclonus and have a natural predisposition to 'non-epileptic myoclonus', which is not accompanied by electrical discharges or seizures. Clinical manifestations do not show any signs of localised origin of the epileptogenic processes, and the PPR are also bilateral and synchronous. However, experimental data document that the origin of PPR and seizures is in the motor cortex.[118-120]

ELECTROENCEPHALOGRAPHY

The resting EEG of patients with idiopathic photosensitive seizures is usually normal or frequently (in 20–30% of cases) shows eye closure-related paroxysms

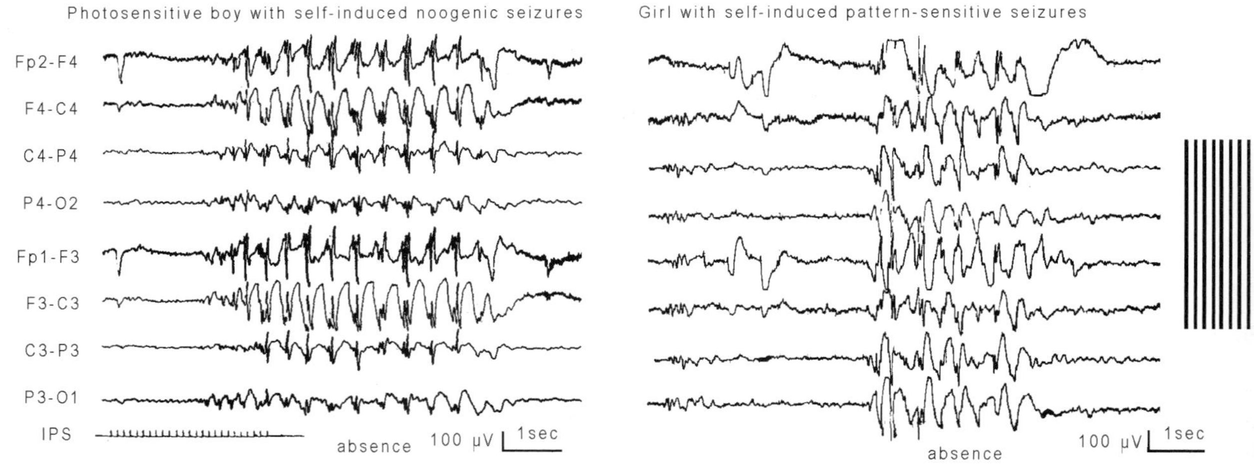

Figure 13.2 Generalised 3-Hz spike or polyspike–wave associated with clinical absence in two patients with self-induced seizures.

Left: Absence seizure induced by IPS. This patient had spontaneous, photically induced and noogenic seizures. He used noogenic processes for self-induction (see ref [52]).

Modified from Koutroumanidis et al.[52] with the permission of the Editor of the *Journal of Neurology, Neurosurgery and Psychiatry.*

Right: Absence seizure induced by a pattern with vertical lines. This patient with learning difficulties had mainly self-induced pattern-sensitive epilepsy. She was also photosensitive (see ref [38]).

Modified from Panayiotopoulos[38] with the permission of the Editor of *Archives of Neurology.*

occurring within 1–3 s of closing the eyes. These are usually brief EEG paroxysms that last for 1–4 s and have similar features to those elicited by IPS for each individual patient. They disappear if eye closure occurs in total darkness.

Properly applied IPS during EEG is the most important test for photosensitivity.[12;15;62;121-123]

OBJECTIVES OF INTERMITTENT PHOTIC STIMULATION

In deciding what is the best method of IPS, the objectives of this activating technique should be determined. My principle is to get as much information as possible for diagnostic and management purposes without endangering the patient to satisfy scientific curiosity. What is the point of continuing photic stimulation after the appearance of abnormal PPR in patients with a clinical history of photosensitive seizures?

A team of experts rightly recommends that:

"*the techniques for detection must use procedures that elicit a clearly defined EEG response in the maximum number of patients who have a history of light-induced seizures, while minimising the chances of inducing such a response in other individuals.*"[122]

The practical objective of IPS is to determine whether:

a. *seizures (of any type) are aetiologically linked to environmental photic stimuli (television, video games and others).* PPR, if they occur, confirm photosensitivity. Whether the particular patient is clinically photosensitive and also has spontaneous seizures relies on taking a good medical history.

b. *photoparoxysmal responses are associated with ictal events.* This can only be determined by video EEG recording; otherwise minor events, such as eyelid or

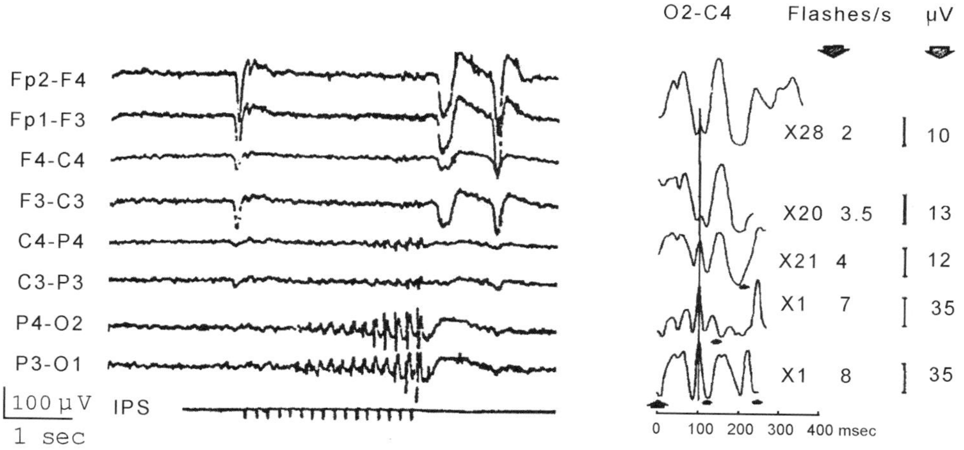

Figure 13.3 Occipital spikes and their relation to the P_{100} component of the visual evoked response (VER) in photosensitive patients with generalised PPR.

Left: Patterned IPS (2 mm x 2 mm graticule superimposed on the grass of the stroboscope) evoked occipital spikes, which are time-locked to flash at 6 flashes/s of a patient with spontaneous and photically elicited GTCS. Higher flash frequencies from 9–30 Hz elicited generalised PPR of spike–wave, briefly preceded by occipital spikes (from ref [109]).

Right: Emergence of occipital spikes from the P_{100} VER component with increasing flash rate. Patient had spontaneous and television-induced GTCS. On EEG, time-locked occipital spikes were apparent only at 5 flashes/s, while higher flash rates from 6–26 Hz elicited generalised discharges of spike–wave briefly preceded by occipital spikes.

The three upper traces show the average VERs to stimulation at 2, 3.5 and 4 flashes/s. The occipital spikes evoked at 7 and 8 flashes/s are shown in the two lower traces. The vertical line crosses the negative component of the occipital spikes and the Vb component of the P_{100} component of the VER. The horizontal line indicates time in ms. The thick arrow indicates the onset of flash.

Modified from Panayiotopoulos et al.[114] with the permission of the Editor of *Nature*.

limb jerks, are likely to escape notice. The presence of these ictal events may have significant implications for the correct syndromic diagnosis and management. This objective by no means indicates the need for prolonged photic stimulation.

Important note

Prolonged photic stimulation that may induce a major convulsive seizure should be totally discouraged. There is nothing to learn and no benefit to the patient from this practice. There are plenty of examples of subjects having an IPS-induced GTCS during an EEG that was performed for reasons other than epilepsy. Management and advice to these subjects is not going to change after this unfortunate discovery of their low seizure-threshold to photic stimulation. To continue a train of photic stimulation after the appearance of EEG ictal discharges or ictal clinical manifestations is unacceptable.

However, problems and their solutions in medicine are not black or white, and IPS is no exception:

- Some patients may have one, two or more seizures always associated with environmental photic stimuli (video games are the best example), but routine IPS fails to reveal EEG photosensitivity. Are these patients photosensitive? Should more potent means of activation be used with sleep deprivation and long IPS/pattern activation?

A team of experts recommends:

"*It is important to include stimulation that is maximally epileptogenic, if patients show no EEG signs of light sensitivity in response to less-provocative stimulation. Failure to do so may result in an underestimation of the contribution of visual stimulation to the seizure problem.*"[122]

But what is *'maximally epileptogenic'* and what are its limitations?

This again is a matter of clinical assessment. In a child who has two GTCS 2 years apart from one another while playing video games for many hours after sleep deprivation and other seizure precipitating factors, IPS confirmation may not be needed, because the association comes from logical deduction. All these facilitating factors were 'maximally epileptogenic' for this particular patient at the particular moment that the seizure occurred. Partial sleep deprivation EEG recording during sleep and awakening is often very informative.

- Some patients have definite epileptic seizures, which appear to occur spontaneously, but EEG demonstrates PPR. Is this relevant to their disease and management? The answer again should be based mainly on the clinical history. For example, patients with juvenile myoclonic epilepsy often have EEG photosensitivity, though they may never have clinical seizures provoked by environmental photic stimulation.

FACTORS THAT INFLUENCE THE RESPONSE TO INTERMITTENT PHOTIC STIMULATION

The epileptogenic properties of flickering lights "depend on the size of the retinal image of the source, its time-averaged luminance, the modulation of the light, the frequency of the modulation, the colour of the light (spectral power distribution) and the part of the retina receiving stimulation."[13]

The epileptogenic properties of flickering lights and its spatial and directional relation with the subject's eyes (retina)

Intensity, frequency and duration of the IPS are of crucial importance and the most significant determinants of the response. An abnormal PPR is more likely to occur with light of high intensity, frequency of mainly 12–20 Hz and longer trains of IPS. Combining light IPS with appropriate geometric patterns makes it much more potent[109;124] than diffused or white light. Colour may not be an important provocative factor for PPR, though it is often emphasised by some authors[15] and certain patients improve with the appropriate use of tinted glasses;[13;125] this has been critically reviewed by Harding and Jeavons (see ref [12]).

Binocular is far more effective than monocular stimulation. This is why it is recommended that photosensitive patients cover one eye when in epileptogenic environmental photic conditions such as discotheques.

Stimulating central vision (fixating on the light source) is much more potent than stimulating peripheral vision. This is because photosensitivity is mainly mediated through central vision and fixation.[126] This is also the reason for the recommendation that, in IPS testing, "a central marker on the diffuser to aid fixation is specified, as photosensitivity is unlikely to be demonstrable in the eyes-open state unless the stimulator is in central vision".[122]

Distance and ambient light mainly influence the intensity of the photic stimuli.

Flicker frequency

The photosensitive range lies between the lowest and highest frequency of IPS that consistently evokes a PPR. Several advantages have been emphasised of defining the photosensitive range, such as that: (a). it defines the degree of photosensitivity in a specific patient; (b). it enables qualitative comparisons over time, as in studies of prognosis or effectiveness of drug therapy in both acute and chronic administration; and (c). it allows identification of the visual stimuli present in the environment that represent a provocative risk (e.g. television viewing).[12] The photosensitive range is, however, often variable.

Internal factors altering the effectiveness of IPS

The effectiveness of IPS in provoking EEG abnormalities depends on a large number of internal and external factors. Alertness, attention, emotion, menstrual cycle, hormones, electrolytes and ingestion of drugs are some of the internal factors that alter the photoconvulsive threshold of the subject.

In patients subjected to identical trains of IPS under constant experimental conditions over a period of several minutes, the EEG responses varied considerably from no detectable abnormality to self-sustained spike–wave discharges of 10-s duration. Cyclical changes were observed when the length of the spike–wave discharge was plotted over the time period.[127-129]

Furthermore, in AED trials the antiepileptic effect on PPR may last for several days after the AED has been eliminated.

Differentiation between eye-closure and eyes-closed state (Figure 13.4)

EEG abnormalities suggesting photosensitive, scotosensitive and FOS epilepsies are often seen in the resting EEG before any other specific test is carried out. It is important to differentiate between eyes closed (Figure 13.4) and eye closure (Figure 13.4) EEG abnormalities, because of their different properties and their different response to intermittent light, darkness and fixation-off.

Eyes closed is the state that lasts as long as the eyes remain closed. FOS is a typical example of eyes closed-related seizures and EEG abnormalities.

Eye closure is the transient state, which immediately follows closing of the eyes, lasts less than 3 s and does not persist in the remaining period of eyes closed. Eye closure is much more potent than 'eyes open' or 'eyes closed' in inducing abnormalities during IPS. Jeavons syndrome is a typical example of eye closure-related seizures and EEG abnormalities. In some photosensitive patients, PPR occur only after eye closure.

Eyes open, eyes closed and eye closure

The state of the eyes during IPS is probably the most significant internal factor that modifies the response. There is a great confusion about this.

Eye closure (closing of the eyes while IPS continues) is by far the most potent factor in eliciting PPR, regardless of patterned, unpatterned or diffuse IPS.[12;109;132] This should be expected, because many of these patients have GSWD in their resting EEG only immediately after closing of the eyes.[12;109]

The effectiveness of IPS when the eyes are opened or closed depends on the physical properties of the light (direct, appropriately patterned or diffuse).

Eyes open is more provocative than eyes closed when patterned IPS is used.

Eyes closed is more provocative than eyes open when direct unpatterned light is used.

When IPS is applied through a diffuser, eyes open become more effective than eyes closed, because of the reduction in light intensity caused by the closed eyelids.[133] This may be the first publication to explain the contradictory findings in the literature as to whether IPS is more effective with eyes-open or closed. Reports that IPS is more provocative when the eyes are closed than when they are open are

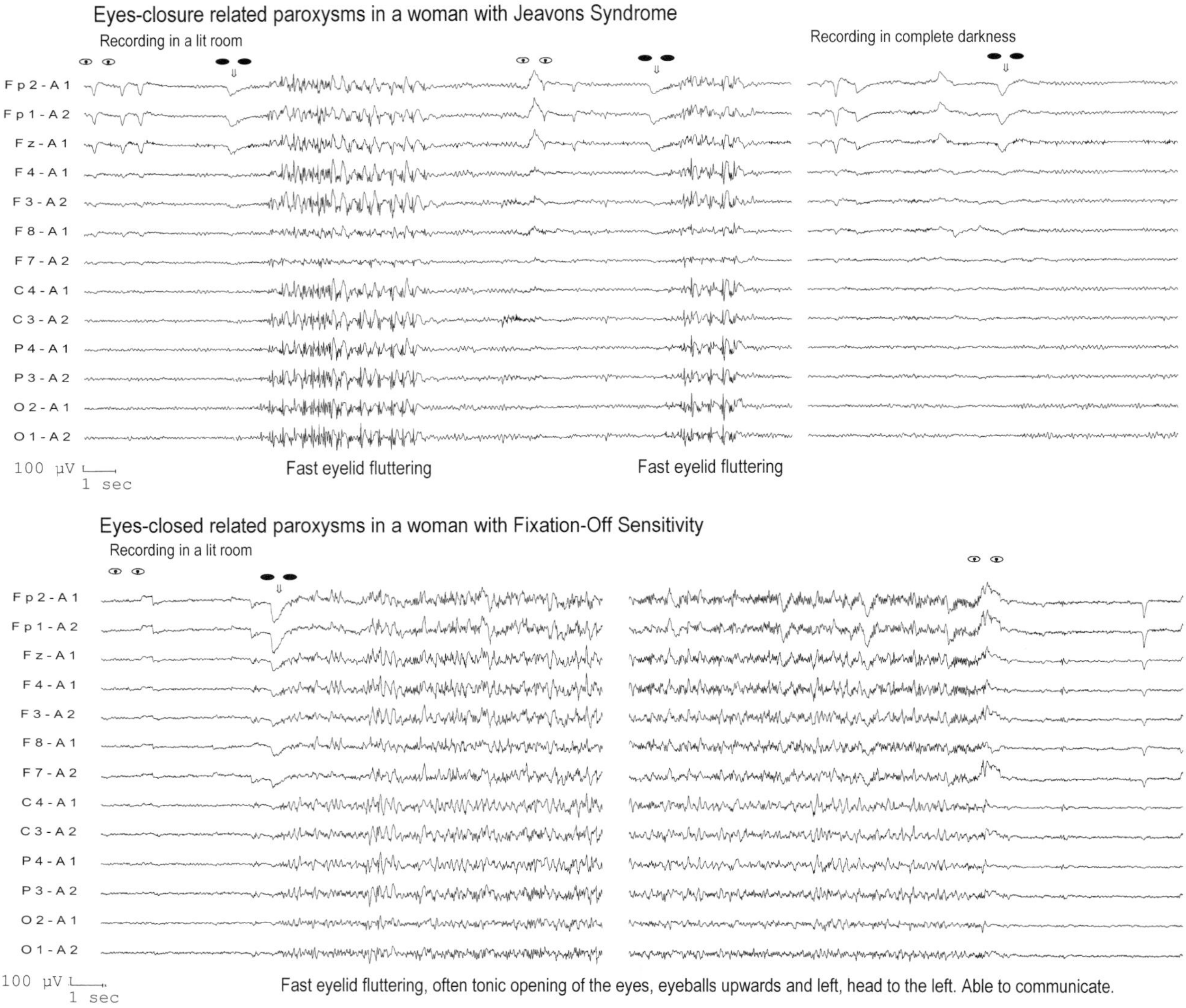

Figure 13.4 Samples from video EEG to illustrate the differentiation between eyes-closed (top) and eye-closure (bottom) abnormalities.

Top: Eye closure-related abnormalities in a patient with Jeavons syndrome.[130] High amplitude generalised discharges occur within 1–3 s after closing the eyes in a lit room. These are of brief duration, do not continue in the resting period while the eyes are closed and are totally inhibited in complete darkness.

Bottom: Eyes closed-related abnormalities in a woman who probably has cryptogenic generalised epilepsy and seizures related to FOS (case report in refs [39;131]). The EEG paroxysms last as long as the eyes are closed. They are abruptly inhibited when the eyes are opened. The responses to fixation off and on were similar irrespective of the means by which they were achieved (eyes closed, darkness, +10 spherical lenses, Ganzfeld stimulation). The best practical means for testing FOS is with underwater goggles covered with opaque tape.

partly due to methodological problems, such as: (a). eyes closed is often equated with eye closure; (b). eyes closed is tested for the same train of IPS after eyes open, thus after longer exposure to IPS; and (c) testing with unpatterned or non-diffused IPS.[133] Eyes open is much more photoparoxysmal than eyes closed when 'appropriately' patterned IPS is used. I emphasise 'appropriately' patterned, because not all patterns are appropriate.

Appropriate patterns: "Quadrilled patterns of thin lines are more effective than similar patterns consisting of thick lines."[128;129] "An optimally epileptogenic pattern consists of black and white stripes of equal width and sharp contour (a square-wave luminance profile)."[36]

Inappropriate pattern: The checkerboard pattern used by some authors[134] is not only a weak stimulus itself, but also greatly reduces the intensity of the light stimulus, because its alternate solid-black squares black out approximately half the lamp.

INTERMITTENT PHOTIC STIMULATION TECHNIQUE

To achieve maximum provocation, IPS has to apply all the potent physical characteristics of the stimulus (intensity, frequency, contrast) and combine flash with linear patterns. The patient should look at the centre of the stroboscope and IPS on eye closure should be tested.[12;121;122] Monocular stimulation is usually ineffective.

There is a great diversity of techniques and photostimulators used for IPS in EEG as detailed in an experts' consensus on the standardisation of IPS screening methods.[122] IPS standardisation is unlikely to have universal success unless the manufacturers of stimulators agree to a standard device. Most of the modern photostimulators are unsuitable for proper IPS testing.

The most comprehensible procedure for photic stimulation is that of Jeavons:[12;135]

1. The procedure is explained to the patient.
2. The same photostimulator that was used initially is used in all repeat tests.
3. Illumination of the room is standardised by drawing blinds and using artificial light.
4. The lowest intensity light is used initially, increased if there is no abnormality, and standardised in subsequent tests.
5. A pattern of small squares with narrow black lines (0.3 mm), with spacing of 2 mm x 2 mm or a pattern of parallel, 1-mm lines spaced 1.5 mm apart, is placed behind the glass of the lamp (dry print transfers are cheap and easily available).
6. A circle, 3 cm in diameter, is drawn in the centre of the glass and the patient looks at this circle.
7. The lamp is placed 30 cm from the eyes.
8. Testing is carried out with the eyes kept open or kept closed and then, only if no PPR is evoked, the effect of eye closure tested.
9. An initial test frequency of 16 Hz can be used to identify the photosensitive patient. If no PPR is elicited, testing starts at 1 Hz and is increased in increments of 2 Hz up to 25 Hz, followed by 30, 40 and 50 Hz.
10. In the photosensitive patient, the duration of the stimulus should not usually exceed 2 s.
11. In the photosensitive patient, testing starts at 1 Hz and increases in steps of 1 Hz until a PPR is evoked. The upper limit is then established by starting at 60 Hz and reducing in steps of 10 Hz.
12. The sensitivity limit is defined as the lowest or highest flash rate that consistently evokes a PPR. The sensitivity range is obtained by subtracting the lower from the upper limit.

The recent consensus recommendations[121;122] are very similar to those of Jeavons.[12;135]

1 For screening purposes, IPS should not be performed during or less than 3 min after hyperventilation.
2. Patients should be positioned at a distance of 30 cm from the photic stimulator (nasion to lamp) with dim surrounding illumination just sufficient to observe the patient.
3. Flashes should be delivered in separate trains of 10 s for each frequency, with minimum intervals of 7 s. During the 10-s stimulation, the eyes should be initially open with the patient gazing directly at the centre of the lamp. After 5-s stimulation, the patient should be asked to close the eyes and should keep them closed until the stimulation ceases. The following frequencies are used: 1, 2, 3, 4, 6, 8, 10, 12, 14, 16, 18 and 20 Hz, in that order. If generalised epileptiform discharges are evoked, the stimulator should be turned off immediately, and the sequence aborted. Next, a second sequence should be presented, beginning at 60 Hz and decreased as follows: 60, 50, 40, 30, 25 and 20 Hz. Again, the stimulator must be turned off immediately if a generalised response is seen, and the sequence stopped at that point.
4. For clinical purposes, it is important to know whether the response is self-sustaining (i.e. whether it can outlast the stimulus); this may not be established unless the stimulator is switched off as soon as a generalised discharge is seen. The issue is not whether the discharge is self-limiting: a self-sustaining discharge may well cease spontaneously if the stimulator is left on. It should be noted whether clinical signs and symptoms are elicited. The alertness of the patient should be noted both at the beginning of the recording and also, specifically, during IPS. It should be determined whether the patient is, for any reason, in a sleep-deprived state. Medication should also be documented.
5. This procedure lasts a maximum of 6 min. If there is insufficient time to perform this IPS screening procedure, it is advisable to omit photic stimulation altogether, because the results may be misleading.

There are some limited practical reservations about some aspects of these recommendations:

"with dim surrounding illumination just sufficient to observe the patient"[121]

This is to increase the relative intensity of IPS that can be achieved through the photostimulators. Most patients feel uncomfortable in dim surroundings. Further, this makes detection of clinical ictal events, particularly if minor, difficult and the video pictures are disturbed.

"For clinical purposes, it is important to know whether the response is self-sustaining (i.e. whether it can outlast the stimulus); this may not be established unless the stimulator is switched off as soon as a generalised discharge is seen."[121]

The clinical significance of this is probably overemphasised. Further, 'as soon as' depends on a variety of factors. Even the same EEG technologist, during the same test, can have different reaction times, and thus make a self-sustaining response outlast the stimulus response and vice versa. The fact that the technologist has to observe for clinical ictal symptoms simultaneously makes this even more difficult.

"This procedure lasts a maximum of 6 min. If there is insufficient time to perform this IPS screening procedure, it is advisable to omit photic stimulation altogether, because the results may be misleading."

The upper and lower limits of photosensitivity may not be of any clinical significance, and may vary considerably in the same patient and even in the same untreated state. For routine purposes, the test can be reliably performed in half the allocated time without the need to define the photosensitive range.

PHOTOPAROXYSMAL RESPONSES

PPR are broadly categorised as follows:[12;35;72]

- Generalised PPR consist of spike/polyspike–waves in various combinations and intra-discharge frequencies. They may be identical with the discharges associated with typical absence seizures or myoclonic jerks. They may be brief or long. They are of higher amplitude in the anterior regions, but their onset, particularly if patterned IPS is employed, is often with occipital spikes. They are highly associated (90%) with clinical photosensitivity, particularly if they outlast the stimulus train (Figure 13.1). Generalised PPR often (60%) associate with clinical events such as jerks, impairment of cognition or subjective sensations, but video EEG may be needed to detect them.[72]

- Posterior (temporo-parieto-occipital with occipital emphasis) spike/polyspike–waves. This is the mildest form of PPR and does not spread to the anterior regions.[136] It consists of occipital spikes, polyspikes or slow waves intermixed with small, larval spikes (Figures 13.1, 13.2, and 13.5). Occipital spikes are often time-locked to the flash with a latency of approximately 100 ms, coinciding with the positive P_{100} of the VER (Figure 13.2). Occipital spikes and other posterior abnormalities induced by IPS are considered of much lower epileptogenic capacity than generalised PPR. Half of the subjects with posterior PPR have epileptic seizures (spontaneous, photically elicited or both).[12]

Occipital spikes precede generalised PPR in 90% of photosensitive patients when IPS is patterned (combined light and pattern; Figure 13.3).[11;12;108-110;110;136]

Note on the duration of PPR and their relation to the IPS train

Emphasis is often placed on whether photoparoxysmal discharges outlast the stimulus train or whether they are self-limited, that is they stop before or with the end of the IPS (Figure 13.1).[121;122] The rationale is that PPR that outlast the stimulus train may strengthen their association with epilepsy. This may be artificial, because the duration of the PPR as a rule depends on the duration and strength of the IPS, and the time that this was stopped after the appearance of the PPR.

Ictal clinical manifestations during PPR are the most important factor with respect to the risk of clinical epilepsy, but this has been neither studied adequately nor emphasised in the expert consensus reports.[121;122]

Photomyoclonic responses

Photomyoclonic responses are not cerebral responses. They are spike or polyspike-like muscle activity that appears in the frontal-central EEG electrodes.[137-140] They occur only when the eyes are closed and are inhibited by opening of the eyes. Provocation of photomyoclonic responses requires very high intensity IPS with the stroboscope positioned very close to the eyes. They are unlikely to occur when IPS is applied at recommended levels.

Photomyoclonic responses are a non-specific finding reported in normal people (0.3%), psychiatric patients (17%), epileptic patients (3%) and patients with brain stem lesions.[137]

Clinically, they manifest with predominant jerking of the facial muscles, especially around the eyes (eyelid fluttering) – a phenomenon called photomyoclonus.[138;139] They may end in generalised convulsions if the stimulation is continued and the eyes of the subject are kept closed.[137]

PROGNOSIS OF PHOTOSENSITIVE EPILEPSY

The overall view is that photosensitive epilepsy as a whole has a good prognosis for seizure control with or without AED treatment but PPR persist in adult life. [105;141] In one of the largest (100 photosensitive patients) and longest follow-up studies

(14 years average duration of follow-up and 27 mean age) [105] the following results were obtained:

- 77 patients became seizure free.
- of 46 untreated patients , photosensitivity disappeared in 14 (30%) patients but persisted in the other 32 (70%).
- of 54 patients who were treated, 31 (57%) showed evidence of PPR or degraded PPR, but 23 (43%) patients no longer showed evidence of photosensitivity.

However, see different prognoses in syndromes of photosensitive epilepsy such as Jeavons syndrome (page 480) and idiopathic photosensitive occipital lobe epilepsy (page 474).

MANAGEMENT OF PHOTOSENSITIVE EPILEPSY

In patients with pure photosensitive seizures (that is with no spontaneous seizures), avoidance of the provocative stimulus may be adequate.[12] For example, patients with television-induced seizures should be advised to watch television in a well-lit room, maintain a maximum comfortable viewing distance (typically, more than 2.5 m from a 19-inch screen), use the remote control and, if necessary, approach the screen by covering one eye with their palm, and avoid prolonged watching particularly if sleep deprived and tired. Occlusion of one eye is also advised when photosensitive subjects are suddenly exposed to flickering lights, as in discotheques, for example.

Patients with VGS can often do without video games or significantly restrict the time spent playing. They should not play when sleep deprived or tired.
Conditioning treatment or wearing appropriate tinted glasses[125] has been recommended. Small doses of valproate may be needed in patients with possible spontaneous seizures or coexisting spontaneous EEG discharges.

Patients with distinct IGE syndromes and photosensitivity need anti-epileptic drug (AED) treatment (see treatment of IGE, pages 333).

Valproate controls all types of seizure in more than 80% of patients. Clonazepam controls myoclonic jerks, while ethosuximide controls absence seizures.

Levetiracetam appears to be the most superior of all the new AEDs controlling all types of seizure (see Chapter 4 and pages 430–8).[142] It is the only new AED with well-established efficacy in EEG and clinical photosensitivity.[143-145] Levetiracetam reduces or eliminates both the photoparoxysmal responses and the myoclonic jerks elicited by IPS.[143]

Lamotrigine also appears to be effective [146] but it may exaggerate jerks. In an old report, suppression of PPR with lamotrigine has been seen in five patients, of whom four were also taking valproate.[147] These results have not been replicated.

All other new and old AEDs are probably contraindicated in photosensitive epilepsy with generalised seizures.

Self-induced seizures are difficult to control and may need psychiatric or behavioural intervention.[90] On anecdotal evidence, fenfluramine (a serotonin-releasing drug) has been recommended for the treatment of self-induced epilepsy in combination with valproate.[148]

EPILEPTIC SYNDROMES OF PHOTOSENSITIVITY

Photosensitive epilepsy was classified among the generalised epilepsies by the ILAE Commission.[2] This is because:

- photoparoxysmal responses were considered to be primarily generalised, despite the fact that the discharge often has an occipital onset

- a quarter of patients with spontaneous seizures and EEG photosensitivity belong to a variety of epileptic syndromes of IGE, such as juvenile myoclonic epilepsy.

Occipital photosensitivity only recently came into prominence with the recognition of 'idiopathic photosensitive occipital lobe epilepsy' (IPOE) as a distinct reflex epilepsy syndrome.[3;140]

Eyelid myoclonia with absences (Jeavons syndrome) despite its distinctive clinical and EEG features has not been formally recognised by the ILAE.

IDIOPATHIC PHOTOSENSITIVE OCCIPITAL LOBE EPILEPSY

Idiopathic photosensitive occipital lobe epilepsy[3;11;149;150] is a newly recognised syndrome of reflex epilepsy with an age-related onset.[3]

Occipital seizures precipitated by photic stimuli have been well described by Gowers (1881)[151] and Holmes (1927),[152] but have only recently attracted interest. The reason for this is that they were overshadowed by the prevailing view that photosensitive epilepsies are mainly generalised. This is because, with the application of IPS as a provocation method in EEG, it was discovered that the majority of photosensitive patients have generalised discharges.[153;154] Reports of photically induced occipital seizures with or without secondarily generalisation were scarce.[108-110;127;155-160] The traditional view that photosensitive occipital seizures are rare contrasts with recent findings.[9;79;161-167] In one report alone, 45 of 95 patients had occipital seizures precipitated by visual stimuli.[85]

Depending on severity, there may be three significant groups of patients with photosensitive occipital seizures:[11]

1. *Patients with low occipital epileptogenic threshold to IPS that manifest with seizures only under extreme exposure to the offending stimulation.* These are classified among 'seizures that do not require a diagnosis of epilepsy';[3] accidental single isolated occipital seizures in normal young persons[166] or patients with migraine[166] during IPS. These people most likely have a low threshold to such events.
2. *Patients with idiopathic occipital (lobular) epileptogenicity that may comprise the majority of IPOE.* Patients, usually children, have clinical occipital seizures elicited by various sources of environmental light stimulation (video games are far more common than television).
3. *Patients, usually children, with idiopathic focal or generalised epilepsies* who also have photosensitive occipital seizures. These are often demanding cases in terms of diagnosis and management.

Considerations on classification:
The boundaries of this syndrome of IPOE are genuinely uncertain. Photosensitive occipital seizures may start in adulthood,[168] may be part of Gastaut-type COE,[11;162] may develop later in children with Rolandic seizures[11;169] or occur accidentally during IPS of normal or migraine subjects.[11] Gastaut[162] included photosensitive patients with or without IPOE in his syndrome. Thus, of 63 patients 7 had IPS-evoked occipital spikes, "not seen in the resting EEG" and 'unrelated to eye opening and closing' and another 7 patients with typical occipital paroxysms had generalised PPR, which were sometimes associated myoclonus (see also case 11 in ref [162]). Also, one-third of the patients reported by Terasaki et al. (1987)[170] had photosensitivity. Contrary to this is the view that "reflex triggering of seizures has not been reported in Gastaut-type COE".[149]

DEMOGRAPHIC DATA

Of 39 patients (18 were boys and 21 girls) with occipital photosensitivity that I reviewed from the literature,[11] age at onset of the first provoked seizure ranged from 15 months to 19 years with a mean at around 12 years of age. Adult onset IPOE has been recently documented.[168] The prevalence is low and comprises about 0.4% of all epilepsies.[11]

CLINICAL MANIFESTATIONS

Occipital seizures are induced by video games and less often by television or other photic stimuli. These reflex seizures contain all the elements detailed in the spontaneous seizures of occipital lobe epilepsy (see page 469).[165;167;171;172] Commonly, they manifest with visual hallucinations, blurring of vision or blindness, alone or in combination. Less often, they may follow other ictal occipital manifestations, such as deviation of the eyes and head, eyelid fluttering and orbital pain.

Visual seizures are the commonest. They usually consist of elementary hallucinations of multicoloured and circular spots (circles or spheres), though other shapes (square, triangular) may occur. They may be stationary, flashing, moving or expanding and appear on one side or the centre of the visual field.

Visual hallucinations may be the only ictal manifestations.[167] They usually last for seconds, frequently 1–3 min and rarely longer 5–15 min, in which case other occipital or extra-occipital symptoms also occur.[165;167] Consciousness is not impaired during the phase of visual symptoms.

Blurring of vision and blindness may be the first ictal symptom reported by almost one-fifth of patients. More often, ictal symptoms appear after the visual hallucinations. Metamorphopsia and sensations of objects moving around are rarely reported.[165]

Eyelid flickering with pallinopsia as an occipital seizure manifestation at onset is uncommon:

> An intelligent student, aged 17 years, had a single seizure provoked after 5 min exposure to stroboscopic lights in a dark room. He vividly remembers his eyelids flickering at the same rate of 15 Hz as the flash of the strobe: "These were time-locked to each flash". At his request, his friends switched the stroboscope off, but he continued to see the flash and he had the eyelid flickering as if the stroboscope was still on. This lasted for another 5 s followed by GTCS. The EEG was otherwise normal, but IPS provoked occipital spikes when his eyes were closed.

Progression of visual seizures to other ictal symptoms

Visual and purely occipital seizures may progress to autonomic symptoms, mainly retching and ictal vomiting, like those occurring in Panayiotopoulos syndrome. Ending with secondarily GTCS is common.[11;167]

Postictal symptoms

Occipital seizures are more likely than any other type of focal seizures to be followed by headache, nausea and vomiting. The headache is usually mild and diffuse, but may also be severe and throbbing, occurring 10–20 min after the end of the visual hallucinations. Postictal headache may also be associated with vomiting lasting for several hours.[167]

OTHER TYPE OF SEIZURES

Patients with IPOE may have exclusively occipital seizures that are only photically induced. Others may also have spontaneous visual or other types of seizures, such as myoclonic jerks, absences and GTCS that may also be photically induced or spontaneous.

In some cases, spontaneous secondarily GTCS occur only during sleep.[11]

Brief photically induced visual seizures started at the age of 9 years. They consist of a flashing light, "like a flash of a camera switching on and off" in the left visual field. In addition, he has three or four nocturnal secondarily GTCS every year. These are stereotyped. He wakes up with the same visual hallucination of a flashing light on the left, he calls his parents and within a minute he has the convulsions (case 12.4 in ref [172]).

A few patients with Rolandic seizures may later develop photosensitive occipital seizures.[11;171]

He had 15 typical nocturnal Rolandic seizures from the age 11 years and the EEG revealed centrotemporal spikes. At the age of 14, he had a single diurnal seizure while playing a television video game. This started with visual hallucinations on the left of his vision with "small multicoloured concentric circles of mainly blue, green and yellow, which gradually within seconds multiplied not allowing him to see through them". These were, within half a minute, followed by a GTCS (case 12.5 in ref [172]).

Occipital seizures with bizarre ictal symptomatology mimicking hysterical attacks or migraine are well reported.[11;167] That these symptoms, even the very prolonged and unusual ones, are ictal has been documented by ictal EEG in the eminent report by Guerrini et al. [167]

PRECIPITATING FACTORS

By definition, all patients with IPOE are sensitive to flickering lights, but the severity of the photosensitivity varies. Some patients have seizures on minimal photic provocation, others following combined pattern and photic provocation or prolonged exposure and, in the majority, photic stimuli are effective only if combined with other facilitating factors, such as excitement, frustration, fatigue and sleep deprivation.[10;11]

Occipital seizures caused by animated cartoons on television reached epidemic proportions in December 1997, when 700 children in Japan developed 'vomiting and convulsions' while watching a popular program called 'Pokemon (Pocket Monsters)'.[85] Of 95 affected children, 31 had generalised seizures and 49 patients had focal seizures. All but four of the focal seizures were occipital and consisted of "visual symptoms such as flickering spots, fogging, visual hallucination, or blindness". Vomiting and headache were common. Focal seizures occurred more frequently than generalised seizures in the younger age group.

Some of the photosensitive patients with VGS suffer from IPOE.[9;79]

AETIOLOGY

IPOE, by definition, is idiopathic and may constitute a small part of the benign childhood seizure susceptibility syndrome. Some patients have a family history of similar seizures elicited by photic stimuli.[150] Symptomatic occipital photosensitivity was already known to Holmes (1927)[152] in patients with gunshot wounds but this by definition is not part of IPOE.

PATHOPHYSIOLOGY

IPOE is a purely occipital reflex epilepsy by virtue of the onset of the clinical seizures (mainly visual seizures), and EEG interictal and ictal localisation. Photosensitive occipital epileptogenesis was first documented by Clementi (1929),[174] who described light-induced seizures with photic stimulation (effective triggering stimuli had to be repetitive) in dogs after application of strychnine to the visual cortex (see review in ref [149]).

DIAGNOSTIC PROCEDURES

All tests apart from the EEG and VER are normal.

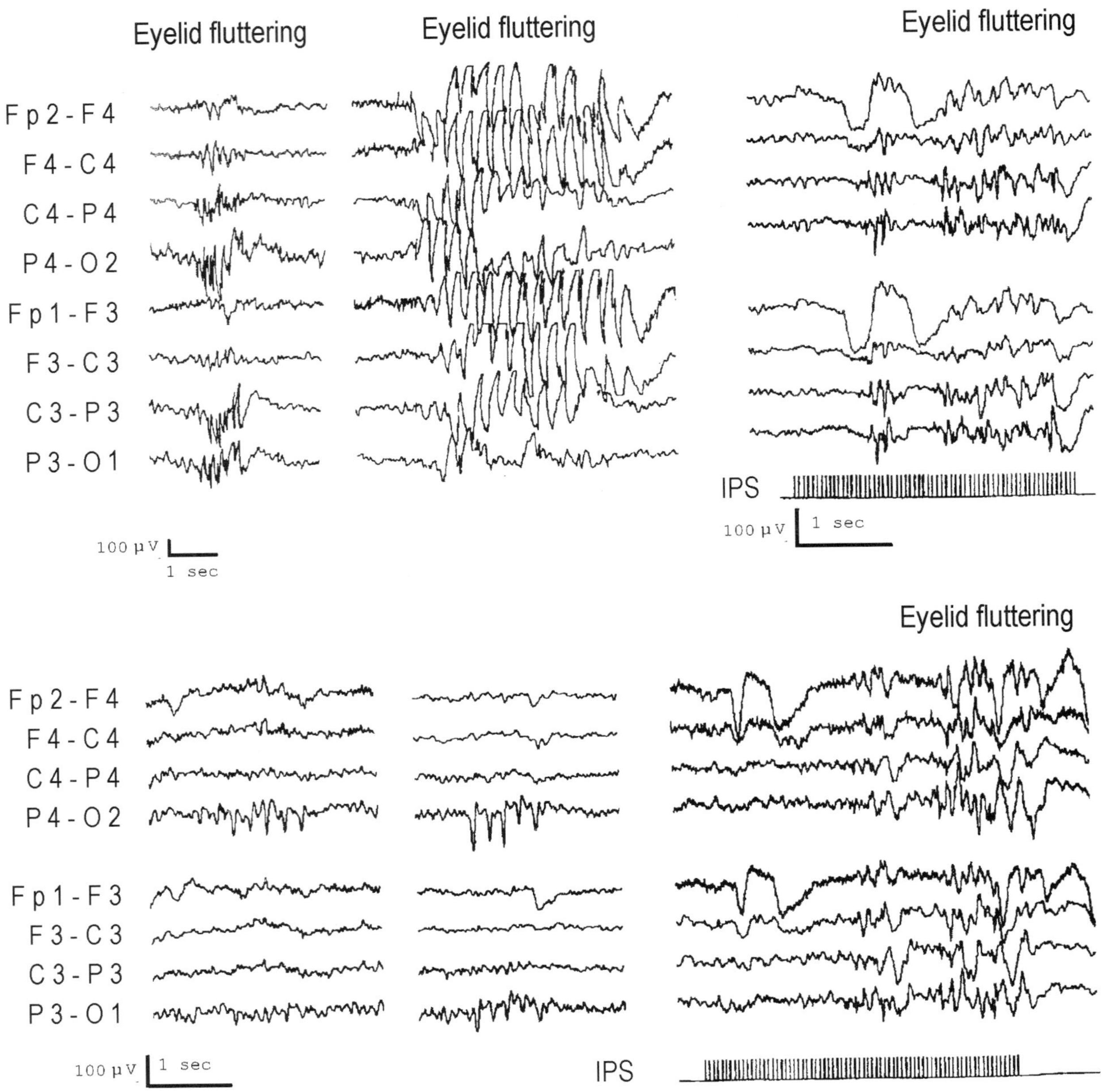

Figure 13.5 Video EEG samples of spontaneous EEG paroxysms and photically induced posterior or maximum posterior PPR in two children with photically induced occipital seizures. They probably have IPOE. Top is case 12.1 and bottom is case 12.2 in ref [11].

Top left and middle: Spontaneous occipital spikes/polyspikes and generalised discharges are associated with eyelid fluttering, which is conspicuous on video EEG. Neither the patient nor her relatives were aware of these.
Top right: IPS consistently elicited posterior spikes, which were also associated with ictal eyelid fluttering.
This patient had typical multicoloured visual seizures from the age 5 years (case 12.1 in ref [11]). They were elicited by environmental lights and occasionally progressed to GTCS. She improved over the years, but at 20 years of age and while on medication with valproate, she had a visual seizure with GTCS while watching TV from nearly touching distance. High resolution MRI was normal.
Bottom left and right: Spontaneous occipital paroxysms without discernible clinical manifestations.
Bottom right: IPS consistently elicited PPR with maximum posterior emphasis. These were often associated with conspicuous eyelid fluttering.
This patient illustrated the links between IPOE and the benign childhood seizure susceptibility syndrome (case 12.2 in ref [11]). She initially had typical Rolandic seizures and then developed frequent visual seizures often with secondarily GTCS. These were sometimes photically induced, but more often occurred during sleep. High resolution MRI was normal.

From Panayiotopoulos (1999)[11] with the permission of the Publisher John Libbe

ELECTROENCEPHALOGRAPHY

By definition, all patients are photosensitive. IPS elicits: (a). PPR spikes or polyspikes entirely confined in the occipital regions; or (b) generalised PPR of spikes or polyspikes that predominate in the posterior regions (Figures 13.5, and 13.6).

Spontaneous, mainly posterior spikes often appear in the resting EEG. Centrotemporal spikes may coexist.

Ictal EEGs document an occipital origin with mainly fast spikes in one or both the occipital electrodes. This may end spontaneously or spread to the temporal regions.[149]

In my experience, most patients with IPOE also have other type of seizures induced by IPS, such as eyelid flickering and myoclonia, myoclonic jerks of the limbs, body or fingers, and brief absences that are occasionally mild, which may escape detection if video EEG is not employed (Figure 13.5).[11]

VISUAL EVOKED RESPONSES

VER are always of abnormally high amplitude,[149] as indeed happens in any type of photosensitive epilepsy.[109;114;173]

DIFFERENTIAL DIAGNOSIS

The differential diagnosis of IPOE includes migraine (rarely an actual problem if symptoms are appropriately analysed), Gastaut-type COE (of no prognostic

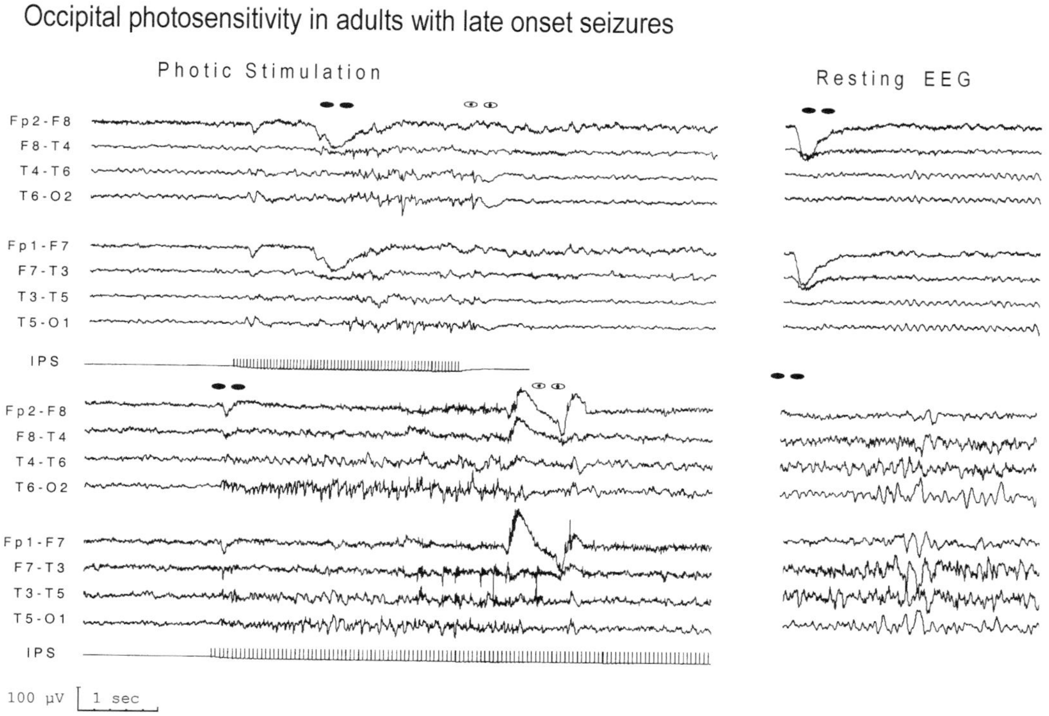

Figure 13.6 Adult onset IPOE.

Top: Sample from an EEG of a man who had his first seizure at the age of 35 years while in a lift cradle at work. His vision became blurred, he felt dizzy and, within 2 min, he had a GTCS. No further seizures occurred in the next 6 months of follow up. MRI was normal.
Bottom. Sample from an EEG of a woman who had her first seizure at the age of 31 years. There was a cluster of precipitating factors. She had consumed a few alcoholic drinks, was sleep deprived, 4 months pregnant and dancing exposed to flickering discotheque lights until the early hours of the next day. She first experienced whirling lights in front of her eyes, visual perception became disturbed and within a minute she had a GTCS. She was well in the next 4 months of follow up. MRI was normal.

significance other than classification and avoidance of precipitating factors), idiopathic generalised epilepsies (probably important in management) and pseudo-seizures (sometimes very difficult).

The differential diagnosis of visual seizures from all types of migraine with visual aura is not different for IPOE. Some seizures of IPOE may be prolonged and also progress from visual symptoms to nausea and vomiting with altered consciousness.[167;175] The spread of the discharge from the occipital cortex can be slow and responsiveness may be maintained while the patient is vomiting.[167;175] These seizures may be erroneously diagnosed as migraine proper.

In children and adolescents, differentiation of IPOE from the Gastaut-type COE is not of any prognostic significance. IPOE may be part of this syndrome.

Differentiation of IPOE from generalised photosensitive epilepsies should rely on clinical criteria. Occipital spikes often precede generalised PPR in photosensitive epilepsies.

Occipital photosensitivity has recently been documented in adults (Figure 13.6).[168] The patients were about 30 years of age and presented with a late onset first GTCS (often preceded by visual symptoms).[168] Of 1550 patients with seizures, three women and two men (0.3%) had EEG occipital photosensitivity and onset of solitary (three patients) or infrequent seizures in adulthood (median age 31 years; range 26–35 years). All five of these patients had generalised convulsions, which were preceded by blurring of vision or elementary visual hallucinations in four cases. Precipitation by lights, alone or in combination with other factors, was apparent in only two patients. Seizures were diurnal in all but one patient. According to the inclusion criteria, all the patients had EEG occipital spikes elicited by IPS (Figure 13.6). Neurological and intellectual state as well as brain imaging was normal.

PROGNOSIS

The frequency of seizures and overall prognosis varies significantly among affected individuals. It depends on the severity of the photosensitivity and exposure to offending visual stimuli.[11;149;167]

There are rare case reports of normal young people[166] or patients with migraine[166;176] having an occipital seizure only during potent IPS in EEG testing. Some patients may have only one or two occipital seizures in their life despite exposure to precipitating factors and no drug treatment.[11;149;167] Others, particularly those who also have spontaneous seizures, may need medication for 1–3 years together with strict avoidance or cautious exposure to insulting stimuli. However, other patients may have frequent spontaneous and reflex occipital fits alone or in combination with other types of seizures, which may include myoclonic jerks, often of the eyelids, infrequent absences and GTCS.[11]

MANAGEMENT

Advice regarding avoidance of precipitating factors is essential and is similar to that for patients with any type of photosensitivity. Particular emphasis is needed regarding video games and television.

Though valproate is the drug of choice in generalised photosensitive epilepsies, it is uncertain whether this is also the case for IPOE. Patients with IPOE resistant to valproate became seizure free with the addition of carbamazepine.[11] Clobazam may be effective.[162]

Levetiracetam may be an effective alternative particularly in view of its broad action in focal and generalised seizures, and photosensitivity. [142-145]

JEAVONS SYNDROME
EYELID MYOCLONIA WITH ABSENCES

Jeavons syndrome is one of the most distinctive reflex IGE syndromes with well-defined clinico-EEG manifestations.[130;177;178] However, it is not recognised by the ILAE Commission[2] and not listed in the new ILAE diagnostic scheme,[3] although vividly described by Jeavons[179;180] and documented in numerous reports.[177;181-183] Jeavons syndrome is characterised by the triad of:

1. eyelid myoclonia with and without absences
2. eye closure-induced seizures, EEG paroxysms or both
3. photosensitivity.

DEMOGRAPHIC DATA

Onset is typically in childhood with a peak at 6–8 years of age (range 2–14 years). There is a twofold preponderance of girls. In our studies all adult patients with EMA were women.[130;178] However, recently I saw a 32-year-old man with eyelid myoclonia from the age of 3 years. He never had any other type of seizure and his disease would have gone unnoticed if he had not been curious to find out about this 'embarrassing tic'. I also saw another man in his late 20s, who had Jeavons syndrome as a child, but whose symptoms subsided in his late teens. Based on this experience, I am of the reasonable opinion that Jeavons syndrome is not only less frequent, but also less potent in men than women.

The prevalence of Jeavons syndrome is around 3% among adult patients with epileptic disorders and 13% among IGEs with absences.[130]

CLINICAL MANIFESTATIONS

Eyelid myoclonia, not the absences, is the hallmark of Jeavons syndrome (Figures 13.7, and 13.8).[130;178]

Eyelid myoclonia consists of marked jerking of the eyelids often associated with jerky upward deviation of the eyeballs and retropulsion of the head *(eyelid myoclonia without absences)*. This may be associated with or followed by mild impairment of consciousness *(eyelid myoclonia with absences)*. The seizures are brief (3–6 s), and occur mainly after eye closure and consistently many times per day.

Considerations on classification:

The new ILAE diagnostic scheme[3] has not recognised Jeavons syndrome. Instead, a new seizure type 'eyelid myoclonia with and without absences' has been accepted.[3;178] These seizures occur in many epileptic conditions of idiopathic, symptomatic or possibly symptomatic causes.[178;184] They are the defining seizure symptom in Jeavons syndrome, which has unique clinical and EEG features and often genetic clustering.[130;178;185;186]

In the absence of any ILAE definition, I propose the following: Jeavons syndrome (eyelid myoclonia with absences) is an idiopathic epileptic syndrome manifested with frequent (pyknoleptic) seizures, consisting of eyelid myoclonia often associated with absences. Onset is usually in early childhood. The seizures are brief (3–6 s) and occur mainly after eye closure. They consist of eyelid myoclonia, which persists throughout the attack with or without absences. Absences without eyelid myoclonia do not occur. The eyelid myoclonia consists of marked, rhythmic and fast jerks of the eyelids, often associated with jerky upward deviation of the eyeballs and retropulsion of the head. There is probably an associated tonic component of the involved muscles. If the seizure is prolonged, impairment of consciousness occurs. The latter is mild or moderately severe without associated automatisms. Milder seizures of eyelid myoclonia without absences are common, particularly in adults and treated patients, and may occur without EEG accompaniments. All patients are highly photosensitive in childhood, but this declines with age. Infrequent GTCS, either induced by lights or spontaneous, are probably inevitable in the long term and are likely to occur after sleep deprivation, fatigue and alcohol indulgence. Myoclonic jerks of the limbs may occur, but are infrequent and random. The eyelid myoclonia of Jeavons syndrome is resistant to treatment and may be lifelong. However, clinical absences may become less frequent with age.

The EEG ictal manifestations consist mainly of generalised polyspike–waves at 3–6 Hz, which are more likely to occur after eye closure in an illuminated room. Total darkness abolishes the abnormalities related to eye closure. PPR are recorded from all untreated young patients.

All patients are photosensitive.

Generalised tonic clonic seizures, either induced by lights or spontaneous, are probably inevitable in the long term and are particularly provoked by precipitating factors (sleep deprivation, alcohol) and inappropriate AED modifications. Typically, GTCS are sparse and avoidable.

Myoclonic jerks of the limbs may occur, but are infrequent and random.

Eyelid myoclonic status epilepticus either spontaneous, mainly on awakening, or photically induced occurs in one-fifth of patients. It consists of repetitive and discontinuous episodes of eyelid myoclonia with mild absence, rather than continuous non-convulsive absence status epilepticus (Figure 13.8).

Precipitating factors

The most potent precipitating factor is eye closure, whether it be voluntary, involuntary or reflex. The majority and, in some patients, all of the seizures are induced immediately after closure of the eyes in the presence of uninterrupted light. Eye closure in total darkness is ineffective.

Contrary to other forms of photosensitive epilepsies that are sensitive only to flickering lights (IPS), patients with Jeavons syndrome are also sensitive to bright, non-flickering lights. This is probably due to the enhancing effect of bright light on eye-closure sensitivity.

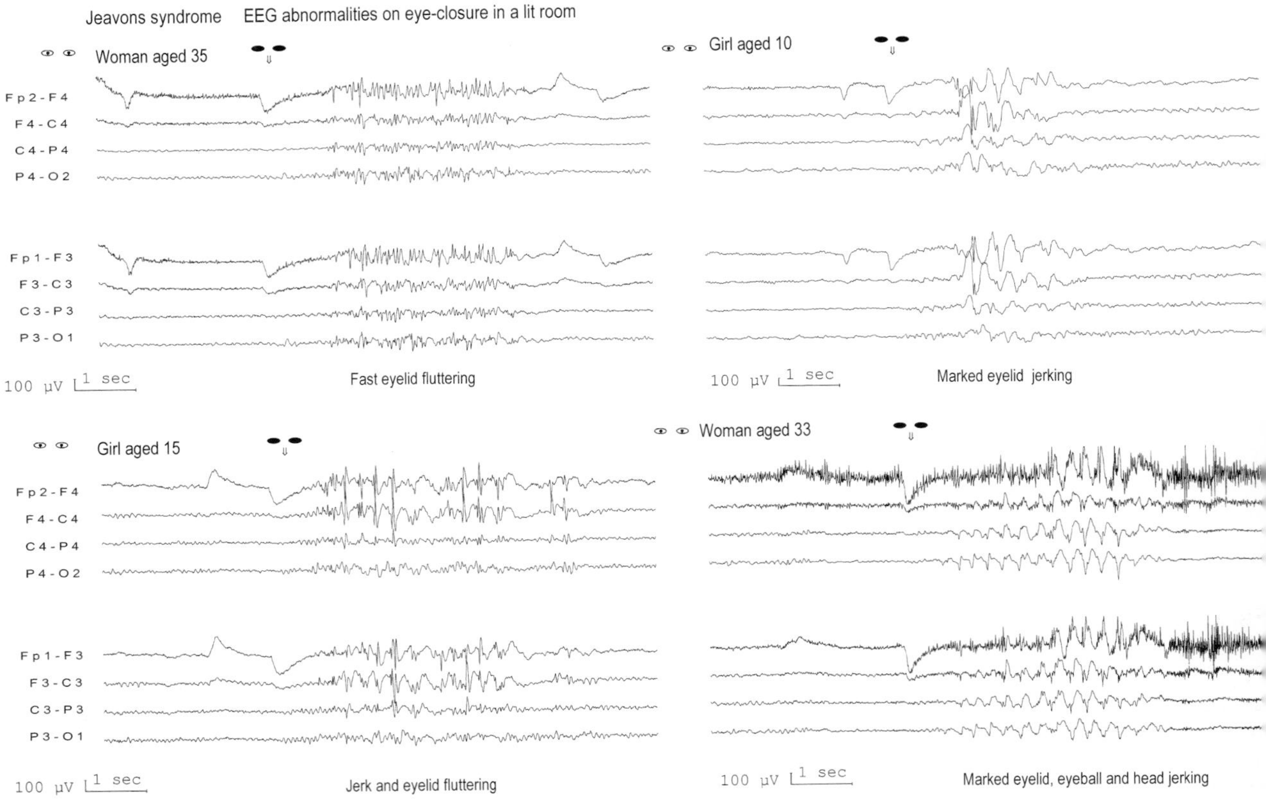

Figure 13.7 Video EEG samples of four women with Jeavons syndrome.[35;130]

Brief generalised discharges of spikes/polyspike–waves in various combinations occur immediately after eye closure in a lit EEG recording room. They are associated with ictal eyelid manifestations with no discernible impairment of consciousness.

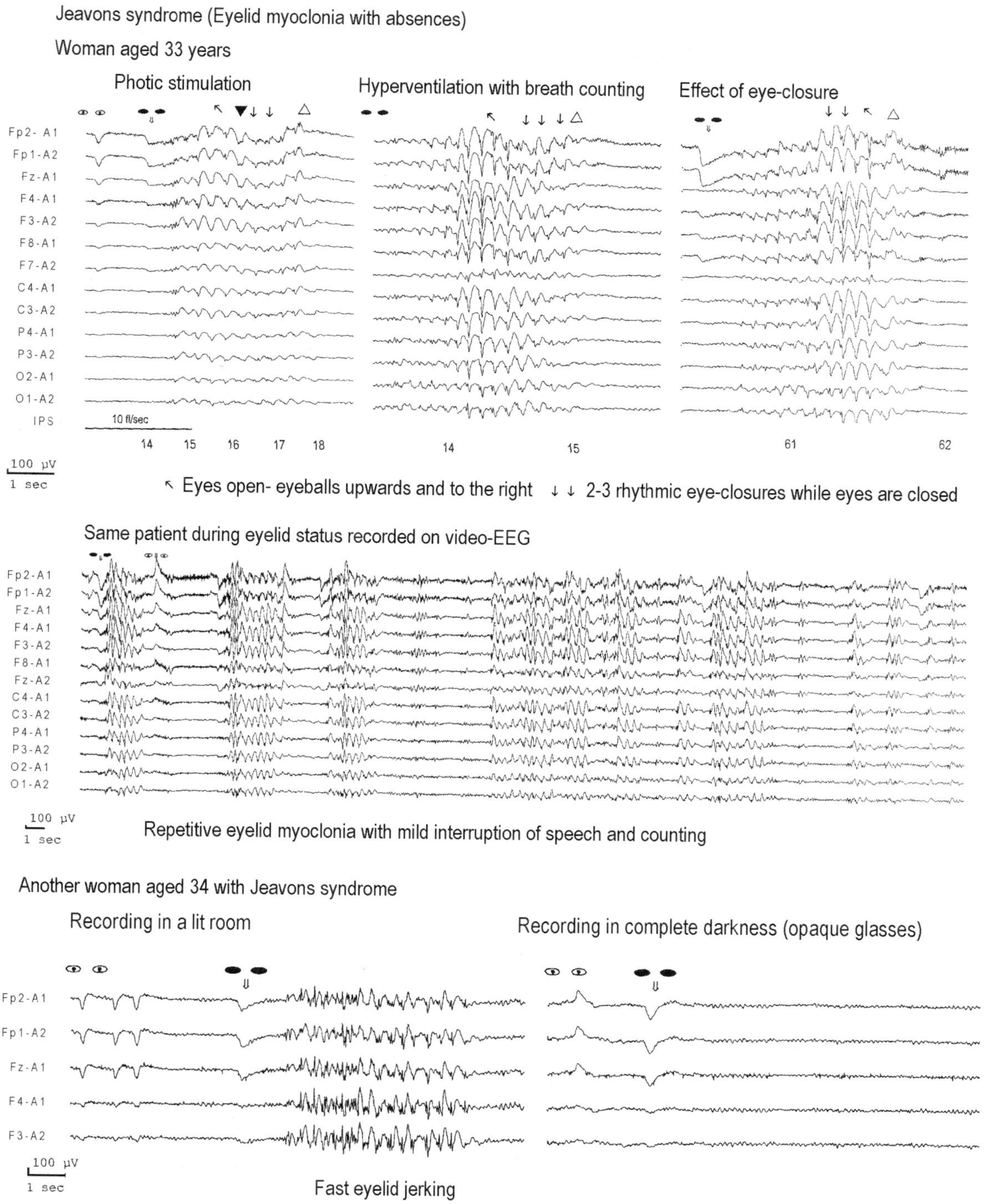

Figure 13.8 Video EEG samples from two women with Jeavons syndrome.[35;130]

Top: Brief GSWD with similar characteristics are induced by IPS (left) or eye closure (right). They occasionally occur spontaneously (middle). In all illustrated occasions, these GSWD were associated with marked eyelid myoclonia denoted by various symbols. Also note that there is no impairment of counting (numbers).
Middle: Repetitive discontinuous seizures of eyelid myoclonia occurred on awakening when the patient was erroneously treated with carbamazepine. These lasted for more than half an hour. There was only mild interruption of speech and counting during the GSWD. The patient was fully aware of her condition.
Bottom: Long video EEG of a woman with Jeavons syndrome while taking valproate. There were frequent eye-closure related GSWD of mainly polyspikes, often associated with fast eyelid jerking, which could be mild or violent. The GSWD occurred only in the presence of light. They were totally inhibited in complete darkness (complete darkness implies that any form of possible light was totally eliminated).
Symbols of eyes indicate when the eyes were open or closed.

Self-induction in Jeavons syndrome

Most relevant reports and most epileptologists unquestionably consider the eyelid myoclonia of Jeavons syndrome as a manoeuvre used by patients to self-induce IPS and elicit seizures. Our view, based on numerous video EEG recordings and interviews with 17 patients, is that eyelid myoclonia is an ictal event (15 patients) and that self-induced seizures in Jeavons syndrome are rare (possibly two patients).[35;178] After all, these patients do not need IPS to induce seizures. Closing of the eyes (there is no need for forceful slow eye-closure) in the presence of uninterrupted light may be more powerful than IPS in provoking a seizure. In physiological terms, these clinical manifestations are likely to be similar to an 'attraction movement' to light and other manifestations of the 'optic fixation reflexes', when volitional movements of the eyes are unattainable or weak.[99]

> My eyes flicker as a reflex to the light.

Patients consider eyelid myoclonia as a socially embarrassing condition, they are relieved when the seizures improve with AEDs and they show excellent compliance with their treatment.

Of two patients suspected of self-induction, one had frequent slow eye-closure EEG abnormalities, but she never admitted self-induction. She insisted:

> I do not know when I am doing it. . . . It gives me no pleasure, and it is a social embarrassment.

The other patient admitted that she occasionally does it voluntarily:

> Yes, I can do it on purpose like that (she imitates rapid eyelid blinking with upwards deviation of the eyes). But that is because there are times that my eyes start to want to go … because they are strained and sore and they will sting, and so if I just do it, it relaxes them. . . .That is a rare occasion. But other than that, I do not know. There have been incidences I have walked into a pole, or into a car. I did not do that on purpose.

However, in a study of six children with Jeavons syndrome, five were found to demonstrate various compulsive or tic-like symptoms including premonitory sensations, compulsive, difficult to resist urges and a sense of relief associated with the attacks.[181] Separate facial tics not associated with absences were also evident in at least two children.[181] Therefore, these patients may not be deliberate 'self-inducers', but may suffer from compulsive 'self-induction' similar to the phenomenology described in Tourette's syndrome.[181]

AETIOLOGY

Jeavons syndrome is a genetically determined homogeneous syndrome.[185;186] In one study of 18 patients with Jeavons syndrome, 14 had a family history of epilepsy and four patients had other family members affected by the same syndrome.[186]

PATHOPHYSIOLOGY

In Jeavons syndrome, as opposed to other photosensitive epilepsies, eye closure is more potent than photic stimulation as a triggering factor.[35;130;178] However, eye closure requires the presence of light, and it is entirely ineffective in darkness, which may explain that continuous light also triggers seizures in patients with Jeavons syndrome. Another intriguing feature is that some patients may manifest with both features of photosensitivity and FOS, which have opposing characteristics.

Eye-closure mechanisms and photosensitivity may be linked, the one enhances the other, and they often coexist, but they can also occur independently and one may persist without the other. A similar situation may exist between eye closure, which is mainly linked with photosensitivity and eyes-closed mechanisms, which are mainly linked to FOS. It is fascinating that two apparently opposite conditions (photosensitivity and FOS) can have synergistic actions as demonstrated in some patients with Jeavons syndrome.

It is possible that, in patients with Jeavons syndrome, the alpha-rhythm generators malfunction, and that both the magnocellular and parvocellular systems are functionally disturbed.[35;178]

We do not know the physiology of the epileptic phenomena and the alterations that may occur in the brain of patients with Jeavons syndrome, under the continuous bombardment from electrical discharges nearly every time that they close their eyes. Age at onset may be significant.

DIAGNOSTIC PROCEDURES

All tests apart from the EEG are normal.

ELECTROENCEPHALOGRAPHY

Video EEG is the single most important procedure for the diagnosis of eyelid myoclonia with or without absences. It shows frequent high amplitude 3–6 Hz GSWD of mainly polyspikes (Figures 13.7, and 13.8). These typically are:

- related to eye closure, that is they occur immediately (within 0.5–2 s) of closing the eyes in an illuminated recording room and they are eliminated in total darkness
- brief (1–6 s, commonly 2–3 s).

GSWD are also enhanced by hyperventilation. Eyelid myoclonia of varying severity often occurs with the GSWD.

PPR are recorded from all untreated young patients, but may be absent in older patients or those on medication. Photosensitivity and FOS may coexist.[39]

Sleep EEG patterns are normal. GSWD are more likely to increase during sleep, but may also decrease. In sleep, the GSWD are shorter and devoid of discernible clinical manifestations of any type, even in those patients who have numerous seizures during alert states.

The EEG and clinical manifestations deteriorate consistently after awakening.

A normal EEG is rare, even in well-controlled patients.

DIFFERENTIAL DIAGNOSIS

The diagnosis of Jeavons syndrome is simple because the characteristic eyelid myoclonia, if seen once, will never be forgotten or confused with other conditions.[187] Furthermore, the EEG with the characteristic eye-closure related discharges and photosensitivity leaves no room for diagnostic error.

As a simple rule of the thumb, eyelid myoclonia is highly suggestive of Jeavons syndrome. This becomes more likely when eyelid myoclonia is combined with photosensitivity, and it is pathognomonic of the syndrome when it also occurs after eye closure.

Nevertheless, eyelid myoclonia is often misdiagnosed as facial tics, sometimes for many years. Also, eyelid myoclonia should not be confused with: (a). the rhythmic or random closing of the eyes, often seen in other forms of IGE with absences; or (b). the eyelid jerking that may occur at the opening or the initial stage of the GSWD in typical absence seizures of childhood absence epilepsy.

Persistent, frequent, nonepileptic paroxysmal eyelid movements that occur in patients with PPR are a source of diagnostic confusion which can be avoided with video-EEG recordings.[188]

The main diagnostic problem, which is probably iatrogenic, is self-induction, but this is a diagnosis that should not be made unquestionably because it is often wrong. However, some photosensitive patients may self-induce seizures by repetitive opening and closing of the eyes in front of a bright light source. These patients are simply photosensitive patients imitating Jeavons syndrome.[35;178]

The symptom/seizure of eyelid myoclonia alone is not sufficient to characterise Jeavons syndrome, because it may also occur in symptomatic and cryptogenic epilepsies, which are betrayed by developmental delay, learning difficulties, neurological deficits, abnormal MRI and abnormal background EEG.[178;184;189]

PROGNOSIS

Jeavons syndrome is a lifelong disorder, even if seizures are well controlled with AEDs. Men have a better prognosis than women. There is a tendency for photosensitivity to disappear in middle age but eyelid myoclonia persists. It is highly resistant to treatment and occurs many times per day, often without apparent absences, and even without demonstrable photosensitivity.[130]

MANAGEMENT

Based on anecdotal evidence, the drugs of choice are those used for other IGEs.[194] Valproate alone or most likely in combination with clonazepam or ethosuximide appears to be the most effective regimen. The choice of the second drug depends on the main seizure type. Clonazepam is highly efficacious in eyelid myoclonia and myoclonic jerks; some patients achieve relatively good control with clonazepam monotherapy.

Of the new AEDs, levetiracetam may be the most effective, because of its antimyoclonic and antiphotosensitive properties). Lamotrigine may exaggerate myoclonic jerks.

Carbamazepine, gabapentin, oxcarbazepine, phenytoin, tiagabine and vigabatrin are contraindicated.

Lifestyle and avoidance of seizure precipitants are important.

Non-pharmacological treatments used for photosensitive patients (such as wearing special glasses) often have a beneficial effect and should also be employed in Jeavons syndrome when photosensitivity persists.[195]

Misconceptions

A main misconception in Jeavons syndrome is that eyelid myoclonia (the seizure) is a self-induced attempt to induce seizures. This belief is so strong that, in nearly all relevant publications, the patient described by Radovici et al. (1932)[190] is erroneously cited as the first reported case of self-induced seizures even by hand waving.[93] No such evidence or mention of self-induced seizures can be found in the original report. *"AA...age de 20 ans, presente des troubles moteurs sous forme de mouvements involontaires de la tete et des yeux sous l' influence des rayons solaires."*[190]

Why have the seizures of eyelid myoclonia been mistaken as a maneuver for self-induction?

The first reports of photosensitive epilepsy concerned patient who had seizures when in bright sunlight or suddenly exposed to bright light, or after exposure to bright sunlight for a period of time.[12;101;109;191-193] However, after the introduction of IPS in EEG activation, the predominant view was that fluctuation of the light stimulus appears necessary t induce an epileptic attack, and that any claims of observing seizure induction by continuous light should probably be discounted as due to interruptions of the light by fluttering of th eyelids.[127] Thus, most epileptologists find it difficult to accept eyelid myoclonia as a seizure elicited by uninterrupted light.

Differential diagnosis of Jeavons syndrome

Non-epileptic conditions, such as tics and exaggerated normal eye movements

Self-induced photosensitive epilepsy

Symptomatic or possibly symptomatic generalised epilepsy

IGE with absences

Idiopathic or symptomatic occipital epilepsy

PATTERN-SENSITIVE EPILEPSY

Pattern-sensitive epilepsy[12;13;36;37;88;128;129;154;196] refers to epileptic seizures induced by patterns; it is not a particular epileptic syndrome. Pattern seizure sensitivity is closely related to photosensitivity. Nearly all patients with clinical pattern sensitivity epilepsy show PPR (Figure 13.9). Conversely, 30% of clinically photosensitive patients are also sensitive to stationary and 70% to appropriately vibrating patterns of stripes. Patterns enhance the effect of photic stimulation, whether under test conditions or in real life. "Whether pattern sensitivity ever occurs in subjects who are consistently insensitive to IPS is uncertain."[36] Pattern sensitivity without photosensitivity,[12] sensitivity to non-geometric patterns[197] and self-induced pattern-sensitive epilepsy are rare. [38;94;198]

DEMOGRAPHIC DATA

Pure pattern-sensitive epilepsy with clinical attacks induced only by patterns is rare.[154] Over 50 years (1950 to 2000) only 73 patients were diagnosed at the Mayo Clinic on the basis of their principal attribute, namely, sensitivity to patterns.[37] In my experience of 442 patients with onset of afebrile seizures between birth and 15 years of age, only one (0.2%) had pattern-sensitive epilepsy.[38;98] This is despite the relatively high incidence of pattern-induced EEG paroxysmal activity in photosensitive patients.[12;13;36;88;128;129;154;196] Nearly all clinically pattern-sensitive patients are also photosensitive.

CLINICAL MANIFESTATIONS

Clinical manifestations have not been well studied in pure pattern-sensitive epilepsy. [37] All types of generalised seizures have been described. My impression is that absences are more common than GTCS and myoclonic jerks, in that order. I am not aware of patterns inducing occipital seizures, though they should exist considering that the visual cortex is the primary target of the pattern stimulus. Self-induced pattern-sensitive epilepsy has been reported (Figure 13.2).[38;94;198]

ENVIRONMENTAL STIMULI

Environmental stimuli that induce seizures in pattern-sensitive patients are those that best match the properties of the provocative patterns used in relevant EEG testing, and best suit and create the conditions of their spatial and directional presentation to the eyes. These are striped clothes, such as shirts, jackets or ties, escalators, wallpaper and furnishings, venetian blinds, air-conditioning grills and radiators. Any activity visually involved with these patterns, such as ironing, is likely to induce seizures. Less direct, but often very significant, is the role of patterns in more complex stimuli, such as television viewing and video games.[12;13;36]

Pattern is recognised as a seizure precipitant less often by patients, caregivers and physicians than are environmental flicker and specific agents, such as the television, discotheque lighting, or video games. Direct questioning implicates pattern as a seizure trigger in 6[71]–30%[88] of photosensitive subjects.

AETIOLOGY

Pattern sensitivity, like photosensitive epilepsy, is a genetically determined trait.

PATHOPHYSIOLOGY

Pattern seizure sensitivity has been extensively studied using elaborate and intelligent methodology, mainly in patients with photically induced seizures. This has revealed many aspects of pattern seizure susceptibility and its pathophysiology:[12;13;36;88;128;129;154;196]

1. The seizures are triggered in the visual cortex.
2. The seizures are triggered by normal neural activity.
3. The trigger involves one cerebral hemisphere or both hemispheres independently.
4. The trigger requires the physiological activation of a critical area of cortical tissue.
5. Synchronisation of neural activity is necessary.

For a more detailed analysis of the pathophysiology of pattern-sensitive epilepsy see ref [13;36].

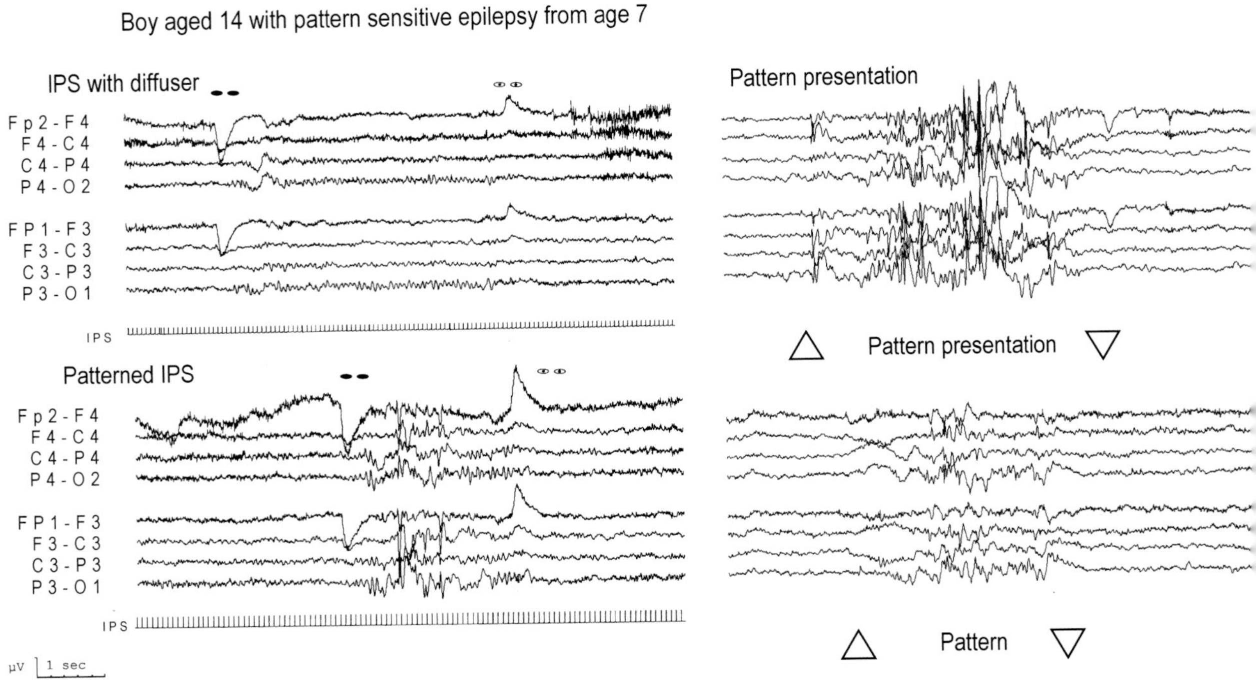

Figure 13.9 Samples from a video EEG of a child aged 14 years with pure pattern-sensitive epilepsy from the age of 7 years.

Left (top and bottom): Only patterned IPS (2 mm x 2 mm graticule superimposed on the glass of the stroboscope)[109;124] elicits PPR.
Right (top and bottom): Paroxysmal discharges were consistently elicited by various linear patterns.
The child is of normal development and scholastic performance. He has brief 4–10-s absence seizures consisting of mild-to-moderate impairment of consciousness and concurrent upwards rolling of the eyeballs with eyelid flickering. The seizures are invariably elicited by patterns with grids or stripes, such as escalators, and the dotted lines of microwaves, radiators or cloths. On five occasions, the absence seizures were followed by GTCS. He is also drawn like a magnet to the television screen, though he is not photosensitive. Spontaneous absence seizures occur only after awakening.
A characteristic feature is that when patterns appear in his visual field, his eyes fixate (freeze) to them and he is unable to break his gaze. He says that he finds patterns "hypnotic," but not pleasant. He would avoid patterns if he could and he does not seek them out.
This behaviour was considered as 'self-induction', but this was not the opinion shared by Dr A. Wilkins and myself who examined him together.

DIAGNOSTIC PROCEDURES

EEG with appropriate pattern presentations is the key test. Pattern sensitivity depends on the spatial frequency, orientation, brightness, contrast and size of the pattern. An optimally epileptogenic pattern consists of black-and-white stripes of equal width and spacing.

The most epileptogenic patterns and their spatial/directional relations to the eyes have been defined by Wilkins and Binnie[13;36] as follows:

1. An optimally epileptogenic pattern consists of black-and-white stripes of equal width and sharp contour (a square-wave luminance profile).
2. The image must be well focused and, if the subject has a refractive error, an appropriate correction must be worn.
3. Spatial frequency is critical; this is the number of cycles of the pattern (pairs of dark and light stripes) per degree of visual angle. For most subjects without a refractive error, a spatial frequency of 2–4 cycles per degree is the most epileptogenic. Thus, each stripe should subtend 7.5–15 minutes of the arc at the eye.
4. The orientation of the lines rarely affects epileptogenicity, except in astigmatic patients.
5. In a susceptible subject, EEG activation is not usually seen at a luminance below 10 cd/rn^2 although exceptions exist. For the purposes of testing, the space-averaged luminance should be at least 200 cd/rn^2. The Michelson contrast (difference in luminance of light and dark stripes expressed as a proportion of their sum) should be more than 0.4.
6. Binocular stimulation should be used.
7. Pattern sensitivity, like visual acuity, depends mainly on central vision. Between a lower threshold and an upper saturation level is an approximately log linear relationship between pattern radius and discharge probability for circular patterns of up to 500 visual angle. To determine whether a subject is pattern sensitive, it is therefore worthwhile using stimuli of at least this size.

PROGNOSIS AND MANAGEMENT

The prognosis and management of pattern-sensitive epilepsy have not been systematically studied.[37] The prognosis may be worse than that of photosensitive epilepsy. Management may be similar to that of photosensitive epilepsy but pattern-sensitive epilepsy may be much more difficult to treat.

FIXATION-OFF SENSITIVITY

Fixation-off sensitivity (FOS) is a term that I coined to denote the form(s) of epilepsy and/or EEG abnormalities, which are elicited by elimination of central vision and fixation.[39;131] 'Elimination of central vision and fixation' is a specific precipitating stimulus, which even in the presence of light, induces high amplitude occipital or generalised paroxysmal discharges.

FOS is suggested in the routine EEG by abnormalities, which consistently occur as long as the eyes are closed, but not when the eyes are opened.

A previous extensive review of all aspects of FOS can be found elsewhere. [39] FOS can be better understood in reviewing the steps followed for their detection and study.

Patients and EEG abnormalities: I first documented FOS in children with occipital paroxysms who clinically had what is now known as Panayiotopoulos syndrome and Gastaut type ICOE. Occipital paroxysms occurred as long as the eyes were closed and disappeared for as long as the eyes were open (Figures 9.7 and 9.12). These children were not photosensitive. Instead, illumination of the closed eyes with a strong light or high frequency IPS sometimes had a partial inhibitory effect on the occipital paroxysms.

Why do the closed eyelids have such a dramatic activating effect on occipital paroxysms?

I considered that these children might be scotosensitive and tested the effect of darkness. Occipital paroxysms would appear on eyes open by switching-off the lights of the recording room but this effect, with some light coming through closed doors and windows, was variable. It was only in *complete* darkness, eliminating any possible light sources, that the occipital paroxysms were invariably activated when the eyes were opened and became continuous whether eyes were open or closed. In complete darkness with the eyes open, the reactivity of the occipital paroxysms could be controlled by switching the light on and off and not by opening or closing of the eyes. Thus light was inhibiting and darkness was activating the occipital paroxysms.

What are the characteristics of a light source responsible for such marked inhibition?

A small spot of low intensity red light, initially produced by the light of an ophthalmoscope shown through a finger from a distance of approximately 3 metres, totally inhibited the occipital paroxysms as long as the patient was fixating on it. Thus, in complete darkness with the eyes open, occipital paroxysms were inhibited by fixation and activated by the absence of fixation.

Fixation-off sensitivity or scotosensitivity?

The behaviour of the occipital paroxysms indicated that it was reactive to fixation-on and -off rather than to the presence of light or its intensity. This I documented by testing the effect of central vision and fixation in a normally lit room. Central vision and fixation were eliminated with +10 spherical lenses or underwater goggles covered with semitransparent tape. Under these conditions of fixation-off in the presence of light, the occipital paroxysms showed the same reactivity as in complete darkness: occipital paroxysms were continuous whether the eyes were open or closed (Figures 9.7 and 9.12). Occipital paroxysms would disappear again if central vision and fixation were restored either binocularly or monocularly. Consequently, the excitatory effect of darkness was in fact due to the elimination of central vision and fixation and that darkness was not a prerequisite for the activation of the occipital paroxysms. Thus, I coined the term *fixation-off sensitivity* to distinguish this from *scotosensitivity*.

Fixation independent of visual cues was not important. There was no inhibition of occipital paroxysms if a patient "looked" at his/her finger in complete darkness. [131;199]

Furthermore, it was not possible to modify the occipital paroxysms by any eye movement or stimulation other than those involving central vision and fixation, suggesting that input from extraocular muscles or other ocular sensory or proprioceptive impulses did not contribute to FOS. Also, the fact that the occipital abnormalities could be inhibited or activated with eyes opened by fixation-off or on was against such a proposition.

CLINICAL AND EEG CORRELATIONS IN PATIENTS WITH FOS

FOS, like photosensitivity, is a non-specific EEG finding despite some preference for certain epileptic conditions.

From clinical and video EEG documentation, there are three types of patients with seizures and EEG abnormalities of FOS:[39;200]

- *The first type* is seen in patients with occipital paroxysms such as those seen in the EEG of some cases with Panayiotopoulos syndrome and more frequently in Gastaut-type COE, which are the model examples of FOS. It was in these cases that FOS was first documented as a new type of activating stimulus in reflex epilepsies (Figures 9.7 and 9.12).[201]

FOS abnormalities are mainly localised *in the occipital regions* and are not associated with overt ictal clinical manifestations.[39;201-203]

- *The second type* may be a 'pure' and distinct clinical form of FOS cryptogenic generalised epilepsy (Figure 13.4 bottom).[131;204-207]

Patients are women of borderline normal intelligence with frequent eyelid myoclonia (with or without atypical absences), absence status epilepticus and GTCS. The eyelid myoclonia manifests with fast, small amplitude clonic movements of the eyelids associated with tonic spasm of the eyelids and eyes that occasionally spread to the neck muscles.[131;202] Absence status epilepticus is preferentially catamenial.[206]

> She also has catamenial absence status epilepticus 'always coming with her menstruation' every month. This lasts for 1-3 days when 'she is vacant, eyes rolling up, feeling slow, drowsy and depressed but also aggressive and not in control of herself'. A diagnosis of temporal lobe epilepsy with fugue-like states was made in a major neurological centre. She has been treated with phenytoin 450 mg and carbamazepine 800 mg daily since the age of 16. The catamenial absence status epilepticus continues every month. She had 4-5 GTCS in her life probably following an absence status and alcohol indulgence. Case in ref [206].

The EEG-FOS abnormalities consist mainly of *diffuse* alpha-like rhythms at 7 Hz, intermixed with bisynchronous sharp and spike/polyspike components. These are often associated with clinical ictal manifestations (Figure 13.4 bottom). The patients are not photosensitive.

These attacks are always related to the eyes being closed. Although initially called 'eyelid myoclonia with absences',[131] this term should be strictly reserved for Jeavons syndrome.[202]

The patient described by Gumnit et al. (1965)[204] had similar clinical and EEG manifestations to the patient of Panayiotopoulos,[131;202] and is probably the first reported patient with FOS in this group, though the authors of that report emphasised the inhibitory effect of patterned vision and not the effect of fixation documented by Panayiotopoulos.

- *The third type* occurs in some patients with IGEs and photosensitivity.[208] The FOS abnormalities are often diffuse and are not associated with overt clinical ictal manifestations.

In the second and third type, the typical abnormalities related to fixation-off are mainly diffuse/generalised, with 'dropout' in sleep stages simultaneous with the alpha rhythm.

FOS may occur in subjects without seizures.[209] In such an asymptomatic adult with FOS, continuous bilateral occipital paroxysms during elimination of central vision were associated with transitory cognitive impairment demonstrated by neuropsychological testing.[209]

The range of EEG abnormalities and clinical manifestations associated with FOS may be extended if testing for it were introduced into routine clinical EEG departments.

PATHOPHYSIOLOGY

The underlying mechanisms of FOS are not known, but they may be related to an abnormality of the alpha-rhythm generators.[39]

FOS has the opposite characteristics of photosensitive epilepsies (Table 13.3) , but conversion from one to the other may rarely occur:[39]

- The resting EEG of photosensitive patients frequently shows abnormalities with eye closure rather than with the eyes closed (Figure 13.7). These are inhibited by total darkness and probably by elimination of central vision and fixation (Figure 13.4 top).
- Photosensitivity is mainly mediated through central vision and fixation. PPR are induced only if the patient 'looks' at the centre of the stroboscope.

  "Sometimes a shift of gaze from the centre of the lamp to the edge (12° or 15°) will inhibit responses, including photic driving".[126]

- In photosensitive epilepsy, PPR are enhanced when IPS is combined with patterns (Figure 13.3).[109;110;114]

FOS has been recently studied with functional MRI.[209;210] In 3 patients with FOS the EEG paroxysmal activity elicited by eliminating central vision correlated significantly with an increased blood oxygen level-dependent signal in the extrastriate cortex (Brodmann areas 19 and 37). [210] Activation of parieto-occipital and frontal brain areas during FOS discharges has been documented in another patient with fMRI and 64-channel EEG source analysis. [209]

Table 13.3 Fixation off sensitivity versus photosensitivity

	FOS	Photosensitive epilepsy
Resting EEG in a lit recording room	Eye-closed abnormalities	Eye-closure abnormalities
Effect of darkness	Activation of abnormalities	Inhibition of abnormalities
Effect of fixation and central vision	Inhibition of abnormalities	Activation of abnormalities
Effect of patterns	Inhibition of abnormalites	Activation of abnormalities
Effect of IPS	None or inhibition	PPR

SCOTOSENSITIVE EPILEPSY

Scotosensitivity (*skotos* in Greek means darkness) denotes forms of epilepsy, seizures or EEG abnormalities that are elicited by the complete elimination of retinal stimulation by light. Pure scotosensitive patients are rare.[211;212]

> A 14-year-old boy had seizures mainly in darkness, which made him sleep with the lights on. Seizures consisted of tonic deviation of the eyes to the left with concomitant clonic movements and left hemianopia. Visual hallucinations of geometric shapes and brilliant colours occurred in the hemianopic field. Secondarily complex focal seizures with déjà vu phenomena or GTCS could occur. A seizure was recorded after 55 s in darkness. Ictal EEG started with occipital spikes, which increased in frequency to 14–16 Hz, followed by high amplitude bi-occipital spike–wave activity.[211]

Most cases described as scotosensitive are probably FOS.[39] All patients with FOS are also sensitive to complete darkness, because of the loss of central vision and fixation. Therefore, the term scotosensitivity should be reserved for only those patients who do not have FOS.

TECHNIQUES FOR DOCUMENTING FOS[39]

Firstly, it is essential to confirm that the EEG abnormalities observed in routine EEG recording are related to the eyes-closed state. The patient is asked to open and close his/her eyes every 5 s six times, consecutively. Instructing the patient to look at a fixed point, such as the tip of a pencil, ensures fixation in the eyes-opened state.

FOS is then evaluated by instructing the patient to perform the same sequence of eyes-opened and eyes-closed states as in conditions described above, which eliminate central vision and fixation. There are many practical ways to achieve this, such as underwater goggles, which are fitted with +10 spherical lenses or covered with semitransparent tape (that allows light in, but obscures any other visual input). It is our practice to test the effect of darkness with the patient wearing another pair of underwater goggles covered with opaque tape. Longer trials of testing may be required for some patients.

Another simple method for testing FOS by producing Ganzfeld stimulation (homogeneous visual field) was introduced by Takahashi.[15;202;202;213] A white paper, 18 x 26 cm, was placed 20 cm before the eyes of a subject, who looked at a central fixation point for 10 seconds. This paper was then quickly replaced by a thin white paper and the subject kept his/her eyes open for 30 seconds. The second situation was considered equivalent to Ganzfeld stimulation.

Important note

Complete darkness, in which the retina is completely deprived of light stimulation, can be difficult to achieve particularly in routine EEG departments. Even a small spot of red light on which the eyes may fixate can totally inhibit EEG abnormalities induced by complete darkness. All possible light sources, such as small indicators on the EEG machine and other equipment, and light coming through door or window openings, must be excluded; if not, central vision and fixation may not be eliminated during testing and the results jeopardised. Switching off the lights in the EEG recording room is not adequate and may explain conflicting results in the literature. Complete darkness can be produced with underwater goggles covered completely with opaque tape.

STARTLE EPILEPSY
STARTLE INDUCED SEIZURES

Startle seizures are induced by sudden and unexpected stimuli.[58;59;214-218]
The startle (unexpected and sudden presentation of the stimulus) is the provoking factor, though rarely patients may be specifically sensitive to one sensory modality. Sudden noise is the main triggering stimulus, but somatosensory and less often visual stimuli are also effective in some patients. Habituation to repetitive stimulation occurs.

DEMOGRAPHIC DATA
Onset is in childhood or early adolescence (1–16 years). Both sexes are equally affected. The prevalence is very low.

CLINICAL MANIFESTATIONS
The majority of patients suffer from static neurological and intellectual handicaps. Infantile hemiplegia predominates.

The startle response is brief (up to 30 s) and consists of axial tonic posturing frequently causing falls, which are often traumatic. The seizures are asymmetrical in one-quarter of patients. In hemiparetic patients, the seizure starts with flexion and abduction of the paretic arm and extension of the ipsilateral leg, which rapidly involve the contralateral side. Concurrent symptoms, such as marked autonomic manifestations, automatisms, laughter and jerks, may occur. Less commonly, startle-induced seizures may be atonic or myoclonic, particularly in patients with cerebral anoxia. Seizures are frequent, occurring many times a day and sometimes progress to status epilepticus.

Spontaneous seizures are common (probably all patients), but are infrequent and may precede or follow the startle-induced seizures.

AETIOLOGY
Startle-induced seizures usually occur in patients with a variety of localised or diffuse static brain pathology (symptomatic startle seizures). Typically, the insults are pre- or perinatal, or occur within the first 2 years of life. Startle-induced seizures appear to be common in Down syndrome.[219]

DIAGNOSTIC PROCEDURES
A variety of focal and diffuse, usually atrophic and often large, cerebral abnormalities are found. Brain MRI is necessary even in those patients with normal neurology.[216] The abnormalities are found predominantly in the lateral sensory-motor cortex.

ELECTROENCEPHALOGRAPHY
Interictal EEG shows a variety of diffuse or focal abnormalities reflecting the underlying brain structural lesions. Ictal EEG consists of an initial vertex discharge followed by diffuse relative flattening or low voltage rhythmic approximately 10 Hz activity, which begins in lesioned motor or premotor cortex and spreads to mesial frontal, parietal and contralateral frontal regions.[58;214;216] On surface EEG, this is often obscured by muscle artefacts.

ILAE classification and definition
The 1989 ILAE definition of startle seizures is: "Epileptic seizures may also be precipitated by sudden arousal (startle epilepsy); the stimulus is unexpected in nature. The seizures are usually generalized tonic but may be partial and are usually symptomatic."[2]

The new ILAE diagnostic scheme considers *'startle epilepsy'* as a syndrome, though most realistically this consists of heterogeneous group of patients with startle-induced seizures. Aetiologies, EEG correlates and brain structural abnormalities are variable.

DIFFERENTIAL DIAGNOSIS

The main diagnostic confusion is with hyperekplexia (also called startle disease), which is a non-epileptic disorder.

Seizures induced by touch, tap or sudden dousing with hot water may have a startle component, but this is not a prerequisite for their provocation. In addition, these reflex seizures are mainly myoclonic, the ictal EEG shows generalised discharges, patients are otherwise normal and there are no structural brain abnormalities.

PROGNOSIS

The prognosis is often bad, particularly for those with severe pre-existing encephalopathies. Mortality is increased compared with the general population. Total control of the seizures is nearly impossible.

MANAGEMENT

There is no established drug of choice, and therapy is often unsatisfactory. Clonazepam, clobazam and carbamazepine are often used. In a study of four patients, adjunctive lamotrigine therapy had a dramatic beneficial effect.[220]

COMPLEX REFLEX EPILEPSIES [4,5]

SEIZURES INDUCED BY THINKING, PROCESSING OF SPATIAL INFORMATION, AND SEQUENTIAL DECISION-MAKING

Thinking-induced seizures occur in response to high cognitive functions; effective triggers include mathematical calculations, drawing, playing cards, chess and other board games, and Rubik's cube.[51;52;221;222] Non-verbal thinking (noogenic epilepsy), decision-making and spatial tasks are essential elements in seizure provocation. Most patients describe more than one effective stimulus.

Thinking-induced seizures usually occur in the context of IGE. They usually start during adolescence and are myoclonic, absences and GTCS; focal seizures are rare. Most patients also suffer from spontaneous seizures. Exceptionally, patients also self-induce seizures by intense thinking:

> "My epilepsy started a few months after my father died. I know when I self-induce the fits. I could self-induce the fits quite easily, if I thought about my father. Like the time that I spent with him, also the time that he was in the hospital or things like these. This could induce the fits. I never did it to gain anything, I did it to get away from other people."[52]

EEG usually shows spontaneous and stimulus-provoked generalised discharges of spike/polyspike–waves at 3–4 Hz. Neuropsychological analysis of the stimuli points to right parietal cortical dysfunction.

ILAE definition

"Seizures precipitated by integration of higher cerebral function such as memory or pattern recognition are most often associated with complex partial epilepsies, but are occasionally observed in generalized epilepsies (such as reading epilepsy). Seizures also occur spontaneously in most such patients."[2]

READING EPILEPSY

Reading (the stimulus) is a well-documented provocative seizure-inducing stimulus in idiopathic and less often cryptogenic/symptomatic epilepsies (Figure 13.10).[40-44;223-226]

Primary (idiopathic) reading epilepsy is a distinctive form of a reflex epilepsy syndrome, which mainly manifests with myoclonic jerks of the masticatory muscles, absences or other type of seizures, and is rare or exceptional.[40;41;44] Conversely, some patients, with mainly symptomatic causes, have prolonged, focal seizures that manifest with alexia and possibly dysphasia.[43]

The following description refers to the idiopathic form of reading epilepsy.

DEMOGRAPHIC DATA

Age at onset is usually 12–19 years with a peak in the late teens that is long after reading skills have been acquired. There is a male preponderance of 1.8/1. The prevalence may be very low. In my experience of 442 patients with onset of afebrile seizures between birth and 15 years of age, only one (0.2%) had primary reading epilepsy.[98]

CLINICAL MANIFESTATIONS

Seizures are elicited by reading silently or aloud, and consist of brief myoclonic jerks mainly restricted to the masticatory, oral and perioral muscles. They are described as clicking sensations and occur a few minutes to hours after reading, particularly after reading aloud texts that are difficult or unusual to read. Jaw myoclonus is by far the commonest manifestation of reading epilepsy. If the patient continues reading despite jaw jerks, these may become more violent, spread to trunk and limb muscles or generate other seizure manifestations before a GTCS develops. This is usually the first and last GTCS in the patient's life, because their condition is effectively treated and the patient learns to stop reading or talking when oral/perioral jerks occur. It is extremely rare for patients with reading epilepsy to have more than 1–5 GTCS or spontaneous seizures unrelated to reading. The majority of the patients have a single GTCS, which is usually self-inflicted because of their curiosity to see what will happen if they continue reading despite jaw jerks or other manifestations. It is also rare for reading epilepsy to present with other types of ictal manifestations (mainly visual hallucinations) in addition to the jaw myoclonic seizures. One of my patients, a 23-year-old normal woman, with primary reading epilepsy, had olfactory hallucinations after repetitive jaw myoclonus induced by prolonged reading or argumentative talking. Hand myoclonic jerking is common among those with writing precipitation of seizures (graphogenic epilepsy).[46]

ILAE classification and definition

Primary reading epilepsy is classified in the 1989 ILAE classification[2] together with 'childhood epilepsy with centrotemporal spikes' and 'childhood epilepsy with occipital paroxysms' in the 'idiopathic, age and localisation-related (partial) epilepsies' and is defined as follows:

"Primary reading epilepsy: All or almost all seizures in this syndrome are precipitated by reading (especially aloud) and are independent of the content of the text. They are simple partial motor-involving masticatory muscles, or visual, and if the stimulus is not interrupted, GTCS may occur. The syndrome may be inherited. Onset is typically in late puberty and the course is benign with little tendency to spontaneous seizures. Physical examination and imaging studies are normal but EEG shows spikes or spike-waves in the dominant parieto-temporal region. Generalized spike and wave may also occur."[2]

This classification was criticised by many experts emphasising that reading epilepsy[41;43;44] had no common links with the benign childhood focal seizures, and that this is a purely reflex epilepsy. The new ILAE diagnostic scheme (Table 1.7) rightly categorises 'reading epilepsy' as a syndrome of reflex epilepsy.[3] Regarding its categorisation as focal or generalised, "From the clinician's point of view, reading- or language-induced myoclonic seizures are neither partial nor generalized, but bilateral and synchronous focal motor resulting from the simultaneous activation of parts of the speech network that expands over both hemispheres, with a potential for rapid spread and secondary generalization if exposure to the stimulus is not interrupted."[43]

Some patients have prolonged, clearly focal, seizures that manifest with alexia and possibly dysphasia, while occasionally absences may occur.

PRECIPITATING FACTORS

Reading silently or aloud is the defining precipitant stimulus. One-quarter of patients may also have similar jaw jerks provoked by talking (particularly if this is

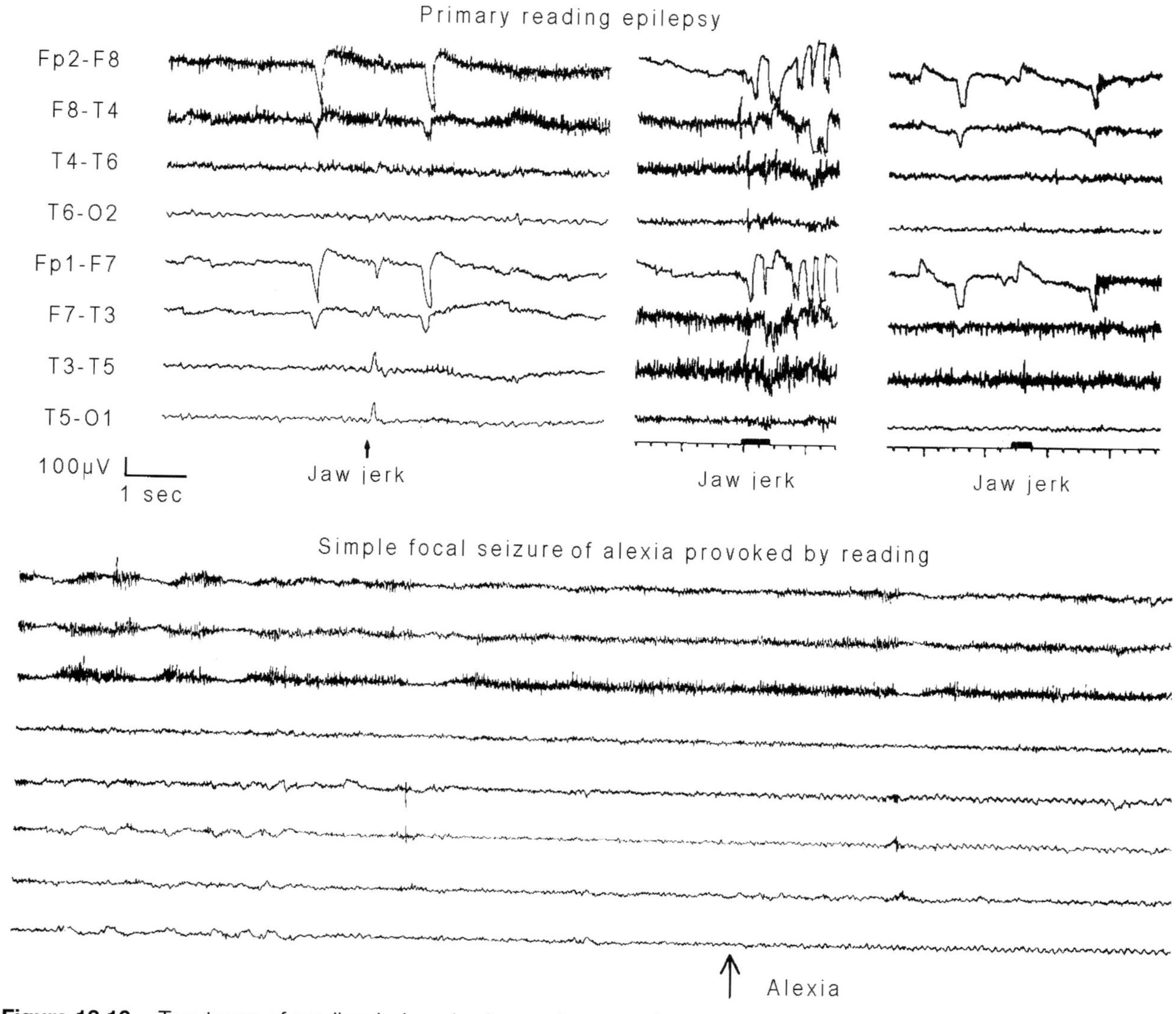

Figure 13.10 Two types of reading-induced seizures; jaw myoclonus and alexia.

Top left: EEG of a woman with jaw jerks (arrow) while reading (case 8 in ref [43]). She is successfully treated with clonazepam 0.5 mg nocte. Her sister also suffered from jaw jerks, mainly when involved in argumentative and fast talk.
Top middle and right: Video EEG of another woman with jaw jerks (bars and arrows) while reading (case 10 in ref [43]). The EEG shows no detectable abnormality during jaw jerks and possible changes are obscured by muscle activity.
Bottom: Video EEG of a 24-year-old man with simple focal seizures manifested with alexia (inability to understand written words) and four nocturnal GTCS (case 17 in ref [43]). Interictal EEG during reading showed sharp and slow waves focused in the left temporal regions (midway between middle and posterior temporal electrode). When the patient indicated his inability to understand text (arrow), the EEG showed low-amplitude fast rhythms (around 10–11 Hz), which were localised in the left middle temporal regions. This lasted 70 s before clinical recovery. MRI and a PET scan were normal. The patient was effectively treated with carbamazepine.

Modified from Panayiotopoulos (1996)[6] with the permission of the Editor S. Wallace and the Publishers Chapman & Hall.

fast or argumentative), writing, reading music or chewing. Clinically identical seizures can also be provoked by the other linguistic activities, justifying the term language-induced epilepsy.[43;46]

AETIOLOGY

Reading epilepsy is probably genetically determined, and has been reported in identical twins and among first-degree relatives. [40]

PATHOPHYSIOLOGY

The main mechanism whereby reading elicits seizures is the transformation, transcoding from written linguistic symbols into phonetic, loud or silent, speech.[40;225] This may be enhanced by other superimposed factors, such as proprioceptive impulses from oral, perioral and eye muscles involved in reading, and difficulty in transcoding script into speech.[40]

According to Koutroumanidis et al.[43] "Ictogenesis in reading or language-induced epilepsy is based on the reflex activation of a hyperexcitable network that subserves the function of speech and extends over multiple cerebral areas in both hemispheres. The parts of this network responding to the stimulus may drive the relative motor areas producing the typical regional myoclonus."[43]

Based on functional MRI findings, Archer et al.[226] postulated that, because of a local structural anomaly (an unusual gyrus branching anteriorly off the left central sulcus), the spikes of reading epilepsy spread from working memory areas into adjacent motor cortex, activating a cortical subcortical circuit.

Brain opioid-like substances may be involved in the termination of reading-induced seizures.[223]

DIAGNOSTIC PROCEDURES

All tests apart from the EEG are normal in primary reading epilepsy. In the symptomatic or probably symptomatic forms that manifest with alexia, brain MRI may show abnormalities in the dominant posterior temporal area.

Ictal functional neuroimaging studies show multiple cortical hyperexcitable areas that are part of the neuronal network, which subserves the function of speech.

ELECTROENCEPHALOGRAPHY

The interictal EEG is usually normal.

Ictal EEG manifestations may be inconspicuous and difficult to detect because of muscle activity from the jaw muscles and head. Ictal EEG changes show considerable heterogeneity in terms of discharge morphology and scalp topography. In the myoclonic variant, discharges are brief and consist of sharp waves, which are bilateral with left side preponderance in the temporo-parietal regions (Figure 13.10). In the focal probably symptomatic variant with alexia, ictal discharges are prolonged and entirely focal in the language dominant temporo-parietal regions.

PROGNOSIS

The prognosis in reading epilepsy appears to be good, because seizures are usually minor and are related to a precipitant stimulus, which can be modified.

MANAGEMENT

Clonazepam 0.5 mg –1 mg nocte is highly effective. Modification of reading and talking habits may be successful. The sister of one of my patients with reading epilepsy, who has never asked medical advice for her condition and never had GTCS, controlled her condition by modifying her way of reading and talking. She never received any medication and, at last follow-up, aged 40 years, was unmedicated and well.

REFERENCES

1. Wieser HG. Seizure induction in reflex seizures and reflex epilepsy. *Adv Neuro.l* 1998;**75**:69-85.
2. Commission on Classification and Terminology of the International League Against Epilepsy. Proposal for revised classification of epilepsies and epileptic syndromes. *Epilepsia* 1989;**30**:389-99.
3. Engel J, Jr. A proposed diagnostic scheme for people with epileptic seizures and with epilepsy: Report of the ILAE Task Force on Classification and Terminology. *Epilepsia* 2001;**42**:796-803.
4. Beaumanoir A, Gastaut H, Roger J, (eds). Reflex seizures and reflex epilepsies. Geneve: Medecine and Hygiene, 1989.
5. Zifkin B, Andermann F, Rowan AJ, Beaumanoir A, (eds). Reflex Epilepsies and Reflex Seizures. New York: Lippincot-Raven, 1998.
6. Panayiotopoulos CP. Epilepsies characterized by seizures with specific modes of precipitation (reflex epilepsies). In Wallace S, ed. *Epilepsy in Children*, pp 355-75. London: Chapman & Hall, 1996.
7. Blume WT, Luders HO, Mizrahi E, Tassinari C, van Emde BW, Engel J, Jr. Glossary of descriptive terminology for ictal semiology: report of the ILAE task force on classification and terminology. *Epilepsia* 2001;**42**:1212-8.
8. Duncan JS, Panayiotopoulos CP. Typical absences with specific modes of precipitation (reflex absences):Clinical aspects. In Duncan JS, Panayiotopoulos CP, eds. *Typical absences and related epileptic syndromes*, pp 206-12. London: Churchill Communications Europe, 1995.
9. Ferrie CD, De Marco P, Grunewald RA, Giannakodimos S, Panayiotopoulos CP. Video game induced seizures. *J Neurol Neurosurg Psychiatry* 1994;**57**:925-31.
10. Ferrie CD, Robinson RO, Giannakodimos S, Panayiotopoulos CP. Video-game epilepsy. *Lancet* 1994;**344**:1710-1.
11. Panayiotopoulos CP. Benign childhood partial seizures and related epileptic syndromes. London: John Libbey & Company Ltd, 1999.
12. Harding GFA, Jeavons PM. Photosensitive epilepsy. London: MacKeith Press, 1994.
13. Wilkins, A. Visual stress. Oxford: Oxford University Press, 1995.
14. Zifkin BG,Kasteleijn-Nolst TD. Reflex epilepsy and reflex seizures of the visual system: a clinical review. *Epileptic Disord.* 2000;**2**:129-36.
15. Takahashi T. Photosensitive epilepsy. EEG diagnosis by low-luminance, visual stimuli and preventive measures. Tokyo: Igaku-Shoin Publication Service Ltd, 2002.
16. Forster FM,.Cleeland CS. Somatosensory evoked epilepsy. *Trans Am.Neurol Assoc* 1969;**94**:268-9.
17. DeMarco P. Parietal epilepsy with evoked and spontaneous spikes: report on siblings with possible genetic transmission. *Clin Electroencephalogr* 1986;**17**:159-61.
18. Fonseca LC,Tedrus GM. Somatosensory evoked spikes and epileptic seizures: a study of 385 cases. *Clin Electroencephalogr* 2000;**31**:71-5.
19. Tedrus GM,.Fonseca LC. Benign focal epilepsy of childhood: epileptic seizure during somatosensory evoked potential: a case report. *Clin EEG Neurosci.* 2004;**35**:94-6.
20. Deonna T. Reflex seizures with somatosensory precipitation. Clinical and electroencephalographic patterns and differential diagnosis, with emphasis on reflex myoclonic epilepsy of infancy. *Adv Neurol* 1998;**75**:193-206.
21. Koutroumanidis M, Pearce R, Sadoh DR, Panayiotopoulos CP. Tooth brushing-induced seizures: a case report. *Epilepsia* 2001;**42**:686-8.
22. Chuang YC, Lin TK, Lui CC, Chen SD, Chang CS. Tooth-brushing epilepsy with ictal orgasms. *Seizure* 2004;**13**:179-82.
23. Satishchandra P, Ullal GR, Shankar SK. Hot water epilepsy. *Adv Neurol* 1998;**75**:283-93.
24. Ioos C, Fohlen M, Villeneuve N, Badinand-Hubert N, Jalin C, Cheliout-Heraut F *et al.* Hot water epilepsy: a benign and unrecognized form. *J Child Neurol* 2000;**15**:125-8.
25. Incecik F, Herguner MO, Elkay M, Altunbasak S. Hot water epilepsy - a report of three cases. *Indian Pediatr.* 2004;**41**:731-3.
26. Grosso S, Farnetani MA, Francione S, Galluzzi P, Vatti G, Cordelli DM *et al.* Hot water epilepsy and focal malformation of the parietal cortex development. *Brain Dev* 2004;**26**:490-3.
27. Dreifuss FE. Classification of reflex epilepsies and reflex seizures. *Adv Neurol* 1998;**75**:5-13.
28. Duncan JS, Panayiotopoulos CP. The differentiation of 'eye-closure' from 'eye-closed' EEG abnormalities and their relation to photo- and fixation-off sensitivity. In Duncan JS, Panayiotopoulos CP, eds. *Eyelid myoclonia with absences*, pp 77-87. London: John Libbey & Company Ltd, 1996.
29. Beaumanoir A, Mira L, van Lierde A. Epilepsy or paroxysmal kinesigenic choreoathetosis? *Brain Dev.* 1996;**18**:139-41.
30. Spinnler H,Valli G. Micturition "reflex" epilepsy. Presentation of a clinical case. *Riv Patol Nerv Ment.* 1969;**90**:212-20.
31. Yamatani M, Murakami M, Konda M, Konishi T, Suzuki Y, Okada T *et al.* An 8-year-old girl with micturition-induced epilepsy. *No To Hattatsu* 1987;**19**:58-62.
32. Senanayake N. 'Eating epilepsy'—a reappraisal. *Epilepsy Res.* 1990;**5**:74-9.
33. Remillard GM, Zifkin BG, Andermann F. Seizures induced by eating. *Adv Neurol* 1998;**75**:227-40.
34. Tassinari CA, Rubboli G, Rizzi R, Gardella E, Michelucci R. Self-induction of visually-induced seizures. *Adv Neurol* 1998;**75:179-92**:179-92.
35. Panayiotopoulos CP, Giannakodimos S, Agathonikou A, Koutroumanidis M. Eyelid myoclonia is not a manoeuvre for self-induced seizures in eyelid myoclonia with absences. In Duncan JS, Panayiotopoulos CP, eds. *Eyelid myoclonia with absences*, pp 93-106. London: John Libbey & Company Ltd, 1996.
36. Binnie CD, Wilkins AJ. Visually induced seizures not caused by flicker (intermittent light stimulation). *Adv Neurol* 1998;**75**:123-38.
37. Radhakrishnan K,Klass DW. Half a century of visual pattern-sensitive epilepsy. *Mayo Clin Proc.* 2004;**79**:269-70.
38. Panayiotopoulos CP. Self-induced pattern-sensitive epilepsy. *Arch Neurol* 1979;**36**:48-50.
39. Panayiotopoulos CP. Fixation-off, scotosensitive, and other visual-related epilepsies. *Adv Neurol* 1998;**75**:139-57.
40. Wolf P. Reading epilepsy. In Roger J, Bureau M, Dravet C, Dreifuss FE, Perret A, Wolf P, eds. *Epileptic syndromes in infancy, childhood and adolescence*, pp 281-98. London: John Libbey & Company, 1992.
41. Radhakrishnan K, Silbert PL, Klass DW. Reading epilepsy. An appraisal of 20 patients diagnosed at the Mayo Clinic, Rochester, Minnesota, between 1949 and 1989, and delineation of the epileptic syndrome. *Brain* 1995;**118**:75-89.
42. Koepp MJ, Hansen ML, Pressler RM, Brooks DJ, Brandl U, Guldin B *et al.* Comparison of EEG, MRI and PET in reading epilepsy: a case report. *Epilepsy Res* 1998;**29**:251-7.
43. Koutroumanidis M, Koepp MJ, Richardson MP, Camfield C, Agathonikou A, Ried S *et al.* The variants of reading epilepsy. A clinical and video-EEG study of 17 patients with reading-induced seizures. *Brain* 1998;**121**:1409-27.
44. Ramani V. Reading epilepsy. *Adv Neurol* 1998;**75**:241-62.
45. Cirignotta F, Zucconi M, Mondini S, Lugaresi E. Writing epilepsy. *Clin Electroencephalogr* 1986;**17**:21-3.
46. Oshima T, Hirose K, Murakami H, Suzuki S, Kanemoto K. Graphogenic epilepsy: a variant of language-induced epilepsy distinguished from reading- and praxis-induced epilepsy. *Seizure* 2003;**12**:56-9.
47. Martinez-Manas R, Daniel RT, Debatisse D, Maeder-Ingvar M, Meagher-Villemure K, Villemure JG *et al.* Intractable reflex audiogenic epilepsy successfully treated by peri-insular hemispherotomy. *Seizure* 2004;**13**:486-90.
48. Wieser HG, Hungerbuhler H, Siegel AM, Buck A. Musicogenic epilepsy: review of the literature and case report with ictal single photon emission computed tomography. *Epilepsia* 1997;**38**:200-7.
49. Zifkin BG, Zatorre RJ. Musicogenic epilepsy. *Adv Neurol* 1998;**75:273-81**:273-81.
50. Michelucci R, Gardella E, de Haan GJ, Bisulli F, Zaniboni A, Cantalupo G *et al.* Telephone-induced seizures: a new type of reflex epilepsy. *Epilepsia* 2004;**45**:280-3.
51. Andermann F, Zifkin BG, Andermann E. Epilepsy induced by thinking and spatial tasks. *Adv Neurol* 1998;**75:263-72**:263-72.
52. Koutroumanidis M, Agathonikou A, Panayiotopoulos CP. Self induced noogenic seizures in a photosensitive patient. *J Neurol Neurosurg Psychiatry* 1998;**64**:139-40.
53. Forster FM, Richards JF, Panitch HS, Huisman RE, Paulsen RE. Reflex epilepsy evoked by decision making. *Arch Neurol* 1975;**32**:54-6.
54. Mutani R, Ganga A, Agnetti V. Reflex epilepsy evoked by decision making: report of a case. *Schweiz Arch Neurol Neurochir Psychiatr.* 1980;**127**:61-7.
55. Wiebers DO, Westmoreland BF, Klass DW. EEG activation and mathematical calculation. *Neurology* 1979;**29**:1499-503.
56. Rocand JC, Graveleau D, Etienne M, Le Balle JC, Laplane R. Emotionally precipitated epilepsy. Its relations to hysteroepilepsy and reflex epilepsy. Apropos of a case. *Ann Pediatr.(Paris)* 1965;**12**:434-9.
57. Gras P, Grosmaire N, Giroud M, Soichot P, Dumas R. Investigation via electroencephalogram with sphenoidal electrodes of a case of reading epilepsy: role of the temporal lobe in the emotional evocation of seizures. *Neurophysiol Clin* 1992;**22**:313-20.
58. Vignal JP, Biraben A, Chauvel PY, Reutens DC. Reflex partial seizures of sensorimotor cortex (including cortical reflex myoclonus and startle epilepsy). *Adv Neurol* 1998;**75**:207-26.
59. Zifkin B, Andermann F. Startle epilepsy. In Gilman S, ed. *Medlink Neurology*, San Diego SA: 2004.

60. Doose H, Waltz S. Photosensitivity—genetics and clinical significance. *Neuropediatrics* 1993;**24**:249-55.
61. Waltz S, Stephani U. Inheritance of photosensitivity. *Neuropediatrics* 2000;**31**:82-5.
62. Kasteleijn-Nolst Trenite DG, Guerrini R, Binnie CD, Genton P. Visual sensitivity and epilepsy: a proposed terminology and classification for clinical and EEG phenomenology. *Epilepsia* 2001;**42**:692-701.
63. Dravet C. Dravet syndrome (Severe myoclonic epilepsy in infancy). In Gilman S, ed. *Medlink Neurology*, San Diego SA: Arbor Publishing Corp, 2004.
64. Roger J, Genton P, Bureau M, Dravet C. Progressive myoclonus epilepsies in childhood and adolescence. In Roger J, Bureau M, Dravet C, Dreifuss FE, Perret A, Wolf P, eds. *Epileptic syndromes in childhood and adolescence*, pp 381-400. London: John Libbey & Company Ltd, 1992.
65. De Bittencourt PR. Photosensitivity: the magnitude of the problem. *Epilepsia* 2004;**45 (Suppl 1)**:30-4.
66. Quirk JA, Fish DR, Smith SJ, Sander JW, Shorvon SD, Allen PJ. First seizures associated with playing electronic screen games: a community-based study in Great Britain. *Ann Neurol* 1995;**37**:733-7.
67. Quirk JA, Fish DR, Smith SJ, Sander JW, Shorvon SD, Allen PJ. Incidence of photosensitive epilepsy: a prospective national study. *Electroencephalogr Clin Neurophysiol.* 1995;**95**:260-7.
68. Grecory RP, Oates T, Merry RTC. EEG epileptiform abnormalities in candidates for aircrew training. *Electroencephalogr Clin Neurophysiol.*1993; **86**, 75-7.
69. Agathonikou A, Panayiotopoulos CP, Koutroumanidis M, Rowlinson A. Idiopathic regional occipital epilepsy imitating migraine. *J Epilepsy* 1997;**10**:287-90.
70. Gastaut H, Regis H, Bostem F, Beaussart M. Etude electroencephalographique de 35 sujets ayant presente des crises au cours d' un spectacle televise. *Revue Neurologique* 1960;**102**:533-4.
71. Kasteleijn-Nolst Trenite DG. Photosensitivity in epilepsy:electrophysiological and clinical correlates. Acta Neurol Scandin. 1989 (Suppl.125): 3-149.
72. Kasteleijn-Nolst Trenite DG. Reflex seizures induced by intermittent light stimulation. *Adv Neurol* 1998;**75**:99-121.
73. Kasteleijn-Nolst Trenite DG, Binnie CD, Meinardi H. Photosensitive patients: symptoms and signs during intermittent photic stimulation and their relation to seizures in daily life. *J Neurol Neurosurg Psychiatry* 1987;**50**:1546-9.
74. Benbadis SR, Gerson WA, Harvey JH, Luders HO. Photosensitive temporal lobe epilepsy. *Neurology* 1996;**46**:1540-2.
75. Wilkins AJ. Visual sensitivity and hyperexcitability in epilepsy and migraine. In Andermann F, Lugaresi E, eds. *Migraine and epilepsy*, pp 339-65. Boston: Butterworths, 1987.
76. Kasteleijn-Nolst Trenite DG, Van Der BG, Heynderickx I, Groen P. Visual stimuli in daily life. *Epilepsia* 2004;**45 (Suppl 1)**:2-6.
77. Rushton DN. "Space invader" epilepsy. *Lancet* 1981;**1**:501.
78. Bureau M, Hirsch E, Vigevano F. Epilepsy and videogames. *Epilepsia* 2004;**45 (Suppl 1)**:24-6.
79. Graf WD, Chatrian GE, Glass ST, Knauss TA. Video game-related seizures: a report on 10 patients and a review of the literature. *Pediatrics* 1994;**93**:551-6.
80. Kasteleijn-Nolst Trenite DG, da Silva AM, Ricci S, Binnie CD, Rubboli G, Tassinari CA *et al.* Video-game epilepsy: a European study. *Epilepsia* 1999;**40 (Suppl 4)**:70-4.
81. Kasteleijn-Nolst Trenite DG, Silva AM, Ricci S, Rubboli G, Tassinari CA, Lopes J *et al.* Video games are exciting: a European study of video game-induced seizures and epilepsy. [Published with videosequences]. *Epileptic Disord.* 2002;**4**:121-8.
82. Zifkin BG, Inoue Y. Visual reflex seizures induced by complex stimuli. *Epilepsia* 2004;**45 Suppl 1**:27-9.
83. Harding GF, Jeavons PM. Video material and epilepsy. *Epilepsia* 1994;**35**:1208-16.
84. Millett CJ, Fish DR, Thompson PJ, Johnson A. Seizures during video-game play and other common leisure pursuits in known epilepsy patients without visual sensitivity. *Epilepsia* 1999;**40 (Suppl 4)**:59-64.
85. Takada H, Aso K, Watanabe K, Okumura A, Negoro T, Ishikawa T. Epileptic seizures induced by animated cartoon, "Pocket Monster". *Epilepsia* 1999;**40**:997-1002.
86. Takahashi Y, Fujiwara T. Effectiveness of broadcasting guidelines for photosensitive seizure prevention. *Neurology* 2004;**62**:990-3.
87. Wilkins AJ, Darby CE, Binnie CD, Stefansson SB, Jeavons PM, Harding GF. Television epilepsy—the role of pattern. *Electroencephalogr Clin Neurophysiol.* 1979;**47**:163-71.
88. Wilkins AJ, Darby CE, Binnie CD. Neurophysiological aspects of pattern-sensitive epilepsy. *Brain* 1979;**102**:1-25.
89. Parain D, Zorrilla F, Samson-Dollfus D, Menard JF. Several cases of EEG registration of epilepsy induced by television. *Rev Electroencephalogr Neurophysiol Clin* 1982;**12**:311-4.
90. Ng BY. Psychiatric aspects of self-induced epileptic seizures. *Aust N Z J Psychiatry* 2002;**36**:534-43.
91. Andermann, K. and et al. Self-induced epilepsy. Arch Neurol 6, 49-79. 1962.
92. Ames FR. "Self-induction" in photosensitive epilepsy. *Brain* 1971;**94**:781-98.
93. Binnie CD. Differential diagnosis of eyelid myoclonia with absences and self-induction by eye closure. In Duncan JS, Panayiotopoulos CP, eds. *Eyelid myoclonia with absences*, pp 89-92. London: John Libbey & Company Ltd, 1996.
94. Matricardi M, Brinciotti M, Trasatti G, Porro G. Self-induced pattern-sensitive epilepsy in childhood. *Acta Paediatr Scand.* 1990;**79**:237-40.
95. Guerrini R, Genton P, Dravet C, Viallat D, Bureau M, Horton EJ *et al.* Compulsive somatosensory self-stimulation inducing epileptic seizures. *Epilepsia* 1992;**33**:509-16.
96. Fenwick PB. Self-generation of seizures by an action of mind. *Adv Neurol* 1998;**75**:87-92.
97. Ames FR,Saffer D. The sunflower syndrome. A new look at "self-induced" photosensitive epilepsy. *J Neurol Sci.* 1983;**59**:1-11.
98. Panayiotopoulos CP. Panayiotopoulos syndrome:A common and benign childhood epileptic syndrome. London: John Libbey & Company, 2002.
99. Walsh FB. Clinical Neuro-ophthalmology. Second Edition, pp186-245 Baltimore:The Williams & Wilkins Company,1957.
100. Rafal RD, Laxer KD, Janowsky JS. Seizures triggered by blinking in a non-photosensitive epileptic. *J Neurol Neurosurg Psychiatry* 1986;**49**:445-7.
101. Robertson EG. Photogenic epilepsy:self-precipitated attacks. *Brain* 1954;**77**:232-51.
102. Panayiotopoulos CP. Typical absence seizures. In Gilman S, ed. *Medlink Neurology*, San Diego SA: Arbor Publishing Corp, 2004.
103. Faught E, Falgout J, Nidiffer D, Dreifuss FE. Self-induced photosensitive absence seizures with ictal pleasure. *Arch Neurol* 1986;**43**:408-10.
104. Stephani U, Tauer U, Koeleman B, Pinto D, Neubauer BA, Lindhout D. Genetics of Photosensitivity (Photoparoxysmal Response): A Review. *Epilepsia* 2004;(**45 Suppl 1**):19-23.
105. Harding GF, Edson A, Jeavons PM. Persistence of photosensitivity. *Epilepsia* 1997;**38**:663-9.
106. Pinto D, Westland B, de Haan GJ, Rudolf G, da Silva BM, Hirsch E *et al.* Genome-wide linkage scan of epilepsy-related photoparoxysmal EEG response: evidence for linkage on chromosomes 7q32 and 16p13. *Hum Mol Genet.* 2004.
107. Wilkins AJ, Bonanni P, Porciatti V, Guerrini R. Physiology of human photosensitivity. *Epilepsia* 2004;**45 (Suppl 1)**:7-13.
108. Hishikawa Y, Yamamoto J, Furuya E, Yamada Y, Miyazaki K. Photosensitive epilepsy: relationships between the visual evoked responses and the epileptiform discharges induced by intermittent photic stimulation. *Electroencephalogr Clin Neurophysiol.* 1967;**23**:320-34.
109. Panayiotopoulos CP. A study of photosensitive epilepsy with particular reference to occipital spikes induced by intermittent photic stimulation. PhD Thesis, Aston University in Birmingham,1972.
110. Panayiotopoulos CP, Jeavons PM, Harding GF. Occipital spikes and their relation to visual responses in epilepsy, with particular reference to photosensitive epilepsy. *Electroencephalog Clin Neurophysiol.* 1972;**32**:179-90.
111. Menini C,.Silva-Barrat C. The photosensitive epilepsy of the baboon. A model of generalized reflex epilepsy. *Adv Neurol* 1998;**75**:29-47.
112. Bickford RG, Klass DW. Stimulus factors in the mechanism of television induced seizures. *Trans Amer Neurol Assoc* 1962;**87**:176-8.
113. Gastaut H, Regis H, Bostem F. Attacks provoked by television, and their mechanisms. *Epilepsia* 1962;**3**:438-45.
114. Panayiotopoulos CP, Jeavons PM, Harding GF. Relation of occipital spikes evoked by intermittent photic stimulation to visual evoked responses in photosensitive epilepsy. *Nature* 1970;**228**:566-7.
115. Anyanwu EC, Ehiri JE, Campbell AW. Efficacy of sodium valproate in the treatment of photosensitive epilepsy and the probable reasons for the persistence of occipital spikes. *Scientific World Journal.* 2004;**4**:521-30.
116. Quesney LF, Andermann F, Gloor P. Dopaminergic mechanism in generalized photosensitive epilepsy. *Neurology* 1981;**31**:1542-4.
117. Quesney LF, Andermann F. A dopaminergic mechanism in photosensitive epilepsy and its possible relevance to migraine. In Andermann F, Lugaresi E, eds. *Migraine and epilepsy*, pp 391-404. Boston: Butterworths, 1987.
118. Naquet R, Silva-Barrat C, Menini C. Reflex epilepsy in the Papio-papio baboon, particularly photosensitive epilepsy. *Ital J Neurol Sci.* 1995;**16**:119-25.
119. Teillet MA, Guy N, Fadlallah N, Le Gal LS, Schuler B, Batini C *et al.* Reflex epilepsy of the fowl and its transfer to normal chickens by brain embryonic grafts. *Ital J Neurol Sci.* 1995;**16**:83-9.

120. Naquet RG,.Valin A. Experimental models of reflex epilepsy. *Adv Neurol* 1998;**75**:15-28.
121. Kasteleijn-Nolst Trenite DG, Binnie CD, Harding GF, Wilkins A, Covanis T, Eeg-Olofsson O *et al.* Medical technology assessment photic stimulation—standardization of screening methods. *Neurophysiol Clin* 1999;**29**:318-24.
122. Kasteleijn-Nolst Trenite DG, Binnie CD, Harding GF, Wilkins A. Photic stimulation: standardization of screening methods. *Epilepsia* 1999;**40 (Suppl 4)**:75-9.
123. Rubboli G, Parra J, Seri S, Takahashi T, Thomas P. EEG Diagnostic Procedures and Special Investigations in the Assessment of Photosensitivity. *Epilepsia* 2004;**45 Suppl 1**:35-9.
124. Jeavons PM, Harding GF, Panayiotopoulos CP, Drasdo N. The effect of geometric patterns combined with intermittent photic stimulation in photosensitive epilepsy. *Electroencephalogr Clin Neurophysiol.* 1972;**33**:221-4.
125. Wilkins AJ, Baker A, Amin D, Smith S, Bradford J, Zaiwalla Z *et al.* Treatment of photosensitive epilepsy using coloured glasses. *Seizure* 1999;**8**:444-9.
126. Jeavons PM, Harding GF, Panayiotopoulos CP. Photosensitive epilepsy and driving. *Lancet* 1971;**1**:1125.
127. Bickford RG, Klass DW. Sensory precipitation and reflex mechanisms. In Jasper HH, Ward AA, Pope A, eds. *Basic mechanisms of the epilepsies*, pp 543-64. Boston, Mass: Little, Brown and Co, 1969.
128. Chatrian GE, Lettich E, Miller LH, Green JR, Kupfer C. Pattern-sensitive epilepsy. 2. Clinical changes, tests of responsiveness and motor output, alterations of evoked potenials and therapeutic measures. *Epilepsia* 1970;**11**:151-62.
129. Chatrian GE, Lettich E, Miller LH, Green JR. Pattern-sensitive epilepsy. I. An electrographic study of its mechanisms. *Epilepsia* 1970;**11**:125-49.
130. Giannakodimos S, Panayiotopoulos CP. Eyelid myoclonia with absences in adults: a clinical and video- EEG study. *Epilepsia* 1996;**37**:36-44.
131. Panayiotopoulos CP. Fixation-off-sensitive epilepsy in eyelid myoclonia with absence seizures. *Ann Neurol* 1987;**22**:87-9.
132. Panayiotopoulos CP. Effectiveness of photic stimulation on various eye-states in photosensitive epilepsy. *J Neurol Scienc* 1974;**23**:165-73.
133. Leijten FS, Dekker E, Spekreijse H, Kasteleijn-Nolst Trenite DG, Van Emde BW. Light diffusion in photosensitive epilepsy. *Electroencephalogr Clin Neurophysiol.* 1998;**106**:387-91.
134. Engel J. Selective photoconvulsive responses to intermittent diffuse and patterned photic stimulation. *Electroencephalogr Clin Neurophysiol* 1974;**37**:283-92.
135. Jeavons PM, Harding GFA. Photosensitive epilepsy. London: W. Heinemann Medical Books, 1975.
136. Maheshwari MC. The clinical significance of occipital spikes as a sole response to intermittent photic stimulation. *Electroencephalogr Clin Neurophysiol* 1975;**39**:93-5.
137. Gastaut H, Trevisan E, Naquet R. Diagnostic value of electroencephalographic abnormalities provoked by intermittent photoc stimulation. *Electroencephalogr Clin Neurophysiol* 1958;**10**:194-5.
138. Bickford RG, Sem-Jacobsen CW, White PT, Daly DD. Some observations on the mechanism of photic and photo-metrazol activation. *Electroencephalogr Clin Neurophysiol* 1952;**4**:275-83.
139. Bickford RG, White PT, Sem-Jacobsen CW, Rodin EA. Components of the myoclonic response in man. *Fed Proc Transl.* 1953;**12**:1.
140. Guerrini R,.Genton P. Epileptic syndromes and visually induced seizures. *Epilepsia* 2004;**45 (Suppl 1)**:14-8.
141. Verrotti A, Trotta D, Salladini C, di Corcia G, Latini G, Cutarella R *et al.* Photosensitivity and epilepsy: a follow-up study. *Dev Med Child Neurol.* 2004;**46**:347-51.
142. Kasteleijn-Nolst Trenite DG, Marescaux C, Stodieck S, Edelbroek PM, Oosting J. Photosensitive epilepsy: a model to study the effects of antiepileptic drugs. Evaluation of the piracetam analogue, levetiracetam. *Epilepsy Res* 1996;**25**:225-30.
143. Kasteleijn-Nolst Trenite DG, Marescaux C, Stodieck S, Edelbroek PM, Oosting J. Photosensitive epilepsy: a model to study the effects of antiepileptic drugs. Evaluation of the piracetam analogue, levetiracetam. *Epilepsy Res* 1996;**25**:225-30.
144. Kasteleijn-Nolst Trenite DG, Hirsch E. Levetiracetam: preliminary efficacy in generalized seizures. *Epileptic Disord.* 2003;**5 Suppl 1**:S39-S44.
145. Covanis A, Stodieck SR, Wilkins AJ. Treatment of photosensitivity. *Epilepsia* 2004;**45 (Suppl 1)**:40-5.
146. Gericke CA, Picard F, Saint-Martin A, Strumia S, Marescaux C, Hirsch E. Efficacy of lamotrigine in idiopathic generalized epilepsy syndromes: a video-EEG-controlled, open study. *Epileptic Disord.* 1999;**1**:159-65.
147. Binnie CD, van Emde BW, Kasteleijn-Nolste-Trenite DG, de Korte RA, Meijer JW, Meinardi H *et al.* Acute effects of lamotrigine (BW430C) in persons with epilepsy: *Epilepsia* 1986;**27**:248-54.
148. Casaer P,Boel M. Fenfluramine as a potential antiepileptic drug. *Epilepsia* 2002;**43**:205-6.
149. Guerrini R, Bonanni P, Parmeggiani L, Thomas P, Mattia D, Harvey AS *et al.* Induction of partial seizures by visual stimulation. Clinical and electroencephalographic features and evoked potential studies. *Adv Neurol* 1998;**75**:159-78.
150. Guerrini R, Bonanni P, Parmeggiani A. Idiopathic photosensitive occipital lobe epilepsy. In Gilman S, ed. *Medlink Neurology*, San Diego SA: Arbor Publishing Corp, 2004.
151. Gowers WR. Epilepsies and other chronic convulsive diseases. Their causes, symptoms and treatment. London: Churchill JA, 1881.
152. Holmes G. Sabill memorial oration on focal epilepsy. *Lancet* 1927;**i**:957-62.
153. Gastaut H, Roger J, Gastaut Y. Les formes experimentales de l' epilepsie humaine: 1. L' epilepsie induite par la stimulation lumineuse intermittente rythmee ou epilepsie photogenique. *Rev Neurolog* 1948;**80**:161-83.
154. Bickford RG, Daly DD, Keith HM. Convulsive effects of light stimulation in children. *Am J Dis Child* 1953;**86**:170-83.
155. Lloyd-Smith DL, Henderson LR. Epileptic patients showing susceptibility to photic stimulation alone. *Electroencephalogr Clin Neurophysiol* 1951;378-9.
156. Naquet R, Fegersten L, Bert J. Seizure discharges localised to the posterior cerebral regions in man, provoked by intermittent photic stimulation. *Electroencephalogr Clin Neurophysiol* 1960;**12**:305-16.
157. Davidoff RA, Johnson LC. Photic activation and photoconvulsive responses in a nonepileptic subject. *Neurology* 1963;**13**:617-21.
158. Fischer-Williams M, Bickford RG, Whisnant JR. Occipito-parieto-temporal seizure discharge with visual hallucinations and aphasia. *Epilepsia* 1964;**5**:279-92.
159. Courjon J, Moene Y, Revol M, Genin P. Occipital attacks trigerred by photic stimulation. *Electroencephalogr Clin Neurophysiol* 1968;**25**:587.
160. Delwaide PJ, Barragan M, Gastaut H. Remarks about a partial epilepsy: occipital epilepsy. *Acta Neurol Belg* 1971;**71**:383-91.
161. Aso K, Watanabe K, Negoro T, Takaesu E, Furune A, Takahashi I *et al.* Visual seizures in children. *Epilepsy Research* 1987;**1**:246-53.
162. Gastaut H, Zifkin BG. Benign epilepsy of childhood with occipital spike and wave complexes. In Andermann F, Lugaresi E, eds. *Migraine and epilepsy*, pp 47-81. Boston: Butterworths, 1987.
163. Aso K, Watanabe K, Negoro T, Furune A, Takahashi I, Yamamoto N *et al.* Photosensitive partial seizure:The origin of abnormal discharges. *J Epilepsy* 1988;**1**:87-93.
164. Tassinari CA, Rubboli G, Plasmati R, Salvi F, Ambrosetto G, Bianchedi G *et al.* Television-induced epilepsy with occipital seizures. In Beaumanoir A, Gastaut H, Naquet R, eds. *Reflex seizures and reflex epilepsies*, pp 241-3. Geneve: Editions Medecine & Hygiene, 1989.
165. Michelucci R, Tassinari CA. Television-induced occipital seizures. In Andermann F, Beaumanoir A, Mira L, Roger J, Tassinari CA, eds. *Occipital seizures and epilepsies in children*, pp 141-4. London: John Libbey & Company Ltd, 1993.
166. Ricci S, Vigevano F. Occipital seizures provoked by intermittent light stimulation: ictal and interictal findings. *J Clin Neurophysiol* 1993;**10**:197-209.
167. Guerrini R, Dravet C, Genton P, Bureau M, Bonanni P, Ferrari AR *et al.* Idiopathic photosensitive occipital lobe epilepsy. *Epilepsia* 1995;**36**:883-91.
168. Sharief M, Howard RO, Panayiotopoulos CP, Koutroumanidis M, Rowlinson S, Sanders S. Occipital photosensitivity with onset of seizures in adulthood: an unrecognised condition of good prognosis. *J Neurol Neurosurg Psychiatry* 2000;**68**:257.
169. Panayiotopoulos CP. Benign childhood occipital seizures (Panayiotopoulos syndrome). In Gilman S, ed. *Medlink Neurology*, San Diego, USA: Arbor Publishing Corporation, 2004.
170. Terasaki T, Yamatogi Y, Ohtahara S. Electroclinical delineation of occipital lobe epilepsy in childhood. In Andermann F, Lugaresi E, eds. *Migraine and epilepsy*, pp 125-37. Boston: Butterworths, 1987.
171. Guerrini R, Bonanni P, Parmeggiani L, Belmonte A. Adolescent onset of idiopathic photosensitive occipital epilepsy after remission of benign Rolandic epilepsy. *Epilepsia* 1997;**38**:777-81.
172. Panayiotopoulos CP. Elementary visual hallucinations, blindness, and headache in idiopathic occipital epilepsy: differentiation from migraine. *J Neurol Neurosurg Psychiatry* 1999;**66**:536-40.
173. Anyanwu EC, Ehiri J. Ocular defects in photosensitive epilepsy. *Scientific World Journal* 2004;**4**:159-66.
174. Clementi A. Stricninizzasione della sfera corticale visiva ed epilessia sperimentale da stimuli luminosi. *Arch Fisiol* 1929;**27**:356-87.
175. Guerrini R, Ferrari AR, Battaglia A, Salvadori P, Bonanni P. Occipitotemporal seizures with ictus emeticus induced by intermittent photic stimulation. *Neurology* 1994;**44**:253-9.
176. Donnet A, Bartolomei F. Migraine with visual aura and photosensitive epileptic seizures. *Epilepsia* 1997;**38**:1032-4.

177. Duncan JS, Panayiotopoulos CP, eds.Eyelid myoclonia with absences. London: John Libbey & Company Ltd, 1996.
178. Panayiotopoulos CP. Eyelid myoclonia with or without absences. In Gilman S, ed. *Medlink Neurology*, San Diego SA: Arbor Publishing Corp, 2004.
179. Jeavons PM. Nosological problems of myoclonic epilepsies of childhood and adolescence. *Devell Med Child Neurol* 1977;**19**:3-8.
180. Jeavons PM. Eyelid myoclonia and absences:the history of the syndrome. In Duncan JS, Panayiotopoulos CP, eds. *Eyelid myoclonia with absences*, pp 13-5. London: John Libbey & Company Ltd, 1996.
181. Kent L, Blake A, Whitehouse W. Eyelid myoclonia with absences: phenomenology in children. *Seizure.* 1998;**7**:193-9.
182. Incorpora G, Sofia V, Pavone P, Biondi R, Barone B, Parano E. Clinical heterogeneity in eyelid myoclonia, with absences, and epilepsy. *Eur J Pediatr.* 2002;**161**:175-7.
183. Striano S, Striano P, Nocerino C, Boccella P, Bilo L, Meo R *et al.* Eyelid myoclonia with absences: an overlooked epileptic syndrome? *Neurophysiol Clin.* 2002;**32**:287-96.
184. Ferrie CD, Agathonikou A, Parker A, Robinson RO, Panayiotopoulos CP. The spectrum of childhood epilepsies with eyelid myoclonia. In Duncan JS, Panayiotopoulos CP, eds. *Eyelid myoclonia with absences*, pp 39-48. London: John Libbey & Company Ltd, 1996.
185. Bianchi A, and the Italian LAE Collaborative Group. Study of concordance of symptoms in families with absence epilepsies. In Duncan JS, Panayiotopoulos CP, eds. *Typical absences and related epileptic syndromes*, pp 328-37. London: Churchill Communications Europe, 1995.
186. Parker A, Gardiner RM, Panayiotopoulos CP, Agathonikou A, Ferrie CD. Observations on families with eyelid myoclonia with absences. In Duncan JS, Panayiotopoulos CP, eds. *Eyelid myoclonia with absences*, pp 107-15. London: John Libbey & Company Ltd, 1996.
187. Panayiotopoulos CP. Absence epilepsies. In Engel JJ, Pedley TA, eds. *Epilepsy: A comprehensive Textbook*, pp 2327-46. Philadelphia: Lippincott-Raven Publishers, 1997.
188. Camfield CS, Camfield PR, Sadler M, Rahey S, Farrell K, Chayasirisobbon S *et al.* Paroxysmal eyelid movements: a confusing feature of generalized photosensitive epilepsy. *Neurology* 2004;**63**:40-2.
189. Ferrie CD, Giannakodimos S, Robinson RO, Panayiotopoulos CP. Symptomatic typical absence seizures. In Duncan JS, Panayiotopoulos CP, eds. *Typical absences and related epileptic syndromes*, pp 241-52. London: Churchill Communications Europe, 1995.
190. Radovici MMA, Misirliou VL, Gluckman M. Epilepsy reflex provoquee par excitations optiques des rayons solaires. Revue Neurologique 1932;1: 1305-1307 [Translated in English by Koutroumanidis M. Reflex epilepsy provoked by optic excitation by (means of) sunrays)]. In Duncan JS, Panayiotopoulos CP, eds. *Eyelid myoclonia with absences*, pp 103-5. London: John Libbey & Company Ltd, 1996.
191. Penfield W, Jasper HH. Epilepsy and the functional anatomy of the human brain. Boston: Little, Brown & Co., 1954.
192. Davidson S,Watson CW. Hereditary light-sensitive epilepsy. *Neurology* 1956;**6**:235-61.
193. Livingston S, Torres IC. Photic epilepsy: report of an unusual case and review of the literature. *Clin Pediatr* 1964;**3**:304-7.
194. Panayiotopoulos CP. Treatment of typical absence seizures and related epileptic syndromes. *Paediatr Drugs* 2001;**3**:379-403.
195. Wilkins A. Towards an understanding of reflex epilepsy and absence. In Duncan JS, Panayiotopoulos CP, eds. *Typical absences and related epileptic syndromes*, pp 196-205. London: Churchill Communications Europe, 1995.
196. Wilkins AJ, Andermann F, Ives J. Stripes, complex cells and seizures. An attempt to determine the locus and nature of the trigger mechanism in pattern-sensitive epilepsy. *Brain* 1975;**98**:365-80.
197. Sack G, Feudell P. Pattern-sensitive epilepsy with an unusual triggering mechanism. *Psychiatr Neurol Med Psychol (Leipz)* 1978;**30**:408-13.
198. Sacquegna T, Pazzaglia P, Ambrosetto G, Forti A, Giovanardi RP. Reflex epilepsy self-induced by ocular fixation on finely structured surfaces (pattern sensitive epilepsy). *Riv Neurol* 1976;**46**:431-40.
199. Panayiotopoulos CP. Inhibitory effect of central vision on occipital lobe seizures. *Neurology* 1983;**33**:523-4.
200. Panayiotopoulos CP, Agathonikou A, Koutroumanidis M, Giannakodimos S, Rowlinson S. Fixation-Off Sensitivity in Epileptic Syndromes. *Epilepsia* 1996;**37 (Suppl 4)**:83.
201. Panayiotopoulos CP. Inhibitory effect of central vision on occipital lobe seizures. *Neurology* 1981;**31**:1330-3.
202. Panayiotopoulos CP, Binnie CD, Takahashi T. Fixation-off-sensitive epilepsies:clinical and EEG characteristics. In Wolf P, ed. *Epileptic seizures and syndromes*, pp 55-66. London: John Libbey & Company Ltd, 1994.
203. Silva GE, Coelho ME, Laurentino SG. Clinical and etiological considerations about the symptomatic epileptic syndromes with occipital paroxism blocked when the eyes open . *Arq Neuropsiquiatr.* 2002;**60**:269-73.
204. Gumnit RJ, Niedermeyer E, Spreen O. Seizure activity uniquely inhibited by patterned vision. *Arch Neurol* 1965;**13**:363-8.
205. Barclay CL, Murphy WF, Lee MA, Darwish HZ. Unusual form of seizures induced by eye closure. *Epilepsia* 1993;**34**:289-93.
206. Agathonikou A, Koutroumanidis M, Panayiotopoulos CP. Fixation-off-sensitive epilepsy with absences and absence status: video- EEG documentation. *Neurology* 1997;**48**:231-4.
207. Ming X,.Kaplan PW. Fixation-off and eyes closed catamenial generalized nonconvulsive status epilepticus with eyelid myoclonic jerks. *Epilepsia* 1998;**39**:664-8.
208. Agathonikou A, Koutroumanidis M, Panayiotopoulos CP. Fixation-off (Scoto) sensitivity combined with photosensitivity. *Epilepsia* 1998;**39**:552-5.
209. Krakow K, Baxendale SA, Maguire EA, Krishnamoorthy ES, Lemieux L, Scott CA *et al.* Fixation-off sensitivity as a model of continuous epileptiform discharges: electroencephalographic, neuropsychological and functional MRI findings. *Epilepsy Res* 2000;**42**:1-6.
210. Iannetti GD, Di Bonaventura C, Pantano P, Giallonardo AT, Romanelli PL, Bozzao L *et al.* fMRI/EEG in paroxysmal activity elicited by elimination of central vision and fixation. *Neurology* 2002;**58**:976-9.
211. Pazzaglia P, Sabattini L, Lugaresi E. Occipital seizures precipitated by darkness . *Riv Neurol* 1970;**40**:184-92.
212. Beaumanoir A, Capizzi G, Nahory A, Yousfi Y. Scotogenic seizures. In Beaumanoir A, Gastaut H, Roger J, eds. *Reflex seizures and reflex epilepsies*, pp 219-23. Geneve: Medecine and Hygiene, 1989.
213. Takahashi T. Influence of gazing at a fixation point and total visual field on electroencephalograms . *No To Shinkei* 1976;**28**:95-103.
214. Bancaud J, Talairach J, Lamarche M, Bonis A, Trottier S. Neurophysiopathological hypothesis on startle epilepsy in man. *Rev Neurolog* 1975;**131**:559-71.
215. Wilkins DE, Hallett M, Wess MM. Audiogenic startle reflex of man and its relationship to startle syndromes. A review. *Brain* 1986;**109**:561-73.
216. Manford MR, Fish DR, Shorvon SD. Startle provoked epileptic seizures:features in 19 patients. *J Neurol Neurosurg Psychiatry* 1996;**61**:151-6.
217. Cokar O, Gelisse P, Livet MO, Bureau M, Habib M, Genton P. Startle response: epileptic or non-epileptic? The case for "flash" SMA reflex seizures. *Epileptic Disord.* 2001;**3**:7-12.
218. Cengiz B, Odabasi Z, Ozdag F, Eroglu E, Gokcil Z, Vural O. Essential startle disease may not be a uniform entity. *Clin Electroencephalogr.* 2001;**32**:92-5.
219. Guerrini R, Genton P, Bureau M, Dravet C, Roger J. Reflex seizures are frequent in patients with Down syndrome and epilepsy. *Epilepsia* 1990;**31**:406-17.
220. Faught E. Lamotrigine for startle-induced seizures. *Seizure* 1999;**8**:361-3.
221. Matsuoka H, Takahashi T, Sasaki M, Matsumoto K, Yoshida S, Numachi Y *et al.* Neuropsychological EEG activation in patients with epilepsy. *Brain* 2000;**123**:318-30.
222. Goossens LA, Andermann F, Andermann E, Remillard GM. Reflex seizures induced by calculation, card or board games, and spatial tasks: a review of 25 patients and delineation of the epileptic syndrome. *Neurology* 1990;**40**:1171-6.
223. Koepp MJ, Richardson MP, Brooks DJ, Duncan JS. Focal cortical release of endogenous opioids during reading-induced seizures. *Lancet* 1998;**352**:952-5.
224. Mayer T, Wolf P. Reading epilepsy: clinical and genetic background. In Berkovic SF, Genton P, Hirsch E, Picard F, eds. *Genetics of focal epilepsies*, pp 159-68. London: John Libbey and Company Ltd, 1999.
225. Pegna AJ, Picard F, Martory MD, Vuilleumier P, Seeck M, Jallon P *et al.* Semantically-triggered reading epilepsy: an experimental case study. *Cortex* 1999;**35**:101-11.
226. Archer JS, Briellmann RS, Syngeniotis A, Abbott DF, Jackson GD. Spike-triggered fMRI in reading epilepsy: involvement of left frontal cortex working memory area. *Neurology* 2003;**60**:415-21.

14 PHARMACOPOEIA OF PROPHYLACTIC ANTIEPILEPTIC DRUGS

ACETAZOLAMIDE

Acetazolamide, an heterocyclic sulfonamide, is a carbonic anhydrase-inhibiting drug used mainly for the treatment of glaucoma.[1;2]

CLINICAL APPLICATIONS

Acetazolamide is effective as an adjunctive therapy for a variety of seizures, but mainly absences.[1;3;4] However, it also controls myoclonic jerks, GTCS and focal seizures. It is particularly used for intermittent administration in catamenial epilepsy (8 days before the expected onset of menses and continued until termination of bleeding); it is not recommended if there is a likelihood of pregnancy.

DOSAGE AND TITRATION

Adults: start treatment with 250 mg and increase to 500–750 mg.

Children: 10–20 mg/day.

Dosing: two or three times daily.

Therapeutic range: 40–100 mg/L (300–700 μmol/L).

Therapeutic drug monitoring: not needed.

MAIN ADVERSE REACTIONS

Common: flushing, lethargy, anorexia, paraesthesia and increased diuresis.

Serious: idiosyncratic reactions as for other sulfonamides (rash, aplastic anaemia, Stevens-Johnson syndrome), renal failure, nephrolithiasis in chronic treatment and metabolic acidosis (see also topiramate page 513).

MECHANISM OF ACTION

Acetazolamide is a carbonic anhydrase inhibiting drug and reversibly catalyses the hydration of CO_2 and the dehydration of carbonic acid. It blocks the action of brain carbonic anhydrase resulting in elevation of intracellular CO_2, decrease of intracellular pH and depression of neuronal activity.

PHARMACOKINETICS

Oral bioavailability: > 90%.

Protein binding: 90–95%.

Metabolism: does not undergo metabolic alteration.

Excretion: renal.

Elimination half-life: 12–14 hours.

DRUG INTERACTIONS

Not significant. Reduces carbamazepine levels. Salicylates increase levels of acetazolamide.

MAIN DISADVANTAGES

Unpredictable seizure efficacy, development of tolerance and idiosyncratic reactions that exceptionally may be fatal.

USEFUL NOTE

Risk of withdrawal seizures. Combination with carbamazepine or oxcarbazepine increases the risk of hyponatraemia. It should be withdrawn prior to starting a ketogenic diet.

CARBAMAZEPINE

Carbamazepine is an iminodibenzyl derivative designated chemically as iminodibenzyl (10,11-dihydro-5H-dibenzo[b,f]azepine). It is structurally related to the tricyclic antidepressants. It was synthesised during the development of the antidepressant drug imipramine. Carbamazepine was first introduced in clinical practice in 1962 mainly for the treatment of trigeminal neuralgia prior to becoming the main AED for the therapy of focal epilepsies.

CLINICAL APPLICATIONS

Carbamazepine is the superior drug for the treatment of focal epilepsies of any type (idiopathic or symptomatic) with or without secondarily GTCS. It is also effective in primarily GTCS. In numerous comparative studies, no other drug showed better efficacy than carbamazepine in focal seizures though some of the new AEDs are better tolerated. Other AEDs are only used to treat these conditions when carbamazepine fails, either because of adverse reactions or ineffectiveness.

However, carbamazepine is ineffective and often contraindicated in generalised epilepsies, such as juvenile myoclonic epilepsy, juvenile absence epilepsy and epileptic encephalopathies (e.g. Lennox-Gastaut syndrome). It exaggerates myoclonic jerks, absences and atonic seizures.[3;5] It is ineffective in neonatal and febrile seizures.

DOSAGE AND TITRATION

'Start low and go slow' is important when initiating carbamazepine treatment in order to minimise adverse reactions.

Adults and children over 12 years of age: start treatment with 200 mg/day in two equally divided doses and increase at weekly intervals in increments of 200 mg/day up to 800–1200 mg/day. Rarely, higher doses of up to 1800 mg/day are needed.

Children 6–12 years old: start treatment with 100 mg/day in two equally divided doses and increase at weekly intervals in increments of 100 mg/day up to 600–1000 mg/day.

Children under 6 years: start treatment with 5–10 mg/kg/day in two or three divided doses and increase at weekly intervals in increments of 5–10 mg/kg/day up to a maintenance dose of no more than 35 mg/kg/day.

Dosing: two or three times daily. Four times daily dosing may be needed for children receiving a high dosage.

There is a significant difference in the dose of carbamazepine given as monotherapy and that used in combination with other AEDs. Higher doses may be necessary in polytherapy with enzyme-inducing AEDs, which increase the metabolism of carbamazepine.

Fluctuations in the levels of carbamazepine can be reduced by the use of sustained-release preparations.

The clearance of carbamazepine in children is faster than in adults and therefore three times daily dosing may be required.

Therapeutic drug monitoring: useful, but substantial diurnal variation in plasma concentration are common and symptoms of toxicity due to carbamazepine epoxide may occur without increases in carbamazepine levels.

Therapeutic range: 3–12 mg/L (12–50 μmol/L). Carbamazepine epoxide: up to 9 μmol/L.

Developing diplopia may be a good indicator of maximum tolerated carbamazepine levels or epoxide toxicity when carbamazepine levels are within the target range.

MAIN ADVERSE REACTIONS

Common: sedation, headache, diplopia, blurred vision, rash, gastrointestinal disturbances, ataxia, tremor, impotence, hyponatraemia and neutropenia. CNS-related adverse reactions are usually dose-related and appear on initiation of treatment. These are primarily reversible and can be prevented by slow and careful upward titration following initiation of treatment.

Carbamazepine causes a dose-related reduction in the neutrophil count in 10–20% of patients, but it rarely drops below 1.2 x 10^9 and is seldom of any clinical significance. Hyponatraemia occurs in around 5% of treated patients. Most physicians advise obtaining blood counts at baseline and every 6–8 weeks for the first 6 months of carbamazepine treatment.

Serious: rash, hepatic dysfunction, haematological toxicity and cardiac arrhythmias. Allergic skin rash is the commonest idiosyncratic adverse reaction that occurs in 5–10% of patients. This is usually mild and develops within the first 2–6 weeks of treatment. Carbamazepine should be withdrawn immediately a skin rash develops in order to prevent serious and sometimes life-threatening conditions, such as anticonvulsant hypersensitivity syndrome. Hepatotoxicity usually occurs in the setting of a generalised hypersensitivity response.

There are exceptional instances of aplastic anaemia, agranulocytosis, thrombocytopenia and cardiac conduction disturbances.

CONSIDERATIONS IN WOMEN

Pregnancy: category D. Contrary to previous studies, a recent pregnancy registry study found that the risk of teratogenicity is small.[6] In a UK Epilepsy and Pregnancy Register, serious malformation rates for monotherapy were 2.3% for carbamazepine as opposed to 2.4% with no AED, 2.1% for lamotrigine and 5.9% for valproate.[7]

MAIN MECHANISMS OF ACTION

Carbamazepine inhibits sustained, repetitive high-frequency firing of cortical neurons via use- and frequency-dependent blockade of voltage-gated sodium channels. Other mechanisms may include inhibition of L-type calcium channels and modulations of neurotransmission.

Like other tricyclic compounds, carbamazepine has a moderate anticholinergic action, which is responsible for some of its adverse reactions.

PHARMACOKINETICS

Oral bioavailability: 75–85% and unaffected by food intake. Bioavailability may be reduced by up to 50% when stored in hot humid conditions. After oral administration, absorption is relatively slow and often erratic reaching peak plasma concentrations within 4–24 hours; 75–85% of orally ingested carbamazepine is absorbed. Absorption and bioavailability vary among different carbamazepine formulations. Slow-release formulations have a prolonged absorption phase. Syrup formulations reach maximum plasma concentration faster than chewable or plain tablets.

There are significant diurnal variations in plasma concentrations of carbamazepine. This is greater in children than in adults, which can result in intermittent side effects that demand adjustments to the daily dose.

Protein binding: 66–89%.

Metabolism: carbamazepine is extensively metabolised in the liver. The predominant elimination pathway results in the formation of carbamazepine 10,11-epoxide, which is a stable and pharmacologically active agent with its own antiepileptic activity and adverse reactions.

Carbamazepine-epoxide makes a greater contribution to the pharmacological effects (both beneficial and toxic) of carbamazepine in children than in adults. This is because children metabolise carbamazepine more rapidly than adults and this results in carbamazepine-epoxide concentrations approaching those of carbamazepine.

Carbamazepine is a potent enzyme inducer. It also induces its own metabolism (autoinduction) by simulating the activity of the CYP3A4 component of cytochrome P450. Autoinduction is usually completed within 3–5 weeks. The half-life of carbamazepine decreases considerably from 18–55 hours to 6–18 hours as autoinduction takes place. In practical terms, this means that carbamazepine levels fall significantly (by about 50%) after several weeks of treatment, which may result in seizure recurrence within this period of autoinduction.

Elimination half-life: 5–26 hours. In combination treatment, the elimination half-life of carbamazepine is reduced by enzyme-inducers and increased by enzyme-inhibitors.

DRUG INTERACTIONS[19;20]

Antiepileptic drugs

Carbamazepine metabolism is highly inducible by certain AEDs.

Enzyme-inducing AEDs, such as phenytoin, phenobarbitone and primidone, cause significant reductions in plasma concentrations of carbamazepine. Furthermore, AEDs exacerbate and often double the diurnal variation of plasma carbamazepine concentrations, thus increasing the risk of transient side effects.

Valproate markedly increases carbamazepine epoxide levels (sometimes four-fold) without concurrent changes in carbamazepine plasma concentration.

Co-medication with lamotrigine may cause neurotoxic symptoms of headache, nausea, diplopia and ataxia, probably as the result of a pharmacodynamic interaction and not by increasing carbamazepine epoxide (as originally suggested).

Non-antiepileptic drugs

Major: carbamazepine increases the metabolism and therefore decreases the efficacy of a wide variety of drugs, such as oral contraceptives, theophylline, oral anticoagulants and beta-blockers.

Macrolide antibiotics, such as erythromycin, inhibit carbamazepine metabolism and have been associated with carbamazepine toxicity. Carbamazepine toxicity is observed shortly after starting erythromycin therapy, is rapidly reversed on withdrawal of the antibiotic, but can be severe if not recognised early.

Carbamazepine should not be combined with monoamine oxidase inhibitors because of drug interactions.

Potential: additive cardiotoxicity with calcium channel blockers and beta-blockers.

MAIN DISADVANTAGES

Idiosyncratic and other adverse reactions, drug–drug interactions, need for laboratory testing and relatively narrow spectrum of antiepileptic efficacy.

Although carbamazepine is by far the best AED in the treatment of focal and secondarily GTCS, it offers no benefit in most other epilepsies, because of ineffectiveness or seizure exacerbation; these include absences and myoclonic jerks of IGE, non-convulsive generalised seizures in Lennox-Gastaut syndrome and epileptic encephalopathies.

Pregnancy category C and D drugs: teratogenicity and antiepileptic drugs[8;9]

Pregnancy registries are a new method for assessing the foetal risks from exposure in pregnancy.[6;7;10-15]

The results from these studies are generally encouraging in that, overall, 95% of offspring did not have a major congenital malformation. The risk is increased in polytherapy, which should be avoided if possible.

The Food and Drug Administration categorises AED medications into two classes: D and C.

Category D drugs are those drugs for which teratogenicity was seen in both animal and human pregnancies. Phenytoin, carbamazepine and valproate are category D drugs.

Category C drugs have demonstrated teratogenicity in animals, but the risk in humans is not known.

Of the new AEDs, all of which are classified as category C, it is too early to draw definite conclusions. With the exception of topiramate and vigabatrin, the newer AEDs do not appear to be teratogenic in animals when administered in subtoxic doses.[16] On a preliminary basis in humans, gabapentin,[13] lamotrigine[17] and levetiracetam[18] may be relatively safe, but certainly they should be used very cautiously in women of childbearing age. In both categories C and D, the recommendation remains the same: selection of an AED in pregnancy should be based on the risk:benefit ratio.

Results released from the North American AED pregnancy register refer only to phenobarbitone and valproate.[11;12] Against a background prevalence of major non-syndromic congenital anomalies of 1.62%, the relative risk of having an affected offspring for women exposed to valproate was 5% and to phenobarbitone was 3.8%.[11;12] The results from a similar UK Epilepsy and Pregnancy Register[7] are more informative and showed that the major malformation rate with no AED was 2.4%, with AED monotherapy was 3.4% and with polytherapy was 6.5%. For the individual drugs used in monotherapy, the malformation rates were: carbamazepine 2.3%, valproate 5.9% and lamotrigine 2.1%. Cardiac and neural tube defects, and genitourinary and gastrointestinal tract abnormalities have been reported with all three drugs, and orofacial clefting and skeletal abnormalities have been reported with sodium valproate and carbamazepine.

Exceptionally carbamazepine may exaggerate seizures in Rolandic epilepsy and may induce non-convulsive status and features of serious atypical evolutions.

CLOBAZAM

Clobazam is a benzodiazepine. Clobazam was the first 1,5-benzodiazepine and was designed to have a chemical structure with a different pharmacological profile from that of the 1,4- benzodiazepines.

CLINICAL APPLICATIONS

Based on recent evidence, clobazam is a very useful AED, both as polytherapy and monotherapy.[21-31] It is neglected in current clinical practice mainly because it is considered to induce high dependence/tolerance, it is of similar effectiveness regarding seizure type to clonazepam and it is a benzodiazepine. It is not licensed in the USA.

The main clinical applications of clobazam are as follows.

a. It is used as adjunctive medication in all forms of drug-resistant epilepsy in adults and children.[21-29] It is particularly effective in focal rather than generalised seizures. Clobazam was found to be of equivalent efficacy to carbamazepine and phenytoin as monotherapy in childhood epilepsy.[30;31]

b. Intermittent clobazam administration 5 days prior and during the menses in catamenial epilepsy[32] is the most popular textbook recommendation.

DOSAGE AND TITRATION

Adults and children over 12 years: start treatment with 5–10 mg/day at night and increase at weekly intervals in increments of 5 mg/day up to 40 mg/day. In my experience 10 mg taken before sleep is often therapeutic in focal seizures. I do not use dose of more than 20 mg in children.

Children under 12 years: start with 0.1–0.2 mg/kg/day and slowly increase at weekly intervals in increments of 0.1mg/kg/day up to 0.8 mg/kg/day.

Dosing: once or twice daily; a smaller dose in the day time and a larger dose prior to going to sleep.

Therapeutic range: norclobazam (active metabolite) 60–200 μg/L (200–670 nmol/L).

Therapeutic drug monitoring: not useful except when unusual side effects appear.[34]

MAIN ADVERSE REACTIONS

As for all the benzodiazepines, but much milder than with most of them.[22;29] Somnolence may be partly prevented by administering the drug in small doses 1 hour prior to going to sleep. The cognitive and behavioural effects of clobazam appear to be similar to those of standard monotherapy with carbamazepine or phenytoin.[31]

Severe aggressive outbursts, hyperactivity, insomnia and depression with suicidal ideation may occur, particularly in children.

Tolerance may develop, but this aspect has been largely overemphasised as documented in many recent studies.[22;30] More than one-third of patients do not develop tolerance.[25] When clobazam is effective, most patients continue to benefit for years without drug dependence or unwanted side effects.[25]

MAIN MECHANISM OF ACTION

$GABA_A$ receptor agonist.

PHARMACOKINETICS

Oral bioavailability: 90%.

Protein binding: 85%.

Metabolism: hepatic oxidation and then conjugation.

Elimination half-life: 20 hours, but that of its principal metabolite, norclobazam, is about 50 hours.

DRUG INTERACTIONS

Minor and not clinically significant. Potentiates the effect of CNS depressants such as alcohol, barbiturates and neuroleptics.

MAIN DISADVANTAGES

Sedation and development of tolerance.

A reminder about benzodiazepines

Benzodiazepines are a group of two-ring heterocyclic compounds consisting of a benzene ring fused to a diazepine ring. Many compounds with this structure have psychotropic and neurotropic properties, and are used as sedatives, anticonvulsants, muscle relaxants and in related applications. Of the benzodiazepines,[33] clonazepam, clobazam, clorazepate and nitrazepam are used in the treatment of recurrent seizures. Diazepam, lorazepam and midazolam are exclusively used in the treatment of status epilepticus. Clonazepam and clobazam are the most useful of all benzodiazepines for preventing recurrent seizures. Clonazepam is the main drug used for myoclonic jerks, while clobazam is more effective in focal seizures.

Main adverse reactions of all the benzodiazepines: sedation (sometimes intolerably severe), fatigue, drowsiness, behavioural and cognitive impairment, restlessness, aggressiveness, hypersalivation and coordination disturbances.

Tolerance and withdrawal syndrome: administration of therapeutic doses of benzodiazepines for 6 weeks or longer can result in physical dependence, characterised by a withdrawal syndrome when the drug is discontinued. With larger doses, the physical dependence develops more rapidly.

USEFUL CLINICAL NOTE

a. Clobazam should be tried as adjunctive medication in all drug-resistant epilepsies at a dose of 10–30 mg nocte (half this dose in children > 3 years old). It is more effective in focal than symptomatic epilepsies and can also be used as monotherapy. Probably only 1 out of 10 patients will have a clinically significant improvement, but this may be very dramatic and render the patient seizure-free.

b. Unlike clonazepam, clobazam is much less effective in myoclonic jerks and absences.

c. Avoid overmedication. Small doses of 10–20 mg given 1 hour prior to going to sleep may be therapeutic and well tolerated.

d. Withdrawal should be very slow (months). Rapid discontinuation often leads to withdrawal symptoms, seizures and status epilepticus.

CLONAZEPAM

Clonazepam is a 1,4-benzodiazepine.

CLINICAL APPLICATIONS

Clonazepam[33;35] is the most potent AED in the treatment of myoclonic jerks (superior to valproate), and is also effective in absences (though much inferior to valproate and ethosuximide)[3] and focal seizures (much inferior to carbamazepine and any other appropriate drug for this type of seizure). Opinions about its effectiveness in GTCS are conflicting and range from beneficial[36] to exaggeration.[36;37]

Clonazepam is the main AED for myoclonic jerks in all forms of idiopathic or symptomatic and progressive epilepsies (monotherapy, but mainly adjunctive therapy). Clonazepam monotherapy is probably the first choice in reading epilepsy (better than valproate). It is particularly effective in JME if myoclonic jerks are not controlled by other drugs. Adding small doses of clonazepam (0.5–1 mg prior to going to sleep) to valproate, levetiracetam or lamotrigine is highly beneficial and may prevent an unnecessary increase in the main concomitant drug. It is widely used in epileptic encephalopathies.

DOSAGE AND TITRATION

'Start low and go slow' is essential, both in adults and children.

Adults: initiate treatment with 0.25–8 mg/day._

Start treatment with 0.25 mg/day at night and increase at weekly intervals in increments of 0.25 mg/day up to 8-10 mg/day. In my experience 0.5–1 mg of clonazepam taken before sleep is often highly effective in controlling myoclonic jerks either as monotherapy or as adjunctive therapy.

Children: start with 0.01–0.02 mg/kg/day and slowly increase up to 0.1–0.2 mg/kg/day.

Dosing: once or twice daily; a smaller dose in the day time and a larger dose prior to going to sleep.

Therapeutic range: 20–80 µg/L (80–250 nmol/L).

Therapeutic drug monitoring: not needed.

MAIN ADVERSE REACTIONS

Common: sedation, drowsiness, hypersalivation, hyperactivity, lack of concentration and incoordination. Sedation is more serious than with clobazam. This may be partly prevented by administering the drug in small doses 1 hour prior to going to sleep.

Serious: withdrawal syndrome in chronic use.

MAIN MECHANISM OF ACTION

$GABA_A$ receptor agonist.

PHARMACOKINETICS

Oral bioavailability: > 80%.

Protein binding: 85%.

Metabolism: hepatic.

Elimination half-life: 20–80 hours.

DRUG INTERACTIONS

Minor and not clinically significant. Potentiates the effect of CNS depressants such as alcohol, barbiturates and neuroleptics.

MAIN DISADVANTAGES

Sedation and development of tolerance.

USEFUL NOTE

(a). Clonazepam is the drug of first choice for the control of myoclonic jerks (either as monotherapy if this is the only seizure type as in reading epilepsy or mainly as adjunctive medication).

(b). Avoid overmedication. Small doses 1 hour prior to going to sleep may be effective and well tolerated.

(c). Withdrawal should be very slow in months. Rapid discontinuation often leads to withdrawal symptoms, seizures and status epilepticus.

ETHOSUXIMIDE

Ethosuximide (alpha-ethyl-alpha-methyl-succinimide) is the main survivor of the succinimides.[38-40] It was first introduced in clinical practice in the early 1950s for the treatment of 'petit mal'.[41]

CLINICAL APPLICATIONS

Ethosuximide is still a valuable AED for the treatment of typical absence seizures and has a 70% seizure-free success rate as monotherapy.[3] It does not control GTCS, which on an anecdotal basis may become worse. It is recommended in childhood absence epilepsy (monotherapy) and IGE with intractable absence seizures (adjunctive therapy).

Ethosuximide is also useful as adjunctive treatment in negative myoclonus,[42] drop attacks[43] and certain types of myoclonic epilepsy.[44]

DOSAGE AND TITRATION

Titrate slowly to avoid adverse reactions and mainly gastrointestinal disturbances.

Adults and children over 12 years: start treatment with 250 mg/day and increase slowly in 250 mg increments every 4–7 days to 750–1500 mg.

Children under 12 years: start with 5–10 mg/kg/day increase slowly to 20–35 mg/kg/day.

Dosing: two or three times daily.

Therapeutic range: 40–100 mg/L (300–700 μmol/L).

Therapeutic drug monitoring: mostly not needed.

MAIN ADVERSE REACTIONS

Common: gastrointestinal symptoms include anorexia, vague gastric upset, nausea and vomiting, cramps, epigastric and abdominal pain, weight loss and diarrhoea. Drowsiness, photophobia, euphoria, hiccups, headache and less often behaviour and psychotic disturbances may occur.

Severe: haemopoietic complications (aplastic anaemia), Stevens-Johnson syndrome, renal and hepatic impairment, and systemic lupus erhythematosus.

CONSIDERATIONS IN WOMEN

Pregnancy: category C.

Interaction with hormonal contraception: none.

MAIN MECHANISMS OF ACTION

Ethosuximide exerts its anti-absence effect by either reducing thalamic low threshold calcium currents, probably by a direct channel blocking action that is voltage dependent,[45] or through a potent inhibitory effect in the perioral region of the primary somatosensory cortex.[46;47]

PHARMACOKINETICS

Oral bioavailability: 90–100%.

Protein binding: 85%.

Metabolism: hepatic oxidation and then conjugation.

Elimination half-life: 30–60 hours.

DRUG INTERACTIONS

Commonly, there are no clinically significant drug–drug interactions. Ethosuximide may raise the plasma concentration of phenytoin. Valproate has been reported to both increase and decrease ethosuximide levels.

MAIN DISADVANTAGES

Narrow spectrum of antiepileptic activity limited to absence seizures and certain types of myoclonus (mainly negative myoclonus). It may aggravate GTCS.

It sometimes exhibits severe adverse idiosyncratic reactions.

Abrupt withdrawal in patients with absences may precipitate absence status epilepticus

OTHER AVAILABLE SUCCINIMIDES

(a). Methsuximide is a broader spectrum drug than ethosuximide (but with a weaker action) that is also effective in focal seizures. Adverse reactions are more frequent and may be more serious than with ethosuximide.

(b). Phensuximide is rarely used because its effect is inferior to other succinimides.

FELBAMATE

Felbamate (2-phenyl-1,3-propanediol dicarbamate) is the first AED since 1978 to be approved by the USA Food and Drug Administration in 1993. However, clinical use of felbamate as an AED practically ended 1 year after its release, when it became apparent that felbamate is associated with a high incidence of aplastic anaemia and hepatic failure also with fatalities.[48-51]

Most of the cases of aplastic anaemia occurred in women over the age of 17 years with a history of idiosyncratic reactions to other AEDs. It was not reported in children younger than 13 years.

Hepatic failure mainly occurred in young children.

In addition, felbamate is difficult to use because of a narrow therapeutic window and a high propensity to interact with concomitant drugs.

Currently, the use of felbamate as an AED is cautiously limited to severe cases of Lennox-Gastaut syndrome, mainly with atonic/astatic seizures, in which felbamate is significantly superior to placebo. It should be given for no longer than 2 months in case there is no clear response. In these cases, felbamate should be used with bi-monthly follow-up of transaminases and blood cell counts. However, the risk of using felbamate in Lennox-Gastaut syndrome outweighs any benefits, which even if they occur are short lived.

GABAPENTIN

Gabapentin [GBP-1(aminomethyl)cyclohexaneacetic acid] first received marketing approval for the treatment of focal epilepsies in 1993.[52;53]

CLINICAL APPLICATIONS

Recommendations of gabapentin as an AED are limited to focal seizures. It is the least effective of all other new AEDs even at higher doses of around 3000 mg/day.[54] It has no effect in generalised seizures of any type and may exaggerate them.[55] However, it is considered relatively safe with few side effects. It is mainly used for non-epileptic disorders such as neuropathic pain.

DOSAGE AND TITRATION

Adults: the starting dose is 300mg/day, which can be increased rapidly in increments of 300 mg/day to a typical adult maintenance dose of 900–1800 mg/day given in three divided doses. Doses of up to 3600 mg/day have been used.

Children: start treatment with 15/mg/kg/day and increase to 30 mg/kg/day within a few days. Recommended maintenance dose is 50–100 mg/day. Children require relatively higher doses than adults, because clearance of gabapentin is greater in children than in adults.

Dosing: three times daily.

Therapeutic range: 2–20 mg/L (12–120 μmol/L).

Therapeutic drug monitoring: unnecessary.

MAIN ADVERSE REACTIONS

Gabapentin has a relatively good adverse reaction profile.

Common: increased appetite and weight gain is a problem. Other reactions include dizziness, ataxia, nystagmus, headache, tremor, fatigue, diplopia, rhinitis and nausea. Significant behavioural disturbances, such as aggression, hyperexcitabilty and tantrums, have been reported mainly in children.[56] Caution is recommended in patients with a history of psychotic illness.

Potentially serious adverse reactions: rarely, rash (0.5%), leucopenia (0.2%), and electrocardiographic changes and angina (0.05%).

Gabapentin may unmask myasthenia gravis and should be used with caution in this disease.[57]

Seizure exacerbation: treatment emergent exaggeration of seizures occurs particularly in patients with generalised epilepsies.

CONSIDERATIONS IN WOMEN

Pregnancy: category C.

Breastfeeding: it is excreted in human milk, but the effect on the nursing infant is unknown.

Interaction with hormonal contraception: none.

Others: Weight gain may be of particular importance to women because of the associated risk for polycystic ovary syndrome.*

MAIN MECHANISMS OF ACTION

The mechanism of action is uncertain. Gabapentin was developed because of its structural similarity to GABA and its ability to cross the blood-brain barrier. However, it does not appear to be a GABA-agonist.

The mechanism responsible for its antiepileptic activity and the relief of neuropathic pain is probably due to a modulating action of gabapentin on voltage-gated calcium channels and neurotransmitter release.

PHARMACOKINETICS

Oral bioavailability: low < 60%. Gabapentin is rapidly absorbed reaching peak plasma levels within 2–4 hours after oral ingestion. Bioavailability is less than 60%, but is dose-dependent; absorption is progressively reduced with increasing dosage. Food intake does not influence absorption.

Protein binding: none.

Metabolism: gabapentin is not metabolised and is excreted by the kidneys. Renal impairment reduces drug clearance and raises plasma gabapentin concentrations.

Elimination half-life: 5–9 hours.

DRUG INTERACTIONS

There are no significant interactions with other AEDs.

However, cimetidine reduces the renal clearance of gabapentin and antacids reduce the absorption of gabapentin by 20%.

MAIN DISADVANTAGES

Narrow-spectrum AED limited to the treatment of focal seizures only and with low efficacy.

> Therapeutic efficacy is weak in relation to other AEDs, the number of responders is disappointingly low even when higher doses are used and it is unusual for patients with severe focal epilepsies to derive much benefit.[54;58]

It is ineffective and may exaggerate generalised seizures of any type.

*** Polycystic ovarian morphology versus polycystic ovary syndrome**

Polycystic ovarian morphology has a high prevalence in the adult female population (around 25%). It can be detected with ultrasound, may be found in childhood and persists after the menopause. It is not be associated with any hormonal or clinical abnormalities. When polycystic ovarian morphology is associated with elevated androgen levels, luteinizing hormone concentrations or any clinical symptoms of androgen excess it becomes polycystic ovary syndrome. The prevalence of polycystic ovary syndrome varies from 5–26% of adult women. Weight gain and hyperinsulinaemia can aggravate the features of polycystic ovary syndrome, and may transform polycystic ovarian morphology into polycystic ovary syndrome.

LAMOTRIGINE

Lamotrigine is a 3,5-diamino-6-(2,3-dichlorophenyl)-as-triazine of the phenyltriazine class. Lamotrigine was first licensed for clinical practice in 1993 and is now established as one of the best AEDs of its generation.[59]

CLINICAL APPLICATIONS

Lamotrigine is an effective broad-spectrum AED for the treatment of all types of seizure except myoclonic jerks.[60-67] It has been recommended for all focal or generalised, idiopathic or symptomatic epileptic syndromes of adults,[63-65] children[60;61] and neonates.[68] Exception to this are syndromes with predominantly myoclonic jerks.

In polytherapy, lamotrigine is at its best when combined with valproate, because of very efficacious pharmacodynamic interactions.[69] This combination may be ideal for drug-resistant generalised epilepsies including those with myoclonic seizures.[70] Usually, small doses of lamotrigine added to valproate may render previously uncontrolled patients seizure-free.[3;69;71;72]

Other major advantages of lamotrigine are that it lacks cognitive and behavioural adverse reactions and it is non-sedating with improved global functioning, which includes increased attention and alertness reported in both paediatric and adult trials.[62] Idiosyncratic reactions and mainly rash that can become very serious are a significant disadvantage.[73;74]

DOSAGE AND TITRATION

Slow titration and in small doses is essential in both adults and children.

Dosage and titration vary considerably between monotherapy, co-medication with valproate and co-medication with enzyme-inducing AEDs. For this reason the manufacturers have provided detailed tables to be followed in each of these circumstances in children and adults. The following are some examples of these:

Adults and children over 12 years (monotherapy): start with 25 mg once a day for 2 weeks, followed by 50 mg once daily for 2 weeks. Thereafter, the dose should be increased by a maximum of 50–100 mg every 1–2 weeks until the optimal response is achieved. The usual maintenance dose to achieve optimal response is 100–200mg/day given once daily or as two divided doses. Some patients have required 500 mg/day to achieve the desired response.

Adults and children over 12 years (add-on therapy with valproate): start with 25 mg every alternate day for 2 weeks, followed by 25 mg once daily for 2 weeks. Thereafter, the dose should be increased by a maximum of 25–50 mg every 1–2 weeks until the optimal response is achieved. The usual maintenance dose to achieve optimal response is 100–200 mg/day given once daily or in two divided doses.

Adults and children over 12 years (add-on therapy with enzyme inducing AEDs): start with 50 mg once daily for 2 weeks, followed by 100 mg/day given in two divided doses for 2 weeks. Thereafter, the dose should be increased by a maximum of 100 mg every 1–2 weeks until the optimal response is achieved. The usual maintenance dose to achieve optimal response is 200–400 mg/day given in two divided doses. Some patients have required 700 mg/day to achieve the desired response.

*Children aged 2–12 years (with valproate co-medication):** start with 0.15 mg/kg/day given once daily for 2 weeks, followed by 0.3 mg/kg/day given once daily for 2 weeks. Thereafter, the dose should be increased by a maximum of 0.3 mg/kg every 1–2 weeks until the optimal response is achieved. The usual maintenance dose to achieve optimal response is 1–5 mg/kg/day given once daily or in two divided doses.

*Children aged 2–12 years (with co-medication with enzyme inducing AED):** start with 0.6 mg/kg/day given in two divided doses for 2 weeks, followed by 1.2mg/kg/day for 2 weeks. Thereafter, the dose should be increased by a maximum of 1.2 mg/kg every 1–2 weeks until the optimal response is achieved. The usual maintenance dose to achieve optimal response is 5–15mg/kg/day given in two divided doses.

*Doses should be rounded down to the nearest whole tablet. Only whole tablets should be used for dosing.

Caution: probably, slower dosage titration reduces the risk of skin rash and possibly generalised hypersensitive reaction.[74] Therefore, it is mandatory to follow the recommendations of the manufacturers regarding initial dose and subsequent slow-dose escalation of lamotrigine.

Conversion to monotherapy from polytherapy with valproate or with enzyme-inducing AEDs should follow appropriate guidelines provided by the manufacturers of lamotrigine.

Therapeutic range: 1–15 mg/L (10–60 μmol/L).

Therapeutic drug monitoring: though therapeutic drug monitoring was not recommended initially for lamotrigine, it has recently been recognised that this is particularly useful in pregnancy[75-77] and in conjunction with hormonal contraception.[78]

MAIN ADVERSE REACTIONS

Common: skin rash, headache, nausea, diplopia, dizziness, ataxia, tremor, asthenia and anxiety.

Severe: an allergic skin rash is the commonest and probably the most dangerous adverse effect prompting withdrawal of lamotrigine.[74] Skin rash occurs in approximately 10% of patients, but serious rashes leading to hospitalisation, including Stevens-Johnson syndrome and anticonvulsant hypersensitivity syndrome, occur in approximately 1 out of 300 adults (0.3%) and 1 out of 100 children (< 16 years of age) treated with lamotrigine.[74]

Nearly all cases of life-threatening rashes associated with lamotrigine have occurred within 2–8 weeks of treatment initiation. However, isolated cases have been reported after prolonged treatment (e.g. 6 months). Accordingly, duration of therapy cannot be relied on as a means to predict the potential risk heralded by the first appearance of a rash.

There are suggestions, yet to be proven, that the risk of rash may also be increased by: (1) co-administration of lamotrigine with valproate; (2) exceeding the recommended initial dose of lamotrigine; or (3) exceeding the recommended dose escalation for lamotrigine. However, cases have been reported in the absence of these factors. The incidence of skin rash can probably be reduced by starting treatment with a low dose spread over longer intervals, particularly in patients receiving concomitant valproate, which inhibits lamotrigine metabolism.

Although benign rashes also occur with lamotrigine, it is not possible to predict reliably which rashes will prove to be serious or life threatening. Accordingly, lamotrigine should ordinarily be discontinued at the first sign of rash, unless the rash is clearly not drug related. Discontinuation of treatment may not prevent a rash from becoming life threatening, or permanently disabling or disfiguring.

Patients should be advised to report immediately any symptoms of skin rash, hives, fever, swollen lymph glands, painful sores in the mouth or around the eyes, or swelling of lips or tongue, because these symptoms may be the first signs of a serious reaction.

Other: other adverse experiences have included gastrointestinal disturbance (including vomiting and diarrhoea), irritability/aggression, agitation, confusion and hallucinations. Very rarely, lupus-like reactions have been reported.

There have been reports of haematological abnormalities, which may or may not be associated with the anticonvulsant hypersensitivity syndrome. These have included neutropenia, leucopenia, anaemia, thrombocytopenia, pancytopenia, and very rarely aplastic anaemia and agranulocytosis. Elevations of liver function tests and rare reports of hepatic dysfunction, including hepatic failure, have been reported. Hepatic dysfunction usually occurs in association with hypersensitivity reactions, but isolated cases have been reported without overt signs of hypersensitivity.

Movement disorders such as tics, unsteadiness, ataxia, nystagmus and tremor have also been reported.

Exacerbation of seizures: increase in seizure frequency, mainly myoclonic jerks, has been reported in juvenile myoclonic epilepsy and Dravet syndrome.

CONSIDERATIONS IN WOMEN

Pregnancy: category C.

Breastfeeding: significant amounts of lamotrigine (40%-60%) are excreted in human milk. In breastfed infants, serum concentrations of lamotrigine reached levels at which pharmacological effects may occur.

Interactions with oral hormonal contraception and pregnancy: oral contraceptives are not affected by lamotrigine. However, pregnancy[75-77] and hormonal contraception[78] significantly lower lamotrigine levels (by more than half). Patients may suffer breakthrough seizures, mainly during the first trimester of pregnancy (if lamotrigine levels are not corrected) or toxic effects postpartum (if lamotrigine levels had been adjusted during pregnancy, but not after delivery). Gradual transient increases in lamotrigine levels will occur during the week of no active hormone preparation (pill-free week).

MAIN MECHANISMS OF ACTION

The precise mechanisms by which lamotrigine exerts its antiepileptic action are unknown. The most likely mechanism is inhibition of voltage-gated sodium channels, thereby stabilising neuronal membranes and consequently modulating presynaptic transmitter release of excitatory amino acids (e.g. glutamate and aspartate).

PHARMACOKINETICS

Oral bioavailability: < 100%. Lamotrigine is rapidly and completely absorbed from the gut with no significant first-pass metabolism.

Protein binding: 55%.

Metabolism: hepatic. Uridine diphosphate glucuronosyltransferases (UGT) have been identified as the enzymes responsible for the metabolism of lamotrigine.

Elimination half-life: 29 hours, but this is greatly affected by concomitant medication. Mean half-life is reduced to approximately 14 hours when given with enzyme-inducing drugs and is increased to a mean of approximately 70 hours when co-administered with valproate alone. Valproate is a potent inhibitor of UGT-dependent metabolism of lamotrigine, while enzyme-inducer AEDs are potent inducers of UGT-dependent metabolism of lamotrigine, which is the reason for different schemes of lamotrigine dosage and titration when combined with these AEDS.

Also, the half-life of lamotrigine is generally shorter in children than in adults with a mean value of approximately 7 hours when given with enzyme-inducing drugs and increasing to mean values of 45–50 hours when co-administered with valproate alone.

DRUG INTERACTIONS

The metabolism of lamotrigine is badly affected by concomitant AEDs, which makes its use in polytherapy problematic.

(a). Valproate inhibits lamotrigine metabolism, doubling or tripling its half life,[73] whether given with or without carbamazepine, phenytoin, phenobarbitone or primidone.

(b). Enzyme inducers, such as carbamazepine, phenytoin and phenobarbitone, accelerate its elimination, but lamotrigine itself has no effect on hepatic metabolic processes.[79]

With lamotrigine added to carbamazepine, symptoms of carbamazepine neurotoxicity (headache, diplopia, ataxia) may occur (probably because of pharmacodynamic interactions rather than elevated carbamazepine epoxide levels); this necessitates a reduction in the carbamazepine dose when lamotrigine is introduced.

Oxcarbazepine and levetiracetam do not affect the clearance of lamotrigine

MAIN DISADVANTAGES

(a). High incidence of idiosyncratic adverse reactions, which exceptionally may be fatal.

(b). Slow titration in months.

(c). Significant interactions with other AEDs requiring complex schemes of dosage and titration.

(d). Pregnancy[75-77] and hormonal contraception[78] significantly lower lamotrigine levels (by more than half). This necessitates frequent adjustments of lamotrigine dosage before, during and after pregnancy and hormonal contraception.

(d). Pro-myoclonic effect in syndromes with predominant myoclonic jerks,[80-83] such as juvenile myoclonic epilepsy and Dravet syndrome.

The use of lamotrigine should follow the manufacturer's recommendations regarding titration and include a proper warning to the patient or guardians that immediate withdrawal of the drug is necessary if suspicious rashes appear, unless the rash is clearly not drug-related.

LEVETIRACETAM

Levetiracetam is a single enantiomer (-)-(S)-α-ethyl-2-oxo-1-pyrrolidine acetamide. Levetiracetam, licensed in 1999, is the most promising of all the new AEDs.[84-92] It is chemically unrelated to any of the other current AEDs.

CLINICAL APPLICATIONS

Levetiracetam is probably the major breakthrough in the treatment of epilepsies similar to that of carbamazepine and valproate in the 1960s. It is a highly effective, broad-spectrum, new class of AED with a unique mechanism of action and can be used to treat all focal or generalised, idiopathic or symptomatic epileptic syndromes in all age groups.

Levetiracetam is the first choice AED in polytherapy of focal epilepsies (page 436) and it is the likely candidate to replace valproate in the treatment of JME and IGEs in general (page 317 and 335).

Levetiracetam has a significant proven efficacy for intractable focal seizures with or without secondary generalisation.[93;94] Addition of levetiracetam to standard medication seems to have a positive impact on health-related quality of life.[95]

Its effectiveness in generalised seizures of any type and at any age is promising, because of its profile in experimental and observational studies, and vast postmarketing experience (see treatment of IGE page 335). This includes IGE,[96-98] JME,[99-101] myoclonus[102-105] and photosensitivity.[97;106]

Levetiracetam also appears effective in epileptic encephalopathies, such as Lennox-Gastaut[107] and Landau-Kleffner syndrome.[108]

That levetiracetam is considered as one of drugs most free from adverse reactions[95;109] makes it the most useful of all the new AEDs.[110] Other significant advantages of levetiracetam are:

(a). the starting dose is often therapeutic for all forms of seizures and epilepsies (including the difficult to treat myoclonic seizures)

(b). there are no clinically significant drug–drug interactions. Levetiracetam does not influence other AEDs in a clinically meaningful way and conversely other AEDs do not interfere with the pharmacokinetics of levetiracetam.[111;112] This profile provides a safer and less-complicated therapeutic strategy

(c). it has a wide margin of safety and patient-friendly pharmacokinetics that distinguish it from other currently available AEDs[113]

(d). it does not interfere with liver function (a major problem with most other AEDs that are metabolised in the liver).

DOSAGE AND TITRATION

Adults: start treatment with 1000 mg/day (twice daily dosing), which may be sufficient for seizure control. If needed, levetiracetam can be titrated in steps of 500 mg/week to a maximum of 3000 mg/day. Personally, I recommend starting with 250 mg twice daily and titrate according to the response.

Children: start treatment with 5–10 mg/kg/day, which may be sufficient for seizure control. If needed, levetiracetam can be titrated in steps of 5–10 mg/kg/week to a usual maintenance dose of 20–40 mg/kg/day (a maximum of 60 mg/kg/day has been used) given in two equally divided doses.[85;114-117]

Based on weight, the maintenance dose for children should be 30–40% higher than that for adults. The reason for this is that levetiracetam clearance in children is 30–40% higher than in adults.[118;119] However, it is likely that the increase, compared with adults, is even higher in infants, for whom the data remain insufficient.[120]

The drug is available in tablet form only (250 mg and 500 mg). If a child is unable to swallow tablets, the tablets can be crushed and dissolved in water. The corresponding volume of suspension would then be administered using either a syringe or a 5-mL measuring spoon, often in conjunction with the child's preferred juice or semi-solid food such as yoghurt.

Dosing: twice daily.

Dose adjustment is required for patients with renal dysfunction, but not for patients with liver disease.

Therapeutic range: 6–20 mg/L (35–120 μmol/L).

Therapeutic drug monitoring: not needed. Levetiracetam can be efficacious from the starting dose.

MAIN ADVERSE REACTIONS

Levetiracetam is probably the AED that is most free from adverse reactions. Few major adverse effects were reported in the clinical trials and, overall, their incidence in the levetiracetam groups was little higher than that in the placebo groups.[121]

Common: the most common adverse effects are somnolence, asthenia and dizziness, which are dose-dependent and reversible. Others include headache, infection (common cold, upper respiratory infection which were not preceded by low neutrophil counts that might suggest impaired immunological status), anorexia, pharyngitis and pain. No withdrawal-related adverse events were reported during the cross-titration period.[84;85] Levetiracetam interferes with rapid motor learning in humans due to suppression of excitatory activity in the motor cortex.[122]

Caution should be exercised when administering levetiracetam to individuals who may be prone to psychotic or psychiatric reactions.[87]

In an uncontrolled study, add-on levetiracetam was associated with a paradoxical increase in seizure frequency, particularly in mentally retarded patients and those with difficult-to-treat partial onset seizures treated with high doses of levetiracetam.[123] This may be avoided by using a lower initial dose and a slower dose escalation than that recommended.

CONSIDERATIONS IN WOMEN

Pregnancy: category C. In a small series, three women receiving levetiracetam monotherapy during pregnancy gave birth to normal babies.[18]

Breastfeeding: unknown.

Interaction with hormonal contraception: none.

MAIN MECHANISMS OF ACTION

Levetiracetam has a novel mechanism of action that is distinct from that of other AEDs by targeting a synaptic vesicle protein in presynaptic terminals.[124-126] Its antiepileptic activity does not involve a direct interaction with any of the three main mechanisms of the other AEDs. Thus, levetiracetam does not modulate Na^+ and low voltage-gated (T-type) Ca^{2+} currents, and does not induce any conventional facilitation of the GABAergic system. In contrast, levetiracetam has been observed to exert several atypical electrophysiological actions including a moderate inhibition of high voltage-gated N-type Ca^{2+} currents, reduction of intracellular Ca^{2+} release from the endoplasmic reticulum, as well as suppression of the inhibitory effect of zinc and other negative allosteric modulators of both GABA- and glycine-gated currents.

The apparent absence of any direct interaction with conventional mechanisms involved in the action of other AEDs parallels the discovery of a specific binding site for levetiracetam. Recent experiments have shown that the synaptic vesicle protein 2A (SV2A) is the binding site (Figure 12.21).[127]

Studies in mice lacking SV2A indicate that this protein has a crucial role in the regulation of vesicle function, probably involving a modulation of vesicle fusion. These mice seem normal at birth, but develop unusually severe seizures by 1–2 weeks of age and die within 3 weeks after birth.[127]

Brain membranes and purified synaptic vesicles from mice lacking SV2A did not bind a tritiated derivative of levetiracetam, indicating that SV2A is necessary for levetiracetam binding. Levetiracetam and related derivatives bind to SV2A, but not to the related isoforms, SV2B and SV2C, expressed in fibroblasts, indicating that SV2A is sufficient for levetiracetam binding. In contrast, none of the other AEDs tested revealed any binding to SV2A.[127]

The severe seizures observed in mice lacking SV2A support the interpretation that this protein influences mechanisms of seizure generation or propagation. Furthermore, there is a strong correlation between the binding affinity of a series of levetiracetam derivatives and their anticonvulsant potency in the audiogenic seizure mice model. These results suggest that levetiracetam's interaction with SV2A provides a significant contribution to its antiepileptic activity.

PHARMACOKINETICS

> "The pharmacokinetic profile of levetiracetam closely approximates the ideal characteristics expected of an antiepileptic drug, with good bioavailability, rapid achievement of steady-state concentrations, linear and time-invariant kinetics, minimal protein binding, and minimal metabolism."[113]

"Levetiracetam, comes especially close to fulfilling the desirable pharmacokinetic characteristics for an AED: (1) it has a high oral bioavailability, which is unaffected by food; (2) it is not significantly bound to plasma proteins; (3) it is eliminated partly in unchanged form by the kidneys and partly by hydrolysis to an inactive metabolite, without involvement of oxidative and conjugative enzymes; (4) it has linear kinetics; and (5) it is not vulnerable to important drug interactions, nor does it cause clinically significant alterations in the kinetics of concomitantly administered drugs. Although its half-life is relatively short (6 to 8 hours), its duration of action is longer than anticipated from its pharmacokinetics in plasma, and a twice-daily dosing regimen is adequate to produce the desired response."[112]

Oral bioavailability: 100% and it is unaffected by food. Levetiracetam is rapidly and almost completely absorbed after oral administration with peak plasma concentrations occurring in about 1 hour. The pharmacokinetics are linear and time-invariant, with low intra- and inter-subject variability.

Protein binding: < 10%. Levetiracetam is not appreciably protein-bound nor does it affect the protein binding of other drugs. Its volume of distribution is close to the volume of intracellular and extracellular water.

Metabolism/elimination: the major metabolic pathway of levetiracetam (24% of dose) is an enzymatic hydrolysis of the acetamide group. This is not dependent on the hepatic cytochrome P450 system. Further, levetiracetam does not inhibit or induce hepatic enzymes to produce clinically relevant interactions. Levetiracetam is eliminated from the systemic circulation by renal excretion as unchanged drug, which represents 66% of the administered dose. The mechanism of excretion is glomerular filtration with subsequent partial tubular reabsorption. The metabolites have no known pharmacological activity and are also renally excreted.

Elimination half-life: 6–8 hours. It is shorter in children and longer in the elderly and in subjects with renal impairment.

DRUG INTERACTIONS

Unlike the majority of other AEDs, levetiracetam has no clinically meaningful drug–drug interactions.

Other AEDs: levetiracetam does not influence the plasma concentration of existing AEDs and conversely other AEDs do not influence the pharmacokinetics of levetiracetam. In addition, levetiracetam does not affect the in-vitro glucuronidation of valproate.

Other non-AEDs: levetiracetam has no known interactions with other drugs such as oral contraceptives, warfarin and digoxin. It does not reduce the effectiveness of oral contraceptives.

MAIN DISADVANTAGES

There are some post-marketing reports of increased behavioural abnormalities in children treated with levetiracetam. Though this is not confirmed, one explanation may be fast titration recommended by the manufacturers.

OXCARBAZEPINE

Oxcarbazepine (10,11-dihydro-10-oxo-5H-dibenz[b,f]azepine-5-carboxamide) is a 10-keto derivative of carbamazepine. The antiepileptic activity of oxcarbazepine is primarily exerted through its major metabolite hydroxy-10,11-dihydro-5H-dibenzazepine-5-carboxamide (MHD). Oxcarbazepine was first licensed as an AED in 1990 in Denmark.

CLINICAL APPLICATIONS

Oxcarbazepine is a first class AED for monotherapy, conversion to monotherapy or adjunctive therapy for all types of focal seizures with or without secondarily generalised convulsions in adults and children over the age of 4 years. This has been documented in a series of clinical trials and extensive clinical use from 1980 when it was first licensed in Europe. It is the first AED in 25 years to be approved by the FDA in 2003 for use as monotherapy in children aged 4 years or older with focal epilepsy.

DOSAGE AND TITRATION

Adults: start treatment with 150 mg/day and increase by 150 mg/day every second day until a target dose of 900–1200 mg/day is reached. Others start with 600 mg/day and increase weekly in 600 mg increments until a maintenance dose of between 900–2400 mg/day is reached.

In patients with impaired renal function (creatinine clearance < 30 mL/min), oxcarbazepine should be initiated at one-half the usual starting dose and increased slowly until the desired clinical response is achieved or adverse reactions appear.

Children: start with 10 mg/kg/day in two or three divided doses. The dosage can be increased by 10 mg/kg/day at approximately weekly intervals to a maximum of 30–46 mg/kg/day.

Dosing: twice or three times daily.

Therapeutic range: MHD, 4–12 mg/L (50–140 µmol/L).

Therapeutic drug monitoring: probably not useful.

MAIN ADVERSE REACTIONS

Common: the most common CNS adverse events are headache, dizziness, fatigue, nausea, somnolence, ataxia and diplopia. Most of these are dose–related, they usually occur at the start of therapy and subside during the course of therapy.

Serious: the reported rate of skin rash with oxcarbazepine is around 5% as opposed to 10–15% with carbamazepine. Multiorgan hypersensitivity disorder and Stevens-Johnson syndrome have been reported.

Cross reactivity with carbamazepine is approximately 25% (i.e. of the patients who have skin rash with carbamazepine, 25% will also have skin rash with oxcarbazepine). Therefore, given the availability of other AEDs, oxcarbazepine may not be a good option for patients who developed idiosyncratic reactions with carbamazepine.

Hyponatraemia (serum sodium level < 125 mmol/L) occurs in 3% of patients on oxcarbazepine. This develops gradually during the first few months of treatment. It is usually benign and can be reversed by fluid restriction or a reduction in the dose of oxcarbazepine. Acute water intoxication is rare. Measurement of serum sodium levels are needed for patients with renal disease, those taking medication that may lower serum sodium levels (e.g. diuretics, oral contraceptives or non-steroidal anti-inflammatory drugs) or if clinical symptoms of hyponatraemia develop.

Consumption of large volumes of fluid (e.g. beer) should be discouraged.

Oxcarbazepine is contraindicated in patients with a history of atrioventricular block.

CONSIDERATIONS IN WOMEN

Pregnancy: category C.

Breastfeeding: should be avoided because oxcarbazepine and its active metabolite are secreted in significant amounts in breast milk.

Interaction with hormonal contraception: yes.

MAIN MECHANISMS OF ACTION

Oxcarbazepine exerts its antiepileptic activity primarily via MHD. Like carbamazepine, blockade of voltage-sensitive sodium channels is the main mechanism of action. Others include reduction of the release of excitatory amino acids, probably by inhibiting high voltage-activated calcium currents. An effect on potassium channels might be clinically important.

PHARMACOKINETICS

Oral bioavailability: > 95% and peak concentrations are reached within 4–6 hours. Absorption is unaffected by food.

Protein binding: only 38% of the MHD is bound to serum proteins compared with 67% for the parent compound.

Metabolism: oxcarbazepine is rapidly metabolised in the liver to form the pharmacologically active MHD. This is then conjugated to a glucuronide compound and excreted in the urine as a monohydroxy derivative.

Elimination half-life: 8–10 hours. This is shorter in children and longer in the elderly.

As a neutral lipophilic substance, the active metabolite MHD of oxcarbazepine is able to diffuse rapidly through the various membranes and the blood-brain barrier.

DRUG INTERACTIONS

The oxcarbazepine-MHD complex lowers concentrations of some drugs, such as hormonal contraceptives and lamotrigine, and increases concentrations of others, such as phenytoin. Conversely, strong inducers of the cytochrome P450 enzyme system, such as carbamazepine and phenytoin, lower plasma levels of MHD by 29–40%.

Combination therapy with monoamine oxidase inhibitors should be avoided, because oxcarbazepine has structural similarities with tricyclic antidepressants.

MAIN DISADVANTAGES

(a). Oxcarbazepine is contraindicated in generalised seizures, such as absences or myoclonic jerks in syndromes of IGE.[128] It may not be effective in neonates and children younger than 2 years of age.

(b). One out of four patients have cross sensitivity to idiosyncratic reactions with carbamazepine or other AEDs.

(c) Though probably the first choice AED as monotherapy in focal epilepsies, its use as polytherapy is less satisfactory because of drug–drug interactions.

USEFUL CLINICAL NOTE

Conversion to oxcarbazepine from carbamazepine or phenytoin is complicated by the need for higher

Oxcarbazepine versus carbamazepine

Oxcarbazepine is similar to carbamazepine in its mechanisms of action and antiepileptic efficacy, but is better tolerated and has fewer interactions with other drugs because it does not undergo metabolism to 10,11–epoxide. In contrast to carbamazepine, oxcarbazepine does not induce hepatic drug metabolism and autoinduction is not an issue. Oxcarbazepine has a lower incidence of allergic reactions and is less neurotoxic than carbamazepine; hyponatraemia is more common with oxcarbazepine than carbamazepine.

The profile of oxcarbazepine is more similar to that of the slow-release carbamazepine preparations.

doses of oxcarbazepine initially than needed later as monotherapy.

A carbamazepine dose of 200 mg appears to be equivalent to 300 mg of oxcarbazepine.

On anecdotal evidence, it is possible to change from carbamazepine to oxcarbazepine abruptly, using a dose ratio of 200 mg carbamazepine to 300 mg oxcarbazepine, without the need for titration. A lower ratio of 1:1 or 1:1.25 is commonly better tolerated, especially if the conversion is from slow release preparations of carbamazepine.

Levels of concomitant medication may be affected by the removal of the enzyme-inducing effects of carbamazepine.

PHENOBARBITONE

Phenobarbitone was introduced into clinical practice in 1912[41] and is still a widely used AED, particularly when cost is a problem.[129-132]

It is highly effective in all seizure types except absences.[129-133]

Current main applications: these are neonatal (drug of choice) and febrile seizures (probably first choice if treatment is needed), juvenile myoclonic epilepsy (if absences do not occur) and established convulsive status epilepticus. See also Tables 4.1 and 4.2.

It is useful as adjunctive therapy in small doses at night.

Maintenance dose: adults 50–200 mg nocte (initial 30 mg/day) and children 3–5 mg/kg/day.

Dosing: once daily.

Main adverse reactions: drowsiness, sedation or aggression, depression and impairment of cognition and concentration. Hyperkinesis is a major problem in children.

Pregnancy: category D.

Other available main barbiturate agents: primidone (probably has similar adverse reactions to phenobarbitone and is of no better efficacy) and barbexaclone (of similar effectiveness as phenobarbitone, but less sedative).[134]

Useful clinical note:

(a). Phenobarbitone is unsuitable for children because of age-related serious side effects.

(b). It is erroneous to attempt substitution of phenobarbitone in well-controlled patients unless it is associated with adverse reactions.

(c). Withdrawal should be in very small steps and at long intervals because of the risk of withdrawal seizures.

(d). Always start and titrate slowly with small doses at night (20–30 mg). Avoid high doses (maximum in adults 200 mg).

PHENYTOIN

Phenytoin was introduced into clinical practice in 1938[41] and is probably the most widely used AED.[135] It is highly effective in focal and GTCS.[129-131;133] It is contraindicated in absences and myoclonic jerks, and probably in Lennox-Gastaut syndrome and other childhood epileptic encephalopathies (but may be effective in tonic seizures).

Current main applications: these are neonatal seizures (if phenobarbitone fails), focal and GTCS (none of the other drugs had superior efficacy to phenytoin in recent controlled studies, but drug induced adverse effects are hindering its use) and established convulsive or focal status epilepticus (often considered as the first choice).

Maintenance dose: adults 200–400 mg nocte (initially 50–100 mg/day) and children 5–10 mg/kg/day.

Dosing: once daily.

Main adverse reactions: (a). early non-dose related – anticonvulsant hypersensitivity syndrome that may be fatal (Stevens-Johnson and Lyll's syndrome); (b). dose-related – ataxia, drowsiness, lethargy, sedation and encephalopathy; and (c). chronic use – gingival hyperplasia, hirsutism and dysmorphism.

Other reactions: haematological, neurological (e.g. peripheral neuropathy and cerebellar atrophy) and others, such as systemic lupus erythematosus. Its effect on cognition is probably similar to that of carbamazepine, but much better than that of phenobarbitone.

Pregnancy: category D.

Other available phenytoin-related agents: (a). phosphenytoin for intramuscular and intravenous use, preferred to phenytoin because it does not produce adverse tissue effects;[136-141] and (b). ethotoin and mephenytoin probably offer no advantage over phenytoin.

Useful clinical note:

(a). Phenytoin is a very effective drug in focal and secondarily GTCS, but of little value and often contraindicated in generalised epilepsies.

(b). Acute and long-term adverse reactions hamper its long-term use.

(c). Long-term use of phenytoin is unsuitable for women for aesthetic reasons and because of teratogenic properties.

(d). Therapeutic range is narrow and close to the toxic range requiring frequent monitoring of serum levels. After a certain dose (100–200 mg day), further increases should be small (25 mg) and achieved slowly (every 2–4 weeks).

PREGABALIN

Pregabalin has just (July 2004) been licensed in Europe for the treatment of adults with partial seizures with or without secondarily generalisation and for peripheral neuropathic pain. It has not as yet obtained FDA approval. It is a 3-substituted GABA analogue and is structurally related to gabapentin.

CLINICAL APPLICATIONS

Post-marketing experience is still very limited and it appears that pregabalin is a narrow spectrum AED that exaggerates myoclonus. Therefore pregabalin should be used in rational polytherapy in adults with intractable focal seizures who had failed to respond in other AED combinations as detailed in Chapter 12 (page 433). For these patients, there are insufficient data about withdrawal of concomitant antiepileptic medication, once seizure control with adjunctive pregabalin has been reached, in order to establish monotherapy with pregabalin.

Treatment emergent myoclonic jerks, even in patients with focal seizures,[142;143] may be a warning sign against the use of pregabalin in generalised epilepsies, where myoclonus is often a prominent symptom to treat.

DOSAGE AND TITRATION

Adults: start treatment with 150 mg/day and, based on individual patient response and tolerability, increase to 300 mg/day after an interval of 7 days, and to a maximum dose of 600 mg/day after an additional 7-day interval. The maintenance dose is 150–600/day in either two or three divided doses taken orally.

Dosage adjustments are necessary in patients with renal impairment and probably the elderly.

Therapeutic drug monitoring: probably not needed.

Therapeutic range: not determined.

MAIN ADVERSE REACTIONS

Significant weight gain was noted in 5.6% of pregabalin-treated patients in all trials.

The most commonly (> 10%) reported side effects in placebo-controlled, double-blind studies were somnolence and dizziness. Other commonly (>1% and < 10%) reported side effects were increased appetite, euphoric mood, confusion, decreased libido, irritability, ataxia, attention disturbance, abnormal coordination, memory impairment, tremor, dysarthria, paraesthesia, blurred vision, diplopia, vertigo, dry mouth, constipation, vomiting, flatulence, erectile dysfunction, fatigue, peripheral oedema, feeling drunk, oedema and abnormal gait.

Hypoglycaemic medication may need to be adjusted in diabetic patients who gain weight.

CONSIDERATIONS IN WOMEN

Pregnancy and lactation: pregabalin should not be used during pregnancy unless the benefit outweighs the risk. Effective contraception must be used in women of childbearing potential. Breastfeeding is not recommended during treatment with pregabalin.

Others: Weight gain, which is often significant may be associated with polycystic ovary syndrome.

MAIN MECHANISMS OF ACTION

The precise mechanism of action of pregabalin is still unclear. Though an analogue of GABA, pregabalin is inactive at GABA-A and GABA-B receptors and it has no effect on GABA uptake or degradation. Pregabalin decreases central neuronal excitability by binding to an auxiliary subunit (a_2-delta protein) of a high voltage-gated calcium channel on neurons in the CNS. It reduces the release of certain neurotransmitters including glutamate, noradrenaline and substance P.

PHARMACOKINETICS

Oral bioavailability: > 90%.

Protein binding: does not bind to plasma proteins.

Metabolism: pregabalin is not metabolised in the liver and does not induce hepatic enzymes. It is excreted renally.

Elimination half-life: 6–7 hours.

DRUG INTERACTIONS

Pregabalin does not affect the plasma concentration of other AEDs. In addition, it does not interact with a number of other drug types, including hormonal contraception.

However, pregabalin appears to be additive in the impairment of cognitive and gross motor function when co-administered with oxycodone (an opioid), and potentiates the effect of lorazepam and ethanol.

Patients with galactose intolerance, the Lapp lactase deficiency or glucose-galactose malabsorption should not take pregabalin.

MAIN DISADVANTAGES

As explained on page 438, it is probably too early to make any predictions for the role of pregabalin in the treatment of focal epilepsies. However, the high incidence of weight gain[142] (consider the decline in the use of valproate because of this side effect and its causative relation with polycystic ovary syndrome in women), treatment emergent myoclonic jerks[142;143] and similarities with gabapentin[144] are not promising signs.

SULTHIAME[153-159]

The story of sulthiame's transition from a disgraced to a useful drug is interesting.

Sulthiame is a sulfonamide derivative with carbonic anhydrase inhibiting properties (only one-sixteenth as potent as acetazolamide, which is another sulfonamide drug). It was first introduced as an AED in the 1950s, but its use was abandoned in the 1970s on the assertion that it has little, if any, antiepileptic activity when used alone. Its antiepileptic action was attributed to raised levels of concomitant medication (phenytoin, phenobarbitone and primidone).[153;154] Sulthiame inhibits the metabolism of phenytoin, phenobarbitone and primidone, so these drugs are elevated to 'therapeutic' or 'toxic' levels or rise steeply when sulthiame is introduced.[154] In addition to risks of drug intoxication, sulthiame in polytherapy was adding its own adverse effects, such as hyperventilation, paraesthesias, anorexia, weight loss and renal tubular acidosis. The significant improvement in the disturbed behaviour of mentally handicapped patients was debated and attributed to the sedative effect of sulthiame.[153] Reports that sulthiame, even in monotherapy, was a very effective drug in intractable epilepsies of infancy and childhood,[155] were ignored.

Recently, sulthiame appears to have experienced a revitalisation with reports (including Class 1 evidence) that it is probably the most effective drug in benign childhood epilepsies with regard to its effect in suppressing seizures and EEG abnormalities.[157-159] It may be very useful and should be tried in epileptic encephalopathies,[155] as well as in mainly ECWSS and Landau-Kleffner syndrome. Sulthiame has also re-emerged as an AED in adults.[156]

TIAGABINE

Tiagabine [(R)-N-(4,4-di-(3-methyl-thien-2-yl)-but-3-enyl)nipecotic acid hydrochloride] was first licensed as an AED in 1998.[145]

CLINICAL APPLICATIONS

The antiepileptic efficacy of tiagabine is limited to focal seizures. Its role in clinical epileptology is probably limited to adjunctive medication in severe forms of focal epilepsies that failed to respond to other AED combinations.[146;147] It may also be effective in epileptic spasms of epileptic encephalopathies.

DOSAGE AND TITRATION

Dosage and titration depend on co-medication.

Adults: start treatment with 4–5 mg/day for the first week. Titrate in increments of 4–5 mg/day every week in two divided doses up to 30–45 mg/day (in co-medication with enzyme-inducing drugs) or 15–30 mg/day (with non-enzyme-inducing drugs).

Children: start treatment with 0.1mg/kg/day and titrate in increments of 0.1 mg/kg/day every 1–2 weeks up to 0.5–2 mg/kg/day.

Children eliminate tiagabine more rapidly than adults.

Dosing: twice or preferably three times daily.

Therapeutic range: 50–250 nmol/L (80–450 µg/L).

Therapeutic drug monitoring: not useful.

MAIN ADVERSE REACTIONS

Common: fatigue, headache, dizziness, tremor, cognitive impairment, disturbed concentration, depression and word-finding difficulties.

Severe: none. Concerns that tiagabine like vigabatrin (another GABAergic AED) may cause visual field defects have not been substantiated.[148;149]

Seizure exacerbation: treatment emergent absence status epilepticus has been reported in a significant number of patients. An opinion by a panel of experts that "treatment with tiagabine in recommended doses does not increase the risk of status epilepticus in patients with partial seizures"[150] probably refers to focal status epilepticus and not to the generalised absence status epilepticus where the main risk lies.

CONSIDERATIONS IN WOMEN

Pregnancy: category C.

MAIN MECHANISMS OF ACTION

Tiagabine is an AED specifically designed to increase GABA longevity in the synaptic cleft. It is a potent and selective inhibitor of GABA uptake into neurons and glial cells. This brain GABAergic mediated inhibition of tiagabine explains its antiepileptic effect on focal seizures and also explains its pro-absence effect.

PHARMACOKINETICS

Oral bioavailability: < 96%. High fat meals slow the rate of absorption.

Protein binding: 96%. Salicylic acid and naprofen displace tiagabine.

Metabolism: tiagabine is metabolised by hepatic cytochrome P450 before conjugation to inactive metabolites excreted in the urine and faeces. It is neither an hepatic enzyme inducer nor an inhibitor.

Elimination half-life: 7–9 hours decreasing to 2–3 hours in the presence of hepatic enzyme inducers. The metabolism of tiagabine is reduced in patients with hepatic dysfunction thus prolonging its half-life to 12–16 hours.

DRUG INTERACTIONS

Enzyme-inducing AED (phenytoin, carbamazepine, phenobarbitone) significantly lower the plasma concentrations of tiagabine by a factor of 1.5–3 and shorten its half-life.

Valproate displaces tiagabine from its protein-binding sites.

Tiagabine does not affect other AEDs or hormonal contraception.

MAIN DISADVANTAGES

(a). Narrow spectrum antiepileptic efficacy to focal seizures only.

(b). Tiagabine is a pro-absence drug. Its use is probably prohibited in IGE with absences. The pro-absence effect of tiagabine was expected because it is a GABAergic drug that also increases GABA-B, which is the main activator of absence seizures. This pro-absence effect of tiagabine has been confirmed in animals and humans.[151;152]

TOPIRAMATE

Topiramate is a sulfamate-substituted monosaccharide designated chemically as 2,3:4,5-di-O-isopropylidene-β-D-fructopyranose sulfamate. It was first introduced into clinical practice in 1995.

CLINICAL APPLICATIONS

Topiramate is a highly efficacious new, broad-spectrum AED, but significant adverse effects hinder its clinical use.[160-168] It is the most effective of all the new AEDs in focal seizures. In clinical use, topiramate has been recommended for all types of seizures, focal or generalised, and idiopathic or symptomatic, in adults and children including difficult-to-treat epileptic encephalopathies, such as West and Lennox-Gastaut syndromes.

DOSAGE AND TITRATION

'Start low and go slow' is particularly important in topiramate treatment.

Adults and children over 16 years: start with 25 mg nocte for the first week and then titrate in increments of 25 or 50 mg/day in two equally divided doses at 1 or 2 week intervals. The recommended maintenance dose is 200–400 mg/day. Some authors use a maximum dose of 800 mg/day, but this is rarely tolerated.

Children 6–16 years: start with 25 mg or 1–3 mg/kg/day nocte for the first week. Titrate with increments of 1–3 mg/kg/day in two divided doses at 1 or 2 week intervals to a recommended maintenance dose of 5–9 mg/kg/day in two divided doses.

Children 2–6 years: start with 0.5–1 mg/kg/day nocte for the first week and then titrate as for older children.

Renally impaired patients: half of the usual dose is recommended. Patients with moderate or severe renal impairment may take 10–15 days to reach steady-state plasma concentrations compared with 4–8 days in patients with normal renal function.

Treatment with topiramate should start at a very low dosage and be titrated at a very slow pace. If the patient is unable to tolerate the titration regimen, smaller increments or longer intervals between increments can be used. Maintenance doses are usually reached in 2 months.

Tablets should not be broken.

Therapy should not be withdrawn suddenly because of the risk of aggravating seizures.

Dosing: twice daily.

Therapeutic range: 9–12 mg/L (15–60 μmol/L).

Therapeutic drug monitoring: not useful.

MAIN ADVERSE REACTIONS

Topiramate is an inferior new AED with respect to adverse reactions, which are common, multiple and sometimes severe or potentially fatal.[169;170] Withdrawal rates were low in controlled trials (4.8%), but appear to be much more frequent in non-comparative and post-marketing studies.[160;171] On the positive side, topiramate lacks significant idiosyncratic reactions.

Common: somnolence, anorexia, fatigue and nervousness are common as in other AEDs, but most of the other frequent adverse reactions are of concern.

Abnormal thinking, consisting of mental slowing and word-finding difficulties, has been reported in 31% of patients with titration rates of 100 mg/week.[172;173]

Difficulty with concentration/attention, memory impairment, psychomotor slowing and speech disorders are often very severe even when treatment starts with small doses and titration is slow.

Behavioural and cognitive problems are a limiting factor in some children. Topiramate was reported to have a negative impact on cognition with impairment of performance on tests requiring verbal processing, which was consistent with subjective complaints of patients.[174;175]

Weight loss (10% of patients) may be considered as beneficial by some women, but is sometimes relentless and extremely problematic.[160] A dietary supplement or increased food intake may be considered if the patient is losing weight or has inadequate weight gain while receiving topiramate.

Treatment emergent paraesthesia and abdominal pains may be confused with other systemic disorders.

Metabolic acidosis: hyperchloraemic, non-anion gap, metabolic acidosis (i.e. decreased serum bicarbonate below the normal reference range in the absence of respiratory alkalosis) is associated with use of topiramate. The incidence of persistent treatment-emergent decreases in serum bicarbonate is high and rises significantly with increasing topiramate dosages. Generally, the decrease in bicarbonate occurs early, though it can occur at any time during treatment.

Markedly abnormal low serum bicarbonate (i.e. an absolute value of < 17 mEq/L and > 5 mEq/L decrease from pretreatment levels) occurred in 11% of children receiving topiramate 6 mg/kg/day, and 3% of adults receiving 400 mg/day. In placebo-controlled trials of migraine prophylaxis in adults, markedly abnormally low serum bicarbonate levels occurred in 11% of those receiving 200 mg/day, 9% on 100 mg/day, 2% on 50 mg/day, and < 1% with placebo.

Diseases or therapies that predispose to acidosis, such as renal disease, severe respiratory disorders, status epilepticus, diarrhoea, surgery, ketogenic diet, or certain drugs (e.g. zonisamide) may be additive to the bicarbonate-lowering effects of topiramate.

Manifestations of acute or chronic metabolic acidosis may include hyperventilation, non-specific symptoms, such as fatigue and anorexia, or more severe sequelae including cardiac arrhythmias or stupor.

Depending on the underlying conditions, appropriate evaluation including serum bicarbonate levels is recommended with topiramate therapy.

Chronic, untreated metabolic acidosis may increase the risk of nephrolithiasis or nephrocalcinosis, and may also result in osteomalacia (rickets in paediatric patients) and/or osteoporosis with an increased risk of fractures. Chronic metabolic acidosis in paediatric patients may also reduce growth rates. A reduction in growth rate may eventually decrease the maximal height achieved. The effect of topiramate on growth and bone-related sequelae is unknown and has not been systematically investigated.

Nephrolithiasis: around 1.5% of adults and 0.6% children in clinical trials of topiramate developed renal stones. Risk factors for nephrolithiasis include prior stone formation, a family history of nephrolithiasis and hypercalciuria. None of these risk factors can reliably predict stone formation during topiramate treatment. In addition, patients taking other medication associated with nephrolithiasis, such as zonisamide, may be at increased risk.

Topiramate, like other carbonic anhydrase inhibitors, reduces urinary citrate excretion and increases urinary pH.

Patients receiving topiramate should increase their fluid intake as it may reduce the risk of: (1) developing renal stones; and (2) heat-related adverse events during exercise and exposure to particularly warm environments.

Acute myopia with secondary angle-closure glaucoma is a syndrome reported in adults and children treated with topiramate.[176] Symptoms typically occur within 1 month of the start of treatment and include acute onset of decreased visual acuity and/or ocular pain. Ophthalmological findings include bilateral myopia, anterior chamber shallowing, ocular hyperaemia and increased intra-ocular pressure with or without mydriasis. There may be supraciliary effusion resulting in anterior displacement of the lens and iris. Discontinuation of topiramate should be as rapid as is clinically feasible. Immediate specialist advice should be sought. If left untreated, elevated intra-ocular pressure can lead to serious sequelae including permanent visual loss.

Oligohidrosis and hyperthermia: hypohidrosis or more usually anhidrosis associated with hyperthermia, infrequently resulting in hospitalisation, has been reported in association with topiramate. Symptoms include decreased or absence of sweating, elevation of body temperature, red face and tiredness, which are worse on effort.

The majority of the reports have been in children and have occurred after exposure to hot environmental conditions. Patients, especially children, treated with topiramate should be monitored closely for evidence of such symptoms especially in hot weather.

Caution should be used when topiramate is prescribed with other drugs that predispose patients to heat-related disorders, such as zonisamide (such a combination should probably be avoided), other carbonic anhydrase inhibitors and anticholinergic drugs.

CONSIDERATIONS IN WOMEN

Pregnancy: category C. There is no reliable information on human teratogenicity, but in animals even subtoxic doses of topiramate are teratogenic.[16]

Breastfeeding: breastfeeding is not recommended because of extensive secretion of topiramate into human milk.

Interactions with hormonal contraception: there is a dose-dependent decrease in ethinyl estradiol exposure with topiramate doses between 200–800 mg/day, which may result in decreased efficacy of hormonal contraception and increased breakthrough bleeding.

MAIN MECHANISMS OF ACTION

The antiepileptic effect of topiramate is probably due to multimodal mechanisms of action. These include blockage of voltage-dependent sodium channels, augmentation of the inhibitory activity of GABA at some subtypes of the GABA-A receptor, antagonism with the AMPA/kainate subtype of the glutamate receptor, and inhibition of the carbonic anhydrase enzyme, particularly isozymes II and IV.

PHARMACOKINETICS

Oral bioavailability: > 80%.

Protein binding: 15–41% over the blood concentration range of 0.5–250 μg/mL. The fraction bound decreases as blood concentration increases.

Metabolism: topiramate is not extensively metabolised and is primarily eliminated unchanged in the urine (approximately 70% of an administered dose). Six metabolites have been identified in humans, none of which constitutes more than 5% of an administered dose. The metabolites are formed via hydroxylation, hydrolysis and glucuronidation. There is evidence of renal tubular reabsorption of topiramate.

Elimination half-life: 21 hours.

DRUG INTERACTIONS

The following antiepileptic drug–drug interactions are of clinical significance with topiramate co-medication.

In co-medication, phenytoin plasma levels may increase by 25% and topiramate decrease by 48%. Carbamazepine may decrease topiramate plasma by nearly half.

There is probably no interaction with lamotrigine and levetiracetam, and interactions with valproate are minimal.

Concomitant use with other carbonic anhydrase inhibitors, such as zonisamide, should probably be avoided.

See also interactions with hormonal contraception.

MAIN DISADVANTAGES

Despite high efficacy, the current and future role of topiramate as a major AED is questionable, because of its very poor profile in terms of multiple and severe adverse reactions. The most important of these reactions are those that occur in children, some of which (metabolic acidosis) may have predictable detrimental growth and bone-related sequelae in long-term use.

Its use may be limited to severe epilepsies intractable to other, better tolerated, AEDs.

VALPROATE*

The introduction of valproate as an AED in early the 1960s revolutionised the treatment of generalised epilepsies.[177-179] Valproic acid (2-propyl pentanoic acid, 2-propyl valeric acid) is a short-chain branched fatty acid. Prior to the serendipitous discovery of its antiepileptic activity in 1963, valproic acid was used as an organic solvent.

*Valproate is a general term to include all available forms of valproic acid, such as sodium valproate, magnesium valproate and sodium divalproex.

CLINICAL APPLICATIONS

Valproate is one of the most effective broad-spectrum AEDs for all types of seizures and epilepsies. It has superior efficacy in all types of generalised seizures (idiopathic and symptomatic), all syndromes of IGE and photosensitive epilepsy than any other drug so far, with the probable exception of levetiracetam. The efficacy of valproate has been well documented in long-term and worldwide clinical practice and a few controlled studies.

However, valproate is far inferior to carbamazepine and other newer AEDs in the treatment of focal epilepsies.

Unlike many other AEDs, valproate appears to have a very low potential to aggravate seizures.[180] When seizure aggravation occurs with valproate, it is in a specific clinical context, such as overdose, encephalopathy, or hepatic or metabolic disorders.[180]

DOSAGE AND TITRATION

Adults: start with 200 mg/day in two equally divided doses for 3 days. Titrate in increments of 200 mg/day every 3 days to a maintenance dose of usually 1000–1500 mg/day (maximum 3000 mg/day) given in two equally divided doses. Higher initial dosage and faster titration rates are usually well tolerated.

Children: start with 10/mg/kg/day. Titrate in increments of 10 mg/kg/day every 3 days. The typical maintenance dose in childhood is 20–30 mg/kg/day in two equally divided doses.

Combined therapy: it may be necessary to increase the dose by 30–50% when used in combination with enzyme-inducing AEDs, such as phenytoin, phenobarbitone and carbamazepine. On withdrawal of these AEDs, it may be possible to reduce the dose of valproate.

Dosing: twice or three times daily, and once daily for slow release formulations.

Therapeutic range: 50–100 mg/L (300–700 μmol/L).

Therapeutic drug monitoring: often not useful, because of poor correlation between valproate dose and plasma levels. However, because of significant drug interactions, monitoring of valproate and AEDs given concomitantly may be helpful when enzyme-inducing drugs are added or withdrawn.

MAIN ADVERSE REACTIONS

Valproate is associated with serious adverse reactions particularly in children and women. Acute liver necrosis and acute pancreatitis, which may be fatal, are rare and more likely to occur in children receiving polypharmacy.

An estimated 1–2% risk of neural tube defects, predominantly spina bifida aperta, in babies of women on valproate is well established,[181;182] and the overall risk of major teratogenic effects with valproate is 2–3 times higher than the background prevalence of major non-syndromic congenital anomalies. This together with polycystic ovary syndrome[183] and other endocrine side effects, makes the use of valproate in some women undesirable.[184]

CNS-related adverse reactions: in contrast with other old AEDs, valproate is not usually associated with drowsiness and fatigability or significant dose-related effects on cognition or behaviour. Valproate encephalopathy is exceptional.

Tremor is the more troublesome CNS adverse effect of valproate. There is great individual susceptibility to the development of tremor, which is usually mild, but may become very intense, socially embarrassing and disabling. It is reversible and declines when the dose is lowered.

Systemic: the most serious are fatal hepatotoxicity and acute haemorrhagic pancreatitis.

Hepatic failure resulting in fatalities is primarily age-dependent and occurs mainly in children receiving polypharmacy and with organic brain disease. The risk is 1/600 before the age of 3 years. The incidence of fatal hepatotoxicity decreases considerably in progressively older patient groups (range 1/8000–1/10,000 between 3 and 20 years of age) and in monotherapy with valproate. Hepatic failure has usually occurred during the first 6 months of treatment. The diagnosis depends on clinical criteria with non-specific symptoms, such as malaise, weakness, lethargy, facial oedema, anorexia, vomiting and loss of seizure control. Liver function tests should be performed prior to therapy and at frequent intervals thereafter, especially during the first 6 months. However, this may not be helpful because:

(a). benign elevation of liver enzymes is common during valproate treatment

(b). severe hepatotoxicity is not preceded by progressive elevation of liver enzymes.

Raised liver enzymes are common during treatment with valproate, particularly if used in conjunction with other AEDs. These are usually transient or respond to dose reduction. Patients with such biochemical abnormalities should be reassessed clinically and liver function tests should be performed more frequently. An abnormally low prothrombin level, particularly in association with other relevant abnormalities, requires withdrawal of valproate. Any concomitant use of salicylates should be stopped, since they employ the same metabolic pathway.

Acute haemorrhagic pancreatitis with markedly increased amylase and lipase levels is another rare, but serious, adverse effect of valproate treatment. It develops within the first 3 months of treatment, is more prevalent in children and with polytherapy.

Hyperammonaemic encephalopathy, which is sometimes fatal, has been reported following initiation of valproate therapy in patients with urea cycle disorders. When urea cycle enzymatic deficiency is suspected, metabolic investigations should be performed prior to treatment with valproate.

Thrombocytopenia and other haematological abnormalities:[185] it is recommended that platelet counts and coagulation tests are performed before initiating therapy and at periodic intervals, because of reports of thrombocytopenia, inhibition of the secondary phase of platelet aggregation and abnormal coagulation parameters. Evidence of haemorrhage, bruising or a disorder of haemostasis/coagulation is an indication for reduction or withdrawal of valproate.

Weight gain occurs in 20% of patients and is sometimes marked; women are more vulnerable. This is usually reversible if valproate is withdrawn early.

Hair loss and changes in hair texture or colour are relatively rare, usually occur in the early months of valproate treatment and may resolve spontaneously despite continuation of the drug.

Other adverse effects concern the gastrointestinal system (e.g. anorexia, constipation, dry mouth, stomatitis) and urogenital system (e.g. urinary incontinence, vaginitis, dysmenorrhoea, amenorrhoea, urinary frequency).

CONSIDERATIONS IN WOMEN

Valproate treatment in women raises many issues, see Table 4.3, page 64.

Pregnancy: category D. Valproate crosses the placenta and causes a spectrum of congenital anomalies, such as neural tube defects, craniofacial malformations and skeletal defects. The incidence of these anomalies is much higher when valproate is given as co-medication with other AEDs.

Interaction with hormonal contraception: none.

Other issues: see endocrine abnormalities.

MAIN MECHANISMS OF ACTION[178]

The main mechanism of action is unknown and a combination of several mechanisms may be responsible:

a. Reduction of sustained, repetitive, high frequency firing by inhibiting voltage-sensitive sodium channels, activating calcium-dependent potassium conductance and possibly by direct action on other ion channels.

b Valproate has a GABAergic effect through elevation of brain GABA by various mechanisms, such as inhibiting GABA-transaminase, enhancing GABA synthesising enzymes, increasing GABA release and inhibiting GABA uptake. However, this

GABAergic action is observed only at high valproate levels and may explain its efficacy in other, but not absence, seizures. GABAergic drugs have a pro-absence action because they potentiate absences. Therefore, the most likely explanation for the effect of valproate on absence seizures is that this drug, like ethosuximide, reduces a low threshold (T-type) calcium-channel current,[186] but this effect has not been supported by other studies.[187]

PHARMACOKINETICS

Oral bioavailability: almost complete. Absorption of valproate varies according to the formulation used. Absorption is rapid and peak levels are reached within 2 hours after oral administration of syrup or uncoated tablets. This is longer (3–8 hours) with enteric-coated tablets.

Protein binding: valproate is highly protein bound (about 90%). However, if the plasma level of valproic acid rises above 120 mg/L or if the serum albumin concentration is lowered, the binding sites may become saturated, causing the amount of free drug to rise rapidly, out of proportion to any increase in dosage. Valproate may displace phenobarbitone or phenytoin from plasma protein binding sites.

Metabolism: hepatic. Valproate has a complex metabolism. It is rapidly and nearly totally eliminated by hepatic metabolism as numerous metabolites that contribute to its efficacy and toxicity. The major elimination pathway is via glucuronidation (40–60%). The remainder is largely metabolised via oxidation pathways, beta-oxidation accounting for 30–40% and ω-oxidation, which is cytochrome P450 dependent. Only 1–3% of the ingested dose is excreted unchanged in the urine. Two metabolites of valproate, 2-ene-valproic acid and 4-ene-valproic acid, are among the most pharmacologically active and have a similar potency to the parent drug. They are both produced by the action of cytochrome P450 enzymes induced by other AEDs. They are eliminated primarily in the urine.

Elimination half-life: this is variable, but generally appears to be 8–12 hours (range 4–16 hours). It is shorter in patients receiving enzyme-modifying AEDs or in long-term valproate treatment of children and adults. Many antipsychotic and antidepressants drugs result in competitive metabolism or enzyme inhibition when given as co-medication with valproate.

DRUG INTERACTIONS

There are numerous drug interactions with valproate because:

a. its metabolism is sensitive to enzymatic induction
b. it inhibits the metabolism of other drugs
c. it has a high affinity for serum proteins; it may be displaced or displace other drugs.

Effect of other AEDs on valproate: enzyme inducers particularly those that elevate levels of UGTs, such as phenobarbitone, phenytoin and carbamazepine, may increase the clearance of valproate thus reducing plasma valproate levels by 30–50%.

The addition of ethosuximide may reduce the serum concentration of valproate.

Effects of valproate on other AEDs: valproate does not interact with most of the new AEDs. A notable exception is lamotrigine. Valproate is a potent inhibitor of UGT-dependent metabolism of lamotrigine, and doubles[188] or triples[73] its plasma half-life.

The addition of valproate to ethosuximide or phenobarbitone may double the serum concentration of these AEDs with concomitant toxicity.

There is evidence of severe CNS depression, with or without significant elevations of barbiturate or valproate serum concentrations. All patients receiving concomitant barbiturate therapy should be closely monitored for neurological toxicity. Serum barbiturate concentrations should be measured, if possible, and the barbiturate dosage decreased, if appropriate.

Serum levels of carbamazepine decrease to around 17%, while those of carbamazepine-10,11-epoxide increase by 45% on co-administration with valproate.

Valproate displaces phenytoin from its plasma albumin binding sites and inhibits its hepatic metabolism. Valproate significantly increases the free fraction of phenytoin and reduces total plasma concentrations.

Valproate does not interact with hormonal contraception.

MAIN DISADVANTAGES

The superior efficacy of valproate in generalised seizures is hindered by serious acute and chronic adverse reactions. It is particularly unsuitable for:

(a). women, because of hormonal changes, weight gain and teratogenicity; it is virtually impossible to prescribe valproate to young women today (see Table 4.3, page 64).

(b). young children, particularly those under the age of 2 years, who are at a considerably increased risk of developing fatal hepatotoxicity especially those on multiple anticonvulsants or with congenital metabolic disorders, mental retardation or organic brain disease.

Valproate is the superior AED for generalised epilepsies, but its use in focal epilepsies is of very limited value. In my opinion, valproate is needed in only exceptional cases and only as adjunctive treatment in patients with focal and secondarily

GTCS because:

a. the doses of valproate required to be effective are much higher in focal than generalised epilepsies
b. side effects, particularly in some women, make its use undesirable
c. there are now other more effective and safer drugs for focal seizures.

VIGABATRIN

Vigabatrin (gamma-vilyl-GABA; 4-amino-hex-5-enoic acid) was a result of a rational approach to design compounds that enhance the effect of the inhibitory neurotransmitter GABA. It produces dose-dependent increases in whole-brain levels of GABA.[189]

CLINICAL APPLICATIONS

The use of vigabatrin as an AED is, in practice, limited to infantile (epileptic) spasms for which it is the initial treatment of choice.

Exceptionally vigabatrin may be used cautiously in the treatment of patients with intractable focal seizures that have failed to respond to all other appropriate AED combinations and surgical evaluation.

DOSAGE AND TITRATION

Adults: start with 500 mg/day and titrate in increments of 500 mg/day every week. Typical adult maintenance dose is 1000–3000 mg/day given in two equally divided doses.

Because the excretion is mainly renal, the dose should be reduced in patients with renal insufficiency and creatinine clearance below 60 mL/L.

Children with infantile spasms: start with 50 mg/kg/day and adjust according to the response over 7days up to 150–200 mg/kg/day.

Dosing: despite its short half-life (5–7 hours), vigabatrin may be given once or twice daily, because inhibition of GABA-transaminase (GABA-T) results in a relatively long duration of action, and GABA levels in the CSF can remain elevated for up to 120 hours after a single oral dose.

Therapeutic range: 6–278 μmol/L, which is irrelevant in clinical practice.

Therapeutic drug monitoring: totally unnecessary.

MAIN ADVERSE REACTIONS

Visual field defects are the main concern.[198] Other adverse reactions include sedation, dizziness, headache, ataxia, paraesthesia, memory, cognitive and behavioural disturbances, weight gain and tremor. There is no evidence of idiosyncratic adverse reactions.

Visual field defects: there is a high prevalence of visual field defects occurring in around one-third of patients (adults and children)[199] treated with vigabatrin. Vigabatrin also produces retinal electrophysiological changes in nearly all patients.[148;198;200]

Visual field loss resulting from vigabatrin is not usually reversible. However, visual acuity, colour vision and the loss of amplitude on the electroretinogram may be reversible in patients with minimal or no field loss. There is some evidence that visual field defects remain stable

Lessons to be learned from vigabatrin

Vigabatrin was used as an adjunctive medication in the treatment of focal epilepsies from 1989,[190] when it was first licensed in Europe, until 1997 when a case series report of vigabatrin-emergent irreversible visual field defects was published as a letter to the Editor of the *British Medical Journal*.[191] Prior to this clinical observation (class 4 in the ratings of the so-called 'therapeutics articles'[8;9;192-194] of evidence-based medicine), numerous RCTs (most of class 1 and 2 in the ratings of the so-called 'therapeutics articles'[8;9;192;193] of evidence-based medicine) were all consistent in that vigabatrin was a "relatively safe drug with a relatively benign adverse-effect profile"[190;195;196] and "less effective but better tolerated than carbamazepine".[197]

Concern over neuropathological findings of microvacuolisation of white matter in animals caused trials of vigabatrin to be halted in 1983, but trials were resumed when a lack of evidence (including visual evoked responses) of toxicity in humans was found.

The finding that vigabatrin-emergent irreversible peripheral visual field defects occur in 40% of patients has ended the clinical use of vigabatrin in epilepsies other than infantile spasms. Meanwhile, more than 175,000 patients have been treated with vigabatrin.

Another significant clinical problem with vigabatrin, which also applies to tiagabine, is that these AEDs are pro-absence agents, and are used to induce absences and absence status epilepticus. This alone would prohibit the use of vigabatrin and tiagabine in IGEs with absences. The pro-absence effect of vigabatrin should be expected because it is a GABAergic drug that also increases GABA-B, which is the main activator of absence seizures. Physicians were not appropriately informed of this contraindication and I quote the formal position related to the pro-absence effect of tiagabine:

"*Once again, these suggestions are based on common knowledge, rather than on controlled trial data. We had a great deal of difficulty handling adverse events in an evidence-based fashion. Of course, most adverse-event data of this type derives from case reports rather than randomised controlled trials. We did indicate that tiagabine was associated with spike-wave stupor as an adverse effect. Going beyond the statement would have been going beyond the available evidence.*"[194]

with continuous treatment. It is, therefore, feasible to continue treatment with vigabatrin in these cases, provided visual field monitoring is performed regularly.

In one study involving 24 children treated with vigabatrin, visual field constriction or abnormal ocular electrophysiological studies were seen in over 50% of cases.[199]

The mechanism of vigabatrin-induced visual field defects are probably due to reversible oedema of the myelin in the optic nerves, retinal cone system dysfunction or both.

MAIN MECHANISMS OF ACTION

The mechanism of vigabatrin's antiepileptic action is by selective and irreversible inhibition of GABA-T, thus preventing the breakdown of GABA. Vigabatrin produces dose-dependent increases in GABA concentrations in the CSF, and decreases in GABA-T activity. Raised brain GABA levels inhibit the propagation of abnormal hypersynchronous seizure discharges.

Vigabatrin may also cause a decrease in excitation-related amino acids.

PHARMACOKINETICS

Oral bioavailability: 80–100%.

Protein binding: none.

Metabolism: it is not metabolised and 70% is excreted unchanged in the urine. It is eliminated by the kidneys by glomerular filtration.

Elimination half-life: 5–8 hours (not clinically important).

DRUG INTERACTIONS

There are no drug interactions of any clinical significance except lowering the concentration of phenytoin.

CONSIDERATIONS IN WOMEN

Pregnancy: category C.

Breastfeeding: only small amounts of the drug are excreted in breast milk.

Interactions with hormonal contraception: none.

MAIN DISADVANTAGES

Visual field defects have virtually eliminated vigabatrin from common clinical practice except for infantile spasms.

Aggravation of seizures: vigabatrin is a pro-absence agent which aggravates absence seizures and provokes absence status epilepticus.[201] This alone would prohibit use of vigabatrin in IGEs with absences. The pro-absence effect of vigabatrin should be expected because it is a GABAergic drug that also increases GABA-B, which is the main activator of absence seizures.

Vigabatrin, in addition to its aggravation effect on typical absence seizures, may also exaggerate atypical absences (such as those occurring in Lennox-Gastaut syndrome) and myoclonic seizures (such as those occurring in progressive or non-progressive myoclonic epilepsies).

USEFUL CLINICAL NOTE

Visual field defects may not be clinically detectable. Therefore, patients should be monitored with perimetry prior to and every 6 months during vigabatrin treatment. Electrophysiological testing is considered to be more accurate than perimetry for the direct vigabatrin effect on the outer retina.[202] The manufacturers of vigabatrin provide a procedure for testing children under 9 years of age for visual field defects.

ZONISAMIDE

Zonisamide is a synthetic 1,2-benzisoxazole derivative (1,2-benzisoxazole-3-methanesulfonamide). It is chemically classified as a sulfonamide with a structural similarity to serotonin. It was first introduced as an AED in Japan 1989.[203;204]

Efficacy, dose and mean plasma levels were similar in multicentre Japanese and Caucasian studies.[203;205]

A recent supplement in *Seizure* (December 2004) details "International experiences and perspectives on zonisamide".[204]

CLINICAL APPLICATIONS

Zonisamide appears to be an effective broad-spectrum AED[86;203;205] with extensive clinical use, mainly in Japan.[204] It is efficacious in focal seizures with or without GTCS, primarily and secondarily generalised seizures[86;203;206] including epileptic spasms of West syndrome,[207] other epileptic encephalopathies such as Ohtahara syndrome,[208] and progressive and probably other myoclonic epilepsies such as Unverricht-Lundborg syndrome.

DOSAGE AND TITRATION

'Start low and go slow' is a important part of zonisamide treatment.[204] Significant adjustments are needed in co-medication with hepatic-enzyme inducers.

Adults: start with no more than 100 mg/day for the first week and titrate in increments of 100 mg/day every 1–3 weeks. Usual adult maintenance dose is 400–600 mg/day given in two equally divided doses. Some patients respond well to a smaller maintenance dose of 200 mg/day and some authors recommend one single dose before sleep.

Marked renal impairment (creatinine clearance < 20 mL/min) requires slower dose escalation and lower maintenance doses.

Children: start with 1–2/mg/kg/day for the first week and titrate in increments of 1–2 mg/kg/day every 2 weeks. Usual childhood maintenance dose is 4–8 mg/kg/day (maximum 12 mg/kg/day) in two equally divided doses.

Therapeutic range: 15–40 mg/L (45–180 μmol/L).

Therapeutic drug monitoring: useful, though there is insufficient evidence to support a clear relation between the plasma concentration of zonisamide and the clinical response.[205] Zonisamide monitoring may be needed in order to adjust the dosage in co-medication with phenytoin, phenobarbitone or carbamazepine.

MAIN ADVERSE REACTIONS

Zonisamide causes many adverse reactions.

Common: sedation, somnolence, fatigue, dizziness, agitation, irritability, anorexia, weight loss, nausea, diarrhoea, dyspepsia, dry mouth, slowing of mental activity, depression, ataxia, visual hallucinations, photosensitivity, resting and postural hand tremors.

Serious: some of the adverse reactions are similar to those of topiramate. These are:

(a). cognitive impairment including word-finding difficulty; this is worse in children with plasma concentrations > 140 μmol/L

(b). weight loss and anorexia that may become very severe

(c). nephrolithiasis in 4% of patients on prolonged zonisamide therapy

(d). oligohidrosis and anhidrosis often accompanied by hyperthermia, especially in children and hot environments.

Additional severe adverse reactions are those seen with the sulfonamides, such as rash, Stevens-Johnson syndrome and toxic epidermal necrolysis. The incidence of rash requiring discontinuation of therapy has been approximately 2% in clinical trials.

Zonisamide is contraindicated in patients who have demonstrated hypersensitivity to sulfonamides or zonisamide.[209;210]

Depression and psychosis may be common, particularly in children. In one study, 14 of 74 patients experienced psychotic episodes within a few years of commencement of zonisamide.[211]

Seizure exacerbation: treatment emergent status epilepticus has been reported in 1.1% of treated patients, compared to 0 in placebo-treated individuals.[8;9]

CONSIDERATIONS IN WOMEN

Pregnancy: category C.

Breastfeeding: the transfer rate of zonisamide through the breast milk is high at about 50%.

Interaction with oral hormonal contraception: none.

MAIN MECHANISMS OF ACTION

The antiepileptic mechanism of zonisamide is probably multimodal. Zonisamide blocks the sustained repetitive firing of voltage-sensitive sodium channels and reduces voltage-dependent T-type calcium current without affecting L-type calcium current. It has mild carbonic anhydrase activity and inhibits excitatory glutamatergic transmission. It exhibits free radical scavenging properties.

PHARMACOKINETICS

Bioavailability: 100%.

Protein binding: 40–60%.

Metabolism and route of elimination: zonisamide is metabolised in the liver and eliminated by the kidneys. It undergoes extensive hepatic metabolism to a number of metabolites by cytochrome P450 (CYP 3A4). Its metabolism is markedly increased by enzyme-inducing drugs. It does not induce hepatic enzymes. Nearly half of zonisamide is excreted unchanged in the urine.

Half-life elimination: 63 hours decreasing to 27–38 hours in the presence of hepatic enzyme inducers.

INTERACTION WITH OTHER DRUGS

Serum concentrations of zonisamide are altered by drugs that either induce or inhibit CYP3A4 . Phenytoin, phenobarbitone and carbamazepine increase zonisamide plasma clearance and reduce its half-life to 27–38 hours. Valproate also reduces its half life to 46 hours.

Zonisamide does not appear to affect phenytoin, but significantly increases the plasma concentration of carbamazepine-epoxide when added to carbamazepine.

Concomitant administration of carbonic anhydrase inhibitors, such as acetazolamide or topiramate, is probably ill advised because of the increased potential for renal stone and metabolic acidosis.

MAIN DISADVANTAGES

Zonisamide has significant adverse reactions, some of which may be severe such as cognitive, psychotic episodes, anhidrosis and hyperthermia, nephrolithiasis and Stevens-Johnson syndrome. It also has many interactions with other AEDs in polytherapy.

REFERENCES

1. Gram L. Acetazolamide,benzodiazepines and lamotrigine. In Duncan JS, Panayiotopoulos CP, eds. *Typical absences and related epileptic syndromes*, pp 368-75. London: Churchill Europe Communications, 1995.
2. Neufeld MY. Acetazolamide. In Shorvon S, Perucca E, Fish D, Dodson E, eds. *The treatment of epilepsy (2nd edition)*, pp 334-44. Oxford: Blackwell Publishing, 2004.
3. Panayiotopoulos CP. Treatment of typical absence seizures and related epileptic syndromes. *Paediatr Drugs* 2001;**3**:379-403.
4. Resor SR, Jr,Resor LD. Chronic acetazolamide monotherapy in the treatment of juvenile myoclonic epilepsy. *Neurology* 1990;**40**:1677-81.
5. Kochen S, Giagante B, Oddo S. Spike-and-wave complexes and seizure exacerbation caused by carbamazepine. *Eur J Neurol.* 2002;**9**:41-7.
6. Vajda FJ, O'Brien TJ, Hitchcock A, Graham J, Lander C. The Australian registry of anti-epileptic drugs in pregnancy: experience after 30 months. *J Clin Neurosci.* 2003;**10**:543-9.
7. Morrow JI, Russell AJC, Irwin B, Guthrie E, Morrison P, Parsons L, Robertson I, Craig J. The safety of antiepileptic drugs in pregancy: results of the UK epilepsy and pregnancy register. *Epilepsia* 2004;**45 (Suppl.3)**: 57.
8. French JA, Kanner AM, Bautista J, Abou-Khalil B, Browne T, Harden CL *et al.* Efficacy and tolerability of the new antiepileptic drugs II: treatment of refractory epilepsy: report of the Therapeutics and Technology Assessment Subcommittee and Quality Standards Subcommittee of the American Academy of Neurology and the American Epilepsy Society. *Neurology* 2004;**62**:1261-73.
9. French JA, Kanner AM, Bautista J, Abou-Khalil B, Browne T, Harden CL *et al.* Efficacy and Tolerability of the New Antiepileptic Drugs, II: Treatment of Refractory Epilepsy: Report of the TTA and QSS Subcommittees of the American Academy of Neurology and the American Epilepsy Society. *Epilepsia* 2004;**45**:410-23.
10. Cunnington MC. The international lamotrigine pregnancy registry update for the epilepsy foundation. *Epilepsia* 2004;**45**:1468.
11. Holmes LB, Wyszynski DF, Lieberman E. The AED (Antiepileptic Drug) Pregnancy Registry: A 6-Year Experience. *Arch Neurol.* 2004;**61**:673-8.
12. Wyszynski DF, Holmes LB. The AED (antiepileptic drug) pregnancy registry: a six year experience. *Epilepsia* 2004;**45 (Suppl.3)**: 56.
13. Montouris G. Gabapentin exposure in human pregnancy: results from the Gabapentin Pregnancy Registry. *Epilepsy Behav.* 2003;**4**:310-7.
14. Sabers A, Dam M, Rogvi-Hansen B, Boas J, Sidenius P, Laue FM *et al.* Epilepsy and pregnancy: lamotrigine as main drug used. *Acta Neurol Scand.* 2004;**109**:9-13.
15. Tomson T, Perucca E, Battino D. Navigating toward fetal and maternal health: the challenge of treating epilepsy in pregnancy. *Epilepsia* 2004;**45**:1171-5.
16. Palmieri C, Canger R. Teratogenic potential of the newer antiepileptic drugs: what is known and how should this influence prescribing? *CNS Drugs* 2002;**16**:755-64.
17. Tennis P, Eldridge RR. Preliminary results on pregnancy outcomes in women using lamotrigine. *Epilepsia* 2002;**43**:1161-7.
18. Long L. Levetiracetam monotherapy during pregnancy: a case series. *Epilepsy Behav.* 2003;**4**:447-8.
19. Patsalos PN, Froscher W, Pisani F, van Rijn CM. The importance of drug interactions in epilepsy therapy. *Epilepsia* 2002;**43**:365-85.
20. Patsalos PN, Perucca E. Clinically important drug interactions in epilepsy: interactions between antiepileptic drugs and other drugs. *Lancet Neurol.* 2003;**2**:473-81.
21. Montenegro MA, Cendes F, Noronha AL, Mory SB, Carvalho MI, Marques LH *et al.* Efficacy of clobazam as add-on therapy in patients with refractory partial epilepsy. *Epilepsia* 2001;**42**:539-42.
22. Barcs G, Halasz P. Effectiveness and tolerance of clobazam in temporal lobe epilepsy. *Acta Neurol Scand.* 1996;**93**:88-93.
23. Sheth RD, Ronen GM, Goulden KJ, Penney S, Bodensteiner JB. Clobazam for intractable pediatric epilepsy. *J Child Neurol* 1995;**10**:205-8.
24. Singh A, Guberman AH, Boisvert D. Clobazam in long-term epilepsy treatment: sustained responders versus those developing tolerance. *Epilepsia* 1995;**36**:798-803.
25. Remy C. Clobazam in the treatment of epilepsy: a review of the literature. *Epilepsia* 1994;**35 (Suppl 5)**:S88-S91.
26. Schmidt D. Clobazam for treatment of intractable epilepsy: a critical assessment. *Epilepsia* 1994;**35 (Suppl 5)**:S92-S95.
27. Buchanan N. Clobazam in the treatment of epilepsy: prospective follow-up to 8 years. *J R Soc Med* 1993;**86**:378-80.
28. Munn R, Farrell K. Open study of clobazam in refractory epilepsy. *Pediatr Neurol* 1993;**9**:465-9.
29. Canadian Clobazam Cooperative Group. Clobazam in treatment of refractory epilepsy: the Canadian experience. A retrospective study. *Epilepsia* 1991;**32**:407-16.
30. Canadian Study Group for Childhood Epilepsy. Clobazam has equivalent efficacy to carbamazepine and phenytoin as monotherapy for childhood epilepsy. *Epilepsia* 1998;**39**:952-9.
31. Bawden HN, Camfield CS, Camfield PR, Cunningham C, Darwish H, Dooley JM *et al.* The cognitive and behavioural effects of clobazam and standard monotherapy are comparable. Canadian Study Group for Childhood Epilepsy. *Epilepsy Res* 1999;**33**:133-43.
32. Feely M, Gibson J. Intermittent clobazam for catamenial epilepsy: tolerance avoided. *J.Neurol Neurosurg Psychiatry* 1984;**47**:1279-82.
33. Farell K. Benzodiazepines. In Pellock JM, Dodson WE, Bourgeois BFD, eds. *Pediatric epilepsy*, pp 373-83. New York: Demos, 2001.
34. Parmeggiani A, Posar A, Sangiorgi S, Giovanardi-Rossi P. Unusual side-effects due to clobazam: a case report with genetic study of CYP2C19. *Brain Dev.* 2004;**26**:63-6.
35. Sato A, Malow BA. Clonazepam. In Shorvon S, Dreifuss F, Fish D, Thomas D, eds. *The treatment of epilepsy*, pp 378-90. London: Blackwell Science, 1996.
36. Naito H, Wachi M, Nishida M. Clinical effects and plasma concentrations of long-term clonazepam monotherapy in previously untreated epileptics. *Acta Neurol Scand.* 1987;**76**:58-63.
37. Obeid T, Panayiotopoulos CP. Clonazepam in juvenile myoclonic epilepsy. *Epilepsia* 1989;**30**:603-6.
38. Richens A. Ethosuximide and valproate. In Duncan JS, Panayiotopoulos CP, eds. *Typical absences and related epileptic syndromes*, pp 361-7. London: Churchill Comunications Europe, 1995.
39. Posner EB, Mohamed K, Marson AG. Ethosuximide, sodium valproate or lamotrigine for absence seizures in children and adolescents. *Cochrane.Database.Syst.Rev.* 2003;CD003032.
40. Glauser TA. Ethosuximide. In Shorvon S, Perucca E, Fish D, Dodson E, eds. *The treatment of epilepsy (2nd edition)*, pp 391-402. Oxford: Blackwell Publishing, 2004.
41. Scott D F. The history of epileptic therapy. An account of how medication was developed. Langashire, UK:The Parthenon Publishing Group.1993.
42. Oguni H, Uehara T, Tanaka T, Sunahara M, Hara M, Osawa M. Dramatic effect of ethosuximide on epileptic negative myoclonus: implications for the neurophysiological mechanism. *Neuropediatrics* 1998;**29**:29-34.
43. Snead OC, III, Hosey LC. Treatment of epileptic falling spells with ethosuximide. *Brain Dev.* 1987;**9**:602-4.
44. Wallace SJ. Myoclonus and epilepsy in childhood: a review of treatment with valproate, ethosuximide, lamotrigine and zonisamide. *Epilepsy Res.* 1998;**29**:147-54.
45. Coulter DA. Antiepileptic drug cellular mechanisms of action: where does lamotrigine fit in? *J.Child Neurol.* 1997;**12 Suppl 1**:S2-9.
46. Manning JP, Richards DA, Leresche N, Crunelli V, Bowery NG. Cortical-area specific block of genetically determined absence seizures by ethosuximide. *Neuroscience* 2004;**123**:5-9.
47. Manning JP, Richards DA, Bowery NG. Pharmacology of absence epilepsy. *Trends Pharmacol.Sci.* 2003;**24**:542-9.
48. Palmer KJ, McTavish D. Felbamate. A review of its pharmacodynamic and pharmacokinetic properties, and therapeutic efficacy in epilepsy. *Drugs* 1993;**45**:1041-65.

49. Battino D, Estienne M, Avanzini G. Clinical pharmacokinetics of antiepileptic drugs in paediatric patients. Part II. Phenytoin, carbamazepine, sulthiame, lamotrigine, vigabatrin, oxcarbazepine and felbamate. *Clin Pharmacokinet.* 1995;**29**:341-69.

50. French J, Smith M, Faught E, Brown L. Practice advisory: The use of felbamate in the treatment of patients with intractable epilepsy: report of the Quality Standards Subcommittee of the American Academy of Neurology and the American Epilepsy Society. *Neurology* 1999;**52**:1540-5.

51. Leppik IE. Felbamate. In Shorvon S, Perucca E, Fish D, Dodson E, eds. *The treatment of epilepsy (2nd edition)*, pp 403-9. Oxford: Blackwell Publishing, 2004.

52. Morris GL. Gabapentin. *Epilepsia* 1999;**40 (Suppl 5)**:S63-S70.

53. McLean MJ, Gidal BE. Gabapentin dosing in the treatment of epilepsy. *Clin Ther.* 2003;**25**:1382-406.

54. Shorvon SD. The choice of drugs and approach to drug treatments in partial epilepsy. In Shorvon S, Perucca E, Fish D, Dodson E, eds. *The treatment of epilepsy (2nd edition)*, pp 317-33. Oxford: Blackwell Publishing, 2004.

55. Chadwick D, Leiderman DB, Sauermann W, Alexander J, Garofalo E. Gabapentin in generalized seizures. *Epilepsy Res* 1996;**25**:191-7.

56. Wolf SM, Shinnar S, Kang H, Gil KB, Moshe SL. Gabapentin toxicity in children manifesting as behavioral changes. *Epilepsia* 1995;**36**:1203-5.

57. Boneva N, Brenner T, Argov Z. Gabapentin may be hazardous in myasthenia gravis. *Muscle & Nerve* 2000;**23**:1204-8.

58. Shorvon S. Handbook of epilepsy treatment. Malden, MA, USA: Blackwell Science Ltd, 2000.

59. Matsuo F. Lamotrigine. In Shorvon S, Perucca E, Fish D, Dodson E, eds. *The treatment of epilepsy (2nd edition)*, pp 425-42. Oxford: Blackwell Publishing, 2004.

60. Barron TF, Hunt SL, Hoban TF, Price ML. Lamotrigine monotherapy in children. *Pediatr Neurol* 2000;**23**:160-3.

61. Culy CR, Goa KL. Lamotrigine. A review of its use in childhood epilepsy. *Paediatr Drugs* 2000;**2**:299-330.

62. Messenheimer J, Mullens EL, Giorgi L, Young F. Safety review of adult clinical trial experience with lamotrigine. *Drug Saf* 1998;**18**:281-96.

63. Mullens EL. Lamotrigine monotherapy in epilepsy. *Clin Drug Invest* 1998;**16**:125-33.

64. Brodie MJ. Lamotrigine—an update. *Can J Neurol Sci.* 1996;**23**:S6-S9.

65. Messenheimer JA. Lamotrigine. *Epilepsia* 1995;**36 (Suppl 2)**:S87-94.

66. Faught E. Lamotrigine for startle-induced seizures. *Seizure* 1999;**8**:361-3.

67. Frank LM, Enlow T, Holmes GL, Manasco P, Concannon S, Chen C *et al.* Lamictal (lamotrigine) monotherapy for typical absence seizures in children. *Epilepsia* 1999;**40**:973-9.

68. Barr PA, Buettiker VE, Antony JH. Efficacy of lamotrigine in refractory neonatal seizures. *Pediatr Neurol.* 1999;**20**:161-3.

69. Panayiotopoulos CP, Ferrie CD, Knott C, Robinson RO. Interaction of lamotrigine with sodium valproate. *Lancet* 1993;**341**:445.

70. Ferrie CD, Panayiotopoulos CP. Therapeutic interaction of lamotrigine and sodium valproate in intractable myoclonic epilepsy. *Seizure.* 1994;**3**:157-9.

71. Mikati MA, Holmes GL. Lamotrigine in absence and primary generalized epilepsies. *J Child Neurol.* 1997;**12 (Suppl 1)**:S29-37.

72. Brodie MJ, Yuen AW. Lamotrigine substitution study: evidence for synergism with sodium valproate? 105 Study Group. *Epilepsy Res* 1997;**26**:423-32.

73. Faught E, Morris G, Jacobson M, French J, Harden C, Montouris G *et al.* Adding lamotrigine to valproate: incidence of rash and other adverse effects. Postmarketing Antiepileptic Drug Survey (PADS) Group. *Epilepsia* 1999;**40**:1135-40.

74. Guberman AH, Besag FM, Brodie MJ, Dooley JM, Duchowny MS, Pellock JM *et al.* Lamotrigine-associated rash: risk/benefit considerations in adults and children. *Epilepsia* 1999;**40**:985-91.

75. Tran TA, Leppik IE, Blesi K, Sathanandan ST, Remmel R. Lamotrigine clearance during pregnancy. *Neurology* 2002;**59**:251-5.

76. de Haan GJ, Edelbroek P, Segers J, Engelsman M, Lindhout D, Devile-Notschaele M *et al.* Gestation-induced changes in lamotrigine pharmacokinetics: a monotherapy study. *Neurology* 2004;**63**:571-3.

77. Pennell PB, Newport DJ, Stowe ZN, Helmers SL, Montgomery JQ, Henry TR. The impact of pregnancy and childbirth on the metabolism of lamotrigine. *Neurology* 2004;**62**:292-5.

78. Sabers A, Ohman I, Christensen J, Tomson T. Oral contraceptives reduce lamotrigine plasma levels. *Neurology* 2003;**61**:570-1.

79. Fitton A, Goa KL. Lamotrigine. An update of its pharmacology and therapeutic use in epilepsy. *Drugs* 1995;**50**:691-713.

80. Guerrini R, Dravet C, Genton P, Belmonte A, Kaminska A, Dulac O. Lamotrigine and seizure aggravation in severe myoclonic epilepsy. *Epilepsia* 1998;**39**:508-12.

81. Guerrini R, Belmonte A, Parmeggiani L, Perucca E. Myoclonic status epilepticus following high-dosage lamotrigine therapy. *Brain Dev.* 1999;**21**:420-4.

82. Carrazana EJ, Wheeler SD. Exacerbation of juvenile myoclonic epilepsy with lamotrigine. *Neurology* 2001;**56**:1424-5.

83. Biraben A, Allain H, Scarabin JM, Schuck S, Edan G. Exacerbation of juvenile myoclonic epilepsy with lamotrigine. *Neurology* 2000;**55**:1758.

84. Boon P, Chauvel P, Pohlmann-Eden B, Otoul C, Wroe S. Dose-response effect of levetiracetam 1000 and 2000 mg/day in partial epilepsy. *Epilepsy Res.* 2002;**48**:77-89.

85. Glauser TA, Pellock JM, Bebin EM, Fountain NB, Ritter FJ, Jensen CM *et al.* Efficacy and safety of levetiracetam in children with partial seizures: an open-label trial. *Epilepsia* 2002;**43**:518-24.

86. Leppik IE. Three new drugs for epilepsy: levetiracetam, oxcarbazepine, and zonisamide. *J.Child Neurol.* 2002;**17 Suppl 1**:S53-S57.

87. Welty TE, Gidal BE, Ficker DM, Privitera MD. Levetiracetam: a different approach to the pharmacotherapy of epilepsy. *Ann Pharmacother.* 2002;**36**:296-304.

88. Morrell MJ, Leppik I, French J, Ferrendelli J, Han J, Magnus L. The KEEPER trial: levetiracetam adjunctive treatment of partial-onset seizures in an open-label community-based study. *Epilepsy Res.* 2003;**54**:153-61.

89. Ferrendelli JA, French J, Leppik I, Morrell MJ, Herbeuval A, Han J *et al.* Use of levetiracetam in a population of patients aged 65 years and older: a subset analysis of the KEEPER trial. *Epilepsy Behav.* 2003;**4**:702-9.

90. Sadek A, French JA. Levetiracetam. In Shorvon S, Perucca E, Fish D, Dodson E, eds. *The treatment of epilepsy (2nd edition)*, pp 443-50. Oxford: Blackwell Publishing, 2004.

91. Briggs DE, French JA. Levetiracetam safety profiles and tolerability in epilepsy patients. *Expert.Opin.Drug Saf* 2004;**3**:415-24.

92. Patsalos PN. Levetiracetam. *Reviews in Contemporay Pharmacology* 2004;**13**:1-168.

93. Privitera M. Efficacy of levetiracetam: a review of three pivotal clinical trials. *Epilepsia* 2001;**42 (Suppl 4)**:31-5.

94. Chaisewikul R, Privitera MD, Hutton JL, Marson AG. Levetiracetam add-on for drug-resistant localization related (partial) epilepsy (Cochrane Review). *Cochrane.Database.Syst.Rev* 2001;**1**:CD001901.

95. Cramer JA, Arrigo C, Van Hammee G, Gauer LJ, Cereghino JJ. Effect of levetiracetam on epilepsy-related quality of life. N132 Study Group. *Epilepsia* 2000;**41**:868-74.

96. Cohen J. Levetiracetam monotherapy for primary generalised epilepsy. *Seizure* 2003;**12**:150-3.

97. Covanis A, Katsalouli M. Levetiracetam monotherapy in generalised epilepsy and photosensitivity. *Epilepsia* 2003;**44 (Suppl 8)**:80.

98. Kasteleijn-Nolst Trenite DG, Hirsch E. Levetiracetam: preliminary efficacy in generalized seizures. *Epileptic Disord.* 2003;**5 Suppl 1**:S39-S44.

99. Greenhill L, Betts T, Smith K. Effect of levetiracetam on resistant juvenile myoclonic epilepsy. *Epilepsia* 2002;**43 (Suppl 7)**:179.

100. Krauss GL, Betts T, Abou-Khalil B, Bergey G, Yarrow H, Miller A. Levetiracetam treatment of idiopathic generalised epilepsy. *Seizure* 2003;**12**:617-20.

101. Gallagher MJ, Eisenman LN, Brown KM, Erbayat-Altay E, Hecimovic H, Fessler AJ *et al.* Levetiracetam Reduces Spike-Wave Density and Duration during Continuous EEG Monitoring in Patients with Idiopathic Generalized Epilepsy. *Epilepsia* 2004;**45**:90-1.

102. Genton P, Gelisse P. Antimyoclonic effect of levetiracetam. *Epileptic Disord.* 2000;**2**:209-12.

103. Krauss GL, Bergin A, Kramer RE, Cho YW, Reich SG. Suppression of post-hypoxic and post-encephalitic myoclonus with levetiracetam. *Neurology* 2001;**56**:411-2.

104. Schauer R, Singer M, Saltuari L, Kofler M. Suppression of cortical myoclonus by levetiracetam. *Mov Disord.* 2002;**17**:411-5.

105. Gelisse P, Crespel A, Genton P, Baldy-Moulinier M. Dramatic effect of levetiracetam on epileptic negative myoclonus. *Acta Neurol Scand.* 2003;**107**:302-3.

106. Kasteleijn-Nolst Trenite DG, Marescaux C, Stodieck S, Edelbroek PM, Oosting J. Photosensitive epilepsy: a model to study the effects of antiepileptic drugs. Evaluation of the piracetam analogue, levetiracetam. *Epilepsy Res* 1996;**25**:225-30.

107. Huber B, Bommel W, Hauser I, Horstmann V, Liem S, May T *et al. Seizure* 2004;**13**:168-75.

108. Kossoff EH, Boatman D, Freeman JM. Landau-Kleffner syndrome responsive to levetiracetam. *Epilepsy Behav.* 2003;**4**:571-5.

109. Marson AG, Hutton JL, Leach JP, Castillo S, Schmidt D, White S *et al.* Levetiracetam, oxcarbazepine, remacemide and zonisamide for drug resistant localization-related epilepsy: a systematic review. *Epilepsy Res.* 2001;**46**:259-70.

110. Ben Menachem E. Preliminary efficacy of levetiracetam in monotherapy. *Epileptic Disord.* 2003;**5 Suppl 1**:S51-S55.

111. Levetiracetam-a new drug for epilepsy. *Drug Ther Bull.* 2002;**40**:30-2.

112. Perucca E, Johannessen SI. The ideal pharmacokinetic properties of an antiepileptic drug: how close does levetiracetam come? *Epileptic Disord.* 2003;**5 Suppl 1**:S17-S26.

113. Patsalos PN. Pharmacokinetic profile of levetiracetam: toward ideal characteristics. *Pharmacol Ther.* 2000;**85**:77-85.

114. Herranz JL, Rufo-Campos M, Arteaga R. Effectiveness and tolerability of levetiracetam in 43 children and adolescents with epilepsy. *Rev Neurol* 2003;**37**:1005-8.

115. Tan MJ, Appleton RE. Efficacy and tolerability of levetiracetam in children aged 10 years and younger: a clinical experience. *Seizure* 2004;**13**:142-5.

116. Wheless JW, Ng YT. Levetiracetam in refractory pediatric epilepsy. *J Child Neurol.* 2002;**17**:413-5.

117. Lagae L, Buyse G, Deconinck A, Ceulemans B. Effect of levetiracetam in refractory childhood epilepsy syndromes. *Eur J Paediatr Neurol.* 2003;**7**:123-8.

118. French J. Use of levetiracetam in special populations. *Epilepsia* 2001;**42 Suppl 4**:40-3.

119. Pellock JM, Glauser TA, Bebin EM, Fountain NB, Ritter FJ, Coupez RM *et al.* Pharmacokinetic study of levetiracetam in children. *Epilepsia* 2001;**42**:1574-9.

120. Glauser TA, Dulac O. Preliminary efficacy of levetiracetam in children. *Epileptic Disord.* 2003;**5 Suppl 1**:S45-S50.

121. French J, Edrich P, Cramer JA. A systematic review of the safety profile of levetiracetam: a new antiepileptic drug. *Epilepsy Res.* 2001;**47**:77-90.

122. Sohn YH, Kaelin-Lang A, Jung HY, Hallett M. Effect of levetiracetam on human corticospinal excitability. *Neurology* 2001;**57**:858-63.

123. Nakken KO, Eriksson AS, Lossius R, Johannessen SI. A paradoxical effect of levetiracetam may be seen in both children and adults with refractory epilepsy. *Seizure.* 2003;**12**:42-6.

124. Klitgaard H, Pitkanen A. Antiepileptogenesis, neuroprotection, and disease modification in the treatment of epilepsy: focus on levetiracetam. *Epileptic Disord.* 2003;**5 Suppl 1**:S9-16.

125. Klitgaard H, Matagne A, Gobert J, Wulfert E. Evidence for a unique profile of levetiracetam in rodent models of seizures and epilepsy. *Eur J Pharmacol.* 1998;**353**:191-206.

126. Klitgaard H. Levetiracetam: the preclinical profile of a new class of antiepileptic drugs? *Epilepsia* 2001;**42 (Suppl 4)**:13-8.

127. Lynch BA, Lambeng N, Nocka K, Kensel-Hammes P, Bajjalieh SM, Matagne A *et al.* The synaptic vesicle protein SV2A is the binding site for the antiepileptic drug levetiracetam. *Proc Natl Acad Sci.USA* 2004;**101**:9861-6.

128. Gelisse P, Genton P, Kuate D, Pesenti A, Baldy-Moulinier M, Crespel A. Worsening of seizures by oxcarbazepine in juvenile idiopathic generalized epilepsies. *Epilepsia* 2004;**45**:1282-8.

129. Taylor S, Tudur S, Williamson PR, Marson AG. Phenobarbitone versus phenytoin monotherapy for partial onset seizures and generalized onset tonic-clonic seizures. *Cochrane.Database.Syst.Rev.* 2001;CD002217.

130. de Silva M, MacArdle B, McGowan M, Hughes E, Stewart J, Neville BG *et al.* Randomised comparative monotherapy trial of phenobarbitone, phenytoin, carbamazepine, or sodium valproate for newly diagnosed childhood epilepsy. *Lancet* 1996;**347**:709-13.

131. Heller AJ, Chesterman P, Elwes RD, Crawford P, Chadwick D, Johnson *et al.* Phenobarbitone, phenytoin, carbamazepine, or sodium valproate for newly diagnosed adult epilepsy: a randomised comparative monotherapy trial. *J Neurol Neurosurg Psychiatr* 1995;**58**:44-50.

132. O'Connell MT, Patsalos PN. Phenobarbitone. In Shorvon S, Dreifuss F, Fish D, Thomas D, eds. *The treatment of epilepsy*, pp 446-53. London: Blackwell Science, 1996.

133. Mattson RH, Cramer JA, Collins JF, Smith DB, Delgado-Escueta AV, Browne TR *et al.* Comparison of carbamazepine, phenobarbital, phenytoin, and primidone in partial and secondarily generalized tonic-clonic seizures. *N Engl J Med* 1985;**313**:145-51.

134. Reis TT, Maia Filho PC, Cechini PC. Clinical evaluation of the therapeutic value of barbexaclone including determination of plasma levels of the barbiturate. *Arq Neuropsiquiatr.* 1980;**38**:93-8.

135. Browne TR. Phenytoin and other hydantoins. In Engel JJr, Pedley TA, eds. *Epilepsy: A comprehensive Textbook*, pp 1557-79. Philadelphia: Lippincott-Raven Publishers, 1997.

136. Bebin M, Bleck TP. New anticonvulsant drugs. Focus on flunarizine, fosphenytoin, midazolam and stiripentol. *Drugs* 1994;**48**:153-71.

137. Pellock JM. Fosphenytoin use in children. *Neurology* 1996;**46**:S14-S16.

138. Browne TR. Fosphenytoin (Cerebyx). *Clin Neuropharmacol.* 1997;**20**:1-12.

139. Voytko SM, Farrington E. Fosphenytoin sodium: new drug to replace intravenous phenytoin sodium. *Pediatr Nurs.* 1997;**23**:503-6.

140. Luer MS. Fosphenytoin. *Neurol Res.* 1998;**20**:178-82.

141. DeToledo JC, Ramsay RE. Fosphenytoin and phenytoin in patients with status epilepticus: improved tolerability versus increased costs. *Drug Saf* 2000;**22**:459-66.

142. Arroyo S, Anhut H, Kugler AR, Lee CM, Knapp LE, Garofalo EA *et al.* Pregabalin Add-on Treatment: A Randomized, Double-blind, Placebo-controlled, Dose-Response Study in Adults with Partial Seizures. *Epilepsia* 2004;**45**:20-7.

143. Huppertz HJ, Feuerstein TJ, Schulze-Bonhage A. Myoclonus in epilepsy patients with anticonvulsive add-on therapy with pregabalin. *Epilepsia* 2001;**42**:790-2.

144. Fink K, Dooley DJ, Meder WP, Suman-Chauhan N, Duffy S, Clusmann H *et al.* Inhibition of neuronal Ca(2+) influx by gabapentin and pregabalin in the human neocortex. *Neuropharmacology* 2002;**42**:229-36.

145. Kalviainen R. Tiagabine. In Shorvon S, Perucca E, Fish D, Dodson E, eds. *The treatment of epilepsy (2nd edition)*, pp 507-14. Oxford: Blackwell Publishing, 2004.

146. Loiseau P. Review of controlled trials of gabitril (tiagabine): a clinician's viewpoint. *Epilepsia* 1999;**40 (Suppl 9)**:S14-S19.

147. Schmidt D, Gram L, Brodie M, Kramer G, Perucca E, Kalviainen R *et al.* Tiagabine in the treatment of epilepsy - a clinical review with a guide for the prescribing physician. *Epilepsy Res.* 2000;**41**:245-51.

148. Krauss GL, Johnson MA, Sheth S, Miller NR. A controlled study comparing visual function in patients treated with vigabatrin and tiagabine. *J Neurol Neurosurg Psychiatry* 2003;**74**:339-43.

149. Lawden MC. Vigabatrin, tiagabine, and visual fields. *J Neurol Neurosurg Psychiatry* 2003;**74**:286.

150. Shinnar S, Berg AT, Treiman DM, Hauser WA, Hesdorffer DC, Sackellares JC *et al.* Status epilepticus and tiagabine therapy: review of safety data and epidemiologic comparisons. *Epilepsia* 2001;**42**:372-9.

151. Panayiotopoulos CP. Absence status epilepticus. In Gilman S, ed. *Medlink Neurology*, San Diego SA: Arbor Publishing Corp, 2004.

152. Panayiotopoulos CP. Typical absence seizures. In Gilman S, ed. *Medlink Neurology*, San Diego SA: Arbor Publishing Corp, 2004.

153. Green JR, Troupin AS, Halperm LM, Friel P, Kanarek P. Sulthiame: evaluation as an anticonvulsant. *Epilepsia* 1974;**15**:329-49.

154. Houghton GW, Richens A. Phenytoin intoxication induced by sulthiame in epileptic patients. *J Neurol Neurosurg Psychiatry* 1974;**37**:275-81.

155. Lerman P, Nussbaum E. The use of sulthiame- in myoclonic epilepsy of childhood and adolescence. *Acta Neurol Scand.Suppl* 1975;**60**:7-12.

156. Koepp MJ, Patsalos PN, Sander JW. Sulthiame in adults with refractory epilepsy and learning disability: an open trial. *Epilepsy Res.* 2002;**50**:277-82.

157. Kramer U, Shahar E, Zelnik N, Lerman-Sagie T, Watemberg N, Nevo Y *et al.* Carbamazepine versus sulthiame in treating benign childhood epilepsy with centrotemporal spikes. *J Child Neurol.* 2002;**17**:914-6.

158. Bast T, Volp A, Wolf C, Rating D. The influence of sulthiame on EEG in children with benign childhood epilepsy with centrotemporal spikes. *Epilepsia* 2003;**44**:215-20.

159. Engler F, Maeder-Ingvar M, Roulet E, Deonna T. Treatment with Sulthiame (Ospolot) in benign partial epilepsy of childhood and related syndromes: an open clinical and EEG study. *Neuropediatrics* 2003;**34**:105-9.

160. Ormrod D, McClellan K. Topiramate: a review of its use in childhood epilepsy. *Paediatr Drugs* 2001;**3**:293-319.

161. Glauser TA. Topiramate in the catastrophic epilepsies of childhood. *J Child Neurol.* 2000;**15 Suppl 1**:S14-S21.

162. Reife R, Pledger G, Wu SC. Topiramate as add-on therapy: pooled analysis of randomized controlled trials in adults. *Epilepsia* 2000;**41 (Suppl 1)**:S66-S71.

163. Shank RP, Gardocki JF, Streeter AJ, Maryanoff BE. An overview of the preclinical aspects of topiramate: pharmacology, pharmacokinetics, and mechanism of action. *Epilepsia* 2000;**41 Suppl 1**:S3-S9.

164. Perucca E. A pharmacological and clinical review on topiramate, a new antiepileptic drug. *Pharmacol Res.* 1997;**35**:241-56.

165. Rosenfeld WE. Topiramate: a review of preclinical, pharmacokinetic, and clinical data. *Clin Ther.* 1997;**19**:1294-308.

166. Coppola G, Capovilla G, Montagnini A, Romeo A, Spano M, Tortorella G *et al.* Topiramate as add-on drug in severe myoclonic epilepsy in infancy: an Italian multicenter open trial. *Epilepsy Res.* 2002;**49**:45-8.

167. Singh BK, White-Scott S. Role of topiramate in adults with intractable epilepsy, mental retardation, and developmental disabilities. *Seizure.* 2002;**11**:47-50.

168. Wang Y, Zhou D, Wang B, Kirchner A, Hopp P, Kerling F *et al.* Clinical effects of topiramate against secondarily generalized tonic-clonic seizures. *Epilepsy Res.* 2002;**49**:121-30.

169. Dooley JM, Camfield PR, Smith E, Langevin P, Ronen G. Topiramate in intractable childhood onset epilepsy—a cautionary note. *Can J Neurol Sci.* 1999;**26**:271-3.

170. Baeta E, Santana I, Castro G, Goncalves S, Goncalves T, Carmo I *et al.* Cognitive effects of therapy with topiramate in patients with refractory partial epilepsy. *Rev Neurol* 2002;**34**:737-41.

171. Aldenkamp AP, Baker G, Mulder OG, Chadwick D, Cooper P, Doelman J *et al.* A multicenter, randomized clinical study to evaluate the effect on cognitive function of topiramate compared with valproate as add-on therapy to carbamazepine in patients with partial-onset seizures. *Epilepsia* 2000;**41**:1167-78.

172. Crawford P. An audit of topiramate use in a general neurology clinic. *Seizure.* 1998;**7**:207-11.

173. Ojemann LM, Ojemann GA, Dodrill CB, Crawford CA, Holmes MD, Dudley DL. Language Disturbances as Side Effects of Topiramate and Zonisamide Therapy. *Epilepsy Behav.* 2001;**2**:579-84.

174. Thompson PJ, Baxendale SA, Duncan JS, Sander JW. Effects of topiramate on cognitive function. *J Neurol Neurosurg Psychiatry* 2000;**69**:636-41.

175. Mula M, Trimble MR, Thompson P, Sander JW. Topiramate and word-finding difficulties in patients with epilepsy. *Neurology* 2003;**60**:1104-7.

176. Banta JT, Hoffman K, Budenz DL, Ceballos E, Greenfield DS. Presumed topiramate-induced bilateral acute angle-closure glaucoma. *Am J Ophthalmol.* 2001;**132**:112-4.

177. Arroyo S. Valproate. In Shorvon S, Perucca E, Fish D, Dodson E, eds. *The treatment of epilepsy (2nd edition)*, pp 528-39. Oxford: Blackwell Publishing, 2004.

178. Johannessen CU, Johannessen SI. Valproate: past, present, and future. *CNS.Drug Rev.* 2003;**9**:199-216.

179. Loscher W. Valproate: a reappraisal of its pharmacodynamic properties and mechanisms of action. *Prog Neurobiol.* 1999;**58**:31-59.

180. Hirsch E, Genton P. Antiepileptic drug-induced pharmacodynamic aggravation of seizures: does valproate have a lower potential? *CNS.Drugs* 2003;**17**:633-40.

181. Delgado-Escueta AV, Janz D. Consensus guidelines: preconception counseling, management, and care of the pregnant woman with epilepsy. *Neurology* 1992;**42**:149-60.

182. Laegreid L, Kyllerman M, Hedner T, Hagberg B, Viggedahl G. Benzodiazepine amplification of valproate teratogenic effects in children of mothers with absence epilepsy. *Neuropediatrics* 1993;**24**:88-92.

183. Chappell KA, Markowitz JS, Jackson CW. Is valproate pharmacotherapy associated with polycystic ovaries? *Ann Pharmacother.* 1999;**33**:1211-6.

184. Isojarvi JI, Rattya J, Myllyla VV, Knip M, Koivunen R, Pakarinen AJ *et al.* Valproate, lamotrigine, and insulin-mediated risks in women with epilepsy. *Ann Neurol.* 1998;**43**:446-51.

185. Acharya S, Bussel JB. Hematologic toxicity of sodium valproate. *J Pediatr Hematol Oncol.* 2000;**22**:62-5.

186. Macdonald RL,.Kelly KM. Antiepileptic drug mechanisms of action. *Epilepsia* 1995;**36 (Suppl 2)**:S2-12.

187. Coulter DA, Huguenard JR, Prince DA. Characterization of ethosuximide reduction of low-threshold calcium current in thalamic neurons. *Ann Neurol* 1989;**25**:582-93.

188. Yuen AW, Land G, Weatherley BC, Peck AW. Sodium valproate acutely inhibits lamotrigine metabolism. *Br J Clin Pharmacol.* 1992;**33**:511-3.

189. Kramer G. Vigabatrin. In Shorvon S, Perucca E, Fish D, Dodson E, eds. *The treatment of epilepsy (2nd edition)*, pp 540-7. Oxford: Blackwell Publishing, 2004.

190. French JA. Vigabatrin. *Epilepsia* 1999;**40 Suppl 5**:S11-S16.

191. Eke T, Talbot JF, Lawden MC. Severe persistent visual field constriction associated with vigabatrin. *BMJ* 1997;**314**:180-1.

192. French JA, Kanner AM, Bautista J, Abou-Khalil B, Browne T, Harden CL *et al.* Efficacy and tolerability of the new antiepileptic drugs I: treatment of new onset epilepsy: report of the Therapeutics and Technology Assessment Subcommittee and Quality Standards Subcommittee of the American Academy of Neurology and the American Epilepsy Society. *Neurology* 2004;**62**:1252-60.

193. French JA, Kanner AM, Bautista J, Abou-Khalil B, Browne T, Harden CL *et al.* Efficacy and Tolerability of the New Antiepileptic Drugs, I: Treatment of New-Onset Epilepsy: Report of the TTA and QSS Subcommittees of the American Academy of Neurology and the American Epilepsy Society. *Epilepsia* 2004;**45**:401-9.

194. French JA. Response: efficacy and tolerability of the new antiepileptic drugs. *Epilepsia* 2004;**45**:1649-51.

195. Connelly JF. Vigabatrin. *Ann Pharmacoth* 1993;**27**:197-204.

196. French JA, Mosier M, Walker S, Sommerville K, Sussman N. A double-blind, placebo-controlled study of vigabatrin three g/day in patients with uncontrolled complex partial seizures. Vigabatrin Protocol 024 Investigative Cohort. *Neurology* 1996;**46**:54-61.

197. Chadwick D. Safety and efficacy of vigabatrin and carbamazepine in newly diagnosed epilepsy: a multicentre randomised double-blind study. Vigabatrin European Monotherapy Study Group. *Lancet* 1999;**354**:13-9.

198. Hardus P, Verduin WM, Postma G, Stilma JS, Berendschot TT, van Veelen CW. Concentric contraction of the visual field in patients with temporal lobe epilepsy and its association with the use of vigabatrin medication. *Epilepsia* 2000;**41**:581-7.

199. Gross-Tsur V, Banin E, Shahar E, Shalev RS, Lahat E. Visual impairment in children with epilepsy treated with vigabatrin. *Ann Neurol* 2000;**48**:60-4.

200. Duboc A, Hanoteau N, Simonutti M, Rudolf G, Nehlig A, Sahel JA *et al.* Vigabatrin, the GABA-transaminase inhibitor, damages cone photoreceptors in rats. *Ann Neurol* 2004;**55**:695-705.

201. Panayiotopoulos CP, Agathonikou A, Sharoqi IA, Parker AP. Vigabatrin aggravates absences and absence status. *Neurology* 1997;**49**:1467.

202. van der TK, Graniewski-Wijnands HS, Polak BC. Visual field and electrophysiological abnormalities due to vigabatrin. *Doc Ophthalmol.* 2002;**104**:181-8.

203. Glauser TA, Pellock JM. Zonisamide in pediatric epilepsy: review of the Japanese experience. *J Child Neurol.* 2002;**17**:87-96.

204. Willmore LJ, Seino M, eds. International experiences and perspectives:Zonisamide. *Seizure* 2004; 13**(Suppl)**:S1-S72.

205. Chadwick DW, Marson AG. Zonisamide add-on for drug-resistant partial epilepsy. *Cochrane.Database.Syst.Rev.* 2002;CD001416.

206. Leppik IE. Zonisamide. *Epilepsia* 1999;**40 (Suppl 5)**:S23-S29.

207. Suzuki Y, Nagai T, Ono J, Imai K, Otani K, Tagawa T *et al.* Zonisamide monotherapy in newly diagnosed infantile spasms. *Epilepsia* 1997;**38**:1035-8.

208. Ohno M, Shimotsuji Y, Abe J, Shimada M, Tamiya H. Zonisamide treatment of early infantile epileptic encephalopathy. *Pediatr Neurol.* 2000;**23**:341-4.

209. Okumura A, Hayakawa F, Kuno K, Watanabe K. Oligohidrosis caused by zonisamide. *No To Hattatsu* 1996;**28**:44-7.

210. Okumura A, Ishihara N, Kato T, Hayakawa F, Kuno K, Watanabe K. Predictive value of acetylcholine stimulation testing for oligohidrosis caused by zonisamide. *Pediatr Neurol.* 2000;**23**:59-61.

211. Miyamoto T, Kohsaka M, Koyama T. Psychotic episodes during zonisamide treatment. *Seizure* 2000;**9**:65-70.

INDEX

Note: Page references in **bold** refer to figures in the text; those in *italics* to tables or boxed material. The letter 'n' following page references refers to material in the footnotes